TABLE II.

VIRUSES OF NEUROLOGIC IMPORTANCE IN MAN

A. DNA Viruses

Herpesviruses
  Group A
    Herpesvirus hominis, types 1, 2
    Herpes simiae (B virus)
  Group B
    Varicella-zoster virus
    Cytomegalovirus
    Epstein-Barr virus

Adenoviruses

Poxviruses
  Variola virus
  Vaccinia virus

Papovaviruses

B. RNA Viruses

Myxoviruses
  Influenza viruses
  Parainfluenza viruses
  Mumps virus
  Rubeola (measles) virus

Arboviruses (grouping on an ecological basis)

  Mosquito-borne
    California encephalitis virus
    St. Louis encephalitis virus
    Eastern equine encephalitis virus
    Western equine encephalitis virus
    Venezuelan equine encephalitis virus
    Japanese B encephalitis virus (Australian X)
    Yellow fever virus
    Dengue
    West Nile virus

  Tick-borne
    Colorado Tick Fever virus
    Powassan virus
    Russian spring-summer encephalitis virus
    Louping-ill virus

Picornaviruses
  Enteroviruses
    Polioviruses, types 1, 2, 3
    Coxsackie A virus, type 1–24
    Coxsackie B virus, type 1–6
    Echovirus, type 1–34
  Rhinoviruses (many serotypes)

Togaviruses
  Rubella virus
  Most arboviruses, groups A and B

Arenaviruses
  iomeningitis

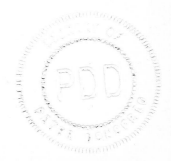

Other monographs in the series, Major Problems in Clinical Pediatrics:

Altman and Schwartz: *Malignant Diseases of Infancy, Childhood and Adolescence* — 1978

Avery, Fletcher and Williams: *The Lung and Its Disorders in the Newborn Infant* — Fourth Edition, 1981

Bell and McCormick: *Increased Intracranial Pressure in Children* — Second Edition, 1978

Brewer: *Juvenile Rheumatoid Arthritis* — 1970

Cornblath and Schwartz: *Disorders of Carbohydrate Metabolism in Infancy* — Second Edition, 1976

Dubowitz: *Muscle Disorders in Childhood* — 1978

Gryboski: *Gastrointestinal Problems in the Infant* — 1975

Hanshaw and Dudgeon: *Viral Diseases of the Fetus and Newborn* — 1978

Harrison and Harrison: *Disorders of Calcium and Phosphate Metabolism in Childhood and Adolescence* — 1979

Lubchenco: *The High Risk Infant* — 1976

Markowitz and Gordis: *Rheumatic Fever* — Second Edition, 1972

Oski and Naiman: *Hematologic Problems in the Newborn* — Second Edition, 1972

Rowe, Freedom and Mehrizi: *The Neonate with Congenital Heart Disease* — Second Edition, 1980

Royer, et al: *Pediatric Nephrology* — 1974

Scriver and Rosenberg: *Amino Acid Metabolism and Its Disorders* — 1973

Smith: *Recognizable Patterns of Human Deformation*

Smith: *Recognizable Patterns of Human Malformation* — Second Edition, 1976

Smith: *Growth and Its Disorders* — 1977

Solomon and Esterly: *Neonatal Dermatology* — 1973

Solomon, Esterly and Loeffel: *Adolescent Dermatology* — 1978

Volpe: *Neurology of the Newborn* — 1981

Forthcoming Monographs

Belman and Kaplan: *Urologic Problems in Pediatrics*
Bluestone and Klein: *Otitis Media in Infants and Children*
Drash: *Juvenile Diabetes*
Glader: *Anemias in Children*
Griffin: *Children's Orthopedics*
Ingelfinger: *Pediatric Hypertension*
Kerns: *Child Abuse and Neglect*

NEUROLOGIC INFECTIONS IN CHILDREN

Second Edition

By

William E. Bell, M.D.

Professor, Departments of Pediatrics and Neurology;
Director, Section of Pediatric Neurology,
The University of Iowa College of Medicine,
Iowa City, Iowa

and

William F. McCormick, M.D.

Professor, Departments of Pathology and Neurology;
Chief, Division of Neuropathology,
University of Texas Medical Branch,
Galveston, Texas

Volume XII in the Series

MAJOR PROBLEMS IN CLINICAL PEDIATRICS

MILTON MARKOWITZ
Consulting Editor

W. B. Saunders Company • Philadelphia • London • Toronto • Sydney • 1981

W. B. Saunders Company: West Washington Square
Philadelphia, Pa. 19105

1 St. Anne's Road
Eastbourne, East Sussex BN21, 3 UN. England

1 Goldthorne Avenue
Toronto, Ontario M8Z 5T9, Canada

9 Waltham Street
Artarmon, N.S.W. 2064, Australia

Listed here is the latest translated edition of this book together with the language of the translation and the publisher.

Spanish *(1st Edition)*—Salvat Editores, Barcelona, Spain

Library of Congress Cataloging in Publication Data

Bell, William Edward, 1929–
    Neurologic infections in children.

    (Major problems in clinical pediatrics; v. 12)

    Includes index.

        1. Nervous system—Infections.   2. Pediatric neurology.
3. Communicable diseases in children.   4. Infection in children.
I. McCormick, William F.   II. Title.   III. Series.   [DNLM: 1. Central
nervous system diseases—In infancy and childhood.   2. Communicable
diseases—In infancy and childhood.   W1 MA492N v. 12 / WS 340 B435n]

RJ496.I53B44 1981   618.92′8   80-52767

ISBN 0-7216-1676-3   AACR2

Neurologic Infections in Children   ISBN   0-7216-1676-3

Last digit is the print number: 9   8   7   6   5   4   3   2   1

Foreword

It is a pleasure to present the second edition of *Neurologic Infections in Children* by Drs. Bell and McCormick, coauthors well known to this monograph series for both the first edition of this book and another volume entitled *Increased Intracranial Pressure in Children.*

The first edition was heralded for its excellence and termed the best book available on the subject. One reviewer stated that "it is hard to think of an infectious disease of the nervous system that is not adequately discussed in this book." The new edition contains the latest diagnostic procedures and therapeutic advances. Like the first edition, it is well organized, equally thorough, beautifully illustrated, and very readable. It contains excellent coverage of the clinical, microbiologic, and pathologic aspects of each topic. There is also a section on nervous system complications of infectious diseases as well as chapters on conditions that may be related to infectious disorders, such as Reye's syndrome and acute cerebellar ataxia. Practitioners will find the detailed discussions of treatment especially useful for quick reference.

MILTON MARKOWITZ, M.D.

Preface

Certain of the disorders included within this volume are among the most dramatic and potentially devastating illnesses that attack infants and children. Acute suppurative meningitis, viral encephalitis, and certain post-viral conditions such as Reye's syndrome often strike suddenly with little warning and can either result in death or leave the child with lasting neurologic deficits. An unfortunate outcome cannot always be prevented but with the advances in knowledge of the spectrum of neurologic infections, with new diagnostic techniques and the current therapeutic modalities, many children can be spared the ravages of these diseases. Effective treatment, however, is dependent upon early recognition, and recognition in turn depends on the practitioner's awareness of the diagnostic possibilities and the selection of the diagnostic tests and procedures most likely to yield useful information. Therein lies the purpose of this book, which is designed to outline the common symptoms and signs as well as the natural course of the various types of infections of the nervous system, and to illustrate the value and pitfalls of the different laboratory methods available for their identification. The historical perspectives and descriptions of pathology are included because it is the authors' belief that knowledge of these aspects can in some instances contribute significantly to the care of a child affected with an infectious disease in which there is neurologic involvement.

We wish to acknowledge the resources provided by Dr. F. Smith and Dr. M. W. Van Allen, and also the advice provided by Dr. A. Menezes, Dr. M. Myers, and Dr. R. Strauss in the development of certain sections in this volume. Dr. R. Caplan deserves thanks for providing us with certain photographs of cutaneous lesions of rare disorders which the authors could not otherwise have found. The assistance of Miss Mary Cowell and the highly professional talents of those persons of the W. B. Saunders Company who convert 1800 pages of typed manuscript and many folders of photographs into a final product are appreciated. Special thanks are extended to Miss Melanie Morris for her many hours of library work and her tireless dedication to the completion of the manuscript.

William E. Bell, M.D.
William F. McCormick, M.D.

Contents

Chapter Twenty-One

Chapter Twenty-Two

Chapter Twenty-Three

Chapter Twenty-Four

Chapter Twenty-Five

Bacterial Infections of the Nervous System

Chapter One

BACTERIAL MENINGITIS— GENERAL CONCEPTS AND MANAGEMENT

BACTERIAL AGENTS

Despite the development of antimicrobial agents and the advent of new diagnostic and treatment methods, bacterial infections of the central nervous system continue to pose a serious threat to the health and welfare of infants and children. Acute suppurative meningitis is the most common type of bacterial infection of the central nervous system in childhood; however, the brain or spinal cord can be affected in a variety of ways in association with bacterial infections (Table 1–1). In addition, the various pathologic types of infection can occur in combination or one can lead to another. For example, untreated focal cerebritis becomes a solitary brain abscess, which eventually may rupture into the ventricle or subarachnoid space provoking acute meningitis.

The incidence of the different etiologic types of bacterial meningitis has gradually changed over the past several decades, as has the epidemiology of certain types of infection. Articles published in the first two decades of this century emphasized the relatively high percentage of cases of meningitis in children that were tuberculous in origin, the infrequent occurrence of *Hemophilus influenzae* meningitis, and the strong association of pneumococcal meningitis with lobar pneumonia (Dunn 1911, Holt 1911, Wollstein 1911). As of 1918, neonatal meningitis was described as an "exceedingly rare disease" (Barron) and one often not identified until postmortem examination was performed. Meningococcal meningitis at that time was best known for its occurrence in epidemics and was referred to as epidemic cerebrospinal meningitis. All types of acute suppurative meningitis were then nearly uniformly fatal, with the exception of meningococcal meningitis, from which some survived with the use of Flexner's antimeningococcal serum. As late as 1933, Fothergill and Sweet found that, of 705 cases of meningitis in children, 41 percent were tuberculous and only 11 percent were influenzal in origin. Tuberculous meningitis subsequently declined considerably over the years and was eventually balanced by the unexplained increased incidence of meningitis due to *Hemophilus influenzae,* type b, which is now the single most common type of meningitis that occurs in the pediatric age range in this country.

Pneumococcal meningitis has stubbornly retained an unyieldingly stable mortality rate for the past two decades and continues to be particularly dangerous in the infant age group. Unlike its previous high association with lobar pneumonia, pneumococcal meningitis is now most often a complication of systemic sepsis in the infant, of suppurative paracranial infections in the older child, of disorders with cerebrospinal fluid fistulae, or secondary to conditions with immune defects

3

Table 1–1.   Types of Bacterial Infections of the Nervous System in Children

---

Meningitis
Vasculitis (thrombotic, embolic, mycotic aneurysm)
Cerebritis
Abscess (parenchymal, epidural, subdural)
Septic cavernous sinus thrombosis
Orbital cellulitis with cerebral thrombophlebitis
Gradenigo's syndrome (apical petrositis)
Spinal epidural or subdural abscess
Acute disc space infection (spondyloarthritis)

---

such as sickle cell disease or following splenectomy. The meningococcus has not recently been a cause of massive civilian epidemics as in past years, but retains its ability to produce life-threatening disease in the child or young adult in the form of sepsis or meningitis. In the newborn infant, staphylococcal meningitis is now much less often encountered than was the case 20 to 30 years ago, whereas group B streptococcal meningitis has recently become as frequent, or in some centers more frequent, than *Escherichia coli* meningitis. Regardless of the causative organism or the age of the patient, bacterial meningitis is an illness in which diagnosis should be confirmed at the earliest possible moment, followed by the immediate initiation of the proper therapeutic agents administered in the correct fashion. These goals can be achieved only if one is armed with considerable knowledge of the disease and its management.

Bacterial meningitis occurs more often in the pediatric age group than in any other period, as exemplified by the series of Jonsson and Alvin that included 476 cases in all age groups, of which three-fourths occurred in patients less than 15 years of age and one-third in those less than one year of age. The first year of life is a time of special risk, not only because of the greater frequency of meningitis at this time but also because the signs of meningeal inflammation may be less distinct and sequelae more frequent when bacterial agents attack the immature brain.

Virtually any bacterium is capable of causing meningitis but different age groups in childhood are predisposed to meningitis due to certain organisms (Table 1–2). During the first month after birth, *Escherichia coli* and group B *Streptococcus* (*Streptococcus agalactiae*) are the leading causes of bacterial meningitis and account for a high percentage of all cases in this age group. Outbreaks of staphylococcal infections in newborn nurseries are now much less common than two to three decades ago but the organism is still important as a cause of shunt infection in infants with hydrocephalus. Other members of the Enterobacteriaceae that can cause meningitis in the newborn infant include *Citrobacter* species (Gwynn and George, Gross et al.), *Klebsiella* species (Hill et al.), *Salmonella* species (Barclay, Rabinowitz and MacLeod), and *Edwardsiella tarda* (Sachs et al.). Members of the division *Klebsiella-Enterobacter-Serratia* show a predisposition to attack the low birth weight neonate or the infant debilitated with extraneural organ system disease requiring respirator care, intravascular catheters, high-dosage antibiotics, or surgical procedures. *Proteus* and *Pseudomonas* species are additional gram-negative organisms that are infrequent causes of neonatal meningitis but result in severe disease when they do occur (Cussen and Ryan, Levy and Ingall). *Flavobacterium meningosepticum,* a pleomorphic gram-negative anaerobic bacillus, can be acquired by the neonate, resulting in meningitis in either sporadic or epidemic form (Cabrera and Davis, George et al., Plotkin and McKitrick, Sugathadasa and Arseculeratne). Of all reported cases of *Flavobacterium* meningitis, the great majority have been in neonates or young infants; rare adult cases have been described in patients with serious underlying illnesses (Rios et al.). Other anaerobic bacilli, including *Bacteroides* species, give rise to neonatal meningitis on rare occasion, usually in infants with predisposing illnesses (Berman et al., Feldman). Many other organisms can, on rare occasion, result in meningitis in the newborn infant, including *Streptococcus pneumoniae, Hemophilus influenzae, Listeria monocytogenes,* and *Campylobacter (Vibrio) fetus.*

The time span from four to 12 weeks after birth represents an interface between the neonatal period and the older infant period in regard to the common causes of bacterial meningitis. Group B *Streptococcus* and *Streptococcus pneumoniae* are the most common offenders in this age group. Meningitis caused by gram-negative rods of the Enterobacteriaceae have become much less common by this time and cases with *Hemophilus influenzae* have begun to appear. *Listeria monocytogenes* and *Salmonella* species account for some examples, and the same is true for *Neisseria meningitidis.*

From three months until three years of age, *Hemophilus influenzae,* type b, is the most common cause of bacterial meningitis by a considerable margin (Floyd et al.). It also rep-

Table 1–2. Etiologic Sources of Bacterial Meningitis Related to Age

BIRTH TO TWO MONTHS
  Main causes
    Escherichia coli
    Streptococcus agalactiae (group B)
  Less frequent causes
    Streptococcus pneumoniae
    Staphylococcus sp.
    Proteus mirabilis, morgani
    Pseudomonas aeruginosa
    Hemophilus influenzae, type b
    Listeria monocytogenes
    Klebsiella sp.
    Aerobacter sp.
    Salmonella sp.
  Rare causes
    Streptococcus sp. (non-group B)
    Citrobacter freundii, diversus
    Flavobacterium meningosepticum
    Pasturella sp.
    Neisseria meningitidis, gonorrhoeae
    Campylobacter (Vibrio) fetus
    Serratia marcescens
    Bacteroides fragilis
    Aeromonas shigelloides
    Edwardsiella tarda
TWO MONTHS TO FOUR YEARS
  Main causes
    Hemophilus influenzae, type b
    Streptococcus pneumoniae
    Neisseria meningitidis
  Less frequent causes
    Mycobacterium tuberculosis
    Staphylococcus sp.
    Proteus mirabilis, morgani
    Pseudomonas aeruginosa
    Escherichia coli
    Listeria monocytogenes
    Klebsiella sp.

Rare causes
    Streptococcus sp.
    Hemophilus parainfluenzae
    Bacteroides fragilis
    Serratia marcescens
    Neisseria catarrhalis, subflava, sicca
    Pasteurella sp.
    Acinetobacter calcoaceticus var. anitratus
    Acinetobacter calcoaceticus var. lwoffi
    Hemophilus influenzae, non-type b
FOUR YEARS AND OLDER
  Main causes
    Streptococcus pneumoniae
    Neisseria meningitidis
  Less frequent causes
    Mycobacterium tuberculosis
    Hemophilus influenzae, type b
    Streptococcus sp.
    Staphylococcus sp.
    Escherichia coli
    Listeria monocytogenes
    Klebsiella sp.
    Pseudomonas aeruginosa
    Proteus mirabilis, morgani
  Rare causes
    Neisseria gonorrhoeae
    Fusobacterium sp.
    Neisseria catarrhalis, subflava, sicca
    Bacillus anthracis (anthrax)
    Pasteurella sp.
    Brucella melitensis, abortus, suis
    Propionibacterium (Corynebacterium) acnes
    Edwardsiella tarda
    Eikenella (Bacteroides) corrodens
    Acinetobacter calcoaceticus var. anitratus
    Acinetobacter calcoaceticus var. lwoffi
    Bacteroides fragilis
    Hemophilus influenzae, non-type b

resents the single most common cause of meningitis in this country between birth and age 16 years, but in Great Britain is exceeded by the meningococcus, which is the most prevalent cause (Goldacre). Between three years and eight years of age, *Hemophilus influenzae* meningitis becomes progressively less common, and thereafter is unusual as a primary type of meningitis in otherwise normal individuals. The great majority of cases of *Hemophilus influenzae* meningitis are caused by type b encapsulated organisms. Strains other than type b have accounted for relatively few cases, and, of the reported cases, the clinical pattern and response to antibiotics have generally been similar to those in cases due to type b organisms (Denis et al., Greene, Hodes and Leidy). There are only a few reports of meningitis resulting from *Hemophilus parainfluenzae* although it is probably more common than is generally assumed (Bachman, Gullekson and Dumoff, Holt et al., Kaufman et al.). The organism is not distinguishable from *Hemophilus influenzae* by the conventionally used laboratory methods and is identified only by special techniques. The age range, clinical features, and response to therapy appear to be similar to those in meningitis caused by *Hemophilus influenzae*. *Neisseria meningitidis* is a rare isolate from cerebrospinal fluid in the first two months after birth but becomes considerably more prevalent between two and 12 months of age. Its peak incidence is in the first year of life and again in late adolescence and early adulthood. From three months until three years of age, *Streptococcus pneumoniae* ranks second only to *Hemophilus influenzae* as a cause of meningitis.

In children over four years of age, *Streptococcus pneumoniae* and *Neisseria meningitidis* are the most common organisms producing suppurative meningeal infection. *Streptococcus pyogenes*, group A, is an uncommon cause of neurologic infection in children but can produce meningitis in otherwise normal children or in those with underlying immunosuppressive disease (Burech et al.). Meningitis due to this organism can also occur in children with predisposing anatomic defects, such as a congenital dermal sinus (Shadravan et al.). Staphylococcal meningitis can occur in children of any age but is seen more often in those who have a ventricular shunt for hydrocephalus, or rarely as a complication of bacterial endocarditis, bronchiectasis, or osteomyelitis. This organism can also cause meningitis in infants with congenital defects such as meningomyelocele and following neurosurgical procedures (Mulcare and Harter). Meningitis resulting from anaerobic bacilli in older children or adults most often occurs as a complication of chronic otitis media or mastoiditis, chronic sinusitis, abdominal trauma, or following neurosurgical operative procedures. Anaerobic streptococci, *Bacteroides* species, and *Fusobacteria* are the most common offenders in such instances.

Air contrast procedures in hydrocephalic children have been complicated by meningitis due to *Staphylococcus* or *Pseudomonas* species, and *Acinetobacter calcoaceticus (Herellea vaginicola)* (Hook and Aase, Kerman et al.). In children with cerebrospinal fluid rhinorrhea or otorrhea, *Streptococcus pneumoniae* is the chief cause of purulent meningitis, although numerous other aerobic or anaerobic organisms are also important offenders. Traumatic pneumocephalus is an additional condition in which there is danger of intracranial bacterial infection with many possible organisms until the communication with the external environment is obliterated by healing or by surgical repair (Kahn and Daywitt). In children with occipital or lumbar dermal sinuses communicating with the subarachnoid space, meningitis can result from a variety of gram-negative or gram-positive organisms and in some cases is recurrent. In addition to the possibility of suppurative meningitis, the child with a dermal sinus terminating in an intracranial dermoid can experience acute aseptic meningitis secondary to leakage of material from the dermoid or its rupture (Shackelford et al.). Bacterial meningitis, as well as spinal epidural abscess, can develop secondary to extension of infected material from a psoas abscess. The latter is usually associated with some other intra-abdominal suppurative process and may not have been identified at the time of the development of meningitis (Orrison et al.).

Members of the tribe Mimeae include *Acinetobacter calcoaceticus* var. *anitratus* (previously called *Herellea vaginicola*) and *Acineto-*

bacter calcoaceticus var. *lwoffi* (previously called *Mima polymorphia*). They are gram-negative diplococci which, on stained preparations, can readily be confused with the meningococcus or other organisms. *Acinetobacter calcoaceticus* var. *lwoffi* has been described as a cause of meningitis in otherwise normal children but is regarded to be rare (Herman and Melnick, Donald and Doak). *Acinetobacter calcoaceticus* var. *anitratus* is more widely known as a human pathogen, and shows a predisposition to colonize or result in invasive disease in hospitalized patients (Glew et al.). Meningitis caused by this organism has been seen following neurosurgical operative procedures (Daly), after air ventriculography (Hook and Aase), and in head injury patients.

Neisseria gonorrhoeae meningitis has been only rarely described but can occur in the newborn infant as well as in older persons (Bradford and Kelly, Taubin and Landsberg). The illness can be associated with hemorrhagic skin lesions and septic shock and thus be clinically identical to meningococcal infection (Swierczewski et al.). Bacteriologic differentiation of gonococcal and meningococcal meningitis is based upon the ability of the gonococcus to ferment dextrose but not maltose or sucrose. The fluorescent antibody technique has also been used to identify the gonococcus in CSF (Sayeed et al.).

Other bacterial agents which cause meningitis on rare occasion include *Neisseria subflava* (Lewin and Hughes), *Neisseria catarrhalis* (Feigin et al.), *Pasteurella* species (Bates et al., Cooper et al.), *Serratia marcescens* (Graber et al.), and *Propionibacterium (Corynebacterium) acnes* (French et al., Graber et al.). Meningitis caused by *Mycobacterium tuberculosis* has gradually diminished in frequency over the past several decades and now is unusual in many parts of this country. It remains a lingering menace, however, and must still be considered in the differential diagnosis in a variety of clinical situations. Nontuberculous (atypical) mycobacteria are very rare causes of meningitis and only a few cases in children or adults have been described (Wolinsky 1979). "Mixed" meningitis, or meningitis due to more than one organism, is not common but is more often found in infancy than in older children (Gromish et al., Herwig et al.).

Recurrent bacterial meningitis is most commonly seen in children with cerebrospinal fluid fistulae with rhinorrhea or otorrhea (Table 1–3). Rhinorrhea is most often secondary to traumatic injuries with fractures through air-containing paracranial sinuses

Table 1–3. Causes of "Recurrent" Meningitis (Bacterial and Aseptic)

Congenital dermal sinus
Cerebrospinal fluid rhinorrhea and otorrhea
Chronic apical petrositis
Ventricular shunts
Recurrent bacterial meningitis—etiology undetermined
Mollaret's meningitis
Behcet's disease
Vogt-Koyanagi-Harada's disease
Systemic lupus erythematosus
Spontaneous leakage from intracranial dermoid or
   epidermoid
Disorders with immunosuppression

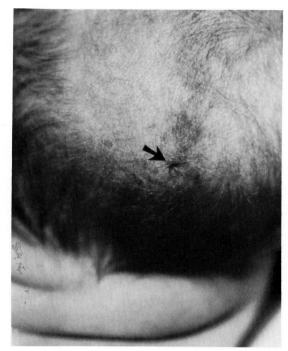

Figure 1–1. Congenital dermal sinus in an infant located in the occipital region (arrow). The cutaneous dimple is in the midline and contains a long tuft of hair. Skull x-ray demonstrated cranium bifidum underlying the occipital skin defect. Infants and children with this congenital lesion are susceptible to the development of bacterial meningitis if the defect communicates with the intracranial contents.

but can also be the result of congenital defects of the anterior cranial fossa or neoplastic erosion of the base of the skull (Brisman et al., Gibson and Kurukchy, Kaufman). CSF otorrhea can follow head injury or surgical trauma, and can also be secondary to congenital defects associated with a fistula through the footplate of the stapes or the oval window (Biggers et al., Carter et al., Skolnik and Ferrer, Stool et al.). The latter disorder is suspected when the child with previously recognized unilateral congenital deafness develops meningitis, and especially when it is recurrent. The precise site of the CSF fistula which predisposes the patient to recurrent meningitis is often difficult to demonstrate but has been simplified somewhat with the development of metrizamide computed tomography (Drayer et al., Maravilla et al.).

Recurrent meningitis is a common complication of occipital or lumbar congenital dermal sinuses (Matson and Jerva, Matson and Ingraham, Shackelford et al.) (Fig. 1–1), and can be a life-threatening complication in patients with transsphenoidal or transethmoidal encephaloceles (Pinto et al., Pollock et al.). Infants and children with intraventricular shunts are at risk for recurrent episodes of meningitis, as are patients with a wide variety of defects of the immune mechanism. There remain a group of children with recurrent meningitis, usually pneumococcal in type, in whom no definite cause can be discovered. The microbiology of recurrent meningitis is diverse, with *Streptococcus pneumoniae* being the most common offender, especially when it is secondary to CSF rhinorrhea. *Staphylococcus* species are the most frequent causes of recurrent meningitis in children with ventricular shunts. With congenital dermal sinuses, multiple episodes of meningitis are caused by many organisms, including *Proteus* and *Pseu-*

domonas species, *Escherichia coli, Streptococcus* species, and *Staphylococcus* species.

Anthrax Meningitis

Anthrax has nearly disappeared from this country, and, as a result, anthrax meningitis is now an exceedingly rare disorder (Fig. 1–2). The illness continues to occur in many other parts of the world, including Asia, Africa, the Middle East, and Mexico. Most cases of anthrax have occurred in workers handling wools or hides and persons directly exposed to animals. The disease is caused by *Bacillus anthracis,* which is a gram-positive, non-motile, encapsulated organism whose spores can survive for years in soil.

Cutaneous anthrax is the most common form of the disease, with inhalation anthrax and a gastrointestinal form occurring much less frequently (Brachman). The cutaneous form is a relatively benign disorder if recognized and treated. The skin lesion is usually solitary and is initially present as a papule,

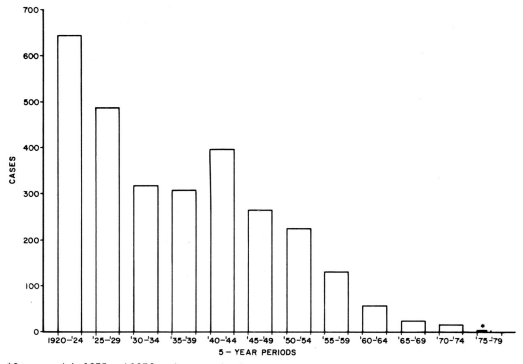

*2 cases each in 1975 and 1976, and no cases in 1977.

Figure 1–2.   Anthrax. Reported human cases by five-year period in United States, 1920–1977. (From: Morbidity and Mortality Weekly Report, Annual Summary, 1977. Volume 26, No. 53, Sept. 1978.)

which progresses to a vesicle and subsequently to a painless ulcerated crater one or two centimeters in diameter. Associated systemic symptoms are mild or absent but tender lymphadenopathy is often present in the region of lymphatic drainage of the cutaneous lesion. Septic dissemination can occur but does so infrequently, and most cutaneous lesions heal with appropriate antibiotic therapy. Inhalation anthrax is a much more serious illness, which begins after a short incubation period of a few days. Initial symptoms consist of mild fever, malaise, and cough. This is followed by precipitous worsening of respiratory function, with high fever, depressed state of responsiveness, and sometimes shock, which rapidly proceeds to death. In some instances, death from progressive respiratory compromise occurs within one or two days of onset of severe symptoms, while in others, the infection is complicated by septic dissemination leading to hemorrhagic meningitis (Plotkin et al.). Gastrointestinal anthrax is a rare form of the disease but also has a high mortality rate. In this form, the organism is introduced by consumption of infected meat. Symptoms are

acute in onset and include fever, vomiting, and bloody diarrhea.

Anthrax meningitis is a rare complication of the cutaneous or visceral forms of the disease, and in a few instances has occurred without a primary source of origin (Haight, Pluot et al.). Previous literature reviews indicate that fewer than 5 percent of cases of anthrax are followed by dissemination to the meninges and that most cases of meningitis complicate the most common, or the cutaneous, form (Haight, Shanahan et al.). Since anthrax is an illness that is occupationally related, most reports of anthrax meningitis have been in adults, although it has been described in children as well (Rangel and González, Tahernia and Hashemi).

Anthrax meningitis is a fulminating illness with rapid emergence of fever and signs of severe, diffuse neurologic involvement. The CSF usually is hemorrhagic and contains a mixture of red blood cells and polymorphonuclear leukocytes, as well as a marked elevation of the protein content. Less often, the CSF is purulent to gross inspection (Tahernia and Hashemi). *Bacillus anthracis* can usually be cultured from the CSF and also from the blood. The neuropathology of the illness includes an inflammatory meningeal exudate which contains both red blood cells and leukocytes. Severe cerebral swelling is usually found, along with cortical or deep nuclear hemorrhages that are evident on observation of gross specimens. Severe and widespread vasculitis is also usually present (Haight, Rangel and González). The hemorrhagic aspect of the meningeal and cerebral reaction is the most distinctive feature of anthrax meningitis. Penicillin in high dosage is recommended for this illness. Survival has been infrequent (Shanahan et al., Tahernia and Hashemi), although many of the reported cases of anthrax meningitis occurred prior to the availability of antibiotic therapy.

Bacteroides *Meningitis*

Bacteroides species are anaerobic, non-sporulating, gram-negative bacilli which are found as part of the normal flora of the upper respiratory and gastrointestinal tracts, as well as the female genital tract. While their role as potential causes of serious disease is now well known, in the first half of this century, *Bacteroides* species were often regarded as nonpathogenic contaminants (McVay and Sprunt). They are uncommon causes of infection in otherwise normal persons but can be important pathogens in patients with chronic debilitating diseases or when there is compromise of the mucous membranes of the respiratory or intestinal tracts. Central nervous system infections with *Bacteroides* species can occur in any age group but are more common in adults than in infants or children. Among the various species included in the group, *Bacteroides fragilis* is the most common cause of infection in children as well as in adults (Dunkle et al., Felner and Dowell).

In past years when chronic suppurative otitis media was common, most cases of *Bacteroides* meningitis or brain abscess were from this source (Sanders and Stevenson, Smith et al.). *Bacteroides* meningitis of otogenic origin still occurs on infrequent occasion, and recent studies have shown that *Bacteroides* species are still a common isolate from middle ear pus in patients with chronic otitis media (Brook and Finegold). Currently, *Bacteroides* meningitis is more often due to septic dissemination from intra-abdominal sepsis or chronic pulmonary disease. *Bacteroides* meningitis has been described in the newborn period following surgical repair of gastric perforation (Feldman)

and as a septic complication of necrotizing enterocolitis (Berman et al.). It has also been seen in early infancy secondary to peritonitis (Cooke) and as a result of an infected ventriculoatrial shunt (Feldman). It is not surprising that *Bacteroides* species, as part of the normal flora of the female genital tract, are sometimes identified as the cause of neonatal septicemia in stressed prematurely born infants or in infants delivered of mothers with amnionitis or endometritis (Harrod and Stevens). Only rarely has *Bacteroides* meningitis been discovered in a child without a clearcut source of origin (Lifshitz et al.).

Antibiotic treatment of *Bacteroides* species infections, as in other anaerobic infections, is best determined by sensitivity data; however, they are not always reliable with this group of organisms. Chloramphenicol is usually the drug of choice for *Bacteroides* meningitis or brain abscess. In some instances, response to treatment with this drug is suboptimal, and metronidazole proves to be more effective (Berman et al., Feldman).

Brucella *Meningoencephalitis*

Brucella species are gram-negative aerobic bacilli that are transmitted to man from infected animals. *Brucella abortus* is found in cattle, *Brucella suis* in swine, and *Brucella melitensis* in goats. Brucellosis, also called Malta fever or undulant fever, has become progressively less common in this country with control of the disease in cattle, and is especially uncommon in children (Street et al.) (Fig. 1–3). In past years, the condition was sometimes acquired by the consumption of unpasteurized milk or other dairy products, but currently it is largely an occupational disease of slaughterhouse workers or farmers (Buchanan et al.). With this gradual transition in the mode of transmission of brucellosis in this country, *Brucella suis* has come to far exceed *Brucella abortus* as the cause of human disease. In Mexico, *Brucella melitensis* is the causative organism in most human cases. In most abattoir-acquired cases, the organism is contracted via breaks in the skin of the hands (Buchanan et al.). Other possible portals of entry include by inhalation, via the conjunctiva, and by oral consumption of infected milk products. Human infections with *Brucella suis* and *Brucella abortus* are clinically similar, while infection with *Brucella melitensis* is likely to be more severe and with a higher incidence of complications.

Brucellosis can be either insidious or acute

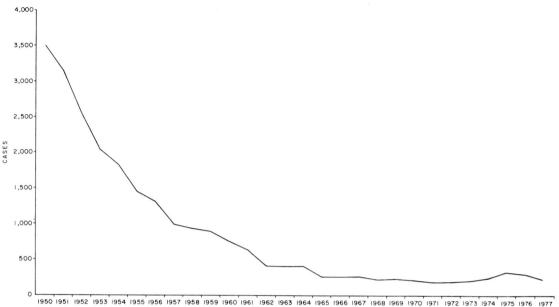

Figure 1–3. Brucellosis. Reported cases by year in the United States, 1950–1977. (From: Morbidity and Mortality Weekly Report, Annual Summary, 1977. Volume 26, No. 53, Sept. 1978.)

in onset with the predominant symptoms of fever, chills, night-sweats, malaise, headache, and arthralgia. Joint pain in unusual cases is severe, and authors have pointed out that so-called pseudoparalysis of an extremity caused by articular pain can be misinterpreted as an indication of poliomyelitis (DeBono). Spleno-megaly and hepatomegaly are present in a relatively small percentage of patients early in the illness. The disease can be subclinical, mild and transient, chronic with relapsing symptoms, or fulminating, leading to death on rare occasion. Leukopenia is a common laboratory finding in the acute stage of bru-cellosis, although leukocytosis or a leukemoid reaction can occur as well (Street et al.).

Neurologic complications of brucellosis are infrequent but can be exceedingly diverse, with involvement of any part of the central, peripheral, or autonomic nervous system. An accurate incidence of occurrence of neuro-logic involvement in this disease is not known and has been estimated at less than 10 per-cent (Spink) but is probably considerably less than this estimate. Meningitis or meningoen-cephalitis can be acute or subacute, and in some cases follows a relapsing course (Bough-ton, Nichols, Poston and Thomason). Signs of meningeal involvement or encephalitis can occur soon after onset of the systemic fea-tures of the illness, or can be delayed for sev-eral weeks thereafter. In rare instances, stiff neck, confusion, seizures, or other signs of cerebral dysfunction can represent the pre-senting signs of brucellosis (Abramsky). With-out treatment, the signs of meningoen-cephalitis will in some cases gradually dimin-ish only to relapse subsequently, or will pro-ceed downhill eventually resulting in death (Nelson-Jones). The CSF findings in *Brucella* meningoencephalitis are almost as protean as are the clinical manifestations (Fincham et al.). CSF pleocytosis usually consists mainly of lymphocytes, but, less often, polymorphonu-clear leukocytes will be more prevalent. The glucose content is usually normal but can be moderately reduced. The protein content of CSF is fairly consistently elevated but to vari-able degrees. Organisms can be isolated from CSF in some cases but this also is quite incon-sistent.

Acute transverse myelitis is a rare neuro-logic manifestation of brucellosis (Abramsky). Either meningitis or myelitis may be compli-cated subsequently by progressive adhesive arachnoiditis which adds further neurologic deficits (Sahadevan et al.). An additional rare complication of brucellosis is acute subarach-noid hemorrhage secondary to rupture of a mycotic aneurysm (Nelson-Jones). Peripheral neuropathy, cranial nerve neuropathy, and intervertebral disk disease producing a sciatic syndrome are other possible manifestations of neurobrucellosis (Abramsky, Aguilar and

Elvidge, Fincham et al.). A variety of ocular complications of brucellosis have been described, including uveitis, a macular retinopathy, optic neuritis, and optic atrophy secondary to adhesive arachnoiditis (Solanes et al.).

Diagnosis of brucellosis is based on the clinical manifestations of the illness, the epidemiologic features, and a significant antibody titer rise on serologic tests. Isolation of *Brucella* species from body fluids, including blood, bone marrow, or CSF, is the definitive diagnostic measure, but is especially difficult in patients who have received prior antibiotic therapy. The brucella skin test can be used as a method to indicate prior infection with the organism but should not be used as a diagnostic test for acute infection. Significant titer rise can result from the application of the skin test, possibly resulting in diagnostic confusion. Buchanan and colleagues have reviewed the value of the available serologic tests for brucellosis which include the standard agglutination test, the complement-fixation test, the indirect fluorescent antibody test, and the card agglutination test. The tube agglutination test was found to detect elevated brucella agglutinins in most infected patients by the end of the first week of illness.

Tetracycline is the drug of choice for treatment of brucellosis or its infectious complications; however, in severe infections, tetracycline and streptomycin in combination are recommended. Buchanan et al. found a lower relapse rate among patients treated with both drugs as compared to those receiving tetracycline alone. Tetracycline should be continued for a minimum of three to four weeks.

Campylobacter fetus *Meningitis*

Campylobacter fetus, classified as *Vibrio fetus* until 1973, is a thin, comma-shaped, mobile, microaerophilic gram-negative rod which has been recognized to be a human pathogen only relatively recently. The designation, *Campylobacter,* is derived from two Greek words meaning "curved" and "rod" (Rettig). The organism was well known to be an important cause of abortion in cattle, sheep, and other animals since the first decade of this century but was not identified to be a cause of human disease until 1947. In that year, Vinzent et al. described a 39-year-old woman with a febrile illness during pregnancy from whom *Vibrio fetus* was isolated on blood cul-

ture. The pregnancy terminated with a stillborn fetus and the placenta was found to have undergone a necrotizing process. In 1962, Eden first reported fatal neonatal meningitis in a premature infant caused by this organism, and subsequently only a few additional cases in the newborn period have been described (Burgert and Hagstrom, Willis and Austin). With improvement in methods of isolation of the organism, *Campylobacter fetus* has recently been established as a frequent cause of enteritis in infants and children.

An analogy has been made between human disease caused by *Campylobacter fetus* and *Listeria monocytogenes.* Like the latter, *Campylobacter fetus* has been shown to have a predisposition to attack the pregnant female and the fetus, the newborn infant in whom there is a decided predilection for the infection to invade the central nervous system, and the adult with pre-existent clinical illness or immunosuppressive conditions. Although this clinical pattern of susceptibility has been demonstrated, the organism is regarded to be a rare cause of invasive disease in the childhood years. Bacteremia is the most common form of *Campylobacter fetus* infection, sometimes associated with gastrointestinal involvement (Guerrant et al.). Meningitis in children beyond the newborn period has only rarely been identified (Willis and Austin). In adults, bacteremia has been associated with diffuse meningitis, localized meningoencephalitis, necrotizing vasculitis resulting in cerebrovascular occlusion, and intracranial hemorrhage (Gunderson and Sack, Zelinger and Vargas).

The method by which humans acquire *Campylobacter fetus* has remained unclear in most cases in that only the minority have had known occupational or environmental exposure to infected animals. Consumption of contaminated food or raw milk has been implicated in some cases (Taylor et al.), and venereal transmission to the female from the male believed to be able to harbor the organism for lengthy periods in asymptomatic fashion has also been postulated (Eden, 1966).

Infection with this gram-negative bacillus has been claimed by some to perhaps be more common than is generally believed because it is easily mistaken for other organisms on stained preparations and is difficult to isolate in culture unless special precautions are taken. At best, several days may be required for its growth on artificial media under microaerophilic conditions (Rettig). Meningitis has been fatal in cases in the neonatal period while recovery is possible with therapy in older patients. There is little available information regarding the optimal antibiotic treatment for *Campylobacter fetus* meningitis although most isolates have been sensitive to chloramphenicol and aminoglycosides.

Eosinophilic Meningitis

A significant eosinophilic pleocytosis in cerebrospinal fluid is a rare finding except in a few foreign regions where certain types of helminthic infections are prevalent. Identification of this cell type in CSF requires a carefully prepared stained slide, as their presence will often not be recognized in the conventional counting chamber (Kuberski). While parasitic infections of the central nervous system are recognized to be the most common international cause of CSF eosinophilia and coccidioidomycosis is most likely the leading cause in this country, there are a few other situations in which this finding has been observed. A transient CSF eosinophilia has been described following intraventricular placement of a rubber catheter for shunting of hydrocephalus (Jeanes, Kessler and Cheek). In these cases, the eosinophilic pleocytosis occurred several weeks after the shunt was installed and at a time when the patients were not ill except for some degree of fever. Eosinophils in the CSF in association with transient signs of meningeal irritation have been observed after Pantopaque myelography (Holley and Al-Ibrahim). Meningeal invasion with lymphoma has been described with an eosinophilic response in CSF; however, this is acknowledged to be very unusual and is not the typical finding in CSF with this disease (Evans and McElwain, King et al.). Demyelinating diseases can also rarely be associated with a significant number of eosinophils in the CSF in the absence of a peripheral blood eosinophilia (Hughes and Adams, Snead and Kalavsky). In all these conditions, the presence of eosinophils in the CSF is believed to be the result of a local hypersensitivity reaction of central nervous system tissue and is usually transient. CSF eosinophilia is not usually observed with viral infections of the central nervous system but has been described in a child with chronic lymphocytic choriomeningitis virus meningitis (Chesney et al.).

Eosinophils in CSF can be found in a number of parasitic diseases with intracranial involvement although it is the exception rather than the rule. The best known examples include cysticercosis (Bickerstaff et al., Nieto), paragonimiasis (Kim, Oh), and toxocara encephalitis (Anderson et al.). Eosinophils in the CSF in these disorders usually constitute a relatively low percentage of the total cell population and in most instances are not present at all. In contrast, however, is a parasitic disorder referred to as eosinophilic meningitis in which eosinophils make up a large percentage of the CSF pleocytosis. This disease has been identified in Tahiti, Hawaii, Taiwan, Thailand, and a few other Pacific islands, and is caused by nematodes, including *Angiostrongylus cantonensis* and *Gnathostoma spinigerum* (Char and Rosen, Yii et al., Punyagupta et al., Rosen et al.). Meningoencephalitis produced by the rat lung-worm, *Angiostrongylus cantonensis,* is much more common of the two, and consists of an acute illness with headache, meningeal signs, variable degrees of lethargy, and cranial nerve signs in some cases. In Taiwan, it has been seen predominantly in children (Yii et al.), while in other areas, young adults are more commonly affected. Spontaneous improvement follows in a few weeks in most instances although fatal cases have been described. The CSF findings vary from case to case and at different times in a single case, but often include the presence of several hundred cells per cu. mm., of which 60 to 100 percent are eosinophils. Since the nematode is rarely isolated from the CSF, diagnosis is presumptive and is assumed on the basis of the epidemiologic features and the natural course of the illness.

Gram-Negative Bacillary Meningitis

Members of the Enterobacteriaceae (enteric bacilli) are best known as causes of meningitis in the neonatal period, discussed in Chapter 3. Meningitis resulting from these organisms is not limited to this age group, however, and can occur in older children and adults. *Escherichia coli, Klebsiella pneumoniae* and other species, *Salmonella* species, and *Proteus* species account for most such cases but the other members of the Enterobacteriaceae can also do so on rare occasion (Table 1–4). Meningitis caused by *Edwardsiella tarda* (Okubadejo and Alausa, Sachs et al.), *Enterobacter* species (Crane and Lerner, Mojtabaee and Siadati), and *Serratia marcescens* (Stamm et al.) has been described but is very unusual. Meningitis beyond the newborn period secondary

Table 1–4. Members of the Enterobacteriaceae

Genus:	Escherichia
Genus:	Edwardsiella
Genus:	Citrobacter
Genus:	Salmonella
Genus:	Shigella
Genus:	Klebsiella
Genus:	Enterobacter
Genus:	Hafnia
Genus:	Serratia
Genus:	Proteus
Genus:	Yersinia
Genus:	Erwinia

to any of these organisms is usually associated with some type of underlying predisposing cause (Gorman et al.). The most common predisposing causes of gram-negative bacillary meningitis in older children and adults include head injuries, neurosurgical procedures, chronic otitis media, and lower respiratory disease. Sickle cell disease is the best known of the conditions that increase the predisposition to *Salmonella* species infections, most of which are bacteremic or osteomyelitic infections (Barrett-Connor, Johnson).

Escherichia coli meningitis in older children or adults is exceedingly rare in otherwise previously normal persons. Most cases have occurred following open craniocerebral trauma or after neurosurgical operations, including ventricular shunts, meningomyelocele repair, and many other types of intracranial procedures (Mangi et al., Robinson et al.). In either setting, the initial manifestations of the illness may be obscured by the presence of obtundation or meningeal signs directly attributable to the injury or the surgical procedure. This form of meningitis has occurred in several adults following septic abortion (Hughes and Manning, Margarey et al.), in patients with genitourinary tract disease (Kunin et al., Rosenfeld), and as a complication of lumbar puncture or spinal anesthesia (Kremer). A number of cases of *Escherichia coli* meningitis have occurred in persons with chronic alcoholism and cirrhosis, especially with pelvic or genitourinary tract infection (Crane and Lerner, Manesis and Stanosheck). It is believed that the presence of cirrhosis with its alterations of portal venous circulation allows circulating bacilli from the pelvis to bypass the phagocytic cells of the liver. *Escherichia coli* meningitis in the older individual is a serious disease, in part because it is almost always a complication of another underlying process,

and also because it is usually associated with a diffuse ependymitis and extensive cerebral phlebitis and arteritis resulting in cerebral vascular compromise (Robinson et al.). The case fatality rate is difficult to estimate because of the limited number of cases reported in older persons but is stated to be approximately 40 to 50 percent (Crane and Lerner, Mangi et al.).

Meningitis caused by *Klebsiella pneumoniae* and other *Klebsiella* species is very uncommon and does not usually occur in otherwise normal persons, regardless of age. Even in the newborn period, *Klebsiella* species are infrequent causes of meningitis. Of 117 cases of neonatal meningitis due to gram-negative bacilli in one series, only four (3 percent) were caused by these organisms (McCracken and Mize). *Klebsiella* infections in newborn intensive care nurseries are nosocomial in type and usually represent the emergence of infection caused by antibiotic-resistant organisms secondary to the widespread use of antibiotic therapy. The occurrence of *Klebsiella* species in this setting can be in the form of nosocomial asymptomatic colonization of a large number of infants (Adler et al.), of outbreaks of pneumonia, sepsis, or meningitis in epidemic fashion (Hable et al., Hill et al.), or a sporadic case of sepsis or meningitis in an infant with prior respiratory or gastrointestinal disease. In older children and adults, the most common predisposing causes of *Klebsiella* meningitis are neurosurgical procedures (Mangi et al., Price and Sleigh) including ventricular shunts (Quintiliani and Lentnek), and recent head injuries (Spivack et al.). In past years more than currently, the primary foci of infection leading to *Klebsiella* meningitis included otitis media, mastoiditis, and lower respiratory infection (Soscia et al., Thompson et al.). In combination with any of the above factors, diabetes mellitus in adults appears to enhance the susceptibility to *Klebsiella* sepsis and meningitis, as is the case with *Escherichia coli*. Authors in the past commented on the gelatinous appearance of the CSF in patients with *Klebsiella* meningitis, but these were usually advanced cases (Thompson et al.).

Meningitis caused by *Proteus mirabilis* and other *Proteus* species is similar epidemiologically to *Klebsiella* meningitis. In the pediatric age group most cases occur in the newborn period whereas in adults it is a complication of head injuries, neurosurgical operations, chronic otitis media, or other underlying diseases (Gorman et al., Mangi et al.). *Proteus* species bear another similarity to *Klebsiella* species in that either can contaminate the nursery environment, residing in humidifiers, suction apparatus, sink traps, or oxygen tubing (Adler et al., Becker). Most cases of *Proteus* species meningitis in children beyond the newborn period have been secondary to chronic otitis media although the disease can be a complication of a congenital dermal sinus, meningomyelocele repair, or other invasive procedures (Scherzer et al.). In infants especially, *Proteus* meningitis is often a destructive process with extensive vascular injury leading to widespread necrotizing cerebral damage (Cussen and Ryan).

Salmonella species meningitis is much more common in infancy than later in life (Henderson, Saphra and Winter). Among the series of 117 cases of neonatal gram-negative bacillary meningitis compiled by McCracken and Mize, *Salmonella* species were second only to *Escherichia coli* as the cause, but still accounted for only seven (6 percent) cases. Unlike *Escherichia coli* meningitis in infancy which occurs mainly in the first six weeks after birth, *Salmonella* meningitis is encountered at any time in infancy or early childhood. Except for the occasional occurrence of preceding diarrhea, infants with *Salmonella* meningitis are usually previously normal (Rabinowitz and MacLeod). The illness can be caused by one of several *Salmonella* serotypes. While *Salmonella* meningitis in this country cannot now be considered to be rare, it is much more common in certain other parts of the world (Barclay). *Salmonella typhi* meningitis can occur during the course of acute typhoid fever but is exceedingly rare (Osuntokun et al.). Abnormalities of neurologic function are common in typhoid fever but are usually attributable to severe dehydration, hyperthermia, and serum electrolyte abnormalities (Zellweger and Idriss).

Listeria *Meningitis*

Neurologic infection caused by *Listeria monocytogenes* is less common than that due to many other bacteria but when human infection does occur with this organism, there is a decided predisposition for central nervous system involvement. Although otherwise normal persons of any age can develop *Listeria* meningitis, the "opportunistic" qualities of this organism have become clear in recent years. Infections caused by *Listeria monocytogenes* are most common in the pregnant female, the fetus, the newborn and young in-

fant, and the immunosuppressed patient with lymphoproliferative malignant disease or following renal transplantation. Other conditions in which there is an increased risk of *Listeria* infection include chronic alcoholism, systemic lupus erythematosus, and chronic corticosteroid therapy. Acute meningitis is the most common type of neurologic infection caused by *Listeria monocytogenes*. In other cases, meningitis occurs in association with cerebral vasculitis or cerebritis. Still less common are focal cerebritis, multiple cerebral microabscesses, a solitary cerebral abscess, and a rare form referred to as rhomboencephalitis. The latter is a pontobulbar syndrome characterized by an acute inflammatory process with vasculitis and microabscesses limited to the pons and medulla.

Listeria monocytogenes is a gram-positive rod with tumbling motility demonstrable by the hanging-drop preparation and shows beta hemolysis on blood agar. The organism is often difficult to find on stained preparations of exudates and is commonly not seen on gram stain of infected CSF. After 24 hours of growth on artificial media, rods may elongate with palisade formation and be indistinguishable from diphtheroids on gram stain, or assume a coccoid appearance and thus be confused with streptococci or pneumococci. If decolorized excessively by alcohol during gram staining, *Listeria* will appear to be gram-negative and can be mistaken for *Hemophilus influenzae*. By far the most frequent error in the past has been the assumption from gram stains that they were diphtheroids, and thus discarded as non-pathogenic contaminants.

Disease caused by the organism now known as *Listeria monocytogenes* was first described by Murray et al. in 1926 in a colony of laboratory rabbits. It was a septicemic illness with a mononuclear leukocytosis and microabscesses in the liver. The organism was called *Bacterium monocytogenes* by Murray et al., the species designation because of the mononuclear cell response observed in infected animals. The first case of human disease was reported by Nyfeldt in 1929 in a patient with an infectious mononucleosis-like illness, and the initial report of listeriosis in this country was by Burn in 1935 who described infection in newborn infants. Pirie in 1940 proposed the name *Listeria monocytogenes*, now the official designation of the organism. *Listeria monocytogenes* is now recognized to cause a wide spectrum of human disease and also affects many animal species.

Fetal and neonatal listeriosis, described in

Chapter 3, occurs in a variety of clinical patterns. Infection during pregnancy can result in abortion or stillbirth, and it has been postulated that persistent maternal genital infection may be a cause of repeated abortion. Early neonatal septicemic forms can result from either intrauterine acquired infection or acquisition of the organism by the infant during the birth process. One type, referred to as granulomatosis infantisepticum, is characterized by multiple abscesses and granulomas in the liver and other organs, pneumonitis, meningitis, and a nearly uniformly fatal outcome (Ahlfors et al.). A second neonatal type of infection resembles group B *Streptococcus* sepsis in the neonatal period and consists of severe illness with cardiorespiratory collapse, meningitis in some cases, and also a high mortality rate. Infants with either of the early onset types of listeriosis are commonly premature (Albritton et al.). The later onset variety of neonatal disease with *Listeria monocytogenes* is more common, with onset between one week and two months of age, and manifested by acute meningitis. Affected infants are much less often of low birth weight, and prognosis is better than with the early onset form (Visintine et al.).

In 1967, Louria and colleagues drew attention to the predisposition of patients with malignant disease to sustain infection with *Listeria monocytogenes*. Subsequent reports emphasized the susceptibility to *Listeria* infection of persons with lymphoreticular malignancies (Buchner and Schneierson, Kalis et al., Simpson et al.), of post-renal transplant patients (Isiadinso, Schröter and Weil, Watson et al.), and of individuals receiving chronic corticosteroid therapy (Johnson and Colley). In addition, many other chronic debilitating disorders, such as alcoholism, immune deficiency states, and systemic lupus erythematosus (Rosengarten and Bourn), can be complicated by serious infection with this organism. Disturbed cellular resistance in immunocompromised patients or in persons on corticosteroid therapy results in defective handling of facultative intracellular pathogens such as *Listeria* which freely multiply within cells of the reticuloendothelial system of the host. The intracellular location of organisms of this type serves to protect them against circulating antibody.

Meningitis is the most common manifestation of *Listeria* infection in the debilitated or immunosuppressed patient, although the illness is often associated with focal or multi-focal neurologic signs, suggesting that *Listeria* cerebritis or vasculitis is a common component of the neurologic infection. Solitary brain abscess in this group of patients has now been described on several occasions, further illustrating the broad spectrum of neurologic involvement that can be produced by this organism (Buchner and Schneierson, Crocker and Leicester, Dykes et al., Lechtenberg et al.). Johnson and Colley reported an elderly woman on chronic corticosteroid therapy who developed fever and hemiplegia which resulted from multiple microabscesses confined to one cerebral hemisphere. *Listeria monocytogenes* was isolated from the blood and was visualized at autopsy within the cerebral lesions. In cases with *Listeria* meningitis, the CSF findings are somewhat more variable than with the "common" organisms that cause meningitis. The cell count is usually a variable mixture of polymorphonuclear leukocytes and lymphocytes, while the glucose content is frequently normal initially only to drop at a later time. The most significant aspect of the CSF examination is the infrequency with which the organism can be found on gram stain and the danger of mistaken interpretation of the growth on artificial media.

A rare manifestation of *Listeria* cerebritis is referred to as rhomboencephalitis, which has been described in previously normal persons as well as in patients immunosuppressed (Duffy et al., Ford et al., Mahony et al.). The process is a necrotizing infection limited to the brain stem and is manifested by an acute onset of vomiting, vertigo, and signs of pontomedullary dysfunction including cranial nerve deficits, ataxia, and long tract signs. The CSF may be normal (Ford et al.) or contain a moderate number of white blood cells. The pathology includes an inflammatory exudate in the pons and medulla but sparing the meninges, along with widespread fibrinoid necrosis of blood vessel walls, perivascular cuffing, and multiple petechial hemorrhages. Still less common is a chronic leptomeningeal infection with *Listeria monocytogenes* in which the clinical features are those of a dementing illness associated with progressive communicating hydrocephalus (Heck et al.). In addition to the predisposition for *Listeria monocytogenes* to give rise to neurologic infection in persons with a variety of immunocompromised conditions and in the newborn infant, the organism can also be the cause of meningitis in otherwise normal children and adults (Medoff et al., Nichols and Woolley).

Ampicillin is usually considered to be the drug of choice for *Listeria* infection of the central nervous system. Most strains are also sensitive to penicillin and tetracycline. A synergistic effect of ampicillin or penicillin and gentamicin resulting in more rapid in vitro killing of *Listeria* has been postulated (Gordon et al., Wiggens et al.), although ampicillin alone is usually deemed adequate for treatment of meningitis.

Pasteurella *Meningitis*

Pasteurella multocida is a non-motile gram-negative coccobacillary organism, which is primarily a pathogen in the animal world. It is a common inhabitant of the upper respiratory tract of dogs, cats, cattle, and other animals, and most human infections are localized lesions at the site of an animal bite or scratch. Central nervous system infection caused by this organism is infrequent but can occur under certain circumstances. Isolated cases of acute meningitis have occurred in all age groups, ranging from the newborn period (Bates et al., Repice and Neter), to the elderly (Swartz and Kunz). In some but not all these cases, the patient had been in close contact with a family pet found to harbor *Pasteurella multocida* in the mouth or respiratory tract (Bhave et al., Frutos et al.). Skull fractures with CSF fistulae have also been implicated as a route of entry of *Pasteurella multocida* from the respiratory pathways into the meninges (Whitmore and Whelan). In addition, the organism has been isolated from a cerebellar abscess of otogenic origin (Larsen et al.) and from a cerebral abscess which followed a penetrating cranial dog bite in a child (Klein and Cohen). The infrequent occurrence of serious human infection by this organism and its similarity on gram stain to *Hemophilus influenzae* and *Mimae* species often delays its laboratory identification (Controni and Jones). Unlike most similar gram-negative bacilli, *Pasteurella multocida* is usually highly sensitive to penicillin.

Meningitis caused by other *Pasteurella* species has been reported on rare occasion. Cooper et al. described two patients with acute meningitis resulting from *Pasteurella pneumotropica*, the first being a child who had been in close contact with sick kittens prior to his illness. *Pasteurella ureae*, an organism without known animal hosts, has been the cause

of acute meningitis in patients with basilar skull fractures (Kolyvas et al., Wang and Haiby).

Plague meningitis was recognized prior to the turn of the century but has been an exceedingly rare complication of bubonic or pneumonic plague. This has been especially true in this country owing to the limited number of cases of plague that occur annually, even though a reservoir exists in the ground squirrel and other animals in the Southwest. Almost all cases of plague meningitis have been in patients with the bubonic form of the disease. There have been rare descriptions of *Yersinia (Pasteurella) pestis* meningitis as a primary illness (Landsborough and Tunnell), although it has been doubted by some that this ever occurs (Martin et al., Pollitzer). Among cases of plague meningitis that have been described, the illness has been acute in onset and clinically similar to other, more common, forms of bacterial meningitis (Feeley and Kriz). The CSF is cloudy or turbid with a polymorphonuclear pleocytosis and reduction in glucose content, and the organism can usually be found on gram stain and culture. Martin et al. in 1963 reported three children in New Mexico with plague meningitis, all of whom recovered with antibiotic therapy. *Yersinia (Pasteurella) pestis* is sensitive to streptomycin and chloramphenicol but not to penicillin. Streptomycin is the drug of choice for the common types of plague but the addition of chloramphenicol would be indicated in cases with meningitis because of its ability to gain entrance into the CSF.

Pertussis Encephalopathy and Pertussis Vaccine Complications

Pertussis is an acute respiratory illness which can affect susceptible persons of any age but is most serious and has its highest mortality rate in young infants. The incubation period can extend from six to 20 days but is most often in the range of seven to eight days. The illness has been classically divided into three stages but this pattern is less distinct when the disease occurs in the young infant or the older person previously immunized who becomes infected at a time when immunity has waned. The initial, or *catarrhal*, stage of the symptomatic illness is characterized by rhinorrhea, low-grade fever, and mild cough, and generally lasts for one to two weeks. As the *catarrhal* stage merges into the *paroxysmal* stage, the frequency and intensity of coughing increases until the patient experiences attacks characterized by a series of explosive coughs with the paroxysm being followed by forceful inspiration against an edematous glottis, which provokes the characteristic "whoop." The attack can be followed by vomiting and, if severe, will exhaust the child. Intense coughing spasms become associated with facial and ocular congestion, subconjunctival hemorrhages, and signs of acute air hunger. The *paroxysmal* stage can persist for two to four weeks and is the period when acute, severe airway obstruction can result in convulsions or cardiac arrest. The length of the *convalescent* stage of gradual recovery in part depends on the severity of the illness but can extend for several weeks. Intermittent coughing will sometimes linger even longer. One of the most notable features of pertussis which develops late in the *catarrhal* stage and extends into the *paroxysmal* stage is leukocytosis with counts between 20,000 and 60,000 per cu. mm., of which lymphocytes constitute a high percentage of the total white blood cell count.

Bordetella pertussis, the most common cause of the pertussis syndrome, is not known to cause asymptomatic nasopharyngeal carriage (Linnemann et al.) and thus the infection is sustained in the population by transmission of the organism from symptomatic persons. In past years, infants and children were usually infected by exposure to other children with the symptomatic illness. Currently, however, young adults with mild illnesses attenuated by waning immunity secondary to early childhood immunization are believed to represent the primary reservoir for transmission of the infection to young infants (Nelson 1978). *Bordetella pertussis* is a small, non-motile, aerobic gram-negative rod. It is best isolated from an infected patient with nasopharyngeal swab specimens inoculated on Bordet-Gengou medium on which incubation is required for 72 hours or more for its growth. Colonies are smooth and glistening and are somewhat larger than those of *Hemophilus influenzae.* Despite the best efforts, a significant proportion of patients with pertussis are found to have negative cultures for *Bordetella pertussis.*

Neurologic complications during the acute stage of pertussis were well known before the turn of the century and early descriptions were reviewed by Nelson (1939). Greater awareness of the neurologic aspects of the illness evolved in this country with the publication of a number of articles in the English literature between 1920 and 1950, a time when over 200,000 cases of pertussis were reported annually in the United States with a case fatality rate of 2 to 3 percent (Litvak et al.). Death was attributed to airway obstruction in most instances but it was also widely recognized that in children with pertussis who developed convulsions or other neurologic signs, the mortality rate was dramatically increased (Habel and Lucchesi). There were many different explanations proposed to account for neurologic abnormalities which complicated this disease, including encephalitis, so-called spasmophilia, a neurotoxic encephalopathy, angiospasm, and hypoxia (Askin and Zimmerman, Berg, Dolgopol, Ford, Woolf and Caplin). Acute onset of convulsions or stupor, or the development of spastic hemiplegia or quadriplegia in association with depressed consciousness were the most frequently occurring neurologic signs. Other reports described the sudden onset of blindness, either transient or persistent, and in some cases visual loss was without other signs of neurologic dysfunction (Lazarus and Levine, Litvak).

The reports describing cerebral involvement in children with pertussis were characterized by a number of features which seemed to be reasonably constant in the majority of cases. Severe and recurrent convulsions were the most common initial manifestations of neurologic involvement and their occurrence was strongly associated with the paroxysmal stage of the illness and they were often provoked by acute attacks of violent coughing. The CSF was normal in the majority of instances but, when abnormal, it consisted only of the presence of a small number of lymphocytes. In addition, the majority of children who developed seizures or other signs of acute cerebral dysfunction were those with relatively severe respiratory distress. Among reports of children with neurologic complications of pertussis in which there was an adequate description of the neuropathology, the majority included few if any inflammatory changes (Dolgopol, Ford, Litvak et al.). Most found cerebral swelling in combination with acute neuronal injury, and frequently with cerebral congestion and petechial hemorrhages. Major venous sinus thromboses or subarachnoid hemorrhage was seen in some instances. Reviewing the clinical descriptions, the CSF findings, and the available neuropathologic observations, it seems highly likely that the neurologic complications of pertussis which sometimes were

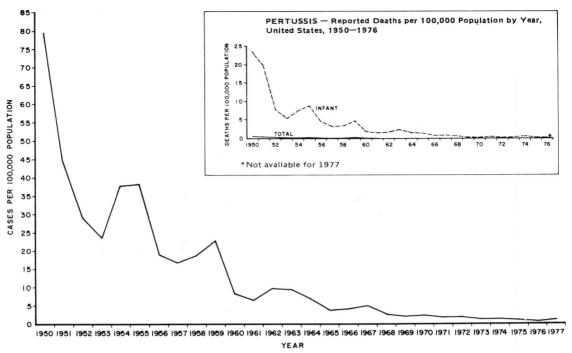

Figure 1–4. Pertussis—reported cases per 100,000 population, United States, 1950–1977. (From: Morbidity and Mortality Weekly Report. Annual Summary, 1977. Vol. 26, No. 52, Sept. 1978.)

referred to as pertussis "encephalitis" were actually the result of acute hypoxic-ischemic cerebral injury compounded by intense venous congestion, sometimes with venous thrombosis. Those pathologic abnormalities were most likely caused by airway obstruction, perhaps associated with acute diminution of cerebral perfusion and with intense venous congestion secondary to increased intrathoracic venous pressure.

Pertussis vaccine was introduced in this country in the early 1930's but did not achieve wide-scale use until almost 20 years later. Although data on the incidence of the disease relative to use of the vaccine would support its effectiveness (Fig. 1–4), no other vaccine has provoked as much controversy regarding its effectiveness and adverse reactions. In the United States, it has been generally accepted that pertussis vaccine does provide protection against the illness but that such protection is less than total and is in the range of 75 to 85 percent (Harrison and Fulginiti, Koplan et al.). In other countries, especially in Great Britain, some investigators have challenged the preventive value of pertussis vaccine and have suggested that the risk of its adverse effects are greater than the risks of the natural illness (Stewart).

While adverse neurologic reactions to pertussis vaccine had been described before, the first being that of Madsen in 1933, it was the report by Byers and Moll in 1948 which brought wide attention to the existence of the problem. They described 15 infants between five and 18 months of age who suddenly developed convulsions beginning between 20 minutes and 72 hours after receiving pertussis vaccine, some with lasting deficits thereafter. In the following years, attempts were made to categorize the types of central nervous system reactions that could result from this immunizing agent and the incidence of their occurrence, and to determine whether pre-existent cerebral disease predisposed to their occurrence. Because the adverse neurologic reactions attributed to pertussis vaccine seemed nearly identical to those associated with the "triple" vaccine (DPT), it has been assumed that those resulting from DPT could be accounted for by the presence of the pertussis component (Kulenkampff et al.). Neurologic reactions that were recognized included "screaming fits" consisting of continuous crying and irritability lasting for several hours, brief convulsions with or without fever but with recovery expected, a "shock-like" syndrome, and an acute vaccine encephalopathy usually manifested by repetitive convulsions, stupor or coma and other abnormal neurologic signs, and often followed by lasting sequelae or even death. Certain authors suggested that the subsequent development of "infantile spasms" with developmental retardation could also be attributed in some instances to prior pertussis vaccine administration, but this has remained unproven and is doubted by some (Melchior). Most reports stressed the high frequency of occurrence of neurologic complications in infants, although this is the age in which the vaccine is most often given, the considerably higher incidence in males than in females, and the onset of neurologic abnormalities within hours or a day or so after the vaccine is administered. The estimated incidence of any of these neurologic complications has varied a great deal in different studies and remains uncertain. Strom (1967) in Sweden found the incidence of adverse neurologic reactions to pertussis vaccine to be one in 3,100 vaccinated children. These consisted mainly of severe encephalopathy, the acute occurrence of convulsions or a shock-like state, and uncontrolled screaming. Others claim that serious reactions are far less frequent and estimate that pertussis vaccine encephalopathy is more in the range of one in 100,000 to one in 500,000 children who receive the vaccine (Prensky, World Health Organization).

It has been widely assumed that infants and children with a history of seizures are much more likely to experience recurrent seizures, and perhaps even more severe adverse neurologic effects, following pertussis immunization. Absolute documentation of this is difficult to identify; however, the recommendation remains that children with a past history of convulsions should not receive pertussis vaccine and those who have had a previous systemic or neurologic reaction to the vaccine should not receive it again (Harrison and Fulginiti, Kulenkampff et al.).

Streptococcus *Meningitis*

In the pediatric age group, the term streptococcal meningitis is now largely equated with group B Streptococcus (*Streptococcus agalactiae*) meningitis in the neonatal period. Neonatal group B *Streptococcus* infection is discussed in detail in Chapter 3 and is not further detailed here except to say that in the past decade, it has emerged as the single most common type of meningitis in the newborn period in many centers. It is characterized by its occurrence in two rather distinct forms, although there is some degree of overlap in the clinical presentation in some cases. The early onset form is an acute, fulminating illness with onset in the first hours or days after birth, with severe septic and respiratory manifestations and a high mortality rate. The late onset variety is usually predominantly meningitic and with a much more favorable prognosis. The current preoccupation with group B *Streptococcus* in the pediatric age range is not inappropriate in view of its prevalence, but is not entirely representative of the total spectrum of neurologic infection caused by streptococcal organisms in children. Numerous other streptococcal serogroups are capable of causing meningitis in the newborn infant as well as in older children.

The basis for classification of streptococci was established in 1933 by Rebecca Lancefield of the Rockefeller Institute. With serologic techniques, she separated streptococci into five groups, designated A through E, on the basis of the carbohydrate antigen in the cell wall. Group A (*Streptococcus pyogenes*) was largely obtained from strains of human origin and the organism was at that time recognized to be the predominant streptococcal pathogen in humans. The group B organisms in Lancefield's study were made up of strains derived from mastitis in cows and from normal milk. Group B *Streptococcus* was known to be a cause of bovine mastitis, thus the term *Streptococcus agalactiae*, but was doubted to be a pathogen in humans. In 1938, however, Fry in London described three fatal cases of infection in the puerperium caused by group B *Streptococcus*, thus establishing the role of the organism as a potential cause of serious human disease. Non-groupable streptococci were referred to as *Streptococcus viridans*, a term that has persisted but one that has acquired less usefulness as many strains previously referred to as *Streptococcus viridans* have subsequently been classified among one of the various subgroups (Duma et al.). There are now 18 streptococcal serogroups, a number of which only rarely cause human disease.

In 1919, the concept of alpha, beta, and gamma hemolysis was introduced by Brown as a laboratory method of classification of streptococcal organisms. Alpha hemolysis on blood sugar agar is green or incomplete, and beta hemolysis is clear or complete, while the gamma reaction is the absence of hemolysis. Many assumed that the pathogenicity of streptococci could be predicted on the basis of the type of hemolysis, and group A *Streptococcus* was equated with beta hemolysis. It is now known that group A *Streptococci* are usually but not always beta-hemolytic, group B are characteristically hemolytic and certain other serogroups may likewise be, and that non-beta-hemolytic *Streptococci* can be pathogenic in humans (Reinarz and Sanford). Alpha hemolysis is characteristic of *Streptococcus viridans* but the alpha reaction is not entirely limited to this group. The bacitracin disc sensitivity described by Maxted in 1953 has been a useful method of differentiation of streptococci, but it also is not an infallible method. Bacitracin sensitivity has been used to imply the presence of group A organisms. Group B *Streptococcus* is ordinarily bacitracin-resistant; however, group C and group G *Streptococcus* isolates can be both beta-hemolytic and bacitracin-sensitive, and thus can be confused with group A organisms unless serologic identification is made. *Streptococcus* species of the types discussed above are gram-positive cocci, which in CSF usually appear in short or long chains. Lerner has emphasized the frequent inability to distinguish these *Streptococcus* species from *Streptococcus pneumoniae* (pneumococcus) on gram stain alone.

Group A *Streptococcus* (*Streptococcus pyogenes*) has never been a common cause of childhood meningitis but is much less frequent now than in the first half of this century. Until approximately 30 years ago, the organism was the leading cause of puerperal and neonatal sepsis but was then replaced by gram-negative organisms and more recently by group B *Streptococcus* (Nyhan and Fousek, Smith et al.). Nursery outbreaks or sporadic neonatal cases of infection with group A *Streptococcus* still occur on occasion, although most are usually mild illnesses with cutaneous involvement (Geil et al.). Unlike the frequent asymptomatic colonization rate of the newborn infant with group B *Streptococcus,* group A colonization of the normal neonate is infrequent, and the introduction of the organism into the newborn nursery is likely to result in clinical disease. Infrequently, the illness will be in the form of sepsis and meningitis (Dillon, Nelson et al.).

Prior to 1940, streptococcal meningitis, presumably group A, was an occasional cause of acute meningitis in older children as well as adults, with most cases being secondary to otitis media or mastoiditis, or complicating injuries to the head or paranasal sinuses. In 1935, Zeligs reported 57 cases of streptococcal meningitis in children, 54 percent resulting from otitis media, mastoiditis, or traumatic injuries. Tripoli, in 1936, tabulated the etiologic causes of bacterial meningitis at Charity Hospital in New Orleans from 1925 to 1934 and found that 5 percent were streptococcal in origin, the specific group not being known. In 1938, Neal reviewed the etiologic causes of 3,502 cases of bacterial meningitis in all age groups in New York City. Eight percent of the cases were streptococcal, presumably most being of group A. Prior to the introduction of the sulfa preparations, streptococcal meningitis had a case fatality rate estimated to be approximately 97 percent (Gray). Streptococcal meningitis of otitic or post-traumatic origin was one of the very first serious diseases in which the curative effect of sulfonamides was clearly demonstrated. Such publications appeared as early as 1937 and became abundant in the years immediately thereafter (Trachsler et al., Weinberg et al.). With eventual control of middle ear infections with antibiotic therapy, the incidence of *Streptococcus* meningitis dropped to a low level, and is now infrequent except for that caused by group B *Streptococcus* in the newborn infant.

Meningitis due to group A *Streptococcus pyogenes* had been previously observed in association with scarlet fever, but was acknowledged to be rare. In 1935, Gordon and Top commented on the observation of 17,311 patients with scarlet fever, among whom were only 19 children who developed streptococcal meningitis. According to these authors, meningitis associated with scarlet fever was invariably a complication of focal infection, either otitis media or suppurative sinusitis. Another form of non-bacterial meningitis was recognized to occur on rare occasion in the child with scarlet fever. It was called acute "serous" meningitis and was recognized in 11 of 1,503 children with scarlet fever by Sweet and Lepper. The illness was characterized by the presence of meningeal signs with a lymphocytic pleocytosis in sterile CSF with a normal glucose content. The illness was benign and the pathogenesis was never understood. In current times, serious group A streptococcal disease in children is not common, except for the non-infectious complications including rheumatic fever and acute glomerulonephritis, although sporadic cases with pneumonia (Molterni), sepsis, or meningitis (Burech et al.) periodically are recorded. The organism can also act as an opportunistic invader, causing meningitis in children with immunosuppressive disorders or with anatomic defects that are associated with CSF fistulae (Shadravan et al.).

Group B *Streptococcus* is subdivided into five serotypes designated types Ia, Ib, Ic, II, and III. It is best known for its role as a cause of serious neonatal disease but can also be an important pathogen in older age groups (Patterson and Hafeez). Most adult infections with group B *Streptococcus* are bacteremic conditions associated with the puerperal period, or occur in patients with underlying illnesses such as diabetes mellitus or genitourinary disorders. The association of group B *Streptococcus* bacteremia in adults with diabetes mellitus is especially strong, and of 24 adults with group B infection reported by Bayer et al., 11 (45 percent) occurred in diabetics. Similar to sepsis in the neonate, that in the adult can be fulminating with shock, respiratory compromise, and early death. Meningitis in bacteremic adults with this organism is infrequent but can occur (Bayer et al.). Group B *Streptococcus* meningitis can also follow surgical procedures, such as laminectomy (Rantz), and can originate from a CSF fistula with rhinorrhea (Lentnek et al.).

Group C *Streptococcus* infrequently gives rise to invasive disease in humans, although it can colonize the female genital tract and is an infrequent cause of wound infection (Duma et al.). Meningitis from this organism is exceedingly rare but has been described in a newborn infant (Stewardson-Krieger and Gotoff) and in an adult without a predisposing cause (Mohr et al.). Because group C *Streptococcus* isolates can be beta-hemolytic and bacitracin-sensitive, it is readily confused with group A organisms unless serologic typing is performed.

Group D *Streptococcus* has been separated into enterococcal and non-enterococcal types. Enterococci include *Streptococcus faecalis,* *Streptococcus faecium,* and *Streptococcus durans,* while members of the non-enterococci are *Streptococcus bovis* and *Streptococcus equinus.* They are important and common human pathogens, especially in patients with chronic debilitating or malignant disease, but are uncommon causes of meningitis (Duma et al.). Bacteremia with group D *Streptococci* is most often related to infection of the intestinal tract, the genitourinary tract, or the cardiac valves. Meningitis and sepsis caused by group D *Streptococcus* in the newborn infant is rare but has been described with a clinical picture identical to early onset group B infection with respiratory distress and shock soon after birth (Alexander and Giacoia, Headings et al.). In other cases of group D streptococcal sepsis and meningitis in the newborn period, the illness is manifested by fever and lethargy

and follows a relatively mild clinical course with a prompt and favorable response to antibiotic therapy (Buchino et al.). Meningomyelocele, other anatomic defects predisposing to neurologic infection, and leukemia have accounted for rare cases of group D *Streptococcus* meningitis in infants and older children (Bayer et al., Skeel et al.). Meningitis caused by group D organisms can complicate endocarditis (Lerner), and brain abscess has been described as a consequence of acute mastoiditis (Rantz). Eradication of group D *Streptococcus* from the CSF is sometimes difficult, requiring intrathecal therapy in some instances. Bayer et al. emphasized the frequent lack of a significant cellular response in CSF with infection caused by this organism, with most recorded samples having less than 200 white cells per cu. mm.

In addition to the above, there are rare descriptions of meningitis in infants or older persons caused by *Streptococci* of groups F, H, K, and R (Duma et al., Lerner, Rantz, Zanen and Engel). Streptococci of Lancefield group R, called porcine *streptococci,* have been known to be an important cause of septic disease in pigs but only recently have been isolated from adults with meningitis (Agass et al.). In most human cases with meningitis, the patient has had occupational exposure to live or slaughtered pigs from which the organism was acquired (Zanen and Engel). Non-groupable *streptococci (Streptococcus viridans)* can produce a variety of infectious conditions, the best known being subacute bacterial endocarditis. In 1950, Hoyne and Herzon summarized the literature available to that date regarding *Streptococcus viridans* meningitis. In contrast to the expected association with subacute bacterial endocarditis, these investigators found only 13 percent of 55 cases of meningitis due to this organism could be attributed to endocarditis. In 31 percent, meningitis due to *Streptococcus viridans* was a complication of otitic or nasopharyngeal infection, and in 35 percent of cases, no primary focus could be found. *Streptococcus viridans* continues to be an important cause of subacute bacterial endocarditis in children and adults, and can give rise with this disease to neurologic complications in the form of infected or bland cerebral emboli, mycotic aneurysms, cerebral vasculitis, and acute meningitis.

SYMPTOMS AND SIGNS

Symptoms and signs in children with bacterial meningitis are variable and depend on several factors, the most important of which are age of the patient and duration of the illness when the child is first seen by the physician. Infants less than one month of age depart most from the conventional manifestations. Irritability, lethargy, vomiting, lack of appetite, and seizures are common in this group, but signs of meningeal irritation are not expected at this age, and even significant fever may not be present. Newborn infants with the early onset type of group B *Streptococcus* sepsis and meningitis commonly exhibit a fulminating illness with apnea, other types of respiratory distress, or shock. The illness can simulate hyaline membrane disease both clinically and roentgenographically. Less often, a similar rapidly progressive disorder in the newborn infant can be caused by *Listeria monocytogenes* (Ahlfors et al.), *Hemophilus influenzae* (Lilien et al.), *Streptococcus pneumoniae* (Bortolussi et al.), and group D *Streptococcus* (Alexander and Giacoia, Headings et al.).

Beyond four months of age, infants with meningitis manifest findings similar to those described in the neonate in addition to a usual febrile response, tenseness of the fontanel, neck rigidity, and other signs of meningeal irritation. In older children, headache, vomiting, mental confusion, and lethargy are the common initial complaints followed by seizures in some, progressive decline of responsiveness, and neck rigidity within 12 to 24 hours after onset. In an occasional child the initiation of the illness is precipitated by a generalized convulsion, which can erroneously be assumed to represent a "febrile" convulsion unless the cerebrospinal fluid is examined (Ratcliffe and Wolf). Less common presenting manifestations include focal cerebral signs of abrupt onset or ataxic gait disturbances (Schwartz, Yabek). Pneumococcal meningitis in the older child is suspected when acute meningeal infection follows a suppurative infection of the middle ear or the paracranial sinuses, or occurs in the child with sickle cell disease or one who has had splenectomy. Meningococcal meningitis is more likely when the onset is abrupt and is followed by the appearance of petechial skin lesions or arthritis. In many cases, no hints regarding the probable offending agent are evident from the clinical findings and one must await laboratory identification of the organism.

Convulsions may be focal or generalized and may become continuous (Fig. 1–5). It has been estimated that seizures occur in up to 30 percent of children with meningitis at some point during the illness and are more common with *Hemophilus influenzae* meningitis than that due to other organisms (Bresnan). With neonatal meningitis, the percentage exhibiting seizures is probably even higher. In some instances, the child is irritable, restless, and somewhat drowsy until the moment of a convulsion, but remains markedly different thereafter, with minimal re-

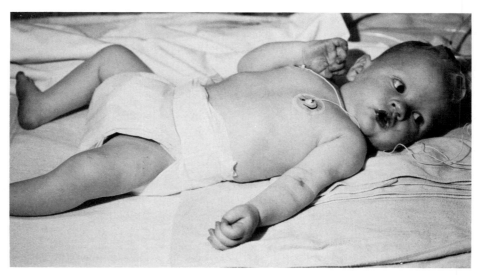

Figure 1–5. *Streptococcus pneumoniae* meningitis in a 3-month-old infant, acute stage. The child is having a focal seizure manifested by forced conjugate ocular deviation to the left, rigid extension of the left arm with repetitive clonic jerking of the fingers of the left hand, and sucking movements of the lips with excessive salivation. This pattern suggests the presence of an irritative focus in the right frontal lobe, sometimes the result of an infarctional lesion or cortical vein thrombosis.

sponse to pain and sometimes with rigid and hyperreflexic limbs, not previously present. Focal neurologic deficits are not common in the early stages of bacterial meningitis and more than minimal papilledema is not usually observed. The presence of high-grade papilledema within the first few days after onset is sufficiently unusual with acute purulent meningitis that the accuracy of diagnosis should be questioned. Other possible considerations under these circumstances include brain abscess with rupture into the ventricle or subarachnoid space, intracranial extradural abscess with extension to the subarachnoid space, and posterior fossa dermoid with congenital dermal sinus and associated meningitis. Focal neurologic signs and papilledema may develop more rapidly in patients with tuberculous or cryptococcal meningitis than with the more common bacterial pathogens.

The rate of progression of clinical signs in the child with acute bacterial meningitis is remarkably variable and unpredictable. For example, the infant with *Hemophilus influenzae* meningitis over 24 to 48 hours commonly has gradual increase of vomiting, irritability, and lethargy after the first signs of illness. Others, however, proceed to deep coma and convulsions within hours after onset. This rapidly progressive form is frequently associated with severe brain swelling, which provokes transtentorial herniation leading to brain stem compression. The clinical correlates of this event are an abrupt drop in blood pressure, abnormality of pupillary size and responsiveness, and respiratory arrest with death soon thereafter. A similar fulminating course is well known with *Neisseria meningitidis* meningitis, resulting either from massive brain swelling or secondary to peripheral vascular collapse from endotoxic shock.

Cutaneous Manifestations with Infections

A variety of cutaneous lesions may be observed in children with sepsis and meningitis, some of which are of diagnostic importance in regard to either the etiologic bacterial agent or a pathologic complication of the septic process. A drug-induced eruption is one of the more commonly observed skin lesions and is usually in the form of a maculopapular or urticarial rash. Tache cérébrale can be seen in some children with bacterial meningitis but is not specific for this disorder (Martin). It is elicited by stroking the skin in linear fashion with a dull object, such as a tongue blade. The stimulus is followed in 30 to 60 seconds by the appearance of a streak of erythema which persists for several minutes. It most likely represents a disturbance of autonomic innervation and is more often seen in infants who are febrile and are seriously ill with meningitis.

The most specific skin lesion for diagnostic purposes is the petechial or hemorrhagic rash that occurs with meningococcemia (Fig. 1–6). This finding is observed in approximately 60 percent of patients with meningococcal dis-

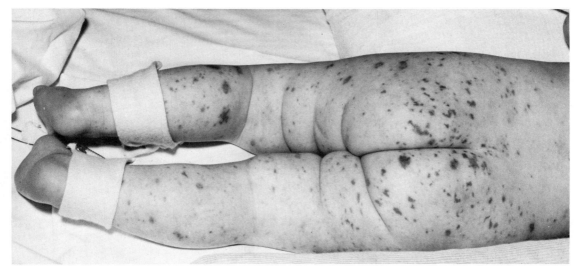

Figure 1–6. Meningococcal meningitis. One-year-old child with an acute febrile illness, convulsions, and cloudy CSF containing gram-negative diplococci. The purpuric rash is typical of meningococcemia.

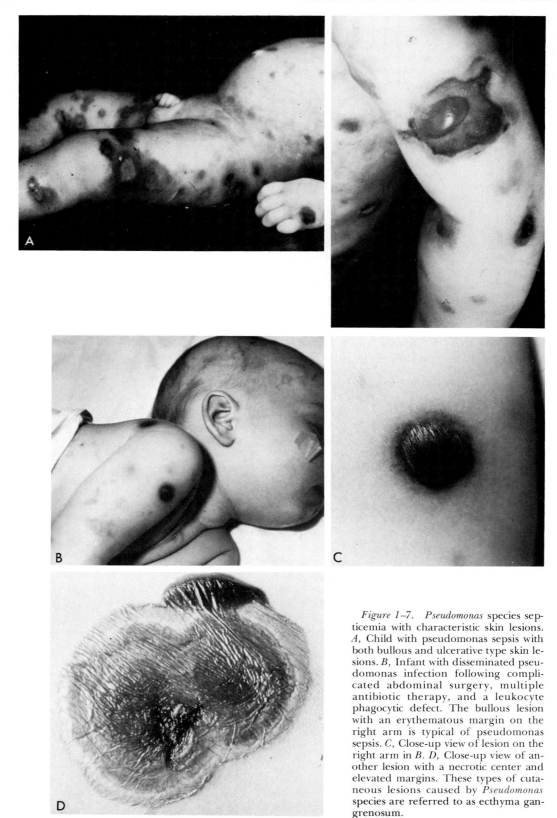

Figure 1–7. Pseudomonas species septicemia with characteristic skin lesions. *A,* Child with pseudomonas sepsis with both bullous and ulcerative type skin lesions. *B,* Infant with disseminated pseudomonas infection following complicated abdominal surgery, multiple antibiotic therapy, and a leukocyte phagocytic defect. The bullous lesion with an erythematous margin on the right arm is typical of pseudomonas sepsis. *C,* Close-up view of lesion on the right arm in *B. D,* Close-up view of another lesion with a necrotic center and elevated margins. These types of cutaneous lesions caused by *Pseudomonas* species are referred to as ecthyma gangrenosum.

ease and is diffuse but frequently most pronounced over the lower extremities and buttocks. An identical eruption may accompany *Neisseria gonorrhoeae* sepsis and meningitis or infections with *Mima polymorpha*. On rare occasion, cutaneous petechiae are seen in children with *Hemophilus influenzae* meningitis. A petechial rash similar to that with meningococcemia can also occur with Echo type 9 (Frothingham) and adenovirus type 7 infections (Sahler and Wilfert). An erythematous maculopapular rash is occasionally noted with meningococcal disease but is less common than lesions of the petechial variety. The other form of cutaneous involvement seen in patients with meningococcal infection, and less often in children with other types of bacterial meningitis, is necrosis or gangrene of the distal extremities (De Fuccio and Dresner), which is usually the result of intravascular coagulation or follows a shock episode.

Pseudomonas species septicemia produces a distinctive type of skin lesion known as ecthyma gangrenosum (Heffner and Smith), which is sufficiently characteristic to suggest the causative agent (Geppert et al.) (Fig. 1–7). The usual sequence of evolution of the cutaneous lesion begins with a well-circumscribed but raised edematous area which quickly becomes flattened and erythematous. Central hemorrhage into the lesion converts it into a purplish-blue bulla, often more than a centimeter in diameter, with a distinct margin but surrounded by a thin zone or erythema. The lesion subsequently becomes necrotic with an excavated central zone surrounded by a violaceous rim (Dorff et al.). The lesions are almost always multiple and are located in an indiscriminate fashion anywhere on the body.

A rare disorder, probably related to disseminated intravascular coagulation, which

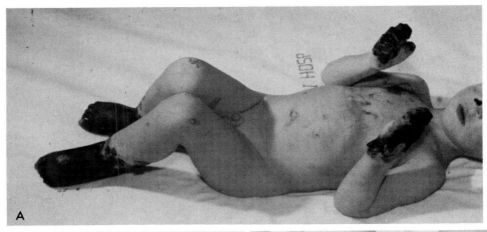

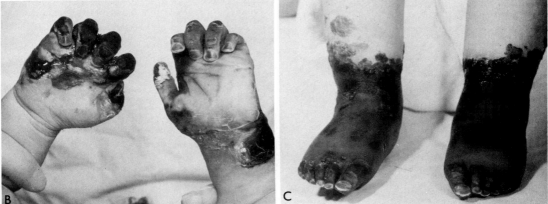

Figure 1–8. Purpura fulminans secondary to bacterial sepsis. Seventeen-month-old child who sustained a burn on the anterior chest from hot coffee. The cutaneous burn was complicated by bacterial sepsis. While recovering on antibiotic therapy, cyanosis of the hands and feet developed and rapidly progressed to the necrotizing soft tissue changes seen in *A*, *B*, and *C*. During the illness, the child had leukocytosis, anemia, and severe thrombocytopenia. He survived but required partial surgical amputation of both hands and both feet.

occurs in the convalescent stage of various infections is referred to as purpura fulminans (Bouhasin, Brown and Nelson, Becker and Buckley, Fishbein). (Fig. 1–8). The condition is a prognostically serious one and has followed streptococcal and meningococcal infections as well as varicella and rubella. The initial stages of the disorder consist of cyanosis and ecchymosis of large areas of the skin, often nearly symmetrically involving the extremities. Any cutaneous region may be affected but points of pressure and more distal parts of the limbs are predisposed. The cyanotic region rapidly becomes hemorrhagic and continued progression leads to eventual gangrene. Systemic symptoms, including chills and fever, coincide with the necrotizing process. Shock and subsequent death has been the outcome in excess of 50 percent of recorded cases (Fishbein). Thrombocyto-

penia and reduction in serum fibrinogen, prothrombin, and factors V and VIII support the concept that purpura fulminans is a manifestation of consumption coagulopathy and should be treated accordingly (Antley and McMillan).

Meningeal Signs

Signs of meningeal irritation of greatest value are limitation of motion with pain on flexion of the neck, Kernig's sign and Brudzinski's sign (Fig. 1–9). The pathogenesis of these signs in the patient with bacterial or viral meningitis is not fully understood but is generally attributed to the inflammatory process within the meninges. The classic signs of meningeal irritation have, however, been described with meningitis in the absence of cells

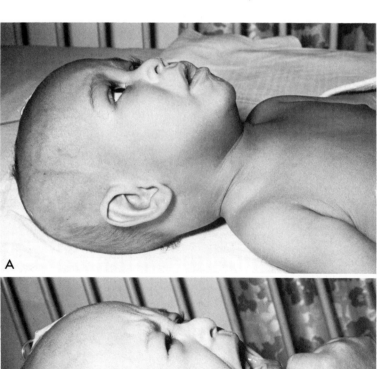

Figure 1–9. Neck stiffness in a 6-month-old child with tuberculous meningitis. *A,* Lying at rest, the child appears to be comfortable. *B,* On attempting to flex the neck there is limitation of forward flexion and the child displays the presence of pain by immediately crying.

in the cerebrospinal fluid (Bernstein et al.). Neck rigidity requires several hours to develop after the entrance of organisms into the cerebrospinal fluid and thus its absence does not exclude the possibility of bacterial meningitis. In addition, neck rigidity is not usually seen in newborn infants with bacterial meningitis or in the first several weeks after birth in infants with the disease. Neck stiffness can also be observed with subarachnoid hemorrhage, aseptic meningitis due to viral agents, in tetanus, and in certain conditions such as upper lobe pneumonia in which the spinal fluid is normal. The latter condition of neck rigidity without cerebrospinal fluid evidence of inflammation is referred to as meningismus and usually requires a diagnostic lumbar puncture to exclude the possibility of meningitis. Pain and limitation of neck flexion may also be found in children with tender posterior cervical adenopathy and with retropharyngeal abscess. Exclusion of meningeal irritation on clinical grounds is sometimes difficult in the child with rheumatoid disease with cervical spine involvement and spiking fever due either to the basic illness or secondary to an incidental viral or bacterial infection. Limitation of neck flexion in such children may require lumbar puncture before one can be satisfied that meningitis is not present.

Kernig's sign, described in 1884 by Vladimir Kernig, is elicited with the patient in the supine position. With the knee flexed, the leg is flexed at the hip so that the thigh is brought to a position perpendicular to the trunk. An attempt is then made to extend the knee, which cannot be done and which results in pain if meningeal irritation is present. The Brudzinski sign, described in 1909, consists of spontaneous flexion of the lower limbs following passive flexion of the neck and has the same significance as the other meningeal signs. Signs of meningeal irritation previously present may disappear if the child's condition deteriorates and if deep coma supervenes.

Pathology and Pathogenesis of Clinical Signs in Acute Bacterial Meningitis

The primary site of the purulent exudate in the infant or child with acute meningitis is within the subarachnoid space and in the basilar cisterns at the base of the brain (Fig. 1–10). In addition to signs of infection and those of meningeal irritation, however, there are commonly a variety of signs of cerebral dysfunction, the most frequent being lethargy or coma, cranial nerve deficits, seizures, and certain types of long tract signs. The pathogenesis of these clinical abnormalities of cerebral involvement is not entirely understood and to some extent is variable from case to case.

The wide variety of pathologic lesions that are found in meningitis is evidence that the explanation for the clinical signs of cerebral dysfunction is on a multifactorial basis. In select instances, some of the clinical abnormalities observed can be explained by secondary events that are associated with or complications of the infectious illness. High fever, dehydration, or hyponatremia might account for some degree of lethargy or the occurrence of seizures. Transient obtundation will follow convulsions regardless of the cause, and airway obstruction producing anoxia will give rise to cerebral functional abnormalities of variable severity. Likewise, disturbance of cerebral perfusion associated with endotoxic shock will itself provoke signs of cerebral dysfunction. While any of these complications can be contributory to the abnormal neurologic signs observed in the child with meningitis, most of the deficits in neurologic function are more directly attributable to the cerebral effects that are primarily associated with the meningeal infection.

As mentioned above, in most cases of acute bacterial meningitis, organisms and exudate are confined to cerebrospinal fluid–containing spaces and the adjacent membranes (Fig. 1–11). As a result of protective barriers, the normal brain parenchyma is relatively impermeable to penetration by bacteria. This is truer in the older child with meningitis and somewhat less so in the young infant in whom the infection is often associated with severe necrotizing effects on the periventricular tissue as well as profound damage of the deep white matter (Fig. 1–12).

The subarachnoid space lies between the arachnoid and the pia, the latter being a discontinuous sheath which can allow tracer substances placed in the subarachnoid space to gain entrance into the extracellular fluid of the underlying brain neuropil (Shabo and Maxwell, Waggener and Biggs). Substances can also gain entrance to the cerebral parenchyma by way of the perivascular extensions of the subarachnoid space referred to as the Virchow-Robin spaces, and between the ependymal cells of the ventricles. The importance of these pathways that allow access of substances from the CSF into the brain in

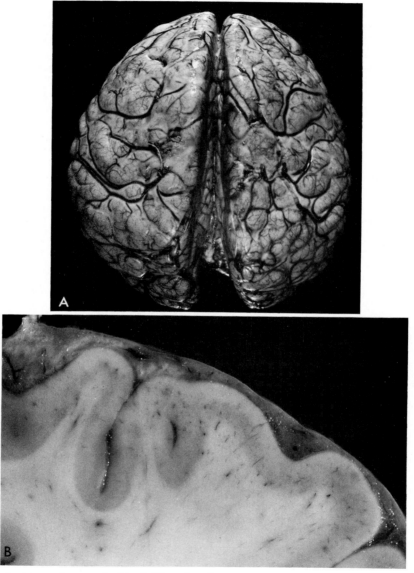

Figure 1–10.   Acute purulent meningitis. *A,* There is a dense subarachnoid exudate over the cerebral convexity. The brain is diffusely swollen and the surface veins are distended. *B,* Coronal section of the brain demonstrates the purulent leptomeningeal exudate in addition to venous congestion within the cortex and underlying white matter.

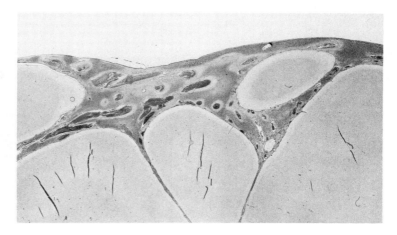

Figure 1–11. Acute purulent meningitis in a 16-month-old child. A dense leptomeningeal exudate composed of inflammatory cells and bacteria is present over the surface of the brain. There is marked distention of meningeal veins enmeshed within the inflammatory exudate and also expansion of Virchow-Robin spaces within the brain caused by invasion of inflammatory cells. Note the confinement of the inflammatory process to the meningeal spaces without evidence, at this power, of direct extension into the cortical layers (H & E, 20×).

the pathogenesis of cerebral swelling or in the production of abnormal neurologic signs is unknown. The decrease in the CSF pH, increase in lactic acid content, and existence of other "toxic" factors from bacterial products in CSF in pyogenic meningitis could well account for certain disturbances in cerebral function, once diffusion into the extracellular fluid of the neuropil has occurred (Bland et al., Brook et al., Ducker and Simmons). Cerebral swelling and encephalopathic manifestations have also been attributed to toxic factors present within granulocytic leukocytes, which are abundant in the CSF in bacterial meningitis (Fishman et al.).

The pathology of acute bacterial meningitis varies considerably, depending on the duration of the illness prior to death, the mechanism accounting for death, and the age of the patient. For example, in the older child with meningococcal sepsis and meningitis who expires soon after onset of endotoxic shock, the neuropathology may include little except for some degree of leptomeningeal exudate along with cerebral congestion and swelling. Likewise, with fulminating sepsis and men-

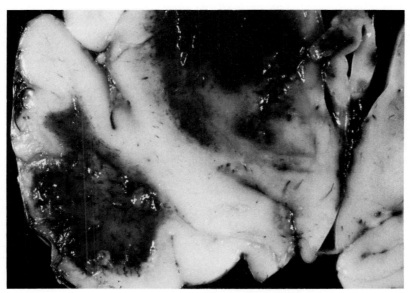

Figure 1–12. Neonatal *Escherichia coli* meningitis. There is widespread hemorrhagic necrosis of the cerebral white matter and the thalamus. These changes are more characteristic of gram-negative meningitis in the newborn infant than of meningitis in older infants or children. Hemorrhagic, necrotizing changes are the result of extensive inflammatory vasculitis, ventriculitis with ependymal disruption, and bacterial invasion into cerebral tissue.

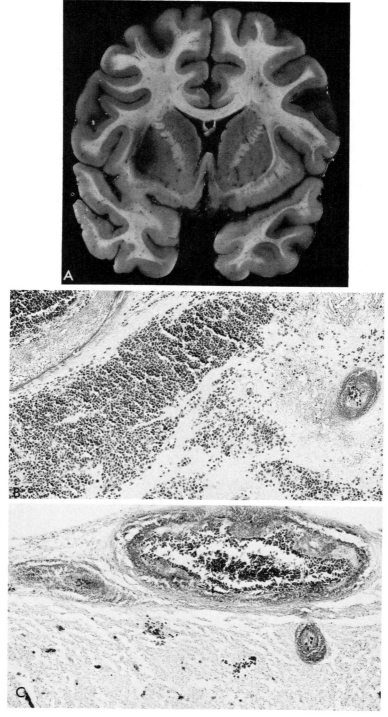

Figure 1–13.   See legend on opposite page

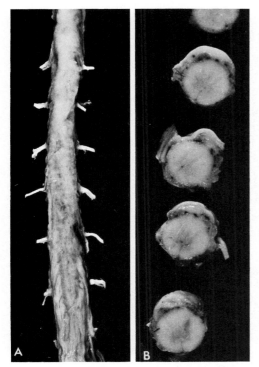

Figure 1–14. *Hemophilus influenzae* meningitis. *A,* Dorsal view of the spinal cord and cauda equina, which are encased within a thick purulent exudate. *B,* Cross-sections of the spinal cord at different levels which demonstrate the inflammatory exudate to be most dense over the dorsal surface.

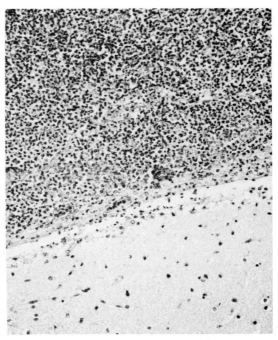

Figure 1–15. Acute purulent meningitis. Heavy inflammatory exudate consists mainly of polymorphonuclear leukocytes in the subarachnoid space over the cerebral cortical surface (H&E, 200×).

ingitis in certain immunosuppressed patients and in those with profound neutropenia, bacteria can be abundant in the subarachnoid space but with little inflammatory exudate, while the cerebral pathology may include vascular invasion by organisms leading to necrotizing changes in vessel walls resulting in thrombotic or hemorrhagic lesions (Fig. 1–13).

The subarachnoid exudate in acute meningitis is distributed over both the brain and the spinal cord (Fig. 1–14) and is usually most extensive in the interpeduncular and chiasmatic cisterns and along the Sylvian and Rolandic sulci. It is also abundant anterior to the brain stem encasing the cranial nerves in the vicinity. Microscopically, it consists largely of granulocytes with a smaller number of lymphocytes and histiocytes, and with leukocytic infiltration of the perivascular spaces of vascular structures in the external layers of the cerebral cortex (Fig. 1–15). Bacteria can usually be found in the subarachnoid space as well as within granulocytes and macrophages

Figure 1–13. Sepsis, necrotizing vasculitis, and cerebral hemorrhage in a 3-year-old child with combined immunodeficiency. *A,* Coronal section of the brain reveals a hemorrhagic lesion in the lateral aspect of the right putamen. *B,* Microscopic section in the region of the lesion in *A* demonstrates extravasation of red blood cells into the brain parenchyma. Note the small vascular structure with necrotic walls to the right of the photograph (H&E, 100×). *C,* Leptomeningeal vessels showing necrotizing vasculitis but with relatively little inflammatory response (H&E, 100×). Bacterial invasion of the arterial wall was abundant.

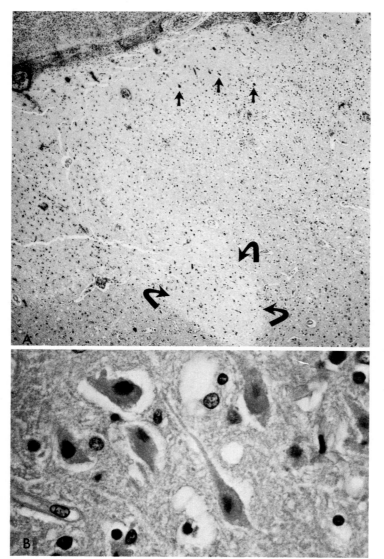

Figure 1–16. Acute purulent meningitis. *A,* Inflammatory leptomeningeal exudate is seen in the upper left corner of the photograph. Note the distended vascular structures within the purulent exudate and the pyknotic neurons in the upper layers of the cerebral cortex (straight arrows). There is an oval pale zone representing an ischemic infarct in the deeper layer of the cortex (curved arrows) (H&E). *B,* Photomicrograph demonstrates anoxic (homogenizing) necrosis of neurons. Neurons are shrunken with eosinophilic changes of the cytoplasm and with pyknotic nuclei (H&E).

Figure 1–17. Acute purulent meningitis. *A,* Photomacrograph shows subarachnoid exudate with distended leptomeningeal vessels, and multiple foci of acute cortical necrosis secondary to vasculitis. The pale areas in the cortex (arrows) represent early ischemic infarction (Trichrome stain, 20×). *B,* Death on the fifth day of acute bacterial meningitis. Leptomeningeal exudate with distended vascular structures. Pale areas (arrows) represent large cerebral cortical infarcts secondary to inflammatory vasculitis (Trichrome, 4×). *C,* Same case as *B* above. Diffuse laminar cortical necrosis (arrows) secondary to hypoxic-ischemic cortical injury (Trichrome, 4×).

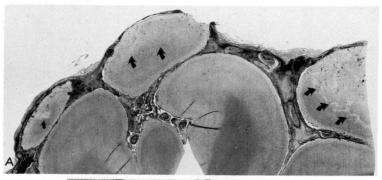

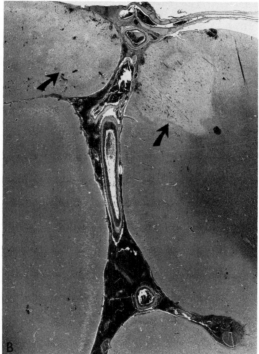

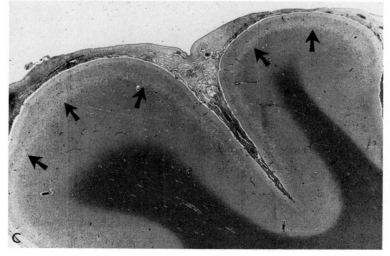

Figure 1–17. See legend on opposite page

in those patients who succumb in the early stages of the illness.

The cerebral pathology in the acute stage of meningitis is exceedingly variable in type and degree. The brain is usually swollen with venous congestion and with pyknotic changes or destruction of cortical neurons and glial cells, and areas of pallor of the neuropil (Fig. 1–16). Neuronal degeneration or necrosis of the basal ganglia is also found and is more striking in children with meningitis than in older persons (Wertham). Pale areas of the cortex and white matter of microscopic or macroscopic size are commonly present, and are attributable to infarctional changes (Adams et al., Wertham) (Fig. 1–17). When severe, the cerebral white matter will show diffuse and extensive necrosis (Buchan and Alvord, Scheinker).

The vascular origin of much of the cortical and white matter pathology in meningitis has generally become apparent since emphasized by Wertham in 1931. Segmental arteritis of meningeal and perforating branches of the carotid artery, compression or collapse of surface veins by purulent meningeal exudate and by cerebral edema, and phlebitis of cortical veins are now recognized to contribute heavily to the clinical manifestations, the pathologic findings, and the long-term sequelae of bacterial meningitis. In cases with necrotizing ependymitis, one finds inflammation, fibrinoid necrosis, and occlusion of small arterioles in the subependymal region (Cairns and Russell) (Fig. 1–18). Brain edema contributes to venous obstruction, and at the same time, venous stasis and phlebitis accelerate cerebral swelling, resulting in a vicious and progressive cycle. Cortical venous thrombosis gives rise to relatively large areas of hemorrhagic cortical infarction that can be visualized grossly (Fig. 1–19), and are especially extensive if cortical vein occlusion is complicated by superior sagittal sinus thrombosis. Segmental narrowing, stenosis, or frank obstruction of major intracranial arteries, especially at the base of the brain, has been repeatedly demonstrated angiographically (Gado et al., Headings and Glasgow, James et al., Lyons and Leeds, Raimondi and DiRocco). These angiographic changes correspond to areas of inflammatory cell infiltration of the media and intima of the arterial wall in addition to intimal hyperplasia, resulting in elevation of the endothelial layer, with either narrowing of the lumen or total arterial obstruction (Fig. 1–20). Infarcted areas of the brain resulting from inflammatory arterial obstruction can eventually become a glial scar, an area of microcystic or macrocystic degeneration (Fig. 1–21), or can be the site of penetration of bacteria, subsequently becoming an abscess if bacteriologic cure is not brought about by antibiotic therapy.

The above-described pathology is also applicable to the newborn infant with bacterial meningitis, but the brain in the neonate often reveals much more severe destructive effects. This is especially true of the newborn with *Escherichia coli* or *Proteus* species meningitis in which vasculitis, ependymal destruction, and hydrocephalus allow penetration of the brain parenchyma with bacteria, leading to a diffuse hemorrhagic and necrotizing encephalitis (Berman and Banker, Cussen and Ryan, Shortland-Webb). The virulent nature of the Enterobacteriaceae, the difficulty in eradicating the organisms from the CSF-containing spaces, and the rapid degeneration of tissue secondary to vascular injury which occurs in the immature brain promptly lead to ependymal and subependymal tissue destruction. The abundant ventricular exudate characteristic of neonatal meningitis is often complicated by hydrocephalus due to aqueductal obstruction or obstruction of CSF flow at the outlet foramina of the fourth ventricle or within the basilar cisterns (Berman and Banker, Kaul et al.) (Fig. 1–22). Increased intracranial pressure secondary to hydrocephalus further compromises cerebral arterial perfusion and venous drainage and adds additional injury to the already damaged ependymal border, with both factors accelerating the destructive effects on the cerebral cortex and white matter.

Infected purulent exudate within the ventricles in neonatal meningitis has been referred to as ventriculitis, which has been defined as greater than 200 leukocytes per cu. mm. in the ventricular fluid in addition to the presence of bacteria (Salmon). Infected ventricular fluid is a common occurrence in all types of meningitis but is of less degree in the older infant or child than in the neonate. In fact, in some instances, bacterial invasion of the cerebrospinal fluid may initially occur by transport of organisms from the blood across the choroid plexuses into the ventricular fluid (Gilles et al.). When the intraventricular infection progresses so that the ventricular fluid becomes frank pus, it is accompanied by lack of flow through the aqueduct and is referred to as pyoventriculitis or ventricular empyema, a condition associated with a very

Text continued on page 39

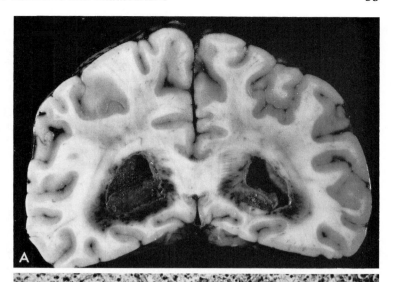

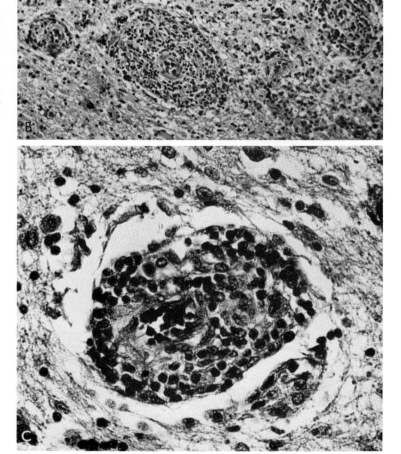

Figure 1–18. *A,* Acute purulent meningitis with hemorrhagic, necrotizing ependymitis. *Pseudomonas* species sepsis and meningitis in a child with extensive cutaneous burns. There is ependymal destruction with hemorrhagic necrosis of the subependymal white matter. These changes are the result of inflammatory vasculitis and bacterial invasion of the subependymal tissue secondary to ependymal damage. *B,* Vasculitis with inflammatory infiltrate in arteriolar walls in the subependymal region (H&E, 80×). *C,* Higher power demonstrating severe subependymal vasculitis with inflammation of the arteriolar wall (H&E, 200×).

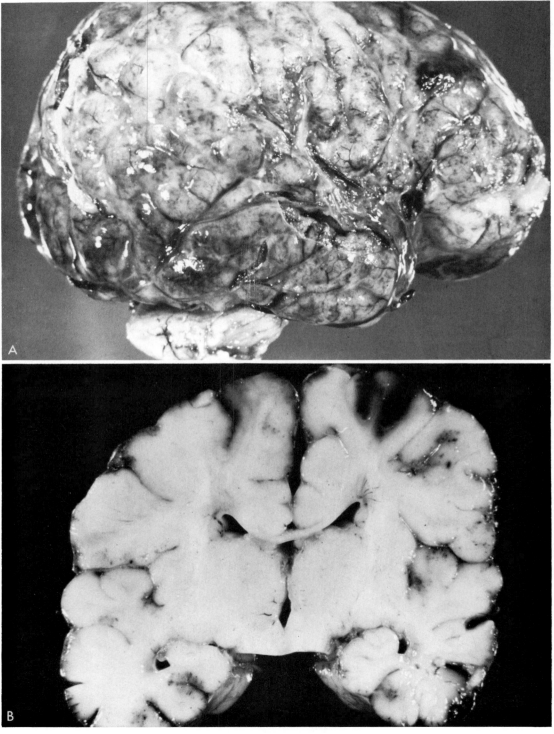

Figure 1–19.   See legend on opposite page

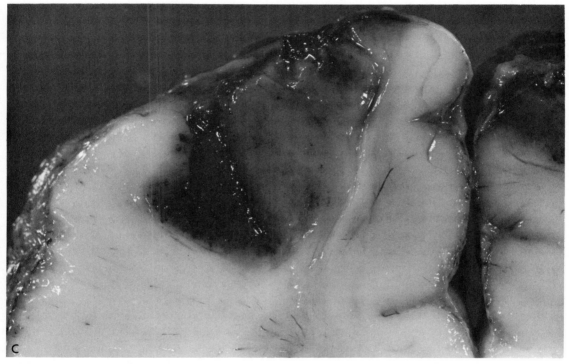

Figure 1–19. Acute purulent meningitis with cortical vein thrombosis. Group B *Streptococcus* meningitis with onset at age nine days and death at 12 days of age. *A,* Lateral surface of the right cerebral hemisphere shows the thick leptomeningeal exudate, cortical venous distention, and areas of cortical hemorrhage. *B,* Coronal section of the brain reveals diffuse swelling resulting in decreased size of the lateral ventricles. Purulent material can be seen within the lateral ventricles, and a hemorrhagic cortical infarct is present in the parasagittal region on the right. *C,* Parasagittal hemorrhagic cortical infarct secondary to septic cortical vein thrombosis.

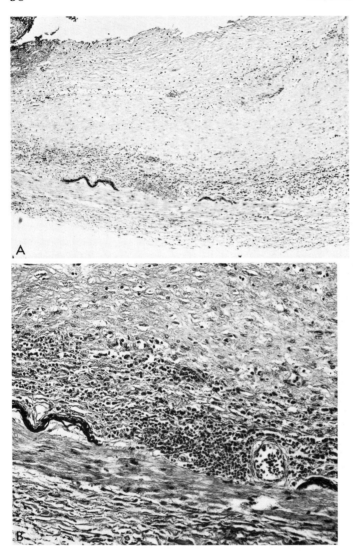

Figure 1–20. Inflammatory vasculitis of intracranial vessels in a child with pyogenic meningitis. *A,* Elastic stain (80×) reveals transmural inflammatory reaction resulting in luminal encroachment. There is fragmentation and disruption of the elastica. *B,* Elastic stain (500×) shows the disruption of the elastic layer and the dense inflammatory infiltrate within the arterial wall.

Figure 1–21. Acute purulent meningitis with obliterative arteritis resulting in multiple cystic infarcts in the thalamus.

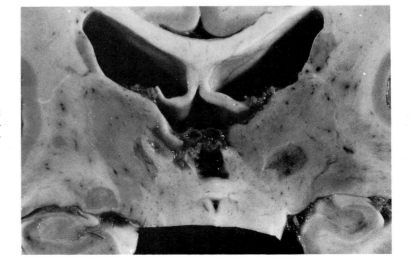

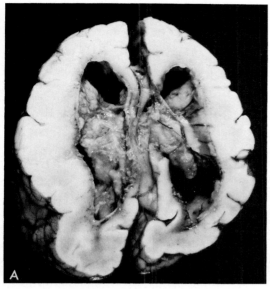
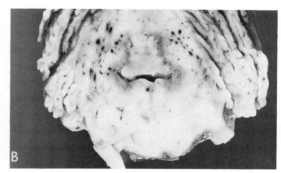

Figure 1–22. Acute gram-negative neonatal meningitis. *A,* Horizontal section of the brain showing severe pyo-ventriculitis. The lateral ventricles are acutely distended and are occupied by a thick purulent exudate. The ependyma is denuded and the adjacent white matter softening is evident from the discoloration in the occipital regions. *B,* The fourth ventricle is almost completely filled with creamy exudate. Note the venous congestion in the region of the cerebellar peduncles bilaterally.

high mortality (Izquierdo et al.) and one that requires direct ventricular drainage.

With understanding of the pathophysiology and pathology of acute bacterial meningitis, it becomes easier to explain many of the clinical signs that accompany the disease. Transmission of leukocyte and bacterial degradation products from the CSF into the neuropil probably accounts for some degree of cerebral swelling and cerebral dysfunction in the form of headache, mental confusion, disorientation, and lethargy. Exudate adjacent to the brain stem (Fig. 1–23) and in the chiasmatic cisterns is associated with an inflammatory reaction of cranial nerves, which can cause pupillary abnormalities, visual deficits, extraocular muscle paresis, facial weakness, and hearing loss. Vascular compromise is one of the most important mechanisms leading to cerebral injury, which is manifested in the form of seizures, coma, or long tract signs. Arteritis of major vessels leading to foci of cerebral ischemic infarction, and venous compression or phlebitis significantly adds to

Figure 1–23. Acute purulent meningitis. There is a thick layer of purulent exudate encasing the medulla. Pus is also present within the fourth ventricle. The fourth ventricle is moderately distended as a result of communicating hydrocephalus secondary to inflammatory adhesions and exudate within the basilar cisterns. The exudate adjacent to the brain stem is a common cause of cranial nerve palsies sometimes seen in the acute stage of bacterial meningitis.

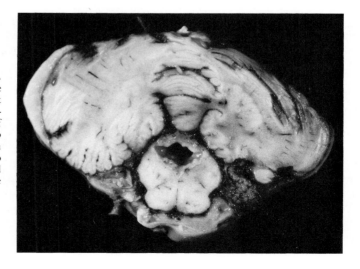

cerebral swelling, with increased pressure itself being capable of provoking many abnormal signs, including vomiting, stupor, and, finally, any of the signs that are a consequence of either transtentorial or cerebellar tonsillar herniation. Cardiorespiratory failure can result from either internal herniation secondary to the above events, or from direct inflammatory or vascular compromise of the medulla.

It is important to recognize how so many of these events can aggravate or accelerate the adverse effects of other pathophysiologic features in bacterial meningitis. Cerebral swelling impairs venous drainage and venous obstruction enhances the degree of swelling and also impedes arterial perfusion, with ischemia provoking further swelling. Complicating the condition by the addition of hydrocephalus further increases intracranial pressure, which itself diminishes arterial perfusion and venous drainage. The eventual occurrence of respiratory compromise with increase in the $PaCO_2$ expands the intracranial vascular volume and precipitously increases intracranial pressure and is frequently the event that precipitates internal herniation, brain stem compression, respiratory failure, and death.

DIAGNOSTIC STUDIES

The value of the white blood cell count as a predictor of bacterial disease in the febrile child has been debated for years (McCarthy et al., Morens, Todd). The test can never be considered to be diagnostic of a bacterial infection, but counts in excess of 15,000 per cu. mm. with a significant increase in band forms (nonsegmented neutrophils) can certainly be accepted to be suggestive of the probability of a bacterial process. Children with acute purulent meningitis are often found to have a marked increase in the total white blood cell count with an increase in immature granulocytes representing a "shift to the left." Although leukocytosis is usually present in children with bacterial meningitis, it does not necessarily differentiate bacterial from viral disease since the latter can also be associated with significant white blood cell count elevations. On occasion, the initial total blood leukocyte count in a child with meningitis is normal, but within 48 hours an increase to 20,000 to 30,000 per cu. mm. can occur. This change may be observed simultaneous to improvement in the child's clinical status with

antibiotic therapy and is not necessarily evidence of worsening or progression of the infectious process. Conversely, persistent leukopenia may represent a poor prognostic sign in a child with acute meningitis of bacterial origin.

The white blood cell count has been assumed to be a less reliable indicator of bacterial infection in the newborn than in the older child because of the wide range of normal values during the first few days of life. In the normal neonate, the white blood cell count in the first day of life has been stated to range from 9,000 to 30,000 per cu. mm. with a mean of 18,100 per cu. mm. (Oski). The healthy newborn infant exhibits a transient neutrophilic leukocytosis, but this is usually limited to the first three or four days after birth. By one week after birth, lymphocytes normally predominate in the peripheral blood, with a normal mean total count being 12,200 per cu. mm. and a normal range of 5,000 to 21,000 per cu. mm. (Gregory and Hey, Oski). After the first four days of life, infants can respond to bacterial infection with changes in the blood neutrophils indicative of infection. While the total white blood cell count in this age group is usually of limited value as an indicator of bacterial disease, a significant increase in band forms and the appearance of toxic granulations and Döhle bodies are supportive evidence of a septic disorder (Gregory and Hey, Xanthou, Zipursky et al.). The absence of these findings, however, does not exclude the possibility of bacterial infection. Leukopenia in the neonate, or a white blood cell count less than 5,000 per cu. mm., is a strong indicator of bacterial infection which alone warrants investigation. Thrombocytopenia, presumably due to peripheral destruction or consumption, is further suggestive evidence of a septic illness in the newborn infant (Zipursky et al.).

Other studies that should be performed when meningitis is considered include determination of serum glucose, electrolytes, urea nitrogen, and blood culture (Table 1–5). When petechial skin lesions are present, punch biopsy can provide material for gram staining, if needed. In children with recurrent meningitis or with a past history of repeated, significant bacterial infections, serum immunoglobulins should be measured, and the presence of and functional status of the spleen should be investigated.

The nitroblue tetrazolium test was introduced by Park et al. in 1968 as a method to aid in the differentiation of bacterial and viral

Table 1–5. Check List of Studies Indicated or To Be Considered in a Child with Bacterial Meningitis

Studies usually indicated
  Complete blood count
  Urinalysis
  Platelet count
  Cultures (blood, urine, nasopharyngeal, CSF)
  Serum electrolytes
  Blood glucose
  Blood urea nitrogen and creatinine
  Tuberculin skin test
  Lumbar puncture and cerebrospinal fluid
    examination
  Skull and chest x-rays
Studies to be considered
  Serum immunoglobulins
  Prothrombin time, partial thromboplastin time,
    serum fibrinogen, and factors V and VIII
  Blood and urine osmolarities
  Electrocardiogram, echocardiogram
  Subdural taps
  Transillumination of the skull (infant)
  Sinus and mastoid x-rays
  Electroencephalogram
  Radioactive brain scan
  Computed cranial tomogram

infections. Increased nitroblue tetrazolium reduction by phagocytic leukocytes is expected with infections of bacterial origin but not with most viral illnesses (Fikrig et al., Humbert et al.). A normal NBT test usually is found in tuberculous meningitis, and abnormal tests in pyogenic meningitis revert toward normal following the introduction of specific antibiotic therapy. False positive and false negative results detract from its potential usefulness. The test has been applied to leukocytes in cerebrospinal fluid, with results suggesting it can be of some value in the differentiation of bacterial from viral meningitis (Zwibel and Schwartzman). The test is of limited value in the newborn as an indicator of bacterial infection because increased reduction has been observed in the absence of infection in this age group (Chandler et al., Humbert et al.). Low or absent nitroblue tetrazolium reduction by neutrophils in the presence of recurrent bacterial infections occurs in children with chronic granulomatous disease (Baehner and Nathan).

Serum hypo-osmolarity with hyponatremia and hypochloremia is not uncommon in children with bacterial meningitis but does not usually create significant management problems, assuming that the cause is identified and proper fluid and electrolyte management ensues (Beisel et al.). Inappropriate antidiuretic hormone secretion has been found to be present in over 50 percent of patients on admission with acute bacterial meningitis (Kaplan and Feigin). This is assumed to be one of the most common causes of serum hypo-osmolarity in the early stages of meningitis, and its presence is documented on the basis of hyponatremia with a significantly elevated urine osmolarity in the absence of systemic dehydration and with intact renal and adrenal function. The pathogenesis of the inappropriate release of ADH is unclear but it is believed to be secondary to the effects of the inflammatory process or vascular compromise of the anterior portion of the hypothalamus. Hypothalamic dysfunction in the form of diabetes insipidus is much less common in the acute stage of meningitis and generally is regarded to be a rare event (Lam et al.). When it does occur, it is usually in seriously ill children and implies necrotizing damage to the hypothalamus or the infundibular stalk.

Additional procedures not to be overlooked are the application of the tuberculin skin test, transillumination of the skull of the infant if subdural effusions are a consideration, and electrocardiogram and echocardiogram when there is clinical evidence of cardiac dysfunction. Serious arrhythmias can occur in children with meningitis although they are not common (Morriss et al.). Electrocardiographic changes of many types have been described in meningitis, most of which are not of major clinical importance (Mehta et al.). Although clinically significant pericardial effusion or pericarditis is unusual in children with acute bacterial meningitis, Laird and colleagues have shown that small pericardial effusions which resolve with antibiotic therapy are quite common, especially in infants and young children with meningitis. Echocardiography is the most sensitive noninvasive method to detect pericardial fluid and should be done when fever is persistent or recurrent or when clinical signs suggest cardiac dysfunction.

Skull and chest x-rays are usually indicated at some point in the illness, and judgment dictates the need for sinus and mastoid views. Obtaining x-rays of children with meningitis is not usually urgent. It is generally wiser to obtain the initial laboratory studies, initiate appropriate therapy and delay the roentgenographic examinations for two or three days until improvement has occurred. Evidence suggesting the possibility of acute suppurative sinusitis, orbital cellulitis, or petrositis would warrant more urgent accomplishment of diagnostic roentgenographic examinations. In young children whose anterior fontanel has closed, repeating skull films 10 to 14 days after the initial series may be helpful if clinical signs are suggestive of subdural effusions. Suture spread more marked on the second set of x-rays despite improvement in the infectious process indicates the probability of either post-meningitic subdural effusions or hydrocephalus.

Computed cranial tomography can provide important information in some instances in the acute stage of meningitis (Cockrill et al.). In the newborn infant, demonstration of adequate ventricular size is useful if intraventricular antibiotic therapy is considered. The technique is also useful to demonstrate the presence or absence of focal intracranial suppurative collections, of subdural effusions, or of progressive ventricular enlargement which may require shunt therapy. Certain findings on computed tomography, such as evidence of diffuse microcystic degeneration with associated cortical atrophy, can have prognostic value, enhancing the subsequent care of the child as well as the parents' comprehension of the nature of the cerebral injury.

A further point worthy of consideration in the febrile child with meningitis as well as other infectious conditions is the possibility that certain of the clinical signs might be secondary to salicylates administered prior to hospitalization. Rising fever is sometimes assaulted with increasing doses of aspirin, resulting in salicylate intoxication with signs therefrom intermixed with those of the underlying disease which caused fever. Thus, the blood salicylate level should be determined if hyperventilation, metabolic acidosis, or a history of salicylate administration is present.

Cerebrospinal Fluid Examination

The honor for the performance of the first lumbar puncture for the purpose of obtaining cerebrospinal fluid goes to Heinrich Quincke, whose report in 1891 added a new dimension to neurologic diagnosis. His initial subject for this procedure was a child with advanced hydrocephalus which had resulted from meningococcal meningitis. Quincke did the procedure to remove fluid with the hope that temporary relief of pressure might initiate function of the absorptive mechanisms. Although the method of doing lumbar puncture became widely known, cerebrospinal fluid was often obtained by cisternal tap in the early part of this century. The cisterna magna was recognized as a readily available site for percutaneous puncture but the procedure was initially considered too hazardous to perform in humans. It was used for laboratory experiments on cerebrospinal fluid in animals (Dixon and Halliburton) until 1919 when Wegeforth, Ayer, and Essick introduced the technique in humans. Cisternal puncture rapidly became popular, and in 1923 Ayer reported its use in 450 patients, illustrating the relative safety of the procedure. It was mainly done at that time for purposes of irrigation of the spinal subarachnoid space in cases of suppurative meningitis, and for instillation of medications for treatment of central nervous system syphilis.

Cisternal tap was also frequently performed to obtain cerebrospinal fluid for diagnostic analysis. The procedure was fairly simple, and the rate of success in obtaining fluid was higher than with lumbar puncture (Levinson et al.), but with the potential hazard of penetration of the distal part of the medulla, possibly resulting in respiratory arrest. Cisternal tap is still occasionally indicated for a variety of purposes but should not be done in the child believed to have the Arnold-Chiari malformation or cerebellar tonsillar herniation. The most common indication currently for cisternal tap in patients with neurologic infection is the suspected case of fungal meningitis in whom the organism cannot be identified or isolated in CSF specimens obtained by lumbar puncture.

There is a wide variety of indications for the performance of a spinal tap in children. The procedure should be done with some specific reason in mind and with the desire to obtain certain types of information that will be of diagnostic value and which might influence or alter the therapeutic approach. The most obvious indications for diagnostic lumbar puncture are for the diagnosis and management of neurologic infections, and for the recognition of subarachnoid hemorrhage in the child with sudden onset of headache, coma, or certain types of focal neurologic dysfunction.

Serious adverse effects of lumbar puncture are largely related to its performance in the presence of high-grade increase in intracranial pressure, the presence of internal herniation, or the injudicious application of the Queckenstedt test in circumstances in which it is contraindicated. Infection by direct contamination of the cerebrospinal fluid or the epidural space, giving rise to an epidural abscess (Rangell and Glassman), is possible but is very unusual and should not occur if precautions are taken. The danger of mechanical restriction of ventilation resulting from positioning of the infant for a lumbar puncture when there is already severe respiratory distress has been pointed out (Margolis and Cook). Post-lumbar puncture postural headache can occur in children and sometimes does not become symptomatic until two or three days after the procedure. It is a temporary complaint in the majority of cases but can create a problem when its origin is not recognized by the physician who assumes it represents progression of the disorder for which the spinal tap was done. A rare but interesting complication of lumbar puncture is the occurrence of a sixth nerve palsy (Bryce-Smith and MacIntosh). It also does not usually appear until a few days after the procedure and may be preceded by headache and dizziness. A postulated but unproved complication of repeated lumbar punctures in the infant is the later development of an intraspinal epidermoid tumor (Manno et al., Shaywitz). The concept implies that implantation of epidermal tissue into the spinal canal occurs during needle penetration and that it remains viable, subsequently forming a mass lesion.

The greatest concern of the complications of lumbar puncture, however, is when the procedure is done in the presence of increased intracranial pressure. Whether or not to perform a lumbar puncture when one suspects a syndrome associated with increased pressure must be determined by the circumstances surrounding each individual situation. In certain instances, lumbar puncture is not only contraindicated because of the hazard of tentorial or tonsillar impaction but also because little useful information will become available from its performance. For example, if one suspects an acute epidural hematoma from the clinical data, the danger of lumbar puncture far outweighs any possible benefit that will come from the procedure. When this diagnosis has been made clinically, it is extremely doubtful that management of the patient would be altered regardless of the findings of a lumbar puncture.

There are other situations in which lumbar puncture is necessarily performed despite the presence of increased intracranial pressure. A reasonable possibility of a central nervous system infection requires the accomplishment of the examination for diagnostic reasons.

Tuberculous meningitis and cryptococcal meningoencephalitis cause a multiplicity of abnormal neurologic signs, often including papilledema. If such disorders are seriously considered in the differential diagnosis, one must examine the cerebrospinal fluid regardless of the presence of clinical evidence of increased pressure. Subarachnoid hemorrhage, if suspected from the history and physical findings, should be confirmed or excluded by careful lumbar puncture. When lumbar puncture is deemed necessary despite evidence of increased intracranial pressure, logic would suggest that in some instances the procedure might be more safely performed immediately after or during an intravenous mannitol infusion. This approach would necessarily nullify the significance of the opening pressure measurement, but would presumably allow other examinations of the cerebrospinal fluid while diminishing the hazard of internal herniation.

Interpretation of the Findings of Lumbar Puncture and Cerebrospinal Fluid Examination

The normal cerebrospinal fluid pressure is generally regarded as not exceeding 180 mm. of water with the patient lying in the lateral recumbent position. This assumes that the child is relaxed and no external pressure is being exerted upon the abdomen or neck vessels. Most accept an opening pressure of 180 to 200 mm. of water as suggestive and over 200 mm. of water as indicative of increased intracranial pressure. When the spinal tap is performed with the patient in the sitting position, these values are no longer valid. In this position, the fluid column more commonly rises to approximately the level of the foramen magnum, and thus the reading on the manometer, if normal, is more dependent on the length of the patient's trunk. Normal values for the spinal fluid pressure in the newborn infant have largely been derived from indirect, non-invasive methods that measure the anterior fontanel pressure. It is believed, however, that there is a good correlation between measurements of the anterior fontanel pressure and measurements obtained by direct recording of the ventricular or subarachnoid space with the infant in the horizontal position (Vidyasagar et al.). Estimates by these methods have generally revealed the CSF pressure in healthy newborn infants to be somewhere between 90 and 110 mm. H_2O

(Salmon et al., Vidyasagar and Rajo, Vidyasagar et al.).

The previously held concept of "normal" spinal fluid pressure in regard to the pressure's effect on the ventricular walls has recently been revised as the result of better understanding of certain physiologic principles (Hakim et al.). Studies have shown that the effect of pressure on the ventricular wall is not only related to the absolute level of pressure but also is dependent on the surface area of the ventricles and probably other factors. Adams et al. have pointed out that the force on the walls of a fluid-filled container is equal to the product of pressure and surface area over which the pressure is exerted. Thus, with markedly enlarged ventricles, a recorded cerebrospinal fluid pressure one ordinarily would consider normal might be sufficient to produce progressive ventricular enlargement by its damaging effect on the surrounding brain.

The contents of the cerebrospinal fluid in the low-birth-weight and full-term newborn infant without evident disease differ considerably from the normal findings in the older child or the adult (Table 1–6). The amount of cerebrospinal fluid in the premature infant with a normal ventricular system has been estimated to be 10 to 30 ml., depending on body weight (Otila). The CSF volume in the term infant is approximately 40 ml. compared to that in adults of 110 to 140 ml. Fluid is continuously being formed and absorbed in the normal individual, with a rate of formation in the older child or adult estimated to be approximately 0.35 ml. per minute, or 500 ml. per day (Cutler et al.). Thus, in the

Table 1–6. Normal Cerebrospinal Fluid Findings

Term newborn infant
Quantity	– approximately 40 milliliters
Appearance	– clear to xanthochromic
WBC's	– 0–32 per cu. mm. (mean = 8)
RBC's	– 0–several hundred per cu. mm.
Glucose	– 70–80% of serum glucose
Protein	– 60–150 mg. per 100 ml. (mean = 90)
Smear and culture	– negative

Premature newborn infant
Quantity	– 10–30 milliliters
Appearance	– clear to xanthochromic
WBC's	– 0–15 per cu. mm. (mean = 7)
RBC's	– 0–several hundred per cu. mm.
Glucose	– 70–80% of serum glucose
Protein	– 60–200 mg. per 100 ml. (mean = 115)
Smear and culture	– negative

older person, the total volume of cerebrospinal fluid is renewed almost five times per day.

The cerebrospinal fluid of the premature child often shows varying degrees of xanthochromia (Glaser), especially when there is indirect hyperbilirubinemia. The degree of xanthochromia of the cerebrospinal fluid is not always parallel to the level of the serum indirect bilirubin in the jaundiced child, a finding assumed to be due to individual variations in the blood-CSF permeability in the newborn period (Stempfel and Zetterström). Normal values of the CSF white blood cell count have not been established in the neonate although there is general agreement that a greater number of cells can be present in the first few days after birth than in the older child. Otila found the mean CSF white count in "normal" premature infants in the first day after birth to be 7 per cu. mm. and the highest count observed was 15 per cu. mm. Sarff et al. found the mean CSF white cell count in premature infants without meningitis to be 9 per cu. mm. and for term infants, the mean CSF white count was 8.2 cells per cu. mm. with a range of 0 to 32 per cu. mm. Polymorphonuclear leukocytes accounted for approximately 60 percent of the white cells in the cerebrospinal fluid. Red blood cells are very frequently present in the cerebrospinal fluid in the neonate, especially the low-birth-weight child, with a wide range from none to several hundred per cu. mm.

The cerebrospinal fluid glucose content in the neonate is usually approximately 75 to 80 percent of the serum glucose level (Sarff et al.), compared to values of 50 to 60 percent in normal children and adults. The protein content of cerebrospinal fluid is normally much higher in the neonate than in the older child and is higher in the premature than the full-term infant. This difference also has been attributed to increased permeability of the blood–cerebrospinal fluid barrier in the immature child. In the study of Bauer et al., the mean CSF protein value in infants less than 1500 grams was 180 mg. per 100 ml., while other authors have found average protein content of approximately 115 mg. per 100 ml. for premature infants and 90 mg. per 100 ml. for term neonates (Wolf and Hoepffner, Sarff et al.). We may assume from these studies that the protein content of cerebrospinal fluid may be as high as 200 mg. per 100 ml. in the low-birth-weight neonate and 150 mg. per 100 ml. in the full-term newborn infant in the absence of disease. At any age, the protein content of ventricular fluid is normally lower than the protein content of the lumbar cerebrospinal fluid. In regard to acid-base balance, the normal newborn infant compared to the older child is said to have an increased pCO_2 in the CSF resulting in a slightly lower pH in CSF than in arterial blood (Krauss et al.). The CSF findings in the normal infant come to approximate those of the older child sometime between one and three months after birth (Naidoo).

Within a few months after birth and in childhood, cerebrospinal fluid is normally crystal clear and colorless, and contains a protein content of 45 mg. per 100 ml. or less. Up to 5 cells per cu. mm. of the mononuclear type can be found in normal CSF. The appearance of CSF on gross observation will change from clear to slightly opalescent when it contains approximately 500 white blood cells per cu. mm. A very large number of white cells are required to produce turbid or cloudy fluid. Yellow discoloration of cerebrospinal fluid in the child can be caused by indirect hyperbilirubinemia or a marked increase in the protein content, but usually is the result of bleeding. Spinal fluid containing up to 360 red blood cells per cu. mm. remains clear but becomes visibly discolored and hazy with 500 red blood cells per cu. mm. and turns pink to red with increasing numbers of erythrocytes (McMenemy, Tourtellotte et al.). It is estimated that the CSF protein is raised approximately 1.5 mg. per 100 ml. for every 1000 red blood cells per cu. mm. (Tourtellotte et al.).

When the CSF obtained by lumbar puncture is bloody, it is important to distinguish whether bleeding was induced by the penetration of the needle or was present before the tap was performed. In the newborn or small infant, the needle tip can easily enter the venous plexus on the posterior surface of the vertebral body. Venous blood exudes from the needle hub indicating that the needle tip is not within the lumbar subarachnoid space. In the older child, more frequently one obtains spinal fluid mixed with blood that may result either from trauma of the procedure or from pre-existent subarachnoid bleeding. If fluid is collected sequentially in each of three or four tubes, the fluid will remain equally bloody in each tube if due to pre-existent bleeding but will usually become progressively clearer if due to needle-induced trauma. One tube should be centrifuged and the supernatant fluid observed. Xanthochromia of the supernatant fluid adds further evidence of preceding subarachnoid bleeding, whereas cystal-clear supernatant fluid indicates that the bleeding is fresh.

Microscopic examination of the fluid to determine if red blood cells are fresh or crenated cannot be considered to be a reliable way to distinguish subarachnoid hemorrhage from needle-induced bleeding because of the rapidity with which crenation occurs. With CSF cytomorphology, using the sedimentation technique or cytocentrifugation, the presence of hemosiderin-laden macrophages indicates subarachnoid bleeding occurred at least 18 hours before the lumbar puncture, since this period of time is required for the formation of these cells (Dyken). When the fluid is definitely hemorrhagic following spontaneous subarachnoid bleeding, xanthochromia of the supernatant fluid obtained by centrifugation becomes apparent within four to six hours after onset. The yellow appearance is believed to be from bilirubin formed from hemoglobin that is released from hemolyzed red blood cells (Roost et al.).

The sodium content of cerebrospinal fluid is approximately the same as that in the serum, while the chloride content is somewhat greater and the potassium slightly less (Lups and Haan). Regulation of cerebrospinal fluid acid-base balance is a complex process but is an important factor in certain metabolic derangements. In addition, the cerebrospinal fluid is not entirely homogeneous in regard to acid-base balance, and minor differences have been observed between lumbar and cisternal fluid (Plum and Price, Kalin et al.). Publications by Posner and Plum have shown that the normal CSF pH is approximately 0.1 unit lower than that in arterial blood and that carbon dioxide diffuses rapidly across the blood-CSF barrier but that hydrogen ions and bicarbonate enter much more slowly. Up to a point, adjustments protect CSF pH changes in the patient with systemic metabolic acidosis, and neurologic signs may be minimal. Carbon dioxide retention with respiratory acidosis is associated with a rapid decline in CSF pH and gives rise to neurologic dysfunction at serum pH levels not expected with metabolic acidosis (Fisher and Christianson, Bulger et al.).

Cerebrospinal Fluid Examination— Bacterial Meningitis

Confirmation of the diagnosis of bacterial meningitis depends on a proper and thorough examination of a cerebrospinal fluid specimen. Lumbar puncture, therefore, must be done whenever there is a reasonable consideration of the possibility of bacterial meningitis from the clinical findings. Performance of the procedure is generally regarded to be safe; however, there have been recurring reports in the literature that, on rare occasion, lumbar puncture in the septic child may itself provoke bacterial meningitis. As early as 1919, investigators provided clinical and experimental evidence that lumbar puncture *might* contribute to the development of acute meningitis (Weed et al., Wegeforth and Latham). The postulate has never been documented but subsequent reports have continued to suggest that it is possible that local damage of meningeal tissue or contamination of CSF by infected blood at the time of lumbar puncture might be a causative factor giving rise to meningitis on rare occasion (Fischer et al., Petersdorf et al., Pray). It is important to stress that this is an unproven theoretical consideration which in no way should prevent one from performing a lumbar puncture whenever the possibility of bacterial meningitis is entertained.

In addition, there are instances in which a child with clinical features suggestive of meningitis will show progression of signs in the hours following a normal CSF examination. This is an indication for a second CSF examination soon after the first, which sometimes will now document the presence of suppurative meningitis (Kindley and Harris, Rapkin). It can be assumed in most such cases that CSF infection existed at the time of the first lumbar puncture but a significant inflammatory reaction had not yet occurred and the concentration of bacteria was insufficient to allow their identification.

While it is true that the so-called "classic" CSF abnormalities in meningitis are present in most instances, it is important to recognize that there can be many variations in the CSF findings in the child with bacterial meningitis. The reasons for unexpected CSF findings in the presence of meningitis are often not apparent but in some instances can be explained by the time relationship between onset of the illness and when the lumbar puncture is done, the administration of prior antibiotic therapy, the concentration of bacteria in the CSF, or the host's ability to mount an inflammatory meningeal reaction. The CSF can be normal or with only minimal abnormalities, with subsequent cultural proof of the presence of bacterial infection (Moore and Ross).

Much more common is the finding of a CSF glucose content which is normal or nearly so, with other features of the fluid examination entirely consistent with acute meningitis. Because of the relationship of the blood sugar level with that in the CSF, a simultaneous blood sugar determination should be obtained when the lumbar puncture is performed.

In addition to the occasional absence of certain expected findings in the CSF when meningitis exists, there are rare instances of false positive findings indicative of meningitis when it is not present (Musher and Schell). Positive CSF gram stains have resulted from contamination of specimen tubes in lumbar puncture trays with non-viable bacteria (Weinstein et al.). Positive gram stains of CSF have also been described when a lumbar puncture was performed with a needle without a stylet, which then harbored within its lumen a small core of bacteria-laden skin tissue that contaminated the collected fluid (Joyner et al.). Finally, false positive findings can represent laboratory error or mislabeling of laboratory slips so that the results of one patient's CSF findings are placed within the record of another.

The characteristic CSF findings in the infant or child with bacterial meningitis include a cloudy or turbid appearance of the fluid on gross observation, a cellular response composed primarily of polymorphonuclear leukocytes, reduction of the sugar content, a variable degree of elevation of the protein content, and identification of the causative organism on gram stain, methylene blue stain, and cultural techniques. Considering only the cell composition and the glucose content, the CSF profile allows the design of the more likely differential diagnostic considerations, although considerable overlap does exist (Table 1–7).

In addition to the established methods of examination of CSF mentioned above, the recent development of new techniques has provided added dimensions that enhance the recognition of bacterial meningitis. Additional methods of analysis of the CSF are of importance, since in only 60 to 80 percent of cases of acute bacterial meningitis is the causative organism rapidly identified by gram stain (Carpenter and Petersdorf, Swartz and Dodge). Furthermore, differentiation of viral and bacterial infections of the central nervous system continues to be a commonly encountered problem and often cannot rapidly be done with the routine CSF studies. The most

Table 1–7. Cerebrospinal Fluid Profiles: Cellular Content and Glucose Value

---

Polymorphonuclear pleocytosis, reduced glucose
  Bacterial meningitis
  Parameningeal suppuration (subdural abscess)
  Primary amebic meningoencephalitis
Polymorphonuclear pleocytosis, normal glucose
  Bacterial meningitis
  Viral encephalitis (early stages)
  Eastern equine encephalitis
  Tuberculous or fungal meningitis (early stages)
Acute hemorrhagic leukoencephalitis
Lymphocytic pleocytosis, reduced glucose
  Tuberculous meningitis
  Fungal meningoencephalitis (certain types)
  Partially treated bacterial meningitis
  Viral aseptic meningitis (rare cases of mumps, HVH, LCM, enterovirus)
  Meningeal leukemia, carcinomatosis
  Meningeal sarcoidosis
  Cerebral cysticercosis
  Laboratory error
Lymphocytic pleocytosis, normal glucose
  Viral aseptic meningitis, encephalitis
  Partially treated bacterial meningitis
  Brain abscess
  Parameningeal suppuration
  Rocky Mountain spotted fever
  Lead encephalopathy
  Tuberculous or fungal meningitis (early)
  "Chemical" meningitis
  Leptospira, mycoplasma meningitis
  Meningeal leukemia
  Cerebral granulomatous angiitis
  Vogt-Koyanagi-Harada disease
  Behcet's disease
Hemorrhagic fluid
  Spontaneous subarachnoid hemorrhage
  Dural sinus—cortical vein thrombosis
  Herpes simplex encephalitis (infrequent cases)
  Ruptured mycotic aneurysm
  Anthrax meningitis
  "Traumatic" tap

---

applicable of these newer methods include latex particle agglutination, countercurrent immunoelectrophoresis, the Limulus lysate test, and the determination of CSF lactic acid content.

Latex particle agglutination is based on specific agglutination of antibody-coated latex particles by bacterial antigens released into the CSF. The test has been shown to be a reliable method for diagnosis of pneumococcal, meningococcal, and *Hemophilus influenzae* meningitis (Ward et al., Whittle et al.), and of group B, type III, streptococcal meningitis (Edwards et al.). It is more sensitive than counterimmunoelectrophoresis, and has the distinct advantage of rapid performance with results available within a few minutes. Neither highly specialized equipment nor de-

tailed technical expertise is required to accomplish the examination. The CSF content of muramidase is elevated in the early stages of bacterial meningitis but not with viral infections of the brain and has been proposed as an additional useful diagnostic procedure (Ansari et al.). Gas-liquid chromatography to detect certain chemical differences between bacteria in CSF, and thus establish an etiologic diagnosis, is in the investigative stage and may eventually become a useful technique (Brice et al., LaForce et al.). These tests should not be thought of as substitutes for the conventional methods of examination of CSF. They can complement the routine studies, enhancing the information obtained from CSF examination.

Countercurrent immunoelectrophoresis (CIE) is a widely used and reasonably reliable technique for detecting bacterial antigen in body fluids, including CSF (Coonrod and Rytel, Greenwood et al., Fossieck et al.). Commercially obtained antisera to the common causes of bacterial meningitis are used, with results of the test usually available within an hour or so after the CSF specimen is obtained. In addition to its applicability in the detection of antigens of *Hemophilus influenzae, Streptococcus pneumoniae,* and *Neisseria meningitidis,* CIE has recently been shown to be useful for the recognition of neonatal group B streptococcal meningitis (Edwards and Baker). The procedure may be positive in cases in which the fluid remains culture-negative owing to previously administered antibiotics. False negative tests are well known and thus a negative CIE on cerebrospinal fluid does not exclude the possibility of meningitis due to one of the common causative organisms. Quantitation of the antigen content by CIE may have some prognostic value in that children with meningitis with higher antigen levels have been found to have a higher incidence of sequelae than those with lower levels (Shackelford et al.). The diagnostic effectiveness of CIE is improved in children with bacterial meningitis by extending the examination to include blood and urine as well as CSF (Feigin et al.). Detectable antigen may persist in CSF for four to five days (Granoff et al.), but can generally be found in urine longer than in CSF (Shackelford et al.).

The Limulus lysate test is a technique by which a lysate prepared from the blood cells, or amebocytes, of the horseshoe crab, *Limulus polyphemus,* undergoes gelation in the presence of minute amounts of endotoxin derived from gram-negative bacteria. The test performed on CSF, thus, provides a rapid morphologic diagnosis of gram-negative meningitis but does not identify the specific etiologic agent (Nachum et al.). It has also been used on serum specimens to attempt to demonstrate endotoxemia indicative of gram-negative sepsis (Levin et al.), although some investigators have found it to be unreliable for this purpose (Elin et al., Feldman and Pearson). The Limulus lysate test on CSF has been shown to be a highly reliable indicator of the presence of gram-negative meningitis and is almost always negative in those with meningitis caused by gram-positive bacteria (Berman et al., Dyson and Cassady, Tuazon et al.). The procedure can be done rapidly, with results available within an hour after the lumbar puncture is done. It requires considerable laboratory expertise and can be complicated by false positive results from contamination of laboratory equipment with endotoxin (McCracken 1976).

Cerebrospinal Fluid Cell Count. Quantitative and qualitative analysis of the cellular composition of CSF is exceedingly important in neurologic infections, both for the initial diagnosis and as an indicator of progress of the illness during treatment. If done skillfully, the cell count determined by use of the Fuchs-Rosenthal counting chamber provides accurate results, but differentiation of the type of cells present cannot be accurately done with this preparation. When cells are abundant, their type can be identified by the slide method using Wright's stain; however, newer techniques for cytologic examination are far superior. Recently developed methods for concentrating cells in CSF with little alteration in cellular morphology include sedimentation and centrifugation, the latter utilizing the cytocentrifuge (Hansen et al., Sörnäs, Woodruff). The sedimentation method has the advantage of slightly less cellular distortion but the use of the cytocentrifuge (Cytospin) is more rapid and is better suited to clinical needs. The study can be done with one ml. of fluid or less.

The end-result of these techniques is the concentration of formed elements in the CSF on a glass slide which are then prepared with Wright's stain, gram stain, or other stains, allowing precise identification of the cellular and, often, bacterial content of the fluid (Choi and Anderson). The ability of the cytocentrifuge to concentrate cells allows a differential count of at least 25 cells on CSF which contains one to five cells per cu. mm., determined by the counting chamber (Hoeltge et al.).

Experience with sedimentation or cytocentrifuge methods for CSF examination has clarified the normal cellular composition of CSF and also enables identification of cell types which previously were less commonly recognized in abnormal CSF, such as plasma cells, eosinophils, histiocytic macrophages, and ependymal-choroidal cells. In normal CSF containing five or less white blood cells per cu. mm., the cell composition includes 60 to 100 percent lymphocytes; cells other than lymphocytes are monocytes, a rare neutrophil, and occasional pia-arachnoid cells (Kolar and Zeman, Woodruff).

The Wright-stained cells in CSF are differentiated by their morphologic characteristics. Certain types of cells are easily identified but others require considerable experience and skill. Normal lymphocytes are usually less than 10 microns in diameter and contain oval, densely-stained nuclei and a relatively small amount of light blue cytoplasm. Monocytic (monocytoid) cells include blood monocytes and reticulomonocytes. They are larger than lymphocytes, contain an indented nucleus with one or more nucleoli, and have abundant, pale cytoplasm, which is often vacuolated. Polymorphonuclear leukocytes are seen only sparsely in normal CSF. Their presence in significant numbers correlates well with neurologic infections of various types, but they can be seen in other disorders, such as acute hemorrhagic leukoencephalitis. They are easily recognized by their dark-stained multilobed nuclei and the ample, bluish cytoplasm. On the initial CSF examination in previously untreated bacterial meningitis, polymorphonuclear leukocytes are the predominant cell type and many times represent nearly the total cell population. After several days of effective therapy, their number has usually decreased both in absolute value and in relative value, with an increase in the number of lymphocytes. Macrophages can often be found at this time, and sometimes an occasional plasma cell as well as ependymal-choroidal cells.

Eosinophils are infrequently observed in CSF and are identified by their dark-stained bilobed nuclei embedded in cytoplasm with abundant eosinophilic granules. Their occurrence in large numbers in CSF is seen in certain parasitic infections of the nervous system, such as cysticercosis or meningoencephalitis caused by the lung worm, *Angiostrongylus cantonensis.* An eosinophilic cell response in CSF has also been described following the instillation of rubber catheters for ventricular shunting (Jeanes, Kessler and Cheek).

Basophils are rarely found in CSF under any condition. Glasser et al. described a basophilic pleocytosis in a child with non-Hodgkin's lymphoma with meningeal invasion. Basophils are considered to represent a cellular marker indicative of a cell-mediated immune response. Their presence in CSF with meningeal tumor might be explained on the basis of the tissues' immune reaction to the presence of cells foreign to that location. Basophils are characterized by the presence of large, coarse, darkly stained granules which often obscure the lighter-stained nucleus.

Macrophages of reticuloendothelial origin are large cells characterized by evidence of phagocytosis and are seen in CSF only under abnormal conditions. Macrophages containing erythrocyte fragments or hemosiderin are seen following subarachnoid hemorrhage, while lipomacrophages are seen in certain conditions with necrotizing parenchymal changes, such as traumatic or ischemic injuries or following Pantopaque myelography.

Plasma cells are not found in normal CSF but have been described in subacute or chronic inflammatory disorders including viral infections of the nervous system, cysticercosis, certain fungal infections, and demyelinating disorders (Glasser et al., Peter). They are identified by their oval shape, intensely basophilic cytoplasm, eccentric position of the nucleus, and spoke-like arrangement of the nuclear chromatin.

Ependymal-choroidal cells, likewise, have generally been regarded to be an abnormal cell type in CSF although some investigators have stated otherwise (Stokes et al.). They can be found in CSF following craniocerebral trauma, ischemic injuries, and after certain neurosurgical procedures. Ependymal-choroidal cells may also be exfoliated into the CSF in children with hydrocephalus (Wilkins and Odom). They are cuboidal to columnar in shape, fairly uniform in size and shape, and contain a well-defined, round or oval dark-stained nucleus. One of the most characteristic features of ependymal-choroidal cells is their occurrence in clusters, which can result in the possibility of confusing them with clumps of neoplastic cells.

Cerebrospinal Fluid Glucose. Hypoglycorrhachia, or abnormal reduction of the CSF glucose content, is an important indicator of one of a variety of disease states. The normal content of glucose in CSF is a range of values and to a certain degree is related to the blood sugar level, which itself is normally quite variable. Abnormally low CSF values have been defined in absolute concentrations measured in mg. per 100 ml., and in the form of a CSF glucose to blood glucose ratio. To this date, however, there is no universally accepted definition of what constitutes hypoglycorrhachia even though it has been a topic of consideration since the early decades of this century (Grayzel and Orent, Wilcox and Lyttle).

CSF glucose levels below which levels are considered abnormal have been placed at 40 mg. per 100 ml. by some investigators (Kelley), at 45 mg. by others (Goodwin and Shelley), and at 50 mg. by still others (Silver and Todd). Lups and Haan claimed the normal CSF glucose content ranges from 45 to 70 mg. per 100 ml., thus implying that levels below 45 mg. are abnormal. CSF glucose to blood glucose ratios that have been considered to be abnormal have varied from less than 0.40 (Fishman) to less than 0.50 (Silver and Todd). A summary of the past literature would allow one to conclude that a CSF glucose content below 40 mg. per 100 ml. can be considered to be abnormal and 40 to 45 mg. is borderline low. The CSF glucose to blood glucose ratio which seems most acceptable to represent an abnormality is a value of less than 0.50.

One of the major problems in interpretation of the CSF to blood glucose ratio is the time required for glucose equilibration to occur in CSF following fluctuations in the serum level. For example, if an ill child experiences a convulsion which provokes an acute rise in the blood glucose content from 100 mg. to 140 mg. per 100 ml., a CSF examination soon thereafter may demonstrate an unchanged glucose concentration of 50 mg. per 100 ml. Because there has been insufficient time for equilibration to occur between the two compartments, the resulting CSF glucose to blood glucose ratio of 0.37 would be within the abnormal range, despite the normal CSF glucose content. Following an acute rise in the blood glucose level, the latent period before there is a significant rise in CSF glucose has been estimated to be from a few minutes up to 39 minutes in some studies (Myers and Netsky), and as long as two hours in others (Grayzel and Orent). Because of this lag time, which must vary considerably under different circumstances, simultaneous blood and CSF glucose determinations may provide misleading information.

Depression of the cerebrospinal fluid glucose is one of the most reliable indicators of bacterial meningitis, assuming that the blood glucose is not reduced. There are many exceptions to this rule, however, and a normal cerebrospinal fluid glucose content by no means excludes the possibility of acute bacterial meningitis. With the more common bacterial agents the cerebrospinal fluid glucose is usually between zero and 20 mg. per 100 ml. when the initial tap is performed. In tuberculous and cryptococcal meningitis the glucose level is often somewhat higher, but even with these infections profound reduction of the glucose content may be encountered. The glucose content in the spinal fluid is normal or elevated in most viral infections of the nervous system although a modest reduction can occur in certain types of viral meningoencephalitis, including those caused by mumps (Wilfert), Herpes simplex (Sarubbi et al.), and lymphocytic choriomeningitis viruses (Adair et al.), as well as the enteroviruses (Silver and Todd). Low CSF glucose has also been described with *Mycoplasma pneumoniae* meningoencephalitis (Klimek et al.).

Hypoglycorrhachia can occur following subarachnoid hemorrhage in older children and adults. The cause of glucose reduction with subarachnoid bleeding remains unclear. Troost et al. suggested increased glycolysis by red cell enzymes and interference with glucose transport into the cerebrospinal fluid as possible pathogenetic mechanisms. In newborn infants with significant intraventricular hemorrhage, hypoglycorrhachia is frequently observed several days thereafter and may persist for several weeks (Deonna et al.). The degree of reduction of the CSF glucose in this instance can be striking, sometimes to levels less than 10 mg. per 100 ml. (Nelson et al.).

Reduction in the CSF glucose content can also occur in patients with meningeal leukemia and other types of neoplastic meningeal invasion.

Many explanations have been proposed for the reduced cerebrospinal fluid glucose in bacterial meningitis. Petersdorf and Harter demonstrated that both white cells and bacteria exhibited relatively slow glycolytic activity alone but when cells and organisms were incubated together, utilization of glucose was markedly accelerated. Studies with tritium-labeled glucose have indicated an increased glucose consumption by actively phagocytic leukocytes in purulent cerebrospinal fluid (Bretz and Mauer). Menkes emphasized other factors, including increased glucose utilization by the brain due to increased glycolysis and a disturbance of glucose transport from blood to cerebrospinal fluid. Thus, the regulatory factors affecting glucose metabolism within the nervous system appear complex and several mechanisms seem operative in accounting for the reduced cerebrospinal fluid glucose content in meningitis.

Cerebrospinal Fluid Lactic Acid Content. As early as 1917, it was shown that there is a depression of the cerebrospinal fluid pH with acute bacterial meningitis (Levinson). In 1924, Nishimura demonstrated an elevation of the lactic acid content in the CSF in this disease, and studies soon thereafter confirmed this observation (Killian, Osnato and Killian). How much the CSF acidosis contributes to disturbances of responsiveness or other neurologic signs remains uncertain, but in recent years, with the improvement in the precision and accuracy of the methodology, the diagnostic value of the CSF lactic acid content in neurologic infections has been stressed (Bland et al., Brook et al., Controni et al., Ferguson and Tearle). Increased CSF lactic acid is not specific for bacterial or fungal infections of the brain, in that it can occur with acute hypoxic or ischemic cerebral injuries and with certain types of cerebral neoplasms (Komorowski et al., Paulson et al. 1971).

Studies by Bland et al. in 1974 revealed that the CSF lactic acid content in viral aseptic meningitis remains normal or is only slightly elevated above the mean level of the controls, the latter being approximately 14 mg. per 100 ml., which corresponds closely to the normal serum level. In untreated bacterial meningitis, the mean CSF lactic acid content was 75 mg. per 100 ml., while in partially treated meningitis, it was 49.5 mg. per 100 ml. A gradual return toward normal occurred during the course of treatment. Brook and colleagues found that all patients studied with acute pyogenic meningitis had a CSF lactic acid content of greater than 35 mg. per 100 ml. on the day of diagnosis, while those with aseptic meningitis had levels less than 35 mg. per 100 ml. The latter report included a single case with cryptococcal meningitis before treatment in whom the CSF lactic acid content was increased to 43 mg. per 100 ml. Elevation of CSF lactic acid has also been found by Komorowski et al. in three patients with fungal meningitis prior to treatment.

The rise in CSF lactic acid in suppurative meningitis occurs independent of the lactic acid blood level. The mechanism for its occurrence remains unclear. Increased CSF lactic acid content has been described with intracranial hypertension and decreased cerebral blood flow, and these factors may be contributory to the increased levels found in bacterial meningitis (Kjallquist et al., Paulson et al. 1972, Zwetnow). It has also been proposed that the high lactic acid values in CSF in pyogenic meningitis may be the result of anaerobic glycolysis by polymorphonuclear leukocytes associated with tissue anoxia (Brook et al.). In an experimental study of pneumococcal meningitis in rabbits, McAllister et al. found that both the maximal level of CSF lactic acid and the maximal degree of inflammation occurred at the same time, at approximately 72 hours after onset, suggesting that granulocytes may contribute to the lactic acid content.

Cerebrospinal Fluid Enzymes. The content of certain enzymes normally present in brain and cerebrospinal fluid may be elevated in patients with bacterial meningitis. These determinations have not proved to be of clinical usefulness, however, because of the variability of results in patients with bacterial infections of the nervous system and owing to the lack of specificity of abnormally high enzyme values. The CSF glutamic oxaloacetic transaminase content is normally 5 to 21 units (Katzman et al.). Belsey studied the CSF content of this enzyme in 95 pediatric patients with purulent meningitis and found a positive correlation between degree of its elevation and prognosis. Patients with levels below 24 units generally did well, whereas those with levels greater than 24 units had a higher incidence of complications or sequelae from the disease.

The CSF lactic dehydrogenase content is increased in the presence of bacterial meningitis (Feldman, Williams and Hawkins) but has also been found to be elevated in viral central nervous system disease (Beaty and Oppenheimer) as well as in other disorders associated with injury to cerebral tissue. Studies of the different lactic dehydrogenase isoenzyme fractions by Beaty and Oppenheimer have suggested that the increased CSF lactic dehydrogenase in meningitis is derived primarily from granulocytes. Different isoenzymes have been found to be elevated in patients with viral encephalitis, although the source of the enzyme in viral disease remains unclear. Creatine phosphokinase activity in the CSF has also been investigated in children with meningitis but without distinctive findings (Katz and Liebman). Elevated levels were found in 8 of 16 patients and could not be correlated with the blood levels of this enzyme.

Cerebrospinal Fluid and Preliminary Treatment. Children with meningitis frequently receive antibiotics orally or by injection before the diagnosis is suspected or established. It is estimated that approximately 50 percent of patients with meningitis receive antibiotics of some form before the diagnosis is made (Dalton and Allison, Harter). In two-thirds of these, penicillin or a penicillin derivative is the antibiotic administered (Converse et al.). The effect of partial treatment on the ability to establish the diagnosis of bacterial meningitis has been debated with conflicting results in the literature but it is generally agreed that it can alter the CSF findings in some instances and can make identification of some organisms difficult. It is important to know what antibiotics have been used, the dose, and the method and duration of administration. One or two oral doses of an antibiotic in the amount usually given for out-patients presumably would have little effect on the CSF findings (Davis et al.), while more prolonged use in higher dosage of an antibiotic that penetrates into the CSF would be expected to alter the CSF abnormalities to a certain degree.

Preliminary antibiotic therapy can suppress the infection to the degree that the cerebrospinal fluid pleocytosis is mainly lymphocytic and the glucose content is normal. When this occurs, the cerebrospinal fluid abnormalities resemble those in viral aseptic meningitis, enhancing the possibility of diagnostic error. Immunofluorescent techniques employing specific fluorescent antisera have been used in an effort to enhance bacterial identification in partially treated cases but without spectacular results (Grossman et al., Page et al.). Cerebrospinal fluid IgM content may prove to be a helpful measure for differentiation of bacterial from viral disease even though overlapping results occur in some cases. Smith and colleagues demonstrated that the CSF IgM was usually elevated in the acute phase of purulent meningitis and suggested that a concentration greater than 3 mg. per 100 ml. weighs heavily against a viral etiology. Countercurrent immunoelectrophoresis and latex particle agglutination are more practical methods that can provide a rapid diagnosis of the common causes of bacterial meningitis in some cases when the gram stain is negative.

Dalton and Allison studied the effects of partial antibiotic treatment before diagnosis of bacterial meningitis and found that it reduced the number of positive cultures from spinal fluid by approximately 30 percent and reduced identification of the organism on gram stain by about 20 percent. Preliminary, partial antibiotic therapy had little effect on recovery of *Hemophilus influenzae* but considerable effect when meningitis was caused by the meningococcus. Davis et al., likewise, have found that preliminary antibiotic therapy for *Hemophilus influenzae* meningitis seldom alters the CSF findings enough to interfere with establishment of the diagnosis. The concentration of bacteria in CSF has been found to be decreased following prior antibiotic therapy for *Hemophilus influenzae* meningitis and meningococcal meningitis, but not in those with meningitis caused by *Streptococcus pneumoniae* (Feldman). The reduction in bacterial concentration in this study did decrease the diagnostic effectiveness of the gram stain but did not alter the results of CSF cultures.

Considering all methods of inquiry, although certain cerebrospinal fluid changes may follow partial preliminary treatment, the alterations are not usually sufficient to alter laboratory confirmation of a diagnosis of bacterial meningitis (Dalton and Allison, Winkelstein). There remains a small but perplexing group of patients with bacterial meningitis in whom preliminary antibiotic therapy alters the cerebrospinal fluid findings to the degree that it is difficult to distinguish acute bacterial meningitis from viral aseptic meningitis or encephalitis. When one cannot distinguish partially treated bacterial meningitis from viral aseptic meningitis, it is advisable to provide adequate therapy for the most likely bacterial agent in the age group the child is in. In addition, unless the fluid is frankly purulent and organisms are identified on gram stain, appropriate cultures for acid-fast bacilli and fungi should be requested.

MORTALITY AND SEQUELAE

Factors related to morbidity and mortality in childhood meningitis are complex, but the age of the child, the rapidity of diagnosis after onset, the state of responsiveness at the time of diagnosis, and the adequacy of the therapeutic regimen are of cardinal importance. The mortality rate of gram-negative neonatal meningitis is in the range of 40 to 60 percent in most series. With neonatal *Escherichia coli* meningitis, morbidity and mortality have been shown to be related to the presence or absence of *Escherichia coli* K1 capsular polysaccharide antigen, an antigen chemically and immunologically similar to meningococcal Group B polysaccharide (Robbins et al.). The detection of K1 capsular antigen in CSF is associated with a worse outcome, and survival tends to be related to the amount of antigen and the period of time of its persistence in body fluids (McCracken et al., 1974). Of the two forms of neonatal group B streptococcal infection, the early onset type, which may or may not be associated with meningitis, has a mortality rate in excess of 50 percent, while the late onset or "meningeal" type is associated with a case fatality rate of 15 to 20 percent (Baker et al., Barton et al.). With *Hemophilus influenzae* and meningococcal meningitis the case fatality rate is approximately 5 to 10 percent, and with pneumococcal meningitis in the pediatric age group it is about 20 percent but would be considerably higher if one restricted the consideration to the first six months of life. Tuberculous meningitis continues to carry a mortality rate of 20 percent.

Post-meningitic sequelae are most frequent when meningitis occurs in the first two months of life and are least frequent in older children with meningococcal meningitis. The high frequency of sequelae in infants is in part related to the more common occurrence of communicating hydrocephalus due to a cisternal block and to the greater adverse effects of cerebritis on the immature brain. Residual deficits in some children following bacterial meningitis are secondary to the inflammatory process itself, and in others, to vasculitis associated with the bacterial infection. The type of neurologic deficits that follow bacterial meningitis is determined by the location, character, and severity of the neuropathologic injury, factors which are widely variable from case to case (Fig. 1–24). Sequelae are mild in some instances, and involve only one type of neurologic function, such as hearing or vision. In others, the deficits are more severe, with a combination of different types of abnormalities. Still others are profoundly affected and regain little functional ability in either the intellectual or motor spheres after the acute stage of the illness. The most common types of neurologic

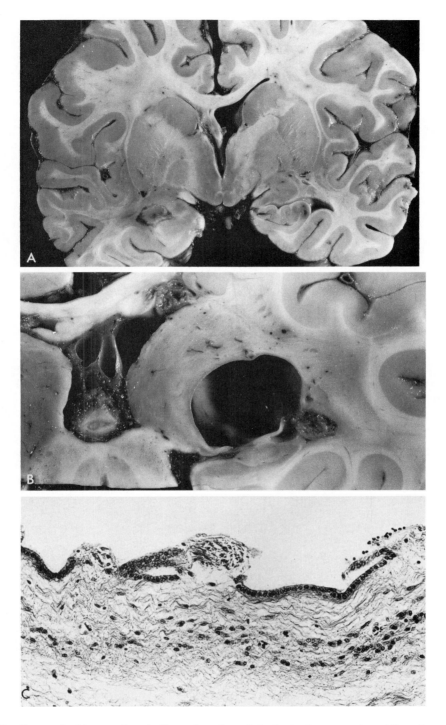

Figure 1–24. Postmeningitic sequelae. *A,* Coronal section of the brain demonstrating obliteration of the right lateral ventricle by ependymal adhesions. The left lateral ventricle is mildly enlarged. *B,* Chronic ependymitis and adhesive arachnoiditis with a postinflammatory arachnoidal cyst in the left hippocampal fissure. *C,* Ependymal granulations secondary to acute pyogenic meningitis three years previously (H&E, 200×).

sequelae following acute bacterial meningitis include hearing loss, behavior disorders, mental retardation, recurrent seizures, hydrocephalus, long tract signs of either the hemiparetic or quadriparetic type, and visual deficits secondary to optic nerve or cerebral cortical injury (Figs. 1–25, 1–26). Unusual long-term sequelae include cerebellar ataxia without other neurologic abnormalities, hypothalamic dysfunction manifested by diabetes insipidus, precocious puberty, and profound hyperphagia leading to obesity (Fig. 1–27).

Hemophilus influenzae is the most common cause of meningitis in the childhood age range and most cases involve infants between four and 24 months of age. The incidence of significant neurologic sequelae among survi-

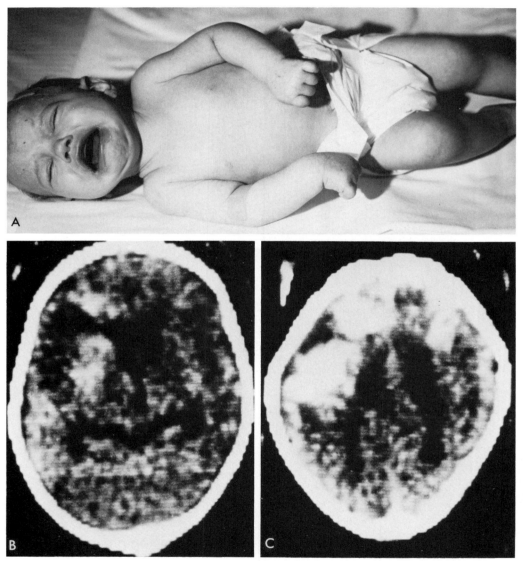

Figure 1–25. Postmeningitic sequelae. *A,* Five-month-old child one month after onset of *Hemophilus influenzae* meningitis. At the time of hospital admission in the acute stage of the illness, she was febrile, minimally responsive, and had recurrent generalized convulsions. CSF became sterile on the third day of antibiotic therapy, although the child remained irritable and poorly responsive to verbal stimuli. Four weeks after onset of the illness, she is irritable and is hypertonic and hyperreflexic in all four extremities. Her hands are held partially fisted and limbs are in partial flexion. *B,* Computed tomogram without contrast infusion reveals mild ventricular enlargement. The lateral ventricles are poorly outlined because of bilateral diffuse microcystic degeneration of the white matter. Patchy areas of increased density in the left cerebral hemisphere represent hemorrhagic softening. *C,* Computed tomogram with contrast enhancement shows two large irregular enhanced areas on the left and one on the right, which suggests disruption of the vascular integrity in these areas. A transfontanel tap of the large enhanced area on the left side yielded only a small amount of sterile, xanthochromic fluid.

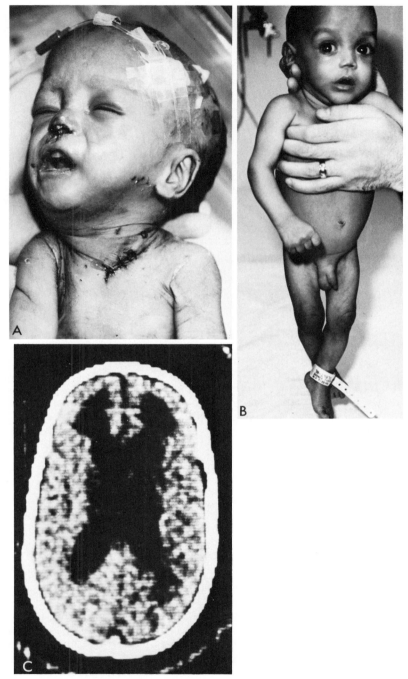

Figure 1–26. Postmeningitic sequelae. *A,* Seven-week-old child with acute coliform meningitis, sepsis, and disseminated intravascular coagulation. Birth weight was 1690 grams, and the neonatal period was complicated by respiratory distress syndrome. At four weeks of age, he had decreased food intake and vomiting but was afebrile. At six weeks of age, there was progressive lethargy, followed by irritability, increased vomiting, and hypothermia. CSF examination soon thereafter revealed cloudy fluid containing gram-negative rods. He developed thrombocytopenia, other laboratory evidence of consumption coagulopathy, and clinical bleeding evident in figure *A. B,* At eight months of age, the child exhibits spastic quadriparesis. Note the extension and adduction of the lower extremities when elevated above the examining table. Growth has been poor; head circumference is large compared to length and weight measurements, and the anterior fontanel is full. *C,* Computed tomogram demonstrates symmetrical hydrocephalus, which was treated with a ventriculoperitoneal shunt.

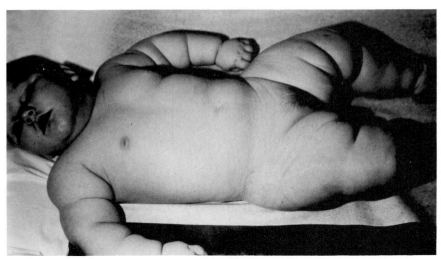

Figure 1–27. Postmeningitic sequelae. Twelve-month-old child with severe hypothalamic injury secondary to Group B *Streptococcus* meningitis at age 30 days. The child has periodic vaginal bleeding, pubic hair, and profound obesity resulting from hyperphagia. She has had marked temperature instability with wide swings in body temperature. Her development is delayed, head circumference is abnormally small, and she is blind with bilateral optic atrophy.

vors with this type of meningitis cannot be clearly delineated from the literature because of different criteria that are used to define sequelae. Of a series of 50 children with *Hemophilus influenzae* meningitis, Feigin et al. found severe neurologic deficits in only 8 percent although an additional 28 percent had IQ scores between 70 and 90. Others have found an even higher incidence of permanent neurologic deficits in children with this illness (Sell et al., Sproles et al.). Summarizing the information available, it appears that either death or significant sequelae will occur in the range of 35 to 45 percent of all children who develop *Hemophilus influenzae* meningitis.

Hydrocephalus complicating bacterial meningitis can occur at any age but is more common in the newborn and young infant. Shunt procedures are often required in such cases although shunt failure due to occlusion of the tube often necessitates several revisions. Most surgeons now favor a ventriculoperitoneal shunt as the preferred method of treatment of post-meningitic hydrocephalus.

TREATMENT

Bacterial meningitis should be regarded as a medical emergency from the standpoint of accomplishment of the diagnostic tests and the initiation of antibiotic therapy. Unnecessary delay in beginning treatment may alter the outcome of such infectious illnesses in re-

gard to both sequelae and mortality. It is usually advisable to obtain blood for culture and to perform the lumbar puncture before starting intravenous antibiotic therapy, although exceptions do exist. The physician in practice who clearly suspects meningitis from the clinical signs may find it desirable or necessary to transport the child to a treatment center for definitive care. When the trip will require more than a few minutes, it is advisable to provide intravenous antibiotic therapy during this period, even though the CSF examination has not yet been accomplished. Such therapy may be life-saving, while the possibility of significant interference with subsequent diagnostic tests is usually negligible. In other instances, the practicing physician who suspects meningitis will perform the lumbar puncture, initiate intravenous therapy, and transport the child *and* the cerebrospinal fluid specimens to a medical center where rapid analysis of the fluid will confirm the diagnosis and identify the causative organism.

Although the mainstay of therapy for bacterial meningitis is the administration of antibiotics, attention must be devoted to a variety of other treatment considerations. Of primary importance is the presence of an adequate airway or the establishment of one in those with ventilation difficulty. In many, intermittent gentle suction of the upper airway will suffice, but occasionally, intubation or even ventilatory support may be required. In the deeply lethargic or comatose child, a nasogastric tube should be placed and the gastric contents removed. This lessens the danger of vomiting and aspiration, and also will improve respiratory function if gastric distention is present. Diligent nursing care is always necessary but is especially important in the child with repetitive seizures, the unconscious child, or the one who is agitated and irrational. Prevention of aspiration, the monitoring of blood pressure and other vital signs, and the recording of observations regarding seizures or behavior in general are all critical aspects of the nursing management. Attention to the control of hyperthermia is imperative, in part because of the greater tendency of seizures to occur in the febrile child and also because of the possible adverse effects of the increased cerebral metabolic rate associated with fever in the child with cerebral swelling and cerebral vascular compromise. Methods of combating fever include the use of an electric fan directed toward the unclothed child, the use of an air-conditioned room for the febrile patient, gentle sponging with appropriately cooled towels, and the administration of antipyretic agents by either the rectal or oral route.

Fluid and electrolyte administration is of paramount importance and should be carefully designed on the basis of daily requirements and the results of serum electrolyte determinations. Administration of an excessive quantity of fluid intravenously can aggravate already-present cerebral edema, enhancing the possibility of tentorial or cerebellar herniation. Because of the common occurrence of cerebral swelling in children with meningitis as well as the relatively high incidence of inappropriate antidiuretic hormone secretion in the early stages of the illness (Kaplan and Feigin), it is advisable to restrict total fluid administration at the initiation of therapy to approximately two-thirds of maintenance needs or 1.5 ml. per kilogram per hour. This is assuming that the child is not severely dehydrated at this point. Should inappropriate ADH secretion be documented, even further fluid restriction might be necessary. With periodic determinations of the serum electrolytes, serum and urine osmolarities, and body weight, the required fluid volume can be determined with the passage of time. In most instances, fluid administration can be liberalized to the usual maintenance requirements of approximately 1800 ml. per square meter per day, or 2.5 ml. per kilogram per hour, after three to four days. The electrolyte content of the fluids given intravenously will vary depending on a number of factors, but in most, fluid containing one-third to one-fifth normal saline in 5 percent glucose is adequate. As improvement occurs and liquids are taken orally, the amount given intravenously is gradually reduced so that the total fluid intake does not exceed maintenance needs.

When seizures have occurred during the course of the illness, it is advisable to place the child on anticonvulsant therapy until recovery has occurred. Phenobarbital in a dose of 3 to 4 mg. per kilogram per day for the older child and 4 to 10 mg. per kilogram per day for the infant is often sufficient. Status epilepticus can usually be controlled by the intravenous administration of diazepam (Valium) or phenobarbital. Airway obstruction and hypoxia should be prevented, as this also contributes to further brain swelling. Cerebral edema is a common event in children with meningitis and when severe it can result in transtentorial herniation with brain stem compression and death. The effects of brain swelling are difficult to judge by clinical assessment but a progressive decline of the state of responsiveness, pupillary dilatation, bradycardia, and the development of early papilledema warrants a therapeutic trial with mannitol. Mannitol has a rapid effect and is given intravenously in a dose of 0.5 to 2 grams per kilogram over 30 minutes. The brisk diuresis resulting requires an indwelling urethral catheter if the patient is unresponsive. Corticosteroids are usually ineffective when used for treatment of increased intracranial pressure in acute bacterial meningitis and are best avoided, except for the special instances of septic shock or associated adrenal insufficiency (Migeon et al., Schumer). Corticosteroids as an adjunct to antibiotics for alleged benefits such as prevention of the development of hydrocephalus or a decrease in the inflammatory reaction have not been proved effective (Belsey et al., deLemos and Haggerty).

Sudden, severe and rapidly progressive increased intracranial pressure due to cerebral swelling in children with meningitis is one of the most difficult aspects of treatment of this disease. Its importance in regard to the eventual outcome is no doubt often underestimated, and it is perhaps the one area of management that is most often ignored or dealt with inadequately. This is true in part because of the difficulty in distinguishing signs indicative of significant intracranial hypertension from those that can be attributed to the cerebral effects of meningitis that occur independent of increased pressure, and also because of the rapidity with which decisions must be made if aggressive treatment is to be initiated. While the need for aggressive treatment is not applicable to every case, there are cases in which one's ability to control increased intracranial pressure determines survival or death of the patient (Nugent et al.). This can pertain to the older infant but is more often a factor in the older child in whom the anterior fontanel and cranial sutures have closed and the system's ability to compensate for a rapid increase in intracranial pressure is limited.

When increase in intracranial pressure is clearly a factor accounting for progressive obtundation judged on the basis of clinical features, the lumbar puncture pressure, and the results of computed cranial tomography, treatment methods are sometimes indicated beyond fluid restriction, control of hyperthermia, and the unmonitored use of mannitol. More aggressive treatment includes intubation with controlled ventilation so that the $PaCO_2$ is maintained below 30 mm. Hg, and the use of central arterial and venous lines for pressure measurements which allow precise administration of fluid volume. This is accompanied by the instillation of a device for continuous intracranial pressure monitoring.

Continuous monitoring of intracranial pressure can be done with the use of an indwelling intraventricular catheter or a subdural or subarachnoid bolt placed through a burr hole. The advantage of an intraventricular catheter is that it allows periodic aspiration of small amounts of ventricular fluid, which is a rapid and effective method for control of acute pressure spikes. The disadvantage in the patient with meningitis is that the catheter must be passed through infected spaces to enter the ventricle, and its placement can be very difficult when the ventricles are small because of cerebral swelling. With continuous monitoring of intracranial pressure, it is possible to regulate blood gases and fluid intake, and to give mannitol intermittently in doses of 0.5 gram per kilogram by bolus so that the intracranial pressure can be maintained within the safe range. The method also provides a guide to the possible danger of certain nursing techniques, such as orotracheal suctioning, which can provoke acute elevations in the intracranial pressure. When it is recognized that suctioning or other manipulations significantly raise intracranial pressure, these procedures should be curtailed to the extent possible and done at a

time when the patient is hyperventilated or is receiving mannitol. When intracranial pressure is not adequately controlled by the above measures, large-dose pentobarbital therapy can be added to the regimen. Systemic hypothermia is still another approach that has been used to control cerebral swelling with head trauma and Reye's syndrome (Boutros et al.) but it has not been extensively used in neurologic infections.

Treatment of endotoxic shock, which sometimes complicates acute bacterial meningitis, continues to be a perplexing and debatable subject. At least it is agreed that appropriate antibiotic therapy is necessary and that early initiation of therapy is more apt to be successful than that started after profound shock has developed. Restoration of blood volume and correction of electrolyte deficits may be necessary if vomiting or diarrhea has occurred. Intravenous fluids may suffice but, in certain instances, fresh whole blood may be desirable. Bicarbonate therapy in conjunction with measures to correct dehydration is useful if metabolic acidosis is present. Central venous and arterial catheters for pressure monitoring facilitate fluid and drug administration if hypotension or shock is present. Dopamine is the most widely used preparation to combat septic shock, and is given in a dose of 2 to 10 μg per kilogram per minute. Since dopamine is inactivated in alkaline solution, it should not be given in the same IV bottle with sodium bicarbonate. The primary effect of dopamine is to increase myocardial contractility, enhancing cardiac output and thus improving tissue perfusion. The use of corticosteroids in septic shock remains questionable although there is little established evidence that supports worsening of this condition therefrom. Large or "pharmacologic" doses of corticosteroids appear justified in view of the seriousness of this condition (Hodes, Schumer). Intravenous hydrocortisone is recommended, with potential beneficial effects including its enhancement of the microcirculation, counteraction of glycogen depletion by endotoxin, reduction of lactic acid formation, and its protective effect in lysosomes, preventing rupture.

Laboratory evidence of intravascular coagulation warrants heparin therapy in some cases although there is controversy regarding the indications unless clinical bleeding has occurred. Heparin is administered intravenously in a dose of 100 units per kilogram and is repeated every 4 hours in an amount sufficient to lengthen the partial thromboplastin time or thrombin time to 2 to 3 times normal. The duration of heparin therapy is variable and is determined by clinical judgment plus evidence of improvement of laboratory data regarding clotting factors and platelets.

Antimicrobial Therapy

Selection of specific antimicrobial therapy before identification of the etiologic agent is on the basis of the most likely organism present relative to the age of the child and the presence or absence of other associated disorders. In addition, the antibiotic(s) chosen must be capable of gaining entrance into the CSF in quantities significantly greater than the minimum inhibitory concentration of the causative organism if it is to be effective (Table 1–8). Appropriate changes in therapy are made, if necessary, after the organism is isolated and sensitivities to various antibiotics are determined.

Antibiotic sensitivity testing has gradually become important for almost all of the bacterial organisms that cause acute meningitis. *Neisseria meningitidis* can still be assumed to be effectively treated with penicillin, although if sulfadiazine is considered for prophylactic therapy, testing of its antimicrobial sensitivity is necessary. Routine testing of *Streptococcus pneumoniae* for its susceptibility to penicillin has not been considered necessary in the past but this, too, may be changing. The recent reports of pneumococci with decreased sensitivity to penicillin suggest that in the future one will not be able to assume that this antibiotic will be consistently effective without laboratory confirmation (Ahronheim et al.). Following the emergence of ampicillin-resistant strains of *Hemophilus influenzae* type b, antibiotic sensitivity testing became vital for the determination of the best method of treatment of meningitis caused by this organism. The capricious behavior of *Hemophilus influenzae* on disc plate testing became widely recognized but this has been resolved by

more reliable methods, including the determination of β-lactamase activity.

The meaning of the terms "sensitive" and "resistant" has been succinctly summarized by Arnold Smith who stated that "sensitive" refers to organisms whose growth is inhibited by antibiotic concentrations readily achieved in blood while "resistant" organisms are those not inhibited by the same concentrations. The antibiotic sensitivities, therefore, provide valuable information regarding the effect upon the microorganism of various antibiotics in vitro, and, to a certain degree, the information is transferable to the clinical setting. The drug potentially most effective on the basis of sensitivity tests is often not the one of choice for treatment of certain types of infections. The final selection depends on several factors, such as the site of infection, the penetrability into tissues of the various antibiotics under consideration, the possible toxic effects of the various drugs relative to age of the patient, and other factors, as well as the antibiotic sensitivities.

With the exception of the aminoglycosides and the rare instances when trimethoprim-sulfamethoxazole or metronidazole is indicated, antibiotic treatment for bacterial meningitis should be administered intravenously, preferably for the entire course of therapy. The duration of antibiotic therapy varies from case to case but in most instances it is not less than 12 to 14 days. Neonatal meningitis usually requires a minimum of two to three weeks of therapy. Pneumococcal meningitis should be treated for not less than 14 days. The rare cases of brucella meningoencephalitis require therapy for a minimum of three weeks. Otherwise, antibiotics should be administered for 12 days or longer, depending on the clinical response and the results of certain laboratory examinations. Most children with meningitis due to the common organisms require isolation for only one or two days after therapy is begun. Neonates with gram-negative meningitis and children with tuberculous meningitis may warrant isolation precautions for longer periods.

The advisability of repeating the lumbar puncture to monitor the effectiveness of antibiotic therapy after the initial tap is a variable matter and depends on the age of the child, the causative organism and its sensitivities to antimicrobial agents, and the rate of clinical improvement. In early infancy, repeating the lumbar puncture after one or two days of therapy is indicated because other parameters of assessing improvement in this

Table 1–8. Antibiotics with Poor CSF Penetration

Aminoglycosides (Streptomycin, Gentamicin, etc.)
Erythromycin
Cephalosporins
Lincomycin
Clindamycin
Polymyxins (Colistin, Polymyxin B)

age group are not distinct. With meningitis caused by enterococcal group D *Streptococci,* repeat lumbar puncture should be done 24 to 48 hours after beginning therapy because of the variable degree of antibiotic sensitivity of these organisms. Older children with *Hemophilus influenzae* or meningococcal meningitis who show prompt, marked, and progressive improvement often need not have repeated lumbar punctures because one can be reasonably certain of the course of the illness from other areas of inquiry. There is no doubt that repeating the lumbar puncture during the course of treatment is sometimes necessary on the basis of lack of anticipated response or the appearance of unexpected symptoms or signs. However, the decision to re-tap should be dictated by the presence of reasonable indications from clinical and laboratory analysis.

Guidelines for discontinuation of antibiotic therapy have been proposed which have included a CSF examination with a white cell count below a certain number, such as 30 or 50 cells per cu. mm. If the CSF is examined after an adequate duration of therapy, one would expect less than 10 to 15 percent of the cells present to be polymorphonuclear leukocytes; however, it is not unusual for the total count to include well over 50 white cells per cu. mm. in children who have shown a rapid and marked clinical response. Jacob and Kaplan found that 50 percent of 38 children with bacterial meningitis had more than 50 white cells per cu. mm. at the end of therapy, while Chartrand and Cho reported that 62 percent of 21 children with *Hemophilus influenzae* meningitis still had more than 60 white cells per cu. mm. in the CSF when treatment was terminated. None experienced a relapse after discontinuation of antibiotics. The CSF glucose is sometimes still less than 40 mg. per 100 ml. at the end of adequate therapy and with a favorable clinical and bacteriologic response (Jacob and Kaplan). More appropriate guidelines for discontinuation of treatment include the rate and degree of improvement after initiation of treatment, knowledge of the causative organism and its sensitivities, the rapidity of sterilization of the CSF in the early stages of treatment, and the pattern of the temperature response along with the white blood cell count and its differential.

A problem commonly encountered during the course of antibiotic therapy is the occurrence of "secondary" fever. This is defined as the re-emergence of temperature to 38.8°C or higher at a point after the child has become afebrile for 24 hours or longer. "Secondary" fever was found in 28 percent of 88 children with bacterial meningitis described by Balagtas et al., and in 22 percent of 106 cases reported by Lipiridou et al. Relapse of fever in such cases most often occurs between three and six days after initiation of treatment. It can be due to one of many causes, but when the organism causing meningitis is sensitive to the antibiotic being used and the treatment regimen is appropriate, recurrence of fever is not usually explained by inadequate response of the meningeal infection (Balagtas et al.). Relapse of fever is often, however, an indication for re-examination of the CSF and reconsideration of the accuracy of the antibiotic sensitivity studies unless its source of origin is quickly identified. When fever persists longer than is expected or relapses after initial improvement, one should first check the accuracy of the patient's recorded body weight on which antibiotic doses are being calculated, recheck the calculations on which the dosage is determined, and finally ascertain for certain that the amount ordered is actually being administered.

The most common causes of recurrent fever include infection of IV or cutdown sites, pneumonitis, otitis, or an incidental viral illness with a short incubation period (Table 1–9). Drug fever has been described more often with ampicillin than with chloramphenicol, and becomes a more likely possibility if a rash appears with or soon after the temperature elevation. The occurrence of "secondary" fever requires repeated careful physical examinations with emphasis in certain areas. Bandages which obscure sites for intravenous infusions should be removed; observation of the ear canals and tympanic membranes should be accomplished, and a

Table 1–9. "Secondary"* Fever During Treatment of Meningitis: Most Common Identified Causes

Phlebitis (IV or cutdown site)
Pneumonitis, otitis, sinusitis, mastoiditis
Hospital-acquired viral infection
Drug fever
Septic arthritis, osteomyelitis
Pericarditis
Infected subdural effusions
Inadequate response to treatment of meningitis
Intracranial abscess

*Recurrence of fever to 38° C or 101° F after afebrile for 24 hours

search made for pain on passive motion of joints or erythema and swelling over joint surfaces. One should look for the presence of new focal signs on neurologic examination and determine the state of tenseness of the anterior fontanel. The blood count and urinalysis should be repeated, and possibly a chest x-ray obtained if fever remains unexplained. Persistence of fullness of the fontanel or abnormal transillumination of the head of the infant usually are indications for subdural taps to identify or exclude infected subdural effusions. When recurrent fever does not abate and is of significant degree, computed cranial tomography is considered, especially if the child has developed signs of increased intracranial pressure or focal neurologic signs.

When no cause for "secondary" fever can be found and the child has shown improvement otherwise, it is not advisable to alter the antibiotic regimen. Unexplained, persistent fever at the end of the treatment regimen is not a contraindication to discontinuation of antibiotic therapy when the child has otherwise done well. Careful observation should follow thereafter, until the temperature elevation has subsided.

Infants under two months of age with meningitis in which the cause is not yet determined are treated with ampicillin, 150 to 200 mg. per kilogram per day intravenously, plus gentamicin, 5 to 7.5 mg. per kilogram per day intramuscularly. The lower ampicillin dosage would be appropriate for the premature infant less than one week of age and in instances where there is significant compromise in renal function above and beyond what would be considered physiologic renal immaturity. When group B *Streptococcus* is proved to be the cause, the regimen consists of penicillin G, the minimum dose being 250,000 units per kilogram per day. Experience with group B *Streptococcus* meningitis in the newborn period has demonstrated that higher penicillin doses are required than for most other conditions in this age group. Current recommendations include penicillin G in a dosage of 300,000 to 400,000 units per kilogram per day in divided doses.

Because of the development of increased resistance of *Escherichia coli* to kanamycin, most authors now prefer gentamicin as the initial aminoglycoside of choice for neonatal, coliform infections (McCracken 1971). Studies by Nelson and McCracken (1972) have shown that therapeutic blood levels of gentamicin can be achieved by an intramuscular dose of 5 mg. per kilogram per day given every 12 hours during the first week of life. From one week until two months of age, the dose recommended for serious bacterial infections is 7.5 mg. per kilogram per day, administered every eight hours (McCracken 1972, McCracken and Nelson 1977). These authors have demonstrated that doses in the above range result in effective serum levels of 2.5 to 7.5 μg per ml., well below postulated ototoxic levels of approximately 12 μg per ml. Gentamicin can also be administered intravenously by constant infusion over 20 minutes and is given by this route when thrombocytopenia is present. Because gentamicin

Table 1–10. Antibiotic Dosages for Bacterial Meningitis (Birth to Two Months)

Ampicillin	150–200 mg./kilogram/day, IV
Penicillin G	
Less than one week	150,000 units/kilogram/day, IV
One week to two months	150,000–250,000 units/kilogram/day, IV
Group B Streptococcus	300,000–400,000 units/kilogram/day, IV
Methicillin	100 mg./kilogram/day, IV
Carbenicillin	400 mg./kilogram/day, IV
Kanamycin	
Less than one week	20 mg./kilogram/day, IM (q12h)
One week to two months	30 mg./kilogram/day, IM (q8h)
Gentamicin	
Less than one week	5 mg./kilogram/day, IM (q12h)
One week to two months	7.5 mg./kilogram/day, IM (q8h)
Tobramycin	
Less than one week	5 mg./kilogram/day, IM (q12h)
One week to two months	5 mg./kilogram/day, IM (q8h)
Amikacin	
Less than one week	15 mg./kilogram/day, IM (q12h)
One week to two months	22.5 mg./kilogram/day, IM (q8h)
Chloramphenicol	
Premature (birth to 1 month)	25 mg./kilogram/day, IV
Full term (1st 7 days)	25 mg./kilogram/day, IV
Full term (7 to 30 days)	50 mg./kilogram/day, IV
Full term (1 to 2 months)	50–100 mg./kilogram/day, IV
Intrathecal agents—administered daily or every second day	
Gentamicin	1–3 mg.
Amikacin	1–3 mg.
Methicillin	10–25 mg.
Erythromycin	3–10 mg.
Polymyxin B	1.0–2.5 mg. (10,000–25,000 units)

Table 1–11. Antibiotic Dosages for Bacterial Meningitis (Over 2 Months)

Ampicillin	300–400 mg./kilogram/day, IV (q4h)
Penicillin G	250,000 Units/kilogram/day, IV (q4h)
Methicillin	200–300 mg./kilogram/day, IV (q4h)
Nafcillin	200 mg./kilogram/day, IV (q4h)
Carbenicillin	400–600 mg./kilogram/day, IV (q4h)
Chloramphenicol	100 mg./kilogram/day, IV (q6h)
Tobramycin	4 mg./kilogram/day, IM (q8h)
Amikacin	15 mg./kilogram/day, IM (q8h)
Streptomycin	20–40 mg./kilogram/day, IM (not over 1 gram) (q12h)
Vancomycin	40–60 mg./kilogram/day, IV (q6h)
Tetracycline	20–50 mg./kilogram/day, IV (q8–12h)
Sulfadiazine	150 mg./kilogram/day, IV (q8h)
Metronidazole	30–40 mg./kilogram/day, po (q6–8h)

is inactivated in vitro by the penicillin preparations, the drugs should not be mixed together in the same IV bottle. Since the peak blood levels and half-life are approximately the same as equivalent doses given intramuscularly, there is little advantage to the intravenous route unless the child is thrombocytopenic. The optimal dosage schedule for gentamicin is arrived at by determination of peak and trough blood levels (Paisley et al.). Blood level determinations are important because of the individual variations in the metabolism of gentamicin and also because of the narrow ratio between therapeutic and toxic serum levels characteristic of this class of antibiotics.

When neonatal meningitis results from gram-negative rods that are resistant to gentamicin as well as to ampicillin, the alternative antimicrobial drugs include amikacin or chloramphenicol. Because of the danger of high serum levels of chloramphenicol in the young infant and because the dose:serum level relationship is not predictable, use of this drug in this age group requires the performance of serum level determinations so that therapeutic levels between 15 and 25 μg per ml. can be attained and to be certain that potentially toxic levels over 50 μg per ml. are avoided (Black et al.).

The major difficulty with treatment of gram-negative neonatal meningitis is that the sensitivity of gram-negative rods to ampicillin is not invariable, and that gentamicin, like other aminoglycosides, penetrates into the cerebrospinal fluid rather poorly with serum levels that can be safely achieved. For this reason, the cerebrospinal fluid should be re-examined 24 and 48 hours after initiation of therapy and, if still positive for bacteria, intraventricular gentamicin should then be considered, although the beneficial effect of

this method of therapy in the neonate has not been documented. Lumbar intrathecal therapy does not result in adequate concentration of the antibiotic within the ventricles (McCracken and Mize). For this reason, if this method of treatment is chosen, direct injection of the drug into the lateral ventricle is necessary (Lee et al., McCracken 1977); however, this may be difficult in the initial stages of the illness because of cerebral swelling, which reduces the size of the lateral ventricles.

All of the above factors account for the gloomy outlook for the child with gram-negative meningitis in the newborn period. Rapid eradication of enteric bacilli from the CSF seems not to occur with ampicillin, while the aminoglycosides penetrate poorly into the CSF when given systemically, and direct intraventricular injection is often difficult at a stage in the illness when the optimal effect is likely to be appreciated. In addition, the use of chloramphenicol alone as an alternative is less than adequate despite its excellent CSF penetrability because it is stated to be bacteriostatic against enteric bacilli in concentrations that can be safely achieved (Rahal and Simberkoff). The combination of chloramphenicol and gentamicin is ill-advised in that there is evidence that chloramphenicol inhibits the bactericidal action of gentamicin against gram-negative rods (Paisley and Washington, Strausbaugh and Sande). The most reasonable approach at the present time for the treatment of neonatal *Escherichia coli* meningitis is the combination of ampicillin and gentamicin in locations where chloramphenicol serum levels are not available. Should rapid improvement in the CSF findings not occur, cranial computed tomography should be performed to determine ventricular size, and intraventricular gentamicin should be added to the regimen if the ventricular capacity is adequate. In centers where accurate determinations of serum chloramphenicol levels can be performed, an alternate method of treatment of this illness is the combination of ampicillin and chloramphenicol, with both drugs given by the intravenous route.

In children older than two months of age, treatment is initiated with ampicillin intravenously in a dosage of 300 to 400 mg. per kilogram per day (not over 16 grams) in addition to chloramphenicol in a dosage of 100 mg. per kilogram per day (not over 6 grams). This combination is now recommended because of the recent emergence of ampicillin-resistant *Hemophilus influenzae*.

This dosage of ampicillin is considerably higher than that recommended by certain authors and beyond doubt is more than would be necessary to eradicate sensitive organisms from the cerebrospinal fluid in the majority of instances (Greene et al.). The increased expense of the higher dose regimen would seem to be of little consequence in the individual case in view of the potentially life-threatening character of bacterial meningitis. In addition, it has not been clearly documented that adverse effects are more frequent or greater with the higher doses than with the lower dose regimen, assuming that renal function is adequate. Among reported cases of *Hemophilus influenzae* meningitis with relapse during treatment that could not be attributed to ampicillin-resistant organisms, almost all received ampicillin in a dose of 200 mg. per kilogram per day or less (Coleman et al., Gold et al., Young et al.). It is possible, however, that this is only a reflection of the most common dosage chosen.

It is desirable to have a single dose recommendation which is both reasonably safe from the standpoint of adverse effects and reasonably adequate under varying circumstances. Since a significant percentage of children with meningitis are managed by physicians in practice with different degrees of experience with this disease, it is not realistic to assume that all will recall all of the complex details regarding such factors as the poor stability of ampicillin in certain solutions or the brief half-life of the drug. The larger dosage of 300 to 400 mg. per kilogram per day, while still safe, provides a buffer which helps assure adequacy of therapy when certain other aspects of the regimen are necessarily a bit less than the optimal standards of the specialist in infectious disease. It is the authors' opinion that it is acceptable to somewhat overtreat the majority, assuming that the higher dose does not significantly add to side effects, if the higher dose has the possibility of being more effective even very infrequently for the child with bacterial meningitis.

Because of the instability of ampicillin in solution and its short half-life, it should be given by rapid intravenous infusion over 20 minutes every four hours. If the organism is shown to be ampicillin-sensitive *Hemophilus influenzae*, chloramphenicol is discontinued. If *Streptococcus pneumoniae* or *Neisseria meningitidis* is identified as the cause of meningitis, ampicillin is adequate but penicillin G is preferable. Chloramphenicol is the second choice with any of these infections when the penicillins cannot be used because of drug allergy. Of the rare cases of acute meningitis caused by group A *Streptococcus (Streptococcus pyogenes)* or *Streptococcus viridans,* penicillin G is the drug of choice, as these organisms are highly penicillin-sensitive. Among group D Streptococci, non-enterococcal strains *(Streptococcus bovis)* are usually penicillin-sensitive, while the antibiotic sensitivity of the enterococcal group is more variable.

In vitro sensitivity studies must be used for selection of antibiotic treatment of enterococcal meningitis, which usually includes ampicillin in combination with an aminoglycoside. If clinical and CSF improvement is not rapid, intrathecal gentamicin should be considered (Bayer et al.). In patients allergic to penicillin, a combination of vancomycin and gentamicin can be used. Enterococci are not usually highly sensitive to vancomycin (Geraci), and if this regimen is chosen, gentamicin should probably be given intrathecally. Vancomycin administered intrathecally in combination with oral rifampin has been successfully used for the treatment of enterococcal meningitis (Ryan et al.), although there is little available information regarding the intrathecal use of vancomycin.

Meningitis developing in a child known to have a ventricular shunt is managed differently because of the greater possibility of penicillinase-producing staphylococcal infection. A combination of ampicillin and methicillin or other antistaphylococcal penicillinase-resistant drugs is recommended until the organism is identified. When methicillin-resistant *Staphylococcus* species are encountered, one must depend on in vitro sensitivity studies to determine the best alternate drug. Rifampin in combination with gentamicin has been effective in such instances; the latter drug is given both systemically and by intraventricular injection (Archer et al.). Vancomycin has an important role in such cases, and achieves adequate CSF concentrations according to some authors (Cook and Farrar, Hawley and Gump), although this has been questioned by others. Its primary side effects are ototoxicity and nephrotoxicity, and it must be used with caution in patients with renal insufficiency. The dosage of vancomycin is adjusted to achieve peak serum levels in the therapeutic and safe range of 25 to 40 μg per ml. (Schaad et al.). To avoid phlebitis, the drug is administered intravenously over a period of 60 minutes every six hours. Sepsis and meningitis in children with intravascular shunts are difficult to overcome, and in most cases, removal of the prosthesis is necessary in addition to intensive antibiotic therapy (Shurtleff et al.).

Treatment of *Escherichia coli* or *Klebsiella* species meningitis in the older person secondary to head trauma, neurosurgical procedures, or other predisposing diseases is determined by the results of sensitivity testing. Chloramphenicol administered intravenously in addition to gentamicin given intraventricularly is the most satisfactory initial approach (Kaiser and McGee, Mangi et al.). Combined antibiotic therapy is important because of the possible occurrence of acquired resistance of these organisms to chloramphenicol during treatment (Kaiser and McGee). When *Klebsiella* species are resistant to gentamicin, amikacin is the preferred alternative in most instances. Amikacin is most effectively used when peak and trough serum levels are determined, with the desirable peak serum concentration being 15 to 20 μg per ml. (Cleary et al.).

Ampicillin is the drug of choice for *Proteus mirabilis* meningitis but other, indole-positive *Proteus* species, including *Proteus morganii, Proteus vulgaris,* and *Proteus rettgeri,* are usually resistant to this antibiotic. Carbenicillin and gentamicin are usually given in combination for indole-positive *Proteus* infections (Ross et al.).

Invasive *Salmonella* species infections are treated with ampicillin or chloramphenicol, depending on the age of the child and the results of sensitivity testing.

Pseudomonas species meningitis usually requires combined therapy with carbenicillin and gentamicin or tobramycin, with the aminoglycoside often given by intrathecal injection (Moellering and Fischer).

Anaerobic bacteria are not common causes of meningitis in children but are notable among the microflora isolated from brain abscesses. The majority of anaerobic organisms are sensitive to penicillin or chloramphenicol, but in certain instances, their occurrence requires the use of antimicrobials uncommonly used in the treatment of meningitis. For example, *Flavobacterium meningosepticum* is a gram-negative anaerobe which is usually highly resistant to the aminoglycosides and the penicillins, but is often sensitive to rifampin, vancomycin, and erythromycin (Aber et al., Rios et al.). Rifampin given orally adequately gains entrance into the CSF. Erythromycin administered systemically penetrates CSF poorly and its use for meningitis probably requires intraventricular injection (Maderazo et al.). Because of the possible development of resistance of the organism to erythromycin during the course of therapy, either both drugs should be used or frequent monitoring of the minimum inhibitory concentration against the organism should be accomplished (Rios et al.). *Bacteroides* is a difficult organism to eradicate from the CSF even though it is usually susceptible to chloramphenicol. Metronidazole has been found to be effective in vitro against most anaerobic bacteria and penetrates well into the CSF (Ralph et al.). It has been used successfully in the treatment of *Bacteroides* meningitis and shows promise as an important drug for this category of infection (Berman et al., Feldman).

Treatment of tuberculous meningitis in past years usually included isoniazid, streptomycin, and para-aminosalicylic acid. Isoniazid was, and remains, the mainstay of therapy because of its excellent penetration into the CSF as well as its relative safety. Para-aminosalicylic acid has largely been abandoned from the treatment regimen because of its relatively low antituberculous activity, its lack of ability to gain entrance into the CSF, and the intolerance to the drug exhibited by certain patients (Fallon). The current combination of drugs commonly recommended for treatment of tuberculous meningitis includes isoniazid in dosage of 20 mg. per kilogram per day orally (up to 500 mg. per day), streptomycin, 20 mg. per kilogram per day IM (up to one gram per day), and rifampin, 15 mg. per kilogram per day orally (up to 600 mg. per day). Streptomycin and rifampin are continued for approximately eight weeks after there is clinical and laboratory improvement, and isoniazid is thereafter continued for an additional 18 to 24 months.

Rifampin has been shown to be a highly effective antituberculous drug, which is well absorbed from the gastrointestinal tract and has adequate penetration into the CSF. The CSF concentration in the acute stage of the illness is approximately 20 percent of the serum concentration, which represents the fraction of the drug in serum that is not protein-bound (D'Oliveira). Possible side effects include rash, hepatitis, hemolytic anemia, and diarrhea. So-called "second line" antituberculous drugs, including ethambutol and ethionamide, are a consideration in cases in which isoniazid-resistant organisms are encountered (Bonforte et al.). Both drugs are available only in oral preparations, and either will enter the CSF adequately in the acute stage of the illness. Ethambutol has relatively low antituberculous activity and can cause acute optic nerve toxicity. Ethionamide is an unpalatable drug and also is beset with problems with toxicity. For these reasons, both ethambutol and ethionamide are reserved for the unusual occurrence in which tuberculous meningitis is caused by isoniazid-resistant organisms.

The value of corticosteroids in the treatment of tuberculous meningitis has been debated for years and remains unsettled. Some have suggested that steroid therapy reduces the inflammatory reaction, thereby decreasing the probability of development of hydrocephalus. Others have provided evidence that the mortality is similar with or without steroid therapy but that sequelae among survivors is higher in those who received corticosteroids. In view of our present concepts of the pathogenesis of the disorder, it would not seem advisable to include corticosteroids as part of the routine treatment of tuberculous meningitis. Corticosteroid therapy would seem logical in cases with rather acute onset in which there is rapid deterioration of the state of responsiveness. Experimental and clinical observations support the concept that brain swelling in such cases can represent a cerebral reaction to tuberculoprotein, and that such response might be inhibited by corticosteroid therapy (Dastur and Udani, Feldman et al.). When used in this fashion, steroid therapy should be relatively brief in duration and the drug should be stopped when improvement occurs.

REFERENCES

Aber, R. C., Wennersten, C., and Moellering, R. C., Jr.: Antimicrobial susceptibility of Flavobacteria. Antimicrob. Agents Chemother. 14:483–487, 1978.

Abramsky, O.: Neurological features as presenting manifestations of brucellosis. Eur. Neurol. 15:281–284, 1977.

Adair, C. V., Gauld, R. L., and Smadel, J. E.: Aseptic meningitis, a disease of diverse etiology: Clinical and etiologic studies on 854 cases. Ann. Intern. Med. 39:675–704, 1953.

Adams, R. D., Fisher, C. M., Hakim, S., Ojemann, R. G., and Sweet, W. H.: Symptomatic occult hydrocephalus with "normal" cerebrospinal fluid pressure. New Eng. J. Med. 273:117–126, 1965.

Adams, R. D., Kubik, C. S., and Bonner, F. J.: The clinical and pathological aspects of influenzal meningitis. Arch. Pediat. 65:354–376, 408–441, 1948.

Adler, J. L., Shulman, J. A., Terry, P. M., Feldman, D. B., and Skalsy, P.: Nosocomial colonization with kanamycin-resistant Klebsiella pneumoniae, types 2 and 11, in a premature nursery. J. Pediat. 77:376–385, 1970.

Agass, M. J. B., Willoughby, C. P., Bron, A. J., Mitchell, C. J., and Mayon-White, R. T.: Meningitis and endophthalmitis caused by Streptococcus suis type II (group R). Brit. Med. J. 2:167–168, 1977.

Aguilar, J. A., and Elvidge, A. R.: Intervertebral disk disease caused by the Brucella organism. J. Neurosurg. 18:27–33, 1961.

Ahlfors, C. E., Goetzman, B. W., Halsted, C. C., Sherman, M. P., and Wennberg, R. P.: Neonatal listeriosis. Am. J. Dis. Child. 131:405–408, 1977.

Ahronheim, G. A., Reich, B., and Marks, M. I.: Penicillin-insensitive pneumococci. Case report and review. Am. J. Dis. Child. 133:187–191, 1979.

Albritton, W. L., Wiggins, G. L., and Feeley, J. C.: Neonatal listeriosis: Distribution of serotypes in relation to age at onset of disease. J. Pediat. 88:481–483, 1976.

Alexander, J. B., and Giacoia, G. P.: Early onset non-enterococcal group D streptococcal infection of the newborn infant. J. Pediat. 93:489–490, 1978.

Anderson, D. C., Greenwood, R., Fishman, M., and Kagan, I. G.: Acute infantile hemiplegia with cerebrospinal fluid eosinophilic pleocytosis: An unusual case of visceral larva migrans. J. Pediat. 86:247–249, 1975.

Ansari, A., Lipsey, A., and Nachum, R.: Cerebrospinal fluid muramidase levels in meningitis. J. Pediat. 94:752–755, 1979.

Antley, R. M., and McMillan, C. W.: Sequential coagulation studies in purpura fulminans. New Eng. J. Med. 276:1287–1290, 1967.

Archer, G. L., Tenenbaum, M. J., and Haywood, H. B., III.: Rifampin therapy of Staphylococcus epidermidis. Use in infections from indwelling artificial devices. J.A.M.A. 240:751–753, 1978.

Askin, J. A., and Zimmerman, H. M.: Encephalitis accompanying whooping cough. Clinical history and report of postmortem examination. Am. J. Dis. Child. 38:97–102, 1929.

Ayer, J. B.: Puncture of the cisterna magna. Report on one thousand nine hundred and eighty-five punctures. J.A.M.A. 81:358–360, 1923.

Bachman, D. S.: Hemophilus meningitis: Comparison of H. influenzae and H. parainfluenzae. Pediatrics 55:526–530, 1975.

Baehner, R. L., and Nathan, D. C.: Quantitative nitroblue tetrazolium test in chronic granulomatous disease. New Eng. J. Med. 278:971–976, 1968.

Baker, C. J., Barrett, F. F., Gordon, R. C., and Yow, M. D.: Suppurative meningitis due to streptococci of Lancefield group B: A study of 33 infants. J. Pediat. 82:724–729, 1973.

Balagtas, R. C., Levin, S., Nelson, K. E., and Gotoff, S. P.: Secondary and prolonged fevers in bacterial meningitis. J. Pediat. 77:957–964, 1970.

Barclay, N.: High frequency of salmonella species as a cause of neonatal meningitis in Ibadan, Nigeria. Acta Pediat. Scand. 60:540–544, 1971.

Barrett-Connor, E.: Bacterial infection and sickle cell anemia. An analysis of 250 infections in 166 patients and a review of the literature. Medicine 50:97–112, 1971.

Barron, M.: Meningitis in the newborn and in early infancy. Am. J. Med. Sci. 156:358–369, 1918.

Barton, L. L., Feigin, R. D., and Lins, R.: Group B beta hemolytic streptococcal meningitis in infants. J. Pediat. 82:719–723, 1973.

Bates, H. A., Controni, G., Elliott, N., and Eitzman, D.

V.: Septicemia and meningitis in a newborn due to *Pasteurella multocida*. Clin. Pediat. 4:668–670, 1965.

Bauer, C. H., New, M. I., and Miller, J. M.: Cerebrospinal fluid protein values of premature infants. J. Pediat. 66:1017–1022, 1965.

Bayer, A. S., Chow, A. W., Anthony, B. F., and Guze, L. B.: Serious infections in adults due to group B streptococci. Clinical and serotypic characterization. Am. J. Med. 61:498–503, 1976.

Bayer, A. S., Seidel, J. S., Yoshikawa, T. T., Anthony, B. F., and Guze, L. B.: Group D enterococcal meningitis. Clinical and therapeutic considerations with report of three cases and review of the literature. Arch. Intern. Med. 136:883–886, 1976.

Beaty, H. N., and Oppenheimer, S.: Cerebrospinal-fluid lactic dehydrogenase and its isoenzymes in infections of the central nervous system. New Eng. J. Med. 279:1197–1202, 1968.

Becker, A. H.: Infection due to Proteus mirabilis in newborn nursery. Am. J. Dis. Child. 104:355–359, 1962.

Beisel, W. R., Sawyer, W. D., Ryll, E. D., and Crozier, D.: Metabolic studies in human subjects during intracellular infections. Ann. Intern. Med. 67:744–779, 1967.

Belsey, M. A.: CSF glutamic oxaloacetic transaminase in acute bacterial meningitis. Am. J. Dis. Child. 117:288–293, 1969.

Belsey, M. A., Hoffauir, C. W., and Smith, M. H. D.: Dexamethasone in the treatment of acute bacterial meningitis: The effect of study design on the interpretation of results. Pediatrics 44:503–513, 1969.

Berg, J. M.: Neurological sequelae of pertussis with particular reference to mental defect. Arch. Dis. Childh. 34:322–324, 1959.

Berman, B. W., King, F. H., Jr., Rubenstein, D. S., and Long, S. S.: Bacteroides fragilis meningitis in a neonate successfully treated with metronidazole. J. Pediat. 93:793–795, 1978.

Berman, N. S., Siegel, S. E., Nachum, R., Lipsey, A., and Leedom, J.: Cerebrospinal fluid endotoxin concentrations in gram-negative bacterial meningitis. J. Pediat. 88:553–556, 1976.

Berman, P. H., and Banker, B. Q.: Neonatal meningitis: A clinical and pathological study of 29 cases. Pediatrics 38:6–24, 1966.

Bernstein, J. G., Slater, L., and Serpick, A. A.: Klebsiella meningitis without pleocytosis. Lancet 2:111–112, 1968.

Bhave, S. A., Guy, L. M., and Rycroft, J. A.: Pasteurella multocida meningitis in an infant with recovery. Brit. Med. J. 2:741–742, 1977.

Bickerstaff, E. R., Small, J. M., and Woolf, A. L.: Cysticercosis of the posterior fossa. Brain 79:622–634, 1956.

Biggers, W. P., Howell, N. N., Fischer, N. D., and Himadi, G. M.: Congenital ear anomalies associated with otic meningitis. Arch. Otolaryngol. 97:399–401, 1973.

Black, S. B., Levine, P., and Shinefield, H. R.: The necessity for monitoring chloramphenicol levels when treating neonatal meningitis. J. Pediat. 92:235–236, 1978.

Bland, R. D., Lister, R. C., and Ries, J. P.: Cerebrospinal fluid lactic acid level and pH in meningitis. Aids in differential diagnosis. Am. J. Dis. Child. 128:151–156, 1974.

Bonforte, R. J., Karpas, C. M., Gribetz, I., and Shanzer, S.: Tuberculous meningitis due to primary drug-resistant *Mycobacterium tuberculosis* hominis. Pediatrics 42:969–975, 1968.

Bortolussi, R., Thompson, T. R., and Ferrieri, P.: Early-onset pneumococcal sepsis in newborn infants. Pediatrics 60:352–355, 1977.

Boughton, C. R.: Brucella meningoencephalitis. Med. J. Aust. 2:993–995, 1966.

Bouhasin, J. D.: Purpura fulminans. Pediatrics 34:264–270, 1964.

Boutros, A., Hoyt, J., Menezes, A., and Bell, W.: Management of Reye's syndrome. A rational approach to a complex problem. Critical Care Medicine 5:234–238, 1977.

Brachman, P. S.: Anthrax. *In:* Hoeprich, P. D.: Infectious Diseases. Harper and Row, Hagerstown, Md. 1972, pages 757–762.

Bradford, W. E., and Kelly, H. W.: Gonococci meningitis in a newborn infant. Am. J. Dis. Child. 46:543–549, 1933.

Bresnan, M. J.: Bacterial meningitis. IV. Neurological aspects. Their diagnosis and treatment. Pediatrics 52:594–597, 1973.

Bretz, G., and Mauer, A. M.: Glucose consumption by polymorphonuclear leukocytes in the cerebrospinal fluid of patients with bacterial meningitis. J. Pediat. 70:767–771, 1967.

Brice, J. L., Tornabene, T. G., and LaForce, F. M.: Diagnosis of bacterial meningitis by gas-liquid chromatography. I. Chemotyping studies of *Streptococcus pneumoniae, Haemophilus influenzae, Neisseria meningitidis, Staphylococcus aureus*, and *Escherichia coli*. J. Infect. Dis. 140:443–452, 1979.

Brisman, R., Hughes, J. E. O., and Mount, L. A.: Cerebrospinal fluid rhinorrhea. Arch. Neurol. 22:245–252, 1970.

Brook, I., and Finegold, S. M.: Bacteriology of chronic otitis media. J.A.M.A. 241:487–488, 1979.

Brook, I., Bricknell, K. S., Overturf, G. D., and Finegold, S. M.: Measurement of lactic acid in cerebrospinal fluid of patients with infections of the central nervous system. J. Infect. Dis. 137:384–389, 1978.

Brown, J. H.: The use of blood agar for the study of streptococci. The Rockefeller Institute for Medical Research. Monograph #9, 1919, New York.

Brown, L. B., and Nelson, A. R.: Postinfectious intravascular thrombosis with gangrene. Arch. Surg. 94:652–656, 1967.

Brudzinski, J.: Un signe nouveau sur les membres inferieurs dans les meningites chez les enfants (signe de la nuque). Arch. Med. 12:745–752, 1909.

Bryce-Smith, R., and MacIntosh, R. R.: Sixth-nerve palsy after lumbar puncture and spinal analgesia. Brit. Med. J. 1:275–276, 1951.

Buchan, G. C., and Alvord, E. C., Jr.: Diffuse necrosis of subcortical white matter associated with bacterial meningitis. Neurology 19:1–9, 1969.

Buchanan, T. M., Farber, L. C., and Feldman, R. A.: Brucellosis in the United States, 1960–1972. An abattoir-associated disease. Part I. Clinical features and therapy. Medicine 53:403–413, 1974.

Buchanan, T. M., Hendricks, S. L., Patton, C. M., and Feldman, R. A.: Brucellosis in the United States, 1960–1972. An abattoir-associated disease. Part III. Epidemiology and evidence for acquired immunity. Medicine 53:427–439, 1974.

Buchanan, T. M., Sulzer, C. R., Frix, M. K., and Feldman, R. A.: Brucellosis in the United States, 1960–1972. An abattoir-associated disease. Part II. Diagnostic aspects. Medicine 53:415–425, 1974.

Buchino, J. J., Ciambarella, E., and Light, I.: Systemic group D streptococcal infection in newborn infants. Am. J. Dis. Child. 133:270–273, 1979.

Buchner, L. H., and Schneierson, S. S.: Clinical and laboratory aspects of Listeria monocytogenes infections. With a report of ten cases. Am. J. Med. 45:904–921, 1968.

Bulger, R. J., Schrier, R. W., Arend, W. P., and Swanson, A. G.: Spinal fluid acidosis and the diagnosis of pulmonary encephalopathy. New Eng. J. Med. 274:433–437, 1966.

Burech, D. L., Koranyi, K. I., and Haynes, R. E.: Serious group A streptococcal diseases in children. J. Pediat. 88:972–974, 1976.

Burgert, W., Jr., and Hagstrom, J. W. C.: Vibrio fetus meningoencephalitis. Arch. Neurol. 10:196–199, 1964.

Burn, C. G.: Clinical and pathological features of an infection caused by a new pathogen of the genus Listerella. Am. J. Path. 12:341–348, 1936.

Byers, R. K., and Moll, F. C.: Encephalopathies following prophylactic pertussis vaccine. Pediatrics 1:437–457, 1948.

Cabrera, H. A., and Davis, G. H.: Epidemic meningitis of the newborn caused by Flavobacteria. I. Epidemiology and bacteriology. Am. J. Dis. Child. 101:289–295, 1961.

Cairns, H., and Russell, D. S.: Cerebral arteritis and phlebitis in pneumococcal meningitis. J. Path. Bact. 58:649–665, 1946.

Carpenter, R. R., and Petersdorf, R. G.: The clinical spectrum of bacterial meningitis. Am. J. Med. 33:262–275, 1962.

Carter, B. L., Wolpert, S. M., and Karmody, C. S.: Recurrent meningitis associated with an anomaly of the inner ear. Neuroradiology 9:55–61, 1975.

Chandler, B. D., Kapoor, N., Barker, B. E., Boyle, R. J., and Oh, W.: Nitroblue tetrazolium test in neonates. J. Pediat. 92:638–640, 1978.

Char, D. F. B., and Rosen, L.: Eosinophilic meningitis among children in Hawaii. J. Pediat. 70:28–35, 1967.

Chartrand, S. A., and Cho, C. T.: Persistent pleocytosis in bacterial meningitis. J. Pediat. 88:424–426, 1976.

Chesney, P. J., Katcher, M. L., Nelson, D. B., and Horowitz, S. D.: CSF eosinophilia and chronic lymphocytic choriomeningitis virus meningitis. J. Pediat. 94:750–752, 1979.

Choi, H-S., H., and Anderson, P. J.: Diagnostic cytology of cerebrospinal fluid by the cytocentrifuge method. Am. J. Clin. Path. 72:931–943, 1979.

Cleary, T. G., Pickering, L. K., Kramer, W. G., Culbert, S., Frankel, L. S., and Kohl, S.: Amikacin pharmacokinetics in pediatric patients with malignancy. Antimicrob. Agents Chemotherap. 16:829–832, 1979.

Cockrill, H. H., Jr., Dreisbach, J., Lowe, B., and Yamauchi, T.: Computed tomography in leptomeningeal infections. Am. J. Roentgenol. 130:511–515, 1978.

Coleman, S. J., Auld, E. B., Connor, J. D., Rosenman, S. B., and Warren, G. H.: Relapse of Hemophilus influenzae type b meningitis during intravenous therapy with ampicillin. J. Pediat. 74:781–784, 1969.

Controni, G., and Jones, R. S.: Pasteurella meningitis. A review of the literature. Am. J. Med. Tech. 33:379–386, 1967.

Controni, G., Rodriquez, W. J., Hicks, J. M., Ficke, M., Ross, S., Friedman, G., and Khan, W.: Cerebrospinal fluid lactic acid levels in meningitis. J. Pediat. 91:379–384, 1977.

Converse, G. M., Gwaltney, J. M., Jr., Strassburg, D. A., and Hendley, J. O.: Alteration of cerebrospinal fluid findings by partial treatment of bacterial meningitis. J. Pediat. 83:220–225, 1973.

Cook, F. V., and Farrar, W. E.: Vancomycin revisited. Ann. Intern. Med. 88:813–818, 1978.

Cooke, R. W. I.: *Bacteroides fragilis* septicaemia and meningitis in early infancy. Arch. Dis. Childh. 50:241–244, 1975.

Coonrod, J. D., and Rytel, M. W.: Determination of etiology of bacterial meningitis by countercurrent immunoelectrophoresis. Lancet 1:1154–1157, 1972.

Cooper, A., Martin, R., and Tibbles, J. A. R.: Pasteurella meningitis. Neurology 23:1097–1100, 1973.

Crane, L. R., and Lerner, A. M.: Non-traumatic gram-negative bacillary meningitis in the Detroit Medical Center, 1964–1974 (With special mention of cases due to *Escherichia coli*). Medicine 57:197–209, 1978.

Crocker, E. F., and Leicester, J.: Cerebral abscess due to Listeria monocytogenes. Med. J. Aust. 1:90–92, 1976.

Cussen, L. J., and Ryan, G. B.: Hemorrhagic cerebral necrosis in neonatal infants with enterobacterial meningitis. J. Pediat. 71:771–776, 1967.

Cutler, R. W. P., Page, L., Galicich, J., and Watters, C. V.: Formation and absorption of cerebrospinal fluid in man. Brain 91:707–720, 1968.

Dalton, H. P., and Allison, M. J.: Modification of laboratory results by partial treatment of bacterial meningitis. Am. J. Clin. Path. 49:410–413, 1968.

Daly, A. K., Postic, B., and Kass, E. H.: Infections due to organisms of the genus Herellea. Arch. Intern. Med. 110:580–591, 1962.

Dastur, D. K., and Udani, P. M.: The pathology and pathogenesis of tuberculous encephalopathy. Acta Neuropath. 6:311–326, 1966.

Davis, S. D., Hill, H. R., Feigl, P., and Arnstein, E. J.: Partial antibiotic therapy in *Haemophilus influenzae* meningitis. Its effect on cerebrospinal fluid abnormalities. Am. J. Dis. Child. 129:802–807, 1975.

DeBono, J. E.: Brucellosis simulating acute anterior poliomyelitis. Lancet 1:1132–1133, 1964.

DeFuccio, C. P., and Dresner, E. E.: Meningococcemia with meningitis accompanied by bilateral gangrene of the lower extremities (Waterhouse-Friderichsen syndrome). Pediatrics 3:837–838, 1949.

deLemos, R. A., and Haggerty, R. J.: Corticosteroids as an adjunct to treatment in bacterial meningitis. Pediatrics 44:30–34, 1969.

Denis, F. A., Chiron, J. P., and Cadoz, M.: Meningitis caused by *Hemophilus influenzae* type C. J. Pediat. 93:1064–1065, 1978.

Deonna, T., Calame, A., van Melle, G., and Prod'hom, L-S.: Hypoglycorrhachia in neonatal intracranial hemorrhage. Helv. Paediat. Acta. 32:351–361, 1977.

Dillon, H. C.: Group A type 12 streptococcal infection in a newborn nursery. Successfully treated neonatal meningitis. Am. J. Dis. Child. 112:177–184, 1966.

Dixon, W., and Halliburton, W.: The cerebrospinal fluid: I. Secretion of the fluid. J. Physiol. 67:215–242, 1913.

Dolgopol, V. B.: Changes in the brain in pertussis with convulsions. Arch. Neurol. Psychiat. 46:477–503, 1941.

D'Oliveira, J. J. G.: Cerebrospinal fluid concentrations of rifampin in meningeal tuberculosis. Am. Rev. Respir. Dis. 106:432–437, 1972.

Donald, W. D., and Doak, W. B.: Mineae meningitis and sepsis. J.A.M.A. 200:287–289, 1967.

Dorff, G. J., Feimer, N. F., Rosenthal, D. R., and Rytel, M. W.: Pseudomonas septicemia. Illustrated evolution of its skin lesion. Arch. Intern. Med. 128:591–595, 1971.

Drayer, B. P., Wilkins, R. H., Boehnke, M., Horton, J.

A., and Rosenbaum, A. E.: Cerebrospinal fluid rhinorrhea demonstrated by metrizamide CT cisternography. Am. J. Roentgenol. 129:149–151, 1977.

Ducker, T. B., and Simmons, R. L.: The pathogenesis of meningitis. Systemic effects of meningococcal endotoxin within the cerebrospinal fluid. Arch. Neurol. 18:123–128, 1968.

Duffy, P. E., Sassin, J. F., Summers, D. S., and Lourie, H.: Rhomboencephalitis due to *Listeria monocytogenes.* Neurology 14:1067–1072, 1964.

Duma, R. J., Weinberg, A. N., Medrek, T. F., and Kunz, L. J.: Streptococcal infections. A bacteriologic and clinical study of streptococcal bacteremia. Medicine 48:87–127, 1969.

Dunkle, L. M., Brotherton, M. S., and Feigin, R. D.: Anaerobic infections in children: A prospective study. Pediatrics 57:311–320, 1976.

Dunn, C. H.: Cerebrospinal meningitis, its etiology, diagnosis, prognosis and treatment. Am. J. Dis. Child. 1:95–112, 1911.

Dyken, P. R.: Cerebrospinal fluid cytology: Practical clinical usefulness. Neurology 25:210–217, 1975.

Dykes, A., Baraff, L. J., and Herzog, P.: Listeria brain abscess in an immunosuppressed child. J. Pediat. 94:72–74, 1979.

Dyson, D., and Cassady, G.: Use of Limulus lysate for detecting gram-negative neonatal meningitis. Pediatrics 58:105–109, 1976.

Eden, A. N.: Vibrio fetus meningitis in a newborn infant. J. Pediat. 61:33–38, 1962.

Eden, A. N.: Perinatal mortality caused by Vibrio fetus. Review and analysis. J. Pediat. 68:297–304, 1966.

Edwards, M. S., and Baker, C. J.: Prospective diagnosis of early onset group B streptococcal infection by countercurrent immunoelectrophoresis. J. Pediat. 94:286–288, 1979.

Edwards, M. S., Kasper, D. L., and Baker, C. J.: Rapid diagnosis of type III group B streptococcal meningitis by latex particle agglutination. J. Pediat. 95:202–205, 1979.

Elin, R. J., Robinson, R. A., Levine, A. S., and Wolff, S. M.: Lack of clinical usefulness of the Limulus test in the diagnosis of endotoxemia. New Eng. J. Med. 293:521–524, 1975.

Evans, R. J. C., and McElwain, T. J.: Eosinophilic meningitis in Hodgkin's disease. Brit. J. Clin. Pract. 23:382–384, 1969.

Fallon, R. J.: The treatment of tuberculous meningitis. J. Antimicrob. Chemother. 4:1–2, 1978.

Feeley, E. J., and Kriz, J. J.: Plague meningitis in an American serviceman. J.A.M.A. 191:412–413, 1965.

Feigin, R. D., Joaquin, V. S., and Middelkamp, J. N.: Purpura fulminans associated with *Neisseria catarrhalis* septicemia and meningitis. Pediatrics 44:120–123, 1969.

Feigin, R. D., Wong, M., Shackelford, P. G., Stechenberg, B. W., Dunkle, L. M., and Kaplan, S.: Countercurrent immunoelectrophoresis of urine as well as of CSF and blood for diagnosis of bacterial meningitis. J. Pediat. 89:773–775, 1976.

Feigin, R. D., Stechenberg, B. W., Chang, M. J., Dunkle, L. M., Wong, M. L., Palkes, H., Dodge, P. R., and Davis, H.: Prospective evaluation of treatment of *Hemophilus influenzae* meningitis. J. Pediat. 88:542–548, 1976.

Feldman, S., Behar, A. J., and Weber, D.: Experimental tuberculous meningitis in rabbits. II. Effect of hydrocortisone on the hypersensitivity reaction of the meninges. Arch. Neurol. 3:420–424, 1960.

Feldman, S., and Pearson, T. A.: The *Limulus* test and

Gram-negative bacillary sepsis. Am. J. Dis. Child. 128:172–174, 1974.

Feldman, W. E.: Cerebrospinal fluid lactic acid dehydrogenase activity. Levels in untreated and partially antibiotic-treated meningitis. Am. J. Dis. Child. 129:77–80, 1975.

Feldman, W. E.: *Bacteroides fragilis* ventriculitis and meningitis. Report of two cases. Am. J. Dis. Child. 130:880–883, 1976.

Feldman, W. E.: Effect of prior antibiotic therapy on concentrations of bacteria in CSF. Am. J. Dis. Child. 132:672–674, 1978.

Felner, J. M., and Dowell, V. R., Jr.: "Bacteroides" bacteremia. Am. J. Med. 50:787–796, 1971.

Ferguson, I. R., and Tearle, P. V.: Gas liquid chromatography in the rapid diagnosis of meningitis. J. Clin. Path. 30:1163–1167, 1977.

Fikrig, S. M., Berkovich, S., Emmett, S. M., and Fordon, C.: Nitroblue tetrazolium dye test and differential diagnosis of meningitis. J. Pediat. 82:855–857, 1973.

Fincham, R. W., Sahs, A. L., and Joynt, R. J.: Protean manifestations of nervous system brucellosis. J.A.M.A. 184:269–275, 1963.

Fischer, G. W., Brenz, R. W., Alden, E. R., and Beckwith, J. B.: Lumbar punctures and meningitis. Am. J. Dis. Child. 129:590–592, 1975.

Fishbein, R. H.: Purpura fulminans: An analysis of the lesion and its treatment. J. Pediat. Surg. 4:320–329, 1969.

Fisher, V. J., and Christianson, L. C.: Cerebrospinal fluid acid-base balance during changing ventilatory state in man. J. Appl. Physiol. 18:712–716, 1963.

Fishman, R. A.: Carrier transport and the concentration of glucose in cerebrospinal fluid in meningeal disease. Ann. Intern. Med. 63:153–155, 1965.

Fishman, R. A., Sligar, K., and Hake, R. B.: Effects of leukocytes on brain metabolism in granulocytic brain edema. Ann. Neurol. 2:89–94, 1977.

Floyd, R. F., Federspiel, C. F., and Schaffner, W.: Bacterial meningitis in urban and rural Tennessee. Am. J. Epidemiol. 99:395–407, 1974.

Ford, F. F.: Degeneration of the cerebral cortex in the course of pertussis. Resume of the literature and report of a case with anatomic observations. Am. J. Dis. Child. 37:1046–1050, 1929.

Ford, P. M., Herzberg, L., and Ford, S. E.: Listeria monocytogenes: Six cases affecting the central nervous system. Quart. J. Med. 37:281–290, 1968.

Fossieck, B., Jr., Craig, R., and Paterson, P. Y.: Counterimmunoelectrophoresis for rapid diagnosis of meningitis due to *Diplococcus pneumoniae.* J. Infect. Dis. 127:106–109, 1973.

Fothergill, L. D., and Sweet, L. K.: Meningitis in infants and children with special reference to age-incidence and bacteriologic diagnosis. J. Pediat. 2:696–710, 1933.

French, R. S., Ziter, F. A., Spruance, S. L., and Smith, C. B.: Chronic meningitis caused by Propionibacterium acnes. A potentially important clinical entity. Neurology 24:624–628, 1974.

Frothingham, T. H.: Echo virus type 9 associated with three cases simulating meningococcemia. New Eng. J. Med. 259:484–485, 1958.

Frutos, A. A., Levitsky, D., Scott, E. G., and Steele, L.: A case of septicemia and meningitis in an infant due to Pasteurella multocida. J. Pediat. 92:853, 1978.

Fry, R. M.: Fatal infections by haemolytic streptococcus group B. Lancet 1:199–201, 1938.

Gado, M., Axley, J., Appleton, D. B., and Prensky, A. L.: Angiography in the acute and post-treatment phases of *Hemophilus influenzae* meningitis. Radiology 110:439–444, 1973.

Geil, C. C., Castle, W. K., and Mortimer, E. A., Jr.: Group A streptococcal infections in newborn nurseries. Pediatrics 46:849–854, 1970.

George, R. M., Cochran, C. P., and Wheeler, W. E.: Epidemic meningitis of the newborn caused by Flavobacteria. II. Clinical manifestations and treatment. Am. J. Dis. Child. 101:296–304, 1961.

Geppert, L. J., Baker, H. J., Copple, B. I., and Pulaski, E. J.: Pseudomonas infections in infants and children. J. Pediat. 41:555–561, 1952.

Geraci, J. E.: Vancomycin. Mayo Clin. Proc. 52:631–634, 1977.

Gibson, R. M., and Kurukchy, T.: Neurosurgical aspects of recurrent meningitis. Proc. Roy. Soc. Med. 67:1150–1153, 1974.

Gilles, F. H., Jammes, J. L., and Berenberg, W.: Neonatal meningitis. The ventricle as a bacterial reservoir. Arch. Neurol. 34:560–562, 1977.

Glaser, J.: Cerebrospinal fluid of premature infants. Am. J. Dis. Child. 40:741–752, 1930.

Glasser, L., Corrigan, J. J., Jr., and Payne, C.: Basophilic meningitis secondary to lymphoma. Neurology 26:899–902, 1976.

Glasser, L., Payne, C., and Corrigan, J. J., Jr.: The in vivo development of plasma cells: A morphologic study of human cerebrospinal fluid. Neurology 27:448–459, 1977.

Glew, R. H., Moellering, R. C., Jr., and Kunz, L. J.: Infections with *Acinetobacter calcoaceticus* (*Herellea vaginicola*): Clinical and laboratory studies. Medicine 56:79–97, 1977.

Gold, A. J., Lieberman, E., and Wright, H. T., Jr.: Bacteriologic relapse during ampicillin treatment of Hemophilus influenzae meningitis. J. Pediat. 74:779–781, 1969.

Goldacre, M. J.: Acute bacterial meningitis in childhood. Incidence and mortality in a defined population. Lancet 1:28–31, 1976.

Goodwin, G. M., and Shelley, H. J.: The sugar content of the cerebrospinal fluid and its relation to the blood sugar. Arch. Intern. Med. 35:242–258, 1925.

Gordon, J. E., and Top, F. H.: Streptococcus meningitis in scarlet fever. J. Pediat. 6:770–783, 1935.

Gordon, R. C., Barrett, F. F., and Clark, D. J.: Influence of several antibiotics, singly and in combination, on the growth of Listeria monocytogenes. J. Pediat. 80:667–670, 1972.

Gorman, C. A., Wellman, W. E., and Eigler, J. O. C.: Bacterial meningitis. II. Infections caused by certain gram-negative enteric organisms. Mayo Clin. Proc. 37:703–712, 1962.

Graber, C. D., Higgens, L. S., and Davis, J. S.: Seldom-encountered agents of bacterial meningitis. J.A.M.A. 192:956–960, 1965.

Granoff, D. M., Congeni, B., Baker, R., Jr., Ogra, P., and Nankervis, G. A.: Countercurrent immunoelectrophoresis in the diagnosis of *Haemophilus influenza* type b infection. Am. J. Dis. Child. 131:1357–1362, 1977.

Gray, H. J.: Streptococcic meningitis. Report of case with recovery. J.A.M.A. 105:92–95, 1935.

Grayzel, H. G., and Orent, E. R.: Blood and cerebrospinal fluid sugar. Am. J. Dis. Child. 34:1007–1012, 1927.

Greene, G. R.: Meningitis due to *Hemophilus influenzae* other than type b: Case report and review. Pediatrics 62:1021–1025, 1978.

Greene, G. R., Overturf, G. D., and Wehrle, P. F.: Am-

picillin dosage in bacterial meningitis with special reference to *Hemophilus influenzae*. Antimicrob. Agents Chemother. 16:198–202, 1979.

Greenwood, B. M., Whittle, H. C., and Dominic-Rajkovic, O.: Countercurrent immunoelectrophoresis in the diagnosis of meningococcal infections. Lancet 2:519–521, 1971.

Gregory, J., and Hey, E.: Blood neutrophil response to bacterial infection in the first month of life. Arch. Dis. Childh. 47:747–753, 1972.

Gromisch, D. S., Gordon, S. G., Bedrosian, L., and Sall, T.: Simultaneous mixed bacterial meningitis in an infant. Am. J. Dis. Child. 119:284–286, 1970.

Gross, R. J., Rowe, B., and Easton, J. A.: Neonatal meningitis caused by *Citrobacter koseri*. J. Clin. Path. 26:138–139, 1973.

Grossman, M., Sussman, S., Gottfried, D., Quock, C., and Ticknor, W.: Immunofluorescent techniques in bacterial meningitis. Am. J. Dis. Child. 107:356–362, 1964.

Guerrant, R. L., Lahita, R. G., Winn, W. C., Jr., and Roberts, R. B.: Campylobacteriosis in man: Pathogenic mechanisms and review of 91 bloodstream infections. Am. J. Med. 65:584–592, 1978.

Gulleks on, E. H., and Dumoff, M.: Haemophilus parainfluenzae meningitis in a newborn. J.A.M.A. 198:1221, 1966.

Gunderson, C. H., and Sack, G. E.: Neurology of Vibrio fetus infection. Neurology 21:307–309, 1971.

Gwynn, C. M., and George, R. H.: Neonatal citrobacter meningitis. Arch. Dis. Childh. 48:455–458, 1973.

Habel, K., and Lucchesi, P. F.: Convulsions complicating pertussis. A clinical study. Am. J. Dis. Child. 56:275–286, 1938.

Hable, K. A., Matsen, J. M., Wheeler, D. J., Hunt, C. E., and Quie, P. G.: Klebsiella type 33 septicemia in an infant intensive care unit. J. Pediat. 80:920–924, 1972.

Haight, T. H.: Anthrax meningitis: Review of literature and report of two cases with autopsies. Am. J. Med. Sci. 224:57–69, 1952.

Hakim, S., Venegas, J. G., and Burton, J. D.: The physics of the cranial cavity, hydrocephalus and normal pressure hydrocephalus: Mechanical interpretation and mathematical model. Surg. Neurol. 5:187–210, 1976.

Hansen, H. H., Bender, R. A., and Shelton, B. J.: The cyto-centrifuge and cerebrospinal fluid cytology. Acta Cytol. 18:259–262, 1974.

Harrison, H. R., and Fulginiti, V. A.: Bacterial immunizations. Am. J. Dis. Child. 134:184–193, 1980.

Harrod, J. R., and Stevens, D. A.: Anaerobic infections in the newborn infant. J. Pediat. 85:399–402, 1974.

Harter, D. H.: Preliminary antibiotic therapy in bacterial meningitis. Arch. Neurol. 9:343–347, 1963.

Hawley, H. B., and Gump, D. W.: Vancomycin therapy of bacterial meningitis. Am. J. Dis. Child. 126:261–264, 1973.

Headings, D. L., and Glasgow, L. A.: Occlusion of the internal carotid artery complicating *Haemophilus influenzae* meningitis. Am. J. Dis. Child. 131:854–856, 1977.

Headings, D. L., Herrera, A., Mazzi, E., and Bergman, M. A.: Fulminant neonatal septicemia caused by Streptococcus bovis. J. Pediat. 92:282–283, 1978.

Heck, A. F., Hameroff, S. B., and Hornick, R. B.: Chronic Listeria monocytogenes meningitis and normotensive hydrocephalus. Case report and review. Neurology 21:263–270, 1971.

Heffner, R. W., and Smith, G. F.: Ecthyma gangrenosum

in pseudomonas septicemia. Am. J. Dis. Child. 99:524–528, 1960.

Henderson, L. L.: Salmonella meningitis. Report of three cases and review of one hundred and forty-four cases from the literature. Am. J. Dis. Child. 75:351–375, 1948.

Hermann, G., and Melnick, T.: Mima polymorpha meningitis in the young. Am. J. Dis. Child. 110:315–318, 1965.

Herweg, C., Middlekamp, J. N., and Hartman, A. F.: Simultaneous mixed bacterial meningitis in children. J. Pediat. 63:76–83, 1963.

Hill, H. R., Hunt, C. E., and Matsen, J. M.: Nosocomial colonization with Klebsiella, type 26, in a neonatal intensive-care unit associated with an outbreak of sepsis, meningitis, and necrotizing enterocolitis. J. Pediat. 85:415–419, 1974.

Hodes, D. S., and Leidy, G.: Meningitis caused by *Hemophilus influenzae* type e. J. Pediat. 91:844–845, 1977.

Hodes, H. L.: Care of the critically ill child: Endotoxin shock. Pediatrics 44:248–260, 1969.

Hoeltge, G. A., Furlan, A., and Hoffman, G. C.: The differential cytology of cerebrospinal fluids prepared by cytocentrifugation. Cleveland Clin. Quart. 43:237–246, 1976.

Holley, H. P., and Al-Ibrahim, M. S.: CSF eosinophilia following myelography. J.A.M.A. 242:2432–2433, 1979.

Holt, L. E.: Observations on three hundred cases of acute meningitis in infants and young children. Am. J. Dis. Child. 1:26–35, 1911.

Holt, R. N., Taylor, C. D., Schneider, H. J., and Hallock, J. A.: Three cases of Hemophilus parainfluenzae meningitis. Clin. Pediat. 13:666–668, 1974.

Hook, E. B.: Central nervous system infection in hydrocephalic children following ventriculography. Clin. Pediat. 4:481–483, 1965.

Hook, E. B., and Aase, J. M.: Herellea meningitis following ventriculography. Am. J. Dis. Child. 108:452–453, 1964.

Hoyne, A. L., and Herzon, H.: *Streptococcus viridans* meningitis. A review of the literature and report of nine recoveries. Ann. Intern. Med. 33:879–902, 1950.

Hughes, E. W., and Manning, G. C.: Bact. coli meningitis in adults. Brit. Med. J. 1:333–334, 1955.

Hughes, I. E., and Adams, J. H.: Eosinophilic meningitis. Lancet 1:1187–1188, 1962.

Humbert, J. R., Kurtz, M. L., Hathaway, W. E.: Increased reduction of nitroblue tetrazolium by neutrophils of newborn infants. Pediatrics 45:125–138, 1970.

Humbert, J. R., Marks, M. I., Hathaway, W. E., and Thoren, C. H.: The histochemical nitroblue tetrazolium reduction test in the differential diagnosis of acute infections. Pediatrics 48:259–267, 1971.

Isiadinso, O. A.: Listeria sepsis and meningitis. A complication of renal transplantation. J.A.M.A. 234:842–843, 1975.

Izquierdo, J. M., Sanz, F., Coca, J. M., Vila, F., and Dierssen, G.: Pyocephalus of the newborn child. Child's Brain. 4:161–169, 1978.

Jacob, J., and Kaplan, R. A.: Bacterial meningitis. Limitations of repeated lumbar punctures. Am. J. Dis. Child. 131:46–48, 1977.

James, A. E., Jr., Hodges, F. J., III, Jordan, C. E., Mathews, E. H., and Heller, R., Jr.: Angiography and cisternography in acute meningitis due to *Hemophilus influenzae*. Radiology 103:601–605, 1972.

Jeanes, A. L.: Cerebrospinal eosinophilia following Torkildsen's operation. Guy's Hosp. Report 114:28–31, 1965.

Johnson, M. L., and Colley, E. W.: *Listeria monocytogenes* encephalitis associated with corticosteroid therapy. J. Clin. Path. 22:465–469, 1969.

Johnson, R. B., Jr.: Increased susceptibility to infection in sickle cell disease: Review of its occurrence and possible causes. South. Med. J. 67:1342–1348, 1974.

Jonsson, M., and Alvin, A.: A 12-year review of acute bacterial meningitis in Stockholm. Scand. J. Infect. Dis. 3:141–150, 1971.

Joyner, R. W., Idriss, Z. H., and Wilfert, C. M.: Misinterpretation of cerebrospinal fluid gram stain. Pediatrics 54:360–362, 1974.

Kahn, R. J., and Daywitt, A. L.: Traumatic pneumocephalus. Am. J. Roentgen. 90:1171–1175, 1963.

Kaiser, A. B., and McGee, Z. A.: Aminoglycoside therapy of gram-negative bacillary meningitis. New Eng. J. Med. 293:1215–1220, 1975.

Kalin, E. M., Tweed, W. A., Lee, J., and MacKeen, W. L.: Cerebrospinal fluid acid-base and electrolyte changes resulting from cerebral anoxia in man. New Eng. J. Med. 293:1013–1016, 1975.

Kalis, P., LeFrock, J. L., Smith, W., and Keefe, M.: Listeriosis. Am. J. Med. Sci. 271:159–169, 1976.

Kaplan, S. L., and Feigin, R. D.: The syndrome of inappropriate secretion of antidiuretic hormone in children with bacterial meningitis. J. Pediat. 92:758–761, 1978.

Katz, R. M., and Liebman, W.: Creatine phosphokinase activity in central nervous system disorders and infections. Am. J. Dis. Child. 120:543–546, 1970.

Katzman, R., Fishman, R. A., and Goldensohn, E. S.: Glutamic-oxalacetic transaminase activity in spinal fluid. Neurology 7:853–855, 1957.

Kaufman, B., Nulsen, F. E., Weiss, M. H., Brodkey, J. S., White, R. J., and Sykora, G. F.: Acquired spontaneous nontraumatic normal-pressure cerebrospinal fluid fistulas originating from the middle fossa. Radiology 122:379–387, 1977.

Kaufman, S. R., Hambly, F., Dyke, J. W., and Gordon, R. C.: Hemophilus parainfluenzae meningitis. Report of two cases. Clin. Pediat. 13:661–663, 1974.

Kaul, S., D'Cruz, J., Rapkin, R., Glista, B., and Behrle, F. C.: Ventriculitis, aqueductal stenosis and hydrocephalus in neonatal meningitis: Diagnosis and treatment. Infection 6:8–11, 1978.

Kelley, A. G.: Sugar findings in normal and pathological spinal fluids. South. Med. J. 16:407–411, 1923.

Kerman, W. Z., Perlstein, M. A., and Levinson, A.: Bacillus pyocyaneus meningitis following pneumoencephalography. Am. J. Dis. Child. 65:912–915, 1943.

Kernig, V.: Ueber ein wenig bemerktes meningitis-symptom. Berlin Klin. Wschr. 21:829–832, 1884.

Kessler, L. A., and Cheek, W. R.: Eosinophilia of the cerebrospinal fluid of noninfectious origin. Report of 2 cases. Neurology 9:371–374, 1959.

Killian, J. A.: Lactic acid of normal and pathological spinal fluids. Proc. Soc. Exp. Biol. Med. 23:255–257, 1925.

Kim, S. K.: Cerebral paragonimiasis. A report of forty-seven cases. Arch. Neurol. 1:30–37, 1959.

Kindley, A. D., and Harris, F.: Repeat lumbar puncture in the diagnosis of meningitis. Arch. Dis. Childh. 53:590–592, 1978.

King, D. K., Loh, K. K., Ayala, A. G., and Gamble, J. F.: Eosinophilic meningitis and lymphomatous meningitis. Ann. Intern. Med. 82:228, 1975.

Kjallquist, A., Siesjo, B. K., and Swetnow, N.: Effects of

increased intracranial pressure on cerebral blood flow and on cerebral venous pO_2, pCO_2, pH, lactate and pyruvate in dogs. Acta Physiol. Scand. 75:267–275, 1969.

Klein, D. M., and Cohen, M. E.: Pasteurella multocida brain abscess following perforating cranial dog bite. J. Pediat. 92:588–589, 1978.

Klimek, J. J., Russman, B. S., and Quintiliani, R.: Mycoplasma pneumoniae meningoencephalitis and transverse myelitis in association with low cerebrospinal fluid glucose. Pediatrics 58:133–135, 1976.

Kolar, O., and Zeman, W.: Spinal fluid cytomorphology. Description of apparatus, technique, and findings. Arch. Neurol. 18:44–51, 1968.

Kolyvas, E., Sorger, S., Marks, M. I., and Pai, C. H.: Pasteurella ureae meningoencephalitis. J. Pediat. 92:81–82, 1978.

Komorowski, R. A., Farmer, S. G., Hanson, G. A., and Hause, L. L.: Cerebrospinal fluid lactic acid in diagnosis of meningitis. J. Clin. Microbiol. 8:89–92, 1978.

Koplan, J. P., Schoenbaum, S. C., Weinstein, M. C., and Fraser, D. W.: Pertussis vaccine—an analysis of benefits, risks and costs. New Eng. J. Med. 301:906–911, 1979.

Krauss, A. N., Thibeault, D. W., and Auld, P. A. M.: Acid-base balance in cerebrospinal fluid of newborn infants. Biol. Neonate 21:25–34, 1972.

Kremer, M.: Meningitis after spinal analgesia. Brit. Med. J. 2:309–313, 1945.

Kuberski, T.: Eosinophils in the cerebrospinal fluid. Ann. Intern. Med. 91:70–75, 1979.

Kulenkampff, M., Schwartzman, J. S., and Wilson, J.: Neurological complications of pertussis inoculation. Arch. Dis Childh. 49:46–49, 1974.

Kunin, C. M., Bender, A. S., and Russell, C. M.: Meningitis in adults caused by Escherichia coli 04 and 075. Arch. Intern. Med. 115:652–658, 1965.

LaForce, F. M., Brice, J. L., and Tornabene, T. G.: Diagnosis of bacterial meningitis by gas-liquid chromatography. II. Analysis of spinal fluid. J. Infect. Dis. 140:453–464, 1979.

Laird, W. P., Nelson, J. D., and Huffines, F. D.: The frequency of pericardial effusions in bacterial meningitis. Pediatrics 63:764–770, 1979.

Lam, A., Sibbald, W. J., and Boone, J.: Transient diabetes insipidus as a complication of Haemophilus meningitis. Pediatrics 61:785–788, 1978.

Lancefield, R. C.: A serologic differentiation of human and other groups of hemolytic streptococci. J. Exper. Med. 57:571–595, 1933.

Landsborough, D., and Tunnell, N.: Observations on plague meningitis. Brit. Med. J. 1:4–7, 1947.

Larsen, T. E., Harris, L., and Holden, F. A.: Isolation of Pasteurella multocida from an otogenic cerebellar abscess. Canad. Med. Assoc. J. 101:114–115, 1969.

Lazarus, S. D., and Levine, G.: Blindness in whooping cough. Am. J. Dis. Child. 47:1310–1317, 1934.

Lechtenberg, R., Sierra, M. F., Pringle, G. F., Shucart, W. A., and Butt, K. M. H.: Listeria monocytogenes: Brain abscess or meningoencephalitis? Neurology 29:86–90, 1979.

Lee, E. L., Robinson, M. J., Thong, M. L., Puthucheary, S. D., Ong, T. H., and Ng, K. K.: Intraventricular chemotherapy in neonatal meningitis. J. Pediat. 91:991–995, 1977.

Lentnek, A. L., Ferguson, R., and Fierer, E.: Group B streptococcal meningitis associated with a CSF fistula. Arch. Neurol. 35:114–115, 1978.

Lerner, P. I.: Meningitis caused by Streptococcus in adults. J. Infect. Dis. 131 (Suppl.):9–16, 1975.

Levin, J., Poore, T. E., Young, N. S., Margolis, S., Zauber, N. P., Townes, A. S., and Bell, W. R.: Gram-negative sepsis: Detection of endotoxemia with the limulus test. Ann. Intern. Med. 76:1–7, 1972.

Levinson, A.: The hydrogen-ion concentration of cerebrospinal fluid: Studies in meningitis. I. J. Infect. Dis. 21:556–570, 1917.

Levinson, A., Greengard, J., and Lifvendahl, R.: Cerebrospinal fluid in the newborn. Am. J. Dis. Child. 32:208–218, 1926.

Levy, H. L., and Ingall, D.: Meningitis in neonates due to Proteus mirabilis. Am. J. Dis. Child. 114:320–324, 1967.

Lewin, R. A., and Hughes, W. T.: Neisseria subflava as a cause of meningitis and septicemia in children. J.A.M.A. 195:821–823, 1966.

Lifshitz, F., Liu, C., and Thurn, A. N.: Bacteroides meningitis. Am. J. Dis. Child. 105:487–489, 1963.

Lilien, L. D., Yeh, T. F., Novak, G. M., and Jacobs, N. M.: Early-onset Haemophilus sepsis in newborn infants: Clinical, roentgenographic, and pathologic features. Pediatrics 62:299–303, 1978.

Linnemann, C. C., Jr., Bass, J. W., and Smith, M. H. D.: The carrier state in pertussis. Am. J. Epidemiol. 88:422–427, 1968.

Lipiridou, O., Lazaridou, S., and Manios, S.: Recurrent and persistent fever in bacterial meningitis with adequate response to antimicrobial therapy. Scand. J. Infect. Dis. 5:23–27, 1973.

Litvak, A.: Temporary amaurosis complicating pertussis. Am. J. Dis. Child. 36:789–796, 1928.

Litvak, A. M., Gibel, H., Rosenthal, S. E., and Rosenblatt, P.: Cerebral complications in pertussis. J. Pediat. 32:357–379, 1948.

Louria, D. B., Hensle, T., Armstrong, D., Collins, H. S., Blevins, A., Krugman, D., and Buse, M.: Listeriosis complicating malignant disease. Ann. Intern. Med. 67:261–281, 1967.

Lups, S., and Haan, A. M. F. H.: The Cerebrospinal Fluid. Elsevier Publishing Co., Amsterdam, 1954.

Lyons, E. L., and Leeds, N. E.: The angiographic demonstration of arterial vascular disease in purulent meningitis. Radiology 88:935–938, 1967.

Maderazo, E. G., Bassaris, H. P., and Quintiliani, R.: Flavobacterium meningosepticum meningitis in a newborn infant. Treatment with intraventricular erythromycin. J. Pediat. 85:675–676, 1974.

Madsen, T.: Vaccination against whooping cough. J.A.M.A. 101:187–188, 1933.

Mahoney, J. F., Tambyah, J. A., Dalton, V. C., and Wolfenden, W. H.: Pontomedullary listeriosis in renal allograft recipient. Brit. Med. J. 2:705, 1974.

Manesis, J. G., and Stanosheck, J.: Escherichia coli meningitis in adults. Arch. Neurol. 13:214–216, 1965.

Mangi, R. J., Holstein, L. L., and Andriole, V. T.: Treatment of gram-negative bacillary meningitis with intrathecal gentamicin. Yale J. Biol. Med. 50:31–41, 1977.

Mangi, R. J., Quintiliani, R., and Andriole, V. T.: Gram-negative bacillary meningitis. Am. J. Med. 59:829–836, 1975.

Manno, N. J., Uihlein, A., and Kernohan, J. W.: Intraspinal epidermoids. J. Neurosurg. 19:754–765, 1962.

Maravilla, K. R., Neuwelt, E. A., and Diehl, J. T.: Application of metrizamide in the radiographic evaluation of the neurologically diseased patient. Neurosurgery 5:389–406, 1979.

Margarey, R., West, L. R., and Pellow, R. A.: Cerebrospinal meningitis due to bacillus coli infection following abortion: recovery. Med. J. Aust. 2:86, 1935.

Margolis, C. Z., and Cook, C. D.: The risk of lumbar puncture in pediatric patients with cardiac and/or pulmonary disease. Pediatrics 51:562–564, 1973.

Martin, A. R., Hurtado, F. P., Plessala, R. A., Hurtado, E. G., Chapman, C. E., Callahan, E. L., and Brutsche, R. L.: Plague meningitis. A report of three cases in children and review of the problem. Pediatrics 40:610–616, 1967.

Martin, G. I.: The significance of tache cerebrale in neonatal meningitis. J. Pediat. 87:321–322, 1975.

Matson, D. D., and Ingraham, F. D.: Intracranial complications of congenital dermal sinuses. Pediatrics 8:463–474, 1951.

Matson, D. D., and Jerva, M. J.: Recurrent meningitis associated with congenital lumbo-sacral dermal sinus tract. J. Neurosurg. 25:288–297, 1966.

Maxted, W. R.: The use of bacitracin for identifying group A haemolytic streptococci. J. Clin. Path. 6:224, 1953.

McAllister, C. K., O'Donoghue, J. M., and Beaty, H. N.: Experimental pneumococcal meningitis. II. Characterization and quantitation of the inflammatory process. J. Infect. Dis. 132:355–360, 1975.

McCarthy, P. L., Jekel, J. F., and Dolan, T. F., Jr.: Temperature greater than or equal to 40C in children less than 24 months of age: A prospective study. Pediatrics 59:663–668, 1977.

McCracken, G. H., Jr.: Changing pattern of the antimicrobial susceptibilities of Escherichia coli in neonatal infections. J. Pediat. 78:942–947, 1971.

McCracken, G. H., Jr.: Clinical pharmacology of gentamicin in infants 2 to 24 months of age. Am. J. Dis. Child. 124:884–887, 1972.

McCracken, G. H., Jr.: Rapid identification of specific etiology in meningitis. J. Pediat. 88:706–708, 1976.

McCracken, G. H., Jr.: Intraventricular treatment of neonatal meningitis due to gram-negative bacilli. J. Pediat. 91:1037–1038, 1977.

McCracken, G. H., Jr., and Mize, S. G.: A controlled study of intrathecal antibiotic therapy in gram-negative enteric meningitis of infancy. Report of the neonatal meningitis cooperative study group. J. Pediat. 89:66–72, 1976.

McCracken, G. H., Jr., and Nelson, J. D., Jr.: Antimicrobial Therapy for Newborns. Practical Application of Pharmacology to Clinical Usage. Grune and Stratton, New York, 1977.

McCracken, G. H., Jr., Sarff, L. D., Glode, M. P., Mize, S. G., Schiffer, M. S., Robbins, J. B., Gotschlich, E. C., Orskov, I., and Orskov, F.: Relation between Escherichia coli K1 capsular polysaccharide antigen and clinical outcome of neonatal meningitis. Lancet 2:246–250, 1975.

McMenemey, W. H.: The significance of subarachnoid bleeding. Proc. Roy. Soc. Med. 47:701, 1954.

McVay, L. V., Jr., and Sprunt, D. H.: Bacteroides infections. Ann. Intern. Med. 36:56–76, 1952.

Medoff, G., Kunz, L. J., and Weinberg, A. N.: Listeriosis in humans: An evaluation. J. Infect. Dis. 123:247–250, 1971.

Mehta, S. S., Kronzon, I., and Laniado, S.: Electrocardiographic changes in meningitis. Isr. J. Med. Sci. 10:748–752, 1974.

Melchior, J. C.: Infantile spasms and early immunization against whooping cough. Danish survey from 1970 to 1975. Arch. Dis. Childh. 52:134–137, 1977.

Menkes, J. H.: The causes for low spinal fluid sugar in bacterial meningitis: Another look. Pediatrics 44:1–3, 1969.

Migeon, C. J., Kenny, F. M., Hung, W., and Voorhess, M. L.: Study of adrenal function in children with meningitis. Pediatrics 40:162–182, 1967.

Moellering, R. C., Jr., and Fischer, E. G.: Relationship of intraventricular gentamicin levels to cure of meningitis. Report of a case of Proteus meningitis successfully treated with intraventricular gentamicin. J. Pediat. 81:534–537, 1972.

Mohr, D. N., Feist, D. J., Washington, J. A., II, and Hermans, P. E.: Meningitis due to group C streptococci in an adult. Mayo Clin. Proc. 53:529–532, 1978.

Mojtabaee, A., and Siadati, A.: Enterobacter hafnia meningitis. J. Pediat. 93:1062–1063, 1978.

Molteni, R. A.: Group A β-hemolytic streptococcal pneumonia. Clinical course and complications of management. Am. J. Dis. Child. 131:1366–1371, 1977.

Moore, C. M., and Ross, M.: Acute bacterial meningitis with absent or minimal cerebrospinal fluid abnormalities. A report of three cases. Clin. Pediat. 12:117–118, 1973.

Morens, D. M.: WBC count and differential. Value of predicting bacterial diseases in children. Am. J. Dis. Child. 133:25–27, 1979.

Morriss, J. H., Gillette, P. C., and Barrett, F. F.: Atrioventricular block complicating meningitis: Treatment with emergency cardiac pacing. Pediatrics 58:866–869, 1976.

Mulcare, R. J., and Harter, D. H.: Changing patterns of staphylococcal meningitis. Arch. Neurol. 7:114–120, 1962.

Murray, E. G. D., Webb, R. A., and Swann, M. B. R.: A disease of rabbits characterized by large mononuclear leukocytosis, caused by a hitherto undescribed bacillus Bacterium monocytogenes (n. sp.). J. Path. Bact. 29:407–439, 1926.

Musher, D. M., and Schell, R. F.: False-positive gram stains of cerebrospinal fluid. Ann. Intern. Med. 79:603–604, 1973.

Myers, G. G., and Netsky, M. G.: Relation of blood and cerebrospinal fluid glucose. Experiments in the dog. Arch. Neurol. 6:18–26, 1962.

Nachum, R., Lipsey, A., and Seigel, S. E.: Rapid detection of gram-negative bacterial meningitis by the limulus lysate test. New Eng. J. Med. 289:931–934, 1973.

Naidoo, B. T.: The cerebrospinal fluid in the healthy newborn infant. S. Afr. Med. J. 42:933–935, 1968.

Neal, J. B.: The treatment of acute infections of the central nervous system with sulfanilamide. J.A.M.A. 111:1353–1356, 1938.

Nelson, J. D.: The changing epidemiology of pertussis in young infants. The role of adults as reservoirs of infection. Am. J. Dis. Child. 132:371–373, 1978.

Nelson, J. D., and McCracken, G. H., Jr.: The current status of gentamicin for the neonate and young infant. Am. J. Dis. Child. 124:13–14, 1972.

Nelson, J. D., Dillon, H. C., Jr., and Howard, J. B.: A prolonged nursery epidemic associated with a newly recognized type of group A streptococcus. J. Pediat. 89:792–796, 1976.

Nelson, R. L.: The neurological complications of whooping cough. A review of the literature with the reports of two cases of pertussis encephalitis. J. Pediat. 14:39–47, 1939.

Nelson, R. M., Bucciarelli, R. L., Nagel, J. W., Beale, E. F., and Eitzman, D. V.: Hypoglycorrachia associated with intracranial hemorrhage in newborn infants. J. Pediat. 94:800–803, 1979.

Nelson-Jones, A.: Neurological complications of undulant fever. The clinical picture. Lancet 1:495–498, 1951.

Nichols, E.: Meningo-encephalitis due to brucellosis with the report of a case in which B. abortus was recovered from the cerebrospinal fluid, and a review of the literature. Ann. Intern. Med. 35:673–693, 1951.

Nichols, W., Jr., and Woolley, P. V., Jr.: Listeria monocytogenes meningitis. J. Pediat. 61:337–350, 1962.

Nieto, D.: Cysticercosis of the nervous system. Diagnosis by means of the spinal fluid complement fixation test. Neurology 6:725–738, 1956.

Nishimura, K.: The lactic acid content of blood and spinal fluid. Proc. Soc. Exp. Biol. Med. 22:322–324, 1924.

Nugent, S. K., Bausher, J. A., Moxon, R., and Rogers, M. C.: Raised intracranial pressure. Its management in *Neisseria meningitidis* meningoencephalitis. Am. J. Dis. Child. 133:260–262, 1979.

Nyfeldt, A. A.: Etiologie de la mononucleose infectieuse. C. R. Soc. Biol. 101:590–591, 1929.

Nyhan, W. L., and Fousek, M. D.: Septicemia of the newborn. Pediatrics 22:268–278, 1958.

Oh, S. J.: Cerebral paragonimiasis. J. Neurol. Sci. 8:27–48, 1968.

Okubadejo, O. A., and Alausa, K. O.: Neonatal meningitis caused by Edwardsiella tarda. Brit. Med. J. 3:357–358, 1968.

Orrison, W. W., Labadie, E. L., and Ramgopal, V.: Fatal meningitis secondary to undetected bacterial psoas abscess. J. Neurosurg. 47:755–760, 1977.

Oski, F. A.: Hematologic Problems: *In:* Avery, G. B.: Neonatology. Pathophysiology and Management of the Newborn. J. B. Lippincott. Philadelphia, 1975. Page 414.

Osnato, M., and Killian, J. A.: Significant chemical changes in the spinal fluid in meningitis. Arch. Neurol. Psychiat. 15:738–750, 1926.

Osuntokun, B. O., Bademosi, O., Osunremi, K., and Wright, S. G.: Neuropsychiatric manifestations of typhoid fever in 959 patients. Arch. Neurol. 27:7–13, 1972.

Otila, E.: Studies on the cerebrospinal fluid in premature infants. V. Success of lumbar puncture and amount of cerebrospinal fluid in the premature infant. Acta Paediat. 35 (Suppl. 8):1–100, 1948.

Otila, E.: Studies on the cerebrospinal fluid in premature infants. VII. Cell count in the cerebrospinal fluid of the premature infant. Acta Paediat. 35 (Suppl. 8):1–100, 1948.

Otila, E.: Studies on the cerebrospinal fluid in premature infants VIII. Tests for proteins in the cerebrospinal fluid of the premature infant. Acta Paediat. 35 (Suppl. 8):1–100, 1948.

Page, R. H., Caldroney, G. L., and Stulberg, C. S.: Immunofluorescence in diagnostic bacteriology. Am. J. Dis. Child. 101:155–159, 1961.

Paisley, J. W., and Washington, J. A., III.: Susceptibility of *Escherichia coli* K1 to four combinations of antimicrobial agents potentially useful for treatment of neonatal meningitis. J. Infect. Dis. 140:183–191, 1979.

Paisley, J. W., Smith, A. L., and Smith, D. H.: Gentamicin in newborn infants. Comparison of intramuscular and intravenous administration. Am. J. Dis. Child. 126:473–477, 1973.

Park, B. H., Fikrig, S. M., and Smithwick, E. M.: Infection and nitroblue tetrazolium reduction by neutrophils. Lancet 2:532–534, 1968.

Patterson, M. J., and Hafeez, A. E. B.: Group B streptococci in human disease. Bact. Rev. 40:774–792, 1976.

Paulson, G. W., Locke, G. E., and Yashon, D.: Cerebral spinal fluid lactic acid following circulatory arrest. Stroke 2:565–568, 1971.

Paulson, O. B., Hansen, E. L., Kristensen, H. S., and Brodersen, P.: Cerebral blood flow, cerebral metabolic rate of oxygen and CSF acid base parameters in patients with acute pyogenic meningitis and with encephalitis. Acta Neurol. Scand. 28 (Suppl. 51):407–408, 1972.

Peter, A.: The plasma cells of the cerebrospinal fluid. J. Neurol. Sci. 4:227–239, 1967.

Petersdorf, R. G., and Harter, D. H.: The fall in cerebrospinal fluid sugar in meningitis. Arch. Neurol. 4:21–30, 1961.

Petersdorf, R. G., Swarner, D. R., and Garcia, M.: Studies on the pathogenesis of meningitis. II. Development of meningitis during pneumococcal bacteremia. J. Clin. Invest. 41:320–327, 1962.

Pinto, R. S., George, A. E., Koslow, M., and Barasch, G.: Neuroradiology of basal anterior fossa (transethmoidal) encephaloceles. Radiology 117:79–85, 1975.

Pirie, J. H. H.: Listeria: Change of name for a genus of bacteria. Nature 145:264, 1940.

Plotkin, S. A., and McKitrick, J. C.: Nosocomial meningitis of the newborn caused by Flavobacterium. J.A.M.A. 198:662–664, 1966.

Plotkin, S. A., Brachman, P. S., Utell, M., Bumford, F. H., and Atchison, M. M.: An epidemic of inhalation anthrax, the first in the twentieth century. I. Clinical features. Am. J. Med. 29:992–1001, 1960.

Plum, F., and Price, R. W.: Acid-base balance of cisternal and lumbar cerebrospinal fluid in hospitalized patients. New. Eng. J. Med. 289:1346–1351, 1973.

Pluot, M., Vital, C., Aubertin, J., Croix, J. C., Pire, J. C., and Poisot, D.: Anthrax meningitis. Report of two cases with autopsies. Acta Neuropath. 36:339–345, 1976.

Pollitzer, R.: Plague. WHO Monogr. Ser. No. 22, 1954.

Pollock, J. A., Newton, T. H., and Hoyt, W. F.: Transsphenoidal and transethmoidal encephaloceles. Radiology 90:442–453, 1968.

Posner, J. B., and Plum, F.: Spinal-fluid pH and neurologic symptoms in systemic acidosis. New Eng. J. Med. 277:605–613, 1967.

Posner, J. B., Swanson, A. G., and Plum, F.: Acid-base balance in cerebrospinal fluid. Arch. Neurol. 12:479–496, 1965.

Poston, M. A., and Thomason, R. H.: Meningitis due to brucella in a child. Am. J. Dis. Child. 52:904–906, 1936.

Pray, L. G.: Lumbar puncture as a factor in the pathogenesis of meningitis. Am. J. Dis. Child. 62:295–308, 1941.

Prensky, A. L.: Pertussis vaccination. Develop. Med. Child Neurol. 16:539–543, 1974.

Price, D. J. E., and Sleigh, J. D.: Klebsiella meningitis—report of nine cases. J. Neurol. Neurosurg. Psychiat. 35:903–908, 1972.

Punyagupta, S., Juttijudata, P., and Bunnag, T.: Eosinophilic meningitis in Thailand. Clinical studies of 484 typical cases probably caused by *Angiostrongylus cantonensis*. Am. J. Trop. Med. 24:921–931, 1975.

Quincke, H.: Die lumbalpunktion des hydrocephalus. Berl. Klin. Wschr. 28:929–933, 965–968, 1891.

Quintiliani, R., and Lentnek, A.: Polymyxin B in the treatment of Klebsiella pneumoniae meningoventriculitis. Intraventricular and intrathecal administration. Am. J. Dis. Child. 121:239–242, 1971.

Rabinowitz, S. G., and MacLeod, N. R.: Salmonella meningitis. A report of three cases and review of the literature. Am. J. Dis. Child. 123:259–262, 1972.

Rahal, J. J., Jr., and Simberkoff, M. S.: Bactericidal and bacteriostatic action of chloramphenicol against meningeal pathogens. Antimicrob. Agents Chemother. 16:13–18, 1979.

Raimondi, A. J., and Di Rocco, C.: The physiopathogenetic basis for the angiographic diagnosis of bacterial infections of the brain and its covering in children. I. Leptomeningitis. Child's Brain. 5:1–13, 1979.

Ralph, E. D., Clarke, J. T., Libke, R. D., Luthy, R. P., and Kirby, W. M. M.: Pharmacokinetics of metronidazole as determined by bioassay. Antimicrob. Agents Chemother. 6:691–696, 1974.

Rangel, R. A., and González, D. A.: *Bacillus anthracis* meningitis. Neurology 25:525–530, 1975.

Rangell, L., and Glassman, F.: Acute spinal epidural abscess as a complication of lumbar puncture. J. Nerv. Ment. Dis. 102:8–18, 1945.

Rantz, L. A.: Streptococcal meningitis. Four cases treated with sulfonamides in which the etiological agent was an unusual streptococcus. Ann. Intern. Med. 16:716–726, 1942.

Rapkin, R. H.: Repeat lumbar punctures in the diagnosis of meningitis. Pediatrics 54:34–36, 1974.

Ratcliffe, J. C., and Wolf, S. M.: Febrile convulsions caused by meningitis in young children. Ann. Neurol. 1:285–286, 1977.

Reinarz, J. A., and Sanford, J. P.: Human infections caused by non-group A or D streptococci. Medicine 44:81–96, 1965.

Repice, J. P., and Neter, E.: Pasteurella multocida meningitis in an infant with recovery. J. Pediat. 86:91–93, 1975.

Rettig, P. J.: Campylobacter infections in human beings. J. Pediat. 94:855–864, 1979.

Rios, I., Klimek, J. J., Maderazo, E., and Quintiliani, R.: *Flavobacterium meningoseptum* meningitis: Report of selected aspects. Antimicrob. Agents and Chemother. 14:444–447, 1978.

Robbins, J. B., McCracken, G. H., Jr., Gotschlich, E. C., Ørskov, F., Ørskov, I., and Hanson, L. A.: *Escherichia coli* K1 capsular polysaccharide associated with neonatal meningitis. New Eng. J. Med. 290:1216–1220, 1974.

Robinson, F., Lamarche, J. B., and Solitare, G. B.: Escherichia coli meningitis in adults: Neurosurgical and neuropathological considerations. J. Neurosurg. 28:452–458, 1968.

Roost, K. T., Pimstone, N. R., Diamond, I., and Schmid, R.: The formation of cerebrospinal fluid xanthochromia after subarachnoid hemorrhage. Neurology 22:973–977, 1972.

Rosen, L., Chappell, R., Laqueur, G. L., Wallace, G. D., and Weinstein, P. P.: Eosinophilic meningoencephalitis caused by a metastrongylid lung-worm of rats. J.A.M.A. 179:620–624, 1962.

Rosenfeld, H.: Hypernephroma of the kidney terminating in colon bacillus meningitis. New York St. J. Med. 42:1490–1494, 1942.

Rosengarten, R., and Bourn, J. M.: Listeria septicemia and meningitis in a case of lupus erythematosus. Neurology 9:704–706, 1959.

Ross, S., Kraybill, E. N., and Khan, W.: Treatment of *Proteus* meningitis with carbenicillin: A report of four cases. J. Infect. Dis. 122 (Suppl.):S62–S70, 1970.

Ryan, J. L., Pachner, A., Andriole, V. T., and Root, R. K.: Enterococcal meningitis: Combined vancomycin and rifampin therapy. Am. J. Med. 68:449–451, 1980.

Sachs, J. M., Pacin, M., and Counts, G. W.: Sickle hemoglobinopathy and *Edwardsiella tarda* meningitis. Am. J. Dis. Child. 128:387–388, 1974.

Sahadevan, M. G., Singh, M., Joseph, P. P., and Hoon, R. S.: Meningomyelitis due to brucellosis. Brit. Med. J. 4:432–433, 1968.

Sahler, O. J. Z., and Wilfert, C. M.: Fever and petechiae with adenovirus type 7 infection. Pediatrics 53:233–235, 1974.

Salmon, J. H.: Ventriculitis complicating meningitis. Am. J. Dis. Child. 124:35–40, 1972.

Salmon, J. H., Hajjar, W., and Bada, H. S.: The fontogram: A non-invasive intracranial pressure monitor. Pediatrics 60:721–725, 1977.

Sanders, D. Y., and Stevenson, J.: Bacteroides infections in children. J. Pediat. 72:673–677, 1968.

Saphra, I., and Winter, J. W.: Clinical manifestations of salmonellosis in man: An evaluation of 7,779 human infections identified at the New York Salmonella Center. New Eng. J. Med. 256:1128–1134, 1957.

Sarff, L. D., Platt, L. H., and McCracken, G. H., Jr.: Cerebrospinal fluid evaluation in neonates: Comparison of high-risk infants with and without meningitis. J. Pediat. 88:473–477, 1976.

Sarubbi, F. A., Jr., Sparling, P. F., and Glezen, W. P.: Herpesvirus hominis encephalitis. Virus isolation from brain biopsy in seven patients and results of therapy. Arch. Neurol. 29:268–273, 1973.

Sayeed, Z. A., Bhaduri, U., Howell, E., and Meyers, H. L.: Gonococcal meningitis. J.A.M.A. 219:1730–1731, 1972.

Schaad, U. B., McCracken, G. H., Jr., and Nelson, J. D.: Clinical pharmacology and efficacy of vancomycin in pediatric patients. J. Pediat. 96:119–126, 1980.

Scheinker, L. M.: Leukoencephalitis associated with purulent leptomeningitis (meningoleukoencephalitis). J. Neuropath. Exper. Neurol. 4:164–171, 1945.

Scherzer, A. L., Kaye, D., and Shinefield, H. R.: Proteus mirabilis meningitis: Report of two cases treated with ampicillin. J. Pediat. 68:731–740, 1966.

Schröter, G. P. J., and Weil, R., III: *Listeria monocytogenes* infection after renal transplantation. Arch. Intern. Med. 137:1395–1399, 1977.

Schumer, W.: Steroids in the treatment of clinical septic shock. Ann. Surg. 184:333–341, 1976.

Schwartz, J. F.: Ataxia in bacterial meningitis. Neurology 22:1071–1074, 1972.

Sell, S. H. W., Merrill, R. E., Doyne, E. O., and Zimsky, E. P., Jr.: Long-term sequelae of *Hemophilus influenzae* meningitis. Pediatrics 49:206–211, 1972.

Shabo, A. L., and Maxwell, D. S.: The subarachnoid space following the introduction of a foreign protein. An electron microscopic study with peroxidase. J. Neuropath. Exper. Neurol. 30:506–524, 1971.

Shackelford, G. D., Shackelford, P. G., Schwetschenau, P. R., and McAlister, W. H.: Congenital occipital dermal sinus. Radiology 111:161–166, 1974.

Shackelford, P. G., Campbell, J., and Feigin, R. D.: Countercurrent immunoelectrophoresis in the evaluation of childhood infections. J. Pediat. 85:478–481, 1974.

Shadravan, I., Fishbein, J., and Hebert, L. J.: Streptococcal meningitis with an unusual portal of entry. Am. J. Dis. Child. 130:214–215, 1976.

Shanahan, R. H., Griffin, J. R., and von Aversperg, A. P.: Anthrax meningitis. Report of a case of internal anthrax with recovery. Am. J. Clin. Path. 17:719–722, 1947.

Shaywitz, B. A.: Epidermoid spinal cord tumors and previous lumbar punctures. J. Pediat. 80:638–640, 1972.

Shortland-Webb, W. R.: Proteus and coliform meningoencephalitis in neonates. J. Clin. Path. 21:422–431, 1968.

Shurtleff, D. B., Foltz, E. L., Weeks R. D., and Loeser, J.: Therapy of Staphylococcus epidermidis: Infections associated with cerebrospinal fluid shunts. Pediatrics 52:55–62, 1974.

Silver, T. S., and Todd, J. K.: Hypoglycorrhachia in pediatric patients. Pediatrics 58:67–71, 1976.

Simpson, J. F., Leddy, J. P., and Hare, J. D.: Listeriosis complicating lymphoma. Report of four cases and interpretive review of pathogenic factors. Am. J. Med. 43:39–49, 1967.

Skeel, R. T., Wright, L. J., Leventhal, C. M., and Henderson, E. S.: Group D streptococcal meningitis masked by meningeal leukemia. Am. J. Dis. Child. 117:334–337, 1969.

Skolnik, E. M., and Ferrer, J. L.: Cerebrospinal otorrhea. Arch. Otolaryngol. 70:795–799, 1959.

Smith, A. L.: Antibiotics and invasive Hemophilus influenzae. New Eng. J. Med. 294:1329–1331, 1976.

Smith, H., Bannister, B., and O'Shea, M. J.: Cerebrospinal fluid immunoglobulins in meningitis. Lancet 2:591–593, 1973.

Smith, R. T., Platou, E. S., and Good, R. A.: Septicemia of the newborn. Current status of the problem. Pediatrics 17:549–575, 1956.

Smith, W. E., McCall, R. E., and Blake, T. J.: Bacteroides infections of the central nervous system. Ann. Intern. Med. 20:920–932, 1944.

Snead, O. C., III., and Kalvsky, S. M.: Cerebrospinal fluid eosinophilia. A manifestation of a disorder resembling multiple sclerosis in childhood. J. Pediat. 89:83–84, 1976.

Solanes, M. P., Heatley, J., Arenas, F., and Ibarra, G. G.: Ocular complications in brucellosis. Am. J. Ophthal. 36:675–689, 1953.

Sörnäs, R.: The cytology of the normal cerebrospinal fluid. Acta Neurol. Scand. 48:313–320, 1972.

Soscia, J. L., Dibenedetto, R., and Crocco, J.: Klebsiella pneumoniae meningitis. Report of a case and review of the literature. Arch. Intern. Med. 113:569–572, 1964.

Spink, W. W.: The Nature of Brucellosis. Minnesota Press, Minneapolis, 1956.

Spivack, A. P., Eisenberg, G. M., Weiss, W., and Flippin, H. F.: Klebsiella meningitis. Am. J. Med. 22:865–871, 1957.

Sproles, E. T., III., Azerrad, J., Williamson, C., and Merrill, R. E.: Meningitis due to Hemophilus influenzae: Long-term sequelae. J. Pediat. 75:782–788, 1969.

Stamm, W. E., Kolff, C. A., Dones, E. M., Javariz, R., Anderson, R. L., Farmer, J. J., III., and de Quinones, H. R.: A nursery outbreak caused by Serratia marcescens—scalp-vein needles as a portal of entry. J. Pediat. 89:96–99, 1976.

Stempfel, R., and Zetterström, R.: Concentration of bilirubin in cerebrospinal fluid in hemolytic disease of the newborn. Pediatrics 16:184–193, 1955.

Stewardson-Krieger, P., and Gotoff, S. P.: Neonatal meningitis due to group C beta hemolytic streptococcus. J. Pediat. 90:103–104, 1977.

Stewart, G. T.: Vaccination against whooping-cough. Efficacy versus risk. Lancet 1:234–237, 1977.

Stokes, H. B., O'Hara, C. M., Buchanan, R. D., and Olson, W. H.: An improved method for examination of cerebrospinal fluid cells. Neurology 25:901–906, 1975.

Stool, S., Leeds, N. E., and Shulman, K.: The syndrome of congenital deafness and otic meningitis: Diagnosis and management. J. Pediat. 71:547–552, 1967.

Strausbaugh, L. J., and Sande, M. A.: Factors influencing the therapy of experimental Proteus mirabilis meningitis in rabbits. J. Infect. Dis. 137:251–260, 1978.

Street, L., Grant, W. W., and Alva, J. D.: Brucellosis in childhood. Pediatrics 55:416–421, 1975.

Ström, J.: Further experience of reactions, especially of a cerebral nature, in conjunction with triple vaccination: A study based on vaccinations in Sweden 1959–65. Brit. Med. J. 4:320–323, 1967.

Sugathadasa, A. A., and Arseculeratne, S. M.: Neonatal meningitis caused by new serotype of Flavobacterium meningosepticum. Brit. Med. J. 1:37–38, 1963.

Swartz, M. N., and Dodge, P. R.: Bacterial meningitis—a review of selected aspects. I. General clinical features, special problems and unusual meningeal reactions mimicking bacterial meningitis. New Eng. J. Med. 272:725–731, 1962.

Swartz, M. N., and Kunz, L. J.: Pasteurella multocida infections in man. Report of two cases—meningitis and infected cat bite. New Eng. J. Med. 261:889–893, 1959.

Sweet, L. K., and Leeper, M. H.: Acute serous meningitis in scarlet fever. J. Pediat. 24:295–309, 1944.

Swierczewski, J. A., Mason, E. J., Cabrera, P. B., and Liber, M.: Fulminating meningitis with Waterhouse-Friderichsen syndrome due to Neisseria gonorrhoeae. Am. J. Clin. Path. 54:202–204, 1970.

Tahernia, A. C., and Hashemi, G.: Survival in anthrax meningitis. Pediatrics 50:329–333, 1972.

Taubin, H. L., and Landsberg, L.: Gonococcal meningitis. New Eng. J. Med. 285:504–505, 1971.

Taylor, P. R., Weinstein, W. M., and Bryner, J. H.: Campylobacter fetus infection in human subjects: Association with raw milk. Am. J. Med. 66:779–783, 1979.

Thompson, A. J., Williams, E. B., Jr., Williams, E. D., and Anderson, J. M.: Klebsiella pneumoniae meningitis. Review of the literature and report of a case with bacteremia and pneumonia, with recovery. Arch. Intern. Med. 89:405–420, 1952.

Todd, J. K.: Childhood infections: Diagnostic value of peripheral white blood cell and differential cell counts. Am. J. Dis. Child. 127:810–816, 1974.

Tourtellotte, W. W., Metz, L. N., Bryan, E. R., and DeJong, R. N.: Spontaneous subarachnoid hemorrhage. Factors affecting the rate of clearing of the cerebrospinal fluid. Neurology 14:301–306, 1964.

Tourtellotte, W. W., Somers, J. F., Parker, J. A., Itabashi, H. H., and DeJong, R. N.: A study on traumatic lumbar punctures. Neurology 8:129–134, 1958.

Trachsler, W. H., Frauenberger, G. S., Wagner, C., and Mitchell, A. G.: Streptococcic meningitis. With special emphasis on sulfanilamide therapy. J. Pediat. 11:248–269, 1937.

Tripoli, C. J.: Bacterial meningitis. A comparative study of various therapeutic measures. J.A.M.A. 106:171–177, 1936.

Troost, B. T., Walker, J. E., and Cherington, M.: Hypoglycorrhachia associated with subarachnoid hemorrhage. Arch. Neurol. 19:438–442, 1968.

Tuazon, C. V., Perez, A. A., Elin, R. J., and Sheagren, J. N.: Detection of endotoxin in cerebrospinal and joint fluids by Limulus assay. Arch. Intern. Med. 137:55–56, 1977.

Vidyasagar, D., and Raju, T. N. K.: A simple noninvasive technique of measuring intracranial pressure in the newborn. Pediatrics 59 (Suppl.): 957–961, 1977.

Vidyasagar, D., Raju, T. N. K., and Chiang, J.: Clinical

significance of monitoring anterior fontanel pressure in sick neonates and infants. Pediatrics 62:996–999, 1978.

Vinzent, R., Dumas, J., and Picard, N.: Septicemie grave au cours de la gross esse, due a un vibrion. Avortement consecutif. Bull. Acad. Natl. Med. 131:90, 1947.

Visintine, A. M., Oleske, J. M., and Nahmias, A. J.: *Listeria monocytogenes* infection in infants and children. Am. J. Dis. Child. 131:393–397, 1977.

Waggener, J. D., and Beggs, J.: The membranous covering of neural tissue. An electron microscopic study. J. Neuropath. Exper. Neurol. 26:412–426, 1967.

Wang, W. L. V., and Haiby, G.: Meningitis caused by *Pasteurella ureae*. Am. J. Clin. Path. 45:562–565, 1966.

Ward, J. I., Siber, G. R., Scheifele, D. W., and Smith, D. H.: Rapid diagnosis of Hemophilus influenzae type b infections by latex particle agglutination and counterimmunoelectrophoresis. J. Pediat. 93:37–42, 1978.

Watson, G. W., Fuller, T. J., Elms, J., and Kluge, R. M.: *Listeria* cerebritis. Relapse of infection in renal transplant patients. Arch. Intern. Med. 138:83–87, 1978.

Weed, L. H., Wegeforth, P., Ayer, J. B., and Felton, L. D.: The production of meningitis by release of cerebrospinal fluid during an experimental septicemia: Preliminary note. J.A.M.A. 72:190–193, 1919.

Wegeforth, P., and Latham, J. R.: Lumbar puncture as a factor in the causation of meningitis. Am. J. Med. Sci. 148:183–202, 1919.

Wegeforth, P., Ayer, J. B., and Essick, C. R.: The method of obtaining cerebrospinal fluid by puncture of the cisterna magna (cisternal puncture). Am. J. Med. Sci. 157:789–797, 1919.

Weinberg, M. H., Mellon, R. R., and Shinn, L. E.: Two cases of streptococcic meningitis. Treated successfully with sulfanilamide and prontosil. J.A.M.A. 108:1948–1951, 1937.

Weinstein, R. A., Bauer, F. W., Hoffman, R. D., Tyler, P. G., Anderson, R. L., and Stamm, W. E.: Factitious meningitis. Diagnostic error due to nonviable bacteria in commercial lumbar puncture trays. J.A.M.A. 233:878–879, 1975.

Wertham, F.: The cerebral lesions in purulent meningitis. Arch. Neurol. Psychiat. 26:549–582, 1931.

Whitmore, D. N., and Whelan, M. J.: Pasteurella septica meningitis with survival. Postgrad. Med. J. 39:98–100, 1963.

Whittle, H. C., Tugwell, P., Egler, L. J., and Greenwood, B. M.: Rapid bacteriological diagnosis of pyogenic meningitis by latex agglutination. Lancet 2:619–621, 1974.

Wiggins, G. L., Albritton, W. L., and Feeley, J. C.: Antibiotic susceptibility of clinical isolates of *Listeria monocytogenes*. Antimicrob. Agents Chemotherap. 13:854–860, 1978.

Wilcox, H. B., and Lyttle, J. D.: The diagnostic value of sugar concentration in spinal fluid. Arch. Pediat. 40:215–255, 1923.

Wilfert, C. M.: Mumps meningoencephalitis with low cerebrospinal-fluid glucose, prolonged pleocytosis and elevation of protein. New Eng. J. Med. 280:855–859, 1969.

Wilkins, R. H., and Odom, G. L.: Ependymal-choroidal cells in cerebrospinal fluid. Increased incidence in hydrocephalic infants. J. Neurosurg. 41:555–560, 1974.

Williams, R. D. B., and Hawkins, R.: The clinical value of cerebrospinal fluid lactic dehydrogenase determinations in children with bacterial meningitis and other neurological disorders. Develop. Med. Child Neurol. 10:711–714, 1968.

Willis, M. D., and Austin, W. J.: Human *Vibrio fetus* infection. Report of two dissimilar cases. Am. J. Dis. Child. 112:459–462, 1966.

Winkelstein, J. A.: The influence of partial treatment with penicillin on the diagnosis of bacterial meningitis. J. Pediat. 77:619–624, 1970.

Wolf, H., and Hoepffner, L.: The cerebrospinal fluid in the newborn and premature infant. World Neurology 2:871–878, 1961.

Wolinsky, E.: Nontuberculous mycobacteria and associated diseases. Am. Rev. Resp. Dis. 119:107–159, 1979.

Wollstein, M.: Influenzal meningitis and its experimental production. Am. J. Dis. Child. 1:42–58, 1911.

Woodruff, K. H.: Cerebrospinal fluid cytomorphology using cytocentrifugation. Am. J. Clin. Path. 60:621–627, 1973.

Woolf, A. L., and Caplin, H.: Whooping cough encephalitis. Arch. Dis. Childh. 31:87–91, 1956.

World Health Organization. Immunization against whooping cough. WHO Chronicle 29:365, 1975.

Xanthou, M.: Leukocyte blood picture in ill newborn babies. Arch. Dis. Childh. 47:741–746, 1972.

Yabek, S. M.: Meningococcal meningitis presenting as acute cerebellar ataxia. Pediatrics 52:718–720, 1973.

Yii, C-Y., Chen, C-Y., Chen, E-R., Hsieh, H-C., Shih, C-C., Cross, J. H., and Rosen, L.: Epidemiologic studies of eosinophilic meningitis in southern Taiwan. Am. J. Trop. Med. 24:447–454, 1975.

Young, L. M., Haddow, J. E., and Klein, J. O.: Relapse following ampicillin treatment of acute Hemophilus influenzae meningitis. Pediatrics 41:516–518, 1968.

Zanen, H. C., and Engel, H. W. B.: Porcine streptococci causing meningitis and septicemia in man. Lancet 1:1286–1288, 1975.

Zeligs, M.: Streptococcic meningitis. Report of two cases with recovery. Am. J. Dis. Child. 50:1497–1501, 1935.

Zelinger, K. S., and Vargas, R. D.: Central nervous system infection by *Vibrio fetus*. Neurology 28:968–971, 1978.

Zellweger, H., and Idriss, H.: Encephalopathy in salmonella infections. Am. J. Dis. Child. 99:770–777, 1960.

Zipursky, A., Palko, J., Milner, R., and Akenzua, G. I.: The hematology of bacterial infections in premature infants. Pediatrics 57:839–853, 1976.

Zwetnow, N.: Effects of intracranial hypertension: Acid base changes and lactate changes in CSF and brain tissue. Scand. J. Clin. Lab. Invest. 22 (Suppl. 102): 1968.

Zwibel, H. L., and Schwartzman, R. J.: Evaluation of the nitroblue tetrazolium test as applied to polymorphonuclear leukocytes in the cerebrospinal fluid. Neurology 24:995–998, 1974.

Chapter Two

ANTIBIOTIC THERAPY— NEUROLOGIC INFECTIONS

Historical Landmarks in Treatment of Acute Bacterial Meningitis

Treatment of bacterial meningitis, in fact, even the recognition of its presence in life, was not possible until the procedure of lumbar puncture was introduced by Heinrich Quincke in 1891. Within a year thereafter, Wynter in Great Britain introduced the technique of CSF drainage via a lumbar trocar for the treatment of tuberculous meningitis. For many years thereafter, spinal drainage accomplished by one method or another represented the basis of treatment of many types of bacterial meningitis. Initially, drainage was accomplished by repeated spinal taps with the intermittent removal of various quantities of CSF, but soon a variety of ingenious methods were devised to enhance the effectiveness of the procedure. One technique was to insert large-bore needles into the subarachnoid space in both the lumbar and the cisternal regions and to irrigate the canal with Ringer's solution from top to bottom (Ayer, Wegeforth et al.). Another method utilized needles in both positions and, with the patient in the upright position, air was injected under pressure through the lumbar needle, which presumably would dissect arachnoidal adhesions and thereby facilitate spinal drainage (Cornwall). Investigators even resorted to surgical lumbar laminectomy so that a trocar could be visually inserted into the subarachnoid space, allowing continuous drainage of CSF (Rainey and Alford). Although the results were generally not dramatic, there were occasional cases in which the course of the illness appeared to have been favorably altered by such drastic measures. Experiences with these procedures led at least one pair of investigators to conclude that "streptococcus meningitis is a surgical disease, just as acute purulent peritonitis is a surgical disease" (Leighton and Pringle 1915).

The first significant advance in the treatment of one specific type of acute bacterial meningitis occurred in 1906 when Dr. Simon Flexner in New York and Dr. Jochmann in Germany independently but nearly simultaneously introduced the use of antimeningococcal horse serum for meningococcal meningitis. The initial trials were with subcutaneous injection of the material, which proved ineffective, but this was soon followed by intrathecal administration (Dunn) and later by cisternal (Wright et al.) and even intraventricular injection (Heiman). Because meningococcal meningitis was the most common type of acute pyogenic meningitis at that time, workers had no hesitation in proceeding with the first intrathecal instillation of 20 to 30 ml. of serum when the initial lumbar puncture revealed cloudy or purulent CSF, even before identification of the organism. If gram-negative diplococci were then found, the intrathecal injections were continued at daily intervals for several days.

By 1913, treatment with antimeningococcal serum had brought about a reduction of the mortality rate of meningococcal meningitis to approximately 30 percent (Flexner). Serum therapy remained the mainstay of treatment of this illness for 30 years when it was eventually supplanted by the sulfonamide preparations. In the mid-1930's, there were attempts to improve the treatment of meningococcal meningitis by the addition of a meningococcal antitoxin to the previously used antiserum (Hoyne). This substance was referred to as Ferry's antitoxin subsequent to its isolation by Ferry et al. in 1931 in bouillon filtrates of the four meningococcal serotypes recognized at that time. Toxic reactions were common and beneficial effects from its use were never clearly documented.

The apparent success of antimeningococcal horse serum spurred the development of a specific antiserum for the treatment of *Hemophilus influenzae* meningitis. Fothergill, in 1931, introduced an immune horse serum for use in this disease; however, for reasons that never became clear, it was found to have little effect on the course of the illness (Ward and Fothergill, Wilkes-Weiss and Huntington). In 1939, Alexander was able to produce a *Hemophilus influenzae* antiserum in rabbits which did seem to have some degree of beneficial effect against the clinical illness. Alexander's rabbit antiserum was subsequently extensively used in combination with sulfonamides, and by 1942 this combination was reported to have reduced the mortality rate of *Hemophilus influenzae* meningitis to 26 percent (Alexander et al.). An antipneumococcal antiserum was also used in an attempt to alter the consistently fatal course of pneumococcal meningitis (Hoyne, Tripoli), although little appeared to change the virulent nature of this illness until the sulfonamides became available.

Between 1910 and 1935, in addition to spinal drainage by one method or another and sometimes in conjunction with this procedure, various chemical agents were administered to attempt to control bacterial meningitis but with nearly uniform lack of success. Substances administered by intraspinal injection included gentian violet (Royster), mercurochrome (Tripoli), and ethylhydrocupreine hydrochloride, the latter with rare reports of survival (Kolmer 1929). Around 1930, another method of treatment

achieved temporary popularity, which consisted of the bilateral intracarotid injection of Pregl's solution of iodine (Crawford, Kolmer 1931). This also was usually performed as an adjunct to spinal drainage or serotherapy, and one can now only speculate as to the adverse effects on the brain that must have resulted from the sudden intra-arterial infusion of such toxic substances. The trials with these various modalities led Dr. John Kolmer in 1931 to predict future developments by stating that "if money and interested workers are available, chemotherapeutic research will ultimately discover chemical agents capable of specifically destroying pneumococci and streptococci in the tissues as efficiently as arsphenamine and its congeners act in the destruction of *Spirochaeta pallida*." Despite his foresight, it is not likely that Kolmer in 1931 would have guessed that the future antimicrobials he predicted would begin to emerge into clinical practice within a period of less than one decade and that their antibacterial effect would far exceed that of the arsenicals against the spirochete.

The sulfonamides were the first effective antimicrobial preparations to become available in this country and were introduced here in 1935. Carithers has provided an elaborate description of the initial treatment with sulfa at the Columbia University Medical Center in New York in 1935. The patient receiving the medication, believed to be the first treated with an antibiotic in the United States, was a 10-year-old girl with *Hemophilus influenzae* meningitis which complicated acute epiglottitis. The antibacterial properties of the sulfonamides had been recognized earlier in Germany and were used in the form of a drug named sulfachrysoidine (Prontosil), the antiseptic component of the drug being sulfanilamide. By 1937, reports began to appear in large number in this country describing the remarkable effect of sulfanilamide on the outcome of meningitis caused by the streptococcus, the meningococcus, and other organisms (Carey, McIntosh et al., McQuarrie, Trachsler et al., Weinberg et al.). The most dramatic response stemming from the use of sulfonamides was in cases of streptococcal meningitis, common then as a complication of head injury or chronic otitic disease, in which the case fatality rate was precipitously reduced from better than 95 percent prior to the use of sulfonamides to less than 20 percent following their utilization (Neal 1938). Within a short period of time, investigations revealed that the drug had excellent penetration into the CSF following oral or intravenous administration (Bigler and Haralambie), although it was commonly given by intrathecal injection. Numerous other sulfa compounds soon were developed and because of the limited antibacterial activity and the high incidence of toxic reactions to sulfanilamide, sulfadiazine eventually became the preferred sulfa preparation by most workers.

Sulfonamides very rapidly became the treatment of choice for meningococcal meningitis, and by 1941 their effect was so dramatic that it was recommended that meningococcal antiserum was no longer necessary (Alexander 1941). Within a few years their use had reduced the mortality rate of this disease to approximately 10 percent (Goldring et al., Jubb). Even after the introduction of penicillin, sulfas remained the mainstay of treatment of meningococcal disease, primarily because it was believed at that time that penicillin did not penetrate the CSF barrier in sufficient concentration to be effective (Rammelkamp and Keefer). That penicillin did gain entrance into the CSF in adequate quantities when given intravenously to patients with inflamed meninges was demonstrated by Rosenberg and Sylvester in 1944. Penicillin finally became more popular for meningococcal infections after Leeper et al. in 1952 demonstrated that it was at least as effective as sulfadiazine if given in sufficient dosage. The final termination of the wide-scale use of sulfadiazine for treatment of this illness and for prophylaxis occurred in 1963 when meningococcal strains exhibiting solid resistance to sulfa were isolated from patients in California (Miller et al.). Control of pneumococcal meningitis with use of the sulfonamides was less dramatic than that of meningococcal infections and the sulfas rapidly gave way to penicillin for this illness once penicillin became available. With *Hemophilus influenzae* meningitis, the sulfonamides alone seemed to have little effect but, when combined with influenzae rabbit antiserum, the mortality rate of the illness was reduced to 25 to 30 percent (Alexander et al. 1942, Sako et al.). Sulfadiazine was later used for treatment of *Hemophilus influenzae* meningitis, combined with streptomycin, but the value of the sulfas in this combination was never clear.

The sulfa preparations thus entered the clinical arena approximately six years before the clinical introduction of a substance which Alexander Fleming in 1928 had fortuitously discovered would inhibit growth of staphylococci on Petri dishes. As a product of a mold, *Penicillium notatum,* Fleming named the antiseptic substance penicillin, and recognized its potential importance to the bacteriologist since it inhibited gram-positive bacteria, allowing luxuriant growth of gram-negative organisms, such as *Bacillus influenzae,* on artificial media. Fleming, a bacteriologist at the St. Mary's Hospital in London, published his findings in the British Journal of Experimental Pathology in 1929. The circumstances surrounding his discovery have recently been eloquently discussed by Sir Ernst Chain (1971), one of the researchers who subsequently performed the experiments which led to the clinical use of the antimicrobial.

By Chain's description, *Penicillium notatum* was commonly present in gardens in London and apparently floated into Fleming's laboratory through an open window to contaminate a Petri dish that had been set aside on a laboratory bench. It was considered no surprise that this had occurred, but the remarkable feature of the event was that Fleming did not promptly remove the dish and send it for cleansing as was the custom when culture plates became contaminated. By allowing the culture plate to remain untouched for several weeks, Fleming unknowingly permitted the contaminating mold to flourish and thus to exert its antibacterial action on the staphylococcus colonies. The inhibitory effect on gram-positive cocci was subsequently observed and recorded by Fleming who then carried out additional experiments with the material, including its injection into laboratory animals to demonstrate its lack of toxicity. Fleming's primary interest in his newfound antiseptic was relative to its potential importance in bacteriologic diagnosis, although he made mention of the possible future use of penicillin in the treatment of bacterial infections. One might assume that the discovery of penicillin was able to occur because of the absence of air-conditioning in the medical facility and because of the less than compulsive nature of the scientist, features which nowadays would be considered to be detrimental to scientific investigation.

The report by Fleming in 1929 interested but did not excite the scientific community until 1940 when Ernst Chain, Lord Florey, and others reported the antibacterial effect of penicillin in the treatment of experimental bacterial infections in mice. It is of interest that in the same year, Abraham and Chain discovered an enzyme in extracts from certain bacteria which destroyed the antibacterial properties of penicillin. They called this enzyme penicillinase and shortly thereafter it was found that penicillin-resistant strains of bacteria produced this enzyme, which opened the β-lactam ring of the penicillin molecule, thus inactivating the antibiotic. In 1941, Abraham and colleagues at Oxford published in Lancet the initial report of the clinical use of penicillin for the treatment of human septic infections. In this initial report in 1941, the authors' extraordinary insight relative to the pharmacokinetics of the drug is exemplified by the statement, "To avoid the uncertainties of intestinal absorption, the first cases were treated with penicillin given intravenously. Since it is rapidly eliminated by the kidneys and probably partially inactivated in the body, it was clear that frequent doses would be necessary."

The drug was in limited supply in the first years after its introduction into clinical medicine, years which corresponded to World War II. Despite its limited availability to the civilian population, penicillin was rapidly shown to be a remarkably effective antibiotic, and reports soon appeared which documented its value in the treatment of many types of infections. With pneumococcal meningitis, penicillin initially resulted in only a mild reduction in the mortality rate; however, the doses used were quite low by modern standards and varied from 50,000 to 400,000 units per day by intramuscular injection and were combined with intrathecal penicillin injections (Sweet et al., White et al.). For older children with meningitis, recommended doses ranged from 30,000 to 80,000 units per day along with daily intrathecal penicillin in doses of 5,000 to 6,000 units (Herrell and Kennedy). Intrathecal penicillin remained a part of the regimen until approximately 1948 when Lowrey and Quilligan showed that systemic penicillin alone was sufficient if a sufficient dosage was used. With doses of penicillin of one million units every two hours for adults given intramuscularly, the mortality of pneumococcal meningitis was reduced to approximately 38 percent (Dowling et al. 1949). With the eventual use of the drug by intravenous administration, the mortality rate was reduced even further, especially in children.

Streptomycin was discovered in 1944 by Schatz, Bugie, and Waksman and promptly acquired an important role in the treatment of tuberculous and *Hemophilus influenzae*

meningitis. For *Hemophilus influenzae* meningitis, streptomycin was customarily given by both the intramuscular and intrathecal routes and usually in combination with sulfonamides or Alexander's rabbit antiserum (Alexander and Leidy). While this regimen brought about an improvement in survival statistics, it did so at the expense of rather common and sometimes severe side effects peculiar to the intrathecal use of streptomycin. When chloramphenicol became available in 1947, it soon supplanted streptomycin for treatment of *Hemophilus influenzae* meningitis, thereby obviating the need for intrathecal medication (Prather and Smith, Ross et al.).

In 1950, so-called "triple" therapy emerged and received broad acceptance for the initial treatment of acute suppurative meningitis in older infants and children until the causative organism was identified. The regimen consisted of penicillin (for the pneumococcus), sulfadiazine (for the meningococcus), and chloramphenicol (for *Hemophilus influenzae*). This remained the standard initial therapy for acute bacterial meningitis until soon after the introduction of ampicillin in 1961. With the demonstration that ampicillin was effective for the treatment of *Hemophilus influenzae* meningitis and was adequate for infections caused by the other two common pathogens which cause meningitis in children beyond three months of age, the single drug approach replaced "triple" therapy. Single drug treatment with ampicillin became firmly established and remained so until 1973 when the first ampicillin-resistant strains of *Hemophilus influenzae* were discovered in this country. Once again, an adjustment was required, and the outcome was the recommendation that ampicillin and chloramphenicol in combination should be the initial method of treatment of acute bacterial meningitis in the child over two months of age, continued until the organism is isolated and its antibiotic sensitivities are predictable or are proved.

Antimicrobial Agents and Their Selection

The selection of an antibiotic regimen for treatment of a child with meningitis or other types of suppurative intracranial infection depends upon a number of factors. In cases of pyogenic meningitis, the primary considerations are the age of the child, which is a predictor of the most probable causative microorganism, and the presence or absence of other factors, such as a ventricular shunt or a prior history of splenectomy, which predispose to infection with certain specific bacteria. Certain physical signs, such as the rash characteristic of meningococcemia and the results of the gram stain on a CSF specimen, also influence the choice of the most optimal antibiotic or combination of antibiotics. Once the organism is isolated and sensitivities are known or predictable, the regimen is altered accordingly. Antimicrobials that are chosen are those most likely to be effective against the probable or proven organism, those which will gain entrance into the CSF in quantities that are sufficient to eradicate the infection, and those that can be given with reasonable safety in regard to the age of the child and the presence or absence of hepatic or renal disease.

To the degree possible, combinations of antibiotics are avoided that might possibly be antagonistic to each other, reducing their effectiveness against the organism that has been isolated and identified. Thus, penicillin and chloramphenicol are best not used simultaneously in proven cases of *Streptococcus pneumoniae* meningitis, and chloramphenicol and gentamicin in combination should probably be avoided in infants with meningitis caused by *Escherichia coli* or *Proteus* species. Conversely, advantage is taken of synergistic activity of ampicillin and gentamicin against enterococcal Group D *Streptococcus* and carbenicillin plus gentamicin, or ticarcillin with tobramycin against *Pseudomonas aeruginosa*.

Attention must be directed to details such as the compatibility of different antibiotics mixed together in solution, the stability of antibiotics in solution, and the rate with which a given antibiotic is injected intravenously. The frequency of administration is largely determined by known pharmacokinetic data peculiar to each antibiotic which is commonly found to be relative to the age of the child. Standard, accepted dosages are administered but sometimes must be altered on the basis of whether the drug is metabolized and how it is excreted, and especially when there is significant compromise in hepatic or renal function. For example, in the patient with acute, severe renal failure, the dose of the penicillins or the aminoglycosides may need to be reduced, while in one with hepatic insufficiency, standard doses of chloramphenicol or nafcillin can result in excessively high serum levels. In the newborn period,

because of physiologic immaturity of hepatic and renal function, and in older infants and children with hepatic or renal disease, serum level monitoring of the concentrations of the aminoglycosides and chloramphenicol can be critical for the optimal dosage selection.

Of the antimicrobials that are currently available, some have few if any indications for the treatment of suppurative neurologic infections; some are prescribed only occasionally but do have specific indications, and a relatively small number are exceedingly important and enjoy widespread use. Among the first group are the cephalosporins, erythromycin, and the tetracyclines. The cephalosporins are chemically closely related to penicillin but are not inactivated by penicillinase and have their greatest value in the treatment of penicillinase-producing staphylococcal infections in patients allergic to penicillin. As a class, the cephalosporins gain entrance poorly into the CSF and therefore are not recommended for the treatment of bacterial meningeal infections. Cefamandole has been found to be an exception in regard to its ability to penetrate into the CSF (Beaty and Walters, Steinberg et al. 1977). Cefamandole is more active against certain Enterobacteriaceae than other available cephalosporins and also is effective against β-lactamase-positive *Hemophilus influenzae*. Clinical trials of treatment of meningitis with cefamandole have had conflicting results (Korzeniowski et al., Steinberg et al. 1978) and the drug cannot be recommended for this purpose at the present time. Cefamandole or an effective analogue might later play a role in select instances in children with meningitis caused by *Hemophilus influenzae* resistant to both ampicillin and chloramphenicol.

Erythromycin is a macrolid antibiotic with very low toxicity; however, it also penetrates inflamed meninges so poorly that it is not effective for treatment of bacterial meningitis (Ginsburg and Eichenwald). Erythromycin along with rifampin and vancomycin are among the few drugs which are active against *Flavobacterium meningosepticum* (Aber et al., Rios et al.). If erythromycin is used for treatment of meningitis caused by this organism, direct instillation into the CSF may be necessary (Maderazo et al.).

The tetracyclines have little role in the treatment of pyogenic or other intracranial infections because other available antibiotics are more effective and more adequately penetrate the CSF. In addition, the adverse effects, including deposition of the drug in immature teeth resulting in discoloration and enamel hypoplasia, and the storage in skeletal structures, are major disadvantages in children (Mull, Olson and Riley). Tetracycline is used by some for the treatment of Rocky Mountain spotted fever, although chloramphenicol is probably preferable in children. Tetracycline in combination with streptomycin is recommended for treatment of the rare cases of brucella meningoencephalitis (Abramsky, Buchanan et al.). An interesting neurologic complication of tetracycline therapy in infants is a bulging fontanel syndrome (Fields, O'Doherty). An increased intracranial pressure syndrome has also rarely been described in older children and adults (Maroon and Mealy, Koch-Weser and Gilmore).

Antimicrobials that are infrequently used but have reasonably specific indications for treatment of suppurative intracranial infections include metronidazole, rifampin, streptomycin, vancomycin, carbenicillin, sulfonamides, and amphotericin B. Metronidazole has found a definite place for the treatment of anaerobic meningitis caused by *Bacteroides fragilis,* when the organism is resistant or inadequately responsive to chloramphenicol. The drug would also be important for the management of *Entamoeba histolytica* brain abscess. Rifampin is now part of the therapeutic regimen for tuberculous meningitis and also is the drug of choice for meningococcal prophylaxis. In addition, it is active against *Flavobacterium meningosepticum* in most instances and is important for treatment of meningitis caused by this organism because of its ability to penetrate into the CSF. Vancomycin can be a valuable alternative in penicillin-allergic patients with penicillinase-producing staphylococcal infections of the central nervous system or in those that are methicillin-resistant. Sulfonamides currently have limited use in the management of neurologic infections. Sulfonamide is used for intracranial infections caused by *Nocardia* species and could conceivably be administered for certain penicillin-allergic patients with meningococcal infections if the isolate has been proved to be sulfa-sensitive. Amphotericin B is the primary drug for treatment of a variety of fungal infections of the central nervous system but also is the drug of choice in patients with primary amebic meningitis caused by free-living amebae.

The antimicrobials that are the basis for treatment of the majority of patients with bacterial infections of the central nervous system include the members of the penicillin class of drugs, chloramphenicol, and the aminoglycosides, either singly or in one of a variety of combinations. This is because of their effectiveness against the commonly occurring causative organisms, their ability to gain entrance through inflamed meninges into the CSF, although this is marginal with the aminoglycosides, and because of the extensive information that has been compiled regarding the pharmacokinetics and biological characteristics of these antibiotics in the neonate, the infant, and older children.

Aminoglycosides

The aminoglycoside antibiotics are widely used in the pediatric age group and for many years have had a major role in the treatment of neonatal infections caused by gram-negative organisms. Antibiotics in this class in common use include streptomycin, neomycin, kanamycin, gentamicin, amikacin, and tobramycin. Those produced by *Streptomyces* species contain the letter "y" (streptomycin, kanamycin), while the ones produced by *Micromonospora* species bear the letter "i" (gentamicin) in their names. The utilization of the aminoglycosides in the treatment of neonatal septic infections has periodically changed over the past 25 years, in part on the basis of increasing knowledge of the pharmacokinetics of the drugs and in part as the result of changes in the resistance factors of the causative organisms. In the 1950's, penicillin and streptomycin were commonly prescribed for neonatal coliform infections, but this combination eventually gave way to the use of a penicillin and kanamycin following the increasing occurrence of organisms resistant to streptomycin. Toward the latter part of the 1960's, coliforms resistant to kanamycin began to be prevalent, leading to the wide-scale use of a combination of ampicillin and gentamicin in many newborn nurseries. This reg-

Table 2–1. Aminoglycosides

Streptomycin
Neomycin
Kanamycin
Gentamicin
Tobramycin
Amikacin
Sisomicin
Netilmicin

imen has continued to be the mainstay of treatment of many gram-negative neonatal infections, but recently gentamicin-resistant enteropathogenic bacteria have also begun to appear.

Bacterial resistance to the aminoglycosides occurs by a variety of mechanisms, the most important being the development of extra-chromosomally controlled (R-factor) enzymes, which are believed to inhibit transport of the antibiotic into the cell (Davies, Davies and Courvalin). Whereas multiple enzymes of gram-negative bacteria are capable of inhibiting certain of the aminoglycosides, only one enzyme, 6-amino acetyltransferase, has been found to inactivate amikacin. Thus, amikacin is sometimes still effective against certain coliform bacilli that are resistant to other aminoglycosides, while amikacin-resistant strains are also resistant to the other antibiotics in this class.

The aminoglycosides penetrate the bacterial cell wall to act upon ribosomes, thereby inhibiting protein synthesis. Binding of the drug to the microbial ribosomes causes incorrect amino acids to be inserted into peptide chains, leading to death of the organism. As a class, the aminoglycosides are characterized by a narrow range between therapeutically effective and toxic serum concentrations, low protein binding in the serum, relatively poor CSF penetration with parenteral doses in the safe range, and potential ototoxic and nephrotoxic properties.

An unusual complication that has been described with several of the aminoglycoside antibiotics is neuromuscular blockade (Argov and Mastaglia, McQuillen et al., Wright and McQuillen). The first such report was in 1956 in which a patient became apneic after the intraperitoneal injection of neomycin sulfate (Pridgen). Most reported examples have followed anesthesia for surgical procedures and are manifested by transient respiratory insufficiency and flaccid paralysis of the extremities. The pathogenesis of antibiotic-induced neuromuscular blockade is unclear, although with certain antibiotics it has been postulated that muscle weakness is the result of a reduced level of serum ionized calcium (Levine). Calcium administered intravenously with caution is the recommended form of therapy although it is not always effective. Aminoglycosides can also increase weakness in patients with myasthenia gravis (Hokkanen) and have been reported to potentiate weakness in infant botulism (L'Hommedieu).

The aminoglycosides are largely excreted by glomerular filtration and, thus, the serum levels of these drugs will become elevated in patients with compromised renal glomerular function unless the dose is appropriately reduced. Aminoglycoside antibiotics are well absorbed after intramuscular injection and can be given by this route unless otherwise contraindicated. When administered intravenously, they should be infused over a 20-minute period of time and should not be mixed in the same infusion bottle with any of the penicillin preparations (Noone and Pattison). The drugs have less bactericidal activity in an acid medium, a factor which may, perhaps, reduce their effectiveness in the treatment of acute meningitis, in which there is characteristically a decline in the CSF pH secondary in part to an increase in the CSF lactic acid content.

Of the available aminoglycosides, kanamycin, gentamicin, amikacin, and tobramycin currently are the ones most widely used. Neomycin, similarly to other aminoglycosides, is poorly absorbed after oral administration. It is sometimes used to sterilize the gastrointestinal tract in children with certain neurologic disorders associated with acute hepatic failure, such as Reye's syndrome, but has no primary use in the treatment of pyogenic meningitis. Streptomycin currently has its primary role in the treatment of tuberculosis and its complications and is also of importance in the treatment of plague. The rare cases of *Yersinia pestis* (plague) meningitis should also receive chloramphenicol owing to the far superior CSF penetration characteristic of the latter drug. Streptomycin combined with sulfisoxazole has recently been considered one alternative for treatment of ampicillin- and chloramphenicol-resistant *Hemophilus influenzae* meningitis (Meade).

Kanamycin enjoyed great popularity for treatment of neonatal sepsis and gram-negative bacterial infections in older children until approximately 10 years ago when resistant organisms became commonplace. With the resulting decline in its use, the passage of time again allowed an increase in the percentage of enteropathogenic strains that are susceptible to its effect (Howard and McCracken). In 1974, Baker et al. found that 95 percent of *Escherichia coli* isolates from pediatric patients were susceptible to kanamycin while 98 percent were inhibited by gentamicin. Kanamycin continues to play an important role in the treatment of infection caused by sensitive organisms, although it has the same limitations and similar toxicities as other aminoglycosides. Kanamycin has little activity against *Pseudomonas aeruginosa* and, like other drugs in this class, is of little value for the treatment of anaerobic infections.

The half-life in serum of kanamycin in early infancy is inversely related to birth weight and chronological age. In term infants one week of age and older, the serum half-life is approximately three to four hours, while in low-birth-weight infants in the first three days after birth, the half-life is approximately nine hours (Howard and McCracken). Peak serum levels are achieved about one hour after intramuscular injection; however, the considerable individual variation in the peak level resulting from a given dose emphasizes the importance of monitoring serum levels when the drug is used in the neonatal period or in patients with renal compromise (McCracken 1974). Howard and McCracken found that the highest CSF values of kanamycin in infants with meningitis were detected three to four hours after intramuscular administration. They identified very wide variations in the CSF concentrations following a constant dosage but with a mean CSF concentration of 43 percent of the peak serum level. The initial dose regimen of kanamycin, pending alterations on the basis of peak and trough serum levels, is 20 mg. per kilogram per day in divided doses every 12 hours in infants less than one week of age, and 30 mg. per kilogram per day in divided doses every eight hours in infants older than one week (Hieber and Nelson). Optimal therapeutic peak serum concentration is 15 to 25 μg./ml. It is believed that ototoxicity secondary to kanamycin is unlikely if the total dosage administered does not exceed 500 mg. per kilogram (Yow et al.).

Tobramycin is one of the more recently available aminoglycosides, having been in clinical use since 1975. The antimicrobial spectrum of the drug is similar to that of gentamicin although it is resistant to some of the bacterial enzymes (R-factors) that inhibit gentamicin. Like other aminoglycoside antibiotics, the drug is little metabolized and is excreted primarily by glomerular filtration (Kaplan et al.). Also as with other aminoglycosides, tissue accumulation of tobramycin occurs during treatment so that urine must be collected for 10 to 20 days to achieve complete recovery of the drug (Schentag et al.). Ototoxic and nephrotoxic effects are generally considered to be similar to those of other members in this class of antibiotics. The most

significant effect of tobramycin is its greater activity against *Pseudomonas aeruginosa* compared to gentamicin (McCracken and Nelson). In a study of adults with severe systemic gram-negative infections, mostly caused by *Pseudomonas aeruginosa,* Parry and Neu found the combination of ticarcillin and tobramycin to be superior to that of carbenicillin and gentamicin. There is little information to the present time regarding the use of tobramycin for the treatment of gram-negative meningitis in any age group, and little data describing CSF penetration of the drug in the presence of inflamed meninges. The dose of tobramycin for infants less than one week of age is 5 mg. per kilogram per day given in divided doses every 12 hours, and for infants one week to two months old the dose is 5 mg. per kilogram per day administered in divided doses every eight hours (Yoshioka et al.). For children older than two months, the dose of tobramycin is 4 mg. per kilogram per day in divided doses every eight hours. Optimal therapeutic peak levels are in the range of 3 to 8 μg./ml.

Netilmicin is a new semisynthetic aminoglycoside which is derived from the parent compound, sisomicin. Interest in the drug resulting in extensive study of its properties derived from the early findings that it might be as effective as gentamicin but with less ototoxicity (Dhawan et al., Eickhoff and Ehert, Jahre et al., Trestman et al.). Netilmicin has been found to be effective against certain gentamicin-resistant Enterobacteriaceae, although nephrotoxicity is similar to that of other aminoglycosides and a rise in liver enzymes has been noted in some treated patients (Panwalker et al., Snydman et al.). Scheld and colleagues evaluated the CSF penetrability in rabbits of netilmicin and gentamicin and found each to be just over 20 percent of the concurrent serum concentration, although netilmicin achieved significantly better bactericidal activity in CSF than was the case with gentamicin. The clinical significance of this finding remains uncertain although, to date, netilmicin has not displaced the previously available aminoglycosides.

Amikacin is a semisynthetic aminoglycoside which has been available for clinical use since 1976. It has pharmacokinetic properties similar to those of kanamycin and is equally as effective as gentamicin against gentamicin-sensitive Enterobacteriaceae and *Pseudomonas* species but is also approximately equally ototoxic and nephrotoxic (Lane et al., Smith et al.). Because amikacin is inactivated by only one of the aminoglycoside-inactivating enzymes, gram-negative organisms resistant to other aminoglycosides may still be susceptible to amikacin. The sensitivity to amikacin of bacilli resistant to other aminoglycosides establishes the primary importance of the drug and its use should be restricted only for this purpose (Meyer et al., Yow 1977). Peak serum concentrations are achieved 30 to 60 minutes after intramuscular injection. The half-life in older children is approximately two hours (Kafetzis et al.) and in early infancy it correlates with postnatal age, ranging from three to nine hours (Howard et al. 1976).

Penetration of amikacin from serum into CSF through uninflamed meninges is very poor, a trait in common with all of the aminoglycosides. Briedis and Robson found no detectable levels of amikacin in CSF one to eight hours after intramuscular injection in patients without meningitis, despite simultaneous serum levels which were in the therapeutic range. Experimental studies with rabbits with meningitis have shown the CSF concentration of amikacin to be approximately 15 to 20 percent of mean serum concentration when the drug was given by a constant intravenous infusion (Hamory et al.). In patients with meningitis, CSF levels have been found to vary considerably following parenteral administration. Howard et al. (1976) found the amikacin CSF level one to 12 hours after a 7.5 mg. per kilogram intramuscular dose to range from 0.8 to 9.2 μg./ml, with a mean of 4.4 μg./ml. In one patient with acute meningitis, Sklaver et al. identified amikacin CSF concentrations of 7 μg./ml. and 6.5 μg./ml. with simultaneous serum levels of 9.7 and 8.6 μg./ml. In a second patient who was receiving intravenous amikacin, an intrathecal injection of 10 mg of the drug resulted in a ventricular fluid level of 19 μg./ml. 24 hours later.

Intrathecal or intraventricular administration of amikacin has been described in several instances in patients with multiply resistant organisms, especially for meningitis following head injuries or neurosurgical procedures (Hamory et al., Sklaver et al., Wirt et al.). In some of these, a trial with parenteral antimicrobials to which the organism was sensitive failed to produce improvement, while intrathecal amikacin rapidly sterilized the CSF. Because of the poor circulation of aminoglycosides throughout the CSF following lumbar intrathecal injection, direct injection into the lateral ventricle or into the ventricle via a reservoir would be preferable.

The dose of amikacin for newborn infants less than one week of age is 15 mg. per kilogram per day given intramuscularly in divided doses every 12 hours. For infants one week to two months of age, the dose is 22.5 mg. per kilogram per day administered every 8 hours. In children beyond two months of age, the intramuscular dose is 15 mg. per kilogram per day given every eight hours. Owing to individual variations, the optimal peak and trough serum levels are best determined by monitoring blood levels. The desired therapeutic peak serum level of amikacin is 15 to 20 μg./ml.

Gentamicin was approved for pediatric use in this country in 1972 and rapidly became the most widely used aminoglycoside in this age group. Despite its very extensive use for almost a decade, it has remained effective against most members of the Enterobacteriaceae, most strains of *Pseudomonas aeruginosa,* and many isolates of *Serratia marcescens* (Appel and Neu). Gentamicin has a synergistic effect in combination with carbenicillin or ticarcillin against *Pseudomonas aeruginosa,* and is synergistic with ampicillin against *Listeria monocytogenes.* Enhanced bacterial killing of Group B *Streptococcus,* enterococcal Group D *Streptococcus,* and *Escherichia coli* has been claimed for gentamicin in combination with ampicillin, presumably explained by the penicillin-induced injury to the bacterial cell wall, increasing the cell's permeability to the aminoglycoside.

Gentamicin is also active against *Staphylococcus aureus* and *Staphylococcus epidermidis* (Richards et al.), although resistant strains have been found with increasing frequency in recent years. In some instances, gentamicin-resistant staphylococci have remained susceptible to amikacin (Faden et al., Vogel et al.). Gentamicin is not considered to be the drug of choice for treatment of invasive staphylococcal infections but the drug can play a role in combination with the semisynthetic penicillins in select circumstances. Chloramphenicol has been shown to have an adverse effect upon the bactericidal activity of gentamicin when both drugs are used simultaneously to treat certain gram-negative infections (Strausbaugh and Sande).

Pharmacokinetic studies of gentamicin have been much more extensive than with other aminoglycosides and have resulted in rational dosage schedules dependent on postnatal age and renal function, as well as optimal methods of utilization of the drug for the treatment of sensitive organisms. Gentamicin is not metabolized and is excreted by glomerular filtration. Peak serum levels are achieved in 30 to 60 minutes following intramuscular injection, with no evidence of significant accumulation in serum after courses of treatment of up to 10 days in duration (McCracken 1972). The drug has been found to accumulate in high concentrations in renal cortical and medullary tissue, a fact which probably accounts for the inability to recover from the urine all of a given dose over a limited time span (Edwards et al.).

The mean half-life of gentamicin in serum is approximately five hours in newborn infants less than 72 hours of age and may be considerably more prolonged in low-birth-weight neonates (McCracken 1974, McCracken and Jones 1970). In infants with normal renal function beyond seven days of age, the mean half-life of gentamicin is approximately three hours (McCracken 1972). A single intramuscular dose of 2 to 2.5 mg. per kilogram results in a peak blood level in the range of 2.5 to 7.5 μg./ml., well below the potentially ototoxic level of 12 μg./ml. (McCracken 1972). The individual variations are sufficiently great, however, that it is not possible to accurately predict what serum level will result from a presumably adequate dose (Kaye et al., Paisley et al.), indicating the high desirability of serum level monitoring. Gentamicin administered to the mother crosses the placenta, with peak cord serum levels being approximately one-third of that in the maternal serum (Yoshioka et al.).

In contrast to gram-positive bacteria against which peak CSF levels of penicillin or ampicillin given systemically will achieve values of 10 to 100 times the minimum inhibitory concentration (MIC), the CSF levels of gentamicin achieved intramuscularly in acceptable doses will be less than or only approximately equal to the MIC of sensitive gram-negative organisms (McCracken 1972). For rapid bacterial killing in CSF, the peak antimicrobial concentration should considerably exceed the MIC of the sensitive organism. With therapeutic doses of gentamicin given intramuscularly, McCracken et al. (1971) found peak CSF levels of 1 to 3 μg./ml., while Chang et al. and Pickering et al. demonstrated that CSF gentamicin levels were undetectable in most instances in children with peak serum concentrations in the therapeutic range. The inadequacy of penetration of gentamicin into the CSF was also documented by Kaiser and McGee, who

showed that with serum levels between 1.9 μg./ml. and 7 μg./ml., simultaneous ventricular, cisternal, or lumbar CSF specimens contained 0 to 0.9 μg./ml., quantities well below the MIC of the infecting organism.

Because of the insufficient entrance of gentamicin from serum into CSF, direct injection of the drug into the lumbar subarachnoid space has been attempted; however, this method has not significantly improved the outcome in infants with gram-negative meningitis (McCracken and Mize). The unidirectional flow of CSF from the ventricular system inferiorly as well as the inadequate diffusion of low-density substances through the densely purulent, sometimes loculated, exudate characteristic of neonatal meningitis accounts for the inability of ventricular entrance of gentamicin instilled by lumbar puncture. In addition, following needle penetration of the dura at the time of lumbar puncture, extra-subarachnoid fluid collections sometimes will develop, and, with subsequent taps, the antimicrobial can be deposited therein, with the erroneous belief that it has been placed in the CSF column. The occurrence of such subdural or epidural "lakes" subsequent to lumbar puncture is well known from experiences with attempted pantopaque myelography within hours or a few days after a lumbar puncture. Among infected infants or children with intraventricular obstructive hydrocephalus, one would anticipate no ventricular entry of gentamicin following injection into the lumbar CSF. Kaiser and McGee administered gentamicin by the lumbar route in doses of 5 to 10 mg. in older children and adults and were able to identify ventricular fluid concentrations therefrom of only 0 to 2.1 μg./ml. Despite the negative results with intralumbar injection of gentamicin for treatment of neonatal meningitis, this approach has been found to be beneficial by some workers for treatment of older persons with gram-negative meningitis (Graybill et al., Mangi et al., Rahal et al.) or with refractory staphylococcal meningitis (Shuman and Smith).

Concentrations of gentamicin within the ventricular system considerably higher than the MIC of sensitive organisms can be obtained by direct intraventricular instillation of the drug. Using doses of 5 mg. in older children and adults, Kaiser and McGee were able to achieve ventricular concentrations of 12.8 to 40 μg./ml. in the first six hours, with levels of 4 to 6 μg./ml. persisting in most for up to 24 hours. Pickering et al. injected 1 mg. of gentamicin intraventricularly in children with shunt meningitis and were able to obtain ventricular concentrations of over 20 μg./ml. in one hour and 8 to 14 μg./ml. 36 hours following its administration. Therapeutic intraventricular levels 20 to 24 hours following ventricular injection of 2 mg. of gentamicin were also demonstrated in neonates with meningitis by Lee et al. These studies, as well as the reported therapeutic responses, clearly indicate the superiority of direct intraventricular injection of aminoglycosides compared to the intralumbar instillation of the drug.

The disadvantages of intraventricular therapy include the technical difficulty in entering the lateral ventricle by transfontanel tap in the infant who, in the early stages of meningitis, is likely to have cerebral swelling. In older children or adults, intraventricular antibiotic treatment requires a burr hole or the placement of a ventricular reservoir, the latter possibly becoming colonized during the course of therapy. Intraventricular injection of antibiotics is less complicated in the previously shunted child in whom the shunt allows ready access to the ventricular system. In general, intraventricular gentamicin has been found to be well tolerated with little evidence of toxicity (Lee et al., Kaiser and McGee, Pickering et al.), although the possibility of adverse effects has not been extensively investigated. Watanabe et al. injected gentamicin with preservative in high dosage (2.5 to 5 mg. per kilogram) intracisternally in rabbits, which provoked seizures and respiratory arrest. The cervical spinal cord in the treated animals revealed myelin and axonal injury in addition to glial cell depletion. Similar pathologic changes in the brain stem of a patient with meningitis treated with intrathecal gentamicin were reported from the same institution (Watanabe et al.).

The most important adverse effects of gentamicin, as with other aminoglycosides, are ototoxicity and nephrotoxicity. Eighth nerve dysfunction is believed to be related to peak serum levels and, perhaps, to the total cumulative dose, but is not believed to occur with short-term therapy in which serum concentrations are kept below 12 μg./ml. Finitze-Hieber et al. evaluated by follow-up a large number of children who received gentamicin in the newborn period and could not find evidence of cochlear or vestibular injury secondary to the drug therapy. Initial damage from gentamicin is believed to be primarily on the vestibular portion of the eighth nerve (McGee et al., Meyers), although cochlear injury resulting in hearing loss has been observed (Dayal et al.).

The precise mechanism by which gentamicin impairs renal function is not known; however, the proximal renal tubule is believed to be the primary site of injury (Cronin). Despite this, the commonly used studies to monitor renal function in treated patients include urinalysis and the serum creatinine and creatinine clearance, methods which provide little early warning of proximal tubular damage (Schentag et al. 1979). Rising trough serum concentrations of gentamicin in a patient on a stable dose without renal insufficiency have also been found to be suggestive evidence of impending nephrotoxicity (Schentag et al. 1978). Signs of nephrotoxicity warrant discontinuation of the drug, which is usually followed by rapid recovery. Of interest are the results of experimental studies which have shown that animals that recover from drug-induced acute renal tubular injury are resistant to a second nephrotoxic insult from the same drug (Luft et al.). The applicability of this observation to humans in uncertain, although it indicates that aminoglycosides are not contraindicated in a child who has had previous nephrotoxicity from this group of drugs.

The dose of gentamicin for infants less than one week of age is 5 mg. per kilogram per day administered intramuscularly in divided doses every 12 hours. Between one week and two months of age, the dose is 7.5 mg. per kilogram per day in divided doses every eight hours. Beyond two months of age, the dose of gentamicin is 5 mg. per kilogram per day given every eight hours. This, like other aminoglycosides, is usually given by intramuscular injection, but when necessary it can be injected intravenously over not less than a 20-minute period. When instilled directly into the ventricular system, the dose in infants and children is 1 to 3 mg., depending on the ventricular capacity. The drug is optimally used in conjunction with serum level determinations, especially in the patient with renal insufficiency (Sirinavin et al.). Peak serum levels should be drawn at the end of an intravenous infusion or 30 to 60 minutes following an intramuscular dose. Trough levels should be assessed just before the administration of the next dose. Optimal therapeutic peak serum levels are between 4 and 10 μg./ml. and should not be allowed to exceed 10 μg./ml. to avoid ototoxicity. Laboratory determinations of renal function should be done before initiation of gentamicin therapy and periodically during its administration.

Chloramphenicol

Chloramphenicol was isolated from *Streptomyces venezuelae* in 1947 and soon thereafter became the first so-called broad-spectrum antibiotic to be synthesized. The drug became commercially available in 1949 and rapidly achieved popularity for use by both the oral and the intravenous route for the treatment of a variety of childhood infections. Its widescale use in all ages in childhood was subsequently curtailed to some degree with the recognition of the possible occurrence of aplastic anemia secondary to oral administration of the drug and the identification of the "gray baby syndrome" caused by excessively high serum levels as a result of diminished hepatic conjugation in the newborn and young infant.

The available parenteral preparation, chloramphenicol sodium succinate, is not adequately absorbed after intramuscular injection and thus should be given only intravenously. The succinate salt itself does not have antibacterial activity and becomes effective only after hydrolysis to chloramphenicol base in the liver and in other tissues. Its antimicrobial activity is largely on the basis of inhibition of bacterial ribosomal protein synthesis. Chloramphenicol is generally classified as a bacteriostatic antibiotic; however, in concentrations readily achievable in tissues and body fluids, it has been shown to be bactericidal against *Hemophilus influenzae, Neisseria meningitidis* and, to a lesser extent, *Streptococcus pneumoniae* (Rahal and Simberkoff). Because the latter two organisms are severalfold more susceptible to the bactericidal action of penicillin than to that of chloramphenicol, the latter drug is considered only an alternative choice when the more effective agent cannot be used.

Following the report by Leeper and Dowling in 1951 which showed that there was antagonism between penicillin and aureomycin when used against *Streptococcus pneumoniae,* there arose the concept that the combined use of an antibiotic considered to be bactericidal with one which is bacteriostatic can result in an antagonistic effect when used against certain organisms. The clinical significance of this type of drug interaction has remained somewhat speculative, although studies have supported the existence of antag-

onism between penicillin and chloramphenicol when used against some strains of the pneumococcus, the meningococcus, and other organisms, but not against *Hemophilus influenzae* (Feldman and Zweighaft, Rahal, Wallace et al.), for which ampicillin and chloramphenicol may even be synergistic in some instances (Feldman). This antagonistic effect appears to be greatest when chloramphenicol administration precedes that of penicillin and can be diminished by the administration of penicillin first to be followed by chloramphenicol one hour or more later.

There is also evidence that chloramphenicol can interfere with the bactericidal effect of gentamicin against certain gram-negative enteropathogens (Paisley and Washington). In addition, drug interactions between chloramphenicol and certain anticonvulsants can be of clinical importance in the management of children with meningitis. Phenobarbital has been stated to enhance chloramphenicol metabolism by induction of hepatic microsomal enzymes, leading to a reduced serum level of the antimicrobial (Bloxham et al.). Conversely, chloramphenicol is believed to retard the biotransformation of phenytoin, increasing its serum level and possibly resulting in phenytoin toxicity (Christensen and Skovsted, Rose et al.).

Chloramphenicol is extensively metabolized within the body so that only a small amount of the unchanged drug is excreted in the urine. Glucuronide conjugation in the liver results in the principal metabolite which is secreted by the kidneys. The presence of hepatic failure can markedly diminish the rate of conjugation and can possibly lead to elevated levels of the drug.

Chloramphenicol readily penetrates brain and CSF, which is one of the characteristics of the drug which makes it attractive for treatment of neurologic infections caused by sensitive organisms. Entrance of the drug into CSF occurs with or without meningeal inflammation, a feature that is sometimes of importance in patients with localized parenchymal or meningeal suppurative lesions without widespread meningeal involvement. It is generally stated that the CSF concentration of chloramphenicol is at least one-half of the simultaneous serum level, although investigations have demonstrated considerable variation from patient to patient. In a series of children, most without meningitis, Friedman et al. found the average CSF concentration of chloramphenicol to be 67 percent of the simultaneous serum concentration, with a range from 45 to 99 percent. Dunkle studied the ventricular and lumbar CSF in infants less than 1,500 grams with meningitis and recorded mean levels of the drug to be 66.5 percent of the peak serum levels. Yogev and Williams observed that peak serum levels occurred 30 minutes after completion of intravenous infusion, while peak ventricular fluid levels of chloramphenicol were achieved three hours after intravenous infusion. They found that it is not possible to accurately predict what ventricular fluid level of chloramphenicol will be achieved from a given serum level, and in some instances, the dose administered must be increased to bring CSF levels within the therapeutic range. That serum levels of chloramphenicol can extend from the subtherapeutic range to a potentially toxic level following a given, presumably adequate, therapeutic intravenous dose has been well documented (Black et al., Robinson et al.). These findings indicate the importance of serum level measurements whenever possible. In patients with meningitis caused by chloramphenicol-sensitive organisms who do not show anticipated clinical or CSF improvement, CSF level determinations of the drug can be an important refinement in the management.

The first serious adverse effects of chloramphenicol to be recognized were those involving the bone marrow. The drug was found to have two different, and presumably unrelated, bone marrow effects, the first being a dose-related, reversible bone marrow suppression and the second an idiosyncratic, delayed aplastic state. Some degree of bone marrow suppression has been found to be almost constant with chloramphenicol therapy after the fifth or sixth day of treatment in patients with serum levels greater than 25 μg./ml. It is a reversible process, with reversion of the laboratory abnormalities back to normal usually within two weeks after the drug is discontinued. Dose-related chloramphenicol bone marrow suppression is initially a depression of erythropoiesis reflected by a drop in the reticulocyte count and later by a decline in the hemoglobin concentration. Bone marrow examination at this time reveals a normocellular marrow or some degree of hypocellularity with vacuoles in erythroid precursors. When treatment is prolonged, the platelet count may decline somewhat but not usually to profoundly low levels. Neutropenia can eventually occur but is infrequent (Oski). This dose-related bone marrow effect of chloramphenicol is believed to be secondary to inhibition of mitochondrial protein synthesis and should be watched for by periodic reticulocyte counts, platelets counts, and hemoglobin determinations in any child receiving the drug. While the pathogenesis of this transient hematopoietic depression is generally believed to be different from that of the rare aplastic state, Daum et al. have described a patient in whom fatal aplastic anemia appeared to be a progression of chloramphenicol dose-related bone marrow suppression.

Aplastic anemia is regarded to be an idiosyncratic reaction which is not related to the dose and has been described in some cases with only very brief exposure to the drug. The onset of bone marrow failure occurs weeks to many months thereafter and is often gradually progressive, leading to death. The danger of this complication and the high fatality rate therefrom was widely recognized as early as 1952 (Claudon and Halbrook, Smiley et al., Rheingold and Spurling, Sturgeon). The estimated risk of development of aplastic anemia secondary to chloramphenicol has varied widely from one in 20,000 to one in 60,000 courses of therapy (Smick et al., Wallerstein et al.).

Holt, in 1967, stated that he could find no recorded case of aplastic anemia caused by chloramphenicol administered other than by the oral route. This led to the speculation that perhaps the toxic effect on the bone marrow is secondary to a degradation product of the drug in the gastrointestinal tract and thus might not be expected to occur in patients who receive the drug only by intravenous administration. This possibility cannot be entirely disregarded, although the recent unusual patient described by Daum et al. in which dose-related bone marrow depression progressed to fatal aplastic anemia did receive chloramphenicol exclusively by the intravenous route. It is, no doubt, true that the great majority of cases of chloramphenicol-induced aplastic anemia have followed the oral use of the drug; however, for a number of years, the vast majority of doses of the drug that were administered were by this route. There are also rare reports of aplastic anemia induced by chloramphenicol that was eventually followed by the development of acute myeloblastic leukemia (Brauer and Dameshek).

The disorder in newborn infants which came to be known as the "gray baby syndrome" was first reported by Sutherland in Cincinnati in 1959. The history and the early identification of this complication of chloramphenicol therapy has recently been summarized by Lietman. Beginning in approximately 1957, it became common practice to give prophylactic antibiotics to premature and full-term newborn infants, especially when there had been premature rupture of membranes or other perinatal complications. Chloramphenicol given orally or intramuscularly was often selected, and the dose range for term as well as for low-birth-weight infants varied from 100 to 264 mg. per kilogram per day. A sharp increase in mortality among neonates managed in this fashion was soon observed. A number of investigators almost simultaneously recognized the association of a shock-like state in infants receiving high-dose chloramphenicol leading to high serum levels, presumably secondary to the limited hepatic capacity to conjugate the drug, characteristic of the neonate (Burns et al., Lambdin et al., Lischner et al., Sutherland). In retrospect, the occurrence of chloramphenicol-induced vascular collapse in newborn infants had probably been observed as early as 1951, although the cause-and-effect relationship could not be made at that early date (Epstein et al.).

With the recognition that the disorder was caused by chloramphenicol and that excessively high serum levels in newborn infants were explained by the immaturity of hepatic glucuronyl transferase, resulting in diminished conjugation of chloramphenicol to the acid glucuronide, the use of the drug was curtailed in the newborn period and a more appropriate dose regimen was designed. In addition, the importance of serum level measurements became obvious whenever the drug is used in early infancy or in patients with hepatic dysfunction. The "gray baby syndrome" was eventually noted to correlate with chloramphenicol serum levels of greater than 50 μg./ml., resulting in the recommendation that peak levels must be maintained well below this value. It is now known that the condition is not limited to the neonatal period but can occur in any age group if serum levels are sufficiently high (Craft et al.). The toxic effect of excessive chloramphenicol serum concentrations, giving rise to shock and other symptoms, is believed to be related to a disturbance of mitochondrial electron transport (Hallman). The restricted use of chloramphenicol in the newborn infant has dramatically reduced the occurrence of this toxic reaction although it is still en-

countered on the basis of errors in dosage calculation.

The first manifestations of the "gray baby syndrome" characteristically begin three to four days after initiation of chloramphenicol therapy and include abdominal distention, vomiting, hypothermia, lethargy, and the appearance of an ashen color. Hypotension, acidosis, and respiratory distress will be followed by death one to three days later unless the drug is discontinued and treatment initiated. Treatment includes the immediate cessation of administration of the drug and efforts to correct acidosis and improve tissue perfusion. Peritoneal dialysis and hemodialysis do not effectively remove chloramphenicol from the circulation, while multiple exchange transfusions have been successful in some instances (Kessler et al.). Mauer et al. demonstrated rapid clearing of chloramphenicol with charcoal-column hemoperfusion in one successfully treated patient.

Other possible adverse effects of chloramphenicol administered intravenously include cutaneous rash and drug fever, although these are considerably less frequent than occurs with the penicillin preparations. Optic neuritis with visual loss has been described from prolonged use of chloramphenicol, as once was customary for children with cystic fibrosis (Chang et al., Cocke et al., Huang et al.).

Chloramphenicol is the drug of choice for treatment of meningitis caused by β-lactamase–positive *Hemophilus influenzae* and for patients with this illness who are allergic to the penicillins and thus cannot be given ampicillin. It is also the preferred drug in those with pneumococcal or meningococcal meningitis who are intolerant of penicillin. It is frequently the most effective antimicrobial for meningitis or intracranial abscesses caused by penicillin-resistant anaerobic infections, especially when caused by *Bacteroides fragilis*. Chloramphenicol in combination with methicillin or nafcillin is often the initial antibiotic regimen in infants and children with brain abscesses, orbital cellulitis, or cavernous sinus thrombosis, until the causative organism is isolated and sensitivity studies are completed. It is the drug of choice for treatment of Rocky Mountain spotted fever in children and is frequently the most effective drug in cases with *Salmonella* species meningitis. The use of chloramphenicol in the treatment of neonatal *Escherichia coli* meningitis is debatable and can only be considered if accurate serum level measurements are available. It is believed to be only bacteriostatic against gram-negative enteropathogens and has been shown to antagonize the bactericidal activity of gentamicin against certain gram-negative rods (Paisley and Washington, Strausbaugh and Sande). Chloramphenicol in combination with ampicillin has been used in some cases in gram-negative neonatal meningitis which showed no response to ampicillin and gentamicin therapy.

The intravenous dose of chloramphenicol is that amount required to obtain peak serum levels in the safe and therapeutic range of 15 to 25 μg./ml. The drug is commonly used in infants beyond two months of age and in children without the assistance of serum level determinations but is hazardous without serum level determinations in newborn infants or in children with significant hepatic dysfunction. For full-term infants in the first seven days after birth and for premature infants in the first month of life, the recommended intravenous dose is 25 mg. per kilogram per day given in divided doses every six hours. For full-term infants one to four weeks of age, the dose is 50 mg. per kilogram per day and after four weeks the dose is 100 mg. per kilogram per day in patients with adequate liver function.

Penicillins

The penicillin preparations have remained the most widely used class of antimicrobials for treatment of septic neurologic infections since their introduction into clinical medicine in 1941 (Abraham et al.). Their remarkable antimicrobial effect, first demonstrated in vitro by Fleming in 1929 against staphylococci, is attributable to interference by the antibiotic with the synthesis of bacterial cell wall mucopeptides. The penicillins contain a β-lactam ring and, except for certain of the semisynthetic preparations, are inactivated by an enzyme (penicillinase) elaborated by a variety of organisms which causes opening of the β-lactam structure. In addition to aqueous penicillin G, the currently available preparations for serious invasive infections include the semisynthetic penicillinase-resistant penicillins, such as methicillin, nafcillin, oxacillin, and dicloxacillin, and the so-called extended spectrum penicillins, such as ampicillin, carbenicillin, ticarcillin, and amoxicillin. Like penicillin G, those in the extended spectrum group are inactivated by penicillinase and thus are not effective against penicillinase-producing staphylococci.

The degree of protein binding in serum of different penicillins has been found to vary widely. Serum protein binding is least with ampicillin (20 to 30 percent) and methicillin (30 to 40 percent), intermediate with penicillin G (60 to 70 percent), high with nafcillin and oxacillin (89 to 95 percent), and highest with dicloxacillin (98 percent) (Kunin). The electrolyte content of the penicillin preparations is also variable and can be an important factor in certain patients when large intravenous doses are given. The potassium salt of benzylpenicillin contains 1.7 mEq. of potassium per one million units and is not a significant factor unless a large amount is given by very rapid intravenous injection. The sodium content of sodium penicillin G is 2.0 mEq. per one million units, of ampicillin is 3.4 mEq. per gram, and of carbenicillin is 4.7 mEq. per gram (Weinstein). Large doses can lead to sodium overload, especially in patients with renal failure or uncontrolled cardiac failure.

Penicillin G is the drug of choice for meningitis caused by Group B *Streptococcus, Streptococcus pneumoniae, Neisseria meningitidis,* Group A *Streptococcus,* nonpenicillinase-producing *Staphylococcus* species, *Treponema pallidum,* and the rare cases caused by *Pasteurella multocida* and *Neisseria gonorrhoeae.* It is effective against most anaerobic bacteria except for *Bacteroides fragilis,* and is active for most strains of non-enterococcal Group D *Streptococcus.* Ampicillin is generally the preferred antibiotic for treatment of meningitis due to β-lactamase-negative *Hemophilus influenzae, Listeria monocytogenes, Proteus mirabilis,* and *Salmonella* species. Ampicillin in combination with an aminoglycoside is synergistic for meningeal infections resulting from sensitive Enterobacteriaceae and enterococcal Group D *Streptococcus* (Kaplan et al. 1974). Methicillin or nafcillin are the drugs of primary importance for penicillinase-producing staphylococcal infections and are often given in combination with chloramphenicol for intracranial abscesses, septic orbital cellulitis, or cavernous sinus thrombosis, until the causative organism is isolated. Carbenicillin in combination with gentamicin or amikacin represents the treatment of choice in most instances for meningitis caused by *Pseudomonas* species and indole-positive *Proteus* species.

While susceptibility of most penicillin-sensitive bacteria that cause meningitis has been retained after many years of utilization of the drug, the biologic behavior of *Streptococcus pneumoniae* has recently begun to change. The pneumococcus was for years found to be invariably sensitive to penicillin with MIC's in the range of 0.01 to 0.1 μg./ml., but in 1967 a relatively less sensitive strain was isolated from a patient in Australia (Hansman and Bullen). Thereafter, additional although infrequent reports appeared of pneumococcal isolates with decreased susceptibility to penicillin from patients with poorly responding or relapsing meningitis (Ahronheim et al., Appelbaum et al., Naraqi et al.). Of these isolates, the MIC's of penicillin were 0.2 to 1 μg./ml., levels approximately equal to the CSF concentrations that could be achieved with conventional intravenous doses, and thus a suboptimal response would be expected. More recently, pneumococcal isolates fully resistant to penicillin with MIC's of 1 to 4 μg./ml. have been identified (Cates et al., Jacobs et al.). The mechanism accounting for penicillin-resistance among pneumococci is unclear but is not on the basis of β-lactamase production.

An additional observation that has been made in recent years is the occasional in vivo failure of penicillin in conventional doses to rapidly eradicate Group B *Streptococcus* from CSF (Edwards et al.). Although Group B *Streptococcus* is known to have a wide range of susceptibilities to penicillin and is less sensitive than Group A *Streptococcus,* it had been assumed that penicillin in sufficient concentration could readily be achieved in CSF to result in bacterial killing. One suggestion to explain the occurrence of unyielding meningeal infection to penicillin therapy is that there may be as much as a 10-fold discrepancy between the MIC and the MBC (minimum bactericidal concentration) of penicillin for Group B *Streptococcus* (Allen and Sprunt). The occurrence of an inadequate response to penicillin therapy has been sufficiently common that higher doses are now recommended for this infection in the newborn infant than are used for other infections in this age group.

Penicillin G (benzylpenicillin), like most other penicillins, undergoes rapid excretion, resulting in a short half-life in serum following intravenous administration. The half-life correlates inversely with postnatal age and creatinine clearance. In newborn infants less than six days of age, the half-life of penicillin was found by McCracken et al. (1973) to be approximately 3.2 hours. In infants beyond 14 days, the half-life is 1.4 hours while in older children it is the range of 30 minutes. Because of its rapid renal excretion, penicillin G should be administered intravenously at intervals of approximately four hours. Each infusion should be over a 20-minute time period. This rate of infusion helps avoid the risk of inactivation of penicillin in solutions that might be alkaline (Simberkoff et al.). Regardless of the infusion rate, penicillin should not be mixed in the same bottle with sodium bicarbonate. Likewise, the penicillins, and especially carbenicillin, should not be mixed with gentamicin, since the latter can be inactivated if combined with large quantities of these drugs (Noone and Pattison).

Rapid, bolus injection of penicillin G can be hazardous because of the electrolyte content of the material. The potassium salt of penicillin which is commonly stocked in hospitals contains 1.7 mEq. of potassium per each one million units. When it is elected to administer a loading dose of penicillin to a child with fulminating meningitis, and especially if there is renal failure, the potassium content of the total dose must be taken into consideration. Excessively rapid infusion of a large quantity of potassium-containing penicillin can result in acute hyperkalemia with cardiac arrest. For this reason, so-called loading doses should be administered over 30 to 60 minutes and conventional intravenous doses should be given over a period of not less than 20 minutes. Loading doses should probably not be used in children with acute renal failure.

Penicillin G is transported from serum to CSF very poorly when the meninges are uninflamed, reaching CSF concentrations only 1 to 2 percent of those in the serum (Plorde et al., Rammelkamp and Keefer, Ruedy). With meningeal inflammation, however, there is considerable enhancement of the penetration of penicillin into the CSF. With intravenous doses of penicillin of 250,000 units per kilogram per day for children with suppurative meningitis, Hieber and Nelson found mean CSF concentrations of 0.8 μg./ml., 0.7 μg./ml., and 0.3 μg./ml. on the first, fifth, and tenth day of treatment respectively. These levels represented 18.4, 9.9, and 3.4 percent of the simultaneous serum levels, and indicate the decline of penicillin entry into the CSF corresponding to the subsidence of the meningeal and vascular inflammatory reaction during the course of treatment. Even by the tenth day, when the CSF concentrations of penicillin had diminished, the amount was still 25 to 50 times the customary MIC of penicillin-sensitive microorganisms (Hieber and Nelson).

The penicillin concentration in the CSF is determined by the equilibrium between the rate of entry and the rate of removal of the drug. The rate of entry of the lipid-insoluble molecule is significantly affected by the structural integrity of the meninges and the meningeal blood vessels. Its clearance is in part on the basis of usual bulk flow of CSF through the arachnoid villi into the venous sinuses and in part the result of an active transport system within the choroid plexuses which clears penicillin and other organic acids (Dixon et al., Spector and Lorenzo). Probenecid, which increases serum levels of penicillin by inhibiting its renal excretion and by competing with penicillin for common binding sites on serum protein, thus increasing the level of freely diffusible penicillin (Fishman), can also block the choroid plexus transport mechanism, resulting in an increase in the CSF penicillin concentration (Craft et al., Dacey and Sande, Walters et al.). The therapeutic implications of probenecid for this purpose are limited, owing to its possible adverse effects; however, the principle may be important and deserves further investigation.

Benzylpenicillin, like all of the penicillins, is a notable cause of allergic reactions, most of which are transient cutaneous rashes of one type or another. Serum sickness and anaphylaxis are considerably less common but are more threatening. Hematologic reactions and nephrotoxicity are more common with the penicillinase-resistant penicillins than with penicillin G. Penicillin neurotoxicity was recognized as early as 1945 when a child with hydrocephalus abruptly developed seizures and coma soon after the direct injection of 50,000 units of penicillin into the lateral ventricle (Johnson and Walker). Similar cases manifested by seizures, coma, and death following large intrathecal doses of penicillin were observed soon thereafter (Cohen, Neymann et al.), although it was not recognized until more recently that penicillin neurotoxic reactions could result from systemic administration.

The circumstances in common in most of the reported cases of penicillin neurotoxicity following intravenous administration of the drug have included very high doses, over 50 million units per day in most instances, the presence of renal insufficiency, or simultaneous treatment with probenicid (Lerner et al., New and Wells, Oldstone and Nelson, Raichle et al.). The encephalopathy is manifested by mental confusion, hyperreflexia, and myoclonus that is usually first observed in the facial muscles. If the disorder progresses, generalized convulsions and coma supervene (Seamans et al.). Myoclonus is considered to be characteristic of penicillin-induced neurotoxicity and may have its origin from multiple sites in the central nervous system, including the caudal brain stem and spinal cord, as well as higher centers (Sackellares and Smith).

The penicillinase-resistant semisynthetic penicillins are of primary importance because of their activity against penicillinase-producing *Staphylococcus* species. They are less effective than benzylpenicillin for most other penicillin-sensitive bacteria and also possess greater toxicity than the parent compound. Except for methicillin, this group of penicillins is more highly protein-bound in serum, one factor that has been claimed to limit their antimicrobial action. Methicillin and nafcillin are the most widely used preparations for treatment of benzylpenicillin-resistant invasive staphylococcal infections, while dicloxacillin is generally reserved for those conditions in which oral therapy is sufficient.

Methicillin (dimethoxyphenyl penicillin) was introduced for clinical use in 1959 and was the first available penicillin preparation effective against penicillinase-producing *Staphylococcus* species. Initially, methicillin-resistant staphylococci were only infrequently discovered but, with the passage of time, their prevalence gradually increased (Parker and Hewitt). *Staphylococcus* species resistant to methicillin are also resistant to benzylpenicillin and usually to other penicillinase-resistant penicillins. Methicillin is rapidly eliminated by renal excretion. Sarff et al. found the serum half-life of methicillin to range from 2.8 to 3.1 hours in premature infants less than two weeks of age, and to be 1.1 hours in term infants three to six weeks of age. The half-life is even shorter in older children with normal renal function. Similar findings of the pharmacokinetics of the drug were described by Axline et al. Little is known regarding penetration of methicillin into CSF with meningitis, although the available information suggests that the concentrations achieved are usually below or barely equal to the MIC of penicillinase-producing staphylococci (Oppenheimer et al.). Methicillin is inactivated in acid solutions and thus should be administered intravenously over a time period of not more than 20 minutes at intervals of every four hours.

The precise incidence of side effects of methicillin in children is not known. Adverse reactions that have been observed include rash, drug fever, eosinophilia, and, rarely, neutropenia (Yow et al. 1976). Nephropathy is the best known of the side effects of methicillin, although its pathogenesis is poorly understood (Feigin and Fiascone). Methicillin nephropathy has been considered to be a direct toxic reaction by some, but its frequent association with rash and eosinophilia, in addition to the results of immune studies on renal tissue, supports the concept that it is a hypersensitivity response (Border et al., Sanjad et al.). Histologic examination of renal biopsy material from patients with methicillin nephropathy has revealed an interstitial nephritis but without glomerular abnormalities or arteritis (Baldwin et al., Sanjad et al.). The disorder is usually manifested by microscopic or gross hematuria, cylindruria, and a rise in blood urea nitrogen. Recovery is expected with termination of methicillin therapy.

Nafcillin was introduced in 1963 and differs from other penicillins in that only 20 percent or less undergoes renal excretion, while the major fraction of an administered dose is excreted by the liver into the biliary system. Renal failure does not significantly affect the half-life of the drug (Diaz et al.), and thus nafcillin may be the drug of choice in the azotemic patient who requires a penicillinase-resistant penicillin. Conversely, the use of nafcillin in the patient with hepatic insufficiency would require dosage adjustments to avoid excessively high serum levels. The half-life of nafcillin in older infants and children with normal liver function has been found to be about 45 minutes (Feldman et al. 1978).

Nafcillin appears to gain entrance into the CSF in greater quantities than other penicillinase-resistant penicillins and has even been found to enter the CSF in measurable amounts when the meninges are uninflamed (Fossieck et al.). With meningeal inflammation, nafcillin administered intravenously has been found to achieve peak CSF levels of 9 percent of the peak serum concentration (Ruiz and Warner). Kane et al. demonstrated that the drug could reach CSF concentrations of three to 100 times the MIC for *Staphylococcus aureus*, findings that may indicate that nafcillin would be superior to methicillin for treatment of penicillinase-producing *Staphylococcus* species meningitis. Possible side ef-

fects of nafcillin include neutropenia, rash, and eosinophilia (Greene and Cohen, Zakhirch and Root), although some feel that such reactions are less common with nafcillin than with methicillin (Kancir et al.). Nephrotoxicity does appear to be decidedly less common with nafcillin.

Oxacillin has been less popular for treatment of meningeal infection caused by benzylpenicillin-resistant staphylococci, in part because there is limited information regarding its pharmacokinetics in infants and children and because there are few data regarding its ability to penetrate into CSF. In addition, the drug appears to have a greater tendency to produce hepatotoxicity than occurs with methicillin or nafcillin (Bruckstein and Attia, Olans and Weiner, Pollock et al.).

Among the so-called extended-spectrum penicillins, ampicillin (alpha-aminobenzyl-penicillin) has been by far the most important for treatment of suppurative meningitis because of the susceptibility of many strains of *Hemophilus influenzae*, *Escherichia coli*, and *Proteus mirabilis*, as well as many of the gram-positive cocci. Until 1974, strains of *Hemophilus influenzae* type b were believed to be consistently sensitive to ampicillin, but the discovery then of resistant isolates compromised the usefulness of the drug as the sole, initial method of treatment of meningitis in patients beyond the neonatal period. The great majority of ampicillin-resistant *Hemophilus influenzae* strains are resistant because of their production of β-lactamase, although recently non-β-lactamase-producing ampicillin-resistant strains have been identified on rare occasion (Bell and Plowman, Markowitz).

Ampicillin in newborn infants results in higher peak serum concentrations in premature than in full-term infants (Kaplan et al. 1974) and has a half-life in serum of 4 hours in infants from birth to 7 days of age, of 2.8 hours from 8 to 14 days of age, and 1.7 hours in infants 15 to 30 days of age (Axline et al.). Kaplan and colleagues (1974) studied the CSF penetration of ampicillin in infants in the early weeks after birth and observed that the highest values in CSF occurred 3 to 7 hours after intravenous administration. CSF concentrations were 11 to 65 percent of the simultaneous serum levels and could not be shown to correlate closely to the degree of meningeal inflammation. In patients two months of age or older, Thrupp et al. (1965) demonstrated that the content of ampicillin in CSF gradually declined during treatment as the CSF returned toward normal. During the first three days of treatment the mean CSF-to-serum ratio was 36 percent, while by the tenth day the mean ratio had decreased to 12 percent.

Adverse reactions to ampicillin are relatively frequent, especially rash and eosinophilia. Of 370 children who received ampicillin reported by Kerns et al. and of 422 patients described by Shapiro and colleagues, rash occurred in approximately 9.5 percent. Macular or maculopapular rashes provoked by ampicillin do not imply that the patient is allergic to the penicillin class of drugs and does not necessarily require termination of ampicillin therapy. This is especially true in patients with infectious mononucleosis in whom there is a very high incidence of rash when exposed to ampicillin. Urticarial rashes or erythema multiforme bullosa secondary to ampicillin occurs much less frequently and indicates penicillin allergy, requiring that the drug be stopped. Interstitial nephritis (Ruley and Lisi) and bone marrow suppression (Graf and Tarlov) have been described with ampicillin therapy but are very unusual complications.

Carbenicillin (disodium alpha carboxybenzylpenicillin) administered intravenously has a spectrum similar to that of ampicillin, except for its activity against *Pseudomonas aeruginosa* and indole-positive *Proteus* species (Bodey et al., Nelson 1970, Ross et al.). It is much more expensive than ampicillin and, like the latter, is inactivated by β-lactamase although at a slower rate. Because of a synergistic effect of carbenicillin in combination with gentamicin against *Pseudomonas aeruginosa*, both drugs are recommended for infections caused by this organism. In the newborn, carbenicillin, like other penicillins, has a serum half-life inversely related to age and weight. For infants under 2000 grams, the mean half-life is approximately 6 hours while in neonates over 2500 grams, the mean half-life is 3.5 hours (Nelson and McCracken 1973). The half-life is shorter in older infants and children owing to rapid renal excretion of the drug. There is little available information regarding how well carbenicillin gains entrance into the CSF. Carbenicillin has been reported to result in anicteric hepatitis on rare occasion (Wilson et al.) and also fairly consistently disturbs platelet aggregation, which can result in clinical bleeding (Brown et al.). Large doses of carbenicillin leading to very high serum levels in patients with renal compromise can result in systemic acidosis (Whelton et al.).

Ticarcillin is very similar to carbenicillin in all respects, including its pharmacokinetics (Nelson et al. 1978) and its activity against *Pseudomonas aeruginosa*. Preliminary studies have indicated that ticarcillin plus tobramycin is, perhaps, superior to the combination of carbenicillin and gentamicin for the treatment of infections caused by *Pseudomonas aeruginosa* (Parry and Neu). Like carbenicillin, ticarcillin can inactivate aminoglycosides if mixed together for intravenous infusion (Murillo et al.).

Metronidazole

Metronidazole (Flagyl) is a nitroimidazole antimicrobial first introduced in 1959 for treatment of *Trichomonas vaginalis* infections. The drug was subsequently shown to be effective against *Entamoeba histolytica* and highly so with bactericidal activity against most obligatory anaerobic microorganisms (Tally et al.). It has been used successfully for serious infections caused by *Bacteroides* species, *Fusobacterium* species, and other anaerobic organisms. *Bacteroides fragilis,* an anaerobe characteristically resistant to penicillin, is almost consistently sensitive to metronidazole. The drug is well absorbed after oral administration with peak serum levels achieved between one and two hours after ingestion. The average serum half-life is approximately eight hours and the drug is minimally protein-bound (Ralph et al.). The compound diffuses well into tissues and has excellent penetration into CSF following oral administration.

Metronidazole is not considered the primary drug for infections of the central nervous system caused by anaerobic organisms and is still considered to be in the investigational stage for this purpose. It has, however, been found to be of considerable value in patients with meningitis or brain abscess caused by *Bacteroides fragilis,* and occasionally other anaerobes, when the organism is resistant to penicillin and the response to chloramphenicol is suboptimal (Feldman, Ingham et al., Peterson et al., Warner et al.). Metronidazole has been used successfully for treatment of *Bacteroides* species meningitis in very-low-birth-weight premature infants by Berman et al. and Warner et al. The drug also has recently been recommended to be the treatment of choice for *Entamoeba histolytica* liver abscess (Harrison et al.) and, perhaps, the same would apply to brain abscess produced by this parasite, in conjunction with surgical management. Amebic brain abscess is a life-threatening condition and would warrant the use of metronidazole despite the caution that has been advanced relative to its use generally. Most strains of *Bacteroides fragilis* have minimum inhibitory concentrations of 6 μg./ml. or lower for metronidazole (Nastro and Finegold), a level easily exceeded in blood and CSF with oral administration. Ralph et al. found CSF concentrations of metronidazole of 13.9 and 11.0 μg./ml. two and eight hours after a single 500 mg. dose in an adult with meningitis.

Metronidazole is generally well tolerated, with serious adverse reactions being infrequent. Side effects that have been described include gastrointestinal disturbances, urticaria, reversible neutropenia, bitter taste, and dark urine (Sanders et al.). There has been concern over experimental studies which have shown that metronidazole is both carcinogenic in some animals and mutagenic in bacteria (Rosenkranz and Speck, Rustia and Shubik). A study in humans failed to confirm carcinogenic effects of the drug, although the follow-up period was not prolonged (Beard et al.). Further investigations will be required to clarify the degree of risk that may be associated with clinical use of the drug. Until there is better understanding of the possible long-term effects of metronidazole, it is advised that the drug be used only when absolutely necessary and after other more commonly used antimicrobial agents have been shown to be inadequate.

The optimal dosage of metronidazole for treatment of invasive neurologic infections has not been well defined but most reports describe adult oral doses of 1,500 to 2,000 mg. per day given in divided doses every six to eight hours. A pediatric dosage likewise has not been established but observations in adults would suggest that an oral dose of 30 to 40 mg. per kilogram per day in divided doses every six to eight hours would be expected to result in CSF levels of better than 10 μg./ml. (Berman et al.). To this date, the drug in this country is available only in an oral preparation.

Rifampin

Rifampin is among the rifamycin group of antimicrobials which are produced by *Streptomyces mediterranei*. Rifampin is a fat-soluble molecule which is chemically unlike other commonly used antibiotics and acts by inhibiting RNA synthesis. It is very well absorbed when taken by the oral route and peak serum levels are achieved approximately two hours after ingestion (Dans et al.). The drug penetrates tissues reasonably well, and in patients with tuberculous meningitis, the CSF concentration has been found to be approximately 20 percent of the serum concentration, which is about equal to the fraction of the drug that is not protein-bound in serum (D'Oliveira). The disadvantages of rifampin include the lack of availability of a parenteral preparation, its expense relative to most other antibiotics, and the rapid emergence of resistant organisms when the drug is used alone.

Rifampin has been clearly shown to be a very effective antituberculous drug and now is included with isoniazid and other drugs for the treatment of tuberculous meningitis. It is particularly important in patients with isoniazid-resistant tuberculous organisms, but here, also, it should be used in combination with other drugs. Rifampin has been found to be useful in treatment of sulfone-resistant cases of leprosy and, unlike other available anti-leprosy drugs, it has bactericidal activity against *Mycobacterium leprae* (Rees et al.).

The drug is now the primary choice for chemoprophylaxis of household and other intimate contacts of a patient with meningococcal disease (McCormick and Bennett) and has recently been considered for prophylaxis for young children directly exposed to a patient with *Hemophilus influenzae* meningitis. While the drug is quite effective for meningococcal prophylaxis, it is important that it not be used for treatment of meningococcal disease so that wide-scale resistance is not brought about. The brief, two-day prophylactic regimen is not believed to significantly contribute to the development of resistant strains.

Rifampin is one of the few drugs to which *Flavobacterium meningosepticum* is susceptible (Aber et al., Rios et al.) and the drug can have a role in combination with erythromycin in the treatment of meningitis caused by this organism. Methicillin-resistant *Staphylococcus* species shunt infection is another condition indicating consideration of rifampin therapy in combination with a second antimicrobial, such as vancomycin (Archer et al., Ring et al.). Most fungi are resistant to rifampin; however, the combination of amphotericin B and rifampin is synergistic against isolates of *Aspergillus* species and certain other fungi (Kitahara et al., Sanders). The clinical significance of this interaction, if any, remains uncertain.

Adverse reactions to rifampin are not infrequent but most are not severe. Mild side effects include nausea, vomiting, abdominal pain, dizziness, and discoloration of the urine (Aquinas et al., Dans et al.). An acute confusional state has been described but is rare (Pratt). Additional infrequent problems include thrombocytopenia and hemolytic anemia (Lakschmanarayan et al., Poole et al.). Hepatic toxicity is the possible adverse effect of rifampin which creates the greatest concern and can be manifested only by biochemical changes or, rarely, in the form of symptomatic hepatitis (Most and Markle, Scheuer et al.). A remarkable condition referred to as the "red man syndrome" has been described secondary to rifampin overdosage. This consists of signs of hepatic toxicity in addition to red discoloration of the urine and tears, and a "boiled lobster-like" appearance of the skin (Newton and Forrest).

The dose of rifampin for treatment of invasive infections is 15 to 20 mg. per kilogram per day but not over 600 mg. per day. The drug is available only in an oral preparation.

Vancomycin

Vancomycin is produced by the soil actinomycete, *Streptomyces orientalis*. The drug was introduced into clinical use just before the penicillinase-resistant penicillins became available and was promptly displaced by these agents because of their lesser degree of toxicity. With the more recent emergence of methicillin-resistant strains of staphylococci, there has been renewed interest in vancomycin (Cook and Farrar, Geraci). Vancomycin has limited indications and should be used only infrequently in children, but it is an important member of the antibiotic armamentarium under certain select circumstances. Its antibacterial effect is believed to be primarily the result of inhibition of cell-wall synthesis but it does so in a manner different from that of penicillin.

Vancomycin is poorly absorbed from the gastrointestinal tract and is highly irritating when given intramuscularly. Thus, it is administered only by the intravenous route for invasive infections. The half-life is approximately six hours and it is excreted mainly via the kidneys. Diminished renal function can result in progressive increase in toxic effects. Vancomycin is not believed to enter the CSF in significant amounts in patients with normal meninges, but with meningeal inflammation Schaad et al. found the CSF concentration to range from 7 to 21 percent of the simultaneous serum concentration, with a mean of 14 percent.

Vancomycin is bactericidal against most gram-positive cocci, including pneumococci, streptococci, and *Staphylococcus* species. Most gram-negative organisms are resistant. Its primary usefulness for neurologic infections is in the treatment of methicillin-resistant *Staphylococcus* species meningitis or shunt infections (Hawley and Gump). Vancomycin has likewise been recommended for penicillin-resistant corynebacteria CSF shunt infections (Cook and Farrar). The drug would also be a consideration in the very rare case of meningitis caused by the pneumococcus resistant to both penicillin and chloramphenicol or in the patient with pneumococcal meningitis who is allergic to penicillin and becomes severely neutropenic from chloramphenicol. Vancomycin combined with gentamicin has been recommended as a consideration for treatment of Group D enterococcal meningitis in patients intolerant of penicillin (Bayer et al.). Vancomycin given intrathecally along with oral rifampin has also been successfully used for treatment of enterococcal meningitis (Ryan et al.). *Flavobacterium meningosepticum* is usually sensitive to vancomycin, although rifampin and erythromycin are the usual choices for treatment of the rare cases of meningitis caused by this organism (Maderazo et al., Rios et al.).

Vancomycin is considered to be a drug with relatively high toxicity, which is the primary factor restricting its use. Maculopapular rash is common, and Schaad et al. described a high incidence of a transient erythema multiforme–like pruritic eruption which developed during infusion of the drug. Chills, fever, and phlebitis at the site of infusion are additional possible side effects. The toxic reactions of greatest concern include ototoxicity and nephrotoxicity. These are believed to be blood-level-related reactions and indicate the importance of monitoring blood levels of the drug if the procedure is available. It is possible that the combined use of vancomycin and an aminoglycoside can result in additive ototoxic and nephrotoxic effects, and would be especially troublesome when used in a child with renal compromise.

Dosage of vancomycin recommended for central nervous system infections by Schaad et al. is 60 mg. per kilogram per day given intravenously over 60 minutes in divided doses every six hours. They advise serum concentration measurements to maintain the peak serum levels in the safe and therapeutic range of 25 to 40 μg./ml. This is most important in children with renal dysfunction, in whom blood levels can rapidly rise to toxic levels unless closely monitored.

REFERENCES

Aber, R. C., Wennersten, C., and Moellering, R. C., Jr.: Antimicrobial susceptibility of Flavobacterium. Antimicrob. Agents Chemother. 14:483–487, 1978.

Abraham, E. P., and Chain, E.: An enzyme from bacteria able to destroy penicillin. Nature 146:837, 1940.

Abraham, E. P., Chain, E., Fletcher, C. M., Gardner, A. D., Heatley, N. G., Jennings, M. A., and Florey, H. W.: Further observations on penicillin. Lancet 2:177–189, 1941.

Abramsky, O.: Neurological features as presenting manifestations of brucellosis. Eur. Neurol. 15:281–284, 1977.

Ahronheim, G. A., Reich, B., and Marks, M. I.: Penicillin-insensitive pneumococci. Case report and review. Am. J. Dis. Child. 133:187–191, 1979.

Alexander, H. E.: Type "B" anti-influenzal rabbit serum for therapeutic purposes. Proc. Soc. Exp. Biol. Med. 40:313–314, 1939.

Alexander, H. E.: Treatment of bacterial meningitis. Bull. N.Y. Acad. Med. 17:100–115, 1941.

Alexander, H. E., and Leidy, G.: The present status of treatment for influenzae meningitis. Am. J. Med. 2:457–466, 1947.

Alexander, H. E., Ellis, C., and Leidy, G.: Treatment of type-specific Hemophilus influenzae infections in infancy and childhood. J. Pediat. 20:673–698, 1942.

Allen, J. L., and Sprunt, K.: Discrepancy between minimum inhibitory and minimum bactericidal concentrations of penicillin for group A and group B β-hemolytic streptococci. J. Pediat. 93:69–71, 1978.

Appel, G. B., and Neu, H. C.: Gentamicin in 1978. Ann. Intern. Med. 89:528–538, 1978.

Appelbaum, P. C., Bhamjee, A., Scragg, J. N., Hallett, A. F., Bowen, A. J., and Cooper, R. C.: Streptococcus pneumoniae resistant to penicillin and chloramphenicol. Lancet 2:995–997, 1977.

Aquinas, M., Allan, W. G. L., Horsfall, P. A. L., Jenkins, P. K., Hung-Yan, W., Girling, D., Tall, R., and Fox, W.: Adverse reactions to daily and intermittent rifampicin regimens for pulmonary tuberculosis in Hong Kong. Brit. Med. J. 1:765–771, 1972.

Archer, G. L., Tenenbaum, M. J., and Haywood, H. B., III.: Rifampin therapy of staphylococcus epidermidis. Use in infections from indwelling artificial devices. J.A.M.A. 240:751–753, 1978.

Argov, Z., and Mastaglia, F. L.: Disorders of neuromuscular transmission caused by drugs. New Eng. J. Med. 301:409–413, 1979.

Axline, S. G., Yaffe, S. J., and Simon, H. J.: Clinical pharmacology of antimicrobials in premature infants. II. Ampicillin, methicillin, oxacillin, neomycin, and colistin. Pediatrics 39:97–107, 1967.

Ayer, J. B.: Puncture of the cisterna magna. Report of one thousand, nine hundred and eighty-five punctures. J.A.M.A. 81:358–360, 1923.

Baker, C. J., Barrett, F. F., and Clark, D. J.: Incidence of kanamycin resistance among Escherichia coli isolates from neonates. J. Pediat. 84:126–130, 1974.

Baldwin, D. S., Levine, B. B., McCluskey, R. T., and Gallo, G. R.: Renal failure and interstitial nephritis due to penicillin and methicillin. New Eng. J. Med. 279:1245–1252, 1968.

Bayer, A. S., Seidel, J. S., Yoshikawa, T. T., Anthony, B. F., and Guze, L. B.: Group D enterococcal meningitis. Clinical and therapeutic considerations with report of three cases and review of the literature. Arch. Intern. Med. 136:883–886, 1976.

Beard, C. M., Noller, K. L., O'Fallon, W. M., Kurland, L. T., and Dockerty, M. B.: Lack of evidence for cancer due to use of metronidazole. New Eng. J. Med. 301:519–522, 1979.

Beaty, H. N., and Walters, E.: Pharmacokinetics of cefamandole and ampicillin in experimental meningitis. Antimicrob. Agents Chemother. 16:584–588, 1979.

Bell, S. M., and Plowman, D.: Mechanisms of ampicillin resistance in Haemophilus influenzae from respiratory tract. Lancet 1:279–280, 1980.

Berman, B. W., King, F. H., Jr., Rubinstein, D. S., and Long, S. S.: Bacteroides fragilis meningitis in a neonate successfully treated with metronidazole. J. Pediat. 93:793–795, 1978.

Bigler, J. A., and Haralambie, J. Q.: Sulfanilamide and related compounds. A review of the literature. Am. J. Dis. Child. 57:1110–1167, 1939.

Black, S. B., Levine, P., and Shinefield, H. R.: The necessity for monitoring chloramphenicol levels when treating neonatal meningitis. J. Pediat. 92:235–236, 1978.

Bloxham, R. A., Durbin, G. M., Johnson, T., and Winterborn, M. H.: Chloramphenicol and phenobarbitone—a drug interaction. Arch. Dis. Childh. 54:76–77, 1979.

Bodey, G. P., Whitecar, J. P., Jr., Middleman, E., and Rodriguez, V.: Carbenicillin for pseudomonas therapy. J.A.M.A. 218:62–66, 1971.

Border, W. A., Lehman, D. H., Egan, J. D., Sass, H. J., Glode, J. E., and Wilson, C. B.: Antitubular basemembrane antibodies in methicillin-associated interstitial nephritis. New Eng. J. Med. 291:381–384, 1974.

Brauer, M. J., and Dameshek, W.: Hypoplastic anemia and myeloblastic leukemia following chloramphenicol therapy. Report of three cases. New Eng. J. Med. 277:1003–1005, 1967.

Briedis, D. J., and Robson, H. G.: Cerebrospinal fluid penetration of amikacin. Antimicrob. Agents Chemother. 13:1042–1043, 1978.

Brown, C. H., III., Natelson, E. A., Bradshaw, M. W., Williams, T. W., Jr., and Alfrey, C. P., Jr.: The hemostatic defect produced by carbenicillin. New Eng. J. Med. 291:265–270, 1974.

Bruckstein, A. H., and Attia, A. A.: Oxacillin hepatitis. Two patients with liver biopsy, and review of the literature. Am. J. Med. 64:519–522, 1978.

Buchanan, T. M., Faber, L. C., and Feldman, R. A.: Brucellosis in the United States, 1960–1972. An abattoir-associated disease. Part I. Clinical features and therapy. Medicine 53:403–413, 1974.

Burns, L. E., Hodgman, J. E., and Cass, A. B.: Fatal circulatory collapse in premature infants receiving chloramphenicol. New Eng. J. Med. 261:1318–1321, 1959.

Carey, B. W., Jr.: The use of para-aminobenzenesulfonamide and its derivatives in the treatment of infections due to the β Streptococcus hemolyticus, the meningococcus, and the gonococcus. Report of 38 cases. J. Pediat. 11:202–211, 1937.

Carithers, H. A.: The first use of an antibiotic in America. Am. J. Dis. Child. 128:207–211, 1974.

Cates, K. L., Gerrard, J. M., Giebink, G. S., Lund, M. E., Bleeker, E. Z., Lau, S., O'Leary, M. C., Krivit, W., and Quie, P. G.: A penicillin-resistant pneumococcus. J. Pediat. 93:624–626, 1978.

Chain, E.: Thirty years of penicillin therapy. Proc. Roy. Soc. Lond. B. 179:293–319, 1971.

Chain, E., Florey, H. W., Gardner, A. D., Heatley, N. G., Jennings, M. A., Orr-Ewing, J., and Sanders, A. G.: Penicillin as a chemotherapeutic agent. Lancet 2:226–228, 1940.

Chang, M. J., Escobedo, M., Anderson, D. C., Hillman, L., and Feigin, R. D.: Kanamycin and gentamicin treatment of neonatal sepsis and meningitis. Pediatrics 56:695–699, 1975.

Chang, N., Giles, C. L., and Gregg, R. H.: Optic neuritis and chloramphenicol. Am. J. Dis. Child. 112:46–48, 1966.

Christensen, L. K., and Skovsted, L.: Inhibition of drug metabolism by chloramphenicol. Lancet 2:1397–1399, 1969.

Claudon, D. B., and Holbrook, A. A.: Fatal aplastic anemia associated with chloramphenicol (chloromycetin) therapy. J.A.M.A. 149:912–914, 1952.

Cocke, J. G., Jr., Brown, R. E., and Geppert, L. J.: Optic neuritis with prolonged use of chloramphenicol. J. Pediat. 68:27–31, 1966.

Cohen, M. M.: Fatality following use of intrathecal penicillin: Case report. J. Neuropath. Exper. Neurol. 11:335–339, 1952.

Cook, F. V., and Farrar, W. E., Jr.: Vancomycin revisited. Ann. Intern. Med. 88:813–818, 1978.

Cornwall, L. H.: Pneumorachioclysis and cervicolumbar irrigation in the treatment of meningococcal meningitis. Arch. Neurol. Psychiat. 29:619–623, 1933.

Craft, A. W., Brocklebank, J. T., Hey, E. N., and Jackson, R. H.: The 'grey toddler.' Chloramphenicol toxicity. Arch. Dis. Childh. 49:235–237, 1974.

Craft, J. C., Feldman, W. E., and Nelson, J. D.: Clinicopharmacological evaluation of amoxicillin and probenecid against bacterial meningitis. Antimicrob. Agents Chemother. 16:346–352. 1979.

Crawford, A. S.: The intracarotid treatment of meningitis. Experiences with Pregl's solution of iodine: A further report. J.A.M.A. 98:1531–1535, 1932.

Cronin, R. E.: Aminoglycoside nephrotoxicity: Pathogenesis and prevention. Clin. Nephrol. 11:251–256, 1979.

Dacey, R. G., and Sande, M. A.: Effect of probenecid on cerebrospinal fluid concentrations of penicillin and cephalosporin derivatives. Antimicrob. Agents Chemother. 6:437–441, 1974.

Dans, P. E., McGehee, R. F., Jr., Wilcox, C., and Finland, M.: Rifampin: Antibacterial activity in vitro and absorption and excretion in normal young men. Am. J. Med. Sci. 259:120–132, 1970.

Daum, R. S., Cohen, D. L., and Smith, A. L.: Fatal aplastic anemia following apparent "dose-related" chloramphenicol toxicity. J. Pediat. 94:403–406, 1979.

Davies, J.: Bacterial resistance to aminoglycoside antibiotics. J. Infect. Dis. 124 (Suppl.):7–10, 1971.

Davies, J., and Courvalin, P.: Mechanisms of resistance to aminoglycosides. Am. J. Med. 62:868–872, 1977.

Dayal, V. S., Whitehead, G. L., and Smith, E. L.: Gentamicin—Progressive cochlear toxicity. Canad. J. Otolaryngol. 4:384–351, 1975.

Dhawan, V., Marso, E., Martin, W. J., and Young, L. S.: In vitro studies with netilmicin compared with amikacin, gentamicin, and tobramycin. Antimicrob. Agents Chemother. 11:64–73, 1977.

Diaz, C. R., Kane, J. G., Parker, R. H., and Pelsor, F. R.: Pharmacokinetics of nafcillin in patients with renal failure. Antimicrob. Agents Chemother. 12:98–101, 1977.

Dixon, R. L., Owens, E. S., and Rall, D. P.: Evidence of active transport of benzyl-^{14}C-penicillin from cerebrospinal fluid to blood. J. Pharm. Sci. 58:1106–1109, 1969.

D'Oliveira, J. J. G.: Cerebrospinal fluid concentrations of rifampin in meningeal tuberculosis. Am. Rev. Respir. Dis. 106:432–437, 1972.

Dowling, H. F., Sweet, L. K., Robinson, J. A., Zellers, W. W., and Hirsh, H. L.: The treatment of pneumococcal meningitis with massive doses of systemic penicillin. Am. J. Med. Sci. 217:149–156, 1949.

Dunkle, L. M.: Central nervous system chloramphenicol concentration in premature infants. Antimicrob. Agents Chemother. 13:427–429, 1978.

Dunn, C. H.: Cerebrospinal meningitis, its etiology, diagnosis, prognosis and treatment. Am. J. Dis. Child. 1:95–112, 1911.

Edwards, C. Q., Smith, C. R., Baughman, K. L., Rogers, J. F., and Lietman, P. S.: Concentrations of gentamicin and amikacin in human kidneys. Antimicrob. Agents Chemother. 9:925–927, 1976.

Edwards, K., Ferrieri, P., Thompson, T. R., and Davis, A. T.: Group B streptococcal meningitis: Delayed response to treatment. Child's Brain 3:343–351, 1977.

Eickhoff, T. C., and Ehret, J. M.: In vitro activity of netilmicin compared with gentamicin, tobramycin, amikacin, and kanamycin. Antimicrob. Agents Chemother. 11:791–796, 1977.

Epstein, H. C., Hochwald, A., and Ashe, R.: Salmonella infections in the newborn infant. J. Pediat. 38:723–731, 1951.

Faden, H., Neter, E., McLaughlin, S., and Giacoia, G.: Gentamicin-resistant Staphylococcus aureus. Emergence in an intensive care nursery. J.A.M.A. 241:143–145, 1979.

Feigin, R. D., and Fiascone, A.: Hematuria and proteinuria associated with methicillin administration. New Eng. J. Med. 272:903–904, 1965.

Feldman, W. E.: *Bacteroides fragilis* ventriculitis and meningitis. Report of two cases. Am. J. Dis. Child. 130:880–883, 1976.

Feldman, W. E.: Effect of ampicillin and chloramphenicol against *Haemophilus influenzae*. Pediatrics 61:406–409, 1978.

Feldman, W. E., and Zweighaft, T.: Effect of ampicillin and chloramphenicol against *Streptococcus pneumoniae* and *Neisseria meningitidis*. Antimicrob. Agents Chemother. 15:240–242, 1972.

Feldman, W. E., Nelson, J. D., and Stanberry, L. R.: Clinical and pharmacokinetic evaluation of nafcillin in infants and children. J. Pediat. 93:1029–1033, 1978.

Ferry, N. S., Norton, J. F., and Steele, A. H.: Studies of the properties of bouillon filtrates of the meningococcus: Production of a soluble toxin. J. Immunol. 21:293–312, 1931.

Fields, J. P.: Bulging fontanel: A complication of tetracycline therapy in infants. J. Pediat. 58:74–76, 1961.

Finitzo-Hieber, T., McCracken, G. H., Jr., Roeser, R. J., Allen, D. A., Chrane, D. F., and Morrow, J.: Ototoxicity in neonates treated with gentamicin and kanamycin: Results of a four-year controlled follow-up study. Pediatrics 63:443–450, 1972.

Fishman, R. A.: Blood-brain and CSF barriers to penicillin and related organic acids. Arch. Neurol. 15:113–124, 1966.

Fleming, A.: On the antibacterial action of cultures of a Penicillium, with special reference to their use in the isolation of B. influenzae. Brit. J. Exper. Path. 10:226–236, 1929.

Flexner, S.: Experimental cerebrospinal meningitis and its serum treatment. J.A.M.A. 47:560–566, 1906.

Flexner, S.: The results of serum treatment in thirteen hundred cases of epidemic meningitis. J. Exper. Med. 17:553–576, 1913.

Fossieck, B. E., Jr., Kane, J. G., Diaz, C. R., and Parker, R. H.: Nafcillin entry into human cerebrospinal fluid. Antimicrob. Agents Chemother. 11:965–967, 1977.

Fothergill, L. D.: Hemophilus influenzae (Pfeiffer bacillus) meningitis and its specific treatment. New Eng. J. Med. 216:587–590, 1937.

Friedman, C. A., Lovejoy, F. C., and Smith, A. L.: Chloramphenicol disposition in infants and children. J. Pediat. 95:1071–1077, 1979.

Geraci, J. E.: Vancomycin. Mayo Clin. Proc. 52:631–634, 1977.

Ginsburg, C. M., and Eichenwald, H. F.: Erythromycin: A review of its uses in pediatric practice. J. Pediat. 89:872–884, 1976.

Goldring, D., Hartmann, A. F., and Maxwell, R.: Diagnosis and management of severe infections in infants and children: A review of experiences since the introduction of sulfonamide therapy. III. Meningococcal infections. J. Pediat. 26:1–31, 1945.

Graf, M., and Tarlov, A.: Agranulocytosis with monohistiocytosis associated with ampicillin therapy. Ann. Intern. Med. 69:91–95, 1968.

Graybill, J. R., Mann, J., and Charache, P.: Intrathecal gentamicin in treatment of bacterial meningitis. Johns Hopkins Med. J. 133:51–56, 1973.

Greene, G. R., and Cohen, E.: Nafcillin-induced neutropenia in children. Pediatrics 61:94–97, 1978.

Hallman, M.: Oxygen uptake in neonatal rats: A developmental study with particular reference to the effects of chloramphenicol. Pediat. Res. 7:923, 1973.

Hamory, B., Ignatiadis, P., and Sande, M. A.: Intrathecal amikacin administration. Use in the treatment of gentamicin-resistant Klebsiella pneumoniae meningitis. J.A.M.A. 236:1973–1974, 1976.

Hansman, D., and Bullen, M. M.: A resistant pneumococcus. Lancet 2:264–265, 1967.

Harrison, H. B., Crowe, C. P., and Fulginiti, V. A.: Amebic liver abscess in children: Clinical and epidemiological features. Pediatrics 64:923–928, 1979.

Hawley, H. B., and Gump, D. W.: Vancomycin therapy of bacterial meningitis. Am. J. Dis. Child. 126:261–264, 1973.

Heiman, H.: Epidemic cerebrospinal meningitis. A review of the recent literature. Am. J. Dis. Child. 2:281–286, 1911.

Herrell, W. E., and Kennedy, R. L. J.: Penicillin: Its use in pediatrics. J. Pediat. 25:505–516, 1944.

Hieber, J. P., and Nelson, J. D.: Re-evaluation of kanamycin dosage in infants and children. Antimicrob. Agents Chemother. 9:899–902, 1976.

Hieber, J. P., and Nelson, J. D.: A pharmacologic evaluation of penicillin in children with purulent meningitis. New Eng. J. Med. 297:410–413, 1977.

Hokkanen, E.: The aggravating effect of some antibiotics on the neuromuscular blockade in myasthenia gravis. Acta Neurol. Scand. 40:346–352, 1964.

Holt, R.: The bacterial degradation of chloramphenicol. Lancet 1:1259–1260, 1967.

Howard, J. B., and McCracken, G. H., Jr.: Reappraisal of kanamycin usage in neonates. J. Pediat. 86:949–956, 1975.

Howard, J. B., McCracken, G. H., Jr., Trujillo, H., and Mohs, E.: Amikacin in newborn infants: Comparative pharmacology with kanamycin and clinical efficacy in 45 neonates with bacterial diseases. Antimicrob. Agents Chemother. 10:205–210, 1976.

Hoyne, A. L.: Meningococcic meningitis. A new form of therapy. J.A.M.A. 104:980–983, 1935.

Hoyne, A. L.: Advances in treatment of meningitis. J. Pediat. 19:778–788, 1941.

Huang, N. N., Harley, R. D., Promadhattavedi, V., and Sproul, A.: Visual disturbances in cystic fibrosis following chloramphenicol administration. J. Pediat. 68:32–42, 1966.

Ingham, H. R., Rich, G. E., Selkon, J. B., Hale, J. H., Roxby, C. M., Betty, M. J., Johnson, R. W. G., and Uldall, P. R.: Treatment with metronidazole of three patients with serious infections due to Bacteroides fragilis. J. Antimicrob. Chemother. 1:235–242, 1975.

Jacobs, M. R., Koornhof, H. J., Robins-Browne, R. M., Stevenson, C. M., Vermaak, Z. A., Freiman, I., Miller, G. B., Witcomb, M. A., Isaacson, M., Ward, J. I., and Austrian, R.: Emergence of multiply resistant pneumococci. New Eng. J. Med. 299:735–740, 1978.

Jahre, J. A., Fu, K. P., and Neu, H. C.: Clinical evaluation of netilmicin therapy in serious infections. Am. J. Med. 66:67–73, 1979.

Jochmann, G.: Versuche zue serodiagnostik und serotherapy der epidemischen genickstarre. Dtsch. Med. Wochenschr. 32:788, 1906.

Johnson, H. C., and Walker, A. E.: Intraventricular penicillin. Note of warning. J.A.M.A. 127:217–219, 1945.

Jubb, A. A.: Chemotherapy and serotherapy in cerebrospinal (meningococcal) meningitis. An analysis of 3,206 case reports. Brit. Med. J. 1:501–504, 1943.

Kafetzis, D. A., Sinaniotis, C. A., Papadatos, C. J., and Kosmidis, J.: Pharmacokinetics of amikacin in infants and pre-school children. Acta Paediat. Scand. 68:419–422, 1979.

Kaiser, A. B., McGee, Z. A.: Aminoglycoside therapy of gram-negative bacillary meningitis. New Eng. J. Med. 293:1215–1220, 1975.

Kancir, L. M., Tuazon, C. U., Cardella, T. A., and Sheagren, J. N.: Adverse reactions to methicillin and nafcillin during treatment of serious Staphylococcus aureus infections. Arch. Intern. Med. 138:909–911, 1978.

Kane, J. G., Parker, R. H., Jordan, G. W., and Hoeprich, P. D.: Nafcillin concentration in cerebrospinal fluid during treatment of staphylococcal infections. Ann. Intern. Med. 87:309–311, 1977.

Kaplan, J. M., McCracken, G. H., Jr., Horton, L. J., Thomas, M. L., and Davis, N.: Pharmacologic studies in neonates given large doses of ampicillin. J. Pediat. 84:571–577, 1974.

Kaplan, J. M., McCracken, G. H., Jr., Thomas, M. L., Horton, L. J., and Davis, N.: Clinical pharmacology of tobramycin in newborns. Am. J. Dis. Child. 125:656–660, 1973.

Kaye, D., Levison, M. E., and Labovitz, E. D.: The unpredictability of serum concentrations of gentamicin: Pharmacokinetics of gentamicin in patients with normal and abnormal renal function. J. Infect. Dis. 130:150–154, 1974.

Kerns, D. L., Shira, J. E., Go, S., Summers, R. J., Schwab, J. A., and Plunket, D. C.: Ampicillin rash in children. Relationship of penicillin allergy and infectious mononucleosis. Am. J. Dis. Child. 125:187–190, 1973.

Kessler, D. L., Jr., Smith, A. L., and Woodrum, D. E.: Chloramphenicol toxicity in a neonate treated with exchange transfusion. J. Pediat. 96:140–141, 1980.

Kitahara, M., Seth, V. K., Medoff, G., and Kobayashi, G. S.: Activity of amphotericin B, 5-fluorocytosine, and rifampin against six clinical isolates of Aspergillus. Antimicrob. Agents Chemother. 9:915–919, 1976.

Koch-Weser, J., and Gilmore, E. B.: Benign intracranial hypertension in an adult after tetracycline therapy. J.A.M.A. 200:345–347, 1967.

Kolmer, J. A.: Pneumococcus and streptococcus meningitis. Chemotherapy and serum therapy with especial reference to newer methods. J.A.M.A. 92:874–877, 1929.

Kolmer, J. A.: The intracarotid method of treatment for meningitis with recoveries. J.A.M.A. 96:1358–1361, 1931.

Korzeniowski, O. M., Carvalho, E. M., Jr., Rocha, H., and Sande, M. A.: Evaluation of cefamandole therapy of patients with bacterial meningitis. J. Infect. Dis. 137(Suppl.):S169–S179, 1978.

Kunin, C. M.: Clinical pharmacology of the new penicillins. I. The importance of serum protein binding in determining antimicrobial activity and concentration in serum. Clin. Pharmacol. Therap. 7:166–178, 1966.

Lakshmanarayan, S., Sahn, S., and Hudson, D.: Massive hemolysis caused by rifampicin. Brit. Med. J. 2:282–283, 1973.

Lambdin, M. A., Waddell, W. W., Jr., and Birdsong, M.: Chloramphenicol toxicity in the premature infant. Pediatrics 25:935–940, 1960.

Lane, A. Z., Wright, G. E., and Blair, D. C.: Ototoxicity and nephrotoxicity of amikacin. An overview of phase II and phase III experience in the United States. Am. J. Med. 62:911–918, 1977.

Lee, E. L., Robinson, M. J., Thong, M. L., Puthucheary, S. D., Ong, T. H., and Ng, K. K.: Intraventricular chemotherapy in neonatal meningitis. J. Pediat. 91:991–995, 1977.

Leeper, M. H., and Dowling, H. F.: Treatment of pneumococcic meningitis with penicillin compared with penicillin plus aureomycin. Studies including observations on an apparent antagonism between penicillin and aureomycin. Arch. Intern. Med. 88:489–494, 1951.

Leeper, M. H., Dowling, H. F., Wehrle, P. F., Blatt, N. H., Spies, H. W., and Brown, M.: Meningococcic meningitis: Treatment with large doses of penicillin compared to treatment with gantrisin. J. Lab. Clin. Med. 40:891–900, 1952.

Leighton, W. E., and Pringle, J. A.: Recovery in two cases of streptococcus meningitis following lumbar laminectomy and drainage. J.A.M.A. 64:2054–2055, 1915.

Lerner, P. I., Smith, H., and Weinstein, L.: Penicillin neurotoxicity. Ann. N. Y. Acad. Sci. 145:310–318, 1967.

Levine, R. A.: Polymyxin B-induced respiratory paralysis reversed by intravenous calcium chloride. J. Mt. Sinai Hosp. 36:380–387, 1969.

L'Hommedieu, C., Stough, R., Brown, L., Kittrick, R., and Polin, R.: Potentiation of neuromuscular weakness in infant botulism by aminoglycosides. J. Pediat. 95:1065–1070, 1979.

Lietman, P. S.: Chloramphenicol and the neonate—1979 view. Clin. Pharmacol. 6:151–162, 1979.

Lischner, H., Seligman, S. J., Krammer, A., and Parmelee, A. H., Jr.: An outbreak of neonatal deaths among term infants associated with administration of chloramphenicol. J. Pediat. 59:21–34, 1961.

Lowrey, G. H., and Quilligan, J. J., Jr.: The treatment of pneumococcal meningitis without intrathecal penicillin. J. Pediat. 33:336–341, 1948.

Luft, F. C., Rankin, L. I., Sloan, R. S., and Yum, M. N.: Recovery from aminoglycoside nephrotoxicity with continued drug administration. Antimicrob. Agents Chemother. 14:284–287, 1978.

Maderazo, E. G., Bassaris, H. P., and Quintiliani, R.: Flavobacterium meningosepticum meningitis in a newborn infant. J. Pediat. 85:675–676, 1974.

Mangi, R. J., Holstein, L. L., and Andriole, V. T.: Treatment of gram-negative bacillary meningitis with intrathecal gentamicin. Yale J. Biol. Med. 50:31–41, 1977.

Markowitz, S. M.: Isolation of an ampicillin-resistant non-β-lactamase-producing strain of Haemophilus influenzae. Antimicrob. Agents Chemother. 17:80–83, 1980.

Maroon, J. C., and Mealy, J., Jr.: Benign intracranial hypertension. Sequel to tetracycline therapy in a child. J.A.M.A. 216:1479–1480, 1971.

Mauer, S. M., Chavers, B. M., and Kjellstrand, C. M.: Treatment of an infant with severe chloramphenicol intoxication using charcoal-column hemoperfusion. J. Pediat. 96:136–139, 1980.

McCormick, J. B., and Bennett, J. V.: Public health considerations in the management of meningococcal disease. Ann. Intern. Med. 83:883–886, 1975.

McCracken, G. H., Jr.: The rate of bacteriologic response to antimicrobial therapy in neonatal meningitis. Am. J. Dis. Child. 123:547–553, 1972.

McCracken, G. H., Jr.: Clinical pharmacology of gentamicin in infants 2 to 24 months of age. Am. J. Dis. Child. 124:884–887, 1972.

McCracken, G. H., Jr.: Pharmacological basis for antimicrobial therapy in newborn infants. Am. J. Dis. Child. 128:407–419, 1974.

McCracken, G. H., Jr., and Jones, L. G.: Gentamicin in the neonatal period. Am. J. Dis. Child. 120:524–533, 1970.

McCracken, G. H., Jr., and Mize, S. G.: A controlled study of intrathecal antibiotic therapy in gram-negative enteric meningitis of infancy. Report of the neonatal meningitis cooperative study group. J. Pediat. 89:66–72, 1976.

McCracken, G. H., Jr., and Nelson, J. D.: Commentary: An appraisal of tobramycin usage in pediatrics. J. Pediat. 88:315–317, 1976.

McCracken, G. H., Jr., Chrane, D. F., and Thomas, M. L.: Pharmacologic evaluation of gentamicin in newborn infants. J. Infect. Dis. 124 (Suppl.):214–223, 1971.

McCracken, G. H., Jr., Ginsberg, C., Chrane, D. F., Thomas, M. L., and Horton, L. J.: Clinical pharmacology of penicillin in newborn infants. J. Pediat. 82:692–698, 1973.

McGee, T. M., Webster, J., and Williams, M.: Histologic and functional changes in ears of cats after subcutaneous administration of gentamicin. J. Infect. Dis. 119:432–439, 1969.

McIntosh, R., Wilcox, D. A., and Wright, F. H.: Results of sulfanilamide treatment at the Babies Hospital, New York City. A survey of 58 cases observed prior to June 10, 1937. J. Pediat. 11:167–182, 1937.

McQuarrie, I.: Report of cases treated with sulfanilamide (Prontosil and Prontylin). J. Pediat. 11:188–194, 1937.

McQuillen, M. P., Cantor, H. E., and O'Rourke, J. R.: Myasthenic syndrome associated with antibiotics. Arch. Neurol. 18:402–415, 1968.

Meade, R. H., III.: Streptomycin and sulfisoxazole for treatment of Haemophilus influenzae meningitis. J.A.M.A. 239:324–327, 1978.

Meyer, R. D., Lewis, R. P., and Finegold, S. M.: Amikacin therapy for gram-negative septicemia. Am. J. Med. 62:930–935, 1977.

Meyers, R. M.: Ototoxic effects of gentamicin. Arch. Otolaryngol. 92:160–162, 1970.

Miller, J. W., Seiss, E. E., and Feldman, H. A.: In vivo and in vitro resistance to sulfadiazine in strains of Neisseria meningitidis. J.A.M.A. 186:139–141, 1963.

Most, J. A., and Markle, G. B.: A nearly fatal hepatotoxic reaction to rifampin after halothane anesthesia. Am. J. Surg. 127:593–595, 1974.

Mull, M. M.: The tetracyclines. Am. J. Dis. Child. 112:483–493, 1966.

Murillo, J., Standiford, H. C., Schimpff, S. C., and Tatem, B. A.: Gentamicin and ticarcillin serum levels. J.A.M.A. 241:2401–2403, 1979.

Naraqi, S., Kirpatrick, G. P., and Kabins, S.: Relapsing pneumococcal meningitis: Isolation of an organism with decreased susceptibility to penicillin. J. Pediat. 85:671–673, 1974.

Nastro, L. J., and Finegold, S. M.: Bactericidal activity of five antimicrobial agents against Bacteroides fragilis. J. Infect. Dis. 126:104–107, 1972.

Neal, J. B.: The treatment of acute infections of the central nervous system with sulfanilamide. J.A.M.A. 111:1353–1356, 1938.

Nelson, J. D.: Carbenicillin—a major new antibiotic. Am. J. Dis. Child. 120:382–383, 1970.

Nelson, J. D., and McCracken, G. H., Jr.: Clinical pharmacology of carbenicillin and gentamicin in the neonate and comparative efficacy with ampicillin and gentamicin. Pediatrics 52:801–812, 1973.

Nelson, J. D., Kusmiesz, H., Shelton, S., and Woodman, E.: Clinical pharmacology and efficacy of ticarcillin in infants and children. Pediatrics 61:858–863, 1978.

New, P. S., and Wells, C. E.: Cerebral toxicity associated with massive intravenous penicillin therapy. Neurology 15:1053–1058, 1965.

Newton, R. W., and Forrest, A. R. W.: Rifampicin overdosage—"the red man syndrome." Scott. Med. J. 20:55–56, 1975.

Neymann, C. A., Heilbrunn, G., and Youmans, G. P.: Experiments in treatment of dementia paralytica with penicillin. J.A.M.A. 128:433, 1945.

Noone, P., and Pattison, J. R.: Therapeutic implications of interaction of gentamicin and penicillins. Lancet 2:575–578, 1971.

O'Doherty, N. J.: Acute benign intracranial hypertension in an infant receiving tetracycline. Develop. Med. Child. Neurol. 7:677–680, 1965.

Olans, R. N., and Weiner, L. B.: Reversible oxacillin hepatotoxicity. J. Pediat. 89:835–838, 1976.

Oldstone, M. B. A., and Nelson, E.: Central nervous system manifestations of penicillin toxicity in man. Neurology 16:693–700, 1966.

Olson, C. A., and Riley, H. D., Jr.: Complications of tetracycline therapy. J. Pediat. 68:783–791, 1966.

Oppenheimer, S., Beaty, H. N., and Petersdorf, R. G.: Pathogenesis of meningitis. VIII. Cerebrospinal fluid and blood concentrations of methicillin, cephalothin, and cephaloridine in experimental pneumococcal meningitis. J. Lab. Clin. Med. 73:535–543, 1969.

Oski, F. A.: Hematologic consequences of chloramphenicol therapy. J. Pediat. 94:515–516, 1979.

Paisley, J. W., and Washington, J. A., III.: Susceptibility of Escherichia coli K1 to four combinations of antimicrobial agents potentially useful for treatment of neonatal meningitis. J. Infect. Dis. 140:183–191, 1979.

Paisley, J. W., Smith, A. L., and Smith, D. H.: Gentamicin in newborn infants. Comparison of intramuscular and intravenous administration. Am. J. Dis. Child. 126:473–477, 1973.

Panwalker, A. P., Malow, J. B., Zimelis, V. M., and Jackson, G. G.: Netilmicin: Clinical efficacy, tolerance, and toxicity. Antimicrob. Agents Chemother. 13:170–176, 1978.

Parker, M. T., and Hewitt, J. H.: Methicillin resistance in Staphylococcus aureus. Lancet 1:800–804, 1970.

Parry, M. F., and Neu, H. C.: A comparative study of ticarcillin plus tobramycin versus carbenicillin plus gentamicin for the treatment of serious infections due to gram-negative bacilli. Am. J. Med. 64:961–966, 1978.

Peterson, D. I., Voorhees, E. G., and Elder, H. A.: Bacteroides meningitis successfully treated with metronidazole. Ann. Neurol. 6:364–365, 1979.

Pickering, L. K., Ericsson, C. D., Ruiz-Palacios, G., Blevins, J., and Miner, M. E.: Intraventricular and parenteral gentamicin therapy for ventriculitis in children. Am. J. Dis. Child. 132:480–483, 1978.

Plorde, J., Garcia, M., and Petersdorf, R. G.: Studies on the pathogenesis of meningitis. IV. Penicillin levels in the cerebrospinal fluid in experimental meningitis. J. Lab. Clin. Med. 64:960–969, 1964.

Pollock, A. A., Berger, S. A., Simberkoff, M. S., and Rahal, J. J., Jr.: Hepatitis associated with high-dose oxacillin therapy. Arch. Intern. Med. 138:915–917, 1978.

Poole, G., Stradling, P., and Worlledge, S.: Potentially serious side-effects of high-dose twice-weekly rifampicin. Postgrad. Med. J. 47:742–747, 1971.

Prather, G. W., and Smith, M. H. D.: Chloramphenicol in the treatment of Hemophilus influenzae meningitis. J.A.M.A. 143:1405–1406, 1950.

Pratt, T. H.: Rifampin-induced organic brain syndrome. J.A.M.A. 241:2421–2422, 1979.

Pridgen, J. E.: Respiratory arrest thought to be due to intraperitoneal neomycin. Surgery 40:571–574, 1956.

Quincke, H.: Die lumbalpunktion des hydrocephalus. Berl. Klin. Wschr. 28:929–933, 965–968, 1891.

Rahal, J. J., Jr.: Antibiotic combinations: The clinical relevance of synergy and antagonism. Medicine 57:179–195, 1978.

Rahal, J. J., Jr., and Simberkoff, M. S.: Bacticidal and bacteriostatic action of chloramphenicol against meningeal pathogens. Antimicrob. Agents Chemother. 16:13–18, 1979.

Rahal, J. J., Jr., Hyams, P. J., Simberkoff, M. S., and Rubinstein, E.: Combined intrathecal and intramuscular gentamicin for gram-negative meningitis. Pharmacologic study of 21 patients. New Eng. J. Med. 290:1394–1398, 1974.

Raichle, M. E., Kuh, H., Louis, S., and McDowell, F.: Neurotoxicity of intravenously administered penicillin G. Arch. Neurol. 25:232–239, 1971.

Rainey, W. R., and Alford, L. B.: The treatment of septic meningitis by continuous drainage. J.A.M.A. 81:1516–1518, 1923.

Ralph, E. D., Clarke, J. T., Libke, R. D., Luthy, R. P., and Kirby, W. M. M.: Pharmacokinetics of metronidazole as determined by bioassay. Antimicrob. Agents Chemother. 6:691–696, 1974.

Rammelkamp, C. H., and Keefer, C. S.: The absorption, excretion, and distribution of penicillin. J. Clin. Invest. 22:425–437, 1943.

Rees, R. J. W., Pearson, J. M. H., and Waters, M. F. R.: Experimental and clinical studies on rifampicin in treatment of leprosy. Brit. Med. J. 1:89–92, 1970.

Rheingold, J. J., and Spurling, C. L.: Chloramphenicol and aplastic anemia. J.A.M.A. 149:1301–1304, 1952.

Richards, F., McCall, C., and Cox, C.: Gentamicin treatment of staphylococcal infections. J.A.M.A. 215:1297–1300, 1971.

Ring, J. C., Cates, K. L., Belani, K. K., Gaston, T. L., Sveum, R. J., and Marker, S. C.: Rifampin for CSF shunt infections caused by coagulase-negative staphylococci. J. Pediat. 95:317–319, 1979.

Rios, I., Klimek, J. J., Maderazo, E., and Quintiliani, R.: *Flavobacterium meningosepticum* meningitis: Report of selected aspects. Antimicrob. Agents Chemother. 14:444–447, 1978.

Robinson, L. R., Seligsohn, R., and Lerner, S. A.: Simplified radioenzymatic assay for chloramphenicol. Antimicrob. Agents Chemother. 13:25–29, 1978.

Rose, J. Q., Choi, H. K., Schentag, J. J., Kinkel, W. R., and Jusko, W. J.: Intoxication caused by interaction of chloramphenicol and phenytoin. J.A.M.A. 237:2630–2631, 1977.

Rosenberg, D. H., and Sylvester, J. C.: The excretion of penicillin in the spinal fluid in meningitis. Science 100:132–133, 1944.

Rosenkranz, H. S., and Speck, W. T.: Mutagenicity of metronidazole: Activation by mammalian liver microsomes. Biochem. Biophys. Res. Commun. 66:520–525, 1975.

Ross, S., Kraybill, E. N., and Khan, W.: Treatment of *Proteus* meningitis with carbenicillin: A report of four cases. J. Infect. Dis. 122(Suppl.): S62–S70, 1970.

Ross, S., Rice, E. C., Burke, F. G., McGovern, J. J., Parrott, R. H., and McGovern, J. P.: Treatment of meningitis due to Haemophilus influenzae. Use of chloromycetin and sulfadiazine. New Eng. J. Med. 247:541–547, 1952.

Royster, L. T.: Report of a case of streptococcic meningitis treated with injections of gentian violet. Am. J. Dis. Child. 28:34–37, 1924.

Ruedy, J.: The concentration of penicillins in the cerebrospinal fluid and brain in rabbits with experimental meningitis. Canad. J. Physiol. Pharmacol. 43:763–772, 1965.

Ruiz, D. E., and Warner, J. F.: Nafcillin treatment of *Staphylococcus aureus* meningitis. Antimicrob. Agents Chemother. 9:554–555, 1976.

Ruley, E. J., and Lisi, L. M.: Interstitial nephritis and renal failure due to ampicillin. J. Pediat. 84:878–881, 1974.

Rustia, M., and Shubik, P.: Induction of lung tumors and malignant lymphomas in mice by metronidazole. J. Natl. Cancer Inst. 48:721–726, 1972.

Ryan, J. L., Pachner, A., Andriole, V. T., and Root, R. K.: Enterococcal meningitis: Combined vancomycin and rifampin therapy. Am. J. Med. 68:449–451, 1980.

Sackellares, J. C., and Smith, D. B.: Myoclonus with electrocerebral silence in a patient receiving penicillin. Arch. Neurol. 36:857–858, 1979.

Sako, W., Stewart, C. A., and Fleet, J.: Treatment of influenzal meningitis with sulfadiazine. Further report. J. Pediat. 25:114–126, 1944.

Sanders, C. V., Hanna, B. J., and Lewis, A. C.: Metronidazole in the treatment of anaerobic infections. Am. Rev. Respir. Dis. 120:337–343, 1979.

Sanders, W. E.: Rifampin. Ann. Intern. Med. 85:82–86, 1976.

Sanjad, S. A., Haddad, G. G., and Nassar, V. H.: Nephropathy, an underestimated complication of methicillin therapy. J. Pediat. 84:873–877, 1974.

Sarff, L. D., McCracken, G. H., Jr., Thomas, M. L., Horton, L. J., and Threlkeld, N.: Clinical pharmacology of methicillin in neonates. J. Pediat. 90:1005–1008, 1977.

Schaad, V. B., McCracken, G. H., Jr., and Nelson, J. D.: Clinical pharmacology and efficacy of vancomycin in pediatric patients. J. Pediat. 96:119–126, 1980.

Schatz, A., Bugie, E., and Waksman, S. A.: Streptomycin, substance exhibiting antibiotic activity against gram-positive and gram-negative bacteria. Proc. Soc. Exper. Biol. Med. 55:66–69, 1944.

Scheld, W. M., Brown, R. S., Jr., and Sande, M. A.: Comparison of netilmicin with gentamicin in the therapy of experimental *Escherichia coli* meningitis. Antimicrob. Agents Chemother. 13:899–904, 1978.

Schentag, J. J., Cumbo, T. J., Jusko, W. J., and Plaut, M. E.: Gentamicin tissue accumulation and nephrotoxic reactions. J.A.M.A. 240:2067–2069, 1978.

Schentag, J. J., Lasezkay, G., Cumbo, T. J., Plaut, M. E., and Jusko, W. J.: Accumulation pharmacokinetics of tobramycin. Antimicrob. Agents Chemother. 13:649–656, 1978.

Schentag, J. J., Gengo, F. M., Plaut, M. E., Danner, D., Mangione, A., and Jusko, W. J.: Urinary casts as an indicator of renal tubular damage in patients receiving aminoglycosides. Antimicrob. Agents Chemother. 16:468–474, 1979.

Scheuer, P. J., Summerfield, J. A., Lal, S., and Sherlock, S.: Rifampicin hepatitis. A clinical and histological study. Lancet 1:421–425, 1974.

Seamans, K. B., Gloor, P., Dobell, A. R. C., and Wyant, J. D.: Penicillin-induced seizures during cardiopulmonary bypass. A clinical and electroencephalography study. New Eng. J. Med. 278:861–868, 1968.

Shapiro, S., Slone, D., Siskind, V., Lewis, G. P., and Jick, H.: Drug rash with ampicillin and other penicillins. Lancet 2:969–972, 1969.

Shuman, R. D., and Smith, C. R.: Intrathecal gentamicin for refractory gram-positive meningitis. J.A.M.A. 240:469–471, 1978.

Simberkoff, M. S., Thomas, L., McGregor, D., Shenkein, I., and Levine, B. B.: Inactivation of penicillins by carbohydrate solutions at alkaline pH. New Eng. J. Med. 283:116–119, 1970.

Sirinavin, S., McCracken, G. H., Jr., and Nelson, J. D.: Determining gentamicin dosage in infants and children with renal failure. J. Pediat. 96:331–334, 1980.

Sklaver, A. R., Greenman, R. L., and Hoffman, T. A.: Amikacin therapy of gram-negative bacteremia and meningitis. Treatment in diseases due to multiple resistant bacilli. Arch. Intern. Med. 138:713–716, 1978.

Smick, K. M., Condit, P. K., Proctor, R. L., and Sutcher, V.: Fatal aplastic anemia. An epidemiological study of its relationship to the drug chloramphenicol. J. Chron. Dis. 17:899–914, 1964.

Smiley, R. K., Cartwright, G. E., and Wintrobe, M. M.: Fatal aplastic anemia following chloramphenicol (chloromycetin) administration. J.A.M.A. 149:914–918, 1952.

Smith, C. R., Baughman, K. L., Edwards, C. Q., Rogers, J. F., and Lietman, P. S.: Controlled comparison of amikacin and gentamicin. New Eng. J. Med. 296:349–353, 1977.

Snydman, D. R., Tally, F. P., Landesman, S. H., Barza, M., and Gorbach, S. L.: Netilmicin in gram-negative bacterial infections. Antimicrob. Agents Chemother. 15:50–54, 1979.

Spector, R., and Lorenzo, A. V.: Inhibition of penicillin

transport from the cerebrospinal fluid after intracisternal inoculation of bacteria. J. Clin. Invest. 54:316–325, 1974.

Steinberg, E. A., Overturf, G. D., Baraff, L. J., and Wilkins, J.: Penetration of cefamandole into spinal fluid. Antimicrob. Agents Chemother. 11:933–935, 1977.

Steinberg, E. A., Overturf, G. D., Wilkins, J., Baraff, L. J., Streng, J. M., and Leedom, J. M.: Failure of cefamandole in treatment of meningitis due to *Haemophilus influenzae* type b. J. Infect. Dis. 137(Suppl.): S180–S186, 1978.

Strausbaugh, L. J., and Sande, M. A.: Factors influencing the therapy of experimental *Proteus mirabilis* meningitis in rabbits. J. Infect. Dis. 137:251–260, 1978.

Sturgeon, P.: Fatal aplastic anemia in children following chloramphenicol (chloromycetin) therapy. Report of four cases. J.A.M.A. 149:918–922, 1952.

Sutherland, J. M.: Fatal cardiovascular collapse of infants receiving large amounts of chloramphenicol. Am. J. Dis. Child. 97:761–767, 1959.

Sweet, L. K., Dumoff-Stanley, E., Dowling, H. F., and Leeper, M. H.: The treatment of pneumococcic meningitis with penicillin. J.A.M.A. 127:263–267, 1945.

Tally, F. P., Sutter, V. L., and Finegold, S. M.: Treatment of anaerobic infections with metronidazole. Antimicrob. Agents Chemother. 7:672–675, 1975.

Thrupp, L. D., Leedom, J. M., Ivler, D., Wehrle, P. F., Portnoy, B., and Mathies, A. W.: Ampicillin levels in the cerebrospinal fluid during treatment of bacterial meningitis. Antimicrob. Agents Chemother. 1965:206–213, 1966.

Trachsler, W. H., Frauenberger, G. S., Wagner, C., and Mitchell, A. G.: Streptococcic meningitis. With special emphasis on sulfanilamide therapy. J. Pediat. 11:248–269, 1937.

Trestman, I., Parsons, J., Santoro, J., Goodhart, G., and Kaye, D.: Pharmacology and efficacy of netilmicin. Antimicrob. Agents Chemother. 13:832–836, 1978.

Tripoli, C. J.: Bacterial meningitis. A comparative study of various therapeutic measures. J.A.M.A. 106:171–177, 1936.

Vogel, L., Nathan, C., Sweeney, H. M., Kabins, S. A., and Cohen, S.: Infections due to gentamicin-resistant *Staphylococcus aureus* strain in a nursery for neonatal infants. Antimicrob. Agents Chemother. 13:466–472, 1978.

Wallace, J. F., Smith, R. H., Garcia, M., and Petersdorf, R. G.: Studies on the pathogenesis of meningitis. VI. Antagonism between penicillin and chloramphenicol in experimental pneumococcal meningitis. J. Lab. Clin. Med. 70:408–418, 1967.

Wallerstein, R. O., Condit, P. K., Kasper, C. K., Brown, J. W., and Morrison, F. R.: Statewide study of chloramphenicol therapy and fatal aplastic anemia. J.A.M.A. 208:2045–2050, 1969.

Walters, I. N., Teychenne, P. F., Claveria, L. E., and Calne, D. B.: Penicillin transport from cerebrospinal fluid. Neurology 26:1008–1010, 1976.

Ward, H. K., and Fothergill, L. D.: Influenzal meningitis treated with specific antiserum and complement. Report of five cases. Am. J. Dis. Child. 43:873–881, 1932.

Warner, J. F., Perkins, R. L., and Cordero, L.: Metronidazole therapy of anaerobic bacteremia, meningitis, and brain abscess. Arch. Intern. Med. 139:167–169, 1979.

Watanabe, I., Hodges, G. R., and Dworzack, D. L.:

Chemical injury of the spinal cord of the rabbit after intracisternal injection of gentamicin. J. Neuropath. Exper. Neurol. 38:104–113, 1979.

Watanabe, I., Hodges, G. R., Dworzack, D. L., Kepes, J. L., and Duensing, G. F.: Neurotoxocity of intrathecal gentamicin: A case report and experimental study. Ann. Neurol. 4:564–572, 1978.

Wegeforth, P., Ayer, J. B., and Essick, C. R.: The method of obtaining cerebrospinal fluid by puncture of the cisterna magna (cisternal puncture). Am. J. Med. Sci. 157:789–797, 1919.

Weinberg, M. H., Mellon, R. R., and Shinn, L. E.: Two cases of streptococcic meningitis. Treated successfully with sulfonilamide and Prontosil. J.A.M.A. 108:1948–1951, 1937.

Weinstein, L.: The penicillins. *In:* The Pharmacological Basis of Therapeutics, 5th Edition. Goodman, L. S., and Gilman, A., Eds. Macmillan, New York, 1975, pages 1130–1166.

Whelton, A., Carter, G. G., Garth, M. A., Darwish, M. O., and Walker, W. G.: Carbenicillin-induced acidosis and seizures. J.A.M.A. 218:1942–1943, 1971.

White, W. L., Murphy, F. D., Lockwood, J. S., and Flippin, H. F.: Penicillin in the treatment of pneumococcal, meningococcal, streptococcal and staphylococcal meningitis. Am. J. Med. Sci. 210:1–17, 1945.

Wilkes-Weiss, D., and Huntington, R. W., Jr.: The treatment of influenzal meningitis with immune serum. J. Pediat. 9:462–466, 1936.

Wilson, F. M., Belamaric, J., Lauter, C. B., and Lerner, A. M.: Anicteric carbenicillin hepatitis. Eight episodes in four patients. J.A.M.A. 232:818–821, 1975.

Wirt, T. C., McGee, Z. A., Oldfield, E. H., and Meacham, W. F.: Intraventricular administration of amikacin for complicated gram-negative meningitis and ventriculitis. J. Neurosurg. 50:95–99, 1979.

Wright, E. A., and McQuillen, M. P.: Antibiotic-induced neuromuscular blockade. Ann. N. Y. Acad. Sci. 183:358–368, 1971.

Wright, I. S., De Sanctis, A. G., and Sheplar, A.: The determination of the value of serum in the treatment for meningococcal meningitis. Report of an illustrative series of cases. Am. J. Dis. Child. 38:730–740, 1929.

Wynter, W. E.: Four cases of tubercular meningitis in which paracentesis of the theca vertebralis was performed for the relief of fluid pressure. Lancet 1:981–982, 1891.

Yogev, R., and Williams, T.: Ventricular fluid levels of chloramphenicol in infants. Antimicrob. Agents Chemother. 16:7–8, 1979.

Yoshioka, H., Monma, T., and Matsuda, S.: Placental transfer of gentamicin. J. Pediat. 80:121–123, 1972.

Yoshioka, H., Takimoto, M., Fujita, K., and Maruyama, S.: Pharmacokinetics of tobramycin in the newborn. Infection 7:180–182, 1979.

Yow, M. D.: An overview of pediatric experience with amikacin. Am. J. Med. 62:954–958, 1977.

Yow, M. D., Taber, L. H., Barrett, F. F., Mintz, A. A., Blankinship, G. R., Clark, G. E., and Clark, D. J.: A ten-year experience of methicillin-associated side effects. Pediatrics 58:329–334, 1976.

Yow, M. D., Tengg, N. E., Bangs, J., Bangs, T., and Stephenson, W.: The ototoxic effects of kanamycin sulfate in infants and children. J. Pediat. 60:230–242, 1962.

Zakhrich, B., and Root, R. K.: Unusually high occurrence of drug reactions with nafcillin. Yale J. Biol. Med. 51:449–455, 1978.

Chapter Three

NEONATAL MENINGITIS

In the first 50 years of this century there were only occasional publications on the topic of bacterial meningitis in the newborn infant, most of which stressed the rareness of the condition, the difficulty in clinical diagnosis of the disease until the advanced stages were reached, and the potential seriousness of the condition, even after chemotherapeutic agents came into use (Koplick 1916, Barron 1918, Greenthal 1921, Neal 1926, Pounders 1934, Barrett et al. 1942, Kagan et al. 1949). From the time of the initial reports, the important role of *Escherichia coli* as an offender in the newborn period was repeatedly described, as was the recognition of the rare occurrence of meningitis caused by this organism later in infancy or in older children.

In the past decade, much greater attention has been directed toward the problem of neonatal meningitis, in part because of interest generated from the emergence of Group B *Streptococcus,* first as a rival to the enteric bacilli as the number one cause of the disease and then as the leading cause. The result of intensified interest and investigation has brought about greater awareness of the early symptoms of the illness, more sophisticated diagnostic techniques, and enhanced understanding of the proper dosage and the pharmacokinetics of the antibiotics used for the treatment of meningitis in the newborn infant. Despite these advances, the mortality and morbidity of neonatal gram-negative meningitis and the early onset type of Group B *Streptococcus* sepsis has not yet been significantly improved in recent years. Many of the reasons for the devastating nature of gram-negative meningitis in the newborn have become clear, including the virulence of the organism resulting in extensive ependymal damage, cerebral injury secondary to vasculitis which allows penetration of bacteria into periventricular white matter, the relatively poor CSF penetrability of aminoglycosides into CSF and brain, the possible reduced bactericidal effect of this group of drugs in an acidic environment, and the common occurrence of a high concentration of bacteria in the CSF in this condition.

Of the several different alternative methods of treatment of gram-negative neonatal meningitis, there are major undesirable aspects with each approach. Systemically administered aminoglycosides are transmitted only poorly into the CSF, while lumbar intrathecal administration is not followed by adequate diffusion of the antibiotic throughout the subarachnoid space and ventricular system. Direct intraventricular injection can be technically difficult in the acute stage when the brain is swollen and requires passage of the needle through infected spaces before traversing the brain. Rapid bacterial killing does not usually occur with the use of ampicillin, and all strains of gram-negative enteric bacilli are not consistently sensitive to this agent. Chloramphenicol has possible significant adverse effects when used in the newborn infant, is believed to be only bacteriostatic against many of the coliform bacilli, and can, perhaps, antagonize the bactericidal action of gentamicin or the combination of ampicillin and gentamicin (Paisley and Washington, Rahal and Simberkoff). As a result of the

105

necrotizing effects of this group of pathogens on the immature brain and the less than adequate available methods of treatment of the infection, the case fatality rate of gram-negative neonatal meningitis in most series has exceeded 40 percent, and among survivors the frequency of neurologic sequelae is distressingly high.

Neonatal meningitis, or meningitis occurring in the first four weeks after birth, is most frequently the result of meningeal localization of a septic infection in which the pathogen is acquired by the infant from the mother's birth canal. For this reason, a high percentage of cases have the onset of illness in the first week to 10 days after birth. Neonatal sepsis and meningitis in most instances can be considered to be opportunistic infections in that the causative organisms are generally those that can be readily isolated from the genitourinary or gastrointestinal tracts of normal persons and because of the immunologic features characteristic of the newborn infant which predispose him to bacterial infection (Feigin and Shearer). Male newborn infants more often contract serious bacterial infections than females (Duggve, Yu and Grauaug, Ziai and Haggerty), and premature infants are at considerably higher risk than those born at term (Kagan et al.). The incidence of bacterial meningitis in full-term neonates has been found to be approximately 1.3 per 1000 live births and in premature infants 2.24 cases per 1000 live births (Groover et al., Overall).

Predisposing Factors

In addition to prematurity, certain obstetrical complications are important factors which increase the predisposition of the newborn infant to the development of sepsis and meningitis. Maternal sepsis, urinary tract infection, endometritis, chorioamnionitis, and other peripartum infections are common complications which predispose the neonate to suppurative disease (Overall). Prolonged rupture of fetal membranes, prolonged or precipitous labor and delivery, and mechanical difficulties with delivery of the child are additional obstetrical problems often associated with neonatal bacterial infection. Approximately 50 to 65 percent of cases of neonatal gram-negative enteric bacillus meningitis occur in infants born with such recognized maternal complications (Berman and Banker, Groover et al., Ziai and Haggerty). The same

obstetrical factors are important in the predisposition of the neonate to the early onset form of Group B *Streptococcus* sepsis, in conjunction with maternal vaginal colonization with the organism and deficiency of maternal antibody against the Group B *Streptococcus* capsular antigen (Baker and Kasper 1976). Abnormal fetal heart tones and meconium-stained amniotic fluid are signs of fetal distress during labor which place the infant in the increased risk category regarding the possible occurrence of neonatal infection.

In the days immediately following birth, septic infections of the infant's respiratory or intestinal tract, infected skin lesions, and sepsis of the umbilical stump provide a potential source for the dissemination of bacteria possibly resulting in meningitis. Catheterization of the umbilical vessels and insertion of a central venous feeding catheter provide further potential routes for entry of bacteria in the newborn. Such procedures as well as endotracheal intubation, respirator care, and other specialized techniques required in the neonatal intensive care unit are associated with a high incidence of nosocomial infections. In one large series, the nosocomial infection rate in a newborn intensive care unit was 24.6 percent (Hemming et al.). Surface infections were the most common infectious complications in this report, followed by pneumonia, bacteremia, surgical wound infections, urinary tract infection, and meningitis. The latter accounted for four percent of nosocomial infections in this series.

Studies have shown that spontaneous colonization of the skin of the neonate with *Staphylococcus aureus* has certain protective effects against the acquisition of an infection from gram-negative organisms (Forfar et al., Light et al.). This example of bacterial interference is also applicable to the use of high-dosage and multiple antibiotics, which alter the normal flora of the respiratory and intestinal tracts with the emergence of gram-negative organisms often resistant to the commonly used antibiotics. Invasive infections with *Proteus* species, *Klebsiella* species, and *Serratia marcescens* are frequently partially explained on this basis. For reasons not entirely clear, infants with galactosemia are significantly predisposed to *Escherichia coli* sepsis, sometimes with meningitis, in the first four weeks of life (Levy et al. 1977).

Neonatal sepsis also can be acquired by the infant from contaminated equipment used for resuscitation, mechanical ventilation, or even from incubators used for infant care.

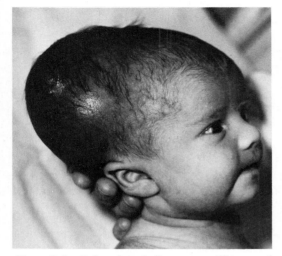

Figure 3–1. Infected cephalhematoma. Three-week-old infant noted to have a right parietal cephalhematoma one day after birth. Lesion remained approximately the same for 2½ weeks when it began to enlarge. Two days before admission cutaneous erythema over the mass was noted, and the day of admission it perforated the skin spontaneously, exuding pus. The lesion was surgically drained, and culture of purulent material, as well as from blood and CSF, was positive for beta-hemolytic *Streptococcus*.

Pseudomonas and *Proteus* species infections in the neonate especially may be acquired in this fashion (Barrie, Becker, Fierer et al.), and *Flavobacterium meningosepticum* meningitis can result from infected water sources or saline used in the newborn nursery (Cabrera and Davis, Plotkin and McKitrick). Congenital anomalies, such as a meningomyelocele, provide an obvious source of bacterial infection of both gram-negative and gram-positive types to the neonate. On rare occasion, a cephalhematoma in the newborn infant may become infected secondary to bacterial sepsis or attempted needle aspiration (Burry and Hellerstein, Levy et al. 1967, Lee and Berg) and can lead to suppurative meningitis by direct extension into the subarachnoid space (Cohen et al.) or osteomyelitis of the calvarium (Ellis et al.) (Fig. 3–1). Suppuration within a cephalhematoma can remain remarkably silent, manifested only by intermittent fever and progressive enlargement of the lesion. Unless diagnosis is made and wide incision with drainage is accomplished, the overlying skin will eventually become erythematous and spontaneous perforation through the skin will occur. In most reports of infected cephalhematomas, the microorganisms isolated have been gram-negative rods although *Staphylococcus* or *Streptococcus*

species can also be at fault. Fetal scalp monitoring during labor with fetal scalp electrodes is an additional factor which on rare occasion leads to serious infection in the neonate. Possible complications of the procedure include scalp abscess, cranial osteomyelitis, CSF leak through the fontanel, sepsis, and meningitis (Feder et al., Overturf and Balfour, Turbeville and McCaffree, Turbeville et al.).

In addition to the exposure to a variety of bacterial pathogens during the birth process and in the newborn period, the defense mechanisms of the neonate provide less protection against infection than in later childhood (Gotoff). Although the full-term newborn infant is provided with immunoglobulin G (IgG) by passive transfer from the mother, the larger immunoglobulin M and A (IgM, IgA) molecules do not pass the placental barrier. Thus, IgM and IgA are undetectable or present in low content in the neonate. Because bactericidal antibodies to gram-negative enteropathogens are largely IgM molecules, this physiologic and transient immunologic deficit probably in part accounts for the increased susceptibility to such infectious illnesses in the newborn period. The low-birth-weight infant may have reduced levels of IgG at birth owing to diminished transplacental passage (Yeung and Hobbs). Risk of invasive disease caused by Group B *Streptococcus* in the newborn infant at least in part can be attributed to deficiency of antibody directed against capsular polysaccharide of the organism in the mother, and thus the child (Baker and Kasper).

Other factors pertinent to defense mechanisms in the newborn are less well established and conflicting results have been reported. Phagocytic function of neutrophils of the newborn has been claimed to be normal by some investigators (Dossett and Quie) and deficient by others (Miller). Coen et al. found that phagocytic function was intact but that in certain newborns defective intracellular bacterial destruction within leukocytes occurred. While most reports have indicated that antibacterial leukocyte function in the healthy newborn infant is normal, there is evidence that in the stressed infant there can be considerable lability in leukocyte function in regard to phagocytosis and intracellular killing (Anderson et al., Wright et al.). The phagocytic process has been divided into four distinct phases (Winkelstein), including chemotaxis, opsonization, ingestion, and digestion or killing. Chemotaxis refers to phagocytic migration toward the bacterial agent. Opsonization is the process during which serum components combine with bacteria making them more susceptible to engulfment by phagocytes. Ingestion of the bacterial agent is followed by intracellular destruction, or digestion, a mechanism which involves rupture of lysosomal contents with their release into the phagocytic vacuole.

Other studies have indicated transient deficiencies of certain components of complement (Fireman et al.) and impaired opsonic activity in newborn infants (Forman and Stiehm). Total complement activity has been found to be subnormal in approximately one-half of healthy term infants, with mean activity in the range of 70 to 90 percent of adult concentrations. Values are somewhat less in preterm newborn infants (Johnston et al.). McCracken and Eichenwald found that both phagocytic and bactericidal function of polymorphonuclear leukocytes of the neonate were normal but that opsonic activity for certain bacteria was deficient.

Clinical Aspects

The symptoms and signs of meningitis in the newborn period are often deceptive and may resemble those of several other disorders. Commonly recognized signs of infection in older children and signs of meningeal irritation are frequently absent in the neonate with purulent meningitis. The initial manifestations of illness are usually those of sepsis, thus indicating the need for lumbar puncture whenever bacterial sepsis is considered in this age group. Irritability, constant crying, abdominal distention, cyanotic or apneic episodes, and unexplained jaundice are frequent initial findings. Other cutaneous abnormalities sometimes observed in infants with neonatal sepsis include pyoderma, petechiae, purpura, and the violet or purple impetiginous or ulcerative lesions characteristic of *Pseudomonas* infection. Vomiting, anorexia, and lethargy are other early symptoms suggestive of an infectious illness.

The early onset type of Group B *Streptococcus* sepsis, with or without meningitis, very often presents in the first few hours after birth with progressive respiratory distress simulating hyaline membrane disease, recurrent apneic attacks, hypotension or shock, and frequently marked neutropenia. A similar clinical course on rare occasion in the neonate can be caused by systemic infection with Group D *Streptococcus* (Alexander and Giacoia), *Streptococcus pneumoniae* (Bortolussi et al.), *Listeria monocytogenes* (Ahlfors et al.), and *Hemophilus influenzae* (Lilien et al.). Some term infants may respond with febrile spikes while premature infants are more prone to have hypothermic episodes with bacterial meningitis. Neck stiffness and other meningeal signs are characteristically absent in this age group and bulging of the fontanel may not be apparent until late in the illness. Seizures, either focal or generalized, can occur early in the disease or be delayed until the process becomes far advanced. The illness often advances rapidly, with death occurring within days after the first symptoms. Infrequently, the illness will progress slowly with signs consisting mainly of irritability and vomiting until abnormal enlargement of the head becomes apparent. Although unusual, such cases can be confused with congenital hydrocephalus due to congenital anomalies of the aqueduct until the spinal or ventricular fluid is examined (Fig. 3–2).

Diagnosis of bacterial meningitis in the newborn or young infant depends on suspicion of the possibility and performance of a lumbar puncture. Because the initial manifestations of bacterial meningitis in the neonate are often those more indicative of septicemia, a lumbar puncture is indicated whenever sepsis is suspected or identified in this age group or when the infant has an otherwise unexplained seizure. Cerebrospinal fluid abnormalities with meningitis in this age group resemble those in older children. The cellular response is largely or entirely polymorphonuclear, the glucose content is usually reduced, and the protein is elevated. Elevation of the CSF protein content is usually much greater in young infants with meningitis than in older children. Levels between 300 and 1,200 mg. per 100 ml. are not uncommon in the neonatal group, especially if the illness has been present for several days. Organisms are usually readily evident on gram stain and are isolated on culture. On rare occasion, the CSF from an infant examined because of signs of systemic sepsis reveals normal chemical values and few or no cells, but bacteria are identified on smear or culture. This is probably explained on a time-relationship basis in which the spinal tap is performed shortly after subarachnoid invasion by the organisms, but before an inflammatory response can occur. The CSF glucose

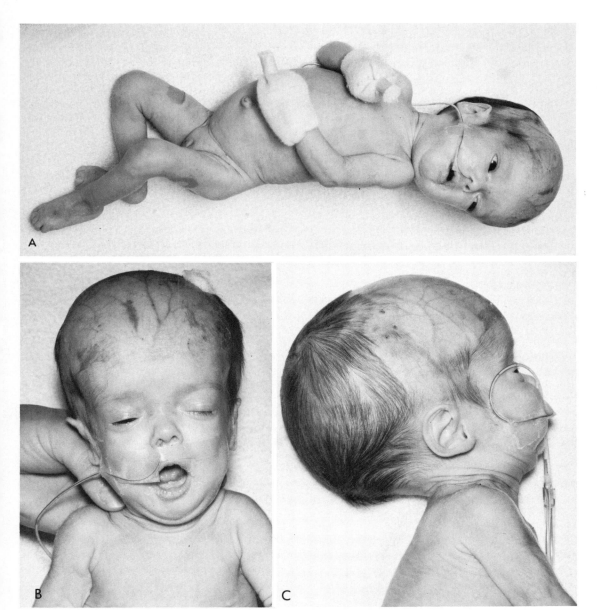

Figure 3–2. Neonatal *Escherichia coli* meningitis. Rapid head enlargement as an early sign. Seven-week-old infant with a birth weight of 1400 grams; head circumference at birth was 27 cm. Membranes ruptured 6 days before delivery and the child received no antibiotics immediately after birth. Feeding and weight gain were described as normal for the first 4 weeks after birth, when rapid rate of head enlargement was noted. When examined at 6 weeks of age, the child was mildly irritable, afebrile, and would feed well. Head circumference then was 37 cm. and the white blood cell count was 26,000 per cu. mm. The tentative diagnosis was congenital hydrocephalus, but a ventricular tap revealed purulent fluid with a protein content of 940 mg. per 100 ml., glucose of 15 mg. per 100 ml., and abundant gram-negative bacilli. Antibiotic therapy was initiated but over the next few days the child deteriorated markedly. Purulent leptomeningitis in this infant was surprisingly silent except for the production of head enlargement secondary to hydrocephalus. The illness was fatal at age 10 weeks. *A,* Infant at 7 weeks of age. She is poorly responsive, hypertonic, somewhat wasted, and the head size is abnormally large compared to her weight and length. *B* and *C,* Scalp veins are distended; the anterior fontanel is enlarged and full, reflecting advanced hydrocephalus.

can be deceptively normal, or even elevated, and is somewhat related to the blood sugar level. For this reason, a simultaneous blood sugar determination should be done when the spinal tap is performed. Blood glucose may be elevated because of infused glucose-containing fluid or may rise following convulsions. Conversely, the septic newborn may be hypoglycemic (Yeung et al.), a factor that can contribute to abnormal signs or possibly even enhance the occurrence of cerebral injury.

A frequently encountered circumstance is the low-birth-weight infant with respiratory distress syndrome treated with ventilatory support and antibiotics and who, for one reason or another, has a lumbar puncture done for the first time at approximately 10 to 15 days of age. The CSF specimen is found to be brown or xanthochromic in color, containing an excessive number of granulocytes and a markedly reduced glucose content with a negative gram stain for bacteria. These CSF findings are entirely compatible with the occurrence of intraventricular bleeding in the first two or three days after birth (Deonna et al., Mathew et al.) but are also consistent with partially treated bacterial meningitis. A normal or only slightly elevated CSF lactic acid value provides some evidence against bacterial infection but, in many instances, the child must again be placed on antibiotic therapy until the CSF and blood cultures are shown to be negative.

Blood cultures should be obtained when meningitis is identified, as positive blood cultures have been found in 70 to 80 percent of cases of neonatal meningitis (Fosson and Fine). Peripheral venous blood is the most reliable specimen for culture but, in newborn infants in whom it is very difficult to obtain venous blood, a sample from an umbilical artery catheter can be used, assuming the catheter has not been in place for more than a few hours (Cowett et al.). Culture of properly collected urine is a frequently overlooked procedure in the septic infant, which may allow the identification of the organism at fault before other cultures become positive. Gastric aspirate obtained immediately after birth, examined by gram stain for polymorphonuclear leukocytes and bacteria, and by cultural techniques, can have some predictive value as an indicator of degree of risk for sepsis, but overlap of positive findings between non-infected and infected infants is considerable (Boyle et al.).

Umbilical cord blood is a poor source of culture, as contaminants frequently result in positive cultures of no clinical significance. The predictive value of histologic evidence of umbilical cord inflammation, so-called funisitis, has been debated for a number of years. Funisitis is not always present when there is perinatal acquisition of bacterial infection, and the presence of funisitis is not invariably followed by clinical or cultural proof of septic infection. The presence of an umbilical cord inflammatory reaction, however, has a strong association with the possibility of perinatal bacterial infection and indicates that the infant is at increased risk for such an illness (Overbach et al.). Navarro and Blanc described an unusual type of necrotizing funisitis with severe endovasculitis in premature infants, which was found to have a very high association with septic ascending antenatal infection.

The white blood cell count is less helpful as an index pointing to bacterial infection in the newborn infant than in the older child because of the wide variation of the normal range that is possible in the neonatal period. On the first day of life, the white blood cell count can normally range from 9,000 to 30,000 per cu. mm., with a mean of 18,100 per cu. mm. (Oski). A neutrophilic leukocytosis is found in the first three days after birth and by one week of age, lymphocytes normally predominate, with the mean total count being 12,200 per cu. mm. by this time. During the first few days after birth, white blood counts less than 4,000 or greater than 30,000 per cu. mm. must be considered very suggestive of infection, especially if there is significant increase in band forms or the appearance of toxic granulations and Döhle bodies (Gregory and Hey, Zipursky et al.).

Thrombocytopenia can result from infections of many types in the newborn infant and provides another fragment of evidence suggesting a suppurative illness. Leukopenia and thrombocytopenia secondary to severe bacterial infection in the neonate are believed to be more likely the result of peripheral consumptive mechanisms than of bone marrow suppression (Squire et al., Zipursky et al.).

The erythrocyte sedimentation rate is not widely used in the newborn period because of its lack of specificity. Normal values in the first month after birth are less than 20 mm. per hour, and few disorders in this age range, other than septic infections, are associated with abnormally elevated levels. A significantly elevated sedimentation rate is usually present in the septic neonate and can be of some diagnostic value in a non-specific way (Adler and Denton).

Hypoosmolarity, with reduced serum sodium and chloride levels resulting from water retention secondary to inappropriate secretion of antidiuretic hormone, has been described in neonatal meningitis (Reynolds et al.). This condition occurs in a variety of neurologic infections in all age groups and is recognized by the combination of reduced serum osmolarity, elevated urine osmolarity, continued renal excretion of sodium, and the expected response to treatment by fluid restriction.

Causative Organisms

The predominant causes of bacterial sepsis and meningitis in the newborn infant have shown many changes over the past 60 years. In 1918, when meningitis in early infancy was claimed to be an "exceedingly rare disease," Barron tabulated the causative organisms in 19 cases of neonatal meningitis and found that seven were caused by *Bacillus coli,* six were said to be mixed staphylococcal and streptococcal infections, two were due to the pneumococcus, and the remaining three were each the result of a different bacillus. For approximately 15 years extending from 1930 through the mid-forties, Group A *Streptococcus* was the leading offender causing septic disease in the neonate (Dunham, Nyhan and Fousek).

For the next decade up to the mid-fifties, *Escherichia coli* came to equal and then to exceed the *Streptococcus* as the cause of neonatal sepsis and its complications, but among *Streptococcus* species, there began to emerge occasional cases of non-Group A strains in infected neonates (Nyhan and Fousek). With the decline of the occurrence of neonatal streptococcal infections, there occurred an increase in those resulting from *Staphylococcus* species. By the late 1950's, coliform bacilli were found to account for 50 to 73 percent of all cases of neonatal sepsis, with *Escherichia coli* the single most commonly isolated organism (Watson, Ziai and Haggerty). This etiologic pattern largely persisted for the next 10 to 15 years, but in 1964, for the first time, in one large eastern medical center, Group B *Streptococcus* was found to be the most common cause of neonatal sepsis over an 18-month period of time (Eickhoff et al.). The significance of this observation as a predictor of future trends did not become immediately apparent as, in most centers, *Escherichia coli* continued to account for 30 to 40 percent of all cases of neonatal meningitis, and Group B *Streptococcus* lagged behind by a considerable margin (Fosson and Fine, Overall). Beginning in approximately 1968, it became apparent that in many major hospitals, Group B *Streptococcus* had become the single leading cause of sepsis and meningitis in the newborn period, with an incidence of neonatal sepsis of 2 to 3 per 1,000 live births (Baker et al. 1973, Barton et al., Franciosi et al.).

Neonatal meningitis can result from a wide variety of gram-negative and gram-positive bacteria but, at present, two organisms account for the majority of cases. *Escherichia coli* and Group B *Streptococcus* are the leading offenders and are currently the cause of the majority of cases of bacterial meningitis in the newborn period. The two have been found in approximately equal frequency in some centers, but in most the balance is in favor of Group B *Streptococcus* as the single leading offender. Among 117 cases of neonatal gram-negative enteric bacillus meningitis, McCracken and Mize found that 82 (70 percent) were caused by *Escherichia coli,* 7 (6 percent) were due to *Salmonella* species, and there were 5 cases (4 percent) each with *Citrobacter* species, *Proteus mirabilis,* and *Serratia* species. *Klebsiella* species and *Enterobacter* species each accounted for 4 cases (3 percent) in this series.

Among streptococcal species, Group B organisms are by far the most important cause of neonatal sepsis and meningitis, although other serotypes on rare occasion are implicated. Occasional cases of Group A *Streptococcus* meningitis continue to occur, although most Group A neonatal infections are benign and primarily involve the skin (Dillon, Nelson et al.). Neonatal meningitis has also been described with Group C (Stewardson-Krieger and Gotoff) and Group D *Streptococcus,* the latter with a clinical course that can resemble the early onset type of Group B *Streptococcus* infection (Alexander and Giacoia, Headings et al.).

The common causes of meningitis beyond three months of age, including *Hemophilus influenzae, Streptococcus pneumoniae,* and *Neisseria meningitidis,* only infrequently give rise to neonatal meningitis. Accumulated cases of *Hemophilus influenzae* meningitis in the neonate reveal that they account for only approximately 1 percent of cases of meningitis in this age span (Fosson and Fine, Groover et al.). The infrequency of invasive disease in the neonate by *Hemophilus influenzae* has been attributed to the rare occurrence of this organism in the maternal genitourinary tract and the presence of protective antibody transplacentally transferred from the mother to the fetus. Notable features of neonatal infection caused by *Hemophilus influenzae* include the higher incidence of non-typable organisms compared to the very high incidence of type b organisms later in infancy (Lilien et al., Khuri-Bulos and McIntosh), and the frequent occurrence of other organ system involvement, such as arthritis, osteomyelitis, pneumonitis, or pericarditis in those with sepsis and meningitis (Collier et al., Granoff and Nankeruis). In some instances, the clinical pattern of neonatal *Hemophilus influenzae* sepsis is identical to the early onset Group B *Streptococcus* infection (Lilien et al.). Even rarer are reports of *Hemophilus parainfluenzae* meningitis in the newborn infant (Gullekson and Dumoff).

Streptococcus pneumoniae meningitis is somewhat more common in the neonate than that resulting from *Hemophilus influenzae* but is still unusual. Among 83 cases of neonatal meningitis reported by Ziai and Haggerty in 1958, 8 percent were pneumococcal in origin while 6.7 percent of 457 cases described by Fosson and Fine (1968) and 5 percent of 211 cases reviewed by Groover et al. (1961) were caused by *Streptococcus pneumoniae*. Recent authors have stressed the similarity of neonatal pneumococcal sepsis or meningitis to the early onset form of Group B streptococcal disease, with features common to both being respiratory distress with onset soon after birth, hypotension, leukopenia, and rapid deterioration (Bortolussi et al., Rhodes et al.). Colonization of the maternal uterine cervix or endocervical infection with pneumococcus has been a common but not invariable finding when the neonate has been found to have invasive disease with this organism (Rhodes et al., Weintraub and Otto). In one report, the mother and the newborn infant simultaneously experienced pneumococcal meningitis (Tempest).

Examples of meningococcal meningitis in the newborn period have been sporadically described for many years (Ravid, Root) although the disease is acknowledged to be rare in this age group. Among cases that have occurred, the organism has been assumed to

have been acquired from the mother's vaginal tract (Sunderland et al.) or by respiratory transmission after the birth process (Stiehm and Damrosch). Gonococcal meningitis in the newborn infant has been described as a complication of gonococcal ophthalmia and sepsis but is quite rare (Bradford and Kelly).

Citrobacter diversus, synonymous with *Citrobacter koseri,* and *Citrobacter freundii* are anaerobic gram-negative members of the Enterobacteriaceae and are occasionally found to be part of the normal bowel flora. *Citrobacter* species represent an infrequent but not rare cause of neonatal meningitis (Gross et al., Gwynn and George) but are better known as causes of brain abscess in the newborn period or in early infancy (Kaplan et al., Vogel). For reasons that are unclear, the literature on brain abscesses in infants under three months of age reveals *Citrobacter* species to be the single most common offender.

Several other members of the Enterobacteriaceae have been incriminated in neonatal meningitis but none can be thought of as common, at least in this country. Among cases of *Salmonella* species meningitis, most occur in young infants (Rabinowitz and MacLeod), but unlike most other gram-negative organisms known to cause neonatal meningitis, *Salmonella* species can result in this disease with almost equal frequency in each of the first several months after birth. The illness in infancy is often preceded or associated with diarrhea and has a high mortality rate (Froeschle et al.), although recovery can occur with appropriate therapy (Burton et al.). Neonatal *Salmonella* species meningitis is more common in certain other parts of the world than in this country (Barclay).

Any of the division *Klebsiella-Enterobacter-Serratia* can colonize and invade infants in a newborn nursery and result in sporadic or epidemic systemic disease, including meningitis (Hable et al., Hill et al., Stamm et al.). This is most likely to occur in an area in which care is directed to premature infants, or those undergoing intensive care requiring procedures which compromise the skin, upper respiratory tract, or intestinal tract in conjunction with the use of antibiotic therapy (Goldmann et al.). Infections with these organisms, and especially nursery outbreaks, commonly are secondary to breakdown in adequate isolation or handwashing techniques of hospital attendants. *Proteus* species can rarely give rise to meningitis in otherwise normal newborn infants but like *Klebsiella* and *Serratia* species, Proteus shows a greater predisposition to attack the low-birth-weight infant or the child debilitated with other conditions (Shortland-Webb). Similarly to *Flavobacterium meningosepticum*, *Proteus* species can colonize water sources or nursery equipment from which transmission to the infant can occur (Becker). *Edwardsiella tarda* is a recent addition to the family Enterobacteriaceae and is an exceedingly rare cause of neonatal meningitis (Okubadejo and Alausa).

A number of cases of meningitis in the newborn infant have resulted from *Flavobacterium meningosepticum*, both in sporadic and epidemic fashion (Cabrera and Davis, George et al.). In some instances, the source of the organism has not been identified (Eykens et al., Rios et al.), while in others contaminated water sources were suspected or identified (Cabrera and Davis, Maderazo et al., Plotkin and McKitrick). *Flavobacterium meningosepticum* is a non-motile, gram-negative rod which is an unusual cause of human disease but, among cases that do occur, there is a decided predilection for invasion of the meninges of the newborn, and especially the premature infant. The organism is known to be a possible contaminant of water sources in a hospital environment and can be transmitted to the newborn infant by this mechanism. Another unusual feature of *Flavobacterium meningosepticum* relates to its antibiotic sensitivities. Most isolates are very resistant to the penicillins, the aminoglycosides, and chloramphenicol, but are sensitive to erythromycin and vancomycin, drugs that penetrate into the CSF poorly (Aber et al., Rios et al.). Rifampin has also been shown to be effective in many instances.

Campylobacter fetus is a curved, microaerophilic, gram-negative rod long known to be a cause of fetal wastage in cattle and sheep. The first case of neonatal meningitis attributed to this organism was described in 1962 by Eden and only a few additional examples have been recognized since (Burgert and Hagstrom, Willis and Austin). The disease has been fatal in reported cases in the newborn period.

Pasteurella species are coccobacillary gram-negative organisms best known for their role in the animal world. Among the rarest of expressions of human disease with these organisms is meningitis in the newborn infant (Bates et al., Frutos et al., Repice and Neter). The organism differs from most gram-negative rods in that it is usually penicillin-sensitive.

Bacteroides species are normal inhabitants of the gastrointestinal tract which are especially likely to invade traumatized or devitalized tissues (Harrod and Stevens). As part of the normal flora of the female genital tract, it is expected that these anaerobes can be found in the infants' intestinal tract soon after birth. They are uncommon causes of neonatal meningitis but the disease has been described secondary to necrotizing bowel lesions and peritonitis, and in infants with open neural tube defects (Berman et al., Cooke, Feldman).

Mycoplasma hominis is an additional rare cause of meningitis in the newborn period. The onset of the illness in most reported cases has been between five and 15 days after birth and the CSF abnormalities are similar to those of bacterial meningitis (Boe et al., Gewitz et al.). The illness usually affects premature infants and, in most, the child is born of a mother with symptomatic perinatal infection or other types of perinatal complications.

Neonatal Gram-Negative Bacillary Meningitis

In the newborn infant meningitis caused by gram-negative pathogens is the most destructive type of bacterial meningitis that occurs in any age group. While numerous gram-negative microorganisms can cause this illness, *Escherichia coli* is by far the most common offender. The disease most often has its onset in the first 10 days after birth but can occur anytime in the first four to six weeks of life. Unlike Group B *Streptococcus* sepsis with meningitis, symptoms of *Escherichia coli* meningitis are infrequently seen in the first 24 hours after birth. The illness is more frequent in premature infants and often has a clear association with premature rupture of fetal membranes, maternal septic infection or other complications of the labor and delivery process, and has a higher incidence in newborn and young infants with galactosemia (Levy et al. 1977). Most cases of *Escherichia coli* meningitis are sporadic although nursery outbreaks have been described (Headings and Overall). Nursery outbreaks of meningitis are more characteristic of *Proteus* species (Becker), *Klebsiella* species (Hill et al.), and *Flavobacterium meningosepticum* (Cabrera et al.), organisms that are known for their propensity to colonize nursery water sources or respiratory equipment, or to emerge in a unit caring for critically ill infants who must receive high-dosage and multiple antibiotic therapy. *Proteus* species meningitis in the newborn infant is a particularly severe process. Most cases are caused by *Proteus mirabilis* (Levy and Ingall, Mikherjee, Scherger et al.), an organism that can attack the otherwise normal infant, the one with a neural tube defect, or the infant debilitated by other major organ system disease. Regardless of the causative organism, the mortality rate of neonatal gram-negative meningitis is high and survivors are commonly disabled with intellectual deficits, hydrocephalus, or other types of neurologic dysfunction.

In 1974, Robbins et al. demonstrated that meningeal invasiveness of *Escherichia coli* is related to the presence or absence of Kl capsular polysaccharide antigen, an antigen with properties similar to those of meningococcal Group B polysaccharide antigen. Over 80 percent of isolates from neonates with *Escherichia coli* meningitis were found to contain Kl antigen, a prevalence much higher than found in isolates from normal children or those with urinary tract infections. In addition, the morbidity and mortality of *Escherichia coli* meningitis was found to correlate with the presence of this antigenic substance in CSF. Among cases with Kl antigen, survival was related to the amount of antigen and the length of time it persisted in body fluids (McCracken et al. 1974).

The neuropathology of neonatal gram-negative meningitis is determined more by the stage of the illness when death occurs than by the causative organism. When death occurs soon after onset, the brain is swollen and hyperemic, and the ventricles are reduced in size (Berman and Banker). The subarachnoid exudate over the convexity and at the base contains primarily polymorphonuclear leukocytes and occasional histiocytes. Bacteria can usually readily be identified within the inflammatory exudate. When survival of the infant extends beyond the initial stages of the illness, severe vasculitis, ependymal disruption, and necrotizing cerebral changes, with bacteria within damaged brain tissue, can often be observed (Fig. 3–3). The ventricular system is frequently distended, in many instances secondary to inflammatory obstruction within the aqueduct or at the outlet foramina of the fourth ventricle. The ventricular exudate may consist of frank pus, a state referred to as pyoventriculitis (Izquierdo et al.) (Fig. 3–4). The constant finding of inflammatory involvement of the ventricular choroid plexuses has suggested to some that the choroid plexus may be the primary site of bacterial invasion of the CSF (Gilles et al.). Fibrous strands or septations rapidly develop within the ventricular system, extending from one denuded ependymal surface to another, leading to irregular, partial compartmentalization of the lateral ventricles (Schultz and Leeds). In some cases, necrotizing vasculitis in combination with bacterial invasion of brain tissue converts the periventricular white matter into a mass of foul-smelling, hemorrhagic, necrotic debris, which leads to extensive multicystic encephalomalacia if the child survives for a period of time (Cussen and Ryan) (Fig. 3–5). Cerebral cortical areas show depletion of the neuronal population, some degree of astrocytic proliferation, and zones of ischemic infarction of variable sizes.

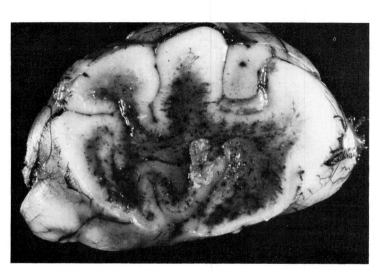

Figure 3–3. Neonatal *Escherichia coli* meningitis. Sagittal section through one cerebral hemisphere. Extensive hemorrhagic necrosis of the cerebral white matter is present, associated with ventriculitis, ependymal destruction, necrotizing vasculitis, and bacterial invasion of brain tissue.

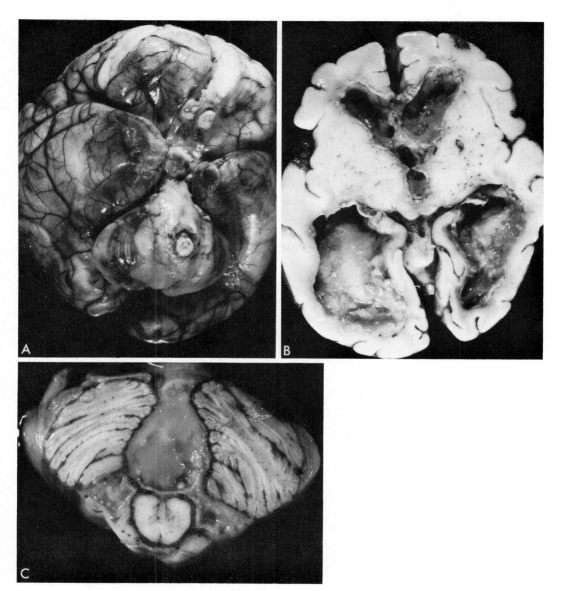

Figure 3–4.   Neonatal *Escherichia coli* meningitis. *A,* The cerebrum is swollen, hyperemic, and softened. A dense purulent exudate at the base coats the cerebellum, encases the brain stem, and extends superiorly into the interpeduncular cistern. *B,* Horizontal section of the brain demonstrates pyoventriculitis with associated ventricular enlargement, necrotizing ependymitis, and periventricular softening. *C,* The medulla is surrounded by a thick purulent exudate which extends over the cerebellum.

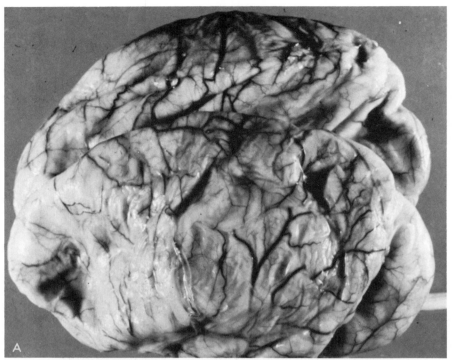

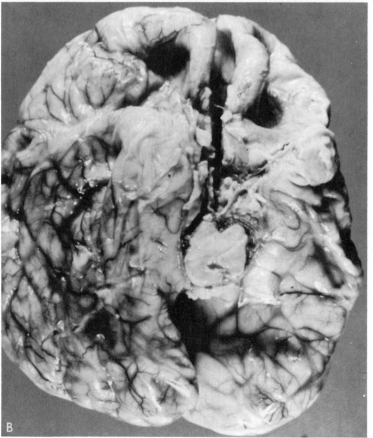

Figure 3–5.   See legend on opposite page

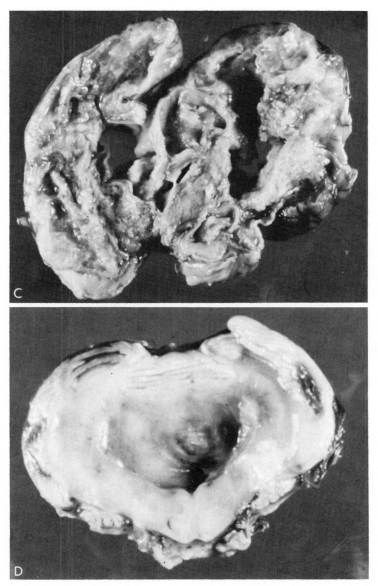

Figure 3–5. Neonatal *Escherichia coli* meningitis. *A,* Dorsal surface of the brain is covered with purulent material. The cerebrum appears to be softened and shows venous congestion. *B,* Ventral surface of the brain with the cerebellum removed. The exudate is thicker at the base than over the cerebral convexity, and the orbital surface of the frontal lobes appears to be necrotic. *C,* Coronal section of the brain demonstrates the severe necrotizing effects of the virulent infection. The cerebral hemispheres have been converted into a necrotic mass with microcystic and macrocystic degeneration. The corpus callosum is necrotic and the lateral ventricles cannot easily be distinguished from cystic cavities within the brain. *D,* Transverse section through the pons looking caudally shows the marked distention of the fourth ventricle, which is completely obstructed distally by purulent material and necrotic debris.

Group B Streptococcus *Meningitis*

When Lancefield established the classification of streptococci on the basis of the cell wall carbohydrate composition in 1933, Group A was the predominant human pathogen and Group B *(Streptococcus agalactiae)* was assumed to be primarily a cause of bovine mastitis but of little significance as a cause of human disease. In 1938, Fry in London reported three fatal cases of puerperal sepsis which resulted from Group B *Streptococcus,* an observation which initiated the awareness of the pathogenic importance of the organism in the human. Soon thereafter, additional examples of invasive disease in adults due to Group B *Streptococcus* were recognized (Rantz and Keefer), and in 1958, Nyhan and Fousek documented the occurrence of Group B *Streptococcus* neonatal meningitis. Hood and colleagues in 1961 showed that Group B *Streptococcus* could be isolated from the genital tract in approximately 5 percent of pregnant women in the absence of symptomatic illness, and in the same report, described three additional cases of neonatal meningitis resulting from this microorganism. The emerging role of Group B *Streptococcus* began to be apparent in 1964 when Eickhoff et al. found it to be the single most common cause of sepsis in the newborn infant over an 18-month period of time. By the end of the decade, the organism was being recognized as the most common isolate in neonates with suppurative meningitis in many hospitals, and by 1973 the two distinct types of neonatal group B *Streptococcus* infection were clearly delineated (Baker et al. 1973, Franciosi et al.). Currently, it is estimated that 12,000 to 15,000 newborn infants in this country contract invasive infection per year caused by Group B *Streptococcus,* making it one of the most dangerous microorganisms to which the neonate is commonly exposed (Baker 1977).

Five serotypes of Group B streptococci are now recognized, designated Ia, Ib, Ic, II, and III. Group B organisms on sheep blood agar have a different appearance from that of Group A and D streptococci. Group B *Streptococcus* is mucoid and gray with a small surrounding zone of beta hemolysis. The great majority of Group B strains are beta-hemolytic although a non-hemolytic strain isolated from a newborn infant has been described (Wilkinson et al.). Identification of an isolate as Group B is on the basis of its customary resistance to bacitracin and its ability to hydrolyze sodium hippurate to benzoate and glycine but its inability to hydrolyze esculin in the presence of bile.

Group B *Streptococcus* is commonly found to colonize the anogenital tract of men and women and, to a lesser degree, the nasopharyngeal region. Likewise, the organism can frequently be isolated from the anal canal, umbilical stump, and nasopharynx of asymptomatic newborn infants. Reported colonization rates have varied considerably, probably reflecting differences in the study populations and lack of standardization of cultural techniques. Baker and Barrett (1973) found vaginal colonization with Group B *Streptococcus* in 22.5 percent of women at the end of pregnancy and colonization of the umbilicus or ear canal in 22.2 percent of neonates. Among nursery personnel, they identified vaginal colonization in 30 percent. Aber et al. did repeated cultures of 297 women in the third trimester of pregnancy and recovered Group B *Streptococcus* at least on one occasion in 28.7 percent. Among 242 infants included in the study, Group B organisms were isolated from throat and umbilical cord specimens obtained in the first two weeks after birth in 37.2 percent. Paredes and colleagues obtained Group B *Streptococcus* from vaginal and throat swab cultures on 27.7 percent of mothers on admission to the labor area and from umbilical and throat cultures from 22.5 percent of neonates in the first 20 hours after birth. Colonization of the infants dramatically increased to 65.4 percent at the time of their hospital discharge. In the series of Speck et al., the colonization rate of asymptomatic infants in the first two weeks after birth was 14 percent, which then declined to 5 percent by age 42 days. These authors demonstrated bacterial antagonism between Group B *Streptococcus* and other bacteria which normally colonize the newborn infant, including *Staphylococcus* species and *Escherichia coli.*

Despite the common prevalence of colonization of newborn infants with Group B *Streptococcus,* the attack rate for sepsis or meningitis is relatively low, being in the range of 2 to 4 cases per 1,000 live births in most series (Aber et al., Baker 1979, Franciosi et al.) and as high as 5.4 per 1,000 live births in the large series reported by Pass et al. Thus, asymptomatic colonization occurs approximately 100 times the incidence of symptomatic infection with this organism in the newborn period. Despite the relatively low attack rate compared to the rate of colonization, Group B *Streptococcus* has clearly become an important potential threat to the newborn infant, and especially the premature infant born under stressful circumstances. If one accepts the conservative figure of two cases per 1,000 live births for the attack rate for the early onset form of Group B *Streptococcus* sepsis, with a mortality rate of 50 percent there would be one death per 1,000 live births from this illness, a figure representing a significant component of total neonatal mortality in this country. Whether the newborn infant is infected in asymptomatic fashion (colonized) or exhibits the early onset form of invasive disease, the fact that the offending organisms isolated from infant and mother are almost invariably of the same serotype indicates that vertical transmission from the maternal genital tract is the source of neonatal infection.

The mode of transmission of the organism to infants who acquire the late onset type of infection is less clear. In some instances, colonization may occur during the birth process, with tissue invasion being delayed for two to six weeks thereafter. In addition, there is good evidence that nosocomial infection is not infrequent, with transmission of Group B *Streptococcus* from other colonized infants via the hands of nursery personnel, as well as the possibility of spread of streptococci from colonized nursery attendants or from maternal nasopharyngeal secretions (Aber et al., Anthony et al., Steere et al.).

The high rate of neonatal colonization compared to the relatively low attack rate with septic disease suggests that other factors must be operative to account for invasive Group B *Streptococcus* infection in the newborn infant. At least one important risk factor identified by Baker and Kasper (1976, 1977) is maternal serum deficiency of type-specific, opsonic antibody directed against the capsular polysaccharide antigen of the organism. These IgG antibodies are transplacentally transmitted and are protective to the infant against invasive disease. The limited transplacental transport of such antibodies prior to 34 weeks of gestation, however, might place the premature infant of very low birth weight at risk despite high maternal antibody titers (Baker 1979). Another determining factor that has been proposed is the degree of colonization of the newborn infant. Pass et al. found that infants heavily colonized in whom Group B *Streptococcus* could be isolated from multiple sites were more likely to develop invasive disease than those in whom positive cultures could be obtained only from a single region.

Soon after Group B *Streptococcus* achieved prominence as a pathogen in the neonatal period, two distinct patterns of infection, referred to as the early and the late onset forms, were delineated (Baker et al. 1973, Franciosi et al.). Most fall clearly into one type or the other, although transitional cases indicate that some overlap does exist. Unlike most other serious bacterial infections in the newborn infant in which there is a predisposition for involvement of the male, Group B *Streptococcus* shows no particular sex preference. The early onset form is predominantly a septic disorder associated with rapidly progressive pulmonary manifestations accompanied by meningitis in approximately 30 percent of cases. The late onset Group B *Streptococcus* infection is primarily a meningeal inflammatory process with onset between 10 days and eight weeks after birth. Investigations by Baker and Barrett (1974) indicate that while all five serotypes are implicated in neonatal asymptomatic colonization and in the early onset illness, the great majority of cases with meningitis with either the early or late onset type are caused by serotype III. This suggests that the type III strains possess a much greater propensity toward meningeal invasion than is true of the other serotypes, although the explanation remains unclear.

The infant with the early onset type of infection frequently has signs of illness within hours after birth and the majority have become manifested by age three days. The term infant born without obvious obstetrical complications can be affected, although the illness shows a decided predilection for the premature infant, especially those of very low birth weight. Prolonged labor, premature rupture of membranes, intrapartum fetal asphyxia, and maternal amnionitis or endometritis are additional risk factors. Respiratory distress, recurrent apneic attacks, and systemic signs of sepsis including hypotension or shock are common signs of the fulminating form of this illness, which can lead to death within hours after onset. Among those with meningitis, it is not infrequent to find that the meningeal inflammatory reaction has remained sparse even though bacteria are abundant within the subarachnoid space (Quirante et al.). Group B *Streptococcus* sepsis in the premature infant is often clinically and roentgenographically identical to idiopathic respiratory distress syndrome. Chest x-ray abnormalities common to both include a diffuse reticulogranular pattern, air bronchograms, and hypoventilation. Much less often, the chest film of the neonate infected with Group B *Streptococcus* reveals localized infiltrates, atelectasis, or pleural effusions, findings more customarily indicative of congenital pneumonia. The latter abnormalities are more likely to be seen in the more mature infant rather than the one of low birth weight, who usually has evidence of hyaline membrane formation on chest x-ray (Lilien et al.).

The pathogenesis of the development of hyaline membranes in infected infants remains uncertain, although it has been suggested that injury to alveolar cells and capillary endothelium by bacteria may allow exudation of plasma constituents into alveolar spaces, leading to membrane formation (Baker 1979). Attempts to find criteria to rapidly differentiate the two disorders have been only partially successful to the present time. Ablow et al. suggested that lower peak inspiratory pressures with mechanical ventilation is required in infants with Group B *Streptococcus* infection compared to infants with surfactant-deficient respiratory distress syndrome, but other investigators have not found this to be consistently true (Menke et al.).

Other findings which are more suggestive of infection but are not invariably reliable include significant neutropenia, abundant gram-positive cocci in the gastric aspirate soon after birth, and pleural effusion on the chest x-ray. The mortality rate with the early onset form of the disease is better than 50 percent, and in many instances, death prevails despite the early initiation of adequate antibiotic therapy.

The late onset type of Group B *Streptococcus* infection occurs from 10 days up to several weeks after birth and is usually expressed as acute meningitis. It is not ordinarily associated with maternal obstetrical complications, as is true of the early onset type. Irritability, fever, bulging fontanel, and seizures are the most common early clinical features, which usually are found in the absence of other organ system involvement or of distinct signs of septicemia. Endophthalmitis (Greene et al.) and osteomyelitis (Ashdown et al.) have been described with Group B neonatal meningitis but are rare associations. Group B *Streptococcus* has recently become the most common cause of osteomyelitis in the first two months of life but most cases do not coexist with meningitis (Edwards et al., Memon et al.). Periorbital cellulitis, scalp abscess at the site of electrodes for fetal monitoring, purulent conjunctivitis, and urinary tract infection are additional possible expressions of neonatal Group B *Streptococcus* infection.

The mortality rate of late onset Group B *Streptococcus* meningitis is approximately 20 percent. The incidence of neurologic sequelae among survivors is not yet established but it is agreed that it is substantially less than that which follows neonatal gram-negative meningitis (Haslam et al.). Sequelae can be mild or devastating, and include hearing loss, hydrocephalus, spastic signs, seizures, or evidence of hypothalamic dysfunction, such as hyperphagia, abnormality of temperature regulation, and diabetes insipidus (Pai et al.).

Proof of Group B *Streptococcus* sepsis or meningitis in the newborn infant is ultimately on the basis of isolation of the organism from cultures of blood or CSF. Presence of the organism on skin or mucosal surfaces cannot be considered to be diagnostically significant. Countercurrent immunoelectrophoresis on body fluids has been found to be highly reliable for the demonstration of Group B *Streptococcus* antigen, especially if the specimens studied include concentrated urine (Edwards and Baker, Siegel and McCracken). Latex particle agglutination has been said to have greater sensitivity than counterimmunoelectrophoresis for the detection of Group B *Streptococcus* antigen in addition to its lesser degree of complexity (Edwards et al.).

Penicillin administered intravenously is the treatment of choice for Group B *Streptococcus* sepsis or meningitis. Group B strains are less sensitive to this antibiotic, however, than are Group A streptococci, and with Group B *Streptococcus,* studies suggest there may be as much as a 10-fold discrepancy between the minimum inhibitory and the minimum bactericidal concentrations (Allen and Sprunt, Deveikis et al.). The not infrequent observation of relapse or recurrence of infection (Broughton et al., Dorand and Adams, Truog et al., Walker et al.), and the demonstration in some cases of delayed eradication of Group B organisms from CSF with penicillin therapy (Edwards et al.) have resulted in elevation of the recommended dose of penicillin to 300,000 to 400,000 units per kilogram per day given in divided doses every 6–8 hours. Whether relapsing meningitis is the result of inadequate CSF concentrations of the antibiotic or a susceptibility for the occurrence of sequestered organisms in subarachnoid microabscesses remains unclear, but its frequency supports the need for at least three weeks of antibiotic therapy for this illness.

The rapidity of Group B *Streptococcus* killing has been shown to be significantly enhanced by a synergistic effect of ampicillin and aminoglycoside (Cooper et al., Deveikis et al.). Because of the limited entrance of the aminoglycosides into the CSF, the value of this synergistic effect is, perhaps, limited in cases with meningeal infection. The combination of penicillin or ampicillin with gentamicin should be considered when the infection is unyielding to single drug therapy in adequate dosage or when more than one relapse has occurred. Because of the variable CSF response to penicillin therapy, CSF examination should be repeated 48 hours after the initiation of treatment and again at the termination of the therapeutic regimen. Should clinical and CSF improvement occur in the early days of treatment only to be followed by worsening or frank relapse, reassessment should include cranial computed tomography to exclude the possibility of infected subdural effusions or ventricular enlargement, possibly indicative of persistent ventricular infection.

The remarkable increase in the incidence of neonatal Group B *Streptococcus* infections in the past decade and the fulminating nature which often characterizes the early onset type have brought about many efforts to design preventive measures. Some have recommended penicillin treatment at the onset of labor of women found to be colonized. Others have suggested that a single injection of penicillin administered to the infant at the time of delivery will prevent Group B *Streptococcus* invasive disease (Steigman et al.) while other reports indicate failure of penicillin therapy to eradicate Group B organisms from mucosal surfaces of newborn infants (Paredes et al.). Yow et al. treated 34 colonized women during labor with a single intravenous injection of 500 mg. of ampicillin and found that none of the offspring were colonized with Group B *Streptococcus* in the first 48 hours after birth. Of 29 women harboring the organism who received no treatment, 58 percent of their newborn infants were colonized.

Much more information must yet be collected before the optimal method of prevention of neonatal disease caused by this organism can be developed. The relatively low attack rate compared to the high rate of asymptomatic colonization of mother and newborn infant, the yet to be proven effectiveness of antibiotic therapy in the eradication of the carrier state, and the potential adverse effects of penicillin when given to large numbers of persons have inclined most to avoid prophylactic antibiotic therapy at the present time (Aber et al., Baker 1979).

Listeria *Meningitis*

Listeria monocytogenes is a gram-positive rod with a clear-cut propensity to attack the fetus and the infant in the newborn period or in the first few weeks after birth. In recent years, the organism has also been shown to be an important cause of serious infection in the immunosuppressed patient or in one with a variety of chronic debilitating disorders. Regardless of the age group affected or the clinical setting in which infection occurs, *Listeria monocytogenes* has a strong predilection to invade the central nervous system.

Maternal infection with *Listeria monocytogenes* early in pregnancy on rare occasion will result in transplacental fetal infection and subsequent abortion. The role of the organism as a cause of repeated abortion has been controversial for a number of years and remains uncertain. In 1960, Rappaport and colleagues found that 25 of 34 women with a history of repeated abortion had positive cervical cultures for *Listeria monocytogenes,* and proposed the possibility that chronic infection could account for repeated fetal wastage. The consideration has been debated on many occasions since, and is still a matter of dispute. It has even been proposed that *Listeria monocytogenes* may have changed the course of history in that some of Queen Anne's approximately 17 pregnancies were perhaps ended by abortion secondary to infection by this organism (Saxbe). Her many pregnancies left no surviving children and, as a result, the British Crown changed hands in the eighteenth century.

Perinatal listeriosis is a spectrum of disease with clinical manifestations and severity of the illness depending to a large extent on when the fetus or newborn infant becomes infected. In many respects, neonatal *Listeria* infection resembles Group B *Streptococcus* infection in the newborn infant in that both are characterized by early and late onset forms. In both conditions, the early onset form is predominantly a septic illness with a high mortality and the late onset variety takes the form of acute meningitis with a much better prognosis.

The one decided difference in neonatal infection with the two organisms is the occurrence of transplacental transmission of *Listeria monocytogenes,* resulting in a disseminated illness of the fetus and neonate, referred to as granulomatosis infantisepticum. The condition is a more common expression of perinatal listeriosis in Europe than in this country and is usually associated with pre-labor maternal fever, malaise, and abdominal pain. Meconium staining of amniotic fluid is common, sometimes with aspiration of infected meconium by the infant at birth. The fetus may be stillborn, or the live neonate will present with apnea or severe respiratory distress, hepatosplenomegaly, leukopenia, or thrombocytopenia (Ahlfors et al., Halliday and Hirata, Ray and Wedgwood). A high percentage of infants with this illness are of low birth weight, and most reveal obvious clinical abnormalities at birth or in the early hours after birth. Blood cultures are positive for *Listeria monocytogenes* and meningitis may or may not coexist. The mortality rate is very high and, at autopsy, multiple microabscesses and granulomata are found in the liver and other organs, including the spleen, adrenals, and lymph nodes.

Neonatal *Listeria* sepsis with pneumonia or meningitis can also result from intravaginal contamination of the infant by the organism. This is also more frequent in the premature infant, and is usually associated with respiratory distress and hematologic abnormalities. Although there is a substantial case fatality rate in this group, the response to early antibiotic therapy is more favorable than when there is multiple organ system involvement due to transplacental infection (Ahlfors et al., Albritton et al.).

The late onset form of neonatal listeriosis has its onset in infants after 10 days of age and is predominantly a meningeal infection. It is more common in this country than the early onset type of illness and can occur any time in the first several weeks after birth. In some centers, *Listeria monocytogenes* is now the third most common cause of meningitis in the first two months of life, exceeded only by Group B *Streptococcus* and *Escherichia coli* (Halliday and Hirata, Visintine et al.). Most infants with the late onset form are term at birth and maternal illness in the pre-delivery period is unusual. The route of acquisition of the organism by the infant is not usually apparent, in contrast to the early onset form. Fever and irritability are the common initial signs of the illness, and the diagnosis is made by isolation of the organism from the CSF. Demonstration of *Listeria monocytogenes* on Gram stain of CSF is not common, regardless of the age group involved (Lavetter et al.). The prognosis for recovery with the late onset form of *Listeria* meningitis is far better than with the early onset form, and is even better than with meningitis caused by most other bacteria in this age group (Nichols and Wooley, Visintine et al.).

Treatment of the early onset form of perinatal listeriosis is optimally begun prenatally when maternal fever is associated with positive cultures of *Listeria* from blood or cervical secretions. The newborn infant with *Listeria* sepsis is usually treated with ampicillin or a combination of ampicillin and gentamicin. The combination of the two drugs has been recommended by some authors because of experimental evidence of synergism, which results in more rapid and more complete killing of the organism in vitro (Gordon et al., Wiggins et al.). In both the early onset and the late onset forms, ampicillin therapy should be continued for a period of three weeks.

Mortality and Sequelae

The seriousness and significance of gram-negative bacterial meningitis in the first month of life is reflected by the mortality and sequelae associated with this disease. The mortality rate remains remarkably high and has been placed at 40 to 60 percent in most reported series (Dyggve, Fosson and Fine, Heckmatt, Lewis and Gupta, Overall, Watson, Yu and Grauaug). With the early onset type of Group B *Streptococcus* sepsis, the case fatality rate exceeds 50 percent, while with the late onset variety, the mortality rate is approximately 20 percent.

Sequelae among survivors with neonatal meningitis have been variously estimated at 31 percent (Watson) to 56 percent (Dyggve), but these figures are probably conservative since little is known about long-term follow-up, with emphasis on seizures beginning later in childhood or mild mental impairment. Fitzhardinge and colleagues studied 37 patients with neonatal meningitis in whom there was a mortality rate of 46 percent. Of 18 survivors who could be evaluated subsequently, only five were completely free of any abnormality. As in preceding studies, these authors found that one bad prognostic sign in neonatal meningitis is a marked increase in the cerebrospinal fluid protein content. While the incidence of permanent neurologic sequelae is high in all types of neonatal meningitis, it is generally agreed that it is substantially greater among those with gram-negative meningitis beginning in the first two weeks after birth as compared to the more favorable outcome in infants with the late onset form of Group B *Streptococcus* meningitis.

The most notable severe residual deficits secondary to neonatal meningitis include hydrocephalus, seizures, mental retardation, hyperactive behavior, and cranial nerve or long tract signs. Specific localized deficits include hearing loss, optic atrophy, and hypothalamic injury manifested by endocrine deficiencies, diabetes insipidus, precocious puberty, and abnormalities of temperature regulation. Lorber and Pickering reviewed the incidence of post-meningitic hydrocephalus in the newborn infant and found it to occur in 31 percent of those who survived the acute illness. Hydrocephalus complicating meningitis can be either communicating in the type owing to disturbance of CSF flow through the basilar cisterns or of absorption over the surface of the brain or in the intraventricular obstructive type secondary to obstruction at the foramen of Monro, within the third ventricle or aqueduct, or at the outlet foramina of the fourth ventricle (Fig. 3–6). In addition to marked ventricular dilatation, air studies may show septations or fibrous bands within the ventricles (Schultz and Leeds), intracerebral cysts (Fig. 3–7), or porencephalic tracts communicating with the ventricle, which result from repeated transfontanel ventricular taps (Lorber and Emery, Salmon) (Fig. 3–8). Injury from the acute effects of the illness can lead to diffuse cerebral atrophy or microcystic degeneration of the cerebral white matter. Large parenchymal clefts within white matter sometimes communicate with the ventricular system and, if not, can result in its displacement. The degree of ventricular enlargement and presence of cystic degeneration of the cerebral

parenchyma can be demonstrated by computed cranial tomography.

Bacterial sepsis or meningitis in the newborn period has been proposed to be a possible mechanism which predisposes the infant to the development of kernicterus with relatively low serum levels of indirect bilirubin (Pearlman et al.). The pathogenesis of this complication is unclear, although neuronal and endothelial injury associated with meningitis could possibly allow more rapid cellular entry of bilirubin than occurs normally. Certain lasting neurologic deficits following neonatal meningitis could possibly be explained on this basis, although it generally would not be possible to distinguish signs of kernicterus from those resulting from other effects of the acute infectious illness.

Treatment

When the newborn infant is found to have CSF abnormalities compatible with bacterial meningitis, antibiotic therapy must usually be initiated before there is positive identification of the causative agent. Because of the spectrum of microorganisms most commonly incriminated in this age group, the customary approach is to start therapy with systemic ampicillin and gentamicin, with appropriate changes being made after the organism is isolated and identified, and antimicrobial sensitivity tests are completed. If Group B *Strep-*

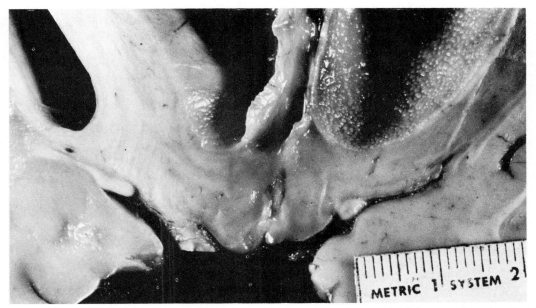

Figure 3–6. Neonatal gram-negative meningitis, late effects. The patient survived for several weeks after the acute stage of the illness, with advanced hydrocephalus and granular ependymitis.

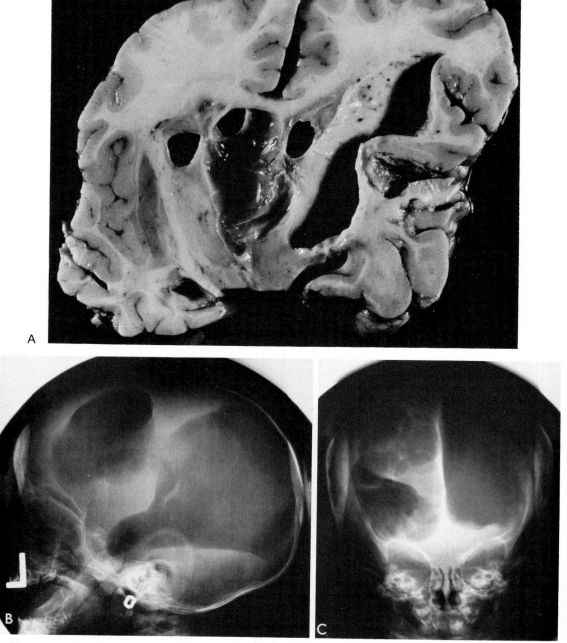

Figure 3–7. Neonatal meningitis, late effects. *A,* Child with severe gram-negative meningitis in the first week of life survived until 9 months of age. Coronal section of the brain shows intraventricular adhesions with partial obliteration of the lateral and third ventricles and cystic degenerative change within the cerebrum. *B,* Ventriculogram, lateral view, of a child several weeks following recovery from neonatal Group B *Streptococcus* meningitis. Advanced hydrocephalus is present with loculation of the left lateral ventricle secondary to intraventricular septations. *C,* The AP view demonstrates more extensive loculation of the right lateral ventricle with septations resulting in a bubble-like appearance of the air within the ventricle.

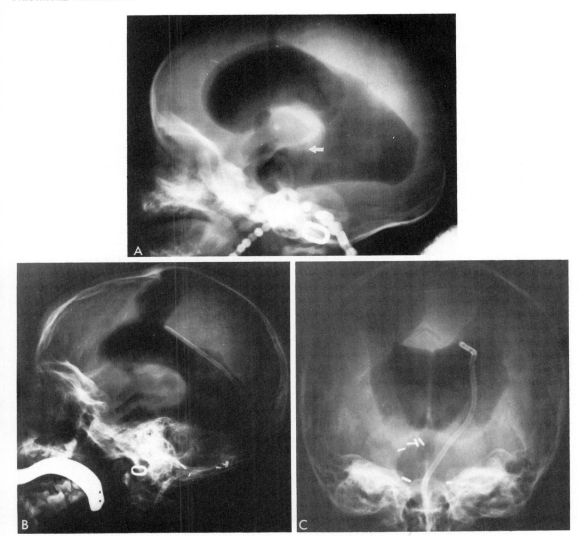

Figure 3–8. Porencephalic lesions resulting from multiple ventricular taps in a child with congenital hydrocephalus. Several ventricular taps were done on each side between 2 and 4 weeks of age. *A,* Ventriculogram at 4 weeks of age shows hydrocephalus secondary to aqueductal obstruction (arrow). Note the small air-filled tract extending from the roof of the lateral ventricle toward the region of the anterior fontanel. The child was treated with a ventriculoatrial shunt. *B* and *C,* The ventriculogram was repeated at age 6 years following shunt failure. The ventricles are mildly enlarged but the porencephalic lesions at the sites of the previous ventricular taps are conspicuous. This illustrates the possible damage that can result from repeated transfontanel ventricular taps in early infancy, with or without infection.

tococcus is isolated, penicillin G is the drug of choice, administered every 6–8 hours over a 20-minute time period. Recent experience with Group B *Streptococcus* meningitis in neonates has led to the recommendation of doses of penicillin G of 300,000 to 400,000 units per kilogram per day, which is greater than is customarily used for other types of penicillin-sensitive infections in this age span. The reported examples of relapsing Group B *Streptococcus* meningitis and the lesser degree of sensitivity to penicillin of this organism compared to Group A strains accounts for

the desirability of the higher dose range, which is, perhaps, best continued for a minimum of three weeks.

The clinical importance of the synergism between ampicillin and gentamicin against Group B *Streptococcus* remains unclear. This combination might be considered in cases not rapidly responsive to penicillin therapy alone or when meningitis has relapsed on more than one occasion despite adequate penicillin doses.

In addition to its use for Group B *Streptococcus*, penicillin is the drug of choice for neonatal meningitis caused by *Streptococcus pneumoniae,* and the infrequent cases resulting from Group A *Streptococcus,* nonenterococcal Group D *Streptococcus,* and *Pasteurella multocida.*

Ampicillin in dosage of 150 to 200 mg per kilogram per day is generally optimal therapy for neonatal meningitis due to *Listeria monocytogenes* (Gordon et al., Lavetter et al., Macnair et al.), *Proteus mirabilis* (Scherzer et al.), and the rare neonatal case of β-lactamase-negative *Hemophilus influenzae.* Synergism has been demonstrated between ampicillin and gentamicin resulting in an increased rate of bacterial killing of *Listeria monocytogenes* (Gordon et al., Wiggins et al.). This combination is seldom used for treatment of infections caused by this organism but might be considered if a suboptimal response occurs with ampicillin alone. Indole-positive *Proteus* species and *Pseudomonas* species meningitis require carbenicillin in combination with gentamicin or tobramycin, and in many instances the aminoglycoside is administered intrathecally because of the intractable nature of meningeal infection with these organisms. Some workers have found ticarcillin and tobramycin to be superior to carbenicillin and gentamicin for non-neurologic *Pseudomonas* species infections in adults but there is little experience to date with ticarcillin in infancy (Parry and Neu).

Enterococcal Group D *Streptococcus,* including *Streptococcus faecalis, Streptococcus faecium,* and *Streptococcus durans,* is often found to exhibit multiple antibiotic resistance, including resistance to penicillin, requiring dependence on sensitivity tests for the best choice of antibiotic therapy. Because of the demonstrated synergism of ampicillin with gentamicin against these organisms, this combination is usually selected (Bavikatte et al., Buchino et al.). Most strains of *Salmonella* species are sensitive to ampicillin or chloramphenicol, although caution is required when the latter is used in the first two months of life. Staphylococcal meningitis in the newborn period is managed with a combination of methicillin and gentamicin until the organism is specifically defined and its sensitivities are known. Should the infected infant have renal failure of one cause or another, nafcillin would be a more appropriate penicillinase-resistant penicillin because of its secretion via the biliary system. *Flavobacterium meningosepticum* is a gram-negative organism which is a very uncommon cause of neonatal meningitis but the character of its antibiotic sensitivities complicates the approach to treatment. This organism is usually highly resistant to the penicillins and the aminoglycosides, but is most often sensitive to rifampin, vancomycin, and erythromycin, the latter two being drugs which gain entrance poorly into the CSF following systemic administration. Treatment would include oral rifampin and systemic erythromycin with frequent CSF examinations to ascertain the response to the antimicrobial regimen. Lack of improvement would warrant consideration of intraventricular erythromycin if the ventricular capacity permits it. *Campylobacter fetus* is an additional gram-negative bacillus which rarely provokes meningitis in the neonate but is usually sensitive to the aminoglycosides and chloramphenicol.

The most perplexing problem at the present time is the method of treatment of neonatal meningitis caused by the gram-negative members of the Enterobacteriaceae, and particularly the most common type, which is *Escherichia coli* meningitis. Systemically administered ampicillin and gentamicin is the most commonly used regimen; however, not all strains are ampicillin-sensitive; rapid eradication of bacteria in the CSF does not usually occur with ampicillin, and gentamicin penetrates CSF only in limited quantity. In addition, the reduced CSF pH characteristically found in bacterial meningitis may decrease the bactericidal action of gentamicin (Strausbaugh and Sande). McCracken (1972) demonstrated that, while rapid eradication of gram-positive bacteria in CSF followed antibiotic therapy, eradication of gram-negative organisms was much more delayed, with positive cultures persisting for a mean of six days. His study showed that CSF levels of penicillin and ampicillin could be achieved which were 10 to 100 times the minimum inhibitory concentration of the commonly encountered gram-positive pathogens, but that CSF levels of gentamicin following systemic doses of 5 to 7.5 mg per kilogram per day only approximately equaled the minimum inhibitory concentration of most strains of *Escherichia coli.*

Aminoglycosides administered intrathecally by the lumbar route do not adequately gain entrance into the ventricular system or over the cerebral convexity (Kaiser and McGee) and have not been found to improve the outcome of this illness in the newborn period (McCracken and Mize). Intraventricular injection of gentamicin results in much more favorable intraventricular levels relative to bacterial killing (Lee et al., Mangi et al.), but the procedure can be very difficult technically in the initial stages of the illness when the ventricles are often reduced in size owing to cerebral swelling.

Chloramphenicol has been proposed as an alternative method of treatment of neonatal gram-negative meningitis, but the drug is believed to be only bacteriostatic against the more common members of the Enterobacteriaceae (Rahal and Simberkoff). Potential serum level–related side effects of chloramphenicol peculiar mainly to the newborn infant make it highly desirable that blood level determinations be available if the drug is used in this age group. In addition, chloramphenicol has been found to significantly antagonize the bactericidal effect of gentamicin against gram-negative rods when the two are used in combination (Paisley and Washington, Strausbaugh and Sande).

Under the best of circumstances, therefore, treatment of neonatal gram-negative meningitis with the currently available antimicrobials is less than optimal and the mortality and morbidity rates remain disturbingly high. In centers in which chloramphenicol serum levels are not available, treatment includes ampicillin and gentamicin administered systemically, with re-examination of the CSF within 24 to 48 hours after onset of therapy. If clinical and CSF improvement has not occurred after a reasonable trial with this regimen, computed tomography should be performed to ascertain if lateral ventricular size permits direct intraventricular administration of gentamicin in conjunction with systemic therapy. When this method is required, the duration of daily intraventricular injections is determined by the rate of CSF improvement and when CSF sterilization occurs. Gentamicin is given by intramuscular injection in a dosage of 5 mg per kilogram per day at 12-hour intervals in infants less than one week of age and 7.5 mg per kilogram per day in divided doses every 8 hours in infants from one to eight weeks of age. Dosage should be adjusted on the basis of peak and trough serum levels, with peak levels optimally maintained between 4 and 10 μg per ml. (Siber et al.). Peak levels are usually achieved 30 to 60 minutes after an intramuscular injection and the mean half-life of the drug is approximately five hours in infants less than 72 hours of age and approxi-

mately three hours in term infants over seven days of age (McCracken 1974). With gentamicin-resistant *Escherichia coli* or *Klebsiella* species, amikacin combined with ampicillin is selected, depending on sensitivity test results (Hamory et al., Sklaver et al.).

An alternative approach to the treatment of neonatal gram-negative meningitis when accurate serum chloramphenicol levels can be measured is the combination of ampicillin and chloramphenicol given intravenously, although this has not been proved superior to the previously described regimen. The therapeutic serum level of chloramphenicol is 15 to 25 μg per ml., while levels greater than 50 μg per ml. have been associated with the "gray baby" syndrome. The dose of chloramphenicol administered intravenously for serious neonatal infections is 25 mg. per kilogram per day every six hours for the premature infant in the first month of life and for the full-term neonate in the first week of life. In the term infant from one week to one month of age, the dose is 50 mg. per kilogram per day given in four divided doses.

Because there is considerable individual variation of the serum level produced by a given intravenous dose of chloramphenicol, serum level determinations are imperative to be certain that an adequate therapeutic concentration is achieved but that it remains well below the potentially toxic level (Black et al.). Although CSF and ventricular fluid penetration of the drug is usually excellent, in most instances in the range of 50 to 70 percent of the simultaneous serum level (Friedman et al.), this also is quite variable from patient to patient and cannot be predicted from the serum level (Yogev and Williams). Measurement of the chloramphenicol CSF or ventricular concentration is an infrequently used refinement of the treatment method, which might significantly improve the usefulness of this antibiotic (Dunkle).

Another important factor to be considered with the use of chloramphenicol is its interaction with phenobarbital, a commonly used anticonvulsant in infants and children with meningitis. Phenobarbital can result in a progressive decline in the chloramphenicol serum level, despite a stable dosage (Bloxham et al.). This effect is believed to be the result of induction of hepatic microsomal enzymes by phenobarbital, leading to an increased rate of glucuronidation of chloramphenicol. Conversely, chloramphenicol has been shown to retard the hepatic biotransformation of phenytoin, possibly resulting in elevation of serum levels of phenytoin and overt drug intoxication (Christensen and Skovsted, Rose et al.).

With most types of neonatal bacterial meningitis, it is advisable to repeat the CSF examination 24 to 48 hours after initiation of treatment and at variable intervals thereafter, depending on the clinical course. Duration of antibiotic therapy is usually longer than is the case in older children with meningitis, and often will need to be in the range of three weeks. Seizures should be controlled to the extent possible with the use of phenobarbital, keeping in mind the interaction with chloramphenicol if the latter drug is being used. Phenobarbital can be initiated with a loading dose of 10 mg. per kilogram intramuscularly followed by a maintenance dose of 5 to 15 mg. per kilogram per day in divided doses in order to achieve serum levels of 15 to 30 μg. per ml.

Increased intracranial pressure does not usually create a threat to the neonate to the degree that it can in the older child with acute meningeal infection. This is partly explained by the presence of a large and patent anterior fontanel and the rapidity with which sutures can separate in the young infant. Extreme tenseness of the fontanel, however, can reflect the possibility of compromise of venous drainage and arterial perfusion of the brain, and warrants consideration of methods of dealing with the problem. The possibility of subdural effusions should first be considered under these circumstances, although subdural fluid collections are less common in neonates with meningitis than later in infancy. In the acute stage of neonatal meningitis, a tense fontanel usually is the result of cerebral swelling and, if marked, is probably best managed by daily or twice daily lumbar punctures, with slow and cautious removal of 4 to 10 ml. of CSF with each tap. Assuming that the ventricular system is not obstructed, this method is reasonably safe in this age group since pathologic evidence of internal herniations is rarely demonstrated in the neonate. The ventricular system can be assumed to be communicating when the fontanel becomes soft or slightly sunken after CSF removal by lumbar puncture. Should little or no change in the fontanel occur, the possibility of hydrocephalus secondary to intraventricular obstruction is an indication for computed tomography to assess ventricular size. Rapidly progressive hydrocephalus complicating the acute stage of neonatal bacterial

meningitis seriously complicates the treatment regimen and temporarily requires periodic ventricular taps. Ventriculoperitoneal shunting is necessarily delayed until the infection is controlled and the ventricular protein content has decreased to a level which will allow adequate shunt function.

Additional general aspects of management of the infant with meningitis include close monitoring of fluid and electrolyte status, methods to support blood pressure and thus cerebral perfusion in those with circulatory compromise, and adequate ventilation of infants with respiratory insufficiency. Nutrition should be maintained by initiation of oral or nasogastric tube feeding as soon as is feasible.

REFERENCES

Aber, R. C., Wennersten, C., and Moellering, R. C., Jr.: Antimicrobial susceptibility of Flavobacteria. Antimicrob. Agents Chemother. 14:483–487, 1978.

Aber, R. C., Allen, N., Howell, J. T., Wilkenson, H. W., and Facklam, R. R.: Nosocomial transmission of group B streptococci. Pediatrics 58:346–353, 1976.

Ablow, R. C., Driscoll, S. G., Effmann, E. L., Gross, I., Jolles, C. J., Uauy, R., and Warshaw, J. B.: A comparison of early-onset Group B streptococcal neonatal infection and the respiratory-distress syndrome of the newborn. New Eng. J. Med. 294:65–70, 1976.

Adler, S. M., and Denton, R. L.: The erythrocyte sedimentation rate in the newborn period. J. Pediat. 86:942–948, 1975.

Ahlfors, C. E., Goetzman, B. W., Halsted, C. C., Sherman, M. P., and Wennberg, R. P.: Neonatal listeriosis. Am. J. Dis. Child. 131:405–408, 1977.

Albritton, W. L., Wiggins, G. L., and Feeley, J. C.: Neonatal listeriosis: Distribution of serotypes in relation to age at onset of disease. J. Pediat. 88:481–483, 1976.

Alexander, J. B., and Giacoia, G. P.: Early onset nonenterococcal group D streptococcal infection in the newborn infant. J. Pediat. 93:489–490, 1978.

Allen, J. L., and Sprunt, K.: Discrepancy between minimum inhibitory and minimum bactericidal concentrations of penicillin for group A and group B β-hemolytic streptococci. J. Pediat. 93:69–71, 1978.

Anderson, D. C., Pickering, L. K., and Feigin, R. D.: Leukocyte function in normal and infected neonates. J. Pediat. 85:420–425, 1974.

Anthony, B. F., Okada, D. M., and Hobel, C. J.: Epidemiology of the group B streptococcus: Maternal and nosocomial sources for infant acquisitions. J. Pediat. 95:431–436, 1979.

Ashdown, L. R., Hewson, P. H., and Suleman, S. K.: Neonatal osteomyelitis and meningitis caused by Group B streptococci. Med. J. Aust. 2:500–501, 1977.

Baker, C. J.: Summary of the workshop on perinatal infections due to group B streptococcus. J. Infect. Dis. 136:137–152, 1977.

Baker, C. J.: Group B streptococcal infections in neonates. Pediatrics (Pediatrics in Review). 1:5–15, 1979.

Baker, C. J., and Barrett, F. F.: Transmission of group B streptococci among parturient women and their neonates. J. Pediat. 83:919–925, 1973.

Baker, C. J., and Barrett, F. F.: Group B streptococcal infections in infants. The importance of the various serotypes. J.A.M.A. 230:1158–1160, 1974.

Baker, C. J., and Kasper, D. L.: Correlation of maternal antibody deficiency with susceptibility to neonatal Group B streptococcal infection. New Eng. J. Med. 294:753–756, 1976.

Baker, C. J., and Kasper, D. L.: Immunological investigation of infants with septicemia or meningitis due to Group B *Streptococcus*. J. Infect. Dis. 136(Suppl.):S98–S104, 1977.

Baker, C. J., Barrett, F. F., Gordon, R. C., and Yow, M. D.: Suppurative meningitis due to streptococci of Lancefield group B: A study of 33 infants. J. Pediat. 82:724–729, 1973.

Barclay, N.: High frequency of salmonella species as a cause of neonatal meningitis in Ibadan, Nigeria. A review of thirty-eight cases. Acta Pediat. Scand. 60:540–544, 1971.

Barrett, G. S., Rammelkamp, C. H., and Worcester, J.: Meningitis due to Escherichia coli. Report of two cases with recovery following chemotherapy; review of the literature and report by experimental studies. Am. J. Dis. Child. 63:41–59, 1942.

Barrie, D.: Incubator-borne Pseudomonas pyocyanea infection in a newborn nursery. Arch. Dis. Childh. 40:555–558, 1965.

Barron, M.: Meningitis in the newborn and in early infancy. Am. J. Med. Sci. 156:358–369, 1918.

Barton, L. L., Feigin, R. D., and Lins, R.: Group B beta hemolytic streptococcal meningitis in infants. J. Pediat. 82:719–723, 1973.

Bates, H. A., Controni, G., Elliott, N., and Eitzman, D. V.: Septicemia and meningitis in a newborn due to Pasteurella multocida. Clin. Pediat. 4:668–670, 1965.

Bavikatte, K., Schreiner, R. L., Lemons, J. A., and Gresham, E. L.: Group D streptococcal septicemia in the neonate. Am. J. Dis. Child. 133:493–496, 1979.

Becker, A. H.: Infection due to Proteus mirabilis in newborn nursery. Am. J. Dis. Child. 104:355–359, 1962.

Berman, B. W., King, F. H., Jr., Rubenstein, D. S., and Long, S. S.: *Bacteroides fragilis* meningitis in a neonate successfully treated with metronidazole. J. Pediat. 93:793–795, 1978.

Berman, P. H., and Banker, B. Q.: Neonatal meningitis: A clinical and pathological study of 29 cases. Pediatrics 38:6–24, 1966.

Black, S. B., Levine, P., and Shinefield, H. R.: The necessity for monitoring chloramphenicol levels when treating neonatal meningitis. J. Pediat. 92:235–236, 1978.

Bloxham, R. A., Durbin, G. M., Johnson, T., and Winterborn, M. H.: Chloramphenicol and phenobarbitone—a drug interaction. Arch. Dis. Childh. 54:76–77, 1979.

Boe, O., Diderichsen, J., and Matre, R.: Isolation of Mycoplasma hominis from cerebrospinal fluid. Scand. J. Infect. Dis. 5:285–288, 1973.

Bortolussi, R., Thompson, T. R., and Ferrieri, P.: Early-onset pneumococcal sepsis in newborn infants. Pediatrics 60:352–355, 1977.

Boyle, R. J., Chandler, B. D., Stonestreet, B. S., and Oh, W.: Early identification of sepsis in infants with respiratory distress. Pediatrics 62:744–750, 1978.

Bradford, W. L., and Kelley, H. W.: Gonococcic meningitis in a newborn infant. Am. J. Dis. Child. 46:543–549, 1933.

Broughton, D. D., Mitchell, W. G., Grossman, M., Hadley, W. K., and Cohen, M. S.: Recurrence of group B streptococcal infection. J. Pediat. 89:183–185, 1976.

Buchino, J. J., Ciambarella, E., and Light, I.: Systemic Group D streptococcal infection in newborn infants. Am. J. Dis. Child. 133:270–273, 1979.

Burgert, W., Jr., and Hagstrom, J. W. C.: Vibrio fetus meningoencephalitis. Arch. Neurol. 10:196–199, 1964.

Burry, V. F., and Hellerstein, S.: Septicemia and subperiosteal cephalhematomas. J. Pediat. 69:1133–1135, 1966.

Burton, B. K., Marr, T. J., Traisman, H. S., and Davis, A. T.: *Salmonella typhi* meningitis in a neonate. Am. J. Dis. Child. 131:1031, 1977.

Cabrera, H. A., and Davis, G. H.: Epidemic meningitis of the newborn caused by Flavobacteria. I. Epidemiology and bacteriology. Am. J. Dis. Child. 101:289–295, 1961.

Christensen, L. K., and Skovsted, L.: Inhibition of drug metabolism by chloramphenicol. Lancet 2:1397–1399, 1969.

Coen, R., Grush, O., and Kauder, E.: Studies of bactericidal activity and metabolism of the leukocyte in full-term neonates. J. Pediat. 75:400–406, 1969.

Cohen, S. M., Miller, B. W., and Orris, H. W.: Meningitis complicating cephalhematoma. J. Pediat. 30:327–329, 1947.

Collier, A. M., Connor, J. D., and Nyhan, W. L.: Systemic infection with Hemophilus influenzae in very young infants. J. Pediat. 70:539–547, 1967.

Cooke, R. W. I.: *Bacteroides fragilis* septicaemia and meningitis in early infancy. Arch. Dis. Childh. 50:241–243, 1975.

Cooper, M. D., Keeney, R. E., Lyons, S. F., and Cheatle, E. L.: Synergistic effects of ampicillin-aminoglycoside combinations on Group B streptococci. Antimicrob. Agents Chemother. 15:484–486, 1979.

Cowett, R. M., Peter, G., Hakanson, D. O., and Oh, W.: Reliability of bacterial culture of blood obtained from an umbilical artery catheter. J. Pediat. 88:1035–1036, 1976.

Cussen, L. J., and Ryan, G. B.: Hemorrhagic cerebral necrosis in neonatal infants with enterobacterial meningitis. J. Pediat. 71:771–776, 1967.

Deonna, T., Calame, A., van Melle, G., and Prod'hom, L-S.: Hypoglycorrhachia in neonatal intracranial hemorrhage. Relationship to posthemorrhagic hydrocephalus. Helv. paediat. Acta 32:351–361, 1977.

Deveikis, A., Schauf, V., Mizen, M., and Riff, L.: Antimicrobial therapy of experimental Group B streptococcal infection in mice. Antimicrob. Agents Chemother. 11:817–820, 1977.

Dillon, H. C., Jr.: Group A type 12 streptococcal infection in a newborn nursery. Successfully treated neonatal meningitis. Am. J. Dis. Child. 112:117–184, 1966.

Dorland, R. D., and Adams, G.: Relapse during penicillin treatment of group B streptococcal meningitis. J. Pediat. 89:188–190, 1976.

Dossett, J. H., and Quie, P. G.: Opsonins and polymorphonuclear leukocyte function in mothers and newborns. Soc. Pediat. Res. 135:1968 (Abs.).

Dunham, E. C.: Septicemia in the newborn. Am. J. Dis. Child. 45:229–253, 1933.

Dunkle, L. M.: Central nervous system chloramphenicol concentration in premature infants. Antimicrob. Agents Chemother. 13:427–429, 1978.

Dyggve, H.: Prognosis in meningitis neonatorum. Acta Pediat. Scand. 51:303–312, 1962.

Eden, A. N.: Vibrio fetus meningitis in a newborn infant. J. Pediat. 61:33–38, 1962.

Edwards, K., Ferrieri, P., Thompson, T. R., and Davis, A. T.: Group B streptococcal meningitis: Delayed response to treatment. Child's Brain 3:343–351, 1977.

Edwards, M. S., and Baker, C. J.: Prospective diagnosis of early onset group B streptococcal infection by countercurrent immunoelectrophoresis. J. Pediat. 94:286–288, 1979.

Edwards, M. S., Kasper, D. L., and Baker, C. J.: Rapid diagnosis of type III group B streptococcal meningitis by latex particle agglutination. J. Pediat. 95:202–205, 1979.

Edwards, M. S., Baker, C. J., Wagner, M. L., Taber, L. H., and Barrett, F. F.: An etiologic shift in infantile osteomyelitis: The emergence of the group B streptococcus. J. Pediat. 93:578–583, 1978.

Eickhoff, T. C., Klein, J. O., Daly, K., Ingall, D., and Finland, M.: Neonatal sepsis and other infections due to Group B beta-hemolytic streptococci. New Eng. J. Med. 271:1221–1228, 1964.

Ellis, S. S., Montgomery, J. R., Wagner, M., and Hill, R. M.: Osteomyelitis complicating neonatal cephalhematoma. Am. J. Dis. Child. 127:100–102, 1974.

Eykens, A., Eggermont, E., Eeckels, R., Vandepitte, J., and Spaepen, J.: Neonatal meningitis caused by Flavobacterium meningosepticum. Helv. paediat. Acta 28:421–425, 1973.

Feder, H. M., Jr., MacLean, W. C., Jr., and Moxon, R.: Scalp abscess secondary to fetal scalp electrode. J. Pediat. 89:808–809, 1976.

Feigin, R. D., and Shearer, W. T.: Opportunistic infection in children. III. In the normal host. J. Pediat. 87:852–866, 1975.

Feldman, W. E.: *Bacteroides fragilis* ventriculitis and meningitis. Report of two cases. Am. J. Dis. Child. 130:880–883, 1976.

Fierer, J., Taylor, P. M., and Gezon, H. M.: Pseudomonas aeruginosa epidemic traced to delivery-room resuscitators. New Eng. J. Med. 276:991–996, 1967.

Fireman, P., Zuchowski, D. A., and Taylor, P. M.: Development of human complement system. J. Immun. 103:25–31, 1969.

Fitzhardinge, P. M., Kazemi, M., Ramsay, M., and Stern, L.: Long-term sequelae of neonatal meningitis. Develop. Med. Child Neurol. 16:3–10, 1974.

Forfar, J. O., Gould, J. C., and Maccabe, A. F.: Effect of hexachlorophene on incidence of staphylococcal and gram-negative infection in the newborn. Lancet 2:177–179, 1968.

Forman, M. L., and Stiehm, E. R.: Impaired opsonic activity but normal phagocytosis in low-birth-weight infants. New Eng. J. Med. 281:926–931, 1969.

Fosson, A. R., and Fine, R. N.: Neonatal meningitis. Presentation and discussion of 21 cases. Clin. Pediat. 7:404–410, 1968.

Franciosi, R. A., Knostman, J. D., and Zimmerman, R. A.: Group B streptococcal neonatal and infant infections. J. Pediat. 82:707–718, 1973.

Friedman, C. A., Lovejoy, F. C., and Smith, A. L.: Chloramphenicol deposition in infants and children. J. Pediat. 95:1071–1077, 1979.

Froeschle, J., Gottfried, D. F., and Grossman, M.: Salmonella oranienburg meningitis in a newborn infant. Am. J. Dis. Child. 108:298–301, 1964.

Frutos, A. A., Levitsky, D., Scott, E. G., and Steele, L.: A case of septicemia and meningitis in an infant due to Pasteurella multocida. J. Pediat. 92:853, 1978.

Fry, R. M.: Fatal infections by hemolytic Streptococcus Group B. Lancet 1:199–201, 1938.

George, R. M., Cochran, C. P., and Wheeler, W. E.: Epidemic meningitis of the newborn caused by Flavobacteria. II. Clinical manifestations and treatment. Am. J. Dis. Child. 101:296–304, 1961.

Gerwitz, M., Dinwiddie, R., Rees, L., Velikas, O., Yuille, T., O'Connell, B., and Marshall, W. C.: Mycoplasma hominis. A cause of neonatal meningitis. Arch. Dis. Childh. 54:231–239, 1979.

Gilles, F. H., Jammes, J. L., and Berenberg, W.: Neonatal meningitis. The ventricle as a bacterial reservoir. Arch. Neurol. 34:560–562, 1977.

Goldmann, D. A., Leclair, J., and Macone, A.: Bacterial colonization of neonates admitted to an intensive care environment. J. Pediat. 93:288–293, 1978.

Gordon, R. C., Barrett, F. F., and Clark, D. J.: Influence of several antibiotics, singly and in combination, on the growth of Listeria monocytogenes. J. Pediat. 80:667–670, 1972.

Gordon, R. C., Barrett, F. F., and Yow, M. D.: Ampicillin treatment of listeriosis. J. Pediat. 77:1067–1070, 1970.

Gotoff, S. P.: Neonatal immunity. J. Pediat. 85:149–154, 1974.

Granoff, D. M., and Nankervis, G. A.: Infectious arthritis in the neonate caused by *Haemophilus influenzae*. Am. J. Dis. Child. 129:730–733, 1975.

Greene, G. R., Carroll, W. L., and Morozumi, P. A.: Endophthalmitis associated with Group-B streptococcal meningitis in an infant. Am. J. Dis. Child. 133:752–753, 1979.

Greenthal, R. M.: Case of meningitis due to the Bacillus acidilactici. Occurring in a premature infant one month old. Am. J. Dis. Child. 21:203–205, 1921.

Gregory, J., and Hey, E.: Blood neutrophil response to bacterial infection in the first month of life. Arch. Dis. Childh. 47:747–753, 1972.

Groover, R. V., Sutherland, J. M., and Landing, B. H.: Purulent meningitis of newborn infants. Eleven-year experience in the antibiotic era. New Eng. J. Med. 264:1115–1121, 1961.

Gross, R. J., Rowe, B., and Easton, J. A.: Neonatal meningitis caused by *Citrobacter koseri*. J. Clin. Path. 26:138–139, 1973.

Gullekson, E. H., and Dumoff, M.: *Haemophilus parainfluenzae* meningitis in a newborn. J.A.M.A. 198:1221, 1966.

Gwynn, C. M., and George, R. H.: Neonatal citrobacter meningitis. Arch. Dis. Childh. 48:455–458, 1973.

Hable, K. A., Matsen, J. M., Wheeler, D. J., Hunt, C. E., and Quie, P. G.: Klebsiella type 33 septicemia in an infant intensive care unit. J. Pediat. 80:920–924, 1972.

Halliday, H. L., and Hirata, T.: Perinatal listeriosis—a review of twelve patients. Am. J. Obstet. Gynecol. 133:405–410, 1979.

Hamory, B., Ignatiadis, P., and Sande, M. A.: Intrathecal amikacin administration. Use in the treatment of gentamicin-resistant *Klebsiella pneumoniae* meningitis. J.A.M.A. 236:1973–1974, 1976.

Harrod, J. R., and Stevens, D. A.: Anaerobic infections in the newborn infant. J. Pediat. 85:399–402, 1974.

Haslam, R. H. A., Allen, J. R., Dorsen, M. M., Kanofsky, D. L., Mellits, E. D., and Norris, D. A.: The sequelae of Group B β-hemolytic streptococcal meningitis in early infancy. Am. J. Dis. Child. 131:845–849, 1977.

Headings, D. L., and Overall, J. C., Jr.: Outbreak of meningitis in a newborn intensive care unit caused by a single Escherichia coli K1 serotype. J. Pediat. 90:99–102, 1977.

Headings, D. L., Herrera, A., Mazzi, E., and Bergman, M. A.: Fulminant neonatal septicemia caused by

Streptococcus bovis. J. Pediat. 92:282–283, 1978.

Heckmatt, J. Z.: Coliform meningitis in the newborn. Arch. Dis. Childh. 51:569–573, 1976.

Hemming, V. G., Overall, J. C., Jr., and Britt, M. R.: Nosocomial infections in a newborn intensive-care unit. Results of forty-one months of surveillance. New Eng. J. Med. 294:1310–1316, 1976.

Hill, H.R., Hunt, C. E., and Matson, J. M.: Nosocomial colonization with Klebsiella, type 26, in a neonatal intensive-care unit associated with an outbreak of sepsis, meningitis, and necrotizing enterocolitis. J. Pediat. 85:415–419, 1974.

Hood, M., Janney, A., and Dameron, G.: Beta hemolytic streptococcus Group B associated with problems of the perinatal period. Am. J. Obstet. Gynec. 82:809–818, 1961.

Izquierdo, J. M., Sanz, F., Coca, J. M., Vila, F., and Dierssen, G.: Pyocephalus of the newborn child. Child's Brain 4:161–169, 1978.

Johnston, R. B., Altenburger, K. M., Atkinson, A. W., Jr., and Curry, R. H.: Complement in the newborn infant. Pediatrics 64:Part2:781–786, 1979.

Kagan, B. M., Hess, J. H., Mirman, B., and Lundeen, E.: Meningitis in premature infants. Pediatrics 4:479–483, 1949.

Kaiser, A. B., and McGee, Z. A.: Aminoglycoside therapy of gram-negative bacillary meningitis. New Eng. J. Med. 293:1215–1220, 1975.

Kaplan, A. M., Itabashi, H. H., Yoshimori, R., and Weil, M. L.: Citrobacter abscesses complicating neonatal Citrobacter freundii meningitis. West. J. Med. 127:418–422, 1977.

Khuri-Bulos, N., and McIntosh, K.: Neonatal Haemophilus influenzae infection. Report of eight cases and review of the literature. Am. J. Dis. Child. 129:57–62,1975.

Koplik, H.: Meningitis in the newborn and in infants under three months of age. Arch. Pediat. 33:481–500, 1916.

Lancefield, R. C.: A serological differentiation of human and other groups of hemolytic streptococci. J. Exper. Med. 57:571–575, 1933.

Lavetter, A., Leedom, J. M., Mathies, A. W., Jr., Ivler, D., and Wehrle, P. F.: Meningitis due to Listeria monocytogenes. A review of 25 cases. New Eng. J. Med. 285:598–603, 1971.

Lee, E. L., Robinson, M. J., Thong, M. L., Puthucheary, S. D., Ong, T. H., and Ng, K. K.: Intraventricular chemotherapy in neonatal meningitis. J. Pediat. 91:991–995, 1977.

Lee, Y., and Berg, R. B.: Cephalhematoma infected with Bacteroides. Am. J. Dis. Child. 121:77–78, 1971.

Levy, H. L., and Ingall, D.: Meningitis in neonates due to Proteus mirabilis. Am. J. Dis. Child. 114:320–324, 1967.

Levy, H. L., O'Conner, J. F., and Ingall, D.: Bacteremia, infected cephalhematoma, and osteomyelitis of the skull in a newborn. Am. J. Dis. Child. 144:649–651, 1967.

Levy, H. L., Sepe, S. J., Shih, V. E., Vawter, G. F., and Klein, J. O.: Sepsis due to Escherichia coli in neonates with galactosemia. New Eng. J. Med. 297:823–825, 1977.

Lewis, B. R., and Gupta, J. M.: Present prognosis in neonatal meningitis. Med. J. Aust. 1:695–697, 1977.

Light, I. J., Sutherland, J. M., Cochran, M. L., and Sutorius, J.: Ecologic relation between Staphylococcus aureus and pseudomonas in a nursery population. New Eng. J. Med. 278:1243–1247, 1968.

Lilien, L. D., Harris, V. J., and Pildes, R. S.: Significance of radiologic findings in early-onset Group B streptococcal infection. Pediatrics 60:360–363, 1977.

Lilien, L. D., Yeh, T. F., Novak, G. M., and Jacobs, N. M.: Early-onset Haemophilus sepsis in newborn infants: Clinical, roentgenographic, and pathologic features. Pediatrics 62:299–303, 1978.

Lorber, J., and Emery, J. L.: Intracerebral cysts complicating ventricular needling in hydrocephalic infants: A clinico-pathologic study. Develop. Med. Child. Neurol. 6:125–139, 1964.

Lorber, J., and Pickering, D.: Incidence and treatment of post-meningitic hydrocephalus in the newborn. Arch. Dis. Childh. 41:44–50, 1966.

Macnair, D. R., White, J. E., and Graham, J. M.: Ampicillin in the treatment of Listeria monocytogenes meningitis. Lancet 1:16–18, 1968.

Maderazo, E. G., Bassaris, H. P., and Quintiliani, R.: Flavobacterium meningosepticum meningitis in a newborn infant. Treatment with intraventricular erythromycin. J. Pediat. 85:675–676, 1974.

Mangi, R. J., Holstein, L. L., and Andriole, V. T.: Treatment of gram-negative bacillary meningitis with intrathecal gentamicin. Yale J. Biol. Med. 50:31–41, 1977.

Mathew, O. P., Bland, H. E., Pickens, J. M., and James, E. J. P.: Hypoglycorrhachia in the survivors of neonatal intracranial hemorrhage. Pediatrics 63:851–854, 1979.

McCracken, G. H., Jr.: The rate of bacteriologic response to antimicrobial therapy in neonatal meningitis. Am. J. Dis. Child. 123:547–553, 1972.

McCracken, G. H., Jr.: Pharmacological basis for antimicrobial therapy in newborn infants. Am. J Dis. Child. 128:407–419, 1974.

McCracken, G. H., Jr., and Eichenwald, H. F.: Leukocyte function and the development of opsonic and complement activity in the neonate. Am. J. Dis. Child. 121:120–126, 1971.

McCracken, G. H., Jr., and Mize, S. G.: A controlled study of intrathecal antibiotic therapy in gram-negative enteric meningitis of infancy. J. Pediat. 89:66–72, 1976.

McCracken, G. H., Jr., Sarff, L. D., Glode, M. P., Mize, S. G., Schiffer, M. S., Robbins, J. B., Gotschlich, E. C., Orskov, I., and Orskov, F.: Relation between Escherichia coli Kl capsular polysaccharide antigen and clinical outcome in neonatal meningitis. Lancet 2:246–250, 1974.

Memon, I. A., Jacobs, N. M., Yeh, T. F., and Lilien, L. D.: Group B streptococcal osteomyelitis and septic arthritis. Its occurrence in infants less than 2 months old. Am. J. Dis. Child. 133:921–923, 1979.

Menke, J. A., Giacoia, G. P., and Jockin, H.: Group B beta hemolytic streptococcal sepsis and the idiopathic respiratory distress syndrome: A comparison. J. Pediat. 94:467–471, 1979.

Mikherjee, S. K., Heilman, K. M., and Rosman, N. P.: An unusual cause of progressive head enlargement following Proteus mirabilis meningitis. Develop. Med. Child Neurol. 11:633–636, 1969.

Miller, M. E.: Phagocytosis in the newborn infant: Humoral and cellular factors. J. Pediat. 74:255–259, 1969.

Navarro, C., and Blanc. W. A.: Subacute necrotizing funisitis. A variant of cord inflammation with a high rate of perinatal infection. J. Pediat. 85:689–697, 1974.

Neal, J. B.: Meningitis caused by bacilli of the colon group. Am. J. Med. Sci. 172:740–748, 1926.

Nelson, J. D., Dillon, H. C., Jr., and Howard, J. B., Jr.:

A prolonged nursery epidemic associated with a newly recognized type of group A streptococcus. J. Pediat. 89:792–796, 1976.

Nichols, W., Jr., and Woolley, P. V., Jr.: Listeria monocytogenes meningitis. J. Pediat. 61:337–350, 1962.

Nyhan, W. L., and Fousek, M. D.: Septicemia of the newborn. Pediatrics 22:268–278, 1958.

Okubadejo, O. A., and Alausa, K. O.: Neonatal meningitis caused by Edwardsiella tarda. Brit. Med. J. 3:357–358, 1968.

Oski, F. A.: Hematologic Problems. In: Avery, G. B.: Neonatology. Pathophysiology and Management of the Newborn. J. B. Lippincott. Philadelphia, 1975, page 414.

Overall, J. C., Jr.: Neonatal bacterial meningitis. Analysis of predisposing factors and outcome compared with matched control subjects. J. Pediat. 76:499–511, 1970.

Overbach, A. M., Daniel, S. J., and Cassady, G.: The value of umbilical cord histology in the management of potential perinatal infection. J. Pediat. 76:22–31, 1970.

Overturf, G. D., and Balfour, G.: Osteomyelitis and sepsis. Severe complications of fetal monitoring. Pediatrics 55:244–247, 1975.

Pai, K. G., Rubin, H. M., Wedemeyer, P. P., and Linarelli, L. G.: Hypothalamic-pituitary dysfunction following group B beta hemolytic streptococcal meningitis in a neonate. J. Pediat. 88:289–291, 1976.

Paisley, J. W., and Washington, J. A., II.: Susceptibility of Escherichia coli Kl to four combinations of antimicrobial agents potentially useful for treatment of neonatal meningitis. J. Infect. Dis. 140:183–191, 1979.

Paredes, A., Wong, P., and Yow, M. D.: Failure of penicillin to eradicate the carrier state of Group B streptococcus in infants. J. Pediat. 89:191–193, 1976.

Paredes, A., Wong, P., Mason, E. O., Jr., Taber, L. H., and Barrett, F. F.: Nosocomial transmission of group B streptococci in a newborn nursery. Pediatrics 59:679–682, 1977.

Parry, M. F., and Neu, H. C.: A comparative study of ticarcillin plus tobramycin versus carbenicillin plus gentamicin for the treatment of serious infections due to gram-negative bacilli. Am. J. Med. 64:961–966, 1978.

Pass, M. A., Gray, B. M., Khare, S., and Dillon, H. C., Jr.: Prospective studies of group B streptococcal infections in infants. J. Pediat. 95:437–443, 1979.

Pearlman, M. A., Gartner, L. M., Lee, K-S., Eidelman, A. I., Morecki, R., and Horoupian, D. S.: The association of kernicterus with bacterial infection in the newborn. Pediatrics 65:26–29, 1980.

Plotkin, S. A., and McKitrick, J. C.: Nosocomial meningitis of the newborn caused by a Flavobacterium. J.A.M.A. 198:662–664, 1966.

Pounders, C. M.: Meningitis in the newborn. J. Pediat. 4:752–756, 1934.

Quirante, J., Ceballos, R., and Cassady, G.: Group B β-hemolytic streptococcal infection in the newborn. I. Early onset infection. Am. J. Dis. Child. 128:659–665, 1974.

Rabinowitz, S. G., and MacLeod, N. R.: Salmonella meningitis. A report of three cases and review of the literature. Am. J. Dis. Child. 123:259–262, 1972.

Rahal, J. J., Jr., and Simberkoff, M. S.: Bactericidal and bacteriostatic action of chloramphenicol against meningeal pathogens. Antimicrob. Agents Chemother. 16:13–18, 1979.

Rantz, L. A., and Keefer, C. S.: The distribution of hemolytic streptococci Groups A, B, and C in human infections. J. Infect. Dis. 68:128–132, 1941.

Rappaport, F., Rabinovitz, M., Toaff, R., and Krochik, N.: Genital listeriosis as a cause of repeated abortion. Lancet 1:1273–1275, 1960.

Ravid, J. M.: Meningococcic and nonmeningococcic meningitis in the newborn and in young infants. Am. J. Dis. Child. 49:1282–1298, 1935.

Ray, C. G., and Wedgwood, R. J.: Neonatal listerosis. Six case reports and a review of the literature. Pediatrics 34:378–392, 1964.

Repice, J. P., and Neter, E.: Pasteurella multocida meningitis in an infant with recovery. J. Pediat. 86:91–93, 1975.

Reynolds, D. W., Dweck, H. S., and Cassady, G.: Inappropriate antidiuretic hormone secretion in a neonate with meningitis. Am. J. Dis. Child. 123:251–253, 1972.

Rhodes, P. G., Burry, V. F., Hall, R. T., and Cox, R.: Pneumococcal septicemia and meningitis in the neonate. J. Pediat. 86:593–595, 1975.

Rios, I., Klimek, J. J., Maderazo, E., and Quintiliani, R.: Flavobacterium meningosepticum meningitis: Report of selected aspects. Antimicrob. Agents Chemother. 14:444–447, 1978.

Robbins, J. B., McCracken, G. H., Jr., Gotschlich, E. C., Ørskov, F., Ørskov, I., and Hanson, L. A.: Escherichia coli Kl capsular polysaccharide associated with neonatal meningitis. New Eng. J. Med. 290:1216–1220, 1974.

Root, J. H.: A case of meningococcus meningitis with obstructive hydrocephalus in the newly born. Am. J. Dis. Child. 21:500–505, 1921.

Rose, J. Q., Choi, H. K., Schentag, J. J., Kinkel, W. R., and Jusko, W. J.: Intoxication caused by interaction of chloramphenicol and phenytoin. J.A.M.A. 237:2630–2631, 1977.

Salmon, J. H.: Puncture porencephaly. Am. J. Dis. Child. 114:72–79, 1967.

Saxbe, W. B.: Listeria monocytogenes and Queen Anne. Pediatrics 49:97–101, 1972.

Scherzer, A. L., Kaye, D., and Shinefield, H. R.: Proteus mirabilis meningitis: Report of two cases treated with ampicillin. J. Pediat. 68:731–740, 1966.

Schultz, P., and Leeds, N. E.: Intraventricular septations complicating neonatal meningitis. J. Neurosurg. 38:620–626, 1973.

Shortland-Webb, W. R.: Proteus and coliform meningoencephalitis in neonates. J. Clin. Path. 21:422–431, 1954.

Siber, G. R., Smith, A. L., and Levin, M. J.: Predictability of peak serum gentamicin concentration with dosage based on body surface area. J. Pediat. 94:135–138, 1979.

Siegel, J. D., and McCracken, G. H., Jr.: Detection of group B streptococcal antigens in body fluids of neonates. J. Pediat. 93:491–492, 1978.

Sklaver, A. R., Greenman, R. L., and Hoffman, T. A.: Amikacin therapy of gram-negative bacteremia and meningitis. Treatment in diseases due to multiple resistant bacilli. Arch. Intern. Med. 138:713–716, 1978.

Speck, W. T., Driscoll, J. M., Polin, R. A., and Rosenkranz, H. S.: Natural history of neonatal colonization with group B streptococci. Pediatrics 60:356–359, 1977.

Squire, E., Favara, B., and Todd, J.: Diagnosis of neonatal bacterial infection: Hematologic and pathologic findings in fatal and nonfatal cases. Pediatrics 64:60–64, 1979.

Stamm, W. E., Kolff, C. A., Dones, E. M., Javariz, R., Anderson, R. L., Farmer, J. J., III., and de Quinones, H. R.: A nursery outbreak caused by Serratia marcescens—scalp-vein needles as a portal of entry. J. Pediat. 89:96–99, 1976.

Steere, A. C., Aber, R. C., Warford, L. R., Murphy, K. E., Feeley, J. C., Hayes, P. S., Wilkinson, H. W., and Facklam, R. R.: Possible nosocomial transmission of group B streptococci in a newborn nursery. J. Pediat. 87:784–787, 1975.

Steigman, A. J., Bottone, E. J., and Hanna, B. A.: Control of perinatal Group B streptococcal sepsis. Efficacy of single injection of aqueous penicillin at birth. Mt. Sinai J. Med. 45:685–693, 1978.

Steigman, A. J., Bottone, E. J., and Hanna, B. A.: Intramuscular penicillin administration at birth: Prevention of early-onset Group B streptococcal disease. Pediatrics 62:842–844, 1978.

Stewardson-Krieger, P., and Gotoff, S. P.: Neonatal meningitis due to group C beta hemolytic streptococcus. J. Pediat. 90:103–104, 1977.

Stiehm, E. R., and Damrosch, D. S.: Neonatal meningococcal meningitis. Report of a case acquired in the nursery. J. Pediat. 68:654–656, 1966.

Strausbaugh, L. J., and Sande, M. A.: Factors influencing the therapy of experimental *Proteus mirabilis* meningitis in rabbits. J. Infect. Dis. 137:251–260, 1978.

Sunderland, W. A., Harris, H. H., Spence, D. A., and Lawson, H. W.: Meningococcemia in a newborn infant whose mother had meningococcal vaginitis. J. Pediat. 81:856, 1972.

Tempest, B.: Pneumococcal meningitis in mother and neonate. Pediatrics 53:759–760, 1974.

Truog, W. E., Davis, R. F., and Ray, C. G.: Recurrence of group B streptococcal infection. J. Pediat. 89:185–186, 1976.

Turbeville, D. F., and McCaffree, M. A.: Fetal scalp electrode complications: Cerebrospinal fluid leak. Obstet. Gynecol. 54:469–470, 1979.

Turbeville, D. F., Heath, R. E., Jr., Bowen, F. W., Jr., and Killam, A. P.: Complications of fetal scalp electrodes: A case report. Am. J. Obstet. Gynecol. 122:530–531, 1975.

Visintine, A. M., Oleske, J. M., and Nahmias, A. J.: *Listeria monocytogenes* infection in infants and children. Am. J. Dis. Child. 131:393–397, 1977.

Vogel, L. C., Ferguson, L., and Gotoff, S. P.: *Citrobacter*

infections of the central nervous system in early infancy. J. Pediat. 93:86–88, 1978.

Walker, S. H., Santos, A. Q., and Quintero, B. A.: Recurrence of group B III streptococcal meningitis. J. Pediat. 89:187–188, 1976.

Watson, D. G.: Purulent neonatal meningitis. A study of forty-five cases. J. Pediat. 50:352–360, 1957.

Weintraub, M. I., and Otto, R. N.: Pneumococcal meningitis and endophthalmitis in a newborn. J.A.M.A. 219:1763–1764, 1972.

Wiggins, G. L., Albritton, W. L., and Feeley, J. C.: Antibiotic susceptibility of clinical isolates of *Listeria monocytogenes*. Antimicrob. Agents Chemother. 13:854–860, 1978.

Wilkinson, H. W., Thacker, L. G., and Facklam, R. R.: Non-hemolytic group B streptococci of human, bovine, and ichthyic origin. Infect. Immunol. 7:496–498, 1973.

Willis, M. D., and Austin, W. J.: Human vibrio fetus infection. Am. J. Dis. Child. 112:459–462, 1966.

Winkelstein, J. A.: Opsonins: Their function, identity, and clinical significance. J. Pediat. 82:747–753, 1973.

Wright, W. C., Jr., Ank, B. J., Herbert, J., and Stiehm, E. R.: Decreased bacterial activity of leukocytes of stressed newborn infants. Pediatrics 56:579–584, 1975.

Yeung, C. Y., and Hobbs, J. R.: Serum-gamma-G-globulin levels in normal, premature, post-mature, and "small-for-dates" newborn babies. Lancet 1:1167–1170, 1968.

Yeung, C. Y., Lee, V. W. Y., and Yeung, M. B.: Glucose disappearance rate in neonatal infection. J. Pediat. 82:486–489, 1973.

Yogev, R., and Williams, T.: Ventricular fluid levels of chloramphenicol in infants. Antimicrob. Agents Chemother. 16:7–8, 1979.

Yow, M. D., Mason, E. O., Leeds, L. J., Thompson, P. K., Clark, D. J., and Gardner, S. E.: Ampicillin prevents intrapartum transmission of Group B Streptococcus. J.A.M.A. 241:1245–1247, 1979.

Yu, J. S., and Grauaug, A.: Purulent meningitis in the neonatal period. Arch. Dis. Child. 38:391–396, 1963.

Ziai, M., and Haggerty, R. J.: Neonatal meningitis. New Eng. J. Med. 259:314–320, 1958.

Zipursky, A., Palko, J., Milner, R., and Akenzua, G. I.: The hematology of bacterial infections in premature infants. Pediatrics 57:839–853, 1976.

Chapter Four

HEMOPHILUS INFLUENZAE MENINGITIS

Hemophilus influenzae type b is the leading cause of purulent meningitis in children between three months and three years of age, with a peak incidence in the second half of the first year and with 95 percent of cases occurring in children less than five years of age (Floyd et al., Peter and Smith). It is estimated that there are at least 10,000 new cases of *Hemophilus influenzae* meningitis per year in this country (Ingram, Mortimer, Parke et al.), with a mortality rate of 5 to 10 percent. The incidence of the disease has been reported to be between 26 and 40 cases per year per 100,000 children less than five years of age (Fraser et al., Tarr and Peter). Smith and Peter (1972) estimated that approximately one in every 2,000 children will develop *Hemophilus influenzae* meningitis between six and 48 months of age, while Tarr and Peter found that in Rhode Island between 1970 and 1974 one of every 1,766 infants acquired the illness during the first year of life. Black children have been found to be at a fourfold greater risk to acquire the illness compared to white children (Tarr and Peter).

The organism was identified by Richard Pfeiffer in 1892 and was erroneously believed to be the cause of the influenza pandemic of 1889–1892, thus accounting for the designation, influenza bacillus. Wollstein credited Pfuhl with the first report of meningitis due to the influenza bacillus in 1892. The organism was identified after death in these cases and it remained for Slawyk, in 1898, to provide the initial report of *Hemophilus influenzae* recovered from purulent spinal fluid during life.

Hemophilus influenzae, or Pfeiffer's bacillus, is a non-motile, non-hemolytic gram-negative pleomorphic organism with both coccoid and bacillary forms on staining. The organism is one of the smaller pathogenic bacteria which, on appropriate agar, results in small, discrete, transparent colonies. Growth on artificial media is best under aerobic conditions and the organism is easily killed by drying or heating. The hemophilic character of the organism refers to the requirement of the presence of blood in the culture medium for its growth. Two factors in blood must be present, designated as X (hematin) and V (nicotinamide dinucleotide). Because V factor is normally entrapped within intact erythrocytes, *Hemophilus influenzae* grows best on media in which red blood cells have been disrupted, such as chocolate agar or Levinthal agar. *Hemophilus parainfluenzae,* assumed to be an unusual cause of meningitis, differs from *Hemophilus influenzae* in the ability of the former organism to grow in the absence of X factor.

In 1911, Wollstein demonstrated the ability to experimentally transmit *Hemophilus influenzae* infection to monkeys, resulting in purulent meningitis. In addition, she appears to have been the first to stress the marked tendency for this infection to occur in infants and young children. Rivers in 1922 drew wide attention to influenzal meningitis by his report of 23 cases. To that date, 220 cases had been published with 17 recoveries, a mortality of 92 percent. Rivers also stressed the occurrence of influenzal meningitis in infancy, pointing out that 79 percent of reported cases had occurred in children under two years of age.

One of the most extensive early studies of *Hemophilus influenzae* meningitis was published by Neal et al. in 1934, in which 111 cases of the disease were reviewed which the authors had seen between the years 1911 and 1934. Ninety-three of the 111 occurred in children less than five years of age and five cases were in persons over 20 years old. The case fatality rate was 96.4 percent. This report helped to establish the concept that this type of acute meningitis was one of the most common in infancy and early childhood but that the disease could occur in any age group. The authors showed that there had been no increase in influenza bacillus meningitis during the influenza epidemic of 1918–1919, dispelling the still prevalent confusion over the possible relationship of the two conditions.

In 1931, Margaret Pittman distinguished six serotypes of encapsulated *Hemophilus influenzae* on the basis of their capsular polysaccharide and designated them a, b, c, d, e, and f. Type b was shown to be responsible for nearly all cases of meningitis due to this organism. Fothergill and Wright in 1933 performed studies to explain the remarkable age relationships which by that time had become evident in regard to *Hemophilus influenzae* meningitis. They showed that only one patient in 276 cases was less than two months of age while the maximum occurrence of the illness was in infants between ages six and nine months. Thereafter, the disease gradually decreased in frequency to become comparatively rare after age four years. Experiments by Fothergill and Wright revealed that passively transferred maternal antibody protected the infant for the first two months after birth but that such protection was largely dissipated by four months of age. From two months to three years of age, little bactericidal activity against the organism was present. Actively acquired immunity evident by bactericidal activity in the blood was found to progressively rise after age three years, accounting for the rapid decline of influenzal meningitis in older children. Once acquired, protective bactericidal activity was believed to be permanent. More recent studies have suggested an increasing susceptibility of neonates to *Hemophilus influenzae* meningitis sec-

ondary to a decrease in transplacentally transmitted protective antibody (Graber et al.).

The next significant advance in regard to knowledge of this disease was related to the development of therapeutic methods for its control. Wollstein in 1911 had used a specific antiserum to treat influenzal meningitis in monkeys, but in 1931 Fothergill introduced an immune horse serum which was used to treat human disease over the next several years. Fothergill's horse antiserum was injected intrathecally but resulted in only slight reduction in mortality from the condition (Fothergill, Ward and Fothergill, Wilkes-Weiss and Huntington).

In 1939, Alexander succeeded in preparing an anti-influenzal antiserum in rabbits which proved to be the first noteworthy step in the development of effective therapeutic agents for the treatment of *Hemophilus influenzae* meningitis. The reason for the greater effectiveness of antiserum prepared in rabbits compared to that previously produced in horses remained unclear, although Alexander suggested that the smaller size of the molecule of rabbit serum permitted better tissue penetration. Sulfonamides alone had been shown to have only a modest effect in reducing mortality. In 1942, however, Alexander et al. described 50 cases of *Hemophilus influenzae* meningitis treated with a combination of sulfonamides and rabbit antiserum with a mortality of only 26 percent. Additional trials over the next four years confirmed the effectiveness of this form of treatment (Edmonds and Neter, Sako et al., Smith et al.). Although a definite reduction in mortality followed the development of serum therapy, the adverse effects of this material prompted the search for other chemotherapeutic agents which might be more safely used. Smith et al. stated that adverse reactions occurred in 12 of 27 patients treated with antiserum, including serum sickness, anaphylaxis, and edema of the conjunctiva and periorbital soft tissues.

Following its introduction in 1944, streptomycin rapidly acquired a place in the treatment of influenzal meningitis with even further improvement in recovery rates (Logan and Herrell, Weinstein). The drug was usually administered both systemically and by intrathecal injection, and often in combination with sulfonamides or anti-influenzal serum. By 1947, Alexander and Leidy stated that the treatment of choice for *Hemophilus influenzae* meningitis was a combination of streptomycin, sulfadiazine, and specific rabbit antiserum. In a series of 90 cases treated with streptomycin and sulfadiazine, Appelbaum and Nelson recorded a recovery rate of 96.6 percent. With the development of chloramphenicol and the demonstration that it passed readily into the cerebrospinal fluid, this antibiotic supplanted streptomycin for treatment of this disease, thus obviating the need for intrathecal medication (Carabelle et al., Prather and Smith, Scott and Walcher). In 1952, Ross and colleagues described the combined use of chloramphenicol and sulfadiazine, a regimen that remained the recommended therapeutic approach for the treatment of *Hemophilus influenzae* meningitis until the introduction of ampicillin in 1961. The next event requiring re-evaluation of the antibiotic therapy occurred in 1973 when ampicillin-resistant strains of *Hemophilus influenzae* were first identified.

Clinical Aspects

Acute meningitis is the most common serious invasive disease caused by *Hemophilus influenzae* in children, although the spectrum of disease this organism can produce is quite extensive (Dajani et al., Todd and Bruhn). In addition, localization of septic infection in more than one site simultaneously is not infrequent, especially in newborn and young infants. Infection with the influenzae bacillus has generally been regarded to be in the form of a localized process in one or another anatomic region but in recent years it has been recognized that this organism can cause a febrile bacteremia without localization, similar to but less common than that secondary to *Streptococcus pneumoniae* (McGowan et al., Todd and Bruhn). Most such cases occur in children less than two years of age and, without treatment, the bacteremic child is at definite risk for the eventual development of serious focal infection, including meningitis (Marshall et al.). Epiglottitis is one of the most life-threatening focal infections caused by *Hemophilus influenzae*. The age range over which epiglottitis occurs is broader and the mean age of occurrence of approximately four years is greater than is the case with *Hemophilus influenzae* meningitis (Faden). In recent years, there has been an increase in the incidence of acute meningitis complicating epiglottitis caused by *Hemophilus influenzae* (Branefors-Helander and Jeppsson, Molteni).

Hemophilus influenzae is the most common cause of orbital and periorbital cellulitis in children under three years of age (Gellady et al., Smith et al. 1978), and this illness also can be concomitant with meningitis (Watters et al.). Orbital cellulitis is usually a complication of acute *Hemophilus influenzae* sinusitis, while periorbital cellulitis is analogous to cellulitis elsewhere. Cellulitis caused by this organism most commonly affects the cheek of the face unilaterally. Most cases occur in children less than 30 months of age and are manifested by fever and a violaceous or purplish-red discoloration with soft-tissue swelling of the affected cheek. The primary importance of early recognition of the disorder is based on the concomitant bacteremia which is almost invariably present (Granoff and Nankervis, Rapkin and Bautista).

Nelson and Ginsburg proposed the hypothesis that acute facial cellulitis in some infants represents lymphatic extension of primary *Hemophilus influenzae* type b infection of the middle ear, which differs from most cases of acute otitis media in infancy caused by this organism that are due to non-typable *Hemophilus influenzae*. The absence of otitis media in other cases suggests that facial cellulitis can also represent bacteremic localization in soft tissues (Dejani et al.). Primary pneumonia in children resulting from *Hemophilus influenzae* type b is one of the more common types of focal infection caused by this organism and is distinguished from *Hemophilus* pneumonia in children with chronic pulmonary disease, which is usually due to non-typable organisms (Jacobs and Harris). Other less common primary focal infections caused by *Hemophilus influenzae* include septic arthritis or osteomyelitis (Granoff et al.), purulent pericarditis (Echeverria et al.), and urinary tract infection (Dajani et al.).

Hemophilus influenzae meningitis can occur at any time of the year, although the illness is more common during the winter months, corresponding to the peak incidence of upper respiratory infections. Among 128 meningitis cases, Koch and Carson found that in 77 percent, an upper respiratory infection or otitis media preceded the onset of meningitis. Type b strains account for the great majority of cases of *Hemophilus influenzae* meningitis but other capsular types can do so on rare occasion. Typing can be determined by several methods, including the use of type-specific antisera by slide agglutination, capsular swelling, fluorescent antibody techniques, and counterimmunoelectrophoresis. Small numbers of cases of meningitis have been described caused by types a, c, e, and f, and a limited number have resulted from unencapsulated (nontypable) *Hemophilus influenzae* (Denis et al., Gray, Greene, Hodes and Leidy). The majority of the recorded examples of non-type b *Hemophilus influenzae* meningitis have had an age spectrum, natural history, and antibiotic sensitivities much like the customary infection caused by type b organisms. Those with meningitis caused by unencapsulated *Hemophilus influenzae* have more often been older children or adults and, in some, have complicated recent head injury.

Hemophilus parainfluenzae is morphologically similar to *Hemophilus influenzae* and is generally regarded to be a normal inhabitant of the nasopharynx. Clinical and laboratory aspects of meningitis caused by these two organisms appear to be identical and only a few examples caused by *Hemophilus parainfluenzae* have been described (Barnshaw and Phillips, Gullekson and Dumoff, Hable et al., Holt et al., Kaufman et al.). Because *Hemophilus parainfluenzae* and *Hemophilus influenzae* are not distinguishable by the customary methods of bacteriologic examination, it is probable that the former organism is a more common cause of meningitis in infants and young children than the available literature suggests (Bachman).

Hemophilus influenzae meningitis in the newborn period and in infants less than two months of age is infrequent but, when it does occur, there is a greater tendency for widespread septic involvement and there is a higher incidence of infection with nontypable organisms. Influenzae meningitis has been found to account for approximately 1 percent of cases of acute suppurative meningitis in the neonatal period (Fosson and Fine, Groover et al.). *Hemophilus influenzae* has been found to colonize the genital tract of normal and pregnant women in less than 1 percent of those sampled; however, in most instances of *Hemophilus influenzae* neonatal sepsis the organism is believed to be acquired by the infant from the mother's birth canal (Khuri-Bulos and McIntosh). The illness in the neonate can be identical to the early onset type of group B *Streptococcus* sepsis (Bale and Watkins, Lilien et al.) and can occur with or without meningitis. The widespread organ system involvement often seen with *Hemophilus influenzae* infection in infants less than two months of age is exemplified by the cases described by Collier et al. in which meningitis was complicated by septic osteomyelitis, pericarditis, or pneumonia with pneumatocele formation. Susceptibility of these infants to this infection resulted from lack of bactericidal activity in maternal blood and thus in fetal blood.

Systemic infections, including meningitis, caused by *Hemophilus influenzae* have gradually increased both relatively and absolutely over the past several decades although the reasons remain unclear (Michaels, Smith and Haynes). The relative increase compared to other types of bacterial meningitis is partially explained by the decline of the tubercle bacillus as a cause of meningitis in children. *Hemophilus influenzae* is now by far the most common cause of bacterial meningitis in children from three months until three years of age, in addition to being the leading cause when the childhood years are considered collectively. After five years of age it becomes infrequent and decidedly so beyond ten years of age.

Recurrent serious infections with this organism or its occurrence in persons over ten years of age can affect previously normal individuals, but many such cases are seen in persons with underlying chronic illnesses, immunologic abnormalities, or those with abnormal communications from the external environment to the subarachnoid space. Fulminating septic infections caused by encapsulated bacteria are well known in post-splenectomized patients and can also occur in children with congenital asplenia (Chilcote et al., Waldman et al.). The young child is particularly susceptible to this condition although no age group is entirely spared. Most such illnesses in the asplenic or hyposplenic patient are due to *Streptococcus pneumoniae*, but *Hemophilus influenzae* is also an important cause and accounts for some cases of rapidly progressive *Hemophilus influenzae* meningitis in the older child and the adult (Nixon and Aisenberg, Weitzman and Aisenberg).

Infections in adults with *Hemophilus influenzae* are believed to have steadily increased in recent years and are most prevalent in persons with an underlying disease. The most prevalent predisposing illnesses in adults include alcoholism, diabetes mellitus, chronic obstructive pulmonary disease, chronic renal disease, the post-splenectomy state, immunoglobulin deficiency syndromes, and conditions with CSF fistulas. *Hemophilus influenzae* pneumonia in adults can occur as lobar consolidation or bronchopneumonia and is frequently associated with pleural disease with effusion or empyema (Levin et al.). Because definitive diagnosis requires isolation of the organism from blood, pleural fluid, or lung aspirate, it is believed that the incidence of *Hemophilus influenzae* pneumonia in adults, and especially in the elderly, is probably significantly underestimated (Hirschmann and Everett). Other infections caused by *Hemophilus influenzae* that have been recognized in adults include acute sinusitis, bronchitis, pericarditis, endocarditis, septic arthritis, and bacteremia (Hirschmann and Everett). Acute epiglottitis, generally considered to be a childhood condition, has also been described on rare occasion in the adult population (Johnstone and Lawy).

Several reports have described *Hemophilus influenzae* meningitis in adults but most have stressed its infrequency compared to pneumococcal or meningococcal meningitis (Eykyn et al., Jervey, Marselis et al.). Stein et al. claimed that, up to 1969, 110 cases of influenzal meningitis had been reported in persons over 20 years of age, of which 66 had some underlying disorder which predisposed them to infection with this organism. Norden and colleagues (1970) described an adult with *Hemophilus influenzae* meningitis in whom lack of bactericidal antibody against the organism was detected. They pointed out that this form of meningitis can occur in otherwise healthy adults and suggested that a significant percent of adults lack sufficient protective antibody. In 1974, Norden reported that among 833 adults over 20 years of age included in his study, only 21 percent were found to have bactericidal antibody to *Hemophilus influenzae* type b, a finding in striking contrast to that of Fothergill and Wright published in 1933.

The initial symptoms and signs of *Hemophilus influenzae* meningitis are often more subtle and less fulminating than those of meningococcal or pneumococcal meningitis in older children. Certain children, however, either convulse or become drowsy within hours after fever or irritability is first observed. Fever and irritability may be the only abnormalities noted on the first day or so, providing little evidence of the localization of the infectious process. At this stage, signs of meningeal irritation may be minimal or absent. Lethargy and vomiting are sometimes apparent early in the illness or can be delayed for two or three days after the initial manifestations. In some, nonspecific signs such as fever, irritability, and anorexia are attributed to otitis media or an upper respiratory infection, but the occurrence of a convulsion leads to lumbar puncture and the identification of meningitis. Unless the illness is recognized and treatment begun, neck stiffness soon develops and in the infant, the fontanel becomes tense. When several days pass between onset of the illness and its diagnosis, lethargy may proceed to coma, recurrent seizures become prominent, and neurologic signs include spasticity of limbs and extraocular or facial palsies. In rare instances, a petechial rash identical to that with meningococcal infection may occur (Warthen).

Sudden development of shock can complicate the clinical course of the illness and is especially common in those with a rapidly progressive downhill course (Lindsay et al.). Alexander (1965) made reference to a particularly fulminating form of *Hemophilus influenzae* meningitis observed during the Asian influenza epidemic in 1957. She suggested that this may have represented an altered host relationship to bacterial infection by the influence of viral disease. The possible influence of an immediately preceding viral illness on the development of *Hemophilus influenzae* meningitis has been supported by experimental studies by Michaels et al. Following intranasal administration of *Hemophilus influenzae* type b to infant rats, these investigators found that the dose required to produce meningitis in the animals was reduced 100-fold among those who first had received influenza virus by the same route. The severity of the illness resulting was not evaluated in these experiments, which were designed to assess the number of animals in each group which became infected and the dose of bacteria required to produce infection.

A rapidly progressive, fulminating clinical course is occasionally observed in children with meningitis due to the influenza bacillus. Within hours after the initial symptoms, the child becomes unresponsive, and deep coma is soon followed by pupillary dilatation and subsequent respiratory failure. Some survive but usually with extensive neurologic damage while many others who follow such a dramatic course appear to show little response to therapy and proceed to death. Those who experience an episode of shock, with its attendant compromise of cerebral perfusion on the already swollen brain, are especially likely to experience a bad outcome. The pathogenesis of this fulminating form of *Hemophilus influenzae* meningitis remains unclear, although profound cerebral swelling plays a significant role and accounts for internal herniations, which are the common cause of death.

There are several possible complications which can develop in the acute stage of *Hemophilus influenzae* meningitis that will sometimes contribute to the clinical findings the child exhibits. Perhaps the most common is inappropriate release of antidiuretic hormone, which leads to fluid retention and a progressive decline in serum sodium and chloride concentrations. Unless prevented by appropriate fluid restriction, this can lead to soft tissue edema and can enhance the probability of occurrence of seizures. Among a series of 50 children with *Hemophilus influenzae* meningitis, Feigin et al. (1976) found that laboratory data suggested the presence of inappropriate secretion of antidiuretic hormone in 88 percent. This metabolic abnormality is most often identified in the first 48 to 72 hours of the illness, and generally abates promptly with management. Acute septic arthritis is a relatively frequent complication of *Hemophilus influenzae* meningitis and is more likely to become symptomatic during the course of therapy than to be present at the time of hospital admission. It is one of many causes of recurrent fever in this illness and can result in so-called pseudoparalysis of an extremity, leading the examiner to the false conclusion that apparent weakness is due to a cerebral or spinal cord insult.

Frank purulent pericarditis producing overt symptoms including acute cardiac tamponade is quite rare with *Hemophilus influenzae* meningitis. Asymptomatic small or moderate pericardial effusions, which are detected only by echocardiography, however, have been found to be relatively common in this illness and were discovered in 19 of 100 cases of Laird et al. None of the 19 patients had a friction rub and only one required pericardiocentesis. The authors assumed that when pericardial involvement occurs in this illness, it is usually secondary to bacterial localization in the pericardium from bacteremia and is most often quickly overcome by antibiotic therapy resulting in a sterile effusion. An infected subdural effusion or subdural empyema is an additional complication of influenzal meningitis which can modify the

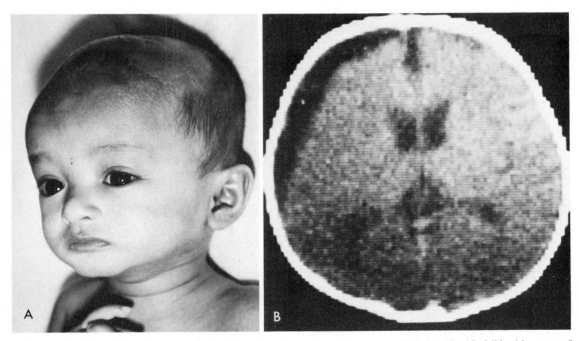

Figure 4–1. Hemophilus influenzae meningitis, infected subdural effusion. *A,* Four-month-old child with onset of symptoms of acute purulent meningitis 6 days prior to photograph. Despite 5 days of intravenous chloramphenicol therapy in adequate dosage, he continued to have temperature spikes, neck stiffness, and irritability. His anterior fontanel had become more tense in the two days prior to the photograph. Repeat CSF examination at this time revealed sterile fluid with improved values; however, the cranial computed tomogram, *B,* reveals a subdural fluid collection over the left cerebral hemisphere. Subdural tap on the left yielded 20 ml. of cloudy fluid with a glucose content of 15 mg. per 100 ml. and positive for *Hemophilus influenzae* on culture. Fever and other signs resolved after the second subdural tap.

clinical features of the illness, resulting in persistent fever, persistence of a bulging fontanel, lethargy, and signs of cortical irritation, including seizures and limb paresis (Fig. 4–1). Endophthalmitis has been much more often associated with meningococcal meningitis and has been seen in children with *Hemophilus influenzae* meningitis only rarely (Sastry and Baker, Ward et al.). Endophthalmitis provokes intense local pain, chemosis, eyelid swelling, and a purulent exudate within the anterior chamber. Unless checked by treatment, it can progress to overt orbital cellulitis or lead to extensive ocular damage followed by permanent visual loss.

Laboratory Studies

Diagnosis of *Hemophilus influenzae* meningitis is established by performance of a lumbar puncture and identification of the organism or its antigen within the CSF. Blood culture is another valuable source of bacteriologic information, as positive cultures have been found in 65 to 75 percent of cases (McGowan et al., Neter). In past years, immediate diagnosis on CSF examination utilized capsular swelling, the Quellung reaction, a method identical to that used by Neufeld for typing pneumococci. The capsular swelling reaction was simple and could be rapidly performed. Specific anti-influenzae serum was added to a spinal fluid specimen colored slightly by the addition of methylene blue, and the preparation was then examined microscopically. The presence of capsular swelling proved not only that the causative agent was *Hemophilus influenzae* but also that it was type b.

Most clinicians now rely on gram stain or methylene blue stain and culture of spinal fluid to establish the diagnosis. On a gram-stained preparation, one sees gram-negative pleomorphic coccobacilli; however, misidentification is not uncommon. The organism may be mistaken for the pneumococcus when it is under-decolorized and because it often contains two dark blue-purple granules that create the false appearance of a diplococcus. Latex particle agglutination has recently been promoted to be a rapid and reliable method to establish the etiologic diagnosis in cases with acute bacterial meningitis (Whittle et al., Ward et al. 1978). Countercurrent immunoelectrophoresis requires much greater technical expertise and is probably more sensitive for the detection of *Hemophilus influenzae* an-

tigen in blood and CSF than of the other common causes of meningitis in children (Shackelford et al.). False negative results do occur, even in patients who have not received preceding antibiotic therapy (Feigin et al. 1976).

The CSF abnormalities are essentially the same with influenzal meningitis as in other forms of acute bacterial meningitis. During the first or second day of the illness, the fluid may be opalescent or turbid but thereafter becomes purulent. The CSF lactic acid content is elevated to levels usually greater than 50 mg per 100 ml. in children with *Hemophilus influenzae* meningitis, as in other types of acute suppurative meningitis, and remains elevated for the first 48 to 72 hours after initiation of treatment (Brook et al., Controni et al.). The cellular response is usually almost entirely composed of polymorphonuclear leukocytes, but with appropriate therapy it reverts to a mixed population, with both mononuclear cells and neutrophils. The glucose content is usually markedly reduced, with levels between zero and 20 mg. per 100 ml. being the common range. The protein content is variably elevated, depending in part on the duration of the illness. As is the case with any type of bacterial meningitis, variations in the CSF abnormalities are not uncommon. A normal CSF glucose content, for example, does not exclude the possibility of *Hemophilus influenzae* meningitis. Even the absence of cells in the cerebrospinal fluid is not inconsistent with the diagnosis (Moore and Ross).

"Mixed" meningitis with two infectious agents present simultaneously in the CSF has been identified in several patients with *Hemophilus influenzae* meningitis. Faber in 1914 described a child with concomitant tuberculous and *Hemophilus* meningitis. Vaden et al. reported cases of influenzal meningitis coexistent with pneumococcal, meningococcal, and streptococcal meningitis. Echo virus type 9 and Herpesvirus hominis have also been isolated from the CSF in children with *Hemophilus influenzae* meningitis (Brunell and Dodd, Wright et al.). Although "mixed" meningitis is rare, it should be considered when the clinical course is decidedly different from that anticipated.

Pathology

The cerebral pathology in fatal cases of *Hemophilus influenzae* meningitis depends on the stage of the disease when death occurs. One of the earliest studies of the neuropathology of influenzal meningitis was that of Davis in 1911 at a time when the disease was still assumed to be a rarity. He commented on the predisposition of the illness to occur in infants less than one year of age and emphasized the abundance of the greenish-yellow leptomeningeal exudate found at the base of the brain in the acute stage but with relatively slight inflammatory infiltrate of the parenchyma of the brain. In one child who probably survived for almost a month after onset of meningitis, subacute fibrinopurulent leptomeningitis at necropsy was accompanied by a large left frontal lobe abscess, which Davis claimed to be the first identified case with brain abscess formation caused by the influenzae bacillus.

In 1948, Adams and colleagues published a study of the neuropathology of 14 fatal cases of *Hemophilus influenzae* meningitis in which there was survival for variable periods of time after onset. In those surviving from one to 14 days, a yellow subarachnoid exudate was usually present over the spinal cord and brain stem, in the basilar cisterns, and over the surface of the cerebrum. When the exudate was sparse in amount, it appeared as yellow streaks along the cerebral veins and within the cortical sulci. Cerebral vessels were congested and convolutions were flattened owing to brain swelling. Gross observation of the sectioned brain revealed few changes in the early cases except for the purulent leptomeningeal exudate. Microscopic examination of the subarachnoid exudate showed a neutrophilic response with scattered lymphocytes enmeshed in strands of fibrin. Even in cases of brief duration, microscopic changes within the brain parenchyma were usually evident. Pallor or pyknosis of nerve cells was evident, at times with large number of rod-shaped microglia present in the cerebral cortex. Endothelial and adventitial proliferation of small vessels within the subarachnoid space and in the cortex was marked. In cases of two to four weeks' duration, the abnormalities were more severe. The amount of purulent exudate over the cortical surface and at the base was greater and generalized ventricular dilatation was often noted. Cerebral changes were profound although the neuronal abnormalities varied from mild alterations to widespread necrosis of the cerebral cortex and subcortical white matter. Microglial proliferation and astrogliosis were usually evident. In the more chronic cases, the ventricles were usually markedly dilated and in large portions of the cerebral cortex there was nearly complete necrosis. Marked proliferation of astroglia and microglia was widespread.

Smith and Landing reported 34 fatal cases of influenzal meningitis and described findings similar to those of Adams et al. Arteritis was noted in certain cases but the authors commented on the surprising rarity of arterial thrombosis in the brain with this type of meningitis. Focal encephalomalacia secondary to venous thrombosis was present in some. Recent angiographic studies, however, have shown that narrowing or occlusion of major intracranial arteries often occurs with severe infection due to this organism, possibly resulting in ischemic damage with subsequent cerebral atrophy (Gado et al., James et al., Thomas and Hopkins). It should be noted that the above description of the cerebral pathology is from patients sufficiently ill to expire from the disease. In patients mildly ill who are diagnosed and treated early and survive without evident neurologic sequelae on follow-up examinations, it is assumed that structural cerebral injury is probably minimal or absent.

Subdural Effusions

Subdural effusions have been recognized as a complication of purulent meningitis in infants since 1950 and are estimated to occur in approximately 30 percent of infants with *Hemophilus influenzae* meningitis (Feigin et al. 1976). McKay and colleagues in Boston first reported meningitic subdural effusions in nine infants, all of whom had *Hemophilus influenzae* meningitis. These authors recognized the possible development of subdural membranes in such patients and described surgical removal in one case (Fig. 4–2). They also described what they believed to be indications for diagnostic subdural taps, which included the persistence of fever after 48 hours of treatment, positive CSF cultures after 48 hours of treatment, convulsions after subsidence of infection, and any gross neurologic abnormality during the immediate convalescent period. Soon after this initial publication, Smith et al. reported 20 cases with subdural effusions in a total of 43 cases of bacterial meningitis in infants under two years of age. Nine of these children had *Hemophilus influenzae* meningitis while 11 had other types of infections, indicating that this complication is not limited to infants with

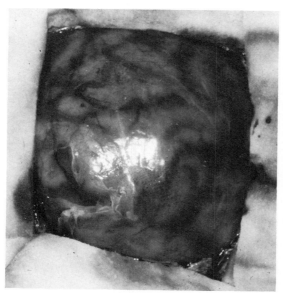

Figure 4–2. Meningitic subdural effusion with well-defined subdural membranes. Four-month-old child with *Hemophilus influenzae* meningitis with onset at age 3 months. The response to antibiotic therapy was satisfactory; however, the illness was complicated by rapid head enlargement and spread of cranial sutures. Multiple subdural taps revealed large quantities of xanthochromic fluid with a high protein content. After numerous taps did not decrease the quantity of the subdural collection, craniotomy was performed to attempt to remove the membranes. The photograph reveals severe venous congestion and thick, adherent subdural membranes. This operative procedure is now rarely, if ever, indicated for this complication.

meningitis due to *Hemophilus influenzae* but can occur in any type of acute bacterial meningitis in the infant age group. The widely recognized association of subdural effusions with *Hemophilus influenzae* meningitis exists probably because this is by far the most common type of pyogenic meningitis in the age group in which there is a predisposition for subdural effusions to occur. The most common indication for subdural taps in the series of Smith et al. was the occurrence of convulsions. Mention was made of a bulging fontanel as a sign warranting diagnostic taps.

The fluid obtained in infants with subdural effusions is usually xanthochromic and may be blood-tinged. Under normal circumstances, a few drops or up to 1 ml. of clear fluid with a slightly higher protein content than normal CSF can be obtained during the performance of transfontanel subdural taps. To be significant, the volume of fluid from the subdural space should be more than 2 ml. (Rabe) although quantities in the range of 2 to 5 ml. almost certainly do not cause significant cerebral compression. The glucose con-

tent in a subdural effusion is often normal, but the protein content is usually elevated and may be as high as 1,000 to 2,000 mg. per 100 ml. Infrequently, the organism can be cultured from the subdural fluid. Most subdural effusions are bilateral and the amount that may be present on each side varies from 4 to 5 ml. up to over 100 ml. Clear or slightly cloudy subdural fluid from which bacteria are isolated is best referred to as an infected subdural effusion, while that in which the fluid is frankly purulent is called a subdural empyema. In some instances, the latter is manifested by induration, erythema, and increased warmth to palpation in the region of the anterior fontanel.

Pathogenesis of Subdural Effusions. The pathogenesis of subdural effusions complicating bacterial meningitis remains unclear. Gitlin studied albumin-to-gammaglobulin ratios in subdural effusions and serum and found the ratio to be higher in the subdural fluid than in concomitantly sampled serum. The assumption from this study was that an effusion forms by passage of fluid through irritated or damaged blood vessel walls. Williams and Stevens proposed the concept that subdural effusions result from removal of excessive amounts of CSF during lumbar puncture. Sagging of the brain and tearing of bridging veins was suggested to result from the diagnostic lumbar puncture, leading to fluid collection within the subdural spaces. This explanation would not account for those effusions found when the initial spinal tap and subdural punctures are done only minutes apart, and does not explain the lack of development of subdural effusions following spinal taps commonly done on infants who do not have meningitis. The concept has not been disproved, however, as a possible factor that enhances reaccumulation of subdural fluid once formed and should enter consideration when one contemplates repeated or multiple spinal taps in infants with post-meningitic effusions. Other studies of the pathogenesis of subdural effusions have utilized I^{131}-labeled albumin injected intravenously and subdurally (Rabe). Following intravenous injection, the material appeared in the subdural space, indicating that albumin within the subdural fluid was derived from plasma. In addition, concentrations of the tagged albumin suggested that in such infants no direct communication existed between plasma, subarachnoid space, and subdural space.

Indications for Subdural Taps. The indications for subdural taps in infants with bacterial meningitis remain poorly defined. Benson et al. suggested that the incidence of effusions is related to the vigor with which they are searched for and stressed the advantages of routine subdural taps on all infants with purulent meningitis. In their large series, 34 percent of the effusions that were identified were discovered during the performance of routine subdural taps. Certain indications proposed in the past have only questionable relationship to the existence of a subdural effusion. Persistence of fever beyond 48 to 72 hours after initiation of therapy or recurrence of fever has many possible explanations in children with meningitis but is difficult to attribute to a sterile subdural effusion. On the other hand, unexplained persistence of fever or recurrence of fever after initial improvement with antibiotic therapy can be secondary to infected subdural effusions and is an indication for subdural taps unless another cause for the febrile response is promptly identified.

Although absolute guidelines remain controversial, certain findings can be accepted as indications for diagnostic subdural taps. The development of a tense, bulging anterior fontanel after two or three days of therapy and with other evidence of improvement is suggestive of subdural effusions. Skull x-rays taken at weekly intervals revealing progressive suture spread likewise suggest a postmeningitic complication, either effusions or hydrocephalus. The occurrence of seizures, especially when focal, evidence of a hemiparesis, or marked obtundation after two or three days of adequate therapy, should warrant diagnostic subdural taps, although these findings are more often the result of inflammatory cerebral vascular involvement than of subdural effusions. An abnormal pattern of skull transillumination with extension of the glow of light more than 3 cm. from the rim of the light source is suggestive of effusions in infants with meningitis (Rabe).

Similar clinical findings suggest the presence of subdural effusions in late infancy or early childhood, although proof of their existence is more difficult after the anterior fontanel is closed. Papilledema, progressive suture spread on serial skull x-rays, focal seizures, and otherwise unexplained lethargy or irritability are indications for computed cranial tomography. Meningitic subdural ef-

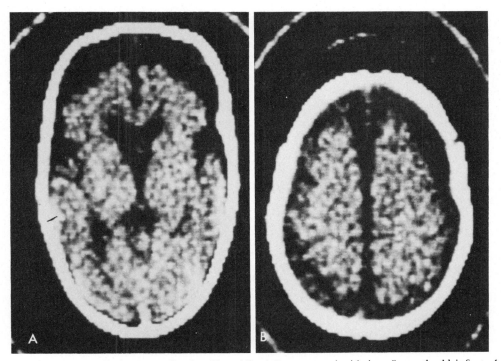

Figure 4–3. Subdural effusions complicating *Hemophilus influenzae* meningitis in a 5-month-old infant. *A,* Computed tomogram at the ventricular level demonstrates large, bilaterally symmetrical subdural effusions, which have a ventricular fluid density. There is mild enlargement of the ventricular system, indicative of early communicating hydrocephalus. *B,* Computed tomogram near the vertex level shows the subdural collections encompassing the cerebral hemispheres, including fluid collection medially, adjacent to the falx cerebri.

fusions are recognized in the form of collections of ventricular fluid density located between the inner surface of the skull and the cerebral convexity and, in most instances, encompass the cerebral hemisphere (Fig. 4–3). Even in younger infants, computed tomography can be used to identify subdural effusions prior to transfontanel taps and, on rare occasion, subdural collections can be present and not found by subdural taps but are identified by computed tomography or radionuclide techniques (Trackler et al.). In addition to demonstrating the presence or absence of subdural effusions, computed tomography can provide other important information, including the status of the ventricular size, demonstration of the site or sites of infarctional lesions when present, and the elimination of the remote possibility of parenchymal abscess.

Treatment of Subdural Effusions. The importance of removal of subdural effusions that complicate bacterial meningitis in infancy is subject to variable opinions. Effusions of small quantity are very likely commonly present and never identified, and most are believed to disappear spontaneously. Large effusions of sufficient volume to result in bulging of the fontanel, or unilateral fluid collections which cause ventricular shift should be aspirated by daily percutaneous transfontanel taps. An infected subdural fluid collection clearly should be removed and those in which the fluid is relatively clear or mildly cloudy can be aspirated by percutaneous taps at daily intervals. A subdural empyema cannot be satisfactorily aspirated through a needle and requires surgical evacuation with irrigation of the infected space, often followed by continuous external drainage for several days.

With large, sterile subdural effusions, some believe that all available fluid should be removed from each side with every tap, while others prefer to restrict the amount aspirated if the volume is greater than 50 ml. In most instances, the total volume from both sides is not greater than 50 to 60 ml., and under these circumstances all available fluid should be removed. The fluid should be permitted to drip freely and not aspirated by applying suction with a syringe. It should be appreciated that when the infant is in the supine position and the needle is inserted at the level of the coronal suture, subdural fluid below that level will not be drained. Thus, "tapping until dry" is not synonymous with complete removal of all fluid from the subdural space.

After a few taps at daily intervals, most become dry and no further procedures are required. When the volume is less than 5 ml., the taps should be discontinued because small quantities of fluid in the subdural space should have no adverse effect on the brain.

The problem of persisting subdural effusions in large volume after multiple daily taps remains the area of greatest controversy in regard to management. Craniotomy and membrane stripping have been done in such cases, although the benefits from this procedure remain unclear and it is now rarely performed. The need for this operation has been based largely on the postulate that adherent membranes formed in association with subdural effusions would restrict continued growth of the brain unless removed. This has remained unproven; however, in the cases studied by Benson et al., those patients in whom membranes were present and were excised did better than those with membranes but not treated surgically. The ultimate fate of membranes not surgically excised is unclear but it is believed that they gradually resolve.

Subdural effusions which do not diminish in volume after multiple subdural taps are sometimes encountered in infants who have experienced severe and diffuse cerebral injury from vasculitis and other effects of acute meningitis. The resulting decrease in cerebral volume which represents cerebral atrophy indicates that a fluid-filled space must exist between the cerebral convexity and the under surface of the skull, unless the skull actually contracts leading to overriding sutures. In such cases, one finds it is not possible to diminish the amount of subdural fluid by periodic subdural taps, but if taps are not done, the persisting effusions do not continue to increase in size and do not give rise to pressure signs, such as tenseness of the anterior fontanel. In this instance, persistent fluid collection in the subdural space is to be expected until either the skull contracts or the brain itself enlarges. No further treatment need be directed toward the fluid collection, but periodic head circumference measurements and periodic computed tomograms would be indicated to be certain that the fluid collections remain stable or gradually diminish.

The generally accepted approach of surgical removal of membranes prevalent two to three decades ago has been largely replaced by more conservative methods (Goodman and Mealey), and such procedures are now rarely, if ever, indicated. In cases with effusions that do not resolve with repeated taps and continue to enlarge in volume or result in pressure signs, a subdural-peritoneal shunt is usually performed (Moyes et al.), although some prefer subdural-pleural shunts for this purpose (Arsalo et al.).

Mortality and Sequelae

Mortality, complications, and sequelae of *Hemophilus influenzae* meningitis have progressively changed with improved methods of treatment. Prior to the introduction of anti-influenzal rabbit antiserum by Alexander in 1939, the case fatality rate from this form of meningitis was estimated to be 90 to 95 percent. Current estimates place the mortality rate at approximately 5 to 10 percent, although there are recent reports of series of cases of *Hemophilus influenzae* meningitis with mortality rates as low as 1.6 percent (Peter and Smith) and 3.5 percent (McGowan et al.). A high percentage of deaths that occur with this disease do so within the first 24 to 36 hours of hospital admission. Younger infants with influenzal meningitis have a higher mortality rate than those over one year of age (Crook et al.). Prognostic signs considered to predict a possible bad outcome of the illness include coma or hypothermia at the time of admission, repetitive seizures before or soon after hospital admission, and an acute episode of shock in the early stages of the disease (Herson and Todd). Prolonged antigenemia or persistence of antigen in CSF as determined by counterimmunoelectrophoresis has been found to correlate with duration of fever and frequency of sequelae (Feigin et al. 1976, Shackelford et al.).

Survivors of this illness may appear entirely normal or can be left with residual sequelae ranging from very mild deficits to severe and incapacitating abnormalities. Hearing loss, facial nerve or other cranial nerve deficits, mental retardation, hydrocephalus, seizures, hyperactive behavior, optic atrophy and motor disturbances in variable combinations remain in some patients (Fig. 4–4). Deafness is one of the most common disabilities complicating *Hemophilus influenzae* meningitis. Subarachnoid exudate in meningitis is believed to extend through the internal auditory canal to the inner ear, resulting in pathologic changes in the labyrinthine structures as well as the divisions of the eighth nerve (Crowe). Auditory impairment occurred in 18 percent

of the 82 survivors evaluated by Lindberg et al. The incidence of hearing loss has been reported by some investigators to be higher among children treated with ampicillin or ampicillin in combination with chloramphenicol as compared to chloramphenicol alone (Gamstorp and Klockhoff), but this has not been confirmed in other studies (Jones and Hanson, Lindberg et al.).

Permanent visual loss can result from damage to the anterior visual pathways and rarely from ocular damage with endophthalmitis or orbital cellulitis. Cortical blindness following meningitis is infrequent but can represent the only manifestation of cerebral injury (Margolis et al., Tepperberg et al.). The pathogenesis of post-meningitic cortical visual loss is presumed to be on the basis of occipital lobe infarction secondary to arterial or venous inflammatory obstruction or the result of posterior cerebral artery compression from transtentorial herniation.

The incidence of such devastating sequelae from *Hemophilus influenzae* meningitis is difficult to judge from the available literature. Bloor et al. reported in 1950 the follow-up findings in 44 children who had influenzal meningitis. Forty-three percent of patients had minimal neurologic abnormalities and 21 percent had major neurologic deficits on examination. Sproles and colleagues examined a series of 40 cases with influenzal meningitis, all treated subsequent to the introduction of chloramphenicol. Mortality rate was 17.5 percent and another 10 percent were seriously handicapped. An additional 27.5 percent had significant neurologic deficits while 45 percent appeared to have recovered without sequelae. Sell et al. studied 86 patients with *Hemophilus influenzae* meningitis which had been treated between 1950 and 1964. The majority of the children (60 of 86) had meningitis in the first year of life, and of the total group, 11 (12.7 percent) had died. Eight of the deaths occurred within 24 hours of hospitalization, and in five of the fatal cases the time between onset of clinical signs of meningitis and death was less than 48 hours. Among survivors in this series, 29 percent had serious or significant neurologic handicaps. Mild residual deficits were found in 14 percent of survivors and 43 percent were judged free of detectable abnormalities. In a more recent study, Herson and Todd (1977) found that 22 percent of a series of 71 survivors of *Hemophilus influenzae* meningitis had sequelae, which ranged from mild to severe.

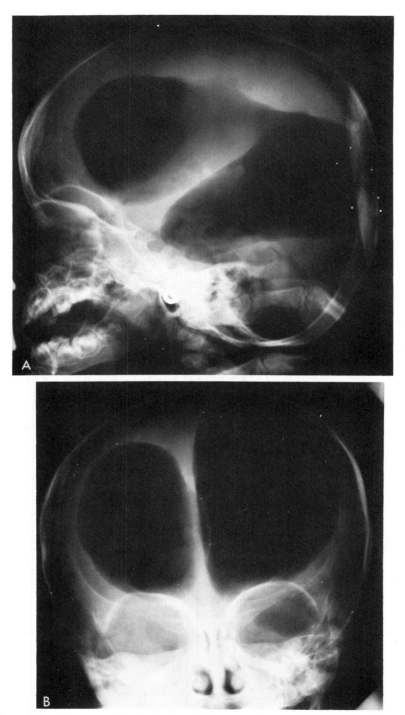

Figure 4–4.   Post-meningitic communicating hydrocephalus. *A* and *B,* Lateral and anteroposterior views of a ventriculogram in a 12-month-old child demonstrate severe hydrocephalus. The child was well until 9 months of age when he developed *Hemophilus influenzae* meningitis. The infant had symptoms of meningitis for 10 days before the diagnosis was established and proper treatment begun. Although the infection was successfully overcome, the child was left with a spastic quadriparesis, blindness, and hydrocephalus, which required a shunt procedure.

Treatment

Treatment of *Hemophilus influenzae* meningitis, as in other types of acute suppurative meningitis in infants and children, requires intravenous antibiotics as well as constant attention to supportive measures. Marked hyperthermia should be prevented and adequate ventilation is mandatory to prevent hypercapnia and hypoxia, which can precipitously lead to internal herniation. Intermittent intravenous doses of mannitol are sometimes indicated when intracranial hypertension is believed to be contributing to the child's downhill course and when increased pressure is not the result of subdural fluid collections. Because of the high frequency of occurrence of inappropriate antidiuretic hormone secretion in the early stages of the illness (Feigin et al. 1976), fluid intake should be restricted to 65 to 70 percent of maintenance needs for the first 48 to 72 hours unless the child is significantly dehydrated or in shock at the time of hospital admission. The presence of shock requires immediate expansion of the blood volume by appropriate means if the child is to survive.

Ampicillin was introduced in 1961 and within a short time it became the drug of choice for treatment of *Hemophilus influenzae* meningitis (Thrupp et al. 1964). The drug was shown to have adequate penetration into the CSF in the presence of inflamed meninges (Barrett et al. 1966, Lithander), with CSF-serum ratios being highest in the first three days of treatment but declining to relatively low levels by 10 days after onset of therapy (Taber et al., Thrupp et al. 1966). Ampicillin and chloramphenicol were found to be equally effective for treatment of *Hemophilus influenzae* meningitis (Barrett et al. 1972, Nelson et al., Schulkind et al.), but the former drug was clearly preferable for the initial treatment of acute meningitis in children over two months of age because of its greater effectiveness against *Streptococcus pneumoniae* and *Neisseria meningitidis*. Disc plate methods of determining antibiotic sensitivities were recognized not to be entirely reliable for *Hemophilus influenzae* (McLinn et al.) but for many years it was found that all isolates were sensitive to ampicillin when properly tested (Yow). Despite the in vitro sensitivity of the organism to ampicillin, a number of cases of meningitis were reported between 1965 and 1972 with treatment failure or relapse of infection, most of which were explained on the basis of insufficient dosage or duration of therapy (Cherry and Sheenan, Coleman et al., Gold et al., Greene, Haltalin and Smith, Kandall et al., Levine et al., Sanders and Garbee, Saxena and Maas, Young et al.).

In December, 1973 the first isolates of ampicillin-resistant *Hemophilus influenzae* in this country were recovered from a child with meningitis in Maryland and from a second in Georgia (Morbidity and Mortality Weekly Report Vol. 23, March 2, 1974) although a previous resistant isolate had been found in Germany in 1972 (Gunn et al.). Soon thereafter, there were additional reports of ampicillin-resistant type b organisms (Morbidity and Mortality Weekly Report, Vol. 23, March 16, June 8, 1974, Turk), and such strains gradually became more prevalent in different parts of the country. The incidence of ampicillin-resistant *Hemophilus influenzae* has shown a step-wise increase in recent years and varies considerably in different geographic regions. Approximately 5 percent of isolates nationwide are now believed to be resistant to ampicillin, although much higher estimates are claimed in certain communities. The highest prevalence of resistant organisms has come from patients with meningitis and bacteremia and the lowest from those with infections of the respiratory tract (Jacobson et al.). In addition, it is possible that a mixed population of bacteria can occur in CSF, composed of both ampicillin-sensitive and ampicillin-resistant organisms (Jubelirer and Yeager). This could conceivably lead to misinterpretation of either the Kirby-Bauer disc method or the β-lactamase determination and result in ampicillin treatment failure of meningitis which is assumed to be caused by ampicillin-sensitive *Hemophilus influenzae*.

Ampicillin resistance is the result of the production of β-lactamase by the resistant strains (Khan et al.), the production of the enzyme being mediated by genes located on a plasmid (Elwell et al., Sykes et al.). The enzyme rapidly hydrolyzes the β-lactam ring of penicillin and closely resembles the β-lactamase produced by enteric bacilli. Reliable laboratory methods have been developed for the rapid determination of the presence of the enzyme, thus predicting from in vitro studies the organism's resistance to ampicillin (Scheifele et al., Thornsberry and Kirven). On rare occasion, ampicillin-resistant strains of *Hemophilus influenzae* have been found which are non-β-lactamase-producing (Markowitz). The mechanism of resistance in these isolates is not understood to the present date.

As a result of the emergence of ampicillin-resistant organisms, it is now recommended that ampicillin and chloramphenicol in combination should be the initial treatment of acute meningitis in the child over two months of age yet to be diagnosed etiologically or for the child with *Hemophilus influenzae* meningitis. Ampicillin is administered intravenously in a dosage of 300 to 400 mg. per kilogram per day and is given every four hours over a 20-minute period of time. Lower doses of ampicillin, in the range of 150 mg. per kilogram per day, are recommended by certain authors, who point out that the great majority of ampicillin-sensitive strains of *Hemophilus influenzae* are killed at concentrations of ampicillin of less than 0.8 μg per ml., a level easily exceeded in the CSF (Greene et al.). The dosage of chloramphenicol is 100 mg. per kilogram per day given every six hours. If laboratory tests prove that the organism is a non-β-lactamase former or otherwise demonstrate the organism to be sensitive to ampicillin, chloramphenicol is discontinued and ampicillin is used for the remainder of the treatment regimen. If studies reveal the isolate to be β-lactamase-positive, or ampicillin-resistant, chloramphenicol is continued as the single drug. Chloramphenicol in concentrations that can be achieved in CSF is bactericidal for *Hemophilus influenzae* and, to this date, only a few examples of chloramphenicol-resistant *Hemophilus influenzae* have been found (Long and Phillips, Morbidity and Mortality Weekly Report, Vol. 25, Aug. 27, 1976, van Klingeren et al.). Antibiotic treatment should be continued for 12 to 14 days and is preferably given by the intravenous route from beginning to the end of the regimen.

The child with *Hemophilus influenzae* meningitis who becomes severely neutropenic from chloramphenicol as well as the future prospect of an increasing prevalence of organisms resistant to both ampicillin and chloramphenicol pose a major problem in regard to antibiotic therapy. Streptomycin intramuscularly and intrathecally in combination with sulfisoxazole represents one alternative for such cases (Barkin et al., Meade). Trimethoprim-sulfamethoxazole has been found to be effective against *Hemophilus influenzae* and has excellent CSF penetration (Pelton et al., Perfect et al.), but the lack of an available intravenous preparation is considered to be a disadvantage for treatment of meningitis. Tetracycline has received consideration although resistant strains of *Hemoph-*

ilus influenzae are not rare (Hansman). The mottling of teeth and deposition of the antimicrobial in bones are major distractions to its use in infants and small children. Rifampin, gentamicin, and erythromycin have also been shown to be effective against this organism (Emerson et al.) but resistance to rifampin is believed to develop rapidly, while gentamicin and erythromycin gain entrance from the serum into CSF quite poorly.

Because of the vital importance of the accuracy of the antimicrobial sensitivity determinations, the physician in practice who cannot be certain of the reliability of his available methods of sensitivity testing should probably depend upon chloramphenicol alone for treatment of meningitis proved to be caused by *Hemophilus influenzae*. When chloramphenicol is used, it is important to take into consideration the possible drug interaction between this antibiotic and phenobarbital or phenytoin, which are often administered to children with meningitis complicated by the occurrence of seizures. Phenobarbital can increase hepatic metabolism, resulting in a reduction of the serum chloramphenicol level (Bloxham), while chloramphenicol can interfere with biotransformation of phenytoin, resulting in an increase in its blood level and possible toxic effects (Rose et al.). When chloramphenicol is given to a patient receiving phenobarbital, a child with parenchymal liver disease, or an infant under two months of age, blood level determinations of the antibiotic are valuable to arrive at the dosage required to maintain the blood level within the therapeutic range.

The combination of ampicillin and chloramphenicol has obvious advantages for the treatment of the child with *Hemophilus influenzae* meningitis until the antimicrobial sensitivities of the organism are known. Studies have failed to show antagonism of this combination against *Hemophilus influenzae* (Ahronheim, Cole et al., Feldman); however, there is evidence to suggest that antagonism does occur between ampicillin and chloramphenicol with *Streptococcus pneumoniae* (Leeper and Dowling, Wallace) and with some strains of *Neisseria meningitidis* (Feldman and Zweighaft). For this reason, chloramphenicol should be stopped as soon as possible once the organism has been positively identified to be either the pneumococcus or the meningococcus.

During the course of treatment of children with *Hemophilus influenzae* meningitis, 20 to 30 percent will experience a recurrence of fever a few days into the regimen, and after fever had subsided on the second or third day of therapy (Balagtas et al., Lipiridou et al.). Relapse of fever has many possible causes but when the organism is sensitive to the antibiotic being used and when the dosage is appropriate, recurrence of fever is not usually found to be the result of unyielding or relapsing meningitis. Nonetheless, recurrent fever is usually an indication to re-examine a CSF specimen unless a cause is immediately found, and, on infrequent occasion, persistent infection or relapse of meningeal infection will be discovered (Feldman et al. 1976). More common explanations include otitis media, pneumonitis, an infected cutdown or intravenous infusion site, septic arthritis, infected subdural effusions, and a hospital-acquired secondary viral illness with a short incubation period. Drug fever is often considered and is more common with ampicillin than with chloramphenicol but is probably overestimated as a cause of fever. Infrequent sources of recurrent fever include pericarditis and brain abscess.

Even after 12 to 14 days of intravenous therapy, an occasional child will continue to have some degree of temperature elevation, which should not deter one from discontinuation of antibiotic therapy if no cause is found after a proper diagnostic search. It is also common that at the end of an adequate course of treatment for *Hemophilus influenzae* meningitis with a favorable clinical response, the CSF will show 50 to 100 white blood cells per cu. mm. (Chartrand and Cho, Jacob and Kaplan), the majority of which are lymphocytes. The persistence of cells in this magnitude likewise is not a contraindication to the termination of antibiotic treatment.

The desirability of prophylactic treatment of children less than five years of age who are household contacts of a patient with *Hemophilus influenzae* meningitis has become apparent as the result of recent observations, although Kline had recommended prophylaxis as early as 1962. Lerman et al. studied 1,084 healthy children four to seven years of age and found that nasopharyngeal cultures for nontypable *Hemophilus influenzae* were positive in 34.2 percent and were positive for type b organisms in 2 percent. Other investigators have found the nasopharyngeal carriage rate of type b organisms in healthy young children to be approximately 6 percent (Peltola et al.). Nasopharyngeal carriage of *Hemophilus influenzae* type b has been shown to increase dramatically among household contacts of an infected patient, and outbreaks of meningitis have been described among persons within an enclosed population (Glode et al., Ward et al. 1978). Ward et al. (1979) have calculated that the risk of severe illness in the next 30 days among household contacts of a patient with influenzal meningitis is 585 times greater than the age-adjusted risk in the general population. The risk, therefore, is almost as great as that of household contacts of a patient with meningococcal disease and would warrant antimicrobial prophylaxis for young children if a safe and consistently effective drug were available. Rifampin and trimethoprim-sulfamethoxazole by the oral route have each been proposed, although their degree of effectiveness remains to be established (Granoff et al., Yogev et al.).

Absolute recommendations for prophylactic therapy have not yet been established and until more information is available close medical surveillance of household contacts and of contacts in day-care centers is warranted and is acceptable in most instances. Progress continues in the development of an effective vaccine to curtail serious infection caused by *Hemophilus influenzae* (Smith et al.). The type b capsular polysaccharide vaccine has been found to be effective when administered to children over 18 months of age, but infants under 18 months—the period of greatest risk for meningitis—do not show an adequate antibody response to vaccination with this preparation (Peltola et al.).

REFERENCES

Adams, R. D., Kubik, C. S., and Bonner, F. J.: The clinical and pathological aspects of influenzal meningitis. Arch. Pediat. 65:354–376, 1948.

Adams, R. D., Kubik, C. S., and Bonner, F. J.: The clinical and pathological aspects of influenzal meningitis. Arch. Pediat. 65:408–441, 1948.

Ahronheim, G. A.: Hemophilus influenzae type b: Lack of in-vitro antagonism between penicillins and chloramphenicol. Pediat. Res. 9:337, 1975.

Alexander, H. E.: Type "B" anti-influenzal rabbit serum for therapeutic purposes. Proc. Soc. Exp. Biol. Med. 40:313–314, 1939.

Alexander, H. E.: The Hemophilus group. *In:* Dubos, R. J., and Hirsch, J. G., Bacterial and Mycotic Infections in Man, 4th Edition. J. B. Lippincott, Philadelphia, 1965.

Alexander, H. E., and Leidy, G.: The present status of treatment for influenzal meningitis. Am. J. Med. 2:457–466, 1947.

Alexander, H. E., Ellis, C., and Leidy, G.: Treatment of type-specific Hemophilus influenzae infections in infancy and childhood. J. Pediat. 20:673–698, 1942.

Appelbaum, E., and Nelson, J.: Streptomycin in the treatment of influenzal meningitis. A study of ninety cases, with 96.6 percent recovery. J.A.M.A. 143:715–717, 1950.

Arsalo, A., Louhimo, I., Santavuori, P., and Valtonen, S.: Subdural effusion: Results after treatment with subdural-pleural shunts. Child's Brain 3:79–86, 1977.

Bachman, D. S.: Hemophilus meningitis: Comparison of H. influenzae and H. parainfluenzae. Pediatrics 55:526–530, 1975.

Balagtas, R. C., Levin, S., Nelson, K. E., and Gotoff, S. P.: Secondary and prolonged fevers in bacterial meningitis. J. Pediat. 77:957–964, 1970.

Bale, J. F., Jr., and Watkins, M.: Fulminant neonatal Hemophilus influenzae pneumonia and sepsis. J. Pediat. 92:233–234, 1978.

Barkin, R. M., Greer, C. C., Schumacher, C. J., and McIntosh, K.: *Haemophilus influenzae* meningitis. An evolving therapeutic regimen. Am. J. Dis. Child. 130:1318–1321, 1976.

Barnshaw, J. A., and Phillips, C. F.: *Haemophilus parainfluenzae* meningitis in a 4-year-old boy. Pediatrics 45:856–857, 1970.

Barrett, F. F., Eardley, W. A., Yow, M. D., and Leverett, H. A.: Ampicillin in the treatment of acute suppurative meningitis. J. Pediat. 69:343–353, 1966.

Barrett, F. F., Taber, L. H., Morris, C. R., Stephenson, W. B., Clark, D. J., and Yow, M. D.: A 12 year review of the antibiotic management of *Hemophilus influenzae* meningitis. Comparison of ampicillin and conventional therapy including chloramphenicol. J. Pediat. 81:370–377, 1972.

Benson, P., Nyhan, W. L., and Shimizu, H.: The prognosis of subdural effusions complicating pyogenic meningitis. J. Pediat. 57:670–683, 1960.

Bloor, B. M., Grant, R. S., and Tabris, J. A.: Sequelae of meningitis due to Hemophilus influenzae. An analysis of forty-four cases. J.A.M.A. 142:241–243, 1950.

Bloxham, R. A., Durbin, G. M., Johnson, T., and Winterborn, M. H.: Chloramphenicol and phenobarbitone—a drug interaction. Arch. Dis. Childh. 54:76–77, 1979.

Branefors-Helander, P., and Jeppsson, P-H.: Acute epiglottitis. A clinical, bacteriological and serologic study. Scand. J. Infect. Dis. 7:103–111, 1975.

Brook, I., Bricknell, K. S., Overturf, G. D., and Finegold, S. M.: Measurement of lactic acid in cerebrospinal fluid of patients with infections of the central nervous system. J. Infect. Dis. 137:384–390, 1978.

Brunell, P. A., and Dodd, M. K.: Isolation of Herpesvirus hominum from the cerebrospinal fluid of a child with bacterial meningitis and gingivostomatitis. J. Pediat. 65:53–56, 1964.

Carabelle, R.W., Mitchell, D. D., and Salmon, G. W.: Influenzal meningitis treated with chloromycetin. A preliminary report. J. Pediat. 37:37–41, 1950.

Chartrand, S. A., and Cho, C. T.: Persistent pleocytosis in bacterial meningitis. J. Pediat. 88:424–426, 1976.

Cherry, J. D., and Sheenan, C. P.: Bacteriologic relapse in *Haemophilus influenzae* meningitis. Inadequate ampicillin therapy. New Eng. J. Med. 278:1001–1003, 1968.

Chilcote, R. R., Baehner, R. L., and Hammond, D.: Septicemia and meningitis in children splenectomized for Hodgkin's disease. New Eng. J. Med. 295:798–800, 1976.

Cole, F. S., Daum, R. S., Teller, L., Goldmann, D. A., and Smith, A. L.: Effect of ampicillin and chloramphenicol alone and in combination on ampicillin-susceptible and -resistant *Hemophilus influenzae* type

b. Antimicrob. Agents Chemother. 15:415–419, 1979.

Coleman, S. J., Auld, E. B., Connor, J. D., Rosenman, S. B., and Warren, G. H.: Relapse of *Hemophilus influenzae* type b meningitis during intravenous therapy with ampicillin. J. Pediat. 74:781–784, 1969.

Collier, A. M., Connor, J. D., and Nyhan, W. L.: Systemic infection with Hemophilus influenzae in very young infants. J. Pediat. 70:539–547, 1967.

Controni, G., Rodriquez, W. J., Hicks, J. M., Ficke, M., Ross, S., Friedman, G., and Khan, W.: Cerebrospinal fluid lactic acid levels in meningitis. J. Pediat. 91:379–384, 1977.

Crook, W. G., Clanton, B. R., and Hodes, H. L.: Hemophilus influenzae meningitis. Observations on the treatment of 110 cases. Pediatrics 4:643–659, 1949.

Crowe, S. J.: Pathologic changes in meningitis of the inner ear. Arch. Otolaryngol. 11:537–568, 1930.

Dajani, A. S., Asmar, B. I., and Thirumoorthi, M. C.: Systemic Haemophilus influenzae disease: An overview. J. Pediat. 94:355–364, 1979.

Davis, D. J.: Influenzae meningitis, with especial reference to its pathology and bacteriology. Am. J. Dis. Child. 1:249–265, 1911.

Denis, F. A., Chiron, J. P., Cadoz, M., and Mar, I. D.: Meningitis caused by Hemophilus influenzae type C. J. Pediat. 93:1064–1066, 1978.

Echeverria, P., Smith, E. W. P., Ingram, D., Sade, R. M., and Gardner, P.: Hemophilus influenzae b pericarditis in children. Pediatrics 56:808–818, 1975.

Edmonds, A. M., and Neter, E.: Appraisal of treatment of hemophilus influenzae type B meningitis with specific rabbit serum and sulfonamides. J. Pediat. 28:462–470, 1946.

Elwell, L. P., DeGraaff, J., Seibert, D., and Falkow, S.: Plasmid-linked ampicillin resistance in *Haemophilus influenzae* type b. Infect. Immun. 12:404–410, 1975.

Emerson, B. B., Smith, A. L., Harding, A. L., and Smith, D. H.: Hemophilus influenzae type b susceptibility to 17 antibiotics. J. Pediat. 86:617–620, 1975.

Eykyn, S. J., Thomas, R. D., and Phillips, I.: *Haemophilus influenzae* meningitis in adults. Brit. Med. J. 2:463–465, 1974.

Faber, H. K.: A case of tuberculous meningitis complicated by influenzal meningitis. Am. J. Dis. Child. 8:150–153, 1914.

Faden, H. S.: Treatment of Haemophilus influenzae type b epiglottitis. Pediatrics 63:402–407, 1979.

Feigin, R. D., Stechenberg, B. W., Chang, M. J., Dunkle, L. M., Wong, M. L., Palkes, H., Dodge, P. R., and Davis, H.: Prospective evaluation of treatment of Hemophilus influenzae meningitis. J. Pediat. 88:542–548, 1976.

Feldman, W. E.: Effect of ampicillin and chloramphenicol against Hemophilus influenzae. Pediatrics 61:406–409, 1978.

Feldman, W. E., and Zweighaft, T.: Effect of ampicillin and chloramphenicol against *Streptococcus pneumoniae* and *Neisseria meningitidis*. Antimicrob. Agents Chemother. 15:240–242, 1979.

Feldman, W. E., Laupus, W. E., and Ledaal, P.: Relapse of Hemophilus influenzae type b meningitis after combined antibiotic therapy: Report of a case. Pediatrics 57:387–391, 1976.

Floyd, R. F., Federspiel, C. F., and Schaffner, W.: Bacterial meningitis in urban and rural Tennessee. Am. J. Epidemiol. 99:395–407, 1974.

Fosson, A. R., and Fine, R. N.: Neonatal meningitis. Presentation and discussion of 21 cases. Clin. Pediat. 7:404–410, 1968.

Fothergill, L. D.: Hemophilus influenzae (Pfeiffer bacillus) meningitis and its specific treatment. New Eng. J. Med. 216:587–590, 1937.

Fothergill, L. D., and Wright, J.: Influenzal meningitis. The relation of age incidence to the bactericidal power of blood against the causal organism. J. Immunol. 24:273–284, 1933.

Fraser, D. W., Henke, C. E., and Feldman, R. A.: Changing patterns of bacterial meningitis in Olmsted County, Minnesota, 1935–1970. J. Infect. Dis. 128:300–307, 1973.

Gado, M., Axley, J., Appleton, D. B., and Prensky, A. L.: Angiography in the acute and post-treatment phases of Hemophilus influenzae meningitis. Radiology 110:439–444, 1973.

Gamstorp, I., and Klockhoff, I.: Bilateral severe, sensorineural hearing loss after Haemophilus influenzae meningitis in childhood. Neuropadiatrie. 5:121–124, 1974.

Gellady, A. M., Shulman, S. T., and Ayoub, E. M.: Periorbital and orbital cellulitis in children. Pediatrics 61:272–277, 1978.

Gitlin, D.: Pathogenesis of subdural collections of fluid. Pediatrics 16:345–351, 1955.

Glode, M. P., Schiffer, M. S., Robbins, J. B., Khan, W., Battle, C. V., and Armenta, E.: An outbreak of Hemophilus influenzae type b meningitis in an enclosed hospital population. J. Pediat. 88:36–40, 1976.

Gold, A. J., Lieberman, E., and Wright, H. T., Jr.: Bacteriologic relapse during ampicillin treatment of Hemophilus influenzae meningitis. J. Pediat. 74:779–781, 1969.

Goodman, J. M., and Mealey, J., Jr.: Postmeningitic subdural effusions: The syndrome and its management. J. Neurosurg. 30:658–663, 1969.

Graber, C. D., Gershanik, J. J., Levkoff, A. H., and Westphal, M.: Changing pattern of neonatal susceptibility to Hemophilus influenzae. J. Pediat. 78:948–950, 1971.

Granoff, D. M., and Nankervis, G. A.: Cellulitis due to Haemophilus influenzae type b. Antigenemia and antibody responses. Am. J. Dis. Child. 130:1211–1214, 1976.

Granoff, D. M., Sargent, E., and Jolivette, D.: Haemophilus influenzae type b osteomyelitis. Am. J. Dis. Child. 132:488–490, 1978.

Granoff, D. M., Gilsdorf, J., Gessert, C., and Basden, M.: Haemophilus influenzae type b disease in a day care center: Eradication of carrier state by rifampin. Pediatrics 63:397-401, 1979.

Gray, B. M.: Meningitis due to Hemophilus influenzae type f. J. Pediat. 90:1031, 1977.

Greene, G. R.: Meningitis due to Haemophilus influenzae other than type b: Case report and review. Pediatrics 62:1021–1025, 1978.

Greene, G. R., Overturf, G. D., and Wehrle, P. F.: Ampicillin dosage in bacterial meningitis with special reference to Haemophilus influenzae. Antimicrob. Agents Chemother. 16:198–202, 1979.

Greene, H. L.: Failure of ampicillin in meningitis. Lancet 1:861, 1976.

Groover, R. V., Sutherland, J. M., and Landing, B. H.: Purulent meningitis of newborn infants. Eleven-year experience in the antibiotic era. New Eng. J. Med. 264:1115–1121, 1961.

Gullekson, E. H., and Dumoff, M.: Haemophilus parainfluenzae meningitis in a newborn. J.A.M.A. 198:1221, 1966.

Gunn, B. A., Woodall, J. B., Jones, J. F., and Thornsberry, C.: Ampicillin resistant Haemophilus influenzae. Lancet 2:845, 1974.

Hable, K. A., Logan, G. B., and Washington, J. A.: Three Hemophilus species. Pathogenic activity. Am. J. Dis. Child. 121:35–37, 1971.

Haltalin, K. C., and Smith, J. B.: Reevaluation of ampicillin therapy for Hemophilus influenzae meningitis. An appraisal based on a review of cases of persistent or recurrent infection. Am. J. Dis. Child. 122:328–336, 1971.

Hansman, D.: Haemophilus influenzae type b resistant to tetracycline. Isolated from children with meningitis. Lancet 2:893–896, 1975.

Herson, V. C., and Todd, J. K.: Prediction of morbidity in Hemophilus influenzae meningitis. Pediatrics 59:35–39, 1977.

Hirschmann, J. V., and Everett, E. D.: Haemophilus influenzae infections in adults: Report of nine cases and a review of the literature. Medicine 58:80–94, 1979.

Hodes, D. S., and Leidy, G.: Meningitis caused by Hemophilus influenzae type e. J. Pediat. 91:844–845, 1977.

Holt, R. N., Taylor, C. D., Schneider, H. J., and Hallock, J. A.: Three cases of Hemophilus parainfluenzae meningitis. Clin. Pediat. 13:666–668, 1974.

Ingram, D. L.: The epidemiology of meningitis in children. Pediatrics 52:586–588, 1973.

Jacob, J., and Kaplan, R. A.: Bacterial meningitis. Limitations of repeated lumbar punctures. Am. J. Dis. Child. 131:46–48, 1977.

Jacobs, N. M., and Harris, V. J.: Acute Haemophilus pneumonia in childhood. Am. J. Dis. Child. 133:603–605, 1979.

Jacobson, J. A., McCormick, J. B., Hayes, P., Thornsberry, C., and Kirvin, L.: Epidemiologic characteristics of infections caused by ampicillin-resistant Hemophilus influenzae. Pediatrics 58:388–391, 1976.

James, A. E., Jr., Hodges, F. J., III, Jordan, C. E., Mathews, E. H., and Heller, R., Jr.: Angiography and cisternography in acute meningitis due to Hemophilus influenzae. Radiology 103:601–605, 1972.

Jervey, L. P.: Adult influenzal meningitis. A report of four cases and review of the recent literature. Arch. Intern. Med. 111:376–383, 1963.

Johnstone, J. M., and Lawy, H. S.: Acute epiglottitis in adults due to infection with Haemophilus influenzae type b. Lancet 2:134–136, 1967.

Jones, F. E., and Hanson, D. R.: H. influenzae meningitis treated with ampicillin or chloramphenicol, and subsequent hearing loss. Develop. Med. Child. Neurol. 19:593–597, 1977.

Jubelirer, D. P., and Yeager, A. S.: Simultaneous recovery of ampicillin-sensitive and ampicillin-resistant organisms in Haemophilus influenzae type b meningitis. J. Pediat. 95:415–416, 1979.

Kandall, S. R., Davis, T. C., and Abramowicz, M.: Ampicillin failure in H. influenzae meningitis. A case report with added commentaries. Clin. Pediat. 11:264–267, 1972.

Kaufman, S. R., Hambly, F., Dyke, J. W., and Gordon, R. C.: Hemophilus parainfluenzae meningitis. Report of two cases. Clin. Pediat. 13:661–663, 1974.

Khan, W., Ross, S., Rodriquez, W., Controni, G., and Saz, A. K.: Haemophilus influenzae type b resistant to ampicillin. A report of two cases. J.A.M.A. 229:298–301, 1974.

Khuri-Bulos, N., and McIntosh, K.: Neonatal Haemophi-

lus influenzae infection. Report of eight cases and review of the literature. Am. J. Dis. Child. 129:57–62, 1975.

Kline, A. H.: Hemophilus influenzae meningitis. Is prophylaxis indicated? Am. J. Dis. Child. 104:595–597, 1962.

Koch, R., and Carson, M. J.: Management of Hemophilus influenzae, type B, meningitis. Analysis of 128 cases. J. Pediat. 46:18–29, 1955.

Laird, W. P., Nelson, J. D., and Huffines, F. D.: The frequency of pericardial effusions in bacterial meningitis. Pediatrics 63:764–770, 1979.

Leeper, M. H., and Dowling, H. F.: Treatment of pneumococcic meningitis with penicillin compared with penicillin plus aureomycin. Arch. Intern. Med. 88:489–494, 1951.

Lerman, S. J., Kucera, J. C., and Brunken, J. M.: Nasopharyngeal carriage of antibiotic-resistant Haemophilus influenzae in healthy children. Pediatrics 64:287–291, 1979.

Levin, D. C., Schwarz, M. I., Matthay, R. A., and LaForce, F. M.: Bacteremic Hemophilus influenzae pneumonia in adults. A report of 24 cases and a review of the literature. Am. J. Med. 62:219–224, 1977.

Levine, M. S., Boxerbaum, B., and Heggie, A. D.: Recrudescence of H. influenzae meningitis after therapy with ampicillin. Late recurrence may result from diminishing levels of ampicillin in the cerebrospinal fluid secondary to decreasing meningeal permeability and too early reduction in dose. Clin. Pediat. 9:54–57, 1970.

Lilien, L. D., Yeh, T. F., Novak, G. M., and Jacobs, N. M.: Early-onset Haemophilus sepsis in newborn infants: Clinical, roentgenographic, and pathologic features. Pediatrics 62:299–303, 1978.

Lindberg, J., Rosenhall, V., Nylen, O., and Ringner, A.: Long-term outcome of Hemophilus influenzae meningitis related to antibiotic treatment. Pediatrics 60:1–6, 1977.

Lindsay, J. W., Rice, E. C., Selinger, M. A., and Robins, L.: The Waterhouse-Friderichsen syndrome. Acute bilateral suprarenal hemorrhage. Am. J. Med. Sci. 201:263–270, 1941.

Lipiridou, O., Lazaridou, S., and Manios, S.: Recurrent and persistent fever in bacterial meningitis with adequate response to antimicrobial therapy. Scand. J. Infect. Dis. 5:23–27, 1973.

Lithander, A.: Ampicillin therapy in experimental *Haemophilus influenzae* meningitis in the rabbit. Acta Path. Microbiol. Scand. 64:335–338, 1965.

Lithander, A.: The passage of parenteral ampicillin to the cerebrospinal fluid in *Haemophilus influenzae* meningitis. Acta. Path. Microbiol. Scand. 64:329–334, 1964.

Logan, G. B., and Herrell, W. E.: Streptomycin in the treatment of influenzal meningitis of children. Mayo Clin. Proc. 21:393–400, 1946.

Long, S. S., and Phillips, S. E.: Chloramphenicol-resistant Hemophilus influenzae. J. Pediat. 90:1030–1046, 1977.

Margolis, L. H., Shaywitz, B. A., and Rothman, S. G.: Cortical blindness associated with occipital atrophy: A complication of H. influenzae meningitis. Develop. Med. Child Neurol. 20:490–493, 1978.

Markowitz, S. M.: Isolation of an ampicillin-resistant, non-β-lactamase-producing strain of *Haemophilus influenzae*. Antimicrob. Agents Chemother. 17:80–83, 1980.

Marshall, R., Teele, D. W., and Klein, J. O.: Unsuspected

bacteremia due to Haemophilus influenzae: Outcome in children not initially admitted to hospital. J. Pediat. 95:690–695, 1979.

McGowan, J. E., Jr., Klein, J. O., Bratton, L., Barnes, M. W., and Finland, M.: Meningitis and bacteremia due to *Haemophilus influenzae*: Occurrence and mortality at Boston City Hospital in 12 selected years, 1935–1972. J. Infect. Dis. 130:119–124, 1974.

McKay, R. J., Jr., Morissette, R. A., Ingraham, F. D., and Matson, D. D.: Collections of subdural fluid complicating meningitis due to *Haemophilus influenzae* (type B). A preliminary report. New Eng. J. Med. 242:20–21, 1950.

McLinn, S. E., Nelson, J. D., and Haltalin, K. C.: Antimicrobial susceptibility of Hemophilus influenzae. Pediatrics 45:827–838, 1970.

Meade, R. H., III: Streptomycin and sulfisoxazole for treatment of Haemophilus influenzae meningitis. J.A.M.A. 239:324–327, 1978.

Merselis, J. G., Jr., Sellers, T. F., Jr., Johnson, J. E., III., and Hook, E. W.: Hemophilus influenzae meningitis in adults. Arch. Intern. Med. 110:837–846, 1962.

Michaels, R. H.: Increase in influenzal meningitis. New Eng. J. Med. 285:666–667, 1971.

Michaels, R. H., Myerowitz, R. L., and Klaw, R.: Potentiation of experimental meningitis due to *Haemophilus influenzae* by influenza A virus. J. Infect. Dis. 135:641–645, 1977.

Molteni, R. A.: Epiglottitis: Incidence of extraepiglottic infection. Report of 72 cases and review of the literature. Pediatrics 58:526–531, 1976.

Moore, C. M., and Ross, M.: Acute bacterial meningitis with absent or minimal cerebrospinal fluid abnormalities. Clin. Pediat. 12:117–118, 1973.

Morbidity and Mortality Weekly Report. Vol. 23, 2 March, 16 March, 8 June, 1974.

Morbidity and Mortality Weekly Report. Vol. 25, Aug. 27, 1976.

Mortimer, E. A., Jr.: Immunization against *Hemophilus influenzae*. Pediatrics 52:633–635, 1973.

Moyes, P. D., Thompson, G. B., and Cluff, J. W.: Subdural peritoneal shunts in the treatment of subdural effusions in infants. J. Neurosurg. 23:584–587, 1965.

Neal, J. B., Jackson, H. W., and Appelbaum, E.: Meningitis due to the influenza bacillus of Pfeiffer (Hemophilus influenzae). A study of one hundred and eleven cases, with four recoveries. J.A.M.A. 102:513–518, 1934.

Nelson, J. D., and Ginsburg, C. M.: An hypothesis on the pathogenesis of Hemophilus influenzae buccal cellulitis. J. Pediat. 88:709–710, 1976.

Nelson, K. E., Levin, S., Spies, H. W., and Lepper, M. H.: Treatment of *Hemophilus influenzae* meningitis: A comparison of chloramphenicol and tetracycline. J. Infect. Dis. 125:459–465, 1972.

Neter, E.: Observations on Hemophilus influenzae (Type B) meningitis of children. J. Pediat. 20:699–706, 1942.

Nixon, D. W., and Aisenberg, A. C.: Fatal *Hemophilus influenzae* sepsis in an asymptomatic splenectomized Hodgkin's disease patient. Ann. Intern. Med. 77:69–71, 1972.

Norden, C. W.: Prevalence of bactericidal antibodies to *Haemophilus* influenzae, type b. J. Infect. Dis. 130:489–494, 1974.

Norden, C. W., Callerame, M. L., and Baum, J.: Haemophilus influenzae meningitis in an adult. A study of bactericidal antibodies and immuno-globulins. New Eng. J. Med. 282:190–194, 1970.

Parke, J. C., Jr., Schneerson, R., and Robbins, J. B.: The attack rate, age incidence, racial distribution, and case fatality rate of Hemophilus influenzae type b meningitis in Mecklenburg County, North Carolina. J. Pediat. 81:765–769, 1972.

Peltola, H., Kayhty, H., Sivonen, A., and Makela, P. H.: Haemophilus influenzae type b capsular polysaccharide vaccine in children: A double-blind field study of 100,000 vaccines 3 months to 5 years of age in Finland. Pediatrics 60:730–737, 1977.

Pelton, S. I., Shurin, P. A., Klein, J. O., and Finland, M.: Quantitative inhibition of Haemophilus influenzae by trimethoprim-sulfamethoxazole. Antimicrob. Agents Chemother. 12:649–654, 1977.

Perfect, J. R., Lang, S. D. R., and Durack, D. T.: Comparison of cotrimoxazole, ampicillin, and chloramphenicol in treatment of experimental Haemophilus influenzae type b meningitis. Antimicrob. Agents Chemother. 17:43–46, 1980.

Peter, G., and Smith, D. H.: Hemophilus influenzae meningitis at the Children's Hospital Medical Center in Boston, 1958 to 1973. Pediatrics 55:523–525, 1975.

Pfeiffer, R.: Vorlaufige mittheilungen uber die erreger der influenza. Deutsch. Med. Wchnschr. 18:28, 1892.

Pittman, M.: Variation and type specificity in bacterial species hemophilus influenzae. J. Exper. Med. 53:471–492, 1931.

Prather, G. W., and Smith, M. H. D.: Chloramphenicol in the treatment of Hemophilus influenzae meningitis. J.A.M.A. 143:1405–1406, 1950.

Rabe, E. F.: Subdural effusions in infants. Pediat. Clin. N. Amer. 14:821–850, 1967.

Rapkin, R. H., and Bautista, G.: Hemophilus influenzae cellulitis. Am. J. Dis. Child. 124:540–542, 1972.

Rivers, T. M.: Influenzal meningitis. Am. J. Dis. Child. 24:102–124, 1922.

Rose, J. Q., Choi, H. K., Schentag, J. J., Kinkel, W. R., and Jusko, W. J.: Intoxication caused by interaction of chloramphenicol and phenytoin. J.A.M.A. 237:2630–2631, 1977.

Ross, S., Rice, E. C., Burke, F. G., McGovern, J. J., Parrott, R. H., and McGovern, J. P.: Treatment of meningitis due to Haemophilus influenzae. Use of chloromycetin and sulfadiazine. New Eng. J. Med. 247:541–547, 1952.

Sako, W., Stewart, C. A., and Fleet, J.: Treatment of influenzal meningitis with sulfadiazine. Further report. J. Pediat. 25:114–126, 1944.

Sanders, D. Y., and Garbee, H. W.: Failure of response to ampicillin in Hemophilus influenzae meningitis. Am. J. Dis. Child. 117:331–333, 1969.

Sastry, R. V., and Baker, C. J.: Endophthalmitis associated with Haemophilus influenzae type b bacteremia and meningitis. Am. J. Dis. Child. 133:606–608, 1979.

Saxena, K. M., and Maas, D.: Relapse of meningitis after ampicillin therapy. Minn. Med. 55:93–96, 1972.

Scheifele, D. W., Syriopoulou, V. P., Harding, A. L., Emerson, B. B., and Smith, A. L.: Evaluation of a rapid β-lactamase test for detecting ampicillin-resistant strains of Hemophilus influenzae type b. Pediatrics 58:382–387, 1976.

Schulkind, M. L., Altemeier, W. A., III., and Ayoub, E. M.: A comparison of ampicillin and chloramphenicol therapy in Hemophilus influenzae meningitis. Pediatrics 48:411–416, 1971.

Scott, J. R., and Walcher, D. N.: Intravenous chloramphenicol in the treatment of meningitis due to He-

mophilus influenzae (type B). J. Pediat. 41:442–444, 1952.

Sell, S. H. W., Merrill, R. E., Doyne, E. O., and Zimsky, E. P., Jr.: Long-term sequelae of Hemophilus influenzae meningitis. Pediatrics 49:206–211, 1972.

Shackelford, P. G., Campbell, J., and Feigin, R. D.: Countercurrent immunoelectrophoresis in the evaluation of childhood infections. J. Pediat. 85:478–481, 1974.

Slawyk, E.: Ein fall von allgemeininfection mit Influenzabacillen. Ztsch. f. Hyg. 32:443–448, 1899.

Smith, D. H., and Peter, G.: Current and future vaccines for the prevention of bacterial diseases. Pediat. Clin. N. Amer. 18:387–412, 1972.

Smith, D. H., Peter, G., Ingram, D. L., Harding, A. L., and Anderson, P.: Responses of children immunized with the capsular polysaccharide of Hemophilus influenzae, type b. Pediatrics 52:637–644, 1973.

Smith, E. W. P., Jr., and Haynes, R. E.: Changing incidence of Hemophilus influenzae meningitis. Pediatrics 50:723–727, 1972.

Smith, J. F., and Landing, B. H.: Mechanisms of brain damage in H. influenzae meningitis. J. Neuropath. Exper. Neurol. 19:248–265, 1960.

Smith, M. H. D., Dormont, R. E., and Prather, G. W.: Subdural effusions complicating bacterial meningitis. Pediatrics 7:34–43, 1951.

Smith, M. H. D., Wilson, P. E., and Hodes, H. L.: The treatment of influenzal meningitis. J.A.M.A. 130:331–335, 1946.

Smith, T. F., O'Day, D., and Wright, P. F.: Clinical implications of preseptal (periorbital) cellulitis in childhood. Pediatrics 62:1006–1009, 1978.

Sproles, E. T., III., Azerrad, J., Williamson, C., and Merrill, R. E.: Meningitis due to Hemophilus influenzae: Long-term sequelae. J. Pediat. 75:782–788, 1969.

Stein, J. A., and DeRossi, R., and Neu, H. C.: Adult Hemophilus influenzae meningitis. A report of nine cases. N.Y. J. Med. 69:1760–1766, 1969.

Sykes, R. B., Matthew, M., and O'Callaghan, C. H.: R-factor mediated β-lactamase production by Hemophilus influenzae. J. Med. Microbiol. 8:437–441, 1975.

Taber, L. H., Yow, M. D., and Nieberg, F. G.: The penetration of broad-spectrum antibiotics into the cerebrospinal fluid. Ann. N.Y. Acad. Sci. 145:473–481, 1967.

Tarr, P. I., and Peter, G.: Demographic factors in the epidemiology of Hemophilus influenzae meningitis in young children. J. Pediat. 92:884–888, 1978.

Tepperberg, J., Nussbaum, E., and Feldman, F.: Cortical blindness following meningitis due to Hemophilus influenzae type b. J. Pediat. 91:434–436, 1977.

Thomas, V. H., and Hopkins, I. J.: Arteriographic demonstration of vascular lesions in the study of neurologic deficit in advanced Haemophilus influenzae meningitis. Develop. Med. Child. Neurol. 14:783–787, 1972.

Thornsberry, C., and Kirven, L. A.: Ampicillin resistance in Haemophilus influenzae as determined by a rapid test for beta-lactamase production. Antimicrob. Agents Chemother. 6:653–654, 1974.

Thrupp, L. D., Leedom, J. M., Ivler, D., Wehrle, P. F., Brown, J. F., Mathies, A. W., and Portnoy, B.: H. influenzae meningitis: A controlled study of treatment with ampicillin. Postgrad. Med. J. 40:(Suppl). 119–126, 1964.

Thrupp, L. D., Leedom, J. M., Ivler, D., Wehrle, P. F., Portnoy, B., and Mathies, A. W.: Ampicillin levels in the cerebrospinal fluid during treatment of bacterial meningitis. Antimicrob. Agents Chemother. 195:206–213, 1966.

Todd, J. K., and Bruhn, F. W.: Severe *Haemophilus influenzae* infections. Spectrum of disease. Am. J. Dis. Child. 129:607–611, 1975.

Trackler, R. T., Miller, K. E., and Cohen, M. L.: The "doughnut sign" in subdural effusion. Am. J. Dis. Child. 129:373–374, 1975.

Turk, D. C.: Ampicillin-resistant Haemophilus influenzae meningitis. Lancet 1:453, 1974.

Vaden, E. B., Rice, E. C., and Stadnichenko, V.: Meningitis due to simultaneous double infections in children. J.A.M.A. 143:1402–1404, 1950.

van Klingeren, B., van Embden, J. D. A., and Dessens-Kroon, M.: Plasmid-mediated chloramphenicol resistance in *Haemophilus* influenzae. Antimicrob. Agents Chemother. 11:383–387, 1977.

Waldman, J. D., Rosenthal, A., Smith, A. L., Shurin, S., and Nadas, A. S.: Sepsis and congenital asplenia. J. Pediat. 90:555–559, 1977.

Wallace, J. F., Smith, R. H., Garcia, M., and Petersdorf, R. G.: Studies on the pathogenesis of meningitis. VI. Antagonism between penicillin and chloramphenicol in experimental pneumococcal meningitis. J. Lab. Clin. Med. 70:408–418, 1967.

Ward, H. K., and Fothergill, L. D.: Influenzal meningitis treated with specific antiserum and complement. Report of five cases. Am. J. Dis. Child. 43:873–881, 1932.

Ward, J. I., Fraser, D. W., Baraff, L. J., and Plikaytis, B. D.: Haemophilus influenzae meningitis. A national study of secondary spread in household contacts. New Eng. J. Med. 301:122–126, 1979.

Ward, J. I., Gorman, G., Phillips, C., and Fraser, D. W.: Hemophilus influenzae type b disease in a day-care center. Report of an outbreak. J. Pediat. 92:713–717, 1978.

Ward, J. I., Siber, G. R., Scheifele, D. W., and Smith, D. H.: Rapid diagnosis of Hemophilus influenzae type b infections by latex particle agglutination and counterimmunoelectrophoresis. J. Pediat. 93:37–42, 1978.

Warthen, R. O.: Hemorrhagic skin manifestations accompanying Hemophilus influenzae meningitis. J. Pediat. 33:489–491, 1948.

Watters, E. C., Waller, H., Hiles, D. A., and Michaels, R. H.: Acute orbital cellulitis. Arch. Ophthalmol. 94:785–788, 1976.

Weinstein, L.: The treatment of meningitis due to *Hemophilus influenzae* with streptomycin. A report of nine cases. New Eng. J. Med. 235:101–111, 1946.

Weitzman, S., and Aisenberg, A. C.: Fulminant sepsis after the successful treatment of Hodgkin's disease. Am. J. Med. 62:47–50, 1977.

Whittle, H. C., Tugwell, P., Egler, L. J., and Greenwood, B. M.: Rapid bacteriological diagnosis of pyogenic meningitis by latex agglutination. Lancet 2:619–621, 1974.

Wilkes-Weiss, D., and Huntington, R. W., Jr.: The treatment of influenzal meningitis with immune serum. J. Pediat. 9:462–466, 1936.

Williams, J. M., and Stevens, H.: Postmeningitic subdural effusions. Int. Surg. 27:590–594, 1957.

Wollstein, M.: Influenzal meningitis and its experimental production. Am. J. Dis. Child. 1:42–58, 1911.

Wright, H. T., Jr., McAllister, R. M., and Ward, R.: "Mixed" meningitis. Report of a case with isolation of *Haemophilus influenzae* type B and ECHO virus type 9 from the cerebrospinal fluid. New Eng. J. Med. 267:142–144, 1962.

Yogev, R., Lander, H. B., and Davis, A. T.: Effect of TMO-SMX on nasopharyngeal carriage of ampicillin-sensitive and ampicillin-resistant Hemophilus influenzae type b. J. Pediat. 93:394–397, 1978.

Yogev, R., Lander, H. B., and Davis, A. T.: Effect of rifampin on nasopharyngeal carriage of Hemophilus influenzae type b. J. Pediat. 94:840–841, 1979.

Young, L. M., Haddow, J. E., and Klein, J. O.: Relapse following ampicillin treatment of acute Hemophilus influenzae meningitis. Pediatrics 41:516–518, 1968.

Yow, M. D.: Ampicillin in the treatment of meningitis due to Hemophilus influenzae: An appraisal after 6 years experience. J. Pediat. 74:848–852, 1969.

Chapter Five

MENINGOCOCCAL MENINGITIS

Meningococcal meningitis is a disease steeped in historical interest because of the devastating epidemics which characterized the illness in past years and because of the dramatic nature of the clinical course and physical signs, including the rash, which often accompany the disorder. In the early part of this century, *Neisseria meningitidis* was reported to rank second only to *Mycobacterium tuberculosis* as a cause of bacterial meningitis in children (Fothergill and Sweet, Holt). It was subsequently surpassed by *Hemophilus influenzae* in the pediatric age group in this country but in Great Britain remains the most common cause of bacterial meningitis in children (Goldacre). Among approximately 600 to 900 annual deaths from meningococcal disease in the United States, more than 60 percent occur in children less than 10 years of age (Vital Statistics of the United States, Volume 2). Of 654 cases of meningococcal meningitis reported by Neal et al. in 1926, 25 percent were children less than one year of age and 71 percent were less than 10 years of age. Banks reviewed 706 cases of meningococcal sepsis or meningitis in 1948, of which 34 percent occurred in children less than five years of age and 47 percent affected patients less than 15 years of age. In 1969 in the United States there were 2,951 reported cases of meningococcal disease, among which 15 percent were in infants less than one year old and 60 percent were in children less than 15 years of age (Morbidity and Mortality Weekly Report, 24 Oct., 1970). The illness is only rarely described in the neonatal period and comprises a very small percentage of cases of acute bacterial meningitis in this age group

(Manginello et al., Root, Stiehm and Damrosch). The prevalence of meningococcal meningitis gradually increases in infants after three months of age to peak in the next 15 to 18 months and then peaks again in adolescence and early adulthood. Among series that report the incidence of types of acute bacterial meningitis in older children and adults, *Neisseria meningitidis* and *Streptococcus pneumoniae* generally rank approximately equal as the leading causes (Allison and Dalton, Carpenter and Petersdorf, Fraser et al.).

In the past two or three decades, there have been gradual changes in the meningococcal serotypes which most often give rise to invasive disease and also changes in the antimicrobial sensitivities of certain serotypes. In addition, there have been certain alterations in the epidemiology of the illness brought about by development of an antimeningococcal polysaccharide vaccine.

Neisseria meningitidis is a gram-negative aerobic coccus which is often arranged in pairs and is therefore referred to as a diplococcus. The diplococci are flattened along their adjacent margins and are morphologically identical to gonococci. Capsules cannot usually be visualized on gram stain but can be demonstrated by the quellung reaction. In CSF, meningococci are characteristically but not invariably intracellular organisms. Specimens of tissue fluids or those obtained from mucosal surfaces for culture should not be allowed to cool below body temperature before inoculation. The organism grows best at a temperature of 35° to 37°C and is readily killed by heating or desiccation. An atmosphere of 10 percent carbon dioxide en-

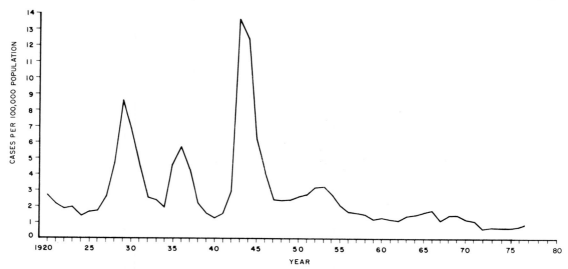

Figure 5–1. Meningococcal infections. Reported cases per 100,000 population in United States, 1920–1977. (From: Morbidity and Mortality Weekly Report, Annual Summary, 1977. Vol. 26, 1978.)

hances growth of the organism, which is accomplished best on blood agar or chocolate agar, on which moist, grayish-white glistening colonies appear. Meningococci were classified into types I through IV by Gordon and Murray in 1915. In 1950, an updated classification included groups A, B, C, and D on the basis of type-specific capsular polysaccharides (Subcommittee on the Family Neisseriaceae). Additional serogroups were described in 1961 by Slaterus (X, Y, Z, Z') and in 1968 by Evans et al. (Bo, 29E, 135). Group Y and group Bo (Boshard) are now believed to be identical (Evans et al. 1968), and serogroup 135 has been designated group W135 to indicate its origin at Walter Reed.

Historical Aspects

Neisseria meningitidis was discovered in purulent cerebrospinal fluid by Weichselbaum in 1887. Known then as *Diplococcus intracellularis*, its role as the agent causing "epidemic cerebrospinal meningitis" was soon recognized. The disease itself had been described long before discovery of the organism. Vieusseux of Geneva, Switzerland, had provided a clear description of "cerebrospinal meningitis" in 1806. Even as early as 1670, an epidemic was described among North American Indians with features highly indicative of a meningococcal outbreak (Plazak). In the early years of this century, meningococcal meningitis was occurring in both epidemic and sporadic forms with a mortality rate between 70

and 90 percent. Massive epidemics in metropolitan areas were characterized by a fulminating illness with death often occurring within 24 hours after the initial symptoms. Such an epidemic in New York in 1904 and 1905 resulted in 6,755 recognized cases (Banks).

In 1906, Dr. Simon Flexner in New York and Dr. Jochmann in Breslau, Germany, almost simultaneously succeeded in the production of antimeningococcal serum which appeared to protect animals against infection with meningococci. Serum was prepared by injecting killed and living organisms into horses, with blood drawn therefrom approximately eight months later. It was administered to humans subcutaneously in the initial trials but was shown to be ineffective by this route and thereafter was given by intraspinal injection (Dunn). In severe cases or those with hydrocephalus, serum was often injected directly into the lateral ventricle (Heiman, Howell and Cohen), and subsequently cisternal administration also became popular (Wright et al.). The initial intrathecal injection of approximately 20 to 30 ml. of serum was made at the time of the first lumbar puncture if the fluid was cloudy and was repeated daily for three or four doses.

In 1913, Flexner reported the results of antimeningococcal serum treatment of 1,294 cases of meningococcal meningitis. The survival rate in this group was 69.1 percent, thus demonstrating this to be the first significant advance in lowering the mortality of the disease. In 1915, Herrick reported the results of serum therapy in 208 young adults with meningococcal meningitis, which included survival in 74 percent. Blackfan subsequently added further evidence of the effectiveness of serum therapy by describing its use in 78 patients under two years of age with meningococcal meningitis. The survival rate in this group was 48 percent, which contrasted with previous death rates which approached 100 percent in this age group.

With World War I, the impact of meningococcal disease on military forces became apparent. During the war years, 2,466 military personnel were admitted to hospitals in the United States with this illness, with a fatality rate of 33 percent (Daniels). The lower death rate again reflected the value of serum therapy introduced earlier. In 1928 and 1929, massive epidemics in civilian populations occurred in several cities in this country, including those in Detroit (Gordon and Norton) and Indianapolis (Kempf et al.). In these outbreaks, there was a striking predisposition for the infection to attack infants less than two years of age, and thus the mortality rate was high (Bell, Norton and Gordon). The experience of the Detroit epidemic resulted in considerable new insight into the epidemiology and contagiousness of the illness. Direct contacts with afflicted patients infrequently became ill, and usually only one member in a family was involved. In 23 of 692 homes containing an ill patient, more than one case occurred, approximately 3.3 percent (Norton and Gordon). The conclusion from this experience was that most persons acquiring meningococcal disease did so from an asymptomatic carrier rather than from exposure to a patient with symptomatic disease. Recent investigations have shown that the attack rate among household contacts of a patient with meningococcal disease is 500 to 800 times greater than that of the population generally, thus indicating the importance of effective prophylactic therapy in this setting (The Meningococcal Disease Surveillance Group, 1976).

An additional therapeutic modality for meningococcal meningitis became available following the demonstration by Ferry et al. in 1931 of soluble exotoxins in filtrates of meningococci. Injection of these toxins into animals resulted in the development of antitoxin, which later was administered intravenously or intrathecally to patients with meningococcal disease (Hoyne). For a period of time, antitoxin was used in combination with sulfonamides with alleged beneficial effects

(Davis et al.), but because of frequent side effects and the eventual favorable experience with sulfadiazine and later with penicillin, the use of antitoxin for the treatment of the disease disappeared.

During World War II, meningococcal disease continued to be a serious problem, although the previous introduction of sulfonamide therapy and prophylaxis resulted in a significantly lower mortality rate. From 1940 to 1945, 14,504 hospital admissions of military personnel were due to this disease, with a fatality rate of only 3.8 percent (Daniels). During the same period, civilian public health problems continued from this illness. From 1939 to 1941, 3,575 reports of meningococcal meningitis from England and Wales were submitted to the Ministry of Health (Beeson and Westerman). Of these cases, 45.5 percent occurred in children under 15 years of age, and the overall mortality rate for all age groups was 15.9 percent. The study documented the previously observed relationship of age of the affected patient to mortality. Among young adults, the case fatality rate was as low as 5.6 percent, but in persons over 60 years of age it was 56 percent, and in infants less than one year of age the mortality rate was 31 percent. One of the most serious epidemics during this period occurred in Santiago, Chile, between 1941 and 1943 (Horwitz and Perroni). There were 4,464 cases of meningococcal meningitis, which amounted to one case per 300 inhabitants. The case fatality rate for all patients in this outbreak was 16.5 percent, but it was 28 percent among children less than four years of age despite the use of sulfonamide drugs.

Sulfonamides were introduced in this country as chemotherapeutic agents in 1935 and soon thereafter were shown to be effective for the treatment of meningococcal meningitis (Schwentker et al.). The first member of the sulfas used for this purpose was Prontosil, a drug developed in Germany in which the active antimicrobial component was sulfanilamide. Other sulfa preparations came into use, but sulfadiazine became the one of choice and was then widely utilized over the next 20 years. In the early part of the 1940's, it was administered orally, subcutaneously, intravenously, or intrathecally, with the common intravenous dose being 400 to 600 mg. per kilogram per day on the first day, then reduced gradually to 100 to 200 mg. per kilogram per day for the balance of the treatment regimen. Side effects were frequently encountered, the most common being hematuria, cutaneous eruptions, and drug fever (Goldring et al.). Agranulocytosis was also described but was infrequent. The impact of the sulfa preparations on the outcome of meningococcal meningitis was evident in a report in 1943 of 2,357 cases so treated in which the mortality rate was only 9.3 percent (Jubb). In 1945, Goldring et al. described a series of 279 children with meningococcal meningitis treated with sulfas, with a similar case fatality rate of 11 percent. Sulfadiazine remained the drug of choice for treatment of meningococcal disease throughout the 1940's because sulfas had been shown to penetrate CSF very well, while penicillin was, at that time, believed not to gain entrance into the CSF and brain (Rammelkamp and Keefer). In 1952, Leeper et al. demonstrated that penicillin given in adequate dosage was at least as effective as sulfonamides for treatment of meningococcal meningitis.

The prophylactic effectiveness of sulfadiazine was clearly demonstrated by a study of military personnel in which 15,000 soldiers were given sulfonamide and only two developed meningococcal meningitis. In the control series of 18,800 men, 40 cases occurred (Kuhns et al.). Although relative resistance of some strains of *Neisseria meningitidis* to sulfa was recognized in the 1940's (Schoenbach and Phair), the important role of sulfadiazine for both treatment and prophylaxis remained unchallenged until 1963 when strains of the organism that were solidly resistant to sulfadiazine were identified in this country in large scale. The first concentration of cases with sulfadiazine-resistant strains of meningococci occurred in the spring of 1963 at the U.S. Naval Training Center in San Diego (Miller et al.), and soon thereafter resistant strains were encountered among Army recruits stationed at Fort Ord in Monterey County, California (Brown and Condit). The resistant organisms were largely group B, and some were found to show in vitro resistance even to high concentrations of sulfadiazine. This experience soon brought forth the recommendation that sulfa preparations could no longer safely be used for treatment of meningococcal disease (Leedom et al.).

The majority of epidemics of meningococcal meningitis in the first four decades of this century were caused by strains of group A meningococci, while group B organisms were responsible for many isolated cases (Cheever). In recent years, only a few sporadic cases of group A meningococcal meningitis have been identified in this country (Morbidity and

Mortality Weekly Report, Dec., 1970), although this serogroup continues to be an important cause of endemic and epidemic meningococcal disease in other countries. During 1966, more than two-thirds of all meningococci submitted to the National Communicable Disease Center were group B (Bennett and Young). During subsequent years, group C organisms that were largely sulfadiazine-resistant gradually increased as a cause of human disease (Evans et al.). Of 306 meningococcal isolates from the United States submitted to the Communicable Disease Center in 1971, 28 percent were group B and 63 percent were group C (Morbidity and Mortality Weekly Report, 16 Oct., 1971). Among 240 isolates from United States civilian cases in 1972, 36 percent were serogroup B, of which 5.7 percent were sulfa-resistant. Serogroup C accounted for 54 percent, of which 82 percent were sulfa-resistant. Only three of the 240 isolates were group A (Morbidity and Mortality Weekly Report, 17 Feb., 1973). Of 324 isolates of *Neisseria meningitidis* obtained from 1973 to 1975 from patients with meningococcal disease, 45 percent were found to be group B, 32 percent were group C, 18 percent were group Y, and 2 percent were group A (The Meningococcal Disease Surveillance Group, 1976). Among the group C isolates in this series, 75 percent were resistant to sulfadiazine.

Group Y *Neisseria meningitidis* was recognized to be a common isolate from asymptomatic carriers following its discovery in 1961 but was then regarded to be of quite low virulence (Artenstein et al. 1971). Almost coincident to the initiation of the use of group C meningococcal polysaccharide vaccine among military recruits in 1971, there occurred a gradual increase in the recognition of disease caused by group Y meningococci (Smilack, Yee et al.). A much higher incidence of primary pneumonia was observed in these cases compared with disease caused by serogroups B and C, although meningococcemia and meningitis were also seen in some instances (Hersh et al., Irwin et al.). Koppes et al. studied 88 cases of group Y meningococcal disease among military recruits between 1971 and 1974. In 68 of the 88 cases, the illness was a primary bacterial pneumonia without obvious manifestations of sepsis or meningitis. Meningococcemia was found in ten cases and meningitis in six. The authors emphasized the striking predisposition for this serogroup to cause pulmonary infection and also suggested, on the basis of the very low case

Table 5–1. Differential Characteristics of *Neisseria* Species

ORGANISM	FERMENTATION		
	Dextrose	*Maltose*	*Sucrose*
Neisseria meningitidis	+	+	–
Neisseria gonorrhoeae	+	–	–
Neisseria catarrhalis	–	–	–
Neisseria flavescens	–	–	–
Neisseria sicca	+	+	+

fatality rate in their series, that perhaps group Y meningococci may be less virulent than group B or C organisms. Workers in Finland have recently recognized an increase in the prevalence of group Y meningococcus among nasopharyngeal isolates and have proposed that it is possibly an outcome of widespread vaccination against serogroups A and C (Nikoskelainen et al.).

Meningitis and meningococcemia caused by serogroup W135 have recently been recognized in Europe with greater frequency than before and cases have also been described in this country (Griffiss and Brandt, Hammerschlag and Baltimore), indicating that this group is fully pathogenic for man. The great majority of cases of meningitis caused by *Neisseria* species are caused by *Neisseria meningitidis*. *Neisseria gonorrhoeae* is an infrequent cause (Sayeed et al., Taubin and Landsberg), while *Neisseria lactamica* (Greenberg and Kleinerman, Lauer and Fisher), *Neisseria catarrhalis* (Feigin et al.), and *Neisseria sicca* (Bansmer and Brem) are very rare causes of acute meningitis.

Clinical Aspects

As is the case with bacterial infections generally, susceptibility to systemic meningococcal disease is determined by the host's deficiency in humoral antibodies to meningococci. Antibody formation occurs with either clinical infection or asymptomatic colonization of the organism in the nasopharynx; thus, in most instances, deficiency of antimeningococcal antibodies is the result of lack of significant exposure to meningococcal antigen in the past. The epidemiology of nasopharyngeal colonization with meningococci has been studied on many occasions and has been found to be remarkably different in infants and children compared with adults, and in military recruits compared with civilian populations. Greenfield et al. investigated the epidemiology of meningococcal nasopharyngeal carriage in an urban population in a nonepidemic period and found the prevalence of carriers to range from 4.9 percent to 10.6 percent, with the median duration of carriage being 9.6 months. In a study restricted to children less than 16 years of age, Marks et al. found the overall carriage rate to be 2.4 percent, based on a single nasopharyngeal culture. The nasopharyngeal carriage rate has been shown to increase markedly among household contacts of an ill patient (Foster et al.) and also has been found to be 60 percent or higher in certain studies involving non-immunized new military recruits (Farrell and Dahl).

Although natural immunity is largely group-specific, Reller et al. have shown that colonization with non-groupable meningococci, which rarely cause systemic disease, may be a potent stimulus to the production of antibody against certain pathogenic strains as well as against the homologous carrier strain. *Neisseria lactamica* is a common inhabitant of the nasopharynx of children but is a rare cause of systemic disease. Gold et al. demonstrated that cross-reactive antibodies to meningococci are induced by carriage of *Neisseria lactamica*, which, thus, contribute to the development of natural immunity to *Neisseria meningitidis*. The infrequency of meningococcal disease in the first few weeks after birth is partially explained by the transient protection from passively transferred maternal antibody. Decline of this antibody level corresponds to the recognized peak occurrence of meningococcal disease in later infancy and early childhood.

Goldschneider et al. found that the percentage of individuals with serum bactericidal activity was inversely proportional to the incidence of meningococcal meningitis during the first 12 years of life. Bactericidal activity declined after the first few months of life to reach its lowest level between six and 24 months of age, followed by a linear increase from two to 12 years. Of young adult recruits entering military service, 67 percent had bactericidal activity against group A, 86 percent against group B, and 76 percent against group C organisms (Goldschneider et al.).

The great majority of persons who contract meningococcal sepsis or meningitis are previously normal individuals in regard to immune mechanisms that protect against infec-

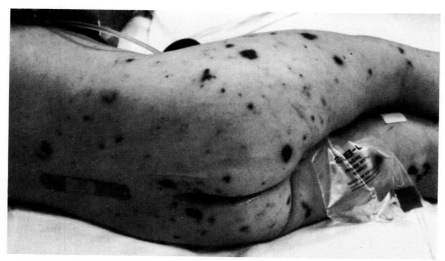

Figure 5–2. Meningococcal meningitis. Extensive purpuric eruption in a child critically ill, with marked hyperthermia, systemic hypotension, and laboratory evidence of consumption coagulopathy.

tion. Predisposition to infection with encapsulated bacteria, including *Neisseria meningitidis* and *Neisseria gonorrhoeae,* has been found in persons with deficiency of the third and fifth components of complement (Alper et al., Snyderman et al.) and is especially striking with deficiency of complement components six, seven, and eight (Lim et al., Petersen et al., Vogler et al.). In some instances with such abnormalities in the complement system, meningococcal meningitis is a repeatedly recurrent process.

It is generally accepted that meningococcal disease results from spread of the organism from the nasopharynx to the blood stream in most instances. Meningitis or meningococcemia, however, is an infrequent complication of nasopharyngeal colonization with this organism. Artenstein and Gold postulated that as few as one of 1,000 patients who acquire group B or C strain will develop symptomatic disease therefrom. Meningococcal conjunctivitis can be the primary site of infection, followed by meningococcal dissemination, but is very infrequent (Nussbaum et al.).

The clinical manifestations of meningococcal disease are those of septicemia with endotoxemia or those that result from dissemination to various organs, including the skin, ears, joints, heart, or central nervous system. Cases have been identified in infancy or childhood in which meningococcal bacteremia is manifested by fever and only mild systemic symptoms, with prompt response to parenteral antibiotic therapy (Baltimore and Hammerschlag). Mild illnesses of this type

are seemingly infrequent and even these would probably proceed to eventual localization of infection were they not identified by blood culture and promptly treated. Meningococcal meningitis can occur at any time of the year but is more common during the winter and in early spring.

Meningococcal sepsis varies greatly in severity but common features include fever, chills, vomiting, headache, myalgia, and rash. An erythematous, maculopapular eruption is occasionally observed but a petechial or hemorrhagic rash is more characteristic. Multiple, small petechial lesions may be present but in some patients are associated with large ecchymotic areas (Figs. 5–2, 5–3, 5–4). The rash is usually most dense over the lower limbs but may be generalized and often involves the palms, soles, ocular conjunctivae, or mucous membranes. The frequency with which a cutaneous eruption occurs has varied in different reports. Kaufman et al. found skin lesions in 65 percent of 238 cases of meningococcal meningitis, and Swartz and Dodge noted their presence in 50 percent of their cases. Of 151 patients with meningococcal infections reported by Toews and Bass, 14 percent had no cutaneous lesions, 75 percent had either maculopapular or petechial lesions, and 11 percent had peripheral purpuric or ecchymotic lesions. Blood obtained from the petechial or purpuric lesions will often reveal the organism on gram stain. Although the rash characteristic of meningococcal sepsis is of considerable diagnostic importance, it may be simulated by eruptions that occur with Rocky Mountain spotted fever (Bell and Las-

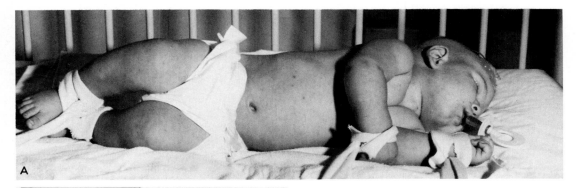

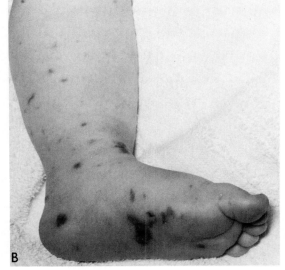

Figure 5–3. Meningococcal meningitis. Five-month-old child with acute, febrile illness with purulent CSF containing gram-negative intracellular diplococci. The child is lethargic, irritable, and has a stiff neck. *A* and *B,* Petechial lesions are sparse on the abdomen and proximal portions of the extremities. Hemorrhagic lesions are more striking distally.

cari), *Neisseria gonorrhoeae* sepsis (Swierczewski et al.), infection due to Echo virus type 9 (Frothingham), adenovirus type 7 (Sahler and Wilfert), and anaphylactoid purpura. Gastrointestinal symptoms including nausea, vomiting, and diarrhea may precede the rash or other more characteristic features of meningococcemia, resulting in delay in diagnosis and thus in the initiation of therapy (Corbett and Brady).

Cardiac involvement associated with meningococcal sepsis is widely recognized and can be a significant factor regarding the outcome of the illness. Death may occur from myocarditis with progressive cardiac decompensation, or even suddenly as a result of asystole due to inflammation of the conduction system (Robboy). Pericarditis is manifested by friction rub, chest pain, or evidence of pericardial effusion on roentgenographic examination. The recurrence of fever during recovery from meningococcal meningitis or the unexpected development of anemia is a

further possible hint of this complication (O'Connell). Meningococcal meningitis has coexisted in most reported examples of meningococcal pericarditis, although exceptions have been described (Herman and Rubin, Naraqi and Kabins). Pericarditis has been considered a rare complication of meningococcal disease (Novak and Samuelson) but recent reports suggest the possibility of an increasing incidence. Meningococcal pericardial effusion is usually serous or serosanguineous but is purulent in some cases identified early in the course of the systemic illness. Cardiac tamponade may require pericardiocentesis (Lebowitz and Nespole) and rarely is complicated by acute constrictive pericarditis (Scott et al.). Corticosteroids in addition to penicillin have been recommended by recent authors for this complication (Beal et al., Morse et al., Pierce and Cooper), although their value remains unestablished. Morse et al. described six patients with meningococcal pericarditis complicating meningitis and speculated that

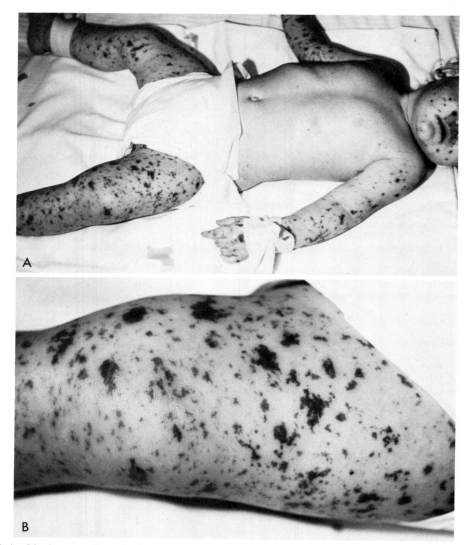

Figure 5–4.   Meningococcal meningitis. Twenty-one-month-old boy who was well until 2 days prior to admission when he developed fever and lethargy. One day before admission he had the onset of a petechial-purpuric rash, which rapidly became extensive over all four extremities and the face. His white blood cell count on hospital admission was 12,800 and platelet count was 60,000. CSF examination revealed cloudy fluid containing 13,800 WBC's per cu. mm., virtually all being polymorphonuclear leukocytes; glucose was 4 mg. per 100 ml., and protein 250 mg. per 100 ml. Gram-negative intracellular diplococci were found on gram stain of the CSF. The child recovered completely with intravenous penicillin therapy. *A,* Dense purpuric eruption over the extremities and on the face. *B,* Close-up view of the rash on the anterior surface of the left thigh.

group C organisms may possess a greater antigenic capacity to produce an inflammatory reaction of an immunologic nature on serosal membranes.

Hardman and Earle studied 200 fatal cases of meningococcal disease and identified interstitial myocarditis of varying severity in 78 percent. Hardman (1968) pointed out that myocarditis was more frequent and usually more severe in adults than in children with this illness. Myocarditis was found to be four times more common in those with septicemia as compared to those with meningitis without significant septicemic manifestations. Endocarditis associated with meningococcal disease is rare (Firestone, Logan), especially since the advent of effective chemotherapeutic agents. Endocarditis at the site of an artificial cardiac valve prosthesis can be caused by *Neisseria meningitidis* but other pathogens are far more frequent (Levin et al.).

Arthritis is occasionally observed but is usually transient and heals without permanent sequelae (Eichner and Deller). The effusion is serous in most cases but can be grossly purulent, especially when arthritic involvement complicates the initial stages of the septic illness. In some children, joint effusion occurs several days after other signs of meningococcal disease have subsided, probably representing a hypersensitivity response rather than bacterial invasion of the joint surfaces. Whittle et al. (1973) observed arthritis in 6.6 percent of 717 patients with meningococcal disease, most of the total series being caused by group A meningococci. The common occurrence of arthritis several days after initiation of successful antibiotic therapy and the relatively high frequency with which multiple joints were affected led the authors to the conclusion that, in most instances, meningococcal arthritis represents an "allergic" response to meningococcal antigen. In a companion paper, Greenwood and colleagues (1973) identified circulating meningococcal antigen in four patients with meningococcal disease complicated by arthritis. Additional evidence of immune complex formation in two of these cases was the presence of meningococcal antigen, immunoglobulin, and complement in synovial fluid white blood cells. The possibility of an inflammatory joint process should be considered in the infant or small child who exhibits marked irritability or apparent tenderness when moved or who develops recurrence of fever after an initial, favorable temperature response to antibiotic therapy.

Endophthalmitis is an unusual complication of meningococcal disease which can be either unilateral or bilateral and which manifests itself with iritis, hypopyon, and vitreous inflammation (Jensen and Naidoff, Mason et al.). This type of ocular inflammatory response is potentially reversible if therapy is begun early but otherwise may progress to vitreous abscess, retinal detachment, and subsequent blindness. Meningococcal endophthalmitis currently is quite infrequent, but prior to the availability of effective antimicrobial agents it was a relatively common complication of meningococcal meningitis (Lazar).

In certain rare cases of meningococcal sepsis, the illness assumes a chronic relapsing pattern. Chronic meningococcemia was first clearly described by Salomon in 1902, and by 1974, Leibel et al. estimated that approximately 150 cases had been reported in the American literature of which only 12 were patients less than 16 years of age. The rash in this form of the illness is more erythematous and maculopapular than petechial, and frequently will coincide with recurrent febrile episodes associated with arthralgia, myalgia, and chills. The illness in childhood can be easily confused with numerous other infectious disorders, Henoch-Schönlein purpura, rheumatoid disease, or an occult neoplasm. Diagnosis of chronic meningococcal sepsis is thus dependent on positive blood cultures. Localization of the infection eventually occurs unless the illness is recognized and treated. After weeks or months of recurrent symptoms, the illness is likely to culminate in meningitis, endocarditis, nephritis, or ocular sepsis (Benoit).

Dissemination of the organism from the vascular compartment into the meninges results in meningococcal meningitis, which is manifested by abrupt onset with headache, vomiting, lethargy, fever, and signs of meningeal irritation. Delirium or a confusional state will occasionally precede a febrile response, sometimes misleading one from the correct diagnosis (Fisher). A petechial or purpuric rash described above will develop early in the illness in many cases and may suggest the likelihood for the illness to assume a rapid and fulminating clinical course. Fulminating involvement with shock followed by death in a matter of hours after onset is well known with meningococcal sepsis and meningitis and results from endotoxemia or disseminated intravascular coagulation. In other cases, the clinical course is acute with rapid deterioration leading to deep coma but without systemic shock (Banks). Massive cerebral swelling is evidenced by a marked increase in the intracranial pressure at the time the lumbar puncture is done, and it is swelling which contributes considerably to the rapid downhill course (Nugent et al.). Unless intracranial pressure can be controlled by therapeutic measures, the process is likely to be followed by early demise of the child. Evidence of meningitis is sometimes minimal at autopsy in such cases, but one finds severe cerebral edema, widespread vascular thromboses in the brain, and sometimes disseminated hemorrhagic lesions.

Laboratory Studies

The blood leukocyte count is usually elevated with an increase in immature forms, although an initial leukopenia is occasionally observed. Proteinuria or microscopic hema-

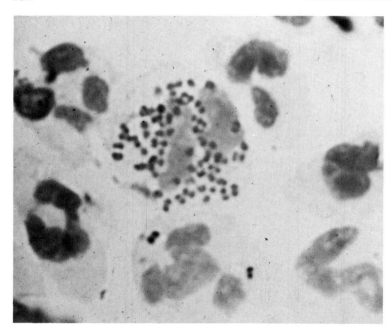

Figure 5–5. Meningococcal meningitis. Gram stain of CSF specimen shows numerous gram-negative intracellular diplococci.

turia is commonly present, at times with a modest elevation of the blood urea nitrogen. Serum electrolytes may either be normal or reveal hyponatremia and hypochloremia, which usually rapidly revert to normal after initiation of intravenous fluids and antibiotic therapy. The blood sugar is frequently elevated in the acute stages of meningococcal meningitis (Wolf and Birbara), especially if the level is measured shortly after seizures have occurred.

Similar to other forms of acute bacterial meningitis, the cerebrospinal fluid in meningococcal meningitis is usually cloudy to purulent, reveals a polymorphonuclear pleocytosis, and has a reduced sugar and an elevated protein content. Rarely, however, the CSF is clear with few or no cells present, with a normal glucose content, but with gram-negative diplococci present on smear and culture (Fig. 5–5). Diagnosis of meningococcal meningitis often is strongly suspected from the clinical findings but must be confirmed by identification of the organism in the CSF or blood. Prior administration of antibiotics, even in relatively small doses, may prevent recovery of the organism by bacteriologic techniques. In addition to the conventional bacteriologic methods, diagnosis of meningococcal meningitis can be aided by the latex agglutination test (Whittle et al. 1974) and by examination of urine and CSF by countercurrent immunoelectrophoresis (Greenwood et al. 1971, Shackelford et al., Whittle et al. 1975).

Waterhouse-Friderichsen Syndrome

The term Waterhouse-Friderichsen syndrome in past years has referred to an acute, fulminating condition with systemic hypotension or shock and with widespread petechial or purpuric skin lesions secondary to an infectious disease (Aegerter, Banks and McCartney, Danciger, Martland). Meningococcal disease is the most widely recognized cause of the Waterhouse-Friderichsen syndrome, but other infections, especially septic states caused by other gram-negative organisms, can give rise to an identical condition. Bilateral adrenal hemorrhage was popularized as the pathologic hallmark of this condition, a finding that suggested to many that shock resulted from acute adrenal insufficiency. Waterhouse in 1911 and Friderichsen in 1918 described cases with death associated with adrenal hemorrhages, but more detailed descriptions had appeared prior to their reports (Andrewes, Little). Waterhouse of London, in his brief report of a single case in Lancet, discussed only the possibility of hemorrhagic smallpox, while Friderichsen of Copenhagen contributed nothing to the etiology of the disorder that had not previously been described. Whether the contribution of either to the understanding of this disorder justified its eponymic designation with their names has been debated but is of little importance at the present time.

In 1948, Ferguson and Chapman reported a detailed analysis of the pathology of 16 patients with fatal meningococcal infections. In addition to adrenal involvement, vascular damage with thromboses in many organs was identified. In certain patients with clinical findings consistent with the "Waterhouse-Friderichsen syndrome," extensive vascular involvement was found in multiple organs but with only slight abnormalities of the adrenal glands. Clinically, cases with and without massive adrenal hemorrhage could not be separated. The authors suggested that adrenal hemorrhage represented but one aspect of multiple organ system involvement in this disease and indicated that adrenal insufficiency was not necessary to account for peripheral vascular collapse that occurred in these cases.

Additonal evidence opposing the concept that shock was secondary to adrenal insufficiency was the often-noted lack of response to replacement corticosteroid therapy. Furthermore, certain patients with circulatory failure due to infection were found to have increased rather than decreased blood corticosteroid levels (Melby and Spink). This finding has not been universal, however, as Migeon et al. found that six of seven patients with meningococcal infection and adrenal hemorrhage had abnormally low cortisol blood levels, consistent with failure of adequate adrenal function. May reviewed the pathogenesis of circulatory failure in meningococcal infection and emphasized the reasons why adrenal failure was not the underlying factor. He supported the concept of bacterial endotoxin altering blood vessel reactivity to epinephrine, leading to peripheral vascular collapse. Dalldorf and Jennette stressed the importance of widespread thrombosis of the pulmonary microcirculation in fatal meningococcemia and postulated that systemic hypotension might in part be secondary to acute cor pulmonale.

Experimental studies of the effect of meningococcal endotoxin in dogs have revealed that hypotension results from an increase in volume of blood in peripheral vessels without significant change in total blood volume (Ebert et al.). The resulting diminution of venous return reduces right atrial and pulmonary pressures, thus decreasing cardiac output. Hodes recently summarized the biologic effects of gram-negative endotoxins. These included the induction of local and generalized Shwartzman reaction, the production of leukopenia followed by leukocytosis, reduction in circulating platelets, injury to vascular endothelium possibly leading to generalized intravascular clotting, and deleterious changes in carbohydrate and protein metabolism. Blood pressure alterations leading to shock have been attributed to release of kallikreins from leukocytes, alterations of the effects of norepinephrine on vessel walls, and the release of histamine from mast cells.

Consumption Coagulopathy. Injury to the vascular endothelium, probably endotoxic in origin, may precipitate a hypercoagulable state followed by diffuse intravascular coagulation with consumption of clotting factors and subsequent hemorrhagic manifestations. Endothelial injury is believed by some to result in activation of Hageman factor (XII), initiating intravascular clotting resulting in fibrin thrombi, and the adhesion of platelets to subendothelial structures. This process was termed "Verbrauchskoagulopathie," or consumption coagulopathy, by Lasch et al. in 1961 and is known to occur in certain patients with severe meningococcal sepsis (Evans et al., McGehee et al., Wilhelm and Cherubin). Although the mechanism of origin of intravascular clotting in meningococcemia remains unproven, the most prevalent opinion has been that endotoxic damage to the endothelium is the initiating factor, and, in addition, phagocytic leukocytes may be induced to release procoagulant factors. Once the clotting process within vessels is initiated, there follows a reduction of plasma fibrinogen, prothrombin, factors V, VIII, and XIII, and platelets. Secondary fibrinolysis may follow, resulting in fibrin split products demonstrable in serum (Merskey et al.). Disseminated fibrin thrombi in small vessels resulting in local tissue necrosis and often with hemorrhage (Fig. 5–6) is the characteristic histologic finding in this disorder.

Prognostic Implications, Complications, and Sequelae

Certain findings early in the course of meningococcal disease have been reputed to be of prognostic significance. Wolf and Birbara claimed the presence of leukopenia at the time of hospital admission to be an ominous sign. Survival beyond 48 hours of initiation of therapy in septicemic cases was judged to be an excellent prognostic sign. Diffuse encephalitic involvement manifested by profound and progressive brain swelling, especially with respiratory compromise, was deemed to be a bad prognostic finding. Stiehm and Damrosch reviewed 63 cases of

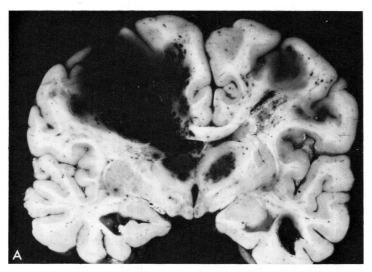

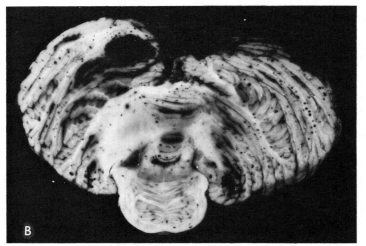

Figure 5–6. Meningococcemia with meningitis and disseminated intravascular coagulation, complicating bacterial endocarditis. *A,* Coronal section of the brain shows a massive hemorrhage in the white matter on the right side with extension into the right lateral ventricle, bilateral thalamic hemorrhages, and multiple other hemorrhagic lesions of variable size elsewhere. There is an area of suppurative cerebritis in the white matter on the left side, just lateral to the caudate nucleus. *B,* The cerebellum demonstrates several hemorrhagic lesions of moderate size in addition to extensive petechial hemorrhages. Bleeding within the brain illustrated in *A* and *B* is the result of a combination of effects, including the enhanced bleeding tendency caused by consumption coagulopathy, stasis associated with hyaline thrombi involved in the consumptive process, and inflammatory vasculitis provoked by the septic infection. *C,* Thrombosed cerebral arteriole whose lumen is packed with bacterial colonies, and with a periluminal inflammatory infiltrate.

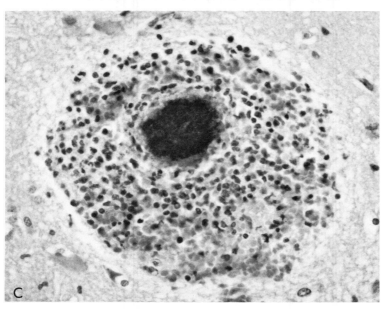

acute meningococcal disease in regard to prognostic factors. They found that of 17 patients with meningitis without signs of septicemia, only one death occurred. Of 46 cases with meningococcemia with or without meningitis, 11 ended fatally. The appearance of a purpuric rash within 12 hours of hospitalization was indicative of a more fulminating process and was associated with a poor prognosis. Leukopenia was suggestive of a poor outcome, as was a low erythrocyte sedimentation rate. As expected, the presence of shock also was found to be a grave prognostic sign, as has been the case in other reports (Lewis).

Niklasson et al. studied 80 patients from the standpoint of prognostic factors with almost identical findings to those of Stiehm and Damrosch. In this series, also, the fatality rate was much higher in those with predominantly septic manifestations compared to those patients with predominantly meningitic features.

The prognostic importance of the type and location of skin lesions in meningococcal disease has been stressed by Toews and Bass. These authors showed that patients with no skin lesions or generalized petechial lesions usually experienced clinical illness which was not fulminant and was associated with signs of a host response to infection. Conversely, the presence of extensive purpuric and ecchymotic lesions primarily of the extremities was much more often associated with a fulminating course with a much higher mortality rate.

The mortality rate of meningococcal meningitis when all cases in all age groups are included is generally estimated to be 5 to 10 percent. It would be expected to be higher if one restricted the considerations to those cases in early infancy or among those with distinct signs of endotoxemia at the time of hospital admission.

Complications during the acute phase and residual sequelae of meningococcal meningitis have received less attention since the introduction of effective antimicrobial agents. Acute otitis media and pneumonia were often mentioned in past years and generally were felt to be due to secondary bacterial invasion rather than of meningococcal origin. Subdural effusion can occur in infants with meningococcal meningitis but appears to be less common than in patients with *Hemophilus influenzae* or pneumococcal meningitis. Vascular thromboses during the septic phase of the illness as a complication of consumption coagulopathy or shock can result in soft tissue necrosis and, in severe cases, can be sufficiently destructive to require amputation of certain fingers or toes.

Residual neurologic sequelae from meningococcal meningitis have been considered infrequent, as most who survived seemed to recover completely. Of the 440 survivors in the pre-chemotherapeutic series studied by Neal et al., 82 percent were believed to have recovered completely and 18 percent showed sequelae. Hearing loss has been found to be the most common residual deficit (Neal et al.), occurring in 5 to 7 percent of surviving cases according to Banks. Cranial nerve palsies persist in certain patients following meningococcal meningitis, with sixth or seventh nerve involvement being the most common (Farmer). Visual deficits and limb paresis remain in a few but have been considered unusual. Even more rare is residual spinal cord damage manifested by weakness of the lower extremities and neurogenic bladder dysfunction (Gotshall). Silverthorne studied 51 patients with meningococcal meningitis treated with anti-meningococcal serum, nine of whom developed postmeningitic hydrocephalus, all being fatal. Seizures may occur as a sequela of any form of bacterial meningitis; however, Swartz and Dodge found no patients with post-meningitic epilepsy among 39 cases of meningococcal meningitis. Pituitary insufficiency with growth failure followed meningitis in one child mentioned by Banks.

Treatment

Penicillin G administered intravenously is the treatment of choice for meningococcal sepsis and meningitis. Because of the well-known potential danger of rapid deterioration that may accompany this disease, it is reasonable to make efforts to achieve an effective antibiotic blood level as soon as possible when the diagnosis is suspected. This can be accomplished by administering intravenously one-half the calculated daily dosage over 30 to 60 minutes at the initiation of treatment. The relatively slower time period for infusion of a loading dose of penicillin is necessary because hospitals commonly stock potassium-containing penicillin, which can be dangerous if a large amount is infused rapidly. A direct intravenous push over a minute or so of the quantity recommended here could result in cardiac arrest. The use of a loading dose is, perhaps, a more important consideration in the child with purpuric skin lesions, systemic hypotension, or thrombocytopenia. The dosage of penicillin G for meningococcal meningitis is 250,000 units per kilogram per day but not over 20 million units per day, given intravenously every four hours over a 20-minute period. Ampicillin is stated to be equally effective (Wehrle et al.) although studies have suggested that penetration of ampicillin into spinal fluid is less with meningococcal meningitis than with pneumococcal or *Hemophilus influenzae* meningitis (Taber et al.).

In persons allergic to penicillin, chloramphenicol provides a satisfactory alternative. Chloramphenicol has been shown to be bactericidal against most strains of *Neisseria meningitidis* (Rahal and Simberkoff); however, ampicillin, and presumably penicillin, in combination with chloramphenicol may be antagonistic to each other against certain strains of meningococci (Feldman and Zweighaft). Since ampicillin in combination with chloramphenicol is now the initial regimen for treatment of meningitis in children beyond the newborn period until the causative organism is identified, it is important to discontinue the chloramphenicol as soon as possible in cases in which the meningococcus is proved to be the cause.

Ten to 14 days of antibiotic therapy is usually sufficient, depending on the degree of illness at the onset of therapy and the rate of improvement after therapy is started. Unless the patient is hypotensive or significantly dehydrated, the volume of intravenous fluids administered should be restricted to approximately two-thirds of maintenance requirements for the first two or three days.

Treatment of fulminating meningococcemia with endotoxic shock continues to be a perplexing and debatable subject. It is generally agreed that appropriate antibiotic therapy is necessary and that early initiation of therapy is more apt to be successful than that started after profound shock has developed. Restoration of blood volume and correction of electrolyte deficits may be necessary if vomiting or diarrhea have occurred. Intravenous fluids may suffice but, in certain instances, plasma expanders or fresh whole blood may be desirable. Bicarbonate therapy in conjunction with measures to correct dehydration is useful if metabolic acidosis is present. Sodium bicarbonate, however, should not be mixed in solution with penicillin or its semisynthetic derivatives. Central venous and arterial catheters for pressure

monitoring will facilitate fluid and drug administration if hypotension or shock is present. Dopamine is the most widely used agent for treatment of septic shock and is given in an intravenous dose of 2 to 10 μg per kilogram per minute (Driscoll et al., Goldberg). Because it is inactivated in alkaline solution, dopamine should not be mixed in the same IV bottle with sodium bicarbonate. The primary effect of this sympathomimetic amine is to increase myocardial contractility, enhancing cardiac output, but it has the additive beneficial effect of selectively increasing renal blood flow.

The value of corticosteroids in septic shock remains questionable and has been a topic of debate. The opponents of corticosteroid therapy in endotoxic shock base their argument on the evidence that an experimental Shwartzman reaction can be elicited after a single dose of endotoxin in animals pretreated with cortisone. The advocates of corticosteroids recommend large or "pharmacologic" doses because of the seriousness of this condition and certain theoretical reasons why they might be beneficial (Hodes, Schumer). Intravenous hydrocortisone is recommended by Hodes with potential beneficial effects, including its action as an adrenergic blocking agent relieving vascular spasm, thus enhancing the microcirculation, its counteraction of glycogen depletion by endotoxin, its reduction of lactic acid formation, and its protective effect in lysosomes, preventing their rupture.

Laboratory evidence of intravascular coagulation is considered an indication for heparin therapy by certain authors, but reports regarding its effectiveness have been quite variable (Gérald et al.). Although most authors have found that laboratory abnormalities indicating intravascular coagulation revert toward normal, it is difficult to ascribe clinical improvement to heparin, and death may still occur in the seriously ill patient (Kisker and Rush). Corrigan has recommended initial treatment with appropriate antishock measures and antibiotics without the addition of heparin. Should laboratory evidence of consumption coagulopathy persist despite these measures, and especially if accompanied by bleeding, heparin is then given in an attempt to abolish intravascular consumption. Heparin is administered intravenously in a dose of 100 units per kilogram and is repeated every 4 hours in an amount sufficient to lengthen the partial thromboplastin time or thrombin time to two to three times normal. The duration of heparin therapy required is variable and is determined by clinical judgment plus evidence of improvement of laboratory data regarding blood clotting factors and platelets.

In bleeding patients it is important to replace depleted clotting factors by transfusion of platelets, cryoprecipitate, or plasma. In addition, plasma infusions will provide antithrombin III (heparin cofactor), a protein that is consumed during intravascular coagulation and which is necessary for an optimal therapeutic effect of heparin. Management of such complex coagulation abnormalities is best encompassed with the consultative aid of a hematologist familiar with the details of the physiology of the coagulation process.

In certain cases of meningococcal meningitis, the course is rapidly progressive, leading to deep coma in the absence of systemic hypotension or shock. Severe cerebral swelling results in high-grade increase in intracranial pressure, which will eventually lead to transtentorial herniation, brain stem compression, and death (Nugent et al.). Immediate recognition of the importance of intracranial hypertension in such cases can be difficult, but survival is likely to be dependent on one's ability to control the intracranial pressure (Bell and McCormick). The use of fluid restriction and mannitol injections may be sufficient in some instances, while others will require a more aggressive approach. When this is necessary, the placement of a subdural bolt or intraventricular catheter to provide a continuous measurement of the intracranial pressure greatly simplifies the development of the most appropriate treatment regimen. Methods used to control intracranial hypertension include control of hyperthermia, restriction of intravenous fluid administration, controlled ventilation to prevent hypercapnea, and intravenous injections of mannitol in doses of 0.5 to 1.0 grams per kilogram at periodic intervals.

When an intraventricular catheter is selected for pressure monitoring and can be successfully inserted into the lateral ventricle, small amounts of CSF can be aspirated at intervals, usually a highly effective means to temporarily reduce intracranial pressure. Sudden pressure spikes can be controlled by intermittent hyperventilation to lower the pCO_2 to less than 30 torr, assuming that cerebral autoregulation has not been lost. An aggressive approach of this type is ordinarily accomplished in an intensive care unit and usually requires intubation, curarization, and

mechanical ventilation. The chances of success of this form of treatment in a patient with meningococcal meningitis with dramatic and progressive cerebral swelling is dependent on early recognition of the significance of increased intracranial pressure. If survival is to occur, treatment must be implemented before the pupils become dilated and fixed and before complete respiratory paralysis has occurred.

The importance of prophylactic treatment among household contacts and others who have been in intimate contact with a patient with meningococcal disease has been emphasized by the recognition that such persons are at risk for an attack at a rate which is at least 500 to 800 times that of the general population (The Meningococcal Disease Surveillance Group, 1976). While penicillin has been highly successful in the treatment of meningococcal disease, it has not proved consistently effective as a prophylactic agent. Dowd et al. found a 65 percent failure rate with penicillin in a small series studied for nasopharyngeal carriage of meningococci. In addition, the emergence of sulfadiazine-resistant meningococci has severely restricted the use of sulfa preparations for prophylaxis. Sulfadiazine can now be recommended only in the event of a meningococcal epidemic documented to be caused by a sulfonamide-sensitive organism. Minocycline, a tetracycline preparation, has shown promise for meningococcal prophylaxis (Guttler et al.); however, the very high incidence of vestibular side effects manifested as vomiting, vertigo, and ataxia prevents its use on a wide-scale basis (Allen, Fanning et al.).

Rifampin has been found to be superior to most other currently available antimicrobial agents for elimination of nasopharyngeal carriage of meningococci (Deal and Sanders, Guttler et al.). Studies by Devine and colleagues (1970) showed that adults given rifampin orally in a dose of 600 mg. four times per day attained salivary concentrations that exceeded the minimal inhibitory concentration for meningococci in vitro, a quality necessary for a drug to effectively eliminate the organism from the nasopharynx (Devine et al., 1971). Owing to the possibility of development of rifampin-resistant strains of meningococci (Weidmer et al.), the drug should not be used for treatment of the disease but should be reserved for its potential value as a prophylactic agent (Ivler et al.).

It is currently recommended that rifampin chemoprophylaxis be administered to all household members of an identified case of meningococcal disease, to other persons who have been in intimate contact with the patient for a given period of time, and to anyone directly exposed to oral secretions of the patient (Jacobson and Fraser, McCormick and Bennett). The latter would apply to hospital attendants who administered mouth-to-mouth resuscitation. Other less direct contacts, such as classmates at school, are not believed to be at significant risk and need not ordinarily receive drug therapy (Jacobson et al.) Because most secondary cases with clinical illness occur within a few days after exposure, the prophylactic regimen should be initiated as soon as possible after diagnosis of the index case. The use of prophylactic measures directed to household contacts does not entirely eliminate the possible occurrence of meningococcal disease (Khuri-Bulos) and, thus, some degree of medical surveillance remains appropriate. The dosage schedule of rifampin for meningococcal prophylaxis is 600 mg. every 12 hours for four doses for adults, 20 mg. per kilogram per day given every 12 hours for four doses for children one to 12 years of age, and 10 mg. per kilogram per day administered every 12 hours for four doses in children less than 12 months of age. The short duration of treatment is not believed to significantly contribute to the development of meningococcal resistance to rifampin.

In the unusual instance in which sulfadiazine can be safely used for prophylaxis, the dose is one gram every 12 hours in adults, 500 mg. every 12 hours for children one to 12 years of age, and 500 mg. once per day for children less than 12 months of age. Treatment is continued for two days. In addition to chemoprophylaxis, group A or C meningococcal vaccine should be considered for household and other intimate contacts over two years of age, especially in epidemic circumstances (McCormick and Bennett).

Meningococcal polysaccharide vaccines against disease caused by *Neisseria meningitidis* serogroups A and C were developed and licensed after it was demonstrated that the polysaccharide antigens of these serogroups were excellent immunogens in man and that the vaccines produced only infrequent and mild adverse effects (Gotschlich et al.). Both monovalent and bivalent vaccines are now available, and the vaccines are highly group-specific, that is, group A vaccine does not provide protection against group C meningococci. Group B polysaccharide preparations are not immunogenic in adults and a satis-factory vaccine against this serogroup has not yet been developed. Group A and group C vaccines have been shown to be highly effective in the control of meningococcal disease in older children and adults caused by the homologous serogroup (Artenstein et al. 1970, Makela et al., Peltola et al. 1976). Antibody responses resulting from vaccine administration to infants under two years of age are less in degree than in older children (Gold et al., Peltola et al. 1977, Lepow et al., Wilkins and Wehrle), and group C vaccine is not recommended in this age group. In addition to its ineffectiveness in this age group, there is concern that group C vaccine, when given to young infants, may give rise to some form of immunologic tolerance by which there results a lesser antibody response to subsequent challenge, perhaps leading to greater risk of disease. Minimal to absent antibody response to meningococcal vaccine in infants less than three months of age is presumed to be due to the suppression of endogenous antibody production by the high levels of maternal antibody possessed by most young infants (Gold et al.).

Group C meningococcal vaccine has resulted in excellent control of group C meningococcal disease among the military forces, although routine vaccination of civilians is not recommended. Serogroup-specific monovalent vaccine is recommended to control outbreaks of meningococcal disease and should be considered as an adjunct to antibiotic chemoprophylaxis for household contacts of meningococcal disease. Protective antibodies have been found to persist in adults for at least five years after a single injection of group C polysaccharide vaccine (Brandt and Artenstein).

REFERENCES

Aegerter, E. E.: The Waterhouse-Friderichsen syndrome. A review of the literature and a report of two cases. J.A.M.A. 106:1715–1719, 1936.

Allen, J. C.: Minocycline. Ann. Intern. Med. 85:482–487, 1976.

Allison, M. J., and Dalton, H. P.: Etiology of bacterial meningitis at the Medical College of Virginia 1961–1965. Virginia Med. Monthly 94:317–319, 1967.

Alper, C. A., Bloch, K. J., and Rosen, F. S.: Increased susceptibility to infection in a patient with type II essential hypercatabolism of C3. New Eng. J. Med. 288:601–606, 1973.

Andrewes, F. W.: A case of acute meningococcal septicemia. Lancet 1:1172–1173, 1906.

Artenstein, M. S., and Gold, R.: Current status of prophylaxis of meningococcal disease. Milit. Med. 135:735–739, 1970.

Artenstein, M. S., Schneider, H., and Tingley, M. D.: Meningococcal infections. I. Prevalence of serogroups causing disease in U.S. Army personnel in 1964–1970. Bull. WHO 45:275–278, 1971.

Artenstein, M. S., Gold, R., Zimmerly, J. G., Wyle, F. A., Schneider, H., and Harkins, C.: Prevention of meningococcal disease by group C polysaccharide vaccine. New Eng. J. Med. 282:417–420, 1970.

Baltimore, R. S., and Hammerschlag, M.: Meningococcal bacteremia. Clinical and serologic studies of infants with mild illness. Am. J. Dis. Child. 131:1001–1004, 1977.

Banks, H. S.: Meningococcosis. A protean disease. Lancet 2:635–640, 1948.

Banks, H. S.: Meningococcosis. A protean disease. Lancet 2:677–681, 1948.

Banks, H. S.: Meningococcal fever. *In*: Modern Practice in Infectious Fevers. Hoeber, New York, 1951, Pp. 303–332.

Banks, H. S., and McCartney, J. E.: Meningococcal adrenal syndromes and lesions. Lancet 1:771–776, 1943.

Bansmer, C., and Brem, J.: Acute meningitis caused by Neisseria sicca. New Eng. J. Med. 238:596–597, 1948.

Beal, L. R., Ustach, T. J., and Forker, A. D.: Meningococcemia without meningitis presenting as cardiac tamponade. Survival with disseminated intravascular coagulation. Am. J. Med. 51:659–662, 1971.

Beeson, P. B., and Westerman, E.: Cerebrospinal fever. Analysis of 3,575 case reports, with special reference to sulphonamide therapy. Brit. Med. J. 1:497–500, 1943.

Bell, A. J.: Epidemic meningitis. (Bacteriology, immunology, complications). J. Pediat. 4:541–547, 1934.

Bell, W. E., and Lascari, A. D.: Rocky Mountain spotted fever. Neurologic symptoms in the acute phase. Neurology 20:841–847, 1970.

Bell, W. E., and McCormick, W. F.: Increased Intracranial Pressure in Children. W. B. Saunders Company, Philadelphia, 1978.

Bennett, J. V., and Young, L. S.: Trends in meningococcal disease. J. Infect. Dis. 120:634–636, 1969.

Benoit, F. L.: Chronic meningococcemia. Case report and review of the literature. Am. J. Med. 35:103–112, 1963.

Blackfan, K. D.: The treatment of meningococcus meningitis. Medicine 1:139–212, 1922.

Brandt, B. L., and Artenstein, M. S.: Duration of antibody responses after vaccination with group C *Neisseria meningitidis* polysaccharide. J. Infect. Dis. 131:S69–S72, 1975.

Brown, J. W., and Condit, P. K.: Meningococcal infections: Fort Ord and California. Calif. Med. 102:171–180, 1965.

Carpenter, R. R., and Petersdorf, R. G.: The clinical spectrum of bacterial meningitis. Am. J. Med. 33:262–275, 1962.

Cheever, F. S.: The meningococci. *In*: Dubois, R. J., and Hirsch, J. G.: Bacterial and Mycotic Infections in Man. J. P. Lippincott Co., Philadelphia, 1965.

Corbett, T. H., and Brody, J. A.: An epidemic in an Eskimo village due to group-B meningococcus. Part 2. Clinical features. J.A.M.A. 196:388–390, 1966.

Corrigan, J. J.: Heparin therapy in bacterial septicemia. J. Pediat. 91:695–700, 1977.

Dalldorf, F. G., and Jennette, C.: Fatal meningococcal septicemia. Arch. Path. Lab. Med. 101:6–9, 1977.

Danciger, J. A.: Fulminating meningococcemia with bilateral adrenal hemorrhage (Waterhouse-Friderichsen syndrome). J. Pediat. 16:495–499, 1940.

Daniels, W. B.: Case of death in meningococci infection. Analysis of 300 fatal cases. Am. J. Med. 8:468–473, 1950.

Davis, J. H., Morrow, W. J., and Toomey, J. A.: Results in the treatment of meningococcic meningitis with antitoxin and sulfonamide drugs. J. Pediat. 26:455–459, 1945.

Deal, W. B., and Sanders, E.: Efficacy of rifampin in treatment of meningococcal carriers. New Eng. J. Med. 281:641–645, 1969.

Devine, L. F., Johnson, D. P., Hagerman, C. R., Pierce, W. E., Rhode, S. L., III, and Peckinpaugh, R. O.: Rifampin. Levels in serum and saliva and effect on the meningococcal carrier state. J.A.M.A. 214:1055–1059, 1970.

Devine, L. F., Rhode, S. L., Pierce, W. E., Johnson, D. P., Hagerman, C. R., and Peckinpaugh, R. O.: Rifampin: effect of two-day treatment on the meningococcal carrier state and the relationship to the levels of drug in sera and saliva. Am. J. Med. Sci. 261 (2):79–83, 1971.

Dowd, J. M., Blink, D., Miller, C. H., Frank, P. F., and Pierce, W. E.: Antibiotic prophylaxis of carriers of sulfadiazine-resistant meningococci. J. Infect. Dis. 116:473–480, 1966.

Driscoll, D. J., Gillette, P. C., and McNamara, D. G.: The use of dopamine in children. J. Pediat. 92:309–314, 1978.

Dunn, C. H.: Cerebrospinal meningitis, its etiology, diagnosis, prognosis and treatment. Am. J. Dis. Child. 1:95–112, 1911.

Ebert, R. V., Borden, C. W., Hall, W. H., and Gold, D.: A study of hypotension (shock) produced by meningococcus toxin. Circ. Res. 3:378–384, 1955.

Eichner, H. L., and Deller, J. J., Jr.: Meningococcal arthritis. Report of two cases. Arthritis Rheum. 13:272–275, 1970.

Evans, J. R., Artenstein, M. S., and Hunter, D. H.: Prevalence of meningococcal subgroups and description of three new groups. Am. J. Epidemiol. 87:643–646, 1968.

Evans, R. W., Glick, B., Kimball, F., and Lobell, M.: Fatal intravascular consumption coagulopathy in meningococcal sepsis. Am. J. Med. 46:910–918, 1969.

Fanning, W. L., Gump, D. W., and Sofferman, R. A.: Side effects of minocycline: A double-blind study. Antimicrob. Agents Chemother. 11:712–717, 1977.

Farmer, T. W.: Neurologic complications during meningococcic meningitis treated with sulfonamide drugs. Arch. Intern. Med. 76:201–209, 1945.

Farrell, D. G., and Dahl, E. V.: Nasopharyngeal carriers of *Neisseria meningitidis*. J.A.M.A. 198:1189–1192, 1966.

Feigin, R. D., Joaquin, V. S., and Middelkamp, J. N.: Purpura fulminans associated with Neisseria catarrhalis septicemia and meningitis. Pediatrics 44:120–123, 1969.

Feldman, W. E., and Zweighaft, T.: Effect of ampicillin and chloramphenicol against *Streptococcus pneumoniae* and *Neisseria meningitidis*. Antimicrob. Agents Chemother. 15:240–242, 1979.

Ferguson, J. H., and Chapman, O. D.: Fulminating meningococcic infections and the so-called Waterhouse-Friderichsen syndrome. Am. J. Path. 24:763–782, 1948.

Ferry, N. S., Norton, J. F., and Steele, A. H.: Studies of the properties of bouillon filtrates of the meningococcus: Production of a soluble toxin. J. Immunol. 21:293–312, 1931.

Firestone, G. M.: Meningococcus endocarditis. Am. J. Med. Sci. 211:556–564, 1946.

Fisher, D. S.: Toxic psychosis without fever as sign of acute meningitis. Arch. Intern. Med. 111:54–57, 1963.

Flexner, S.: Experimental cerebrospinal meningitis and its serum treatment. J.A.M.A. 47:560–566, 1906.

Flexner, S.: The results of the serum treatment in thirteen hundred cases of epidemic meningitis. J. Exp. Med. 17:553–576, 1913.

Foster, M. T., Jr., Sanders, E., and Ginter, M.: Epidemiology of sulfonamide-resistant meningococcal infections in a civilian population. Am. J. Epidemiol. 98:346–353, 1971.

Fothergill, L. D., and Sweet, L. K.: Meningitis in infants and children with special reference to age-incidence and bacteriologic diagnosis. J. Pediat. 2:696–710, 1933.

Fraser, D. W., Henke, C. E., and Feldman, R. A.: Changing patterns of bacterial meningitis in Olmsted County, Minnesota, 1935–1970. J. Infect. Dis. 128:300–307, 1973.

Friderichsen, C.: Nebennierenapoplexie bei kleinen Kindern. Jahrb. Kinswehwilk. 87:109, 1918.

Frothingham, T. H.: Echo virus type 9 associated with three cases simulating meningococcemia. New Eng. J. Med. 259:484–485, 1958.

Gérald, P., Moriau, M., Bachy, A., Malvaux, P., and DeMeyer, R.: Meningococcal purpura: Report of 19 patients treated with heparin. J. Pediat. 82:780–786, 1973.

Gold, R., Goldschneider, I., Lepow, M. L., Draper, T. F., and Randolph, M.: Carriage of *Neisseria meningitidis* and *Neisseria lactamica* in infants and children. J. Infect. Dis. 137:112–121, 1978.

Gold, R., Lepow, M. L., Goldschneider, I., Draper, T. F., and Gotschlich, E. C.: Clinical evaluation of group A and group C meningococcal polysaccharide vaccines in infants. J. Clin. Invest. 56:1536–1547, 1975.

Goldacre, M. J.: Acute bacterial meningitis in childhood. Incidence and mortality in a defined population. Lancet 1:28–31, 1976.

Goldberg, L. I.: Dopamine-clinical use of an endogenous catecholamine. New Eng. J. Med. 291:707–710, 1974.

Goldring, D., Hartmann, A. F., and Maxwell, R.: Diagnosis and management of severe infections in infants and children: A review of experiences since the introduction of sulfonamide therapy. III. Meningococcal infections. J. Pediat. 26:1–31, 1945.

Goldschneider, I., Gotschlich, E. C., and Artenstein, M. S.: Human immunity to the meningococcus. I. The role of humoral antibodies. J. Exp. Med. 129:1307–1326, 1969.

Gordon, J. E., and Norton, J. F.: Meningococcus meningitis in Detroit in 1928–1930. II. Clinical aspects of the epidemic. J. Prev. Med. 4:339–353, 1930.

Gordon, M. H., and Murray, E. G.: Identification of the meningococcus. J. Roy. Army Med. Corps 25:411–423, 1915.

Gotschlich, E. C., Goldschneider, I., and Artenstein, M. S.: Human immunity to the meningococcus. IV. Immunogenicity of group A and group C meningococcal polysaccharides in human volunteers. J. Exp. Med. 129:1367–1384, 1969.

Gotschlich, E. C., Goldschneider, I., and Artenstein, M. S.: Human immunity to the meningococcus. V. The effect of immunization with meningococcal group C polysaccharide on the carrier state. J. Exp. Med. 129:1385–1395, 1969.

Gotshall, R. A.: Conus medullaris syndrome after me-

ningococcal meningitis. New Eng. J. Med. 286:882–883, 1972.

Greenberg, L. W., and Kleinerman, E.: Neisseria lactamica meningitis. J. Pediat. 93:1061–1062, 1978.

Greenfield, S., Sheehe, P. R., and Feldman, H. A.: Meningococcal carriage in a population of "normal" families. J. Infect. Dis. 123:67–73, 1971.

Greenwood, B. M., Whittle, H. C., and Bryceson, A. D. M.: Allergic complications of meningococcal disease. II. Immunological investigations. Brit. Med. J. 2:737–740, 1973.

Greenwood, B. M., Whittle, H. C., and Dominic-Rajkovic, O.: Countercurrent immunoelectrophoresis in the diagnosis of meningococcal infections. Lancet 2:519–521, 1971.

Griffiss, J. M., and Brandt, B. L.: Disease due to serogroup W135 *Neisseria meningitidis*. Pediatrics 64:218–221, 1979.

Guttler, R. B., Counts, G. W., Avent, C. K., and Beaty, H. N.: Effect of rifampin and minocycline on meningococcal carrier rates. J. Infect. Dis. 124:199–205, 1971.

Hammerschlag, M. R., and Baltimore, R. S.: Infections in children due to Neisseria meningitidis serogroup 135. J. Pediat. 92:503–504, 1978.

Hardman, J. M.: Fatal meningococcal infections: The changing pathologic picture in the '60s. Milit. Med. 133:951–964, 1968.

Hardman, J. M., and Earle, K. M.: Myocarditis in 200 fatal meningococcal infections. Arch. Path. 87:318–325, 1969.

Heiman, H.: Epidemic cerebrospinal meningitis. A review of the recent literature. Am. J. Dis. Child. 2:281–286, 1911.

Herman, R. A., and Rubin, H. A.: Meningococcal pericarditis without meningitis presenting as tamponade. New Eng. J. Med. 290:143–144, 1974.

Herrick, W. W.: The intravenous serum treatment of epidemic cerebrospinal meningitis. Arch. Intern. Med. 21:541–563, 1918.

Hersh, J. H., Gold, R., and Lepow, M. L.: Meningococcal group Y pneumonia in an adolescent female. Pediatrics 64:222–224, 1979.

Hodes, H. L.: Care of the critically ill child: Endotoxic shock. Pediatrics 44:248–260, 1969.

Holt, L. E.: Observations on three hundred cases of acute meningitis in infants and young children. Am. J. Dis. Child. 1:26–36, 1911.

Horwitz, A., and Perroni, J.: Meningococcic meningitis in Santiago, Chili, 1941 to 1943. An epidemic of 4,464 cases. Arch. Intern. Med. 74:365–370, 1944.

Howell, W. W., and Cohen, S. A.: Intraventricular and subdural serum treatment of meningococcus meningitis in infancy. Am. J. Dis. Child. 24:427–432, 1922.

Hoyne, A. L.: Meningococcic meningitis. A new form of therapy. J.A.M.A. 104:980–983, 1935.

Irwin, R. S., Woelk, W. K., and Coudon, W. L., III.: Primary meningococcal pneumonia. Ann. Intern. Med. 82:493–497, 1975.

Ivler, D., Leedom, J. M., and Mathies, A. W., Jr.: In vitro susceptibility of Neisseria meningitidis to rifampin. Antimicrob. Agents. Chemother. 1969, Pp. 473–478.

Jacobson, J. A., and Fraser, D. W.: A simplified approach to meningococcal disease prophylaxis. J.A.M.A. 236:1053–1054, 1976.

Jacobson, J. A., Camargos, P. A. M., Ferreira, J. T., and McCormick, J. B.: The risk of meningitis among classroom contacts during an epidemic of meningococcal disease. Am. J. Epidemiol. 104:552–555, 1976.

Jensen, A. D., and Naidoff, M. A.: Bilateral meningococcal endophthalmitis. Arch. Ophthalmol. 90:396–398, 1973.

Jochmann, G.: Versuche zur Serodiagnostik und Serotherapie der epidemischen Genickstarre. Dtsch. Med. Wochenschr. 32:788, 1906.

Jubb, A. A.: Chemotherapy and serotherapy in cerebrospinal (meningococcal) meningitis. An analysis of 3,206 case reports. Brit. Med. J. 1:501–504, 1943.

Kaufman, B., Levy, H., Zaleznak, B. D., and Litvak, A. M.: Statistical analysis of 242 cases of meningococcus meningitis. J. Pediat. 38:705–716, 1951.

Kempf, G. F., Gilman, L. H., and Zerfas, L. G.: Meningococcic meningitis and epidemic meningo-encephalopathy. Reports of one hundred and twenty-two additional cases in the Indianapolis epidemic and of sixty-eight cases of an epidemic meningo-encephalopathy. Arch. Neurol. Psychiat. 29:433–453, 1933.

Khuri-Bulos, N.: Meningococcal meningitis following rifampin prophylaxis. Am. J. Dis. Child. 126:689–691, 1973.

Kisker, C. T., and Rush, R.: Circulating fibrin in meningococcemia. J. Pediat. 82:787–791, 1973.

Koppes, G. M., Ellenbogen, C., and Gebhart, R. J.: Group Y meningococcal disease in United States Air Force recruits. Am. J. Med. 62:661–666, 1977.

Kuhns, D. M., Nelson, C. T., Feldman, H. A., and Kuhn, L. R.: The prophylactic value of sulfadiazine in the control of meningococcic meningitis. J.A.M.A. 123:335–339, 1943.

Lasch, H. G., Krecke, H. J., Rodriguez-Erdman, F., Sessner, H. H., and Schutterle, G.: Verbrauchskoagulopathien. Folia Haemat. 6:325, 1961.

Lauer, B. A., and Fisher, C. E.: Neisseria lactamica meningitis. Am. J. Dis. Child. 130:198–199, 1976.

Lazar, N.: Early ocular complications of epidemic meningitis. Arch. Ophthalmol. 16:847–856, 1936.

Lebowitz, W. B., and Nespole, A. J.: Purulent pericarditis complicating meningococcal meningitis. Report of a child with cardiac tamponade and survival. Am. J. Dis. Child. 113:385–389, 1967.

Leedom, J. M., Ivler, D., Mathies, A. W., Thrupp, L. D., Portnoy, B., and Wehrle, P. F.: Importance of sulfadiazine resistance in meningococcal disease in civilians. New Eng. J. Med. 273:1395–1401, 1965.

Leeper, M. H., Dowling, H. F., Wehrle, P. F., Blatt, N. H., Spies, H. W., and Brown, M.: Meningococcic meningitis: Treatment with large doses of penicillin compared to treatment with gantrisin. J. Lab. Clin. Med. 40:891–900, 1952.

Leibel, R. L., Fangman, J. F., and Ostrovsky, M. C.: Chronic meningococcemia in childhood. Case report and review of the literature. Am. J. Dis. Child. 127:94–98, 1974.

Lepow, M. L., Goldschneider, I., Gold, R., Randolph, M., and Gotschlich, E. C.: Persistence of antibody following immunization of children with groups A and C meningococcal polysaccharide vaccines. Pediatrics 60:673–680, 1977.

Levin, S., Balagtas, R., Susmano, A., Edwards, L., and Dainauskas, J.: Meningococcus endocarditis at the site of Starr-Edwards mitral prosthesis. Arch. Intern. Med. 129:963–966, 1972.

Lewis, L. S.: Prognostic factors in acute meningococcaemia. Arch. Dis. Childh. 54:44–48, 1979.

Lim, D., Gewurz, A., Lint, T. F., Ghaze, M., Sepheri, B., and Gewurz, H.: Absence of the sixth component of complement in a patient with repeated episodes of

meningococcal meningitis. J. Pediat. 89:42–47, 1976.

Little, E. G.: Cases of purpura ending fatally associated with hemorrhage into the suprarenal capsules. Brit. J. Derm. 13:445, 1901.

Logan, W. R.: Meningococcal endocarditis: A review. Edin. Med. J. 52:49–60, 1945.

Makela, P. H., Kayhty, H., Weckstrom, P., Sivonen, A., and Renkonen, O. V.: Effect of group-A meningococcal vaccine in Army recruits in Finland. Lancet 2:883–886, 1975.

Manginello, F. P., Pascale, J. A., Wolfsdorf, J., and Klein, G. M.: Neonatal meningococcal meningitis and meningococcemia. Am. J. Dis. Child. 133:651–652, 1979.

Marks, M. I., Frasch, C. E., and Shapera, R. M.: Meningococcal colonization and infection in children and their household contacts. Am. J. Epidemiol. 109:563–571, 1979.

Martland, H. S.: Fulminating meningococcic infection with bilateral massive adrenal hemorrhage (the Waterhouse-Friderichsen syndrome). With special reference to the pathology, the medicolegal aspects and the incidence in adults. Arch. Path. 37:147–158, 1944.

Mason, W., Igdaloff, S., Friedman, R., and Wright, H. T., Jr.: Meningococcal sepsis with endophthalmitis. Am. J. Dis. Child. 133:1151–1152, 1979.

May, C. D.: Circulatory failure (shock) in fulminant meningococcal infection. An enquiry into the pathogenesis as an approach to rational therapy. Pediatrics 25:316–328, 1960.

McCormick, J. B., and Bennett, J. V.: Public health considerations in the management of meningococcal disease. Ann. Intern. Med. 83:883–886, 1975.

McGehee, W. G., Rapaport, S. I., and Hjort, P. F.: Intravascular coagulation in fulminant meningococcemia. Ann. Intern. Med. 67:250–260, 1967.

Melby, J. C., and Spink, W. W.: Comparative studies on adrenal cortical function and cortisol metabolism in healthy adults and in patients with shock due to infection. J. Clin. Invest. 37:1791–1798, 1958.

The Meningococcal Disease Surveillance Group: Analysis of endemic meningococcal disease by serogroup and evaluation of chemoprophylaxis. J. Infect. Dis. 134:201–204, 1976.

Merskey, C., Kleiner, G. J., and Johnson, A. J.: Quantitative estimations of split products of fibrinogen in human serum. Relations to diagnosis and treatment. Blood 28:1–18, 1966.

Migeon, C. J., Kenny, F. M., Hung, W., and Voorhess, M. L.: Study of adrenal function in children with meningitis. Pediatrics 40:163–182, 1967.

Miller, J. W., Seiss, E. E., and Feldman, H. A.: In vivo and in vitro resistance to sulfadiazine in strains of Neisseria meningitidis. J.A.M.A. 186:139–141, 1963.

Morse, J. R., Oretsky, M. I., and Hudson, J. A.: Pericarditis as a complication of meningococcal meningitis. Ann. Intern. Med. 74:212–217, 1971.

Naraqi, A., and Kabins, S. A.: Acute meningococcal pericarditis without meningitis. Arch. Intern. Med. 135:314–316, 1975.

Neal, J. B., Jackson, H. W., and Appelbaum, E.: Epidemic meningitis. A study of more than six hundred and fifty cases, with especial reference to sequelae. J.A.M.A. 87:1992–1995, 1926.

Niklasson, P. M., Lundbergh, P., and Strandell, T.: Prognostic factors in meningococcal disease. Scand. J. Infect. Dis. 3:17–25, 1971.

Nikoskelainen, J., Leino, A., Lahtonen, E., Kalliomaki, J. L., and Toivanen, A.: Is group-specific meningococcal vaccination resulting in epidemics caused by other groups of virulent meningococci? Lancet 2:403–405, 1978.

Norton, J. F., and Gordon, J. E.: Meningococcus meningitis in Detroit in 1928–1929. I. Epidemiology. J. Prev. Med. 4:207–214, 1971.

Novak, S. F., and Samuelson, C. W.: An unusual case of meningococcal meningitis. J. Pediat. 78:310–312, 1971.

Nugent, S. K., Bausher, J. A., Moxon, E. R., and Rogers, M. C.: Raised intracranial pressure. Its management in Neisseria meningitidis meningoencephalitis. Am. J. Dis. Child. 133:260–262, 1979.

Nussbaum, E., Jeyaranjan, T., and Feldman, F.: Primary meningococcal conjunctivitis followed by meningitis. J. Pediat. 92:784–785, 1978.

O'Connell, B.: Pericarditis following meningococcic meningitis. Am. J. Dis. Child. 126:265–267, 1973.

Peltola, H., Makela, P. H., Elo, O., Pettay, O., Renkonen, O-V., and Sivonen, A.: Vaccination against meningococcal group A disease in Finland 1974–75. Scand. J. Infect. Dis. 8:169–174, 1976.

Peltola, H., Makela, P. H., Kayhty, H., Jousimies, H., Herva, E., Hallstrom, K., Sivonen, A., Renkonen, O-V., Pettay, O., Karanko, V., Ahvonen, P., and Sarna, S.: Clinical efficacy of meningococcus group A capsular polysaccharide vaccine in children three months to five years of age. New Eng. J. Med. 297:686–691, 1977.

Petersen, B. H., Graham, J. A., and Brooks, G. F.: Human deficiency of the eighth component of complement. The requirement of C8 for serum *Neisseria gonorrhoeae* bactericidal activity. J. Clin. Invest. 57:283–290, 1976.

Pierce, H. I., and Cooper, E. B.: Meningococcal pericarditis. Clinical features and therapy in five patients. Arch. Intern. Med. 129:918–922, 1972.

Plazak, D. J.: Epidemic meningitis in 1670. Bull. Hist. Med. 25:457–459, 1951.

Rahal, J. J., Jr., and Simberkoff, M. S.: Bacterial and bacteriostatic action of chloramphenicol against meningeal pathogens. Antimicrob. Agents Chemother. 16:13–18, 1979.

Rammelkamp, C. H., and Keefer, C. S.: The absorption, excretion, and distribution of penicillin. J. Clin. Invest. 22:425–437, 1943.

Reller, L. B., MacGregor, R. R., and Beaty, H. N.: Bactericidal antibody after colonization with *Neisseria meningitidis*. J. Infect. Dis. 127:56–62, 1973.

Robboy, S. J.: Atrioventricular-node inflammation—mechanism of sudden death in protracted meningococcemia. New Eng. J. Med. 286:1091–1092, 1972.

Root, J. H.: A case of meningococcus meningitis with obstructive hydrocephalus in the newly born. Am. J. Dis. Child. 21:500–505, 1921.

Sahler, O. J. Z., and Wilfert, C. M.: Fever and petechiae with adenovirus type 7 infection. Pediatrics 53:233–235, 1974.

Salomon, H.: Ueber meningokakkenseptikamie. Klin. Wochenschr. 29:1045–1048, 1902.

Sayeed, Z. A., Bhaduri, V., Howell, E., and Meyers, H. L., Jr.: Gonococcal meningitis. A review. J.A.M.A. 219:1730–1731, 1972.

Schoenbach, E. B., and Phair, J. J.: The sensitivity of meningococci to sulfadiazine. Am. J. Hyg. 47:177–186, 1948.

Schumer, W.: Steroids in the treatment of clinical septic shock. Ann. Surg. 184:333–341, 1976.

Schwentker, F. F., Gelman, S., and Long, P. H.: The treatment of meningococcic meningitis with sulfanilamide. Preliminary report. J.A.M.A. 108:1407–1408, 1937.

Scott, L. P., Knox, D., Perry, L. W., and Pineros-Torres, F. J.: Meningococcal pericarditis. Report of 2 cases, 1 complicated by acute constrictive pericarditis. Am. J. Cardiol. 29:104–108, 1972.

Schackelford, P. G., Campbell, J., and Feigin, R. D.: Countercurrent immunoelectrophoresis in the evaluation of childhood infections. J. Pediat. 85:478–481, 1974.

Silverthorne, N., FitzGerald, J. G., and Fraser, D. T.: Studies on the meningococcus and meningococcus infection. J. Pediat. 15:491–502, 1939.

Slaterus, K. W.: Serologic typing of meningococci by means of microprecipitation. Antonie van Leeuwenhoek 27:305–315, 1961.

Smilack, J. D.: Group Y meningococcal disease. Twelve cases at an Army training center. Ann. Intern. Med. 81:740–745, 1974.

Snyderman, R., Durack, D. T., McCarty, G. A., Ward, F. E., and Meadows, L.: Deficiency of the fifth component of complement in human subjects. Clinical, genetic, and immunologic studies in a large kindred. Am. J. Med. 67:638–645, 1979.

Stiehm, E. R., and Damrosch, D. S.: Factors in the prognosis of meningococcal infection. Review of 63 cases with emphasis on recognition and management of the severely ill patients. J. Pediat. 68:457–467, 1966.

Stiehm, E. R., and Damrosch, D. S.: Neonatal meningococcal meningitis. Report of a case acquired in the nursery. J. Pediat. 68:654–656, 1966.

Subcommittee on the Family Neisseriaceae. Preliminary report 1950; Interim report 1953. Int. Bull. Bact. Nomencl. Taxonomy 4:95–105, 1954.

Swartz, M. M., and Dodge, P. R.: Bacterial meningitis—a review of selected aspects. New Eng. J. Med. 272:725–731, 779–787, 842–848, 898–902, 954–960, 1003–1010, 1965.

Swierczewski, J. A., Mason, E. J. Cabrera, P. B., and Liber, M.: Fulminating meningitis with Waterhouse-Friderichsen syndrome due to Neisseria gonorrhoeae. Am. J. Clin. Path. 54:202–204, 1970.

Taber, L. H., Yow, M. D., and Nieberg, F. G.: The penetration of broad-spectrum antibiotics into the cerebrospinal fluid. Ann. N.Y. Acad. Sci. 145:473–481, 1967.

Taubin, H. L., and Landsberg, L.: Gonococcal meningitis. New Eng. J. Med. 285:504–505, 1971.

Toews, W. H., and Bass, J. W.: Skin manifestations of meningococcal infection. An immediate indicator of prognosis. Am. J. Dis. Child. 127:173–176, 1974.

Vieusseux, G.: Memoire sur la maladie qui a regne a Geneve au printemps de 1805. J. Med. Chir. Pharm. 11:163, 1806.

Vital Statistics of the United States. Volume 2, Mortality, Part B. National Center for Health Statistics, Division of Vital Statistics, Washington, D.C., 1959–1967.

Vogler, L. B., Newman, S. L., Stroud, R. M., and Johnston, R. B., Jr.: Recurrent meningococcal meningitis with absence of the sixth component of complement: An evaluation of underlying immunologic mechanisms. Pediatrics 64:465–467, 1979.

Waterhouse, R.: A case of suprarenal apoplexy. Lancet 1:577–578, 1911.

Wehrle, P. F., Mathies, A. W., Leedom, J. M., and Ivler, D.: Bacterial meningitis. Ann. N.Y. Acad. Sci. 145:488–498, 1967.

Weichselbaum, A.: Ueber die aetiologie der akuten meningitis cerebrospinalis. Fortschr. Med. 5:573, 1887.

Weidmer, C. E., Dunkel, T. B., Pettyjohn, F. S., Smith, C. D., and Leibovitz, A.: Effectiveness of rifampin in eradicating the meningococcal carrier state in a relatively closed population: Emergence of resistant strains. J. Infect. Dis. 124:172–178, 1971.

Whittle, H. C., Tugwell, P., Egler, L. J., and Greenwood, B. M.: Rapid bacteriological diagnosis of pyogenic meningitis by latex agglutination. Lancet 2:619–621, 1974.

Whittle, H. C., Greenwood, B. M., Davidson, N. M., Tomkins, A., Tugwell, P., Warrell, D. A., Zalin, A., Bryceson, A. D. M., Parry, E. H. O., Brueton, M., Duggan, M., Oomen, J. W. V., and Rajkovic, A. D.: Meningococcal antigen in diagnosis and treatment of group A meningococcal infections. Am. J. Med. 58:823–828, 1975.

Wilhelm, D. J., and Cherubin, C.: Hypofibrinogenemia and thrombocytopenia with meningococcemia. Am. J. Dis. Child. 113:494–497, 1967.

Wilkins, J., and Wehrle, P. F.: Further characterization of responses of infants and children to meningococcal A polysaccharide vaccine. J. Pediat. 94:828–832, 1979.

Wolf, R. E., and Birbara, C.: Meningococcal infections at an army training center. Am. J. Med. 44:243–255, 1968.

Wright, I. S., De Sanctis, A. G., and Sheplar, A.: The determination of the value of serum in the treatment for meningococcal meningitis. Report of an illustrative series of cases. Am. J. Dis. Child. 38:730–740, 1929.

Yee, N. M., Katz, M., and Neu, H. C.: Meningitis, pneumonitis, and arthritis caused by Neisseria meningitidis group Y. J.A.M.A. 232:1354–1355, 1975.

Chapter Six

PNEUMOCOCCAL MENINGITIS

Streptococcus pneumoniae was discovered independently by Pasteur in France and by Sternberg in New York in 1881 and soon thereafter was shown to be the most common cause of lobar pneumonia. The organism is a gram-positive, non-motile coccus which often occurs in pairs in tissue or fluid specimens and has a well-defined capsule. They may be observed to form short chains, thus resembling other streptococci, and occasionally will become decolorized when stained and thereby appear to be gram-negative, allowing them to be confused with *Hemophilus influenzae* on morphologic examination. The presence of capsular material is believed to contribute to the virulence of the organism by inhibiting its phagocytosis and also provides the basis of the bacteriologic diagnostic technique referred to as the quellung, or "capsular swelling," reaction described by Neufeld in 1902. The test is done by mixing encapsulated bacteria with antiserum and methylene blue dye. Capsular swelling is observed microscopically with the addition of type-specific antipneumococcus antiserum but not with heterologous antiserum. *Streptococcus pneumoniae* is typically alpha-hemolytic on blood agar, on which it forms soft, moist, translucent colonies. It is not assigned a listing among the Lancefield groups of streptococci and is set apart primarily because of the spectrum of disease it gives rise to. The organism can be differentiated in the laboratory from other alpha-hemolytic streptococci by its bile solubility.

Streptococcus pneumoniae has now been separated into more than 80 different serotypes on the basis of type-specific capsular polysac-charides. In addition to pneumonia and acute suppurative meningitis, *Streptococcus pneumoniae* is a common cause of many different infections in infants and children, which most notably include otitis media, sinusitis, bacteremia without localization, and asymptomatic nasopharyngeal colonization. Periorbital or facial cellulitis, commonly caused by *Hemophilus influenzae* in infants and children, is only rarely caused by *Streptococcus pneumoniae* (Thirumoorthi et al.). Lobar pneumonia is the classic type of lower respiratory tract infection attributed to the pneumococcus. A number of variations in the type of pulmonary involvement are possible, however, including pneumonia in infants in which there is striking pneumatocele formation, indistinguishable from that associated with staphylococcal pneumonia in this age group (Asmar et al.).

Pneumococcal meningitis is one of the most common forms of suppurative meningitis at any age beyond the newborn period and was the single most common pathogen identified in the series which included all ages studied by Swartz and Dodge and in that of Carpenter and Petersdorf (Fig. 6–1). *Streptococcus pneumoniae* meningitis is also the most lethal among the three common types of meningitis that occur in infants beyond the neonatal period and in older children. In the newborn infant, the pneumococcus has generally been regarded to be a rare cause of invasive disease, and only infrequent reports of meningitis are found in the older literature (Coppolino and Gannone, Hogg and Bradley).

In the past few years, neonatal pneumococcal sepsis and meningitis either have in-

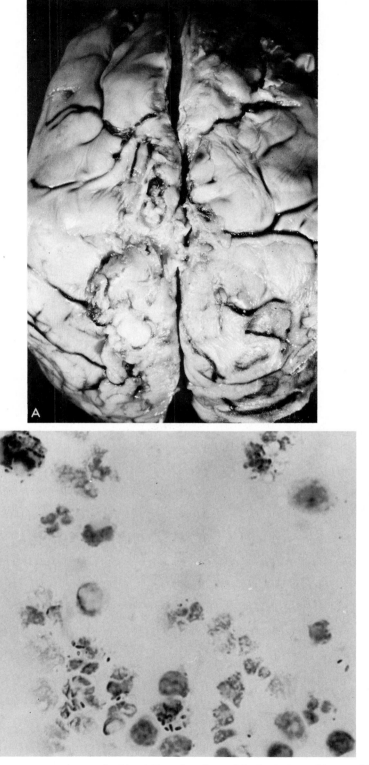

Figure 6–1.   Streptococcus pneumoniae meningitis. *A,* Dorsal surface of the brain in an 11-year-old boy who died in the acute stage of the disease. The fulminating illness in this child occurred several years after splenectomy was done because of hereditary spherocytosis. The surface of the brain is obscured by a dense, green-yellow, purulent exudate. There is marked cortical venous distension. *B,* CSF gram stain reveals many gram-positive diplococci, mostly intracellular in location.

creased in frequency or have been better identified by laboratory techniques. In most cases with onset of illness soon after birth, the infant is believed to acquire the organism from the mother's genital tract where it may be present asymptomatically or, less often, cause symptomatic infection (McCarthy and Cho, Weintraub and Otto). In one report, both the mother and her newborn infant simultaneously experienced pneumococcal meningitis, although the method by which the neonate became infected was not established (Tempest). *Streptococcus pneumoniae* sepsis with or without meningitis in the neonate can be identical to the early onset form of Group B *Streptococcus* sepsis (Bortolussi et al., Rhodes et al.). Clinical features include onset in the first day or so after birth with severe respiratory distress, apneic attacks, and hypotension or shock in some cases.

Streptococcus pneumoniae is one of the most common causes of meningitis in infants between four weeks and three months of age, and from three months until three years of age it ranks second only to *Hemophilus influenzae* as a cause of meningitis. While no age in childhood is spared, pneumococcal meningitis shows a predisposition to occur in the first and second years of life. Of 34 pediatric cases discussed by Hartman et al., 44 percent were in infants less than one year of age, while among 64 cases reported by Ross and Burke 65 percent were in infants under age one year. Laxer and Marks summarized 79 children with pneumococcal meningitis in which the median age at the time of the illness was 11 months and 59 percent of the cases occurred in the first 12 months of life. Of nine deaths from the illness in this series, six occurred in infants less than four months of age, indicative of the virulent nature of the infection in the early months of infancy.

Pneumococcal meningitis is usually rather abrupt in onset and frequently is associated with more rapid progression of symptoms and signs than occurs in most instances with *Hemophilus influenzae* meningitis. The infant as well as the older child may become seriously ill with deep coma, convulsions, and meningeal signs within hours after the very first signs of illness. Convulsions are especially common in infancy and can be the first sign indicative of the neurologic localization of the illness. Of the large series of cases of pneumococcal meningitis in infants and children reported by Laxer and Marks, seizures were described in the acute stage in 31 percent. Mental confusion, disorientation, or other abnormal behavioral characteristics may also be the first evidence of the infection in certain children. In common with all forms of bacterial meningitis, fever, irritability, vomiting, and headache are the most common initial complaints in the older child. Focal signs of cerebral dysfunction to a considerable degree reflect the inflammatory endarteritis and thrombophlebitis of meningeal, cortical, and subependymal vessels, which is commonly present with pneumococcal meningitis (Cairns and Russell).

Gram stain and culture of CSF remain the basis of identification of *Streptococcus pneumoniae* as the cause of acute meningitis. Because of the possibility of confusing *Streptococcus pneumoniae* with other *Streptococcus* species or with *Hemophilus influenzae* on gram-stained preparations, etiologic diagnosis should not be considered to be absolutely established until documentation by an additional confirmatory laboratory test. Latex particle agglutination is a useful and rapid method of demonstration of pneumococcal antigen in CSF (Whittle et al.). Countercurrent immunoelectrophoresis is also a rapid technique to demonstrate bacterial antigen in body fluids but frequently yields false negative results in CSF in patients with *Streptococcus pneumoniae* meningitis (Eckfeldt et al., Feigin et al.).

In many cases, meningitis occurs without an obvious primary focus of suppuration and results from meningeal invasion secondary to pneumococcal bacteremia. In the past few years, pneumococcal bacteremia without localization has been recognized in children with increasing frequency, most likely because of the more widespread use of blood cultures in infants and children with fever of unexplained origin (Burech et al., Burke et al., Heldrich, Torphy and Ray). As with pneumococcal infections in general in children, the majority of those with pneumococcal bacteremia in the absence of localized infection are caused by a relatively limited number of serotypes (Jacobs et al.). This condition, sometimes referred to as "occult" pneumococcal bacteremia, is found most often in infants from four months to two years of age and is characterized by fever of 102° to 105°F, blood leukocyte counts often as high as 20,000 per cu. mm. or greater with an increase in immature forms, and few specific other findings except for the occasional presence of a purulent nasal discharge. Seizures have been described with considerable frequency in such children, even though the

CSF examination reveals no evidence of meningitis. In some cases, a normal CSF examination performed because of unexplained fever is followed within a few days by clinical and CSF evidence of meningitis despite the administration of oral penicillin therapy in the interval (Myers et al., Torphy and Ray).

Myers et al. stressed the potential risk of the child with pneumococcal bacteremia for the eventual localization of the infection in the meninges or elsewhere unless adequate parenteral antibiotic treatment is administered. These observations emphasize the importance of blood culture and CSF examination before initiation of antibiotic therapy in children, and especially those in the infant age group who present with significant unexplained fever and peripheral blood leukocytosis with a shift to the left. Should the blood culture prove to be positive for *Streptococcus pneumoniae*, hospitalization and treatment with parenteral penicillin is indicated (Bratton et al., Klein).

Predisposing Factors

A notable feature in some cases of pneumococcal meningitis is its tendency to be associated with an obvious suppurative focus, a structural defect permitting communication of the subarachnoid space with an air-containing paracranial sinus or the nasopharynx, or an underlying systemic disorder associated with immunosuppression. Cancer patients are predisposed to bacteremia or meningitis from *Streptococcus pneumoniae*, as well as from other gram-positive and gram-negative organisms, especially when severely granulocytopenic (Chernik et al., Kilton et al.). Severe pneumococcal infection, including meningitis, was widely recognized in the past to be a serious threat to children with the nephrotic syndrome. Pneumococcal peritonitis was at one time a common cause of death in this disorder but is now rare because of the effectiveness of antibiotics and the common prompt response of childhood nephrosis to corticosteroid therapy.

In past years, lobar pneumococcal pneumonia was the most common primary focus resulting in meningitis. In his review of childhood meningitis in 1911, Holt included 22 cases due to the pneumococcus, of which 13 had pneumonia. With the decline of lobar pneumonia and its rapid resolution with antibiotic therapy, otitis media has become the most commonly identified primary focus in children with pneumococcal meningitis. Paranasal sinusitis, mastoiditis, and petrositis are other paracranial suppurative infections that may be associated with meningitis due to this organism.

Increased susceptibility to severe septic infection following splenectomy was first described by King and Shumacker in 1952. With further observations, the common features of post-splenectomy infection gradually emerged, which included the most frequent occurrence of the septic illness within two years after removal of the spleen, the age group of greatest risk being children under four years of age, the common occurrence of fulminating infection terminating in death, and the high incidence of infection caused by the pneumococcus (Diamond, Eraklis et al., Erickson et al.). While *Streptococcus pneumoniae* continues to be the most common organism causing fulminating post-splenectomy sepsis or meningitis, the infection can also result from other *Streptococcus* species, *Hemophilus influenzae*, and *Neisseria meningitidis*. The occurrence of fulminating bacterial infections in patients with absence of the spleen is indicative of the spleen's importance as a site for the mechanical filtering of encapsulated bacteria from the circulation as well as its role in the formation of humoral antibody to capsular antigen and in the production of tuftsin and properdin, which serve as opsonins (Eichner).

It has been estimated that the incidence of post-splenectomy sepsis is approximately 25 percent in patients splenectomized with thalassemia major, 10 percent in children whose spleens are removed for staging for Hodgkin's disease, and 2 percent in patients following splenectomy for idiopathic thrombocytopenic purpura (Chilcote et al., Dickerman). Children with congenital asplenia, likewise, are at greater risk than normal, although the degree of danger in this group is unclear (Kevy et al., Waldman et al.). Younger children are especially susceptible to serious and rapidly progressive post-splenectomy septic infection although the condition is now well-known in adults (Gopal and Bisno, Weitzman and Aisenberg). While most such illnesses occur relatively soon after splenic removal, it has been described as late as 25 years following splenectomy (Grinblat and Gilboa).

The typical pneumococcal infection following splenectomy or in the otherwise asplenic patient is manifested by chills, fever, vomiting, and sometimes abdominal pain. Within hours to a day or so, there is rapid deterioration, which may include hypotension, shock, convulsions, and laboratory evidence of disseminated intravascular coagulation (Coonrod and Leach, Wenk and Dutta). The mortality rate is high and the clinical course often is unyielding to antibiotic therapy. Gram-positive diplococci can sometimes be visualized on peripheral blood smear, indicative of the massive bacteremia characteristic of this condition. The CSF will reveal no evidence of meningitis in some cases, but in others the fluid will either be cloudy or appear clear and contain few leukocytes but with abundant microorganisms.

The risk of overwhelming septic infection has been found to be highest in patients undergoing splenectomy for diseases associated with depressed reticuloendothelial function, such as thalassemia major, Wiskott-Aldrich syndrome, and the histiocytoses. It has become clear, however, that there is some degree of increased risk when the spleen is surgically removed because of splenic trauma, for idiopathic thrombocytopenic purpura, renal transplantation, and for staging in patients' with Hodgkin's disease (Balfanz et al., Bourgault et al., Gopal and Bisno, Weitzman and Aisenberg).

Homozygous sickle cell disease is an additional disorder associated with a marked predisposition to pneumococcal sepsis and meningitis (Barrett-Conner, Seeler et al.). Robinson and Watson, in 1966, reported that when meningitis occurs in children with sickle cell disease, it is usually caused by *Streptococcus pneumoniae*. In their series, 87 percent of cases of meningitis complicating sickle cell disease were pneumococcal in origin. The high incidence of the pneumococcus as a cause of meningitis with this disease is especially striking because most cases occur in children between one and five years of age, an age span when *Hemophilus influenzae* is normally the most prevalent cause of meningitis. Pneumococcal meningitis complicating sickle cell disease is remarkably fulminating in some cases (Seeler et al.) and can be a recurrent illness in others (Griesemer et al., Overturf et al.).

There has been abundant speculation as to the nature of the host immunity defect which predisposes children with sickle cell disease to *Streptococcus pneumoniae* sepsis and meningitis. Deficient serum opsonizing activity has been demonstrated in sickle cell patients (Bjornson et al., Winkelstein and Drachman), an abnormality postulated by Johnston to be due to a defect in the function of the com-

plement system. Splenic dysfunction, described as functional asplenia by Pearson et al., in concert with the defect in phagocytosis mentioned above, is presumed to represent the basic defects which predispose children with sickle cell disease to the high incidence of severe pneumococcal infection.

Recurrent Pneumococcal Meningitis

Recurrent attacks of pneumococcal meningitis are particularly common in patients with structural defects that permit communication of certain paracranial air-containing spaces or the nasopharynx to the subarachnoid space. A history of head trauma with skull fracture is important in patients with this condition, as it suggests the possibility of a post-traumatic defect in the cribriform plate, through the floor of the sella turcica into the sphenoid sinus, or in the mastoid region, resulting in otorrhea. The fracture, also, may involve the frontal or ethmoid sinuses, allowing direct access of bacteria into the subarachnoid space (Hand and Sanford) (Fig. 6–2). The identification of intracranial air on x-ray or computed tomography following head injury, so-called traumatic pneumocephalus, implies the presence of a fracture involving an air-containing sinus or mastoid even though the fracture site cannot always be identified (Kahn and Daywitt, Turner) (Fig. 6–3). Pneumocephalus does not necessarily imply a dural tear has occurred, as the air can be confined to an extradural location. Air within the subdural space, within the brain, or in the ventricles usually does indicate the presence of a dural laceration and renders the patient at risk for the development of acute meningitis. *Streptococcus pneumoniae* is the predominant cause of post-traumatic meningitis, followed by a wide variety of gram-positive and gram-negative pathogens. Among 91 cases of bacterial meningitis complicating craniofacial trauma reported by Appelbaum (1960), 47 were pneumococcal in origin.

Congenital defects of the cribriform plate can also be a cause of CSF rhinorrhea and recurrent episodes of bacterial meningitis (Galloway and Chambers). Congenital otic defects can result in CSF leak through the footplate of the stapes (Rice and Wagoner, Schultz and Stool, Stool et al.), giving rise to otorrhea and a syndrome manifested by unilateral deafness and recurrent meningitis. Biggers et al. described an infant with an ac-

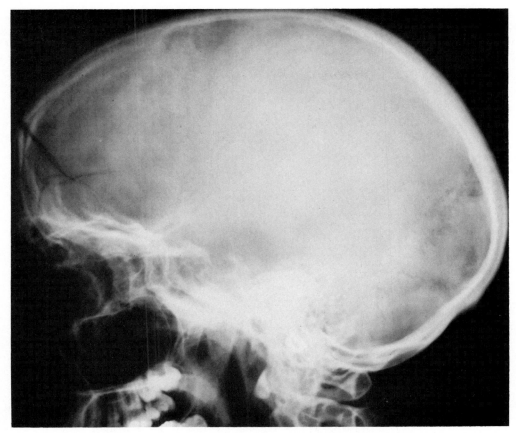

Figure 6–2.   Stellate skull fracture extending into the frontal sinus of a 17-year-old girl who sustained craniocerebral trauma in an automobile accident. She recovered completely but had intermittent CSF rhinorrhea for 2 years after the injury. She then developed severe pneumococcal meningitis, which was complicated by a frontal lobe abscess.

quired facial palsy who subsequently had repeated attacks of pneumococcal meningitis. Although CSF otorrhea was not demonstrated, the child was found to have a fistula of the stapedial footplate and partial labyrinthine agenesis. Surgical correction of the fistula prevented further neurologic infections. A congenital abnormality of the cochlea, the so-called Mondini defect, can be a predisposing cause of recurrent bacterial meningitis. Communication between the subarachnoid space and a persistently large cochlear aqueduct with an anomalous cochlea can lead to CSF accumulation in the middle ear, which is transmitted to the nasopharynx via the eustachian tube if the tympanic membrane is intact (Carter et al.).

Identification of the site of a CSF fistula can be exceedingly difficult in children with recurrent pneumococcal meningitis. Hoyne and Schultz described an adult with five episodes of meningitis, four caused by the pneumococcus, which occurred following head injury. No anatomic defects could be found but postmortem examination revealed two small perforations of the cribriform plate leading to the ethmoid air cells. Barsky reported a child with seven attacks of pneumococcal meningitis preceded by head trauma but without identification of a fistulous site despite an extensive evaluation. An adult who experienced 11 attacks due to five serotypes of *Streptococcus pneumoniae* was discussed by Whitecar et al., also without the establishment of the source of origin of the infectious agent. An unusual source of contamination of the CSF resulting in pneumococcal meningitis is accidental introduction of the organism during myelography or pneumoencephalography (Rose). Although the source of pneumococci in such cases is in question, the presumption is that it is secondary to droplet contamination from the nasopharynx of the operator.

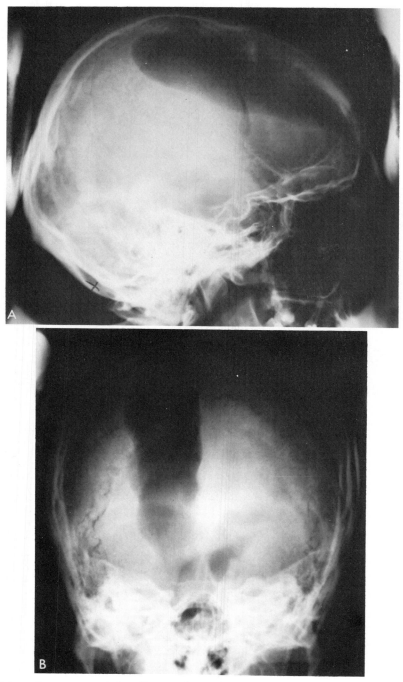

Figure 6–3.   Traumatic pneumocephalus. Young adult male with craniocerebral trauma from a fall. X-rays revealed fractures of the facial bones and the frontal sinus. Plain skull films, *A* and *B*, show intracranial air over the cerebral convexity which presumably gained entrance to the intracranial compartment from the frontal sinus. This roentgen finding usually indicates communication of intracranial structures with one of the air-containing sinuses. Such patients are at risk to develop meningitis, and especially pneumococcal meningitis, until the defect heals or is surgically corrected.

Methods of diagnosis of a CSF fistula include observation for rhinorrhea with the patient in the sitting position, x-rays including stereo views and laminograms when indicated, plus additional more specific studies. Nasal secretions can be tested for glucose with glucose oxidase sticks (Dextrostix), with a positive reaction suggesting the presence of cerebrospinal fluid. Isotope cisternography (Di Chiro et al.) is a useful method for diagnosis of rhinorrhea, and pantopaque basal cisternography has been helpful in cases with otorrhea. Metrizamide computed tomography is probably superior to the above methods for the anatomic localization of an intracranial CSF fistula and is associated with relatively few side effects (Drayer et al.). When the site of a cerebrospinal fluid leak can be demonstrated, it should be surgically corrected with repair of the dural defect. Surgical exploration and search for a previously unidentified fistula, however, is not usually rewarding because of the many locations on either side where such defects may exist.

Mortality

Streptococcus pneumoniae meningitis remains a serious threat to life despite the availability of potentially curative therapy. The mortality rate of the disease has been found to be considerably higher in certain tropical regions than elsewhere, although the reason is uncertain. Baird et al. recorded a mortality rate of 51 percent among 207 patients of all ages with pneumococcal meningitis in Nigeria. Because the outcome of other types of acute meningitis in this geographic region was found to be approximately the same as in the United States, the higher death rate from meningitis caused by the pneumococccus was felt not be be explained on the basis of suboptimal medical care.

The case fatality rate in this country is age-related to a certain degree, with age one to 20 years being the most favorable period regarding survival. Even with modern therapeutic measures, Spink and Su found a mortality rate of 19 percent in children 10 years of age or less, while in adults over age 40 years the mortality was 53 percent. In a study of pneumococcal meningitis extending from 1952 to 1964 which included 130 cases, Weiss et al. established a mortality rate of 21 percent in infants less than one year of age, 17 percent in those one to 29 years, and 53 percent in patients over 50 years of age. The increased fatality rate in the older age group in this series was largely explained by the increased prevalence of associated disease. Of 79 infants and children with pneumococcal meningitis reported by Laxer and Marks, the mortality rate was 10.8 percent, with all deaths occurring in infants less than one year of age and most in those under four months of age.

Although the mortality rate of pneumococcal meningitis remains disturbingly high, it has been favorably influenced by the development of new therapeutic measures. Before the introduction of sulfonamides, only infrequent recoveries from this disease were recorded and in many of those, the accuracy of diagnosis was questioned. With the development of the sulfonamides and their use in conjunction with type-specific antipneumococcal serum, the survival rate was only modestly improved. Ruegsegger reviewed the literature in this regard and stated that the mortality rate with sulfonamide therapy was approximately 73 percent, a figure which correlated well with those in other publications (Dowling et al. 1942, Neal et al.).

Treatment

The introduction of penicillin therapy for pneumococcal meningitis initially resulted in only slight improvement in the outcome, although the dosages used were low and were usually combined with intrathecal penicillin (Hartmann et al. 1945). With penicillin doses of 50,000 to 400,000 units per day plus intrathecal penicillin, the mortality rate remained between 64 and 80 percent (Alexander et al., Sweet et al., White et al.). The presumed requirement for intrathecal penicillin was based on the concept that systemically administered penicillin did not gain entrance into the CSF (Rammelkamp and Keefer). Despite numerous problems with the use of intrathecal penicillin, it remained part of the regimen for pneumococcal meningitis until approximately 1948, when it was shown that results were at least as good with systemically administered penicillin alone (Lowrey and Quilligan). The subsequent use of larger quantities of penicillin, one million units intramuscularly every two hours, resulted in a lower mortality rate of 38 percent in the series of Dowling et al. (1949).

Combinations of antibiotics seemed to offer no further advantage, and in 1951 Lepper and Dowling showed that, with penicillin alone, the mortality rate of pneumococcal meningitis was approximately 30 percent but with a combination of penicillin and chlortetracycline the mortality rate rose to 79 percent. The clinical importance of antagonism by chloramphenicol with the bactericidal action of penicillin against *Streptoccus pneumoniae* has been a debatable topic since that time, but additional studies have indicated that such antagonism can occur (Jawetz et al., Wallace et al.). The antagonistic interaction can, perhaps, be diminished by administering penicillin first, followed by the administration of chloramphenicol. Despite the uncertainty of the significance of this drug interaction, it is advisable not to use the combination of these two antibiotics when the diagnosis of pneumococcal meningitis is definite.

Penicillin administered intravenously is the current drug of choice for pneumococcal meningitis. The dosage is 250,000 units per kilogram per day, up to 20 million units per day, administered every four hours over a 20-minute time period. The tendency for relapse to occur with short-term therapy indicates the need to continue treatment for a minimum of two weeks and occasionally for three weeks. For those who are allergic to the penicillins, chloramphenicol is the most acceptable alternative. The use of corticosteroids has been advocated by some but with little established evidence of benefit.

Streptococcus pneumoniae for many years had been considered to be uniformly highly sensitive to penicillin but in 1967 in Australia, a pneumococcal isolate from a patient with hypogammaglobulinemia was found to be relatively resistant to penicillin (Hansman and Bullen). Reports of poorly responding or relapsing meningitis caused by pneumococcal strains with decreased susceptibility to penicillin subsequently appeared from other countries, including the United States (Appelbaum et al., Naraqi et al.). Unlike the great majority of penicillin-sensitive pneumococcal isolates in which the minimum inhibitory concentration of penicillin has been found to be 0.01 to 0.1 μg per ml., in these initial cases with decreased sensitivity to penicillin the minimum inhibitory concentrations ranged from 0.2 to 1 μg per ml. The "intermediate" sensitivity of these organisms might still allow success with extraneurologic infections treated with higher than usual doses of penicillin. With meningitis, however, penicillin might be expected to be inadequate because the CSF concentration of penicillin with conventional doses would only approximately equal the minimum inhibitory concentration (Hieber and Nelson). Pneumococcal isolates fully resistant to penicillin have more recently been identified with minimum inhibitory concentrations of 1 to 4 μg per ml. (Cates et al., Jacobs et al.).

In the majority of instances, pneumococci found to have decreased sensitivity or frank resistance to penicillin have come from patients who had received long-term antibiotic therapy. The mechanism accounting for the decreased penicillin sensitivity remains unknown, and all isolates have been negative for β-lactamase production. The incidence of penicillin-resistant pneumococci in North America is uncertain, but studies indicate that it is somewhat less than 3 percent of isolates (Dixon et al., Gartner and Michaels). Its occurrence has been sufficiently frequent that certain authors have proposed that in vitro sensitivity testing of *Streptococcus pneumoniae* be performed when the organism causes serious infection or infection not promptly responding to therapy (Ahronheim et al., Cates et al., Gartner and Michaels).

Treatment of pneumococcal meningitis caused by an organism with decreased sensitivity or resistance to penicillin creates an obvious problem in regard to the selection of the drug regimen and depends considerably on the minimum inhibitory concentration. Those only slightly less sensitive than customary can probably be successfully treated with increased doses of penicillin, in the range of 500,000 units per kilogram per day. Penicillin in combination with probenecid, which inhibits transport of penicillin from the CSF, thus raising the CSF level (Craft et al., Dacey and Sande), has also been considered (Ahronheim et al., Hansman et al.). When the organism is more resistant, chloramphenicol is the drug of choice, although isolates resistant to this antimicrobial were identified in France in 1973 (Dang-Van et al.) and have been encountered elsewhere (Appelbaum et al.). Other antibiotics which might be considered with penicillin-insensitive pneumococcal meningitis include rifampin and vancomycin.

A polyvalent pneumococcal polysaccharide vaccine (Pneumovax) was commercially released in February, 1978. The 14-valent vaccine contains capsular polysaccharides derived from the 14 most prevalent types of pneumococci, which account for 75 to 80 percent of pneumococcal disease. The vaccine has been found to be quite safe, although pain and erythema at the site of injection are common. The duration of protection provided by the vaccine is uncertain, but it is believed that elevated antibody titers will persist for at least two years after immunization (Austrian).

Specific indications for the use of pneumococcal vaccine have not been clearly defined, although reasonable guidelines have been established. Mass immunization of the population generally is not advised, nor is the use of the vaccine during pregnancy. It is not recommended for children under two years of age because of the disparate antibody responses in infancy to certain pneumococcal antigens within the vaccine (Cowan et al.). The vaccine is recommended for children with sickle-cell disease and for patients following splenectomy or with functional asplenia (Ammann et al.). Because pneumococcal serotypes not included in the vaccine can result in overwhelming post-splenectomy infection, the use of the vaccine does not entirely replace penicillin prophylaxis, especially in younger children. Immunization is also advised for children over two years of age with certain chronic diseases, including malignant disorders, immune deficiency states, diabetes mellitus, and conditions with impaired renal or hepatic function in which there is an increased risk of pneumococcal infection. Antibody response to pneumococcal vaccine has been found to be impaired in patients with Hodgkin's disease when the vaccine is administered during or soon after treatment with irradiation and chemotherapeutic agents (Minor et al., Siber et al.). For this reason, it is recommended that such patients be immunized before initiation of the therapeutic regimen (Siber et al.). Vaccine-produced antipneumococcal antibodies are not believed to be bactericidal but serve primarily to enhance phagocytosis of bacteria by leukocytes (Austrian). The value of the vaccine, therefore, in children with severe and persistent granulocytopenia or with leukocyte-functional abnormalities is in question.

REFERENCES

Ahronheim, G. A., Reich, B., and Marks, M. I.: Penicillin-insensitive pneumococci. Case report and review. Am. J. Dis. Child. 133:187–191, 1979.

Alexander, J. D., Jr., Flippin, H. F., and Eisenberg, G. M.: Pneumococcic meningitis. Study of one hundred two cases. Arch. Intern. Med. 91:440–447, 1953.

Ammann, A. J., Addiego, J., Wara, D. W., Lubin, B., Smith, W. B., and Mentzer, W. C.: Polyvalent pneumococcal-polysaccharide immunization of patients with sickle-cell anemia and patients with splenectomy. New Eng. J. Med. 297:897–900, 1977.

Appelbaum, E.: Meningitis following trauma to the head and face. J.A.M.A. 173:1818–1822, 1960.

Appelbaum, P. C., Bhamjee, A., Scragg, J. N., Hallett, A. F., Bowen, A. J., and Cooper, R. C.: Streptococcus pneumoniae resistant to penicillin and chloramphenicol. Lancet 2:995–997, 1977.

Asmar, B. I., Thirumoorthi, M. C., and Dajani, A. S.: Pneumococcal pneumonia with pneumatocele formation. Am. J. Dis. Child. 132:1091–1093, 1978.

Austrian, R.: Pneumococcal vaccine: Development and prospects. Am. J. Med. 67:547–549, 1979.

Baird, D. R., Whittle, H. C., and Greenwood, B. M.: Mortality from pneumococcal meningitis. Lancet 2:1344–1346, 1976.

Balfanz, J. R., Nesbit, M. E., Jr., Jarvis, C., and Krivit, W.: Overwhelming sepsis following splenectomy for trauma. J. Pediat. 88:458–460, 1976.

Barrett-Connor, E.: Bacterial infection and sickle cell anemia. An analysis of 250 infections in 166 patients and a review of the literature. Medicine 50:97–112, 1971.

Barsky, P.: Seven recurrent attacks of pneumococcic meningitis with recovery. Canad. Med. Assoc. J. 72:210–216, 1955.

Biggers, W. P., Howell, N. N., Fisher, N. D., and Himadi, G. M.: Congenital ear anomalies associated with otic meningitis. Arch. Otolaryngol. 97:399–401, 1973.

Bjornson, A. B., Gaston, M. H., and Zellner, C. L.: Decreased opsonization for Streptococcus pneumoniae in sickle cell disease: Studies on selected complement components and immunoglobulins. J. Pediat. 91:371–378, 1977.

Bortolussi, R., Thompson, T. R., and Ferrieri, P.: Early-onset pneumococcal sepsis in newborn infants. Pediatrics 60:352–355, 1977.

Bourgault, A-M., Van Scoy, R. E., Wilkowske, C. J., Zincke, H., and Sterioff, S.: Severe infection due to Streptococcus pneumoniae in asplenic renal transplant patients. Mayo Clin. Proc. 54:123–126, 1979.

Bratton, L., Teele, D. W., and Klein, J. O.: Outcome of unsuspected pneumococcemia in children not initially admitted to the hospital. J. Pediat. 90:703–706, 1977.

Burech, D. L., Koranyi, K., Haynes, R. E., and Kramer, R. N.: Pneumococcal bacteremia associated with gingival lesions in infants. Am. J. Dis. Child. 129:1283–1284, 1975.

Burke, J. P., Klein, J. O., Gezon, H. M., and Finland, M.: Pneumococcal bacteremia. Review of 111 cases, 1957–1969, with special reference to cases with undetermined focus. Am. J. Dis. Child. 121:353–359, 1971.

Cairns, H., and Russell, D. S.: Cerebral arteritis and phlebitis in pneumococcal meningitis. J. Path. Bact. 58:649–665, 1946.

Carpenter, R. R., and Petersdorf, R. G.: The clinical spectrum of bacterial meningitis. Am. J. Med. 33:262–275, 1962.

Carter, B. L., Wolpert, S. M., and Karmody, C. S.: Recurrent meningitis associated with an anomaly of the inner ear. Neuroradiology 9:55–61, 1975.

Cates, K. L., Gerrald, J. M., Giebink, G. S., Lund, M. E., Blecker, E. Z., Lau, S., O'Leary, M. C., Krivit, W., and Quie, P. G.: A penicillin-resistant pneumococcus. J. Pediat. 93:624–626, 1978.

Chernik, N. L., Armstrong, D., and Posner, J. B.: Central nervous system infections in patients with cancer. Medicine 52:563–581, 1973.

Chilcote, R. R., Baehner, R. L., and Hammond, D.: Septicemia and meningitis in children splenectomized for Hodgkin's disease. New Eng. J. Med. 295:798–800, 1976.

Coppolino, J. F., and Gannone, P.: Pneumococcic meningitis in the newly born. A case in a two day old infant. Am. J. Dis. Child. 47:378–379, 1934.

Coonrod, J. D., and Leach, R. P.: Antigenemia in fulminant pneumococcemia. Ann. Intern. Med. 84:561–563, 1976.

Cowan, M. J., Ammann, A. J., Wara, D. W., Howie, V. M., Schultz, L., Doyle, N., and Kaplan, M.: Pneumococcal polysaccharide immunization of infants and children. Pediatrics 62:721–727, 1978.

Craft, J. C., Feldman, W. E., and Nelson, J. D.: Clinicopharmacological evaluation of amoxicillin and probenecid against bacterial meningitis. Antimicrob. Agents Chemother. 16:346–352, 1979.

Dacey, R. G., and Sande, M. A.: Effect of probenecid on cerebrospinal fluid concentrations of penicillin and cephalosporin derivatives. Antimicrob. Agents Chemother. 6:437–441, 1974.

Dang-Van, A., Tiraby, G., Acar, J. F., Shaw, W. V., and Bouanchaud, D. H.: Chloramphenicol resistance in *Streptococcus pneumoniae:* Enzymatic acetylation and possible plasmid linkage. Antimicrob. Agents Chemother. 13:577–583, 1978.

Diamond, L. K.: Splenectomy in childhood and the hazard of overwhelming infection. Pediatrics 43:886–889, 1969.

Di Chiro, G., Ommaya, A. K., Asburn, W. L., and Briner, W. H.: Isotope cisternography in the diagnosis and follow-up of cerebrospinal fluid rhinorrhea. J. Neurosurg. 28:522–529, 1968.

Dickerman, J. D.: Splenectomy and sepsis. A warning. Pediatrics 63:938–941, 1979.

Dixon, J. M. S., Lipinski, A. E., and Graham, M. E. P.: Detection and prevalence of pneumococci with increased resistance to penicillin. Canad. Med. Assoc. J. 117:1159–1161, 1977.

Dowling, H. F., Dauer, C. C., Feldman, H. A., and Hartman, C. R.: Pneumococcal meningitis. A study of seventy-two cases. New Eng. J. Med. 226:1015–1018, 1942.

Dowling, H. F., Sweet, L. K., Robinson, J. A., Zellers, W. W., and Hirsh, H. L.: The treatment of pneumococcal meningitis with massive doses of systemic penicillin. Am. J. Med. Sci. 217:149–156, 1949.

Drayer, B. P., Wilkins, R. H., Boehnke, M., Horton, J. A., and Rosenbaum, A. E.: Cerebrospinal fluid rhinorrhea demonstrated by metrizamide CT cisternography. Am. J. Roentgenol. 129:149–151, 1977.

Eckfeldt, J., Ederer, G. M., and Oetjen, R.: Counterimmunoelectrophoresis and bacterial meningitis. J.A.M.A. 239:615–616, 1978.

Eichner, E. R.: Splenic function: Normal, too much and too little. Am. J. Med. 66:311–320, 1979.

Eraklis, A. J., Kevy, S. V., Diamond, L. K., and Gross, R. E.: Hazard of overwhelming infection after splenectomy in childhood. New Eng. J. Med. 276:1225–1229, 1967.

Erickson, W. E., Burgert, E. O., Jr., and Lynn, H. B.: The hazard of infection following splenectomy in children. Am. J. Dis. Child 116:1–12, 1968.

Feigin, R. D., Wong, M., Shackelford, P. G., Stechenberg, B. W., Dunkle, L. M., and Kaplan, S.: Countercurrent immunoelectrophoresis of urine as well as CSF and blood for diagnosis of bacterial meningitis. J. Pediat. 89:773–775, 1976.

Galloway, W. H., and Chambers, W.: Pneumococcal

meningitis. Skull defects as an etiological factor. Lancet 2:68–70, 1953.

Gartner, J. C., and Michaels, R. H.: Meningitis from a pneumococcus moderately resistant to penicillin. J.A.M.A. 241:1707–1709, 1979.

Gopal, V., and Bisno, A. L.: Fulminant pneumococcal infections in 'normal' asplenic hosts. Arch. Intern. Med. 137:1526–1530, 1977.

Griesemer, D. A., Winkelstein, J. A., and Luddy, R.: Pneumococcal meningitis in patients with a major sickle hemoglobinopathy. J. Pediat. 92:82–84, 1978.

Grinblat, J., and Gilboa, Y.: Overwhelming pneumococcal sepsis 25 years after splenectomy. Am. J. Med. Sci. 270:523–524, 1975.

Hand, W. L., and Sanford, J. P.: Posttraumatic bacterial meningitis. Ann. Intern. Med. 72:869–874, 1970.

Hansman, D., and Bullen, M. M.: A resistant pneumococcus. Lancet 2:264–265, 1967.

Hansman, D., Glasgow, H., Sturt, J., Devitt, L., and Douglas, R.: Increased resistance to penicillin of pneumococci isolated from man. New Eng. J. Med. 284:175–177, 1971.

Hartmann, A. F., Love, F. M., Wolff, D., and Kendall, B. S.: Diagnosis and management of severe infections in infants and children: A review of experiences since the introduction of sulfonamide therapy. IV. Pneumococcus meningitis. J. Pediat. 27:115–173, 1945.

Heldrich, F. J., Jr.: Diplococcus pneumoniae bacteremia. Am. J. Dis. Child. 119:12–17, 1970.

Hieber, J. P., and Nelson, J. D.: A pharmacologic evaluation of penicillin in children with purulent meningitis. New Eng. J. Med. 297:410–413, 1977.

Hogg, P., and Bradley, C. D.: Pneumococcus meningitis in the newborn. J. Pediat. 26:406–410, 1945.

Holt, L. E.: Observations on three hundred cases of acute meningitis in infants and young children. Am. J. Dis. Child. 1:26–36, 1911.

Hoyne, A. L., and Schultz, A.: Multiple attacks of meningitis. Report of a case with autopsy. Am. J. Med. Sci. 214:673–676, 1947.

Jacobs, M. R., Koornhof, H. J., Robins-Browne, R. M., Stevenson, C. M., Vermaak, Z. A., Freiman, I., Miller, G. B., Witcomb, M. A., Isaacson, M., Ward, J. I., and Austrian, R.: Emergence of multiply resistant pneumococci. New Eng. J. Med. 299:735–740, 1978.

Jacobs, N. M., Lerdkachornsuk, S., and Metzger, W. I.: Pneumococcal bacteremia in infants and children: A ten-year experience at the Cook County Hospital with special reference to the pneumococcal serotypes isolated. Pediatrics 64:296–299, 1979.

Jawetz, E., Gunnison, J. B., Speck, R. S., and Coleman, V. R.: Studies on antibiotic synergism and antagonism. Arch. Intern. Med. 87:349–359, 1951.

Johnston, R. B., Jr.: Increased susceptibility to infection in sickle cell disease: Review of its occurrence and possible causes. South. Med. J. 67:1342–1348, 1974.

Kahn, R. J., and Daywitt, A. L.: Traumatic pneumocephalus. Am. J. Roentgenol. 90:1171–1175, 1963.

Kevy, S. V., Tefft, M., Vawter, G. F., and Rosen, F. S.: Hereditary splenic hypoplasia. Pediatrics 42:752–757, 1968.

Kilton, L. J., Fossieck, B. E., Jr., Cohen, M. H., and Parker, R. H.: Bacteremia due to gram-positive cocci in patients with neoplastic disease. Am. J. Med. 66:596–602, 1979.

King, H., and Shumacker, H. B., Jr.: Splenic studies. I. Susceptibility to infection after splenectomy performed in infancy. Ann. Surg. 136:239–242, 1952.

Klein, J. O.: Pneumococcal bacteremia in the young child. Am. J. Dis. Child. 129:1266–1267, 1975.

Laxer, R. M., and Marks, M. I.: Pneumococcal meningitis in children. Am. J. Dis. Child. 131:850–853, 1977.

Lepper, M. H., and Dowling, H. F.: Treatment of pneumococcic meningitis with penicillin compared with penicillin plus aureomycin. Arch. Intern. Med. 88:489–494, 1951.

Lowrey, G. H., and Quilligan, J. J., Jr.: The treatment of pneumococcal meningitis without intrathecal penicillin. J. Pediat. 33:336–341, 1948.

McCarthy, V. P., and Cho, C. T.: Endometritis and neonatal sepsis due to *Streptococcus pneumoniae*. Obstet. Gynecol. 53(Suppl.):475–495, 1979.

Minor, D. R., Schiffman, G., and McIntosh, L. S.: Response of patients with Hodgkin's disease to pneumococcal vaccine. Ann. Intern. Med. 90:887–892, 1979.

Myers, M. G., Wright, P. F., Smith, A. L., and Smith, D. H.: Complications of occult pneumococcal bacteremia in children. J. Pediat. 84:656–660, 1974.

Naraqi, S., Kirkpatrick, G. P., and Kabins, S.: Relapsing pneumococcal meningitis: Isolation of an organism with decreased susceptibility to penicillin G. J. Pediat. 85:671–673, 1974.

Neal, J. B., Appelbaum, E., and Jackson, H. W.: Sulfapyridine and its sodium salt. In the treatment of meningitis due to the pneumococcus and Haemophilus influenzae. J.A.M.A. 115:2055–2058, 1940.

Neufeld, F.: Ueber die Agglutination der Pneumokokken und über die Theorien der Agglutination. Z. Hyg. 40:54–72, 1902.

Overturf, G. D., Powars, D., and Baraff, L. J.: Bacterial meningitis and septicemia in sickle cell disease. Am. J. Dis. Child. 131:784–787, 1977.

Pearson, H. A., Spencer, R. P., and Cornelius, E. A.: Functional asplenia in sickle-cell anemia. New Eng. J. Med. 281:923–926, 1969.

Rammelkamp, C. H., and Keefer, C. S.: The absorption, excretion, and distribution of penicillin. J. Clin. Invest. 22:425–437, 1943.

Rhodes, P. G., Burry, V. F., Hall, R. T., and Cox, R.: Pneumococcal septicemia and meningitis in the neonate. J. Pediat. 86:593–595, 1975.

Rice, W. J., and Waggoner, L. G.: Congenital cerebrospinal fluid otorrhea via a defect in the stapes footplate. Laryngoscope 77:341–349, 1967.

Robinson, M. G., and Watson, R. J.: Pneumococcal meningitis in sickle-cell anemia. New Eng. J. Med. 274:1006–1008, 1966.

Rose, H. D.: Pneumococcal meningitis following intrathecal injections. Arch. Neurol. 14:597–600, 1966.

Ross, S., and Burke, F. G.: Pneumococcus meningitis in infants and children. A report on the use of combined sulfonamide and penicillin therapy. J. Pediat. 29:737–757, 1946.

Ruegsegger, J. M.: Pneumococcal meningitis. A review. U. S. Naval Med. Bull. 49:1159–1168, 1949.

Schultz, P., and Stool, S.: Recurrent meningitis due to a congenital fistula through the stapes footplate. Am. J. Dis. Child. 120:553–554, 1970.

Seeler, R. A., Metzger, W., and Mufson, M. A.: *Diplococcus pneumoniae* infections in children with sickle cell anemia. Am. J. Dis. Child. 123:8–10, 1972.

Siber, G. R., Weitzman, S. A., Aisenberg, A. C., Weinstein, H. J., and Schiffman, G.: Impaired antibody response to pneumococcal vaccine after treatment for Hodgkin's disease. New Eng. J. Med. 299:442–448, 1978.

Spink, W. W., and Su, C. K.: Persistent menace of pneumococcal meningitis. J.A.M.A. 173:1545–1548, 1960.

Stool, S., Leed, N. E., and Shulman, K.: The syndrome of congenital deafness and otic meningitis: Diagnosis and management. J. Pediat. 71:547–552, 1967.

Swartz, M. N., and Dodge, P. R.: Bacterial meningitis— a review of selected aspects. New Eng. J. Med. 272:725–731, 779–787, 842–848, 898–902, 954–960, 1003–1010, 1965.

Sweet, L. K., Dumoff-Stanley, E., Dowling, H. F., and Leeper, M. H.: The treatment of pneumococcic meningitis with penicillin. J.A.M.A. 127:263–267, 1945.

Tempest, B.: Pneumococcal meningitis in mother and neonate. Pediatrics 53:759–760, 1974.

Thirumoorthi, M. C., Asmar, B. I., and Dajani, A. S.: Violaceous discoloration in pneumococcal cellulitis. Pediatrics 62:492–493, 1978.

Torphy, D. E., and Ray, C. G.: Occult pneumococcal bacteremia. Am. J. Dis. Child. 119:336–338, 1970.

Turner, J. S., Jr.: Pneumocephalus with facial fractures. Laryngoscope 78:1–15, 1968.

Waldman, J. D., Rosenthal, A., Smith, A. L., Shurin, S., and Nadas, A. S.: Sepsis and congenital asplenia. J. Pediat. 90:555–559, 1977.

Wallace, J. F., Smith, R. H., Garcia, M., and Petersdorf, R. G.: Studies on the pathogenesis of meningitis. VI. Antagonism between penicillin and chloramphenicol in experimental pneumococcal meningitis. J. Lab. Clin. Med. 70:408–418, 1967.

Weintraub, M. I., and Otto, R. N.: Pneumococcal meningitis and endophthalmitis in a newborn. J.A.M.A. 219:1763–1764, 1972.

Weiss, W., Figueroa, E., Shapiro, W. H., and Flippin, H. F.: Prognostic factors in pneumococcal meningitis. Arch. Intern. Med. 120:517–524, 1967.

Weitzman, S., and Aisenberg, A. C.: Fulminant sepsis after the successful treatment of Hodgkin's disease. Am. J. Med. 62:47–50, 1977.

Wenk, R. E., and Dutta, D.: Hyposplenic, coagulopathic, cryptogenetic pneumococcemia. Am. J. Clin. Path. 64:405–409, 1975.

White, W. L., Murphy, F. D., Lockwood, J. S., and Flippin, H. F.: Penicillin in the treatment of pneumococcal, meningococcal, streptococcal and staphylococcal meningitis. Am. J. Med. Sci. 210:1–17, 1945.

Whitecar, J. P., Jr., Reddin, J. L., and Spink, W. W.: Recurrent pneumococcal meningitis. A review of the literature and studies on a patient who recovered from eleven attacks caused by five serotypes of *Diplococcus pneumoniae*. New Eng. J. Med. 274:1285–1289, 1966.

Whittle, H. C., Tugwell, P., Egler, L. J., and Greenwood, B. M.: Rapid bacteriological diagnosis of pyogenic meningitis by latex agglutination. Lancet 2:619–621, 1974.

Winkelstein, J. A., and Drachman, R. H.: Deficiency of pneumococcal serum opsonizing activity in sickle cell disease. New Eng. J. Med. 279:459–466, 1968.

Chapter Seven

TUBERCULOUS MENINGITIS

Robert Whytt of Edinburgh is credited with the first accurate clinical description of the various stages of tuberculous meningitis in 1768. By 1850, pulmonary tuberculosis and its complications were said to account for approximately 25 percent of all deaths in the United States and England (Spink). The widespread nature of the disease led to the belief that it was the explanation of many diverse human maladies, and even mongolism was attributed to tuberculosis of the parents in the original publication by J. Langdon Down in 1886. Both before and for many years after the discovery by Robert Koch in 1882 that "consumption" was caused by *Mycobacterium tuberculosis,* the disease remained one of the most devastating of infectious diseases. The eventual control of bovine tuberculosis, the development of sanatoria which enabled removal of infected patients from the population generally, the wide-scale use of skin testing to detect asymptomatic infection, and the discovery of streptomycin in 1944 and isoniazid in 1952 finally brought the disease under a reasonable degree of control, although it remains far from eliminated.

Mycobacterium tuberculosis, a member of the family *Mycobacteriaceae,* is a narrow, non-motile rod which measures 0.2 to 0.6 μm in diameter and 1 to 4 μm in length (Freeman). The tubercle bacillus is not stained by the usual staining methods used for most other bacteria because the high lipid content of the organism inhibits entrance of dyes into the cell. The high lipid composition of *Myobacterium tuberculosis* not only determines its peculiar staining characteristics but also plays an important role in the pathogenic qualities of the bacillus. A notable feature of the organism is its acid-fast quality, which refers to its resistance to acid decolorization after staining with aniline dyes. The Ziehl-Neelsen staining technique is the customary method used to demonstrate acid-fast organisms microscopically.

Once the leader without rival as the most common form of bacterial meningitis in early childhood, tuberculous meningitis has now become relatively uncommon in this country. In 1911, Holt reviewed 199 cases of bacterial meningitis in children less than three years of age, of which 69 percent were tuberculous. In a series of 642 cases of childhood meningitis seen from 1924 to 1939, Lindsay and colleagues found that 31.9 percent were caused by this organism. In a later series of children which included cases seen from 1930 until 1953, those cases due to the tubercle bacillus had declined to 23 percent (Koch and Carson). Among 248 cases of bacterial meningitis in all age groups observed from 1961 to 1965, only 19, or 7.6 percent, were caused by *Mycobacterium tuberculosis* (Allison and Dalton). Despite this remarkable decline in the incidence of tuberculous meningitis in this country, the disease remains a serious threat to children in urban communities and among many tribes of American Indians as well as in other parts of the world.

There are many reasons for the decrease in this type of meningitis, the most obvious being the reduced frequency of adults with active pulmonary tuberculosis who serve as contacts to the child. Most important also has been the wide-scale use of tuberculin skin testing of children to detect asymptomatic primary pulmonary tuberculosis. This procedure is now recommended for all infants between six and eight months of age and at yearly intervals thereafter. As the greatest risks of complications of primary tuberculosis occur within the first year after acquiring the infection, the use of isoniazid therapy for skin-test-positive children under three years of age has been another important factor in reducing the incidence of meningitis. In addition, the recognition of the hazard to the infant born of a tuberculous mother and the judicious use of BCG vaccine has provided further protection against the danger of meningitis (Avery and Wolfdorf, Kendig).

BCG vaccine was derived from a strain of *Mycobacterium bovis,* and, following several years of serial passage in culture to bring about attenuation, was first administered to humans in 1921 by Calmette and Guérin in France. It is now recommended that its use be considered for skin-test-negative persons, including infants, who have or will have close exposure to patients with sputum-positive pulmonary tuberculosis. It has the disadvantage of converting the tuberculin skin test to a positive reaction, thus largely nullifying its subsequent value. Although BCG vaccine is a reasonably safe immunizing agent, it should not be administered to children with certain immunologic disorders in which disseminated infection may occur. BCG fatalities have been described in patients with chronic granulomatous disease of childhood (Esterly et al.), Swiss-type agammaglobulinemia (Carlgren et al., Matsaniotis and Economou-Mavrou), and other less well-defined defects of cellular immunity (Passwell et al.).

Tuberculous meningitis represents a complication of previous infection elsewhere in the body, with the original focus being in the lung in the overwhelming majority. As bovine tuberculosis has become better controlled, tuberculous cervical adenitis as a source for dissemination of the organism has become rare. Most children are infected with the tubercle bacillus by inhalation of the organism. The primary inflammatory site occurs in the parenchyma of the lung with an accumulation of leukocytes and with epithelioid cell proliferation. Soon thereafter, phagocytes carry the infection to regional hilar lymph nodes, which become enlarged. This stage of tuberculous infection is referred to as primary pulmonary tuberculosis, the primary complex consisting of the primary parenchymal lung lesion, the involved regional nodes, and the interconnected lymphatic channels. Primary

pulmonary tuberculosis, generally considered to be largely a childhood disease in the past, is now seen more often in adults subsequent to the remarkable decline in the disease generally and the change in the epidemiologic patterns (Khan et al.). The majority of children are asymptomatic in the primary stage and are not usually considered to be contagious.

Between two and ten weeks after the initiation of this inflammatory process, tissue hypersensitivity develops and is evidenced by the development of a positive tuberculin skin test. In most cases, spontaneous healing occurs following this sequence, but in some patients, progression may follow, with caseation occurring and one of many complications possibly developing. Hilar lymph nodes may produce bronchial obstruction with distal atelectasis, or can possibly erode through the bronchial wall, resulting in endobronchial tuberculosis with further dissemination of bacteria into the lung parenchyma.

Local progression with caseation of the primary parenchymal focus is unusual in childhood and is referred to as primary progressive pulmonary tuberculosis, also with the risk of widespread dissemination. Generalized dissemination with diffuse pulmonary infiltration in addition to spread to many organs, sometimes including the meninges, is called miliary tuberculosis and progresses to a fatal outcome unless it is recognized and treatment begun (Fig. 7–1). This process in most cases in children is a complication of primary pulmonary tuberculosis within the first three to six months of the illness. Miliary tuberculosis has declined dramatically in children, although it has not yet vanished in this country (Schuit) and is currently more often seen in adults than in the childhood years (Sahn and Neff). The infrequency of the disorder, the non-specific symptoms, including fever, weight loss, cough, and night sweats, plus the occasional negative tuberculin skin tests with this illness render difficult its early diagnosis unless there is a distinct history of exposure.

An additional type of tuberculous involvement in children which has now become rare but is often complicated by neurologic abnormalities is tuberculous otitis or mastoiditis. The pathogenesis of otic localization of the disease is unclear, although it can occur as part of miliary dissemination (Saltzman and Feigin) or by extension to the middle ear by way of the eustachian tubes. The disorder is characterized by chronic watery otorrhea

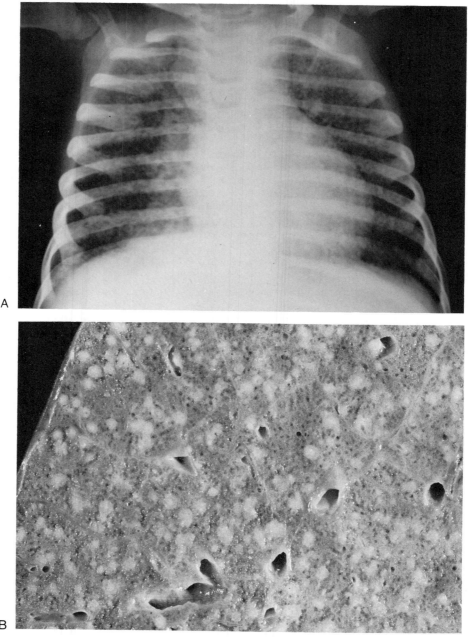

Figure 7–1.   Miliary tuberculosis. *A*, Chest x-ray of a 16-month-old child with massive hematogenous dissemination of infection to the lungs resulting in a "snow-storm" appearance. Paratracheal adenopathy on the right. *B*, Section of the lung with advanced miliary tuberculosis reveals numerous well-defined granulomatous lesions.

and cervical lymphadenopathy and is often associated with severe loss of hearing and peripheral facial paralysis on the affected side (MacAdam and Rubio).

If antituberculous therapy is initiated while the infectious process is limited to the lungs, it is extremely rare that meningitis will develop subsequently, at least during the period that drug therapy is continued. When dissemination does occur during chemotherapy for pulmonary tuberculosis, the possibility of drug-resistance must be suspected (Lintermans and Seyhnaeve).

Pathogenesis

The pathogenesis of tuberculous meningitis and its relation to the stage of pulmonary involvement has long been a matter of debate. The temporal relationship of tuberculous meningitis with miliary tuberculosis has suggested that hematogenous dissemination is an important factor in causation of this disease. Among 297 cases of tuberculous meningitis, Blacklock and Griffin found that miliary tuberculosis coexisted in 68 percent. Direct blood stream spread to the nervous system, however, was doubted to be a common cause of tuberculous meningitis by Rich and McCordock, who published their classic studies in 1933. These authors emphasized the violent nature of the acute phase of tuberculous meningitis which was often observed and suggested that the number of organisms gaining entrance into the subarachnoid space by hematogenous dissemination would be incapable of evoking such a response. In addition, these investigators injected sensitized animals intravenously with heavy doses of tubercle bacilli and were not able to provoke an acute, exudative meningitis. Among 82 cases of tuberculous meningitis, Rich and McCordock found caseous tuberculous foci adjacent to the subarachnoid space in 77 and attributed the diffuse meningitis to discharge of the organisms from these sites. These tubercles were often only 3 to 5 millimeters in diameter and were present either within the meninges or in the substance of the brain adjacent to the subarachnoid space (Fig. 7–2). As the source of acid-fast bacteria resulting in meningitis, these tuberculous foci were believed to have resulted from previous hematogenous spread to the central nervous system, remaining silent for variable periods of time before deposition of organisms into the cerebrospinal fluid. Whether the contiguous tuberculoma explanation of Rich and McCordock accounts for all cases of tuberculous meningitis remains undetermined. It does appear to be an explanation for those cases in children known to have had their exposure and primary illness months or years before, in which no other active tuberculous disease can be identified.

Rich and McCordock stressed the importance of a hypersensitivity or allergic response of the brain and meninges during the initial phase of tuberculous meningitis. Subsequent evidence of nervous tissue hypersensitivity to tuberculoprotein included the finding that intrathecal tuberculin caused no significant response in nonsensitized subjects but resulted in marked cerebrospinal fluid pleocytosis in those previously sensitized (Swinthinback et al.). Furthermore, studies showed that tubercle bacilli injected into the CSF of rabbits produced an immediate inflammatory meningeal response only in those animals previously sensitized to tuberculoprotein (Burn and Finley). Feldman et al. performed similar studies, injecting killed tubercle bacilli into sensitized rabbits. One group of animals was treated with corticosteroids and compared to a similar group who did not receive corticosteroid therapy. Considerable protection, in regard to the cerebrospinal fluid inflammatory response, was provided by corticosteroids, adding further evidence to the hypersensitivity features of the acute meningeal response. Morphologic changes in the brain attributed to this hypersensitivity response in tuberculous meningitis include edema of the white matter with myelin depletion and astrocytic proliferation (Dastur and Udani).

Pathology

The leptomeningeal exudate in tuberculous meningitis consists of a diffuse gray opacity over the cerebral convexity and a thicker, gelatinous infiltrate at the base of the brain extending into the basilar cisterns (Fig. 7–3). Lymphocytes, plasma cells, and giant cells within areas with caseation necrosis are evident (Fig. 7–4). Tubercle bacilli may be present in large numbers but sometimes can be difficult to identify. Meningeal vessel changes are usually prominent in this disease and often result in tissue infarction when the vascular lumen is severely compromised (Rowlatt). Arteries traversing the basilar ex-

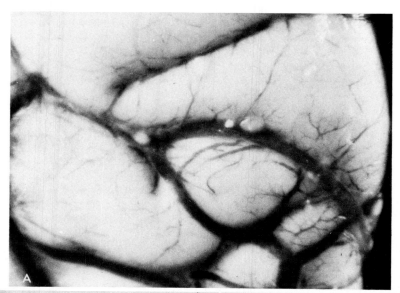

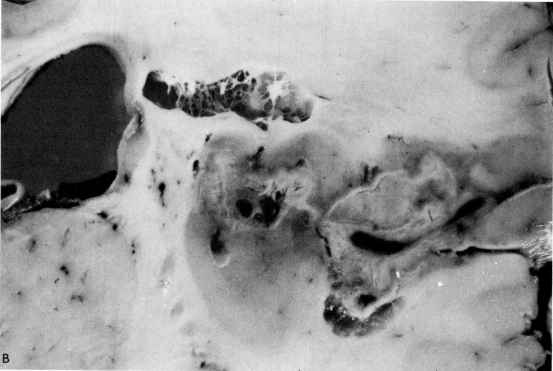

Figure 7–2. Tuberculous meningitis. *A,* Multiple, small tuberculous granulomata adjacent to cortical veins. Tubercles of this type can remain dormant for years after the primary pulmonary infection. Eventual rupture of the lesion and release of organisms into the CSF provokes meningitis, sometimes long after healing of the pulmonary infection. *B,* Larger intracerebral tuberculoma in the region of the Sylvian fissure. The cystic lesion superior and medial to the granulomatous mass is the result of an old infarction secondary to vasculitis.

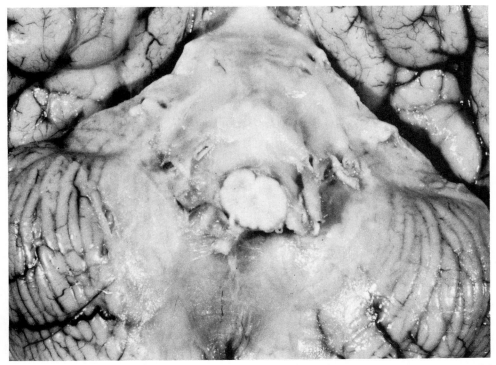

Figure 7–3. Tuberculous meningitis. Thick, gelatinous basilar exudate obscuring the ventral surface of the brain stem and encasing the vertebro-basilar arteries.

udate are most profoundly affected and are usually unaffected where no exudate exists. Swelling of the adventitia results from proliferation of epithelioid cells, while lymphocytic infiltration of the intima narrows the vessel lumen (Doniach) (Fig. 7–5). Veins within meningeal exudate may also show lymphocytic infiltration and epithelioid cell proliferation within their walls. Since the arterial changes described above are virtually limited to areas where vessels pass through thick meningeal exudate, it is assumed that the alterations result from the surrounding inflammatory process (Daniel, Doniach). Narrowing of vessels at the base of the brain, including the supraclinoid portion of the carotid and proximal portions of the anterior and middle cerebral arteries, can be demonstrated angiographically (Mathew et al., Lehrer).

Clinical Aspects

Tuberculous meningitis in children has its highest incidence between six and 24 months of age. Even in past years when it represented a common disease, meningitis due to this organism in infants under three months of age was rare (Blacklock and Griffin), as was congenital tuberculosis of any type (Voyce and Hunt). Among reported cases of infants with congenital tuberculosis, most have been prematurely born and have become symptomatic in the days or weeks after birth (Reisinger et al.). Possible modes of transmission of the infection to the fetus include fetal aspiration of infected amniotic fluid or hematogenous spread from an infected placenta via the umbilical vein (Cashman). As noted earlier, most cases of meningeal tuberculosis in the past occurred in association with miliary tuberculosis and evolved within a year after the child acquired the primary pulmonary form of the disease. Predisposing factors that contribute to the development of this disease include malnutrition, crowded and substandard living conditions, and other infectious illnesses. Severe pertussis may precede the development of tuberculous meningitis, and measles is widely recognized as a potential precipitant of this illness. In a series of 241 cases of tuberculous meningitis, Lincoln et al. found that measles was an immediate antecedent in 9.5 percent. Head trauma may be described in the immediate period before onset of symptoms of meningitis, although the cause-and-effect relationship remains unclear.

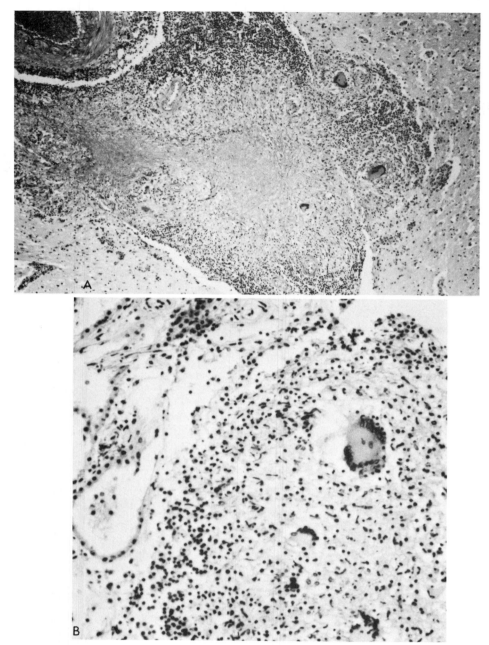

Figure 7–4.   Tuberculous meningitis. *A* and *B,* Meningeal exudate composed of inflammatory cells, Langhans giant cells, and caseation necrosis. In *A,* note the perivascular cuffing and extension of the inflammatory reaction into the brain parenchyma.

Tuberculous meningitis infrequently becomes manifested as an acute illness similar to other forms of bacterial meningitis. Most cases are more gradual in onset, with mild signs of illness present for several days. Fever is the most common initial complaint, followed by listlessness, irritability, headache, and vomiting or abdominal pain in some cases. Rarely, a convulsion or even hemiparesis precedes other abnormalities that lead to a diagnosis of tuberculous meningitis (Udani et al.).

With progression of the illness during the second week after onset, headache and vomiting become more pronounced, neck stiffness and Kernig's sign are found, and other

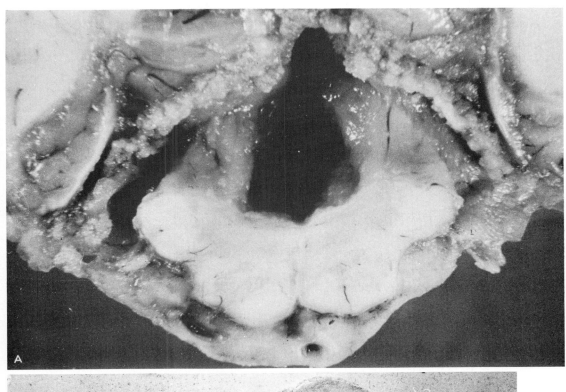

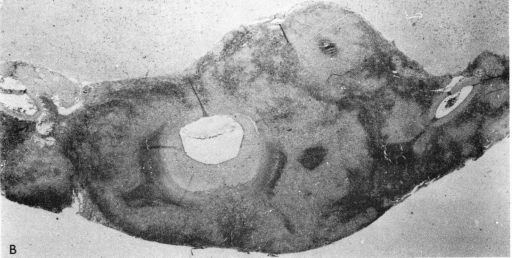

Figure 7–5.   Tuberculous meningitis. *A,* Section through the medulla shows vertebral-basilar artery encasement by tuberculous exudate ventral to brain stem. Note the thick, shaggy exudate dorsolateral to the medulla and the distended fourth ventricle with nodular ependymitis. *B,* Higher power view of the basilar artery engulfed by the dense granulomatous reaction.

Illustration continued on following page

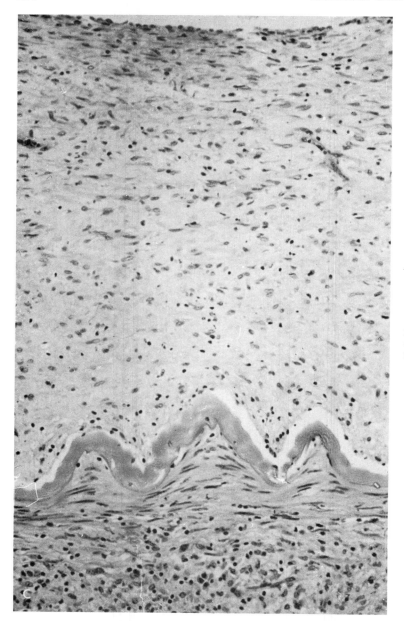

Figure 7–5 Continued. C, Severe intimal thickening of the basilar artery resulting in narrowing of the arterial lumen.

evidence of neurologic involvement is more definite. State of awareness and responsiveness declines and cranial nerve signs, such as facial weakness, ptosis, or extraocular muscle paresis, are often described in this stage. Papilledema can occur relatively early in this form of meningitis, a finding uncommonly present with more common types of acute suppurative meningitis in the early stages. Choroidal tubercles may be seen on fundus examination but are not common. Tache cérébrale was commonly mentioned in the older literature and referred to the presence of a red line which developed and persisted on stroking the skin. This is now known to be a non-specific sign of autonomic dysfunction and is seen in a variety of types of severe, acute suppurative meningitis.

Unless influenced by treatment, the course of the disease is usually relentlessly progressive, with the child passing into a state of deep coma with decerebrate rigidity, convulsions, multiple cranial nerve palsies, and papilledema. The natural course of the untreated disease has been stated to last three to five weeks from onset to death in most cases. Holt found the average duration of the disease from onset to death to be two-and-one-half weeks while Meyers found it to be 17 days in a series of 105 cases. The longest duration before death was 43 days. Both of these reports preceded any effective chemotherapy and thus represented untreated cases. Mild forms with symptoms lasting months before diagnosis have been described but are unusual (Norris et al.). Rare cases have also been reported of benign, transient meningitis due to the tubercle bacillus in which spontaneous recovery occurred without antituberculous therapy (Emond and McKendrick, Zinneman and Hall). It is assumed that the mildness of the illness and the atypical cerebrospinal fluid changes seen in such patients are explained by a relatively small number of organisms gaining entrance into the cerebrospinal fluid.

Intracranial Tuberculoma and Tuberculous Brain Abscess

Intracranial tuberculomas of sufficient size to create a mass effect are now rare in the United States although the lesion continues to represent an important component of series of intracranial mass lesions in certain foreign countries (Anderson and MacMillan). Unlike past experience in foreign lands in which children were more often affected, in this country in recent years intracranial tuberculomas have been found more often among adults (Damergis et al., Mayers et al.).

The tuberculoma is a solid, granulomatous, relatively avascular lesion, which can be round, oval, or lobulated in shape and is usually bounded by a thin capsule. The mass consists of typical tuberculous granulation tissue which includes giant cells and epithelioid cells and varying degrees of caseation necrosis. Calcification within the lesion may be found microscopically but is only infrequently dense enough to be visualized roentgenographically (Sibley and O'Brien). Less than 6 percent of symptomatic intracranial tuberculomas reveal calcium deposition on skull x-ray examination (Anderson and MacMillan). Tuberculomas have been found to be more common in the cerebellum in children (Roedenbeck) and more frequent above the tentorium in adults (Anderson and MacMillan, Sibley and O'Brien). Those in the cerebrum are generally within the depths of the parenchyma, while those in the cerebellum almost always are adjacent to the pial surface, increasing the predisposition to subarachnoid extension of the infection. The lesion can also occur within the parenchyma of the brain stem (Haskett et al., Roedenbeck) and within the spinal cord or the spinal intradural space, causing extrinsic spinal cord compression (Arseni and Samitca, Parsons and Pallis).

Clinical manifestations of intracranial tuberculoma sufficiently large to be symptomatic are exceedingly variable and depend upon the size and location of the lesion. Duration of symptoms prior to medical evaluation can be brief but more often extends into weeks or months. Signs of increased intracranial pressure are common with cerebral or cerebellar lesions, largely resulting from the mass effect of the lesion, but to some extent caused by surrounding inflammation and swelling (Descuns et al.). Seizures, hemiparesis, and visual field defects are common with cerebral hemisphere tuberculomas, while ataxia and pressure signs are customary with cerebellar lesions. Multiple cranial nerve signs and long tract sensory and motor deficits characterize those located within the brain stem. Systemic symptoms, including fever, weight loss, and malaise may be present because of tuberculous disease elsewhere, but in some cases there is no evidence of tuberculosis in other organs and no definite history of exposure (Damergis et al., Mayers et al.). Preoperative diagnosis in such cases is usually that of an intracranial neoplasm, with the true nature of the lesion being established by microscopic examination of the excised lesion.

Computed cranial tomography is of value to localize the lesion and to identify multiple lesions but will not differentiate a tuberculoma from a neoplasm. Surgical excision of large intracranial tuberculomas prior to the availability of effective antituberculous chemotherapy was often followed by the development of tuberculous meningitis and death. When in an accessible location, such lesions can now frequently be safely removed.

Tuberculous brain abscesses are rare lesions compared to intracranial tuberculomas. Most have occurred in adults and the majority have been in association with clear-cut extraneural tuberculosis (Bannister, Whitener). From the clinical and histological standpoint, tuberculous brain abscess more closely resembles pyogenic brain abscess than it does intracranial tuberculoma. The neurologic manifestations are usually acute to subacute and the parenchymal cerebral or cerebellar lesion consists of a central cavity containing purulent material from which tubercle bacilli can be isolated. Solitary abscesses are more common than multiple lesions, and abscess and tuberculoma can coexist at different sites (Whitener).

The cause of abscess formation in these rare instances is unexplained but it is possible that the lesion represents infection within an area of ischemic cerebral softening secondary to vasculitis, which then undergoes progressive necrosis leading to suppuration. Focal neurologic signs, including seizures, and signs of increased intracranial pressure of days to a few weeks' duration, are the usual presenting manifestations. The CSF contains few cells but an increased protein content, and will become more abnormal if perforation of the abscess into the subarachnoid space or ventricle leads to tuberculous meningitis. Treatment includes surgical aspiration or excision, in conjunction with long-term antituberculous drug therapy.

Differential Diagnosis

Differential diagnosis of this disease largely includes those disorders with similar cerebrospinal fluid abnormalities. The most notable of these conditions include acute viral encephalitis, especially that due to Herpes simplex, cryptococcal meningoencephalitis, pyogenic brain abscess, partially treated suppurative meningitis, sarcoidosis, and lead encephalopathy. An ependymoma of the fourth ventricle or medulloblastoma of the cerebellar vermis can rarely be associated with neck stiffness, a lymphocytic pleocytosis in the CSF, and even reduced cerebrospinal fluid glucose, thus resembling tuberculous or granulomatous meningitis. The absence of fever and presence of ataxia should direct one's attention to the consideration of a mass lesion, and cranial computed tomography will generally clarify the problem.

In addition to the cerebrospinal fluid findings described below, other features important in including or excluding the possibility of tuberculosis are the presence or absence of exposure to the illness, the tuberculin skin test, chest x-ray, and gastric washings for identification of acid-fast bacilli. The latter is by far the least rewarding of these various diagnostic methods in children with tuberculous meningitis. It should be stressed, however, that all these ancillary procedures can be negative in a child with tuberculous meningitis. In particularly difficult cases suspected to be tuberculosis in which there is a

localized pulmonary lesion on chest x-ray, percutaneous lung puncture to obtain an aspirate for smear, culture, and guinea pig inoculation has been proposed as a useful diagnostic technique (Schuster et al.).

The purified protein derivative (PPD) skin test is positive in the majority of patients but may be negative in a child seriously ill and markedly emaciated (Harris et al., Holden et al.). In addition, a positive skin test can be depressed by certain viral illnesses, such as measles, influenza, infectious mononucleosis, or varicella (Belsey), following the administration of measles, mumps, and polio virus vaccines (Berkovich and Starr, Kupers et al.) or during the administration of corticosteroids. The sensitivity of the skin test has been improved with the introduction of Tween 80 stabilized tuberculin (Rooney et al.). When interpreted at 48 hours, 10 mm. or more of induration is a positive reaction, 5 to 9 mm. is doubtful, and less than 5 mm. is a negative response.

When meningitis is suspected to be of tuberculous origin, a negative history of pulmonary disease among family members does not exclude them as the possible source of the infection. As many close contacts to the child as possible should have chest x-rays performed in order to find the origin of the disease (Fig. 7–6). In addition to parents and siblings, grandparents, babysitters, and hired help working in or around the home are candidates to be the infected contact and may be identified only by roentgenographic examination.

Tuberculous Osteomyelitis of the Spine

Vertebral osteomyelitis secondary to hematogenous dissemination of tubercle bacilli has become an infrequent complication of childhood tuberculosis in this country. Tuberculous osteomyelitis can implicate any portion of the spine, but the lower thoracic region is the most common site, followed by the upper lumbar region (Bailey et al.) (Fig. 7–7). Several adjacent vertebrae may be affected or multiple areas of one vertebra may show evidence of the disease. The initial location of the process is within the vertebral body in most cases and, less frequently, the site of origin is in the laminar arch. Spread from one vertebral body to another can occur under the anterior spinal ligament or through the intervertebral disc, resulting in a reduction of the disc space diameter. Ex-

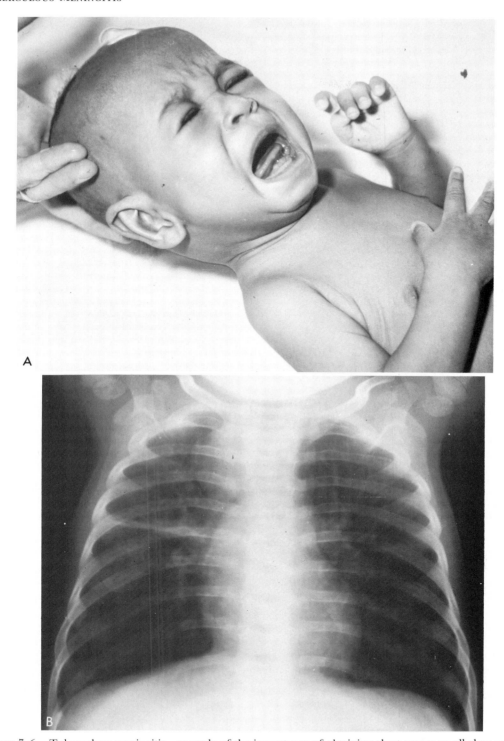

Figure 7–6. Tuberculous meningitis—example of the importance of obtaining chest x-rays on all close contacts of a child with tuberculosis in order to identify the source of the infection. *A,* Six-month-old infant with history of fever and cough with onset at age 4 months. Chest x-ray then showed bilateral infiltrates. Because a Tine test was negative, the diagnosis was "pneumonia" and penicillin was given. Cough and intermittent fever continued until 1 week prior to admission when the child became irritable, listless, and anorectic. Findings on admission included a tense anterior fontanel, neck rigidity, and intense irritability, especially on movement of the head. CSF examination revealed 60 cells per cu. mm., 70 percent being neutrophils. The CSF glucose was 4 mg. per 100 ml. Tubercle bacilli were subsequently isolated from the CSF. *B,* Child's x-ray at age 6 months shows bilateral, diffuse hyperaeration, right paratracheal lymphadenopathy, a small amount of infiltrate in the right upper lobe, and fluid in the minor fissure on the right.

Illustration continued on following page

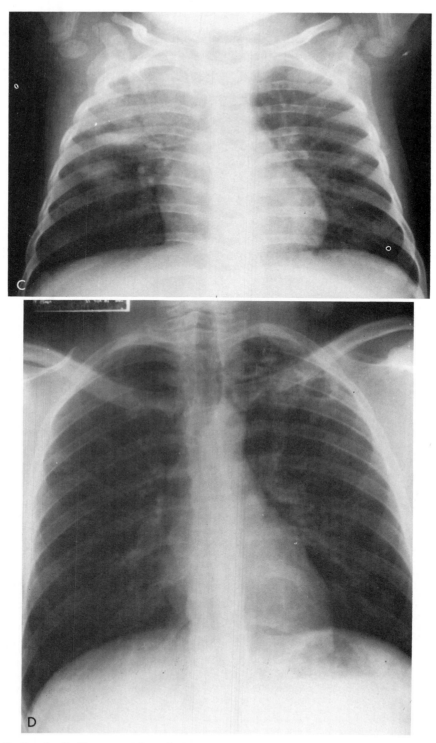

Figure 7–6 Continued. C, Chest x-ray 6 weeks later reveals progressive consolidation of the right upper lobe despite antituberculous therapy. Air bronchogram is visible in the region of consolidation and the minor fissure remains elevated. Adenopathy is now obscured by the parenchymal infiltrate. The family history revealed no source for the child's infection and x-rays of her mother and other close relatives were normal. The origin of her illness became apparent when the mother's boyfriend became available for chest x-ray. *D,* His chest film reveals active "adult" type pulmonary tuberculosis. There is an infiltrate with cavitation in the apical posterior segment of the left upper lobe.

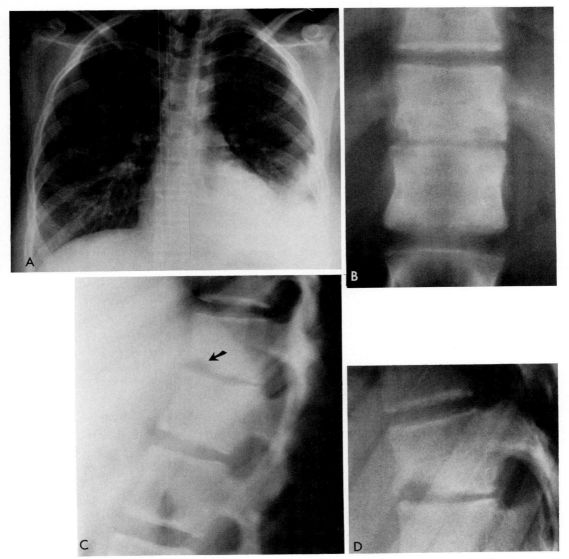

Figure 7–7. Spinal tuberculosis, early stage. Sixteen-year-old girl with a 2-month history of back pain. She developed recurrent nocturnal fever with chills and sweats, cough, and decline in appetite. Her lower extremities were normal on neurologic examination at the time of admission to the hospital. Acid-fast bacilli were obtained from a gastric aspirate. *A,* Chest x-ray on admission reveals a left pleural effusion. *B,* AP tomogram of the spine shows marked narrowing of the T11–12 disc space. *C,* Lateral view of the spine demonstrates the T11–12 disc space collapse in addition to destructive changes of the anterior-inferior portion of the T11 vertebral body (arrow). *D,* Close-up view of the lytic lesion of the anterior portion of the T11 vertebral body.

tension of granulomatous material from the vertebra results in paravertebral soft-tissue abscesses.

Escape of infected material into the epidural space leads to spinal cord dysfunction, either by direct compression of the cord or by compromising its arterial supply. Spinal cord compression occurs in only the minority of patients who develop tuberculous osteomyelitis. Greenfield estimated that approximately 5 to 20 percent of patients with ver-

tebral disease developed paraplegia, while Martin found that among 740 patients with spinal tuberculosis, 16 percent were paraplegic. In addition, tuberculous spinal epidural granulomas can occur in the absence of changes in the adjacent vertebrae, making the diagnosis exceedingly difficult prior to tissue examination (Kocen and Parsons). Spinal cord injury in patients with pulmonary tuberculosis can also be secondary to dissemination of the disease, with vasculitis producing ischemic cord damage. A necrotizing myelopathy characterized by extensive myelin loss without inflammation has been described in adults with pulmonary tuberculosis, although the etiology of the spinal cord lesion is unknown (Hughes and Mair).

Tuberculous disease of the spine with secondary cord compression is primarily a disease of children and young adults (Ginsburg et al.) and currently is also seen in narcotic addicts, who are predisposed to a variety of otherwise uncommon disorders (Forlenza et al.). It is rare in children under two years of age and is infrequent in the elderly. Although the term "Pott's disease" is frequently used to refer to any form of tuberculous spinal involvement, it should be reserved for the association of paraparesis or paraplegia secondary to vertebral tuberculous involvement (Greenfield). Percivall Pott, in 1779, drew attention to the association of paraplegia and progressive spinal deformity but did not recognize the tuberculous nature of the spinal lesion.

Clinical manifestations in the child with tuberculous osteomyelitis depend upon the stage of the disease and the presence or absence of extension of the process to the paraspinal soft tissues or the epidural space. Fever, weight loss, pain and localized spinal tenderness are prominent symptoms of this illness and, in advanced cases, vertebral destruction leads to pronounced gibbus formation with complete paraplegia and sphincter paralysis (Fig. 7–8). Radicular pain usually precedes clinical evidence of spinal cord involvement and, rarely, may even occur before the characteristic roentgenographic vertebral changes become evident. In patients with an epidural granuloma producing a spinal block, the characteristic CSF findings include either no cells or only a few lymphocytes per cu mm. and a normal glucose value but an elevated protein content. Tuberculous spondylitis continues to be a serious complication of tuberculosis but its recognition in earlier stages and the advent of more effective chemotherapeutic agents have reduced the morbidity and mortality of the disorder.

Laboratory Studies

Peripheral blood leukocytosis is usually present in children with tuberculous meningitis, with counts generally between 10,000 and 20,000 per cu. mm. In infants with miliary tuberculosis, a leukemoid reaction with either lymphocytosis or monocytosis, in addition to hepatosplenomegaly, may deceptively resemble acute leukemia. Serum hyponatremia and hypochloremia are not uncommon and result partly from vomiting but may also be present in those without vomiting, probably on the basis of inappropriate release of antidiuretic hormone. It is probable that the reduced cerebrospinal fluid chloride level seen in patients with tuberculous meningitis is largely a reflection of serum hypochloremia.

The cerebrospinal fluid is usually groundglass or opalescent in appearance, is under increased pressure, and contains a variable number of cells. In the first few days of the illness, polymorphonuclear leukocytes frequently predominate, but a lymphocytic pleocytosis soon develops. From 10 to 250 cells per cu. mm. are present in most cases, and only rarely does the CSF cell count exceed 500. On rare occasions, the initial CSF specimen obtained early in the course of the illness will contain few or no inflammatory cells, a finding with obvious misleading diagnostic implications (Wilkinson et al.). The glucose content may be normal initially but declines progressively to reach a level generally between 15 and 35 mg. per 100 ml. and sometimes even lower. Thus, the CSF glucose content is usually lower than that seen with viral meningoencephalitis but is not often reduced to the degree commonly observed with other forms of previously untreated acute bacterial meningitis. In those patients with normal glucose values initially, serial spinal taps may be indicated to show the progressive decline in CSF glucose, which occurs even though the child may have a significant elevation in the blood sugar (Weichsel and Herzger). The CSF protein content also may be normal or only slightly increased in the early stages but later becomes elevated to levels of 100 to 400 mg. per 100 ml.

Acid-fast bacilli may be found on stained smears of the cerebrospinal fluid and should be looked for in the pellicle that forms after the fluid is allowed to stand for a period of time. It is important to perform a Gram stain on all such specimens because the diagnosis regarding the offending organism is usually in doubt at this time. In addition, mixed infections with tubercle bacilli plus other more common bacteria have been described (Levinsky and Wilkinson). Recovery of tubercle bacilli and proof of the etiologic origin are enhanced by culture and guinea pig inoculation of the CSF specimen. Isolation of tu-

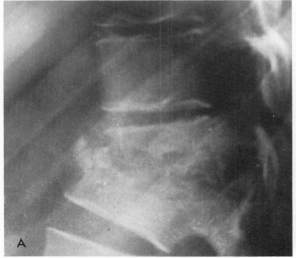

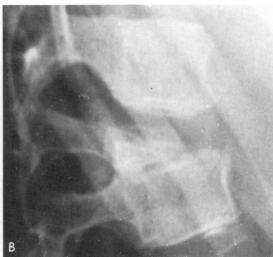

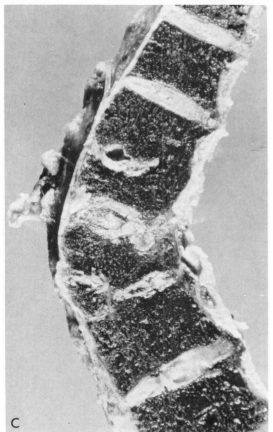

Figure 7–8. Spinal tuberculosis, advanced stages. *A,* Lateral spine x-ray of a young adult female with severe tuberculous osteomyelitis of the lower thoracic region. There is marked destruction and collapse of two adjacent thoracic vertebrae. The greater degree of destructive change of the anterior portion of the vertebral bodies has resulted in a gibbus deformity. *B,* Chronic changes. Nearly complete tuberculous destruction of the vertebral body leaves a wedge-shaped remnant. *C,* Postmortem specimen showing the vertebral body damage which occurs in the thoracic spine by tuberculous spinal involvement. Infection has extended from the vertebral body to the intervertebral disc, which is partially collapsed. The initial lesions in vertebral tuberculosis are usually in the upper and lower margins on the anterior portion of the vertebral bodies. Disc space infection leading to disc space collapse follows, and paravertebral abscess or granuloma then occurs.

bercle bacilli from the CSF is commonly difficult and has been accomplished with variable success, ranging from 55 to 75 percent in reports in the literature (Hinman, Lincoln et al., Todd and Neville, Weiss and Flippin).

Other tests on the CSF were developed in past years as diagnostic aids in tuberculous meningitis but are not widely used. As early as 1917, Kasahara devised a test in which an initial CSF examination was performed and was followed by a subdural injection of tuberculin. After 24 hours, a subsequent CSF study was accomplished. A marked increase in leukocytes and red cells in the fluid indicated the tuberculous nature of the illness. The Levinson test (Giustra, Gleich) was based on variations of hydrogen ion concentration in CSF in different forms of meningitis, with that due to the tubercle bacillus allegedly being more alkaline than other types. The alkaline quality of the CSF was said to result in precipitation of mercuric chloride added to the specimen, providing evidence of tuberculous infection.

The tryptophan test (Lichtenberg) was a color reaction presumed to depend on tryptophan groups present in the CSF. A CSF specimen was added to hydrochloric acid and formaldehyde, and the solution layered with sodium nitrite. A violet ring at the interface of the two fluids represented a positive reaction. These procedures were usually found to be positive in patients with tuberculous meningitis; however, they did not prove to be of consistent value because other inflammatory disorders often would likewise yield positive results.

Of greater interest was the bromide test (Taylor et al.), although the time required to obtain results was a limiting factor. Sodium bromide was given orally in a childhood dose of 0.25 to 0.50 grain three times per day for three days or by a single intravenous dose of two to four grains. Samples of venous blood and CSF were subsequently examined for their bromide contents. The serum-CSF bromide ratio was then determined and in normal controls was found to be 2 or 3 to 1. The ratio in active tuberculous meningitis was depressed to less than 1.5 to 1 and was similarly depressed in those during the intrathecal tuberculin reaction. In recent years, the bromide test as originally devised has received little attention as a useful method for diagnosis of tuberculous meningitis. A modification of the method, which utilizes radioactive bromide, shows promise of restoring this procedure to its earlier value in certain difficult cases (Mandal et al.). It may be particularly useful in the early stages of the illness when the CSF glucose content is still in the normal range and in cases of unspecified lymphocytic meningitis in which tuberculous involvement of other organs is not evident.

Mortality and Sequelae

The mortality of tuberculous meningitis has been markedly reduced since the introduction of chemotherapeutic agents for this disease. Before the discovery of streptomycin in 1944, survival was rare. Mortality rates in recent years in childhood have varied from 60 percent (Todd and Neville), to 41 to 44 percent (Lorber, Tahernia, Wasz-Hockert and Downer), to 32 percent (Lincoln et al.), and even lower with current methods of treatment (Visudhiphan and Chiemchanya 1975). The prognosis for survival is clearly related to the stage of the illness at the time of initiation of treatment, as shown in the series of Idriss et al. in which death occurred in 50 percent of patients admitted in coma but in only 15 to 30 percent of those admitted in a drowsy or lethargic condition. Summarizing the available information, it is assumed that the mortality rate of tuberculous meningitis in childhood is in the range of 20 percent if adequate treatment is initiated before an advanced stage of the illness is reached. The most important single prognostic factor regarding outcome of tuberculous meningitis is the state of responsiveness of the child at the time of hospital admission (Freiman and Geefhuysen).

Complications during the acute phase and long-term sequelae are also related to the stage of the illness at the time diagnosis is established. Subdural effusions may occur in infants as well as in older persons with tuberculous meningitis but are less common than when meningitis is due to certain other bacterial pathogens (Turner). Communicating hydrocephalus is a common occurrence in children with tubercle bacillus meningitis and results from obstruction within the basilar cisterns due to the gelatinous or fibrous exudate so prominent in these regions. This extraventricular block often persists after recovery but can resolve spontaneously. In the past, therapeutic methods advised to prevent or relieve this complication included intrathecal tuberculin and streptodornase or streptokinase injections but with equivocal results.

Permanent neurologic sequelae range from mild facial paresis to severe neurologic defects, including intellectual deficiency, spasticity, convulsions, blindness, and behavioral abnormalities. In the years when repeated intrathecal injections of streptomycin represented the basic treatment method, the subsequent development of intraspinal epidermoid tumors was attributed to the multiple spinal taps (Manno et al.). Among 50 survivors, Lincoln et al. found neurologic sequelae to be present in 24 percent. Lorber studied 100 children who survived the illness, of which 23 percent had various lasting neurologic deficits. Significant neurologic sequelae were found in 22 percent of 103 children studied by Donner and Wasz-Hockert. Infants and young children have been found to have a worse prognosis regarding residual deficits than occurs in older children. It is suspected that the above figures represent conservative estimates regarding permanent sequelae in survivors of tuberculous meningitis.

Eighth nerve dysfunction can result either from the effects of the disease or secondary to the adverse influence of streptomycin. Of 103 children treated for tuberculous meningitis between 1949 and 1954, Ranta and Wasz-Hockert on follow-up examinations found that 63 percent had hearing impairment, either severe in degree or, in 22 percent, total. Streptomycin administered during pregnancy is of concern regarding potential toxic effects to the fetal eighth nerve; however, permanent adverse effects are probably infrequent (Robinson and Cambon).

Hypothalamic damage caused by inflammatory injury or vascular compromise secondary to the basilar exudate can produce diabetes insipidus or hyperphagia with resultant obesity (Hay, Udani et al.). Precocious puberty following tuberculous meningitis likewise probably reflects hypothalamic injury (Lorber). Pituitary insufficiency also can follow recovery from this disease (Haslam et al.).

Intracranial calcification observed on x-ray often develops two to four years following recovery and is believed to represent deposition of mineral within the basilar meningeal fibrotic exudate. Lorber found calcification on skull x-ray in 45 of 99 patients following recovery, while Heikel and Wasz-Hockert found late intracranial calcification in 26 of 101 children following tuberculous meningitis.

Treatment

Treatment of tuberculous meningitis is most effective in a preventive way and includes diagnostic measures for the recognition of the disease, prevention of respiratory droplet spread from infected patients, drug therapy of the symptomatic patient and prophylactic treatment of those with skin test conversion, and the judicious use of BCG vaccine (McConville and Rapoport). Children found to have positive PPD skin tests in the first three to four years of life should be treated for one year with isoniazid (INH) in a daily dose of 10 mg. per kilogram. It is rec-

ommended that periodic monitoring of liver function tests be done in patients receiving INH because of the frequent elevation of SGOT levels associated with the use of this drug and possible occurrence of severe hepatotoxicity (Byrd et al.). Older children who are known to have become skin-test-positive within the previous one year likewise should be treated for a period of one year. Furthermore, a child who is skin-test-positive but not under treatment should receive INH for four weeks after receiving measles vaccine or with occurrence of natural measles. Surveillance and management in this fashion has reduced and will continue to reduce the occurrence of meningitis considerably.

When tuberculous meningitis is a reasonable possibility to account for an acute or subacute meningeal inflammatory reaction, it is advisable to initiate antituberculous therapy in addition to antibiotic therapy appropriate for the more common bacterial pathogens on the basis of the age of the child, while waiting for the results of other diagnostic studies. If a bacterial agent other than the tubercle bacillus is identified, the antituberculous drugs can be discontinued. Bacteriologic proof of tuberculous meningitis may require several weeks, if possible at all, by which time most children with this illness would have expired if therapy were withheld.

Treatment of tuberculous meningitis in past years usually included isoniazid, streptomycin, and para-aminosalicylic acid. Intrathecal therapy was commonly resorted to for many years but is infrequently recommended currently except by a few investigators (Freiman and Geefhuyson). Isoniazid remains the mainstay of therapy because of its excellent penetration into the CSF as well as its relative safety. Para-aminosalicylic acid has largely been abandoned from the regimen because of its relatively low antituberculous activity, its lack of ability to gain entrance into the CSF, and the intolerance to the drug exhibited by certain patients (Fallon).

The current combination of drugs commonly recommended for treatment of tuberculous meningitis includes isoniazid in dosage of 20 mg. per kilogram per day orally (up to 500 mg. per day), streptomycin (20 mg. per kilogram per day IM, up to one gram per day), and rifampin (15 mg. per kilogram per day orally, up to 600 mg. per day). Streptomycin and rifampin are continued for approximately eight weeks after there is clinical and laboratory improvement, and isoniazid is thereafter continued for an additional 18 to 24 months. INH is well absorbed from the gastrointestinal tract, with peak serum levels achieved in one to two hours and with excellent penetrance into the CSF. Isoniazid is known to depress hepatic parahydroxylation of phenytoin, resulting in elevated serum levels of the drug with the possible hazard of drug intoxication (Brennan et al.). For this reason, periodic serum levels of phenytoin should be done in patients who receive both drugs. INH is a drug of low toxicity, although there are rare reports of symptomatic toxic hepatitis and even fatal hepatic necrosis from its use in children (Rudoy et al., Stein and Liang, Vanderhoof and Ament). Elevation of the SGOT is not infrequent in patients on INH, although this rarely requires discontinuation of the drug. Peripheral neuropathy can occur in adults receiving isoniazid and can be prevented by the administration of pyridoxine, 50 mg. per day.

Rifampin has been shown to be a highly effective antituberculous drug which is well absorbed from the gastrointestinal tract and has adequate penetration into the CSF. It must be used in combination with other antituberculous antimicrobials because when given alone there is rapid development of resistant strains (Lester). The CSF concentration in the acute stage of the illness is approximately 20 percent of the serum concentration, which represents the fraction of the drug in serum that is not protein-bound (D'Oliveira). Possible adverse effects that have been described with rifampin include nausea, vomiting, abdominal pain, and dizziness (Aquinas et al.). Transient mental confusion and disorientation have been reported but appear to be rare (Pratt), as is thrombocytopenia (Poole et al.) and acute hemolytic anemia (Lakschmanarayan et al.). Toxic hepatitis is the side effect of greatest concern and can be asymptomatic, manifested only by biochemical alterations, or in the form of severe clinical hepatitis (Most and Markle, Scheuer et al.). Overdose of the drug can result in a curious reaction referred to as the "red man syndrome," associated with hepatotoxicity and red discoloration of the urine, tears, and saliva in addition to a "boiled lobster–like" pigmentation of the skin (Newton and Forrest).

Streptomycin, like rifampin, has the disadvantage of the rapid development of bacterial resistance when used alone. Unlike rifampin, streptomycin is minimally absorbed from the gastrointestinal tract and penetrates CSF poorly, even when meninges are inflamed. Its primary side effect is ototoxicity,

with greater involvement of the vestibular division than of the auditory division of the eighth nerve.

So-called "second line" antituberculous drugs, including ethambutol and ethionamide, are a consideration in cases in which isoniazid-resistant organisms are encountered (Bonforte et al., Steiner and Portualeza) or in the rare instance in which INH hepatotoxicity prevents its use. Both drugs are available only in oral preparations, and either will enter the CSF adequately in the acute stage of the illness. Ethambutol has relatively low antituberculous activity and can cause acute optic nerve toxicity. Periodic visual acuity examinations are advised with the use of the drug but are of limited value in younger children. Recommended dose of ethambutol is 20 mg. per kilogram per day. Ethionamide is an unpalatable drug and also is beset with problems of toxicity. For these reasons, both ethambutol and ethionamide are reserved for the unusual occurrence in which tuberculous meningitis is caused by isoniazid-resistant organisms (Vall-Spinosa et al.).

The value of corticosteroids in the treatment of tuberculous meningitis has been debated for years and remains unsettled (Escobar et al., Ghosh et al., O'Toole et al.). Some have suggested that steroid therapy reduces the inflammatory reaction, thereby decreasing the probability of development of hydrocephalus. Others have provided evidence that the mortality is similar with or without steroid therapy, but that sequelae among survivors is higher in those who received corticosteroids. In view of our present concepts of the pathogenesis of the disorder, it would not seem advisable to include corticosteroids as part of the routine treatment of tuberculous meningitis. Corticosteroid therapy would seem logical in cases with rather acute onset in which there is rapid deterioration of the state of responsiveness. Experimental and clinical observations support the concept that brain swelling in such cases can represent a cerebral reaction to tuberculoprotein, and that such response might be inhibited by corticosteroid therapy (Dastur and Udani, Feldman et al.). When used in this fashion, corticosteroid therapy should be relatively brief in duration, and the drug should be discontinued when improvement occurs.

Progressive hydrocephalus is a frequent complication of tuberculous meningitis and can be a limiting factor regarding outcome unless it is recognized and managed. Hydrocephalus is usually of the communicating type but can also be the result of intraventricular obstruction. The status of the ventricular size can be assessed by computed tomography performed at periodic intervals, and the need for treatment determined by clinical signs as well as the rate and degree of ventricular enlargement. Progressive communicating hydrocephalus has been treated by periodic lumbar punctures for CSF removal along with acetazolamide therapy (Visudhiphan and Chiemchanya 1979), while obstructive hydrocephalus usually requires some type of diversionary procedure.

REFERENCES

Allison, M. J., and Dalton, H. P.: Etiology of meningitis at the Medical College of Virginia, 1961–1965. Virginia Med. Monthly 94: 317–319, 1967.

Anderson, J. M., and MacMillan, J. J.: Intracranial tuberculoma—an increasing problem in Britain. J. Neurol. Neurosurg. Psychiat. 38:194–201, 1975.

Aquinas, M., Allan, W. G. L., Horsfall, P. A. L., Jenkins, P. K., Hung-Yan, W., Girling, D., Tall, R., and Fox, W.: Adverse reactions to daily and intermittent rifampicin regimens for pulmonary tuberculosis in Hong Kong. Brit. Med. J. 1:765–771, 1972.

Arseni, C., and Samitca, D. C.: Intraspinal tuberculosis granuloma. Brain 83:285–292, 1960.

Avery, M. E., and Wolfdorf, J.: Diagnosis and treatment: Approaches to newborn infants of tuberculous mothers. Pediatrics 42:519–522, 1968.

Bailey, H. L., Gabriel, M., Hodgson, A. R., and Shin, J. S.: Tuberculosis of the spine in children. Operative findings and results in one hundred consecutive patients treated by removal of the lesion and anterior grafting. J. Bone Joint Surg. 54A:1633–1657, 1972.

Bannister, C. M.: A tuberculous abscess of the brain. Case report. J. Neurosurg. 33:203–206, 1970.

Belsey M. A.: Tuberculosis and varicella infections in children. Am. J. Dis. Child. 113:444–448, 1967.

Berkovich, S., and Starr, S.: Effects of live type 1 poliovirus vaccine and other viruses on the tuberculin test. New Eng. J. Med. 274:67–72, 1966.

Blacklock, J. W. S., and Griffin, M. A.: Tuberculous meningitis in children. J. Path. Bact. 40:489–502, 1935.

Bonforte, R. J., Karpas, C. M., Gribetz, I., and Shanzer, S.: Tuberculous meningitis due to primary drug-resistant Mycobacterium tuberculosis hominis. Pediatrics 42:969–975, 1968.

Brennan, R. W., Dehejia, H., Kutt, H., Verebely, K., and McDowell, F.: Diphenylhydantoin intoxication attendant to slow inactivation of isoniazid. Neurology 20:687–693, 1970.

Burn, C. G., and Finley, K. H.: The role of hypersensitivity in the production of experimental meningitis. J. Exper. Med. 56:203–221, 1932.

Byrd, R. B., Horn, B. R., Solomon, D. A., and Griggs, G. A.: Toxic effects of isoniazid in tuberculosis chemoprophylaxis. Role of biochemical monitoring in 1,000 patients. J.A.M.A. 241:1239–1241, 1979.

Carlgren, L. E., Hansson, C. G., Henricsson, L., and Wahlen, P.: Fatal BCG infection in an infant with congenital lymphocytopenic agammaglobulinemia. Acta Pediat. Scand. 55:636, 1966.

Cashman, J. M.: Congenital tuberculosis. Proc. Roy. Soc. Med. 52:297, 1959.

Damergis, J. A., Leftwich, E. I., Curtin, J. A., and Witorsch, P.: Tuberculoma of the brain. J.A.M.A. 239:413–415, 1978.

Daniel, P. M.: Gross morbid anatomy of the central nervous system of cases of tuberculous meningitis treated with streptomycin. Proc. Roy. Soc. Med. 42:169–172, 1949.

Dastur, D. K., and Udani, P. M.: The pathology and pathogenesis of tuberculous encephalopathy. Acta Neuropath. 6:311–326, 1966.

Descuns, P., Garre, H., and Pheline, C.: Tuberculomas of the brain and cerebellum. J. Neurosurg. 11:243–250, 1954.

D'Oliveira, J. J. G.: Cerebrospinal fluid concentrations of rifampin in meningeal tuberculosis. Am. Rev. Respir. Dis. 106:432–437, 1972.

Doniach, I.: Changes in the meningeal vessels in acute and chronic (streptomycin-treated) tuberculous meningitis. J. Path. Bact. 61:253–259, 1949.

Donner, M., and Wasz-Hockert, O.: Late neurologic sequelae of tuberculous meningitis. Acta Paediat. Suppl. 141:34–42, 1962.

Down, J. L.: Observations on an ethnic classification of idiots. Clinical Lectures and Reports, London Hospital 3:259–262, 1866.

Emond, R. T. D., and McKendrick, G. D. W.: Tuberculosis as a cause of transient aseptic meningitis. Lancet 2:234–236, 1973.

Escobar, J. A., Belsey, M. A., Duenas, A., and Medina, P.: Mortality from tuberculous meningitis reduced by steroid therapy. Pediatrics 56:1050–1055, 1975.

Esterly, J. R., Sturner, W. Q., Esterly, N. B., and Windhorst, D. B.: Disseminated BCG in twin boys with presumed chronic granulomatous disease of childhood. J. Pediat. 48:141–143, 1971.

Fallon, R. J.: The treatment of tuberculous meningitis. J. Antimicrob. Chemother. 4:1–2, 1978.

Feldman, S., Behar, A. J., and Weber, D.: Experimental tuberculous meningitis in rabbits. II. Effect of hydrocortisone on the hypersensitivity reaction of the meninges. Arch. Neurol. 3:420–424, 1960.

Forlenza, S. W., Axelrod, J. L., and Grieco, M. H.: Pott's disease in heroin addicts. J.A.M.A. 241:379–380, 1979.

Freeman, B. A.: Burrows' Textbook of Microbiology, 21st Edition. W. B. Saunders Company, Philadelphia, 1979.

Freiman, I., and Geefhuysen, J.: Evaluation of intrathecal therapy with streptomycin and hydrocortisone in tuberculous meningitis. J. Pediat. 76:895–901, 1970.

Ghosh, S., Seshadri, R., and Jain, K. C.: Evaluation of corticosteroids in treatment of tuberculous meningitis. Arch. Dis. Childh. 46:51–54, 1971.

Ginsburg, S., Gross, E., Feiring, E. H., and Scheinberg, L. C.: The neurological complications of tuberculous spondylitis. Pott's paraplegia. Arch. Neurol. 16:265–276, 1967.

Giustra, F. X.: A comparative study of the Levinson and tryptophan tests as aids in the diagnosis of tuberculous meningitis. J. Pediat. 11:805–811, 1937.

Gleich, M.: The Levinson test in tuberculous meningitis. Am. J. Dis. Child. 43:1077–1085, 1932.

Greenfield, J. G.: In Greenfield, J. G., Blackwood, W., McMenemey, W. H., Meyer, A., and Norman, R. M.: Neuropathology. Edward Arnold, Publishers, London, 1958.

Harris, V. J., Schauf, V., Duda, F., and White, H.: Fatal tuberculosis in young children. Pediatrics 63:912–914, 1979.

Haskett, J. R., Jr., Branch, C. E., Jr., and Buscemi, J. H.: Brainstem tuberculoma: Value of sequential computed tomography. Ann. Neurol. 6:275–276, 1979.

Haslam, R. H. A., Winternitz, W. W., and Howieson, J.: Selective hypopituitarism following tuberculous meningitis. Am. J. Dis. Child. 118:903–908, 1969.

Hay, D. R.: Diabetes insipidus after tuberculous meningitis. Brit. Med. J. 1:707, 1960.

Heikel, P., and Wasz-Hockert, O.: Late radiological findings after recovery from tuberculous meningitis. Acta Paediat. 51(Suppl. 141):88–92, 1962.

Hinman, A. R.: Tuberculous meningitis at Cleveland Metropolitan General Hospital 1959 to 1963. Am. Rev. Respir. Dis. 95:670–673, 1967.

Holden, M., Dubin, M. R., and Diamond, P. H.: Frequency of negative intermediate-strength tuberculin sensitivity in patients with active tuberculosis. New Eng. J. Med. 285:1506–1509, 1971.

Holt, L. E.: Observations on three hundred cases of acute meningitis in infants and young children. Am. J. Dis. Child. 1:26–36, 1911.

Hughes, R. A. C., and Mair, W. G. P.: Acute necrotic myelopathy with pulmonary tuberculosis. Brain 100:223–238, 1977.

Idriss, Z. H., Sinno, A. A., and Kronfol, N. M.: Tuberculous meningitis in children. Forty-three cases. Am. J. Dis. Child. 130:364–367, 1976.

Kasahara, M.: The specific diagnosis of tuberculous meningitis. Am. J. Dis. Child. 13:141–144, 1917.

Kendig, E. L., Jr.: The place of BCG vaccine in the management of infants born of tuberculous mothers. New Eng. J. Med. 281:520–523, 1969.

Khan, M. A., Kovnat, D. M., Dachus, B., Whitcomb, M. E., Brody, J. S., and Snider, G. L.: Clinical and roentgenographic spectrum of pulmonary tuberculosis in the adult. Am. J. Med. 62:31–38, 1977.

Kocen, R. S., and Parsons, M.: Neurological complications of tuberculosis: Some unusual manifestations. Quart. J. Med. 39:17–30, 1970.

Koch, R.: Die aetiologie der tuberkulose. Berlin Klin. Wchnschr. 19:221–230, 1882.

Koch, R., and Carson, M. J.: Management of Hemophilus influenzae, type B, meningitis. Analysis of 128 cases. J. Pediat. 46:18–29, 1955.

Kupers, T. A., Petrich, J. M., Halloway, A. W., and St. Geme, J. W., Jr.: Depression of tuberculin delayed hypersensitivity by live attenuated mumps virus. J. Pediat. 76:716–721, 1970.

Lakshmanarayan, S., Sahn, S., and Hudson, D.: Massive hemolysis caused by rifampicin. Brit. Med. J. 2:282–283, 1973.

Lehrer, H.: The angiographic triad in tuberculous meningitis. A radiographic and clinicopathologic correlation. Radiology 87:829–835, 1966.

Lester, W.: Rifampin: A semisynthetic derivative of rifamycin—a prototype for the future. Ann. Rev. Microbiol. 26:85–102, 1972.

Levinsky, R. J., and Wilkinson, A.: Mixed pneumococcal and tuberculous meningitis. Arch. Dis. Childh. 49:325–328, 1974.

Lichtenberg, H. H.: The tryptophan test in tuberculous meningitis. Am. J. Dis. Child. 43:32–39, 1932.

Lincoln, E. M., Sordillo, S. V. R., and Davies, P. A.: Tuberculous meningitis in children. J. Pediat. 57:807–823, 1960.

Lindsay, J. W., Rice, E. C., and Selinger, M. A.: The treatment of meningitis due to Hemophilus influenzae (Pfeiffer's bacillus). J. Pediat. 17:220–227, 1940.

Lintermans, J. P., and Sayhnaeve, V.: Tuberculous meningitis developing during the course of chemother-apy for pulmonary tuberculosis. Pediatrics 44:514–517, 1969.

Lorber, J.: Sexual precocity following recovery from tuberculous meningitis with hydrocephalus. Proc. Roy. Soc. Med. 44:726–727, 1951.

Lorber, J.: Long-term follow-up of 100 children who recovered from tuberculous meningitis. Pediatrics 28:778–791, 1961.

Mandal, B. K., Evans, D. I. K., Ironside, A. G., and Pullan, B. R.: Radioactive bromide partition test in differential diagnosis of tuberculous meningitis. Brit. Med. J. 4:413–415, 1972.

Manno, N. J., Uihlein, A., and Kernohan, J. W.: Intraspinal epidermoids. J. Neurosurg. 19:754–765, 1962.

Martin, N. S.: Tuberculosis of the spine. A study of the results of treatment during the last twenty-five years. J. Bone Joint Surg. 52B:613–628, 1970.

Mathew, N. T., Abraham, J., and Chandy, J.: Cerebral angiographic features in tuberculous meningitis. Neurology 20:1015–1023, 1970.

Matsaniotis, N., and Economou-Mavrou, C.: BCG fatalities—new aspects on their etiology. Ann. Paediat. 206:363–378, 1966.

Mayers, M. M., Kaufman, D. M., and Miller, M. H.: Recent cases of intracranial tuberculomas. Neurology 28:256–260, 1978.

MacAdams, A. M., and Rubio, T.: Tuberculous otomastoiditis in children. Am. J. Dis. Child. 131:152–156, 1977.

McConville, J. H., and Rapoport, M. I.: Tuberculosis management in the mid-1970's. J.A.M.A. 235:172–176, 1976.

Meyers, A. E.: A study of 105 cases of tuberculous meningitis. Am. J. Dis. Child. 9:427–445, 1915.

Most, J. A., and Markle, G. B.: A nearly fatal hepatotoxic reaction to rifampin after halothane anesthesia. Am. J. Surg. 127:593–595, 1974.

Newton, R. W., and Forrest, A. R. W.: Rifampicin overdosage—"the red man syndrome." Scott. Med. J. 20:55–56, 1975.

Norris, F. H., Jr., Garvey, P. H., and Swalbach, G. W.: A mild form of tuberculous meningitis. Arch. Neurol. 10:398–401, 1964.

O'Toole, R. D., Thornton, G. F., Mukherjee, M. K., and Nath, R. L.: Dexamethasone in tuberculous meningitis. Relationship of cerebrospinal fluid effects to therapeutic efficacy. Ann. Intern. Med. 70:39–48, 1969.

Parsons, M., and Pallis, C. A.: Intradural spinal tuberculomas. Neurology 15:1018–1022, 1965.

Passwell, J., Katz, D., Frank, Y., Spirer, Z., Cohen, B. E., and Ziprkowski, M.: Fatal disseminated BCG infection. An investigation of the immunodeficiency. Am. J. Dis. Child. 130:433–436, 1976.

Poole, G., Stradling, P., and Worlledge, S.: Potentially serious side-effects of high-dose twice-weekly rifampicin. Postgrad. Med. J. 47:742–747, 1971.

Pott, P.: Remarks on that kind of palsy of the lower limbs which is frequently found to accompany a curvature of the spine and is supposed to be caused by it. Johnson Publications, Ltd., London, 1779.

Pratt, T. H.: Rifampin-induced organic brain syndrome. J.A.M.A. 241:2421–2422, 1979.

Ranta, J., and Wasz-Hockert, O.: Late otological sequelae of tuberculous meningitis. Acta Paediat. 51(Suppl. 141):50–64, 1962.

Reisinger, K. S., Evans, P., Yost, G., and Rogers, K. D.: Congenital tuberculosis: Report of a case. Pediatrics 54:74–76, 1974.

Rich, A. R., and McCordock, H. A.: The pathogenesis

of tuberculous meningitis. Johns Hopkins Med. J. 52:5–38, 1933.

Robinson, G. C., and Cambon, K. G.: Hearing loss in infants of tuberculous mothers treated with streptomycin during pregnancy. New Eng. J. Med. 271:949–951, 1964.

Roedenbeck, S. D.: Tuberculomas of the nervous system in children. A report of 32 cases. World Neurology 3:54–62, 1962.

Rooney, J. J., Crocco, J. A., Kramer, S., and Lyons, H. A.: Further observations on tuberculin reactions in active tuberculosis. Am. J. Med. 60:517–522, 1976.

Rowlatt, V. F.: The effect of prolonged tuberculous meningitis on the brain and spinal cord. Acta Neuropath. 3:532–546, 1964.

Rudoy, R., Stuemky, J., and Poley, J. R.: Isoniazid administration and liver injury. Am. J. Dis. Child. 125:733–736, 1973.

Sahn, S. A., and Neff, T. A.: Miliary tuberculosis. Am. J. Med. 56:495–505, 1974.

Saltzman, S. J., and Feigin, R. D.: Tuberculous otitis media and mastoiditis. J. Pediat. 79:1004–1006, 1971.

Scheuer, P. J., Summerfield, J. A., Lal, S., and Sherlock, S.: Rifampicin hepatitis. A clinical and histological study. Lancet 1:421–425, 1974.

Schuit, K. E.: Miliary tuberculosis in children. Clinical and laboratory manifestations in 19 patients. Am. J. Dis. Child. 133:583–585, 1979.

Schuster, A., Duffau, G., Nicholls, E., and Pino, C. M.: Lung aspirate puncture as a diagnostic aid in pulmonary tuberculosis in childhood. A preliminary study. Pediatrics 42:647–650, 1968.

Sibley, W. A., and O'Brien, J. L.: Intracranial tuberculomas. A review of clinical features and treatment. Neurology 6:157–165, 1956.

Spink, W. W.: Infectious Diseases. Prevention and Treatment in the Nineteenth and Twentieth Centuries. University of Minnesota Press, Minneapolis, 1978.

Stein, M. T., and Liang, D.: Clinical hepatotoxicity of isoniazid in children. Pediatrics 64:499–505, 1979.

Steiner, P., and Portugaleza, C.: Tuberculous meningitis in children. A review of 25 cases observed between the years 1965 and 1970 at the Kings County Center of Brooklyn with special reference to the problem of infection with primary drug-resistant strains of M. tuberculosis. Am. Rev. Respir. Dis. 107:22–29, 1973.

Swinthinback, J., Smith, H. V., and Vollum, R. L.: The intrathecal tuberculin reaction. J. Path. Bact. 65:565–596, 1964.

Tahernia, A. C.: Tuberculous meningitis. Modern diagnosis, treatment and prognosis, as exemplified in 38 cases in southern Iran. Clin. Pediat. 6:173–177, 1967.

Taylor, L. M., Smith, H. V., and Hunter, G.: The blood-CSF barrier to bromide in diagnosis of tuberculous meningitis. Lancet 1:700–702, 1954.

Todd, R. M., and Neville, J. G.: The sequelae of tuberculous meningitis. Arch. Dis. Childh. 39:213–225, 1964.

Turner, L.: Subdural collections of fluid in tuberculous meningitis. Lancet 1:849–852, 1954.

Udani, P. M., Parekh, V. C., and Dastur, D. K.: Neurological and related syndromes in CNS tuberculosis. Clinical features and pathogenesis. J. Neurol. Sci. 14:341–357, 1971.

Vall-Spinosa, A., Lester, W., Moulding, T., Davidson, P. T., and McClatchy, J. K.: Rifampin in the treatment of drug-resistant Mycobacterium tuberculosis infections. New Eng. J. Med. 283:616–621, 1970.

Vanderhoof, J. A., and Ament, M. E.: Fatal hepatic necrosis due to isoniazid chemoprophylaxis in a 15-year-old girl. J. Pediat. 88:867–868, 1976.

Visudhiphan, P., and Chiemchanya, S.: Evaluation of rifampicin in the treatment of tuberculous meningitis in children. J. Pediat. 87:983–986, 1975.

Visudhiphan, P., and Chiemchanya, S.: Hydrocephalus in tuberculous meningitis in children: Treatment with acetazolamide and repeated lumbar puncture. J. Pediat. 95:657–660, 1979.

Voyce, M. A., and Hunt, A. C.: Congenital tuberculosis. Arch. Dis. Childh. 41:299–300, 1966.

Wasz-Hockert, O., and Donner, M.: Results of treatment of 191 children with tuberculous meningitis in the years 1949–54. Acta Paediat.(Suppl. 141):7–25, 1962.

Weichsel, M., and Herzger, G.: Significance of the diminution of the spinal fluid sugar in tuberculous meningitis. J. Pediat. 9:763–770, 1936.

Weiss, W., and Flippin, H. F.: The changing incidence and prognosis of tuberculous meningitis. Am. J. Med. Sci. 250:46–59, 1965.

Whitener, D. R.: Tuberculous brain abscess. Report of a case and review of the literature. Arch. Neurol. 35:148–155, 1978.

Whytt, R.: Observations on the dropsy in the brain. Balfour, Auld and Smellie, Edinburgh, 1768.

Wilkinson, H. A., Ferris, E. J., Muggia, A. L., and Cantu, R. C.: Central nervous system tuberculosis: a persistent disease. J. Neurosurg. 34:15–22, 1971.

Zinneman, H. H., and Hall, W. H.: Transient tuberculous meningitis. Am. Rev. Respir. Dis. 114:1185–1188, 1976.

Chapter Eight

FOCAL SUPPURATIVE INFECTIONS OF THE NERVOUS SYSTEM

BRAIN ABSCESS

Although brain abscesses are not common in the childhood age group, awareness of their possible occurrence is important because they are potentially curable lesions if identified reasonably early in their development. A brain abscess that is not recognized carries the hazard of possible rupture into the ventricular system, leading to fulminating meningitis, or the occurrence of internal herniation, resulting in brain stem compression and death. The latter can happen spontaneously owing to the mass effect of the lesion and the edema surrounding it, or can be provoked by lumbar puncture done for diagnostic reasons when a focal suppurative lesion is not suspected. A brain abscess can be surprisingly silent from the clinical standpoint but most are associated with abnormalities indicative either of infection or of neurologic dysfunction. Fever, focal neurologic signs, or signs of increased intracranial pressure are the common clinical features of a brain abscess, but not all are present in every patient with this lesion.

Focal signs, when present, are determined by the location of the abscess, or abscesses, within the cerebrum or cerebellum, while intracranial hypertension reflects the mass effect of the abscess, the commonly present edema surrounding the mass, or the existence of ventricular obstruction when the lesion is in the posterior fossa. Brain abscesses of otogenic or rhinogenic origin have become less frequent since the introduction of antibiotics; however, the overall incidence of brain abscess has not appreciably decreased in the last three or four decades (Beller et al.). Abscess formation within the parenchyma of the brain can be solitary or multiple, with the lesion being either unilocular or multilocular in configuration. In some cases a parenchymal abscess is associated with epidural abscess, subdural abscess, or an extracranial suppurative focus. In other cases, brain abscess occurs in the absence of evidence of infection elsewhere.

Brain abscesses are less often identified during infancy than in older children (Butler et al., Holt) but have been described in infants in the first few weeks of life (Hoffman et al., Munslow et al., Sanford, Vogel et al.). In most cases in early infancy, the initial presumptive diagnosis has been congenital hydrocephalus because of rapidly progressive head enlargement without obvious focal signs (Fig. 8–1). Diagnosis of cerebral abscess in such instances has often been made unexpectedly at the time of transfontanel cannulation for ventriculography, and more recently, by cranial computed tomography performed for supposed hydrocephalus. With an infant a few weeks of age with progressive head enlargement, a significant elevation of the leukocyte count in the blood may be the first evidence suggestive of an intracranial suppurative process rather than one of the more conventional causes of infantile head enlargement.

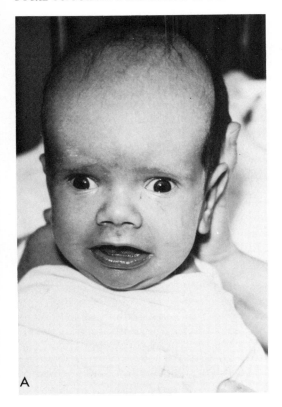

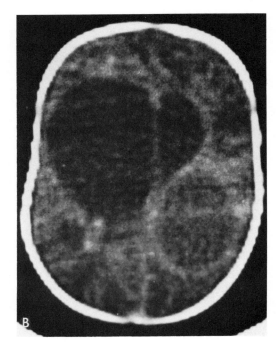

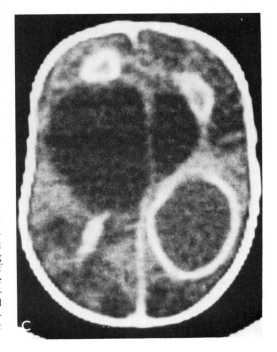

Figure 8–1.   Multiple, pyogenic cerebral abscesses in an 8-week-old infant. The child had a normal birth and delivery and did well in the immediate neonatal period. Head circumference was normal at 37.5 cm. when measured at 3 weeks of age. Eleven days prior to admission, the parents observed the infant to be irritable and thereafter they felt that his head was enlarging at an abnormal rate. *A,* Age 8 weeks at the time of hospital admission. The tentative diagnosis on admission was one of progressive hydrocephalus of undetermined origin. At this time, the head circumference is 45.5 cm. and the anterior fontanel is excessively large and tense. The cranial sutures are palpably separated. There is a mild divergent strabismus and the neck is somewhat stiff. The child is intensely irritable and is hypertonic and hyperreflexic in all four extremities. A wide zone of abnormal transillumination could be observed over the right parietal region. Because of a white blood cell count of 30,000 per cu. mm. on the day of admission, a lumbar puncture was performed which yielded CSF containing 220 WBC per cu. mm. (40 percent polymorphonuclear leukocytes), a glucose of 22 mg. per 100 ml., and protein of 255 mg. per 100 ml. The gram stain of the CSF was negative. *B,* Computed tomogram before contrast infusion shows ventricular enlargement with the left lateral ventricle being much more distended than the right. There are multiple bilateral zones of decreased density of various size. *C,* Computed tomogram after contrast infusion demonstrates two small periventricular frontal abscesses, each with a very thick enhanced ring, and a massive right parieto-occipital abscess with striking ring enhancement. In addition, there are multiple areas of hypodensity within the cerebral parenchyma, believed to be either zones of cerebritis or of softening. Soon after performance of the scan, 80 ml. of thick, yellow pus was drained from the large abscess on the right side. With continued treatment, the child survived but was left with severe neurologic deficits. A ventriculo-peritoneal shunt was required.

At any time in the infant age group, cerebral abscesses are likely to become very large in size before being recognized. A much higher percentage of brain abscesses in infants are caused by gram-negative bacteria than is the case in older children, with the common organisms in the infant group being *Escherichia coli, Citrobacter freundii,* or *Proteus* species. Especially in infants less than two months of age, *Citrobacter* species have been the most common isolates from brain abscesses. Of six cerebral abscesses in infants less than three months of age described by Hoffman et al., all were exceedingly large when discovered, three had ruptured into the ventricle prior to diagnosis, five of the six were caused by gram-negative organisms, and in only one was there an obvious predisposing septic source. Among those who survive with treatment of a cerebral abscess in infancy, the illness is frequently complicated by hydrocephalus, which eventually requires shunting.

In older children, conditions that predispose to the development of brain abscess include chronic otitis media or mastoiditis, sinusitis, suppurative pulmonary infection, bacterial endocarditis, and cyanotic congenital heart disease or pulmonary arteriovenous fistula. Suppurative skin lesions and dental extractions are other potential sources of sepsis which can lead to the formation of a brain abscess. Despite the high incidence of chronic suppurative pulmonary infections in children with cystic fibrosis, brain abscess complicating this disease has only rarely been reported (Duffner and Cohen). Fischer et al. have suggested that, as patients with cystic fibrosis survive into adulthood, the risk of developing a brain abscess may increase. In their three adult patients with intracranial abscesses, the causative organisms were aerobic and anaerobic bacteria of the oral flora rather than from the lungs.

Cerebellar abscess can develop secondary to infection within a dermoid cyst at the termination of a congenital dermal sinus in the posterior fossa. Brain abscess can complicate primary bacterial meningitis in children when diagnosis is delayed and the infection is not properly managed. This is more true of pneumococcal meningitis than other types in children, and perhaps occurs more often with neonatal gram-negative meningitis in which rapid sterilization of the cerebrospinal fluid does not usually occur even with appropriate antibiotic therapy (Kaplan et al.). It should be stressed, however, that parenchy-mal abscess is an unusual complication of meningitis that is promptly recognized and adequately treated. Additional predisposing causes of focal cerebral suppuration provoked by a variety of bacterial agents and certain fungi include disorders associated with immunosuppression or chronic debilitation.

Penetrating cranial injuries can also be the source of entry of bacteria leading to abscess within the brain. Such injuries in children are usually obvious traumatic insults with skull fractures and dural laceration but can be deceptively subtle with evidence of penetration of the skull by a foreign body not initially apparent. Small missiles, such as fragments of wire, may be propelled by power machinery, or an accidental fall on a sharpened pencil can result in transmission of foreign material into the brain, resulting in abscess formation (Horner et al.). Animal bites about the head, especially those of large dogs that attack infants or small children, can introduce bacteria into the brain, leading to abscess formation (Klein and Cohen).

Brain abscess has been described in patients with hereditary hemorrhagic telangiectasia (Dyer), a disorder with a predisposition to intracranial suppuration because of the high incidence of associated pulmonary arteriovenous malformations. In this regard, the vascular shunt within the lung is analogous to the physiology of congenital cardiac defects with right-to-left shunts that are discussed below.

Congenital Heart Disease and Brain Abscess

Congenital heart disease, especially of the cyanotic type, is one of the most important factors predisposing the child to the development of cerebral abscess (Calkins and Bell, Matson and Salam, Raimondi et al.). In children under two years of age with congenital heart disease, acquired neurologic dysfunction is most often due to vascular occlusive disease, while in those over two years abscess must be considered in any cyanotic child who develops headaches, seizures, or other focal neurologic signs. Tetralogy of Fallot is the most common associated cardiac lesion, although brain abscess can develop in any condition with a right-to-left intracardiac shunt or with a pulmonary arteriovenous fistula (Stern and Naffziger). Venous to arterial shunts within the heart allow recirculation of poorly oxygenated venous blood through the systemic circulation, thus bypassing the filtering effects of the lungs. This exposes the brain to bacteria ordinarily present in the circulation only briefly, as in transient bacteremia.

Polycythemia secondary to arterial oxygen desaturation results in increased blood viscosity, leading to a reduction in the rate of cerebral blood flow. These factors are important in the pathogenesis of brain abscess formation in children with cyanotic heart disease, although previous tissue damage from hypoxia may also be necessary. Experiments in animals by Groff in 1934 revealed that bacteremia did not result in the formation of a brain abscess unless preceding brain infarction had occurred. More recent experimental studies by Molinari et al. likewise have shown that normal brain parenchyma exhibits a striking resistance to direct invasion by bloodborne bacteria. A vascular effect with tissue ischemia or infarction is a major predisposing factor allowing penetration of microorganisms into the brain, exciting an inflammatory response and eventual suppuration. In view of the disturbed hemodynamics and alterations in blood flow in children with cyanotic heart disease, ample opportunities exist for hypoxic or ischemic cerebral insults to occur. Bacterial endocarditis is usually not present in those found to have brain abscesses, and preceding infections, including otherwise insignificant bacteremia, are frequently not recognized. Surgical shunt procedures, including the Potts and Blalock anastomoses, do not eliminate the possibility of subsequent development of a brain abscess (Wishingrad et al., Clark and Clarke). These shunt procedures increase pulmonary blood flow, but persistence of the ventricular defect permits venous contamination of systemic blood.

Pathologic Considerations

Abscesses may be located in various positions within the cerebrum or cerebellum (Fig. 8–2). Those associated with cyanotic heart disease are often solitary and are generally found in the distribution of supply of the middle cerebral artery. Brain abscesses in infants with staphylococcal sepsis or with infected meningomyeloceles and secondary ventriculitis are more often multiple than single. Chronic suppurative otitis or mastoiditis results in either temporal lobe or cerebellar hemisphere suppuration, while abscess secondary to sinusitis is more commonly frontal in location. Tarkkanen reported 99 cases of otogenic brain abscesses, of which 78 percent were secondary to chronic otitis and 22 percent resulted from acute otitis media. Children were much less often affected with this complication than adults, and 71 percent of the patients were male. The abscess was located above the tentorium in 54 of the 99 cases, almost all being within the temporal lobe. In 42 patients, the abscess was within the cerebellum and three patients harbored both cerebral and cerebellar lesions. The mortality rate in this series was 66 percent; however, it included cases seen as early as 1930.

Abscesses within the brain stem, basal nuclei, or thalamus are infrequent and those that do occur are generally hematogenous in origin (Law et al.). Abscesses of the pituitary gland are even more unusual and are rarely diagnosed prior to surgery or postmortem examination. Presentation in recorded cases has been either in the form of a syndrome simulating a pituitary tumor with headaches, visual disturbances, and endocrine abnormalities, or with acute meningitis in a patient who is found to have enlargement of the sella turcica on x-ray examination (Domingue and Wilson). In other cases, pituitary abscess occurs in a patient with a previously recognized intrasellar neoplasm, or following surgery for neoplasms in this region.

Streptococcus and *Staphylococcus* species are the organisms most frequently recovered from cerebral abscesses (Raimondi et al., Tarkkanen, Wright and Ballantine), although some are caused by gram-negative bacteria such as *Escherichia coli, Citrobacter* species, *Hemophilus influenzae, Proteus* species, or *Pseudomonas* species (Hoffman et al., Kaplan et al., Munslow et al., Vogel et al.). *Pasteurella multocida* is a rare cause of birth abscess but has been reported in a 19-month-old child following a perforating dog bite (Klein and Cohen) and in an older child with chronic otitis media (Larsen et al.). *Mycoplasma hominis,* an infrequent cause of invasive infection of any type in infancy, was isolated from a cerebral abscess in a three-week-old infant reported by Siber et al.

Anaerobic organisms are important causes of brain abscesses and most likely account for many of the reported cases with negative cultures. *Peptostreptococcus* and *Bacteroides* species are currently the most common anaerobic bacteria isolated from brain abscesses, and, when all age groups are considered, are col-

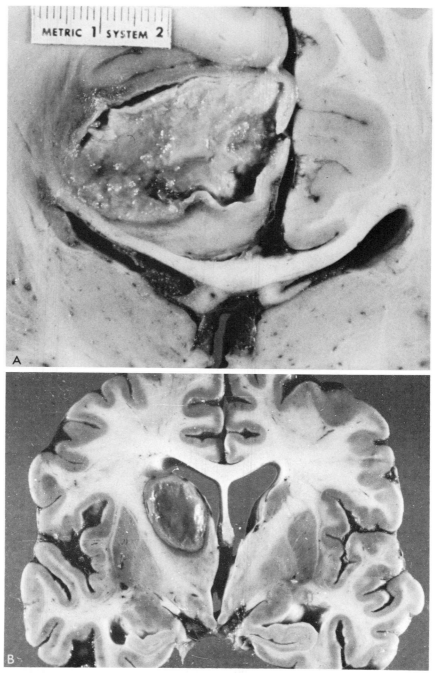

Figure 8–2.   Brain abscesses of variable appearance and location. *A,* Pyogenic abscess in the cingulate gyrus in a child with cyanotic congenital heart disease. The abscess is surrounded by a poorly developed capsule. The lateral margin of the corpus callosum adjacent to the abscess is softened. Purulent material within the underlying lateral ventricle is the result of spontaneous perforation through the corpus callosum. *B,* Solitary encapsulated abscess in the region of the caudate nucleus and internal capsule.

Illustration continued on opposite page

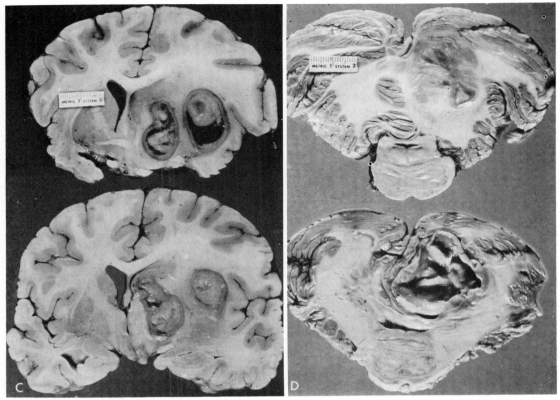

Figure 8–2 Continued. C, Multiple well-encapsulated abscesses. Note the extensive cerebral swelling of the involved hemisphere which results in shift and distortion of the lateral ventricular system. *D,* Large cerebellar abscess, otogenic in origin. The section above shows discolored, softened, and necrotic white matter, while that below reveals a multiloculated abscess surrounded by an incompletely developed capsule.

lectively perhaps the most common cause of this lesion. The increasing prevalence of anaerobes as a cause of focal suppurative intracranial disease emphasizes the need for both aerobic and anaerobic cultures on all such specimens (Heineman and Braude). In addition to culturing purulent material obtained from the confines of an abscess, it is also useful to obtain for culture a small specimen of brain tissue immediately adjacent to the abscess whenever possible. *Bacteroides* species are anaerobic, gram-negative bacilli which are common normal inhabitants of the respiratory and gastrointestinal tracts. These organisms may gain entrance to the blood stream, resulting in a wide range of conditions, including brain abscess (Salibi). *Bacteroides* species brain abscess can also develop secondary to spread of infection from chronic otitis media (Smith et al.). *Hemophilus aphrophilus,* an anaerobic organism with a predilection for a high concentration of carbon dioxide, has been recovered from several brain abscesses in children with cyanotic heart disease (Fischbein).

Neurologic infection with *Listeria monocytogenes* is usually in the form of suppurative meningitis, either in early infancy or in immunosuppressed adults. Brain abscess or focal cerebritis caused by this organism is very uncommon but has been described in renal transplant patients, in chronic alcoholics, or in other immunocompromising conditions (Buchner and Schneierson, Crocker and Leicester, Watson et al.). Another rare disorder with which *Listeria monocytogenes* has been incriminated is focal suppuration and necrosis of the brain stem without infection elsewhere in the nervous system (Duffy et al., Mahony et al.). *Mycobacterium tuberculosis* can cause abscess formation within the brain, although these rare lesions are less common than the more characteristic tuberculous mass lesion referred to as tuberculoma (Whitener). Tuberculous brain abscess grossly resembles a pyogenic abscess and, like the latter, often results in focal symptoms of short duration with fairly rapid progression of clinical signs. The disorder usually occurs in association with other extracranial evidence of tuberculosis. *Toxoplasma gondii* infection of the brain in the immunosuppressed patient is usually either a diffuse meningoencephalitis or multifocal granulomatous lesions but can present as a brain abscess in rare cases (McLeod et al.).

Multiple cerebral microabscesses or even large solitary abscesses can occur with certain fungal infections, including those due to *Cryptococcus neoformans, Blastomyces dermatitidis* (Leers et al.), *Candida* species (Roessman and Friede), *Aspergillus* species (Hughes), and *Allescheria boydii* (Bell and Myers, Forno and Billingham, Rosen et al.). *Nocardia asteroides* is a rare but widely recognized cause of brain abscess, most often seen in patients who are debilitated, or receiving corticosteroids or cytotoxic agents (Rankin and Javid, Shuster et al.). The portal of entry of this organism is by respiratory inhalation in most cases, with hematogenous dissemination resulting in potential abscess formation in multiple organs, including the brain. Nocardia brain abscesses can be either solitary or multiple. Lack of encapsulation is a characteristic feature of cerebral abscess due to this fungus but is not invariable. Brain abscess can also be caused on rare occasion by the dematiacious fungus, *Cladosporium trichoides* (Middleton et al.), and

by *Actinomyces* species (McDowell et al.). Most reported cases have occurred in adults, and immune abnormalities have not been prominent in most instances. Amebic cerebral abscess caused by *Entamoeba histolytica* is an infrequent but catastrophic complication of primary hepatic or intestinal amebic disease. Intracranial suppuration with this parasite is usually in the form of multiple abscesses of various sizes and, in some cases, is associated with diffuse meningeal invasion (Lombardo et al.).

The earliest stage of the development of a cerebral abscess consists of a poorly demarcated area of septic cerebritis with softening, hyperemia, and infiltration of inflammatory cells. Necrotic changes occur centrally, followed by liquefaction and the subsequent formation of purulent material constituting the abscess (Fig. 8–3). Fibroblastic activity around the circumference of the abscess, in addition to gliosis, eventually results in encapsulation of the lesion. In most instances, profound edema of white matter is present in the region of a brain abscess and may extend several centimeters from its periphery (Fig. 8–4). Schurr has stated that a minimum of four to six weeks is required for capsule formation following the initial stage of cerebritis.

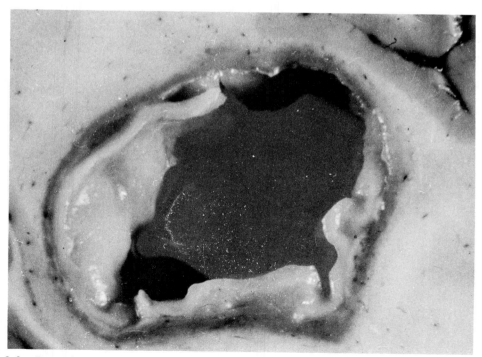

Figure 8–3. Pyogenic cerebral abscess. Purulent material largely escaped from the lesion when the brain was sectioned. Note the hyperemic border and the relative lack of encapsulation.

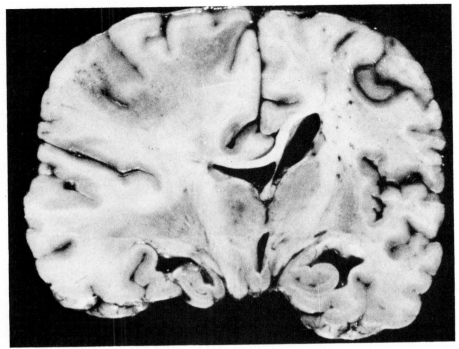

Figure 8–4. Extensive cerebral swelling of one cerebral hemisphere just caudal to an abscess. Note the ventricular shift and flattening of the cingulate gyrus on the side of swelling with herniation of the cingulum beneath the falx.

Symptoms and Signs

Symptoms and signs produced by a brain abscess depend on several factors, including the age of the child, the location and size of the lesion, whether single or multiple, and the degree of associated brain swelling. As a generalization, most of the clinical manifestations and the greatest danger of a brain abscess result from the mass effect of the lesion and the surrounding edema.

During the cerebritis stage, headache, fever, lethargy, or seizures may occur, but more often no clinical evidence of illness is present until the process manifests itself as a mass lesion. In the infant, abnormal head enlargement, vomiting, and seizures are usual manifestations of a brain abscess and can readily be confused with congenital hydrocephalus or other space-taking lesions, including subdural effusions or neoplasm. The older child with a cerebral abscess usually exhibits a progressively worsening clinical course with symptoms and signs being those of focal neurologic dysfunction in conjunction with manifestations of increased intracranial pressure. Headaches, vomiting, and drowsiness are often accompanied by a hemiparesis and a homonymous hemianopsia if the optic radiations are involved. Papilledema is present in many cases and abducens weakness with diplopia frequently develops as a false localizing sign. Posterior frontal or anterior parietal lobe abscesses often cause focal motor or sensory seizures on the opposite side of the body, but generalized convulsions can also occur. An abscess within one cerebellar hemisphere results in papilledema and other increased pressure signs in addition to coordination disturbances. The gait is usually ataxic, and dysmetria is present in the limbs on the homolateral side. Horizontal nystagmus, more marked on gaze to the side of the lesion, provides further evidence of posterior fossa localization.

Abscess within the brain stem has been infrequently reported but may develop either from hematogenous spread or from extension from an otogenic source (Weickhardt and Davis, Van Gilder et al.). Most have been identified after death and clinical signs have been those of focal pontine dysfunction. Fever, headache, facial paresis, nystagmus, ataxia, and long tract signs are the most common findings, in addition to the manifestations of meningeal infection, which often coexists. While most brain abscesses give rise to signs of increased pressure in combination with focal signs, it is important to note that those located in certain areas can be relatively silent. An abscess within the anterior frontal region or the posterior parietal region may produce few overt clinical signs and be manifested for a period of time only by intermittent low-grade fever or headaches.

Sudden deterioration of the clinical status of a patient with a cerebral or cerebellar abscess generally indicates either internal herniation of the medial temporal lobe or cerebellar tonsils or spontaneous rupture of the abscess into the ventricular system or subarachnoid space. Although not invariably fatal, these complications markedly worsen the outlook for the child and indicate the desirability of prompt diagnosis and treatment before such catastrophes occur. Another event that may prove fatal in the patient with a cerebral abscess is massive hemorrhage into the lesion. This can occur spontaneously without obvious explanation or in the child with thrombocytopenia or other coagulation disorders. It has also been described as a complication of inappropriate anticoagulation therapy for presumed cerebrovascular occlusive disease (Abbott and Stern).

Laboratory and Ancillary Studies

Fever and blood leukocytosis are suggestive of an infectious process when present; however, their absence in no way excludes the possibility of a brain abscess. Of 19 patients reported by Raimondi et al., only six had temperature elevation over 101°F. The white blood cell count, likewise, is quite variable and cannot be assumed to be consistently reliable as an indicator of a suppurative lesion in the brain. Marked elevation of the total white blood cell count with an increased number of immature forms is more often seen when meningitis is present in conjunction with an abscess. The cerebrospinal fluid is usually clear, colorless, and without organisms unless rupture of the lesion has produced meningitis. Elevation of the spinal fluid pressure is frequently present and the protein content is usually modestly elevated. The cell count may be normal although 10 to 100 cells per cu. mm. is more characteristic. The cellular response may be either primarily lymphocytic or a combination of lymphocytes and polymorphonuclear leukocytes. As a generalization, the more chronic and encapsulated abscess is associated with a lymphocytic pleocytosis whereas more acute lesions

exhibit a higher percentage of polymorphonuclear cells in the spinal fluid.

Among 23 patients with intracranial abscesses described by Wright and Ballantine, three were found to have completely normal findings on lumbar puncture. Performance of a spinal fluid examination may be of diagnostic assistance; however, when an abscess is strongly suspected and meningitis can be excluded with reasonable certainty from the clinical signs, spinal tap is best avoided because of the potential hazard of the procedure in the presence of a brain abscess. Such patients are in urgent need of additional diagnostic procedures and the results of the lumbar puncture will rarely alter the method of further investigation. The potential danger of lumbar puncture is illustrated by the series of Samson and Clark. Among 22 patients with brain abscess, five exhibited signs of brain stem compression within two hours after the performance of lumbar puncture.

Roentgenograms of the skull in children with brain abscesses are of little definitive help except for evidence of increased pressure manifested by suture spread. An unusual finding on skull x-ray in children with cerebral abscesses is the presence of gas within the abscess cavity (Norrell and Howieson). Most such cases have followed penetrating head wounds, with the abscess being caused by a gas-forming bacillus. Differentiation of a gas-containing abscess from traumatic pneumocephalus may be difficult, although the clinical findings of the two lesions are usually quite dissimilar. Sinus and mastoid films may reveal a potential source of infection and views of the petrous apices are useful to exclude the possibility of osteomyelitis in this region secondary to chronic middle ear disease.

Electroencephalography provides a valuable tool for localization of a cerebral hemisphere abscess. The usual abnormality is in the form of a high-voltage, delta slow focus arising from the region of the suppurative lesion (Fig. 8–5). Radioactive brain scan, like the electroencephalogram, is an additional procedure which can be safely performed and which may localize the site of the lesion with great precision. The available literature does not allow absolute conclusions regarding the percentage of cerebral abscesses that are identified by isotope scanning techniques. Crocker and associates studied diagnostic methods in 18 patients with cerebral abscesses and found abnormal technetium brain scans in all. In five of the 18 cases, the

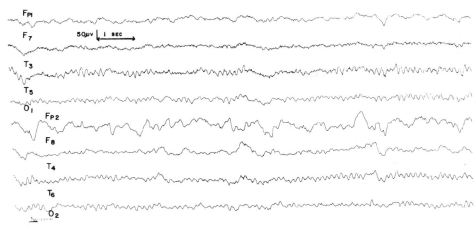

Figure 8–5. Electroencephalogram of a 16-year-old boy with a right frontal lobe abscess secondary to pyogenic orbital cellulitis. The electroencephalogram demonstrates a high-voltage delta focus, primarily right frontal in location.

scan revealed circular isotope uptake surrounding a hollow center, a finding considered characteristic of a cerebral abscess. This and other reports suggest a high degree of localizing value of radioactive scan techniques for brain abscesses, warranting their use whenever the possibility of abscess is entertained.

Computed tomography is of great value for the diagnosis and localization of a brain abscess and for the differentiation of focal cerebritis, which is treated medically, from an abscess, which usually requires surgical drainage. It is also helpful for the identification of multiple lesions and of multiloculation of a solitary abscess (Stephanov). Most abscesses appear in the form of a localized area of decreased density compared to normal brain, sometimes surrounded by a thin rim of increased density (Fig. 8–6). Enhancement of the ring density surrounding a hypodense central zone can usually be accomplished by contrast injection (Fig. 8–7), a finding that helps distinguish abscess from focal cerebritis (New et al., Zimmerman et al.), but also one that can be seen with certain malignant cerebral gliomas.

With cerebritis, the computed tomogram without contrast infusion reveals a low-density lesion in which the zone of hypodensity is nonhomogeneous. The margins are quite irregular and there is usually a mass effect with some degree of shift or distortion of the ventricular system (Weisberg). With contrast infusion, there is enhancement in a diffuse pattern, sometimes with a central zone of hypodensity. In an experimental study of brain abscess formation, Enzmann et al. have

shown that ring enhancement is seen during the late stage of cerebritis, before capsule formation has occurred. The enhanced ring is at its maximum size at this time and some degree of enhanced "filling in" of the necrotic central area occurs in delayed scanning. The diameter of the ring decreases as cerebritis is converted into frank suppuration, at which time the central zone remains hypodense on delayed scans. These observations indicate that the enhanced ring on computed tomography with brain abscess does not simply illustrate the capsule but is determined to some degree by the hyperemia within the zone of inflammation surrounding the degenerating central area.

Confirmation of the presence of a brain abscess may still warrant contrast procedures in select instances before formulating a surgical attack on the lesion. Abscesses involving the cerebral hemispheres in the past were accurately localized by carotid angiography (Fig. 8–8), while cerebellar abscesses were previously localized by air ventriculography. The availability of computed cranial tomography has decreased the need for either ventriculography or angiography but, in certain instances, contrast studies can add important information prior to surgery.

Intracranial Subdural and Epidural Abscess

Subdural abscess is a serious focal suppurative intracranial infection which is characterized by an acute to subacute clinical course manifested by signs of increased intracranial

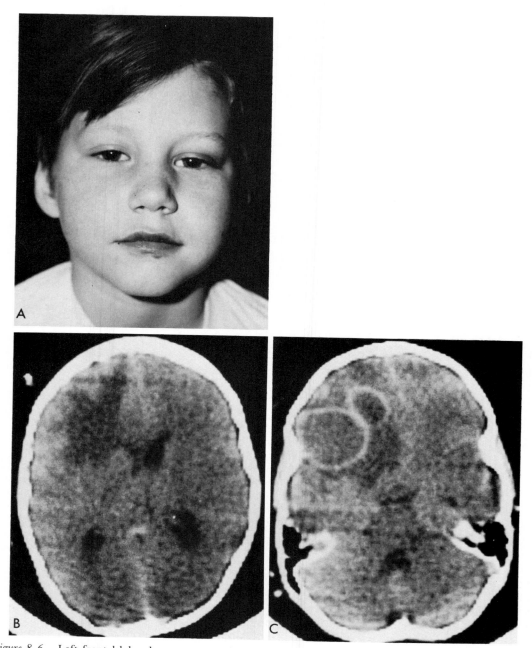

Figure 8–6. Left frontal lobe abscess, computed tomographic diagnosis. *A,* Five-year-old boy who is minimally symptomatic and had a normal neurologic examination. The child had been struck by a moving automobile 4 weeks previously. He was temporarily unconscious and thereafter experienced headache and vomiting for 3 to 4 days. Skull x-rays soon after the injury showed a fracture through the left orbital roof. Three weeks following the accident, he began to have recurrent headaches and vomiting, and became somewhat listless. It was presumed that he had delayed cerebral swelling secondary to trauma and he responded dramatically to corticosteroid therapy. Two days before admission, he again developed headaches, however, only mild in intensity. Following referral, he was admitted to the hospital complaining only intermittently of headache and with a normal neurologic examination. *B,* Computed tomogram before contrast infusion shows a large, irregular hypodense zone in the left frontal area with moderate ventricular distortion. *C,* Computed tomogram after contrast infusion demonstrates a large abscess with ring enhancement and with a smaller "daughter" abscess just anterior to it. Craniotomy was performed for drainage and *Streptococcus pneumoniae* was isolated on culture from pus aspirated from the lesion. Brain abscess was not suspected clinically in this instance until the computed tomogram was performed.

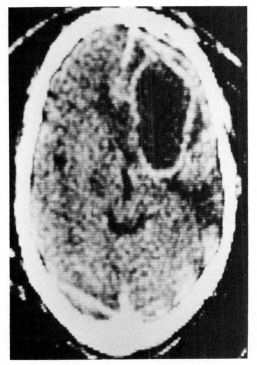

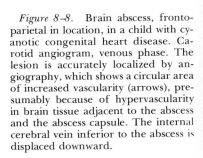

Figure 8–7. Computed tomogram after contrast infusion, large right frontal abscess. There is a fairly regular enhanced ring surrounding a hypodense zone, which represents the pus-filled abscess cavity.

pressure, meningeal irritation, and evidence of focal cortical dysfunction. Subdural abscess is more often seen in males than females and can occur in any age group, although most cases are in children and young adults.

The most common source of infection giving rise to subdural empyema is frontal or ethmoid sinusitis (Bhandari and Sarkari, Hitchcock and Andreadis). In such cases, spread of infection intracranially is secondary to thrombophlebitis of perforating cerebral veins, sometimes resulting in cortical vein thrombosis or even parenchymal abscess formation, in combination with subdural empyema. Direct extension from suppurative sinus disease can also result in frontal osteomyelitis, epidural abscess, and subdural abscess when the dura is penetrated. Subdural abscess can develop secondary to chronic otitis media or mastoiditis, following penetrating head injuries or orbital cellulitis, and rarely, as a complication of septicemia. Another rare cause of subdural empyema is septic contamination of a chronic subdural hematoma (Coonrod and Dans, Lerner et al.).

In infants, the pathogenesis of subdural abscess is usually different from that of older children in that the most common predisposing factor in the child under a year of age is primary leptomeningitis (Farmer and Wise).

Figure 8–8. Brain abscess, frontoparietal in location, in a child with cyanotic congenital heart disease. Carotid angiogram, venous phase. The lesion is accurately localized by angiography, which shows a circular area of increased vascularity (arrows), presumably because of hypervascularity in brain tissue adjacent to the abscess and the abscess capsule. The internal cerebral vein inferior to the abscess is displaced downward.

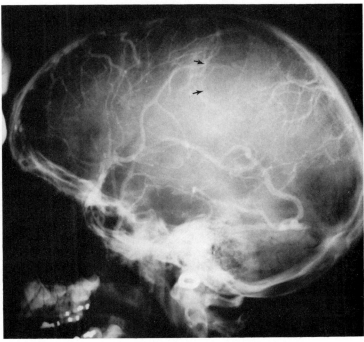

For this reason, bacteria that are isolated from subdural abscesses are somewhat different in infants than in older children or adults. In the infant in whom subdural abscess complicates suppurative meningitis, the usual offenders include *Hemophilus influenzae,* *Streptococcus pneumoniae,* and gram-negative rods among the Enterobacteriaceae. In the older patient with subdural abscess secondary to sinus or mastoid disease, either aerobic or anaerobic streptococci, *Staphylococcus* species and *Proteus* or *Pseudomonas* species are the more frequent pathogens.

Once infection has reached the subdural space, pus is rapidly formed and can spread widely over the cerebral convexity (Fig. 8–9). The entire hemisphere may be enveloped although abscesses arising secondary to frontal sinusitis are often located primarily over the corresponding frontal pole and extending back variable distances over the frontal convexity. A particularly treacherous location of abscess from the diagnostic standpoint is the parafalcine one in which there is accumulation of pus adjacent to the falx cerebri along the medial surface of the cerebral hemisphere. Abscess is sometimes confined to this region or may coexist with subfrontal or convexity accumulation of pus. Subdural abscesses of otitic origin are frequently located primarily in the temporal region or extend subtemporally. Most subdural abscesses are unilateral, although bilateral involvement can occur, especially when the process complicates pyogenic meningitis in the infant.

Clinical manifestations of an intracranial subdural abscess are produced by direct pressure upon the adjacent brain by the mass, and by the effects of thrombophlebitis, arteritis, or cortical venous thrombosis on the underlying brain, giving rise to hemorrhagic infarcts and variable degrees of cerebral swelling. Even major dural sinus thrombosis will occur in certain instances. Meningeal signs arise from irritation provoked by parameningeal suppuration, and meningitis can coexist, further contributing to the neurologic signs. The clinical features of a subdural abscess can be complicated also by the signs of the underlying primary illness, such as those of pansinusitis or suppurative mastoiditis.

Characteristically, the child with subdural empyema is ill for a relatively brief period of time before rapid deterioration ensues. Headache, vomiting, and fever are the usual initial manifestations, followed within hours or days by meningeal signs, irritability, drow-siness, and signs of focal cerebral dysfunction. Mild hemiparesis progresses to definite unilateral motor weakness, and is sometimes associated with seizures of a generalized or focal nature. The time from onset of fever and headache until the occurrence of hemiparesis, focal convulsions, and clear-cut signs of intracranial hypertension may vary from a day or so up to two weeks, but, in general, progression is fairly rapid. By the time the child becomes stuporous or comatose, papilledema has emerged. Unless the lesion is identified and properly treated, death soon follows. The potential seriousness of this disorder is apparent from mortality rates of published series, which range between 30 and 40 percent (Bhandari and Sarkari, Hitchcock and Andreadis, Kaufman et al.). Among 50 cases of subdural empyema observed by Brunner in the pre-antibiotic period, the mortality rate was 65 percent. In the infant in whom an infected subdural effusion complicates primary bacterial meningitis, the lesion is usually identified by subdural taps performed because of persistent or recurrent fever despite appropriate antibiotic therapy, or because of persistent tenseness of the anterior fontanel during the course of therapy.

Diagnosis of subdural abscess depends on recognition of the possibility because of the presence of a predisposing cause, along with signs of intracranial hypertension, fever, and focal neurologic deficits. Skull roentgenograms are helpful in the demonstration of sinusitis, mastoiditis, or even osteomyelitis in unusual cases. In the infant, suture separation is usually present. Cerebrospinal fluid examination reveals variable findings with subdural empyema but only infrequently is normal. The usual abnormality includes a mixed cellular response but with lymphocytic predominance, a moderate elevation of the protein content, a normal glucose value, and the absence of bacteria on gram stain and culture. Lumbar puncture is sometimes necessary when the clinical suspicion is that of bacterial meningitis, but the procedure should be avoided if parameningeal suppuration is strongly suspected. Among seven patients with signs of increased intracranial pressure in the series of Kaufman et al., three developed internal herniation within hours after lumbar puncture was performed. Radioactive brain scan demonstrates positive uptake adjacent to the skull in some cases; however, a normal scan does not exclude the possibility of subdural pus collection.

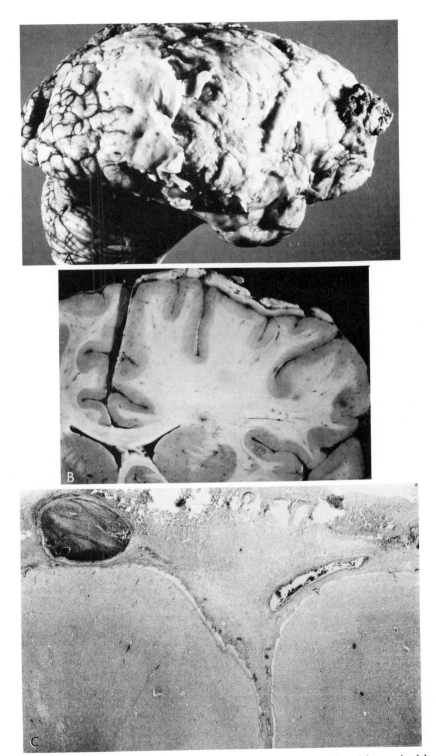

Figure 8–9.   Acute subdural empyema. *A,* Dense subdural exudate covering the right cerebral hemisphere. *B,* Coronal section of the brain showing subdural abscess. *C,* Cortical vein thrombosis within subdural abscess.

The value of computerized tomography for diagnosis of this lesion has recently been documented, and in some instances allows surgical intervention without the use of carotid angiography. Subdural abscess is apparent on computed tomography as a crescent-shaped band of decreased lucency adjacent to the skull, sometimes with an ill-defined zone of increased density medial to the lesion. Ventricular shift is usually present and, with contrast enhancement, the medial rim adjacent to the cerebral cortex is highlighted (Joubert and Stephanov). Epidural abscess can often be distinguished from those in the subdural space by the more restricted extent of the epidural abscess, which is bounded medially by a thick, dense ring, especially with contrast enhancement (Kaufman and Leeds).

In the infant, transfontanel subdural taps can be utilized to identify the presence of pus in the subdural space. Purulent material of high viscosity might not be transmitted through the needle unless one of large caliber is used. Subfrontal and parafalcine abscesses are not identified by this method; however, abscesses in these locations are unusual in infancy. Transillumination of the skull of the infant is positive in some cases in which cloudy subdural fluid is present but is negative when purulent material is of thicker consistency. Carotid angiography was previously the most commonly used technique for diagnosis of subdural abscess prior to the development of computed cranial tomography. Angiography continues to be useful in certain instances, although it is resorted to less often since computed tomography became available. The characteristic angiographic appearance of a convexity subdural abscess is an avascular, semilunar zone with displacement of vessels away from the inner table of the skull (Ferris and Ciembroniewicz, Kim et al.).

Intracranial epidural abscess has diminished considerably in frequency since mastoiditis has become less common. Cases that do occur are either otogenic, secondary to frontal sinusitis, or follow neurosurgical operative procedures (Fig. 8–10). The latter usually occur within four to six weeks after surgery and are frequently associated with subgaleal suppuration. Epidural abscess is generally less aggressive than those in the subdural space. An epidural abscess can remain relatively silent, being identified unexpectedly at surgery or on angiography. Increased intracranial pressure results in headache and vomiting in some cases, but is minimal in others. High-grade pressure signs and striking signs of focal cerebral dysfunction usually indicate the presence of associated cerebral complications, such as parenchymal abscess formation or venous thrombosis. Epidural abscess or suppurative meningitis will complicate the clinical picture with apical petrositis in some cases. Angiographic diagnosis is on the basis of findings similar to those of subdural abscess. With a large convexity epidural abscess, the superior sagittal sinus can be displaced away from the inner table of the skull (Handel et al.).

Treatment

Treatment of a brain abscess or one in the subdural or epidural space includes the intravenous administration of antibiotics, attempts to reduce brain swelling, and surgical removal or evacuation of the lesion by one method or another. Infusion of antibiotics should be started before surgery in any case in which an abscess is a reasonable consideration. Selection of the antibiotic regimen is never precise in this situation since the causative organism is yet unknown. The prominence of the *Staphylococcus* and a variety of anaerobic organisms as causes of brain abscess warrants the use of a combination of one of the penicillinase-resistant penicillins and chloramphenicol until the causative organism is located and sensitivity studies are known. Methicillin in a dose of 300 mg. per kilogram per day intravenously and chloramphenicol, 100 mg. per kilogram per day, are started initially but discontinued in favor of penicillin G if a penicillin-sensitive organism is recovered. Methicillin is less effective than penicillin against most anaerobes. For this reason, if an abscess contains air suggesting an anaerobic infection, or if one develops secondary to chronic otitis media, penicillin and chloramphenicol would be the preferred combination pending bacteriologic diagnosis.

When brain abscess is caused by an unusual bacterium such as *Acinetobacter calcoaceticus* (Waage), one must depend heavily on antibiotic sensitivities. This particular agent is usually found to be susceptible to an aminoglycoside and carbenicillin, the same combination used for *Pseudomonas* species and indole-positive *Proteus* species infections. In some cases with brain abscess caused by *Bacteroides fragilis* that has not responded to therapy with chloramphenicol, improvement has

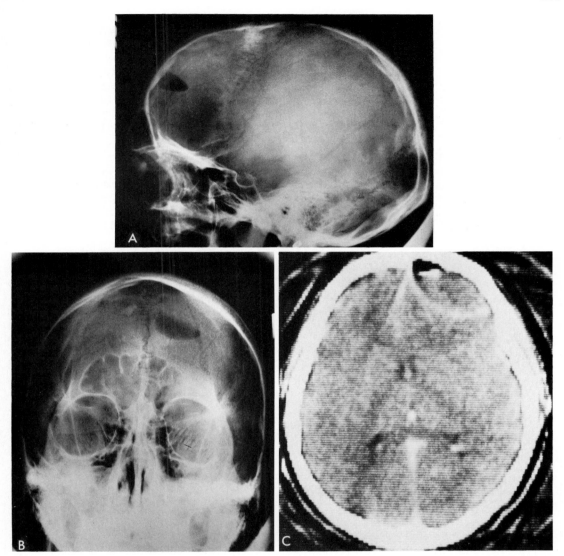

Figure 8–10. Acute epidural abscess secondary to frontal sinusitis. A teenage boy known to be a heavy drug user developed the onset of persistent headache 5 days before hospital admission, followed by chills and fever one day prior to admission. Physical examination at the time of admission revealed him to be febrile, mildly lethargic and disoriented, and with tenderness over the frontal sinuses. His white blood cell count was 15,100 per cu. mm. Lumbar puncture showed an opening pressure of 255 mm. water. The CSF contained 2 cells per cu. mm., glucose of 66 mg. per 100 ml., protein of 80 mg. per 100 ml., and negative gram stain. *A,* Skull x-ray, lateral view, reveals a bullet-shaped collection of intracranial air in the frontal region. *B,* The facial view shows the air collection in the frontal region, in addition to cloudy frontal sinuses bilaterally. *C,* The computed tomogram after contrast infusion demonstrates the right frontal epidural abscess bounded medially by a curvilinear zone of increased density. The intracranial air is visualized in the most anterior and medial aspect of the abscess in the form of a small black area. In other sections of the scan, the mass effect of the abscess resulting in distortion of the frontal horn of the right lateral ventricle could be seen. The posterior wall of the right frontal sinus was found to be necrotic at surgery, allowing entrance of air from the sinus into the frontal epidural space. The patient recovered following antimicrobial therapy and surgical drainage.

been brought about following the administration of metronidazole (Werner et al.). Metronidazole has become the drug of choice for invasive infections caused by *Entamoeba histolytica,* and may be particularly useful for brain abscesses caused by this organism in view of its excellent penetration of the blood-brain barrier. In the rare case in which *Nocardia* species is suspected or identified, sulfadiazine or a combination of sulfadiazine and cycloserine is the treatment of choice. Penicillin is recommended for cerebral abscesses caused by *Actinomyces* species as well as for most anaerobic bacilli other than *Bacteroides* species. If increased pressure signs are marked, such as high-grade papilledema, lethargy, and bradycardia, dexamethasone in a dose of 0.5 mg. per kilogram per day, or mannitol, 2 grams per kilogram intravenously over 30 minutes, would be advisable. Mannitol should be avoided, however, in the child with heart disease if cardiac failure is present or impending. The sudden increase in intravascular volume resulting from use of this preparation may overload the heart, leading to pulmonary edema.

Surgical management of a brain abscess has been a controversial subject for many years. Some have favored aspiration of the contents or drainage by marsupialization, while others have recommended total excision whenever possible. It would appear that no one form of surgical management would be suitable for all cases and that individualization on the basis of size and location of the lesion plus condition of the child would be necessary. The old concept of delaying surgery to permit the abscess to become encapsulated should be abandoned, as this only invites disaster in the form of spontaneous rupture or internal herniation (Wright and Ballantine). Most believe that the clinical diagnosis of an intracranial abscess supported by the typical appearance of the lesion on computed tomography or the demonstration of an avascular mass on angiography or a cerebellar mass on ventriculography should be followed by operation without delay.

Large lesions that are poorly encapsulated are usually best managed by cannula drainage at craniotomy. The same is true of deeply located abscesses which involve the internal capsule or basal ganglia (Law et al.). Wright and Ballantine advocate complete excision of cerebral abscesses and claimed their results were more favorable with this approach than with simple aspiration or drainage. Selker has taken the opposite view and has recommended aspiration of a solitary abscess through a single burr hole, followed by continuous catheter drainage for several days. This approach decreases the surgical morbidity and allows periodic estimation of the size of the lesion by instillation of radiopaque material into the cavity. The condition of the child at the time of surgery is an important factor that must be considered before deciding upon the most appropriate surgical approach. A lengthy operative·procedure may be poorly tolerated by the patient who is in

a precarious state before operation. The rare pituitary abscess is best approached transsphenoidally, allowing open drainage with less chance of cerebrospinal fluid contamination (Dominque and Wilson).

Treatment of brain abscess by non-surgical measures has been described in recent years, although the applicability or the degree of safety of this approach remains to be seen (Berg et al., Heineman et al.). In the report by Berg and colleagues, the diagnosis of brain abscess was on the basis of a compatible clinical course and roentgenographic findings, including cranial computed tomography, consistent with focal suppurative lesions. With intensive antibiotic therapy, there was resolution of the lesion in each of four patients without surgical intervention. Management of brain abscess in this fashion would not be advisable in the child in whom an abscess has resulted in a significant mass effect with definite signs of increased intracranial pressure. The danger of internal herniation in such cases would warrant early surgical drainage. That examples of brain abscess have been successfully treated by nonoperative means is an important observation even though it is generally accepted that surgical treatment continues to be the treatment of choice. There are instances in which other complicating factors preclude immediate surgery and, when the mass effect arising from the presence of an abscess is not great, conservative treatment with close observation of the patient would be acceptable until it is safe to proceed with drainage. If the presumed suppurative lesion is found to resolve on the basis of clinical signs and serial computed tomography, a surgical procedure would then be avoided.

The long-term neurologic sequelae in 16 children who survived a brain abscess treated surgically were studied by Carey et al. Most of the children in this series were able to continue in school but two-thirds had some degree of difficulty with academic achievement. Two children of the total group had severe residual emotional problems. Hemiparesis of severe degree persisted in six of 16 and seizures also developed in six patients. The authors indicated that cerebral abscesses located in the anterior frontal or temporal regions were more likely to be followed by a favorable outcome, while those in the posterior frontal or parietal areas were more often complicated by significant residual deficits.

The frequency with which epilepsy develops as a complication among survivors of ce-

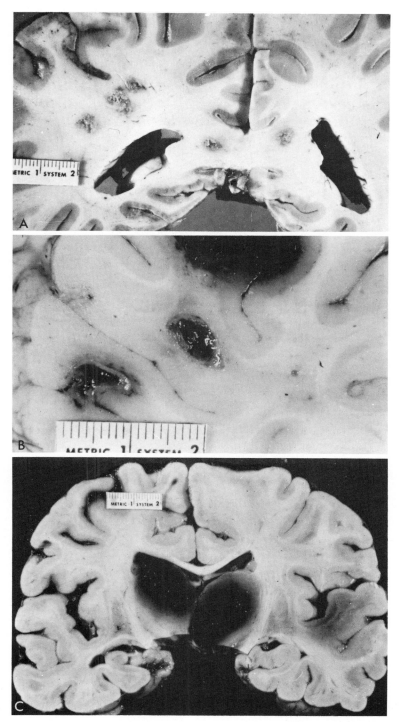

Figure 8–11. Cerebral complications of bacterial endocarditis. *A,* Septic cerebral emboli in a child with endocarditis superimposed on congenital heart disease. There are multiple, small staphylococcal abscesses in the early stage of development. *B,* Multiple hemorrhagic staphylococcal abscesses in a child with bacterial endocarditis. The encapsulation indicates that the lesions are more chronic than those in *A. C,* Septic emboli resulting in massive, bilateral thalamic hemorrhages. Child with subacute bacterial endocarditis complicating rheumatic heart disease.

rebral abscess treated surgically was examined by Legg et al. The series of 70 patients included all age groups followed for variable periods, with a mean of 11 years postoperatively. Seventy-two percent of the 70 patients eventually experienced seizures of one type or another. Interestingly, there was no definite relationship between the development of epilepsy and the age of the patient when abscess occurred, the site of the cerebral abscess, or the mode of surgical treatment. Morgan and colleagues found an incidence of seizures of 55 percent among 31 patients after treatment of cerebral abscess.

NEUROLOGIC COMPLICATIONS OF BACTERIAL ENDOCARDITIS

Although survival from bacterial endocarditis has been greatly improved since the ad-

vent of antibiotics, neurologic complications of the disease continue to pose a serious threat and may even represent the initial clinical manifestations of the disorder. In a series of 218 patients of all ages with bacterial endocarditis, Pruitt and colleagues found that 39 percent had neurologic complications of one type or another. Considering their own series as well as a literature review, Pruitt et al. estimated that approximately 25 percent of all patients with bacterial endocarditis will have a neurologic complication, the most common being cerebral embolization.

The brain can be involved in many ways in children with infectious endocarditis (Fig. 8–11), including the development of meningitis or cerebritis secondary to bacterial seeding, or the subsequent formation of a cerebral abscess. Embolization to the brain may occur with non-infected material, resulting in a cerebral vascular occlusive episode unasso-

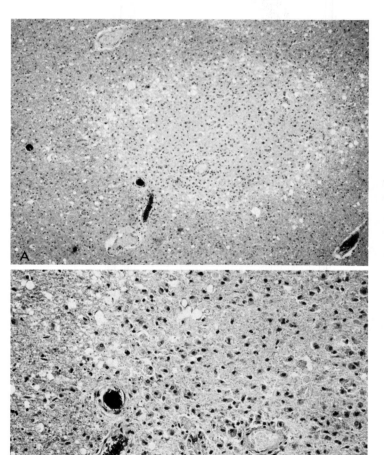

Figure 8–12. Infected cerebral emboli secondary to subacute bacterial endocarditis resulting in cerebral infarction and cerebritis. *A,* Cerebral white matter with multiple vessels occluded with bacteria-laden embolic material (black structures). There is a circular zone of pallor which represents an acute area of infarction (H&E, 80×). *B,* Higher power of the same region shows occluded vessels and macrophage infiltration and some inflammatory cells in the area of white matter necrosis (H&E, 200×). Unless reversed with antibiotic therapy, this infected area of necrosis might proceed to abscess formation.

ciated with other evidence of intracranial infection. Other vascular occlusive episodes precipitating a stroke-like picture are due to infected embolic material from the heart valves with the clinical course subsequently being complicated by symptoms and signs of intracranial suppuration (Fig. 8–12). Venous thrombosis, either of cortical veins or major venous sinuses, is characterized by a variety of neurologic deficits, often associated with convulsions and bilateral signs, and frequently with manifestations of increased intracranial pressure (Figs. 8–13, 8–14). Septic embolization, also, may lead to the formation of intracranial mycotic aneurysms which can either remain silent or subsequently rupture, causing subarachnoid hemorrhage, intracerebral hemorrhage, or both.

Bacterial endocarditis has been divided into acute and subacute types on the basis of the rapidity of progression of the illness and the virulence of the offending organism. This subdivision continues to have clinical application; however, it has become less precise since antibiotics have altered the natural history of the illness so dramatically. What previously would have been an acute, fulminat-

ing process rapidly leading to death before antibiotics were available may now be converted into a more chronic illness with eventual recovery if an effective chemotherapeutic regimen is initiated. Nonetheless, acute bacterial endocarditis indicates a fulminating infection of the endocardium, most often due to *Staphylococcus aureus* and more likely to occur without evidence of pre-existent heart disease. Subacute bacterial endocarditis refers to a more indolent infectious process usually due to an organism of low virulence and most often engrafted upon previously recognized cardiac disease (Panky). *Streptococcus viridans* remains the most commonly identified cause of subacute bacterial endocarditis when all ages are considered (Lerner and Weinstein). In 1965, when Zakrzewski and Keith reviewed their experience with bacterial endocarditis in children, approximately 80 percent were found to be caused by *Streptococcus viridans*, *Streptococcus* group D, and *Staphylococcus* species. More recent studies have shown a decline in gram-positive cocci as causes of childhood endocarditis and an increase in unusual organisms, including fungi (Mendelsohn and Hutchins). *Neisseria*

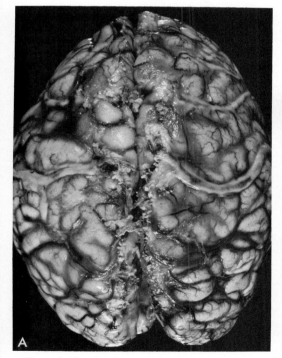
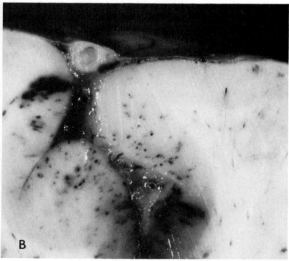

Figure 8–13. Septic cortical vein thrombosis. *A,* Dorsal aspect of the gross brain shows cerebral swelling and distended, blanched cortical venous channels bilaterally, which are completely thrombosed. *B,* Cortical vein lying at the crown of two adjacent gyri contains a premortem thrombus within its lumen. The underlying cerebral cortex reveals congested veins and area of hemorrhagic cortical infarction.

species have become rare causes (Scott, Brodie et al.) and the pneumococcus is now only infrequently identified (Cherubin and Neu). *Corynebacterium* (Merzbach et al.) and *Escherichia coli* (Stanton et al.) cause endocarditis in certain instances, and anaerobic bacteria (Felner and Dowell) are additional occasional offenders. Rheumatic endocarditis was previously recognized to be the most common antecedent for secondary bacterial infection of the endocardium; however, this has now been supplanted in children by congenital heart lesions. Among 50 children with bacterial endocarditis reported by Zakrzewski

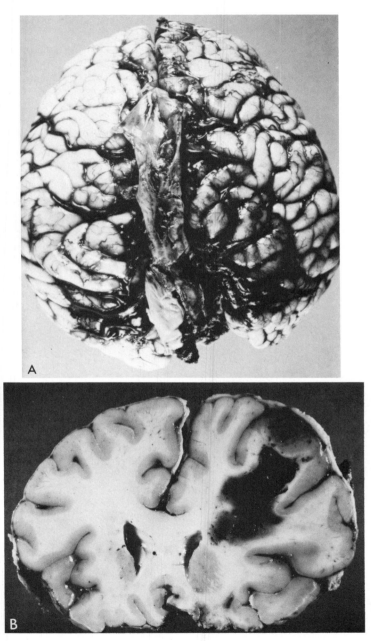

Figure 8–14.   Septic superior sagittal sinus thrombosis secondary to subacute bacterial endocarditis. *A,* Superior sagittal sinus and cortical vein thrombosis results in severe, diffuse cerebral swelling and marked cortical venous distention. Premortem clot is evident within the partially opened superior sagittal sinus. *B,* Septic cortical vein thrombosis with a hemorrhagic infarct in the cortex and adjacent white matter. Suppurative meningitis also complicated the illness, as evident by the diffuse leptomeningeal exudate.

Illustration continued on opposite page

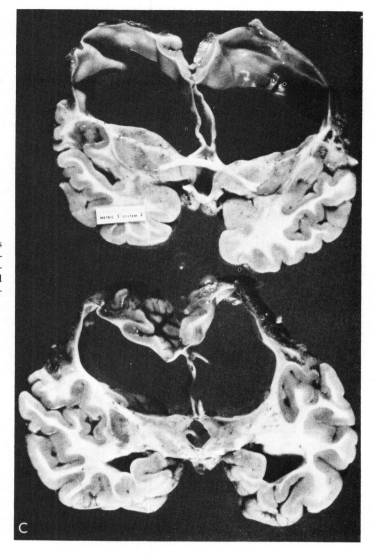

Figure 8–14 Continued. C, Late effects of septic superior sagittal sinus thrombosis. Extreme cerebral atrophy with ventricular distention has replaced infarcted tissue in the region drained by the superior sagittal sinus.

and Keith, 45 had congenital heart disease, with ventricular septal defect and tetralogy of Fallot being the most common types.

The classic symptoms and signs of bacterial endocarditis in children are widely recognized but their absence may deceptively mislead one from consideration of this source as the cause of recurrent fever or a sudden neurologic catastrophe. Fever, weight loss, anorexia, chills, night sweats, arthralgia, petechiae (Fig. 8–15), and splenomegaly are features highly suggestive of endocarditis in a child with cardiac disease, but the absence of any of these signs does not eliminate endocarditis as a possibility. Preliminary antibiotics may mask a febrile response and inhibit recovery of an organism from the blood. Petechiae are diagnostically helpful when

present and are most often observed in the conjunctivae (Fig. 8–16). Among patients studied by Lerner and Weinstein, however, petechiae were identified in only 26 percent and splenomegaly was found in 44 percent of cases of subacute bacterial endocarditis.

A small but significant percentage of children will have their initial manifestation of subacute bacterial endocarditis in the form of an acute neurologic disorder in the absence of many of the other clinical signs usually considered more characteristic of this infection. Thus, any child with heart disease who develops a neurologic deficit of sudden onset that consists either of intracranial hemorrhage or of a cerebral vascular occlusive episode should be considered a candidate for bacterial endocarditis. Likewise, the same

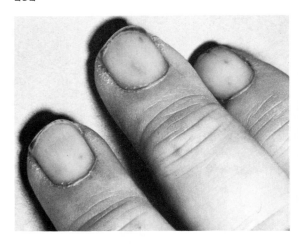

Figure 8–15. Acute staphylococcal endocarditis. Subungual hemorrhages.

neurologic problems in an allegedly previously normal child require appropriate studies to exclude the possibility of previously existent but unrecognized heart disease. The neurologic complications of a left atrial myxoma can mimic precisely those of bacterial endocarditis or rheumatic fever.

Cerebral Mycotic Aneurysm

A mycotic aneurysm is an abnormality of the arterial wall which becomes weakened by invasion by microorganisms, usually bacterial in type. The designation of these lesions as "mycotic" is generally credited to Osler, who used the term in his "Gulstonian Lecture on Malignant Endocarditis" in Lancet in 1885. At that time, "mycotic" referred to infectious processes in a general sense and thus is now

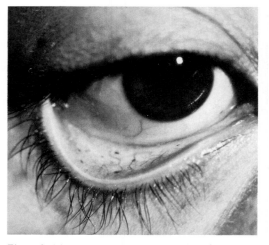

Figure 8–16. Conjunctival petechiae in a young adult female with subacute bacterial endocarditis who had a septic embolus to the left cerebral hemisphere.

somewhat misleading in view of the current usage of the term to imply a fungal infection. For this reason, current authors often favor the designation of bacterial or infectious intracranial aneurysm for this lesion (Bohmfalk et al.). The percentage of all intracranial aneurysms that are infectious in origin has gradually diminished in the past 50 years. Among a series of intracranial aneurysms studied by Fearnsides in 1916, almost 30 percent were of the mycotic variety. In 1939, McDonald and Korb found that 6 percent of 1,125 intracranial aneurysms were infectious in origin. By 1965, mycotic aneurysms accounted for only 2.6 percent of a series of 191 intracranial aneurysms (Roach and Drake).

In the vast majority of mycotic aneurysms bacteria reach the vessel wall as infected emboli which originate from the valves of the heart. In addition to the usual types of cardiac disease complicated by infectious endocarditis, heroin addiction has also been recognized as a predisposing cause of bacterial endocarditis, resulting in intracranial mycotic aneurysms (Gilroy et al.). Rarely, a cerebral mycotic aneurysm can develop secondary to a primary intracranial infection extrinsic to the arterial wall (Heidelberger et al.). Cerebral arterial invasion by microorganisms in the patient with acute bacterial meningitis can lead to aneurysm formation with either hemorrhage or eventual spontaneous healing (Ojemann et al.). The great majority of intracranial mycotic aneurysms are of bacterial origin but fungi can also cause this lesion on rare occasion. *Aspergillus* species, well-known for their predisposition to invade vascular structures, have been the causative organism in most reported cases (Horten et al.). Morriss and Spock described a child with a mycotic aneurysm of the internal carotid artery caused by *Penicillium,* a fungus morphologically similar to *Aspergillus* and a member of the same tribe. An intracranial mycotic aneurysm caused by *Candida albicans* has also been described in a 16-year-old girl with systemic lupus erythematosus (Goldman et al.).

Intracranial mycotic aneurysms may be single or multiple and can be found in association with other cerebral complications of bacterial endocarditis. They may be located anywhere along the arterial tree but are usually found on more distal cerebral vessels, especially in the middle cerebral artery distribution, as compared to the usual location of "berry" aneurysms along the circle of Willis (Noonan et al.). On microscopic examination the wall of a mycotic aneurysm reveals an inflammatory infiltrate with dissolution of the normal architecture and with colonies of bacteria occasionally evident (Fig. 8–17).

Cerebral mycotic aneurysms are usually identified in life by angiography performed on patients with bacterial endocarditis who have experienced either an intracranial hemorrhage or cerebral vascular occlusion resulting in hemiparesis. Not widely recognized, however, is the possibility of intracranial hemorrhage from a ruptured mycotic aneurysm *before* other signs of bacterial endocarditis have become apparent (Bell and Butler, Roach and Drake). Hemorrhage resulting from a ruptured mycotic aneurysm can be either primarily subarachnoid or parenchymal, depending on the location of the aneurysm. Those that bleed directly into brain tissue result in a substantial intracerebral hematoma, giving rise to a combination of focal signs and signs of increased intracranial pressure. An additional cause of subarachnoid hemorrhage in septic patients described by Ray and Wahal resulted from rupture of a "berry" aneurysm secondary to septic embolization to the wall of the lesion.

Treatment of a mycotic aneurysm should be surgical excision if the lesion is single and if it is located on a peripheral cerebral vessel. Angiographic evidence of an intracerebral hematoma adjacent to a ruptured mycotic aneurysm is also an indication for surgical treatment. Intravenous antibiotic therapy should be initiated before the surgical procedure.

Cerebral Bacterial Vasculitis

Emboli from infected heart valves may lodge within a major cerebral artery, obstructing its lumen and producing infarction of brain tissue normally supplied by the involved vessel. The clinical correlate of this event is a sudden onset of a neurologic deficit, with the symptoms and signs resulting being dependent on the anatomic location of the vessel occlusion and its cerebral supply. Hemiparesis and homonymous field defects are the most common clinical signs, but other findings may include dysphasia, seizures, paresis of ocular conjugate deviation, or hemisensory deficits. Ischemic infarction often provokes considerable cerebral edema, with headache, lethargy, or even transtentorial herniation resulting therefrom. Fever, increased sedimentation rate, and other signs of infection usually precede the stroke-like event in children with subacute bacterial endocarditis. In other cases, however, hours or days transpire after the cerebral embolism before signs of sepsis or meningitis become obvious.

Arterial occlusion in these patients may result primarily from enlodgement of the embolic material within the vessel lumen or secondary to intimal proliferation ("arteritis") from bacterial invasion of the vessel wall (Fig. 8–18). The cerebrospinal fluid in children with acute cerebral vasculitis is normal initially in some cases but subsequently reveals findings consistent with meningitis. In other patients, a lymphocytic pleocytosis is present despite the bacterial origin of the process (Wise and Farmer).

Treatment of the child with a "stroke" resulting from septic occlusion of a cerebral artery depends on recognition of the relationship of the vascular occlusive episode to the presence of bacterial endocarditis. The choice of the intravenous antibiotic regimen is determined by the organism either previously identified or suspected on the basis of the clinical findings. Most *Streptococcus* species are sensitive to penicillin and *Staphylococcus aureus* is treated with penicillin or one of the penicillinase-resistant penicillins, on the basis of sensitivity studies. Enterococcal group D *Streptococcus* infection is usually treated with ampicillin (Beaty et al.) or ampicillin and an aminoglycoside. In children with penicillin-sensitive organisms in whom allergic reactions preclude the use of this antibiotic, cephalothin is an alternative (Rahal et al.), although subarachnoid or cerebral penetration of this antibiotic is poor. The irritating effect of this drug on peripheral veins is a significant disadvantage when long-term administration is required. Antibiotics must be given in large doses and should be continued intravenously for four to six weeks.

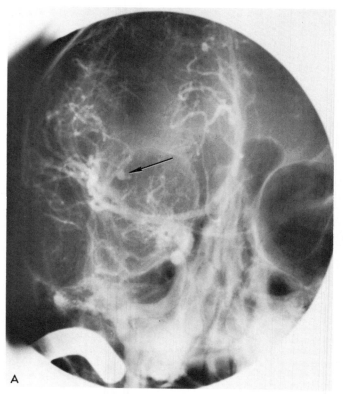

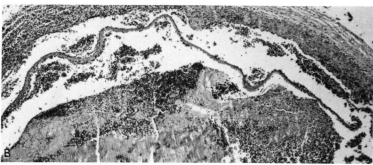

Figure 8–17. Cerebral mycotic aneurysm in an 8-year-old boy with bacterial endocarditis complicating rheumatic heart disease. The first manifestation of bacterial endocarditis in this instance was spontaneous rupture of the intracranial mycotic aneurysm, which resulted in the abrupt onset of headache, lethargy, and left hemiparesis. *A,* Carotid angiogram showing dye trapped within the aneurysm which arose from a branch of the middle cerebral artery. The lesion was surgically removed and an adjacent intracerebral hematoma was evacuated. *B,* Wall of a mycotic aneurysm demonstrating an inflammatory infiltrate and partial destruction of the arterial wall.

ORBITAL CELLULITIS

Sepsis of the orbital contents in children is usually unilateral and is characterized by local pain, tenderness, erythema and swelling of the eyelids. Proptosis develops with progression of the inflammatory condition and is followed by chemosis and systemic signs of infection, such as fever, leukocytosis, and tachycardia. Ocular movements are frequently restricted in those with proptosis. Complete external ophthalmoplegia may develop in severe cases. Resolution of the process can be remarkably prompt after initiation of antibiotic therapy, or gradual worsening may be followed by one of several potential complications described below. In certain cases, cellulitis within the orbit leads to abscess formation located subperiosteally or within the orbital soft tissues.

Orbital cellulitis, described above, refers to a septic process of the orbital contents, and is to be distinguished from periorbital (preseptal) cellulitis, in which the inflammatory process involves the eyelids and surrounding tissues without extension into the orbit itself. The soft tissues of the eyelids are separated from the orbital contents by the orbital septum. This is a reflection of periosteum that inserts into the eyelids and serves as an effective barrier preventing spread of infection from the eyelids into the orbit. Periorbital cellulitis is more common in children than orbital cellulitis, consists of swelling and ery-

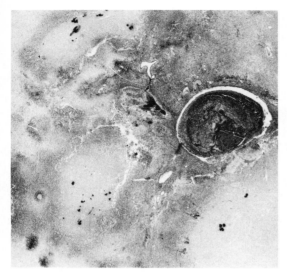

Figure 8–18. Septic cerebral infarction in a patient with subacute bacterial endocarditis. The arterial structure is occluded with embolic material containing bacteria and is surrounded by necrotic brain tissue in which there are many colonies of bacteria.

thema of the periorbital soft tissues, and is not associated with proptosis or ophthalmoparesis. It represents a variety of facial cellulitis and, unlike orbital cellulitis, is not usually secondary to ethmoid sinusitis. Response to antibiotic therapy is usually rapid, and *Hemophilus influenzae* is the most common causative organism (Smith et al.).

Clinical differentiation of diffuse septic inflammation within the orbital contents from an intraorbital abscess is difficult, as the signs with each may be virtually identical. Proptosis with marked displacement of the inflamed globe other than directly forward is more suggestive of abscess formation but is not invariably a reliable sign. Failure of regression of proptosis with appropriate antibiotic therapy is likewise a sign suggestive of the presence of an intraorbital abscess. Orbital computed tomography is a valuable technique to aid in the differentiation of periorbital cellulitis from intraorbital involvement, and also to demonstrate the presence or absence of an intraorbital abscess in the child with orbital cellulitis (Goldberg et al.).

Orbital cellulitis can occur at any age in infancy or childhood and has been described in the newborn period. In the series compiled by Gellady et al., in 80 percent of cases the children were six years of age or younger and the peak incidence was between two and four years of age. In the neonate there are several potential sources of origin, including hema-

togenous spread in a child with neonatal sepsis (Burnard), contiguous extension from suppuration within the ethmoid sinus (Hepner and Hagar) or secondary to osteomyelitis of the adjacent maxilla (Poncher and Blayney) (Fig. 8–19). It is important to note that air cells within the ethmoid and maxillary sinuses are sufficiently developed in the newborn to be a potential site of infection, although the relatively large ostia of the sinuses at this age generally prevents the occurrence of infection. Roentgenographic examination is less valuable in the young infant than in the older child as an indicator of disease of the ethmoid sinuses. Haziness of the ethmoid sinus on x-ray may be observed in the first year of life in the absence of an inflammatory process. Burnard stressed the occurrence of unilateral proptosis as the first sign of septic infection within the orbit in the newborn infant, followed subsequently by more characteristic inflammatory manifestations.

Orbital cellulitis in older children can result from trauma to the eyelids or orbital contents (Fig. 8–20), from metastatic spread of infection during the course of systemic sepsis, or from direct spread of bacteria from nearby structures, including infection of the skin of the face or eyelids, infection of dental structures, or paranasal sinusitis (Jarrett and Gutman, Gamble). Ethmoid sinusitis is the most commonly recognized site of infection leading to orbital cellulitis in children (Haynes and Cramblett) (Fig. 8–21). The orbit is separated from the ethmoid air cells by the thin-walled lamina papyracea, which provides little resistance to spread of a suppurative process. Perforation of this structure leads to extension of infection by contiguity in most instances. In some cases, bacteria are transmitted into the orbit by venous channels draining the ethmoid to the orbit and subsequently into the cavernous sinus.

Complications of suppuration within the orbit are now less common than in the preantibiotic period. Delay in recognition and initiation of therapy may still lead to severe ocular abnormalities, resulting in visual loss or blindness. Panophthalmitis, central retinal artery or retinal vein thrombosis, and ischemic retinal damage due to profound increase in the intraocular pressure are potential ocular complications which deprive the child of useful vision. Intracranial extension of the infection from the orbit can result in epidural, subdural, or cerebral abscess, cavernous sinus thrombosis (Kolmer et al.), cortical vein thrombosis, or bacterial meningitis.

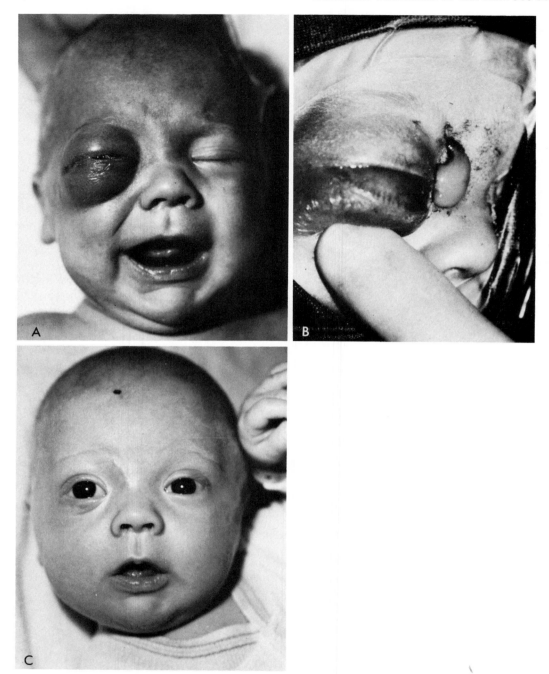

Figure 8–19. Acute septic orbital cellulitis in an 8-week-old infant secondary to ethmoid sinusitis. *A,* Massive swelling and inflammation of the soft tissues of the right orbit. The child had been well until 5 days before hospital admission when he developed intermittent fever and nasal congestion. Two days before admission temperature was 102°F, and parents noted the onset of swelling of the eyelids on the right side. The disorder rapidly progressed and at the time of entrance to the hospital, the swollen eyelids could not be separated. Acute ethmoid sinusitis was demonstrated on x-ray examination. *Staphylococcus aureus* was isolated on culture from the purulent exudate from the eye and from the nasal cavity but not from the blood. *B,* At surgery, mild pressure over the right eye results in the exuding of pus from the right ethmoid sinus and from a subperiosteal orbital abscess. The child also received methicillin intravenously. *C,* By 2 weeks after operation, he was recovered and has only slight proptosis on the right side.

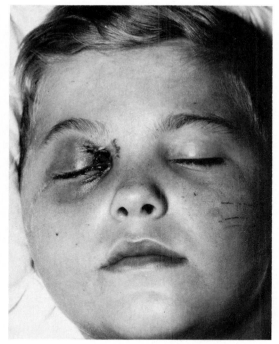

Figure 8–20. Acute, septic orbital cellulitis secondary to trauma to the eyelid. Nine-year-old boy who lacerated his right upper eyelid on a rusty pipe two days before hospital admission. Within 24 hours after the injury, he complained of headache and right orbital pain and developed a temperature of 102°F. On admission, the child had swelling and tenderness of the right periorbital soft tissues. Purulent exudate oozed from between the nearly closed eyelids. Extraocular movements on the right were restricted while the left eye remained normal. Neck stiffness, lethargy, and mild left hemiparesis also were found. Lumbar puncture revealed an opening pressure of 330 mm. H₂O. The fluid was blood-tinged and contained a glucose content of 70 mg per 100 ml. Gram stain and culture of the CSF were negative. Rapid improvement and eventual complete recovery occurred with antibiotic therapy. Certain of the clinical signs and the CSF abnormalities were presumed to be secondary to cerebral thrombophlebitis.

In some patients with orbital cellulitis, meningeal signs, lethargy, convulsions, disorientation, vomiting, and focal neurologic deficits will occur without frank meningitis or the development of a brain abscess. Cerebrospinal fluid in such cases reveals a cellular response plus mild elevation of protein content but with a normal glucose level and without bacteria on smear or culture. This constellation of findings probably results from bacterial cerebritis and generally responds rapidly to antibiotic treatment unless such therapy is delayed. In other children with cellulitis within the orbit, a lymphocytic pleocytosis is found in the spinal fluid without clinical symptoms or signs of intracranial spread of infection. The explanation for this "aseptic meningitis" syndrome remains unclear.

The most troublesome problem in diagnosis is the differentiation of orbital cellulitis from cavernous sinus thrombosis. This is especially true in cases in which orbital cellulitis is bilateral and is associated with cerebral symptoms or signs. Perhaps this diagnostic problem is more apparent than real, as many or perhaps most patients with suppurative thrombosis within the cavernous sinus also have orbital cellulitis owing to spread of infection anteriorly. Thus, the primary diagnostic decision is whether the child has only orbital sepsis or whether the symptoms and signs indicate the presence of both. As a generalization, papilledema is more common in those with cavernous sinus thrombosis, as is pupillary dilatation. Tenderness of the proptosed eye and erythema of the eyelids in the early stages of the illness are more suggestive of orbital sepsis. Severe visual loss with an ischemic-appearing retina on funduscopic examination in a patient who is alert and coherent is also more likely to be due to orbital cellulitis than to cavernous sinus thrombosis. Another condition that may have an abrupt onset with signs resembling those of orbital sepsis is carotid-cavernous fistula. This disorder usually follows head trauma, is generally without fever, and produces pulsating exophthalmos with an audible bruit over the involved globe.

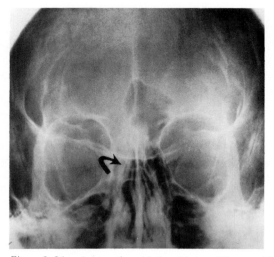

Figure 8–21. Acute ethmoid sinusitis in a 13-year-old boy with right orbital cellulitis. Rapidly progressive illness with headaches and fever of 4 days' duration, and progressive erythema and proptosis of the right eye of two days' duration. X-ray shows opacification of the right ethmoid sinus.

Rhinocerebral phycomycosis caused by fungi of the genus *Rhizopus* or *Mucor* can also be confused with suppurative orbital cellulitis, especially in the early stages of the fungal disease. The usual association of this rapidly progressive mycotic illness with diabetic ketoacidosis, leukemia, or other debilitating conditions is the most noteworthy feature suggestive of the correct diagnosis. The initial site of infection is the nasal cavity or paranasal sinuses in most cases, from where extension occurs to the orbit and subsequently to the brain. Signs include fever, leukocytosis, unilateral proptosis, ptosis, and ophthalmoplegia. Cerebral dysfunction can result from intracranial extension of the infection or massive infarction secondary to mycotic invasion of the carotid artery or other major vascular structures. The similarity to bacterial infection is obvious but is differentiated by the presence of a predisposing cause, the characteristic sequence of events, and histologic identification of the fungus of the Class Phycomycetes on tissue obtained from biopsy.

Treatment

Treatment of orbital cellulitis must be considered urgent and should be approached aggressively from the medical standpoint. Antibiotic administration should be by the intravenous route with the choice of drugs based on the age of the child and probable organism involved. In the child less than eight years of age, the possibility of *Hemophilus influenzae* warrants the use of ampicillin (Londer and Nelson) and chloramphenicol, in addition to methicillin, until the organism is identified and sensitivity studies are available. Other bacteria that cause orbital cellulitis at any age include *Staphylococcus* species, *Streptococcus* species, and *Streptococcus pneumoniae*. A penicillinase-resistant semisynthetic penicillin, such as methicillin or nafcillin, should be used in combination with ampicillin in the child over eight years of age with this disorder. Appropriate changes in the regimen are made when the offending organism is identified and antibiotic sensitivities determined. Nasal decongestants may be helpful or surgical drainage of infected sinuses may be necessary. Surgical procedures on the orbit itself are not usually recommended, although incision and drainage of an abscess is justified whenever discovered. On rare occasion, pressure-induced ischemic retinopathy may warrant an orbital decompressive procedure in an effort to prevent total visual loss.

CAVERNOUS SINUS THROMBOSIS

The cavernous sinuses are located lateral to the sella turcica along the sphenoid bone extending from the superior orbital fissure to the apex of the petrous bone. The sinuses consist of a complex of venous channels and house the carotid siphon in addition to the oculomotor, trochlear, and abducens nerves en route to the extraocular muscles. The first and second divisions of the trigeminal nerve also traverse the cavernous sinus. Ophthalmic veins, veins from the hypophyseal plexus, and certain cerebral veins distribute blood into the cavernous sinuses. Additional communications with the cavernous sinuses exist with the superior petrosal sinus which drains into the transverse sinus, and the inferior petrosal sinus, terminating in the sigmoid sinus or jugular vein. The paired cavernous sinuses communicate freely with one another, accounting for the bilateral ocular signs usually present when infection occurs within this region.

Septic thrombosis of the cavernous sinus is a serious bacterial infection that was nearly uniformly fatal before the availability of antibiotic treatment (Brown). The illness is now sufficiently rare that current mortality statistics are not available, but prognosis is always guarded regarding either survival or residual sequelae. With adequate antibiotic therapy, survival rate in the range of 70 to 80 percent is now expected (Clune). The offending organisms are similar to those that cause orbital sepsis, with most cases resulting from *Staphylococcus aureus* and a lesser number being of streptococcal origin. Infection within the cavernous sinus can develop either from hematogenous seeding from remote suppurative lesions or from direct spread by contiguity or venous dissemination from numerous adjacent structures. Anastomoses of the frontal, angular, or anterior facial veins with the ophthalmic veins may transmit bacteria into the cavernous sinus from focal suppurative lesions of the face or eyelids. Cellulitis of the orbit also is a source of contamination of this intracranial sinus via drainage through the ophthalmic veins or by direct spread. Sphenoid and ethmoid sinusitis or osteomyelitis of the petrous apex secondary to chronic middle ear disease are additional potential sites of origin which may be complicated by cavernous sinus sepsis. Fungal infections, including those caused by *Aspergillus* or Phycomycetes, can result in cavernous sinus thrombosis on rare occasion.

Symptoms and Signs

The child with septic cavernous sinus thrombosis is usually quite ill with a combination of systemic symptoms and local signs. High spiking fever, chills, headache, vomiting, and lethargy may reflect either generalized sepsis or the more localized septic process. Severe, stabbing ocular pain, increased by pressure on the globe, is sometimes present owing to involvement of the first division of the trigeminal nerve within the infected cavernous sinus. Ocular signs are frequently unilateral at first but usually rapidly become apparent on both sides (Fig. 8–22). In rare instances, the ocular signs remain unilateral, in which case it is difficult to be certain whether the infection is intraorbital, within the cavernous sinus, or both. Eyelid and conjunctival edema, exophthalmos, ophthalmoplegia, and pupillary dilatation are ocular hallmarks of this condition, which can worsen precipitously within hours after the very first symptoms. Exophthalmos may be partially due to venous obstruction but coexistent orbital cellulitis appears to be the most important factor accounting for its presence (Brunner, Walsh and Hoyt). Ptosis and extraocular muscle weakness vary in degree, with some cases showing complete external ophthalmoplegia at the peak of the illness. It is unclear whether the ocular palsy is entirely the result of involvement of the nerves to the extraocular muscles within the cavernous sinus or is partly mechanical from the associated swelling and inflammation in the orbits. Retinal venous engorgement is usual and low-grade papilledema is occasionally observed. Visual loss is not primarily attributable to the inflammatory condition within the cavernous sinus but can occur from complications of the process, including ischemic retinopathy or optic neuropathy (Friberg and Sogg), and secondary keratitis.

Symptoms and signs of cerebral involvement have numerous possible sources of origin in children with cavernous sinus thrombosis. Bacterial meningitis or cerebritis may coexist with cavernous sinus thrombosis, with each resulting from dissemination of infection elsewhere. Cerebral venous pathology might be expected in some cases since the

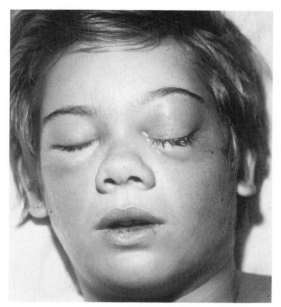

Figure 8–22. Septic cavernous sinus thrombosis secondary to acute ethmoid sinusitis. This 12-year-old boy was well until 2 days prior to admission. Fever, headache, and bilateral retro-orbital pain were the initial symptoms. One day before admission, temperature rose to 105°F, and the patient became confused, and then convulsed. Examination at the time of hospital admission revealed his temperature to be 104°F and the presence of marked lethargy. There was bilateral proptosis and chemosis, left more than right. Extraocular movements became restricted bilaterally, more marked on the left. The white blood cell count was 20,400 per cu. mm. with 82 percent polymorphonuclear leukocytes. With antibiotic therapy, he made an uneventful recovery without sequelae except for ptosis of the left eyelid.

cavernous sinus receives venous blood from certain parts of the brain. Narrowing or occlusion of the carotid artery within the infected cavernous sinus may occur, resulting in cerebral infarction manifested by hemiparesis and other hemisphere signs (Mathew et al.). It is also possible for carotid artery obstruction within the cavernous sinus to result in a vascular steal syndrome, in which the anterior circulation is perfused via the vertebral-basilar artery system. The end-result can be the production of signs of brain stem dysfunction in a child with cavernous sinus thrombosis (Kinnaird et al.). The pituitary gland is often affected in children with cavernous sinus thrombosis (Walsh); however, this does not usually cause clinical abnormalities during the acute stage of the illness. Because of the potential compromise in pituitary function, those who survive should have certain endocrine studies performed at a subsequent date.

Diagnosis of septic cavernous sinus thrombosis is largely on clinical grounds, with hallmarks of the disorder being evidence of acute bacterial infection in conjunction with the characteristic ophthalmologic findings. Spiking fever and increase in the blood leukocyte count are customary. Cerebrospinal fluid examination is normal in some cases, while in others there will be a mild cellular response in the absence of other evidence of meningitis. Carotid angiography may reveal focal arteritis or even obstruction of the cavernous portion of the internal carotid artery. Of greater diagnostic importance is the venous phase, which shows delayed filling or non-visualization of the cavernous sinus and reversal of the normal venous drainage pattern at the base of the skull (Théron and Djindjian).

Except for bilateral orbital cellulitis, the orbitocerebral form of mucormycosis, and carotid-cavernous fistula, there is little in the differential diagnosis of acute septic cavernous sinus thrombosis. The Tolosa-Hunt syndrome of "painful ophthalmoplegia" is a cavernous sinus inflammatory process; however, it has few clinical similarities to acute cavernous sinus sepsis. The disorder was first clearly described with pathologic examination by Tolosa in 1954, although Collier made mention of similar cases as early as 1921. Subsequently, it has been the subject of several reports in both adults and children (Hunt et al., Sondheimer and Knapp, Terrence and Samaha). Largely on the basis of the histologic findings in the case of Tolosa, the illness is believed to be a granulomatous inflammatory disorder with lymphocytic and plasma cell infiltration limited to the cavernous sinus. The precise etiology has not been established to this date.

The onset of painful ophthalmoplegia is either abrupt or gradual and consists of severe, boring retro-orbital pain, or diplopia caused by extraocular muscle weakness. Mild fever and malaise may accompany the initial complaints but a septic-like temperature pattern is not expected. Unlike cavernous sinus sepsis, this disorder is not associated with significant proptosis. Periorbital edema and conjunctival congestion are mild, if present at all. The ocular findings are typically unilateral and vary from mild ophthalmoparesis due to partial third or sixth nerve paresis, to complete ophthalmoplegia associated with pupillary dysfunction. Fifth nerve sensory dysfunction is not common but has been described in some cases. The clinical findings persist for days up to several weeks when remission occurs, followed by recurrences at intervals of several months. In a few cases, orbital venography in the symptomatic stage of the illness has demonstrated occlusion of the superior ophthalmic vein on the involved side and partial obliteration of the cavernous sinus (Sondheimer and Knapp, Takeoka et al.). The response to corticosteroid therapy has been so dramatic in cases of the Tolosa-Hunt syndrome that its use has been proposed as a diagnostic measure as well as the recommended form of treatment.

Treatment

Treatment of septic cavernous sinus thrombosis requires the intravenous administration of high doses of antibiotics in addition to the appropriate supportive measures for a critically ill patient with infectious disease. Lethargy or other manifestations of cerebral involvement would warrant use of anticonvulsants in an effort to prevent seizures. Associated lesions, such as furuncles, chronic otitis, petrositis, or sinusitis, should be searched for and managed appropriately. Ethmoidectomy is important in certain instances when the primary source of the infection is acute suppurative ethmoid sinusitis. Surgical decompression of the orbits is to be considered in cases with severe increase in intraorbital pressure which threatens retinal or optic nerve function. Corticosteroids have been recommended by some to decrease orbital inflammation and also because of the possibility of acute adrenal insufficiency secondary to pituitary involvement (Solomon et al.) but their value remains uncertain. The indications for anticoagulation, likewise, are not completely established. Heparin therapy may be of value in certain patients but probably should be withheld if clinical improvement is evident after two or three days of antibiotic treatment.

COMPLICATIONS OF MIDDLE EAR DISEASE

Cranial and intracranial complications of either acute or chronic inflammatory middle ear disease were precipitously reduced by the development of the antibiotic preparations. In an extensive study of otitic complications from 1928 to 1933, Courville and Nielsen found that approximately 25 of every 1,000 deaths in the Los Angeles County Hospital resulted from an intracranial complication of otitis media (124 fatal cases in 5,227 autopsies). In a comparative study from 1949 to 1954, only 23 cases of fatal intracranial complications were discovered among 9,737 autopsies (Courville). In this latter series in the antibiotic era, approximately 25 in every 10,000 deaths in the same hospital were due to intracranial otitic complications, a decline of 90 percent over the earlier statistics. Furthermore, among the 23 fatal cases in the more recent survey, 18 resulted from meningitis, a complication of acute otitis that remains uncontrolled in younger children.

The prevention of these dreaded neurologic conditions has paralleled the reduction of suppurative mastoiditis and the prevention and control of chronic otitis in children. Although many of the intracranial complications have become unusual, an attitude of complacency in this regard is dangerous because isolated cases continue to occur. Many physicians trained in the past 10 to 15 years have not observed extradural, subdural, or cerebral abscesses secondary to middle ear or mastoid disease in childhood. In addition, the non-specific and poorly localizing signs often associated with these complicating lesions add to the diagnostic complexity, permitting delay in identification and institution of therapy.

Acute bacterial meningitis remains the most common neurologic complication of otitis media in childhood. *Streptococcus pneumoniae* and *Hemophilus influenzae* are the usual offenders in patients with otogenic meningitis (Hara) although numerous other bacterial agents have been implicated, and, infrequently, multiple organisms may be present. In past times when chronic suppurative otitis media was more common, *Bacteroides* species was the most prevalent anaerobic cause of otogenic meningitis or brain abscess (Sanders and Stevenson, Smith et al.), and is still an important cause of such lesions. Cerebral vascular occlusive disease may complicate bacterial infection of the middle ear, resulting in a sudden onset of focal neurologic deficits in a stroke-like fashion (Wise and Farmer). Focal cerebral ischemia in such patients can result either from cerebral arteritis or secondary to thrombophlebitis with hemorrhagic infarction. Cerebrospinal fluid findings in children with bacterial vascular occlusive disease may reveal no abnormalities or exhibit a modest pleocytosis, with lymphocytes predominating. Cerebral venous occlusion is suspected by the presence of red cells or xanthochromia of the spinal fluid, although this also is variable. Smear and culture of the cerebrospinal fluid is usually negative in such cases despite the bacterial origin of the process. Carotid angiography, electroencephalography, radioactive brain scan, and computed tomography are of diagnostic value, but initiation of antibacterial therapy must usually be based on the statistical probability of an association between the suppurative middle ear disease and the acute neurologic syndrome.

Bell's palsy has been attributed to acute otitis in some cases and, on rare occasion, Horner's syndrome may occur in children with acute middle ear infection (Hoefnagel and Joseph, Hubert). The pathogenesis of oculosympathetic paralysis with acute otitis media remains unproven but is believed due to inflammatory involvement of the sympathetic fibers along the carotid artery as it passes by the anterior wall of the tympanic cavity. A benign and transient abducens palsy has been described, which occurs one to three weeks after otherwise uncomplicated otitis media or following other types of non-specific upper respiratory infection in children (Knox et al.). Unlike lateral rectus paresis that is part of the syndrome of apical petrositis or lateral sinus thrombosis, the syndrome of benign sixth nerve palsy is unassociated with other cranial nerve deficits or signs of increased intracranial pressure. The cause is not known and spontaneous recovery is expected.

Other neurologic complications of middle ear disease include extradural or subdural abscess, temporal lobe or cerebellar suppuration, acute bacterial cerebritis, lateral sinus and cortical venous thrombosis, and Gradenigo's syndrome. The identification of extension of infection from the middle ear or mastoid to any intracranial structure should warrant search for other possible intracranial complications. For example, the child with apical petrositis may have an adjacent extradural abscess, or the youngster with septic lateral sinus thrombosis can also harbor a temporal lobe or cerebellar hemisphere abscess. Progression of a focal suppurative intracranial infection may ultimately lead to acute meningitis.

Another form of inflammatory ear disease with neurologic complications is referred to as malignant external otitis, a term coined by Chandler in 1968. The disorder is a subacute or chronic infection of the external ear canal caused by *Pseudomonas aeruginosa,* and occurs almost exclusively in elderly diabetic patients (Chandler, Zaky et al.). It is usually intractable to the common modes of therapy for external otitis. Eventual spread of infection through clefts in cartilage of the floor of the external auditory canal, called the fissures of Santorini, results in necrotizing osteomyelitis of the base of the skull. Local pain in the ear canal is followed by swelling of the face on the involved side, trismus, and unilateral facial paralysis (Schwarz et al.).

Facial nerve involvement is the customary first neurologic sign of malignant external otitis. The seventh nerve is usually affected at its site of exit from the stylomastoid foramen but can be damaged during its course through the facial canal. Progression of the illness in some cases is complicated by involvement of the lower cranial nerves on the same side (Dinapoli and Thomas), with the possible development of meningitis or brain abscess. The development of leptomeningitis or intracranial abscess is a late event in the course of this illness and does not represent a frequent complication. It is not unusual, however, to find a reactive cerebrospinal fluid pleocytosis at a much earlier stage of this disorder, in the absence of organisms in the fluid specimen. Fever is usually minimal or absent, and the white blood cell count is often only mildly increased with this condition. The seriousness of the process is reflected by the mortality rate, which is in the range of 40 to 50 percent (Chandler, Zaky et al.). Successful treatment depends on early diagnosis. Carbenicillin and gentamicin are administered for four to six weeks, in addition to appropriate surgical debridement. Although the great majority of cases of malignant external otitis are found in the older patient with diabetes mellitus, the disorder has been recognized in children with other debilitating conditions (Joachims).

Extradural abscess, now rare, was recognized in past years as a potential threatening complication of middle ear disease but one without distinctive clinical features. Inflammatory bone destruction with pus extending to the dural surface has been unexpectedly identified in certain cases at the time of mastoidectomy. Fever, headache, vomiting, and leukocytosis may be present in children with otogenic epidural abscess but may in part result from the associated ear or mastoid condition. Papilledema may or may not be present but, if high-grade, it suggests an additional intracranial complication, such as a parenchymal brain abscess.

Subdural abscess is even more rare as an otitic complication and also is not characterized by symptoms or signs that permit easy identification. It is more widely recognized as a complication of suppurative paranasal sinus disease, especially secondary to frontal sinusitis (Keith, List, Ray and Parsons). In infants, subdural empyema is more often identified as a complicating feature of bacterial meningitis rather than secondary to sinusitis (Farmer and Wise). Subdural empyema is more likely to result in signs of cerebral cortical irritation and to cause more marked cerebrospinal fluid abnormalities than epidural abscess. The cerebrospinal fluid findings resemble those of partially treated bacterial meningitis or viral encephalitis and thus lead to diagnostic error unless focal suppuration is considered in the differential diagnosis.

Gradenigo's Syndrome

Suppuration of the apex of the petrous portion of the temporal bone is known as Gradenigo's syndrome, following the description by Gradenigo in 1904. The process is a complication of chronic middle ear infection or mastoiditis in the majority of cases although some have occurred days or weeks after mastoidectomy. Only rarely has apical petrositis been described in the absence of significant middle ear or mastoid disease (Allen and Cobb).

The child with apical petrositis is usually obviously ill with spiking fever, anorexia, and local discomfort. Trigeminal nerve irritation results in intense pain in the temporal region, forehead, or orbit, or occasionally in the region of the upper teeth on the affected side. The corneal reflex may be diminished or absent on the same side. Younger children with this disorder are frequently so irritable that accurate corneal sensory testing is not possible. Lateral rectus muscle dysfunction is attributed to involvement of the sixth nerve by either pressure or inflammation as it traverses the petrous apex en route to the lateral rectus muscle. Thus, diagnosis of Gradenigo's syndrome is suspected in the child with middle ear or mastoid disease who develops unilateral fifth and sixth cranial nerve dysfunction manifested by local pain, diplopia, and lateral rectus paresis or paralysis. Roentgenographic examination is usually helpful but requires special views to visualize the petrous ridge and its apex (Fig. 8–23). Both sides should be examined to allow comparison of one with the other. The Stenvers view, or some modification thereof, and the basilar skull film generally provide the most valuable information regarding the presence of bony destruction of the petrous apex.

An adjacent epidural abscess may develop in patients with osteomyelitis or abscess of the petrous apex if destruction of the bony cortex occurs. Venous extension of the infection can lead to cortical vein or cavernous sinus thrombosis. Meningitis is a constant danger in the child with this disorder unless antibiotic therapy and surgical decompression and drainage of the infected bone is accomplished. Lethargy, limb weakness on the opposite side or seizures can be explained on the basis of cerebritis in some cases and may lead to abscess formation unless the progress can be interrupted by intravenous antibiotic treatment.

Lateral Sinus Thrombosis

The most poorly understood and debated condition secondary to otitis media is lateral sinus thrombosis. This effluent venous channel may become obstructed by direct external pressure from an adjacent abscess or granulation tissue, from septic involvement of the vessel wall, or, by mural thrombosis without inflammation within the lumen. Symonds (1931, 1937, 1952) drew attention to lateral sinus thrombosis in patients with otitis media, although the observation had been made many years before (Kalbag and Woolf). He suggested that cases of "otitic hydrocephalus" resulted from extension of venous thrombosis to the superior longitudinal sinus, thereby interfering with cerebrospinal fluid absorption through the arachnoid villi. Following Gardner's demonstration that the lateral ventricles were not distended in these cases, Symonds (1956) agreed that the term "otitic hydrocephalus" was a misnomer and that increased intracranial pressure in such cases was on the basis of brain swelling. He further stressed the variations of the clinical manifestations of lateral sinus thrombosis and pointed out that only a minority of patients developed signs of intracranial hypertension or other neurologic deficits.

The clinical features associated with lateral sinus thrombosis depend on the degree of extension of the clot and the anatomic vari-

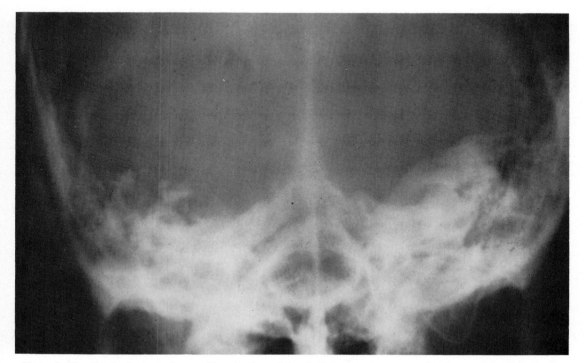

Figure 8–23. Gradenigo's syndrome. Town's view of the skull demonstrates extensive destruction of the petrous ridge on the right compared to the normal appearance on the left. Such advanced roentgenographic changes are unusual with this disorder.

ations of the venous drainage from the brain. When drainage from the superior longitudinal sinus to the torcula Herophili passes freely to both right and left lateral sinuses, obstruction of one lateral sinus usually remains asymptomatic. Not uncommonly, however, venous blood in the superior longitudinal sinus empties predominantly or entirely into the right lateral sinus. In this case, obstruction of the right lateral sinus impedes venous drainage from the cerebral hemispheres, resulting in cerebral edema and subsequent symptoms and signs of increased intracranial pressure. Likewise, extension of the thrombus from one lateral sinus to the torcula Herophili would disturb venous return from the brain regardless of the anatomic arrangement of the venous system. Venous congestion and cerebral edema in such patients resembles the clinical picture of pseudotumor cerebri so precisely that many authors have included lateral sinus thrombosis as one cause of the latter syndrome. Cerebrospinal fluid pressure is elevated while the fluid remains clear to observation and without an increase of cells or protein content.

In more complicated cases where venous thrombosis involves the superior longitudinal sinus and its tributary cortical veins, hemorrhagic infarction produces signs of increased pressure in addition to cortical deficits, including seizures, weakness, and mental disturbances. Cerebrospinal fluid in this situation is more likely to be xanthochromic, and contains an increased protein content and numerous red blood cells.

Symonds (1956) observed abducens nerve paresis so often in patients with increased pressure secondary to lateral sinus thrombosis that he doubted that it could be explained as a false localizing sign due to elevated intracranial pressure. He attributed this to thrombosis of the inferior petrosal sinus with direct compression of the sixth nerve by the occluded sinus at a point where both structures traverse Dorello's canal. The inferior petrosal sinus may become occluded by direct spread of infection from the middle ear or by extension from the lateral sinus. Symonds also suggested that paralysis of the ninth, tenth, and eleventh cranial nerves seen rarely in patients with this disorder may be explained by direct pressure from thrombosis in the jugular bulb.

Diagnosis of lateral sinus thrombosis in children without symptoms or signs there-

from is largely an unexpected finding at the time of surgery. In patients with brain swelling and increased pressure signs, computed tomography or air encephalography reveals normal or even small ventricles. Definitive diagnosis can occasionally be made from the venous phase on carotid angiography (Greer and Berk), although interpretation may be subject to error in this regard owing to normal variations. Diagnosis is generally more by presumption when an increased intracranial pressure syndrome follows significant otitis and when other disorders, including abscess, are excluded by the appropriate studies. Sinography, the injection of contrast material directly into the superior longitudinal sinus, may accurately localize the site of dural sinus obstruction but is not usually indicated or necessary. Tobey and Ayer (1925) applied the Queckenstedt test as a means of diagnosis of lateral sinus thrombosis. With the lumbar puncture needle in place, jugular compression on the side of the occluded sinus results in no elevation of the fluid column in the manometer, while compression of the opposite side produces a normal rise and fall. The Tobey-Ayer test is only rarely utilized now because of the recognized hazard of jugular compression in patients with increased intracranial pressure. Furthermore, it is not always reliable in view of the variations of response to jugular compression related to normal anatomic variations of the cerebral venous system.

Lateral sinus thrombosis is usually regarded to be a benign disorder unless it is associated with other intracranial suppurative complications. Treatment of the causative middle ear condition and prevention of visual loss from chronic papilledema are the major therapeutic considerations. Jugular vein ligation to prevent embolization to the heart or lungs is now rarely performed. Periodic spinal taps at intervals of three or four days with cautious fluid removal may be indicated if papilledema is marked.

ACUTE SPINAL EPIDURAL ABSCESS

Acute epidural abscess within the spinal canal represents a diagnostic and therapeutic emergency somewhat analogous to that of an epidural hematoma within the intracranial space. Although delay in recognition of an intraspinal abscess may not immediately create a life-threatening situation, the longer and the more severe the neurologic deficits are prior to surgery, the greater is the likelihood of residual paraplegia or neurogenic bladder dysfunction (Dandy).

Spinal epidural abscesses are most commonly located in the mid-thoracic or lower lumbar regions, although there are rare reports in which the entire length of the vertebral canal was involved (Hulme and Dott). Suppuration is usually located on the dorsal surface of the spinal dura, a point fortunately enhancing clinical localization and facilitating surgical drainage. The explanation for the dorsal localization of spinal epidural abscesses was proposed by Dandy in 1926. He demonstrated that a definite epidural space exists dorsal to the spinal nerve attachments, but on the ventral surface of the cord, the dura is closely attached to the vertebrae, thus decreasing the likelihood of focal suppuration in this area. He also emphasized that the epidural space in the cervical region is exceedingly shallow but becomes well developed dorsal to the cord at the level of the seventh cervical vertebra. It reaches considerable depth between the fourth and eighth thoracic vertebrae and again becomes narrow from the eleventh thoracic to the second lumbar vertebrae. The epidural space attains its greatest depth below the level of the third lumbar vertebra and in these areas is composed of fatty and loose areolar tissues. Abscess formation within the epidural space appears to occur in areas where the space is largest and contains more abundant areolar tissue.

Most authorities now believe that an epidural abscess results directly from hematogenous spread of bacteria in the majority of instances, and that direct extension from vertebral osteomyelitis is a less common cause. This view departs from that of Browder and Meyers, who in 1937 proposed contiguous spread from infected vertebrae as the usual initiating event. When a source of hematogenous spread is identified, cutaneous furuncle is the most common one, although in many instances no obvious bacterial infection is apparent before the development of symptoms of an acute epidural abscess. Other sites of primary infection mentioned in the past have included pyelonephritis, pneumonia, otitis media or mastoiditis, cellulitis, and dental abscess. Several authors have implicated the studies by Batson as an explanation for epidural abscess formation secondary to in-

tra-abdominal or intrathoracic sepsis. Batson demonstrated that epidural veins have a rich anastomosis at each spinal segment with veins of the abdominal and thoracic cavities. During the Valsalva maneuver, blood is shunted into the low-pressure vertebral venous system and, therefore, could be a source of metastatic spread in this direction. Rangell and Glassman attributed the development of a spinal epidural abscess in one patient to contamination of the epidural space during a diagnostic lumbar puncture. Regardless of the source of origin, the vast majority of cases in recent years have been due to hemolytic *Staphylococcus aureus* (Baker).

Acute spinal epidural abscess is an uncommon lesion and occurs more often in adults than in children, although no age group is completely spared. Most pediatric cases reported have been in older children. The lesion has been identified in early infancy (Aicardi and Lepintre, Miller and Hesch, Rushworth and Martin, Palmer and Kelly) but is considered to be rare in children under ten years of age.

Symptoms and Signs

Certain children with an acute spinal epidural abscess give no history of significant antecedent events, while others describe a preceding bacterial infection or an injury with blunt trauma to the back. Although the pathogenic relationship of trauma to the subsequent development of a spinal epidural abscess remains unclear, the association seems reasonably well established, both from the literature and from personal experience.

Deep, aching pain, at or near the site of the involved level of the spine, is the usual initial symptom of this disease. Fever may be evident simultaneously or may be recorded a day or two subsequent to the onset of symptoms. Local back discomfort rapidly worsens to become agonizing back pain and is made more intense by flexion of the trunk at the hips, by coughing, or by abrupt changes in body position. If the child is examined at this time, localized percussion tenderness over two or three spinous processes in the affected region will be identified. Spinal rigidity is apparent by the presence of tense paraspinus muscles and resistance to forward bending at the hips. Between one and three days after onset, headaches, vomiting, and neck stiffness may occur and can lead one astray diagnostically unless the significance of the back complaints is appreciated.

Within a day or so after the onset of localized back pain, rootlet irritation manifested by radicular pain adds to the child's discomfort. The distribution of the radicular pain varies, depending on the location of the abscess. A thoracic epidural abscess may cause radiating pain to the anterior, lower chest wall or to the upper abdomen and can simulate surgical intra-abdominal disease. An abscess in the lumbar epidural region often produces lancinating pain down one or both legs, into the hip region, or to the external genitalia.

By three to six days after the first complaints, neurologic disturbances begin to appear in the form of weakness of the lower extremities, sensory deficits or hyperesthesia in the legs or feet, and abnormalities of bladder or bowel function. At this stage, the back pain is usually so severe that the child will refuse to walk and may cooperate little on muscle strength testing. In some patients, by the time paralysis of the legs has occurred, the abscess may have dissected under pressure from the spinal epidural space into the paraspinal soft tissues. In advanced cases, tenderness, swelling, and increased heat on palpation may be observed in the involved soft tissues of the back. Although extension of the process may occur externally to involve soft tissues, the dura provides a formidable barrier to infection and usually prevents the development of meningitis, unless the barrier is compromised by the lumbar puncture needle. Bladder retention may be intermittent for a period of time and root pain may have either persisted or disappeared as strength in the legs diminishes progressively.

The findings on neurologic examination are variable at this stage, depending on the location of the lesion, but include the appearance of a child obviously ill, with meningeal signs, and with motor dysfunction in the lower extremities. If the abscess is lumbar in location, deep tendon reflexes are diminished or absent and sensory loss will follow a rootlet pattern without a well-established level. A thoracic epidural abscess can also be associated with reflex loss and flaccidity of the lower extremities or may cause hyperreflexia with pathologic toe signs. Regardless of whether the lesion is thoracic or lumbar in location, an important point on neurologic assessment is that the upper extremities remain essentially normal on examination. Although the distribution of motor and sensory deficits assist in localizing the vertebral level of the abscess, the site of percussion tenderness is often the most highly localizing sign on physical examination. In some children with spinal epidural abscess, systemic sepsis and high fever will be associated with a certain degree of mental confusion or decrease in orientation or alertness. Such "cerebral" signs can be quite misleading in regard to localizing diagnosis, unless attention is directed to the significance of the back signs described above.

Diagnostic Studies

Most children with an acute spinal epidural abscess have a significant blood leukocytosis, with counts ranging from 12,000 to 35,000 per cu. mm. The differential count reveals an increase in immature forms and the erythrocyte sedimentation rate is usually elevated. Blood should be obtained for culture but is frequently negative. X-rays of the spine are useful mainly to eliminate other causes of low back pain, especially that due to lumbar disc space infection, which may bear close clinical similarity to acute epidural abscess. Roentgenographic evidence of osteomyelitis of the spine may be apparent in certain children with epidural suppuration but this is true in only the minority. The absence of x-ray abnormalities, however, does not exclude vertebral involvement because several weeks may be required before such changes become visible.

Lumbar puncture is indicated in most cases in which spinal epidural abscess is suspected but certain precautions and considerations are necessary when the procedure is performed. If the lesion is located in the lumbar region, penetration of the abscess by the needle followed by entrance of the subarachnoid space can result in acute and severe bacterial meningitis (Rosamond). This complication can be avoided by recognition of the possibility and with slow advancement of the needle through the soft tissues. At intervals, the stylet should be removed and gentle suction applied with a syringe to see if pus is encountered. If pus is identified, the diagnosis is established, and after a specimen is obtained for gram stain and culture, the needle should be promptly withdrawn and *not* advanced into the subarachnoid space. Needle drainage of an epidural abscess is never considered adequate and laminectomy will still be necessary.

Epidural abscess located above the level of penetration of the spinal needle causes variable abnormalities in the spinal fluid and only rarely are the findings entirely normal. The absence of a rise in pressure on jugular vein compression (Queckenstedt test) with the needle tip in the subarachnoid space indicates a complete spinal block. The opening pressure below the level of a block can be either elevated or low, but the pressure usually drops precipitously after removal of only a small quantity of cerebrospinal fluid. The protein content is usually increased, and, if the increase is marked, the fluid will be xanthochromic in appearance. A cellular response is commonly present and may include mainly lymphocytes or a combination of lymphocytes and polymorphonuclear leukocytes. The glucose content remains normal and the fluid does not contain bacteria.

When a complete spinal block is present, removal of fluid from the subarachnoid space below the block makes it very difficult to successfully repeat the lumbar puncture in the next few hours or days. This causes considerable difficulty in the performance of myelography, if desired, after a diagnostic tap has been done. This problem can be circumvented if one suspects an epidural abscess by having available an ampule of iophendylate (Pantopaque) when the initial tap is done. If the fluid is xanthochromic, thus indicating a high protein content, and a complete spinal block is present on the Queckenstedt test, the appropriate amount of dye is injected into the subarachnoid space prior to removal of the spinal needle. In the infant 1 ml. of Pantopaque is sufficient and in the older child 3 ml. is adequate to demonstrate the level of the obstruction. After the dye has been injected and the needle withdrawn, the child is promptly transported to the radiology unit where fluoroscopic examination outlines the site of the spinal block. Performance of the spinal tap, interpretation of the results of the manometric studies, and decision to inject Pantopaque in a child suspected of harboring a spinal epidural abscess require considerable skill and judgment. Whenever possible, the procedure should be done by one with a certain degree of experience with this disorder.

Differential Diagnosis

Several disorders share certain clinical findings observed in children with acute spinal epidural abscess, but most can be excluded rapidly on the basis of the physical examination and ancillary studies. Conversion hysteria is sometimes entertained in the early stages of the illness when back discomfort or rootlet pain precedes objective neurologic findings or fever. Back pain of abrupt onset in the childhood years should always be considered organic until proved otherwise. The presence of spinal rigidity, focal percussion vertebral tenderness, or reflex abnormalities in the lower extremities indicates the organic nature of the illness but are signs that can be identified only if properly searched for. Hip synovitis or septic arthritis of the hip is initially suspected because of the location of rootlet pain in some patients but can usually be excluded by the back signs mentioned above.

Flaccid paraparesis and hyporeflexia resulting from a lumbar epidural abscess can be confused with similar findings in children with poliomyelitis or the Guillain-Barré syndrome. Bladder involvement, sensory deficits, the relatively symmetrical motor loss, and the localized back pain all stand in opposition to the diagnosis of polio. Guillain-Barré syndrome is a relatively painless disorder which usually progresses slower than an epidural abscess and generally involves all four limbs and the facial musculature to some extent. Tuberculous spondylitis with spinal cord involvement is usually a more chronic illness which develops in one known to be tuberculous in most cases and with spine roentgenographic changes consistent with the disease.

Acute disc space infection (spondylarthritis) in infants and toddlers may resemble epidural abscess almost precisely but can be recognized and differentiated by the roentgenographic examination of the involved region of the spine. Irritability, fever, exquisite spinal tenderness, and the rapid development of refusal to walk are common to both illnesses in this age group. Furthermore, the intense irritability of the young child with acute disc space infection often precludes a detailed neurologic examination in regard to function of the lower limbs. Thus, being certain that weakness of the legs is not present may be very difficult. A positive diagnosis of disc space infection is usually made from the lateral spine x-ray but lumbar puncture may be necessary to exclude completely epidural suppuration.

Spontaneous spinal epidural hematoma in childhood (Posnikoff) is exceedingly rare but presents in a fashion analogous to that of abscess in the same location except that general signs of infection are not expected. Unless spinal trauma has occurred or the patient is known to have a hemorrhagic disorder such as hemophilia, epidural hematoma causing spinal cord compression is likely to remain unexpected until laminectomy is performed. Additional epidural mass lesions that can manifest themselves with a rapidly progressive course with localizing signs of cord compression include epidural sarcoma, either primary or spread from the retroperitoneal space, and neuroblastoma that has extended medially from its primary site of origin.

The disorder that bears the closest similarity to spinal epidural abscess is acute transverse myelopathy. Rapid progression is characteristic of both, back and rootlet pain may occur with either, and the spinal fluid findings can be identical with the two disorders. Evidence of a spinal block with the Queckenstedt test is usually found with an epidural abscess located above the level of needle penetration but is not inconsistent with acute transverse myelopathy, although most patients with transverse myelopathy have normal manometrics. Altrocchi stressed the clinical similarity of acute transverse myelopathy to epidural abscess and pointed out important features that might permit differential diagnosis. Sudden onset of a transverse cord lesion without prior pain and with progression to maximum neurologic deficit within a few hours is more indicative of acute transverse myelopathy and is unusual with epidural abscess. History of a recent bacterial infection is supportive of the probability of epidural abscess, while no prior infection or a non-specific upper respiratory illness is more often seen with acute transverse myelopathy. Normal spinal fluid findings, including the Queckenstedt test, are more consistent with acute transverse myelopathy although a lymphocytic pleocytosis and increased protein content are not uncommonly found with this disorder. Roentgenographic evidence of vertebral osteomyelitis that corresponds to the level of neurologic involvement would be indicative of epidural abscess, although the absence of x-ray abnormalities in no way excludes the possibility. While overlapping of the clinical symptoms and signs of the two disorders is apparent, in most instances the total evaluation, including the lumbar puncture, permits differentiation of these conditions. Occasionally, the child with acute transverse myelopathy will require myelography before an extramedullary cord compressive lesion can be excluded.

Spinal subdural empyema resembles epidural suppuration from the clinical standpoint, but preoperative differentiation is of little importance since both lesions are managed in similar fashion. Spinal subdural abscess is much less common than epidural abscess but also is characterized by fever, backache, root pain, and a rapidly progressive course with prompt emergence of spinal cord or cauda equina impairment. The cerebrospinal fluid cell count may be higher in subdural than epidural spinal abscess, and vertebral percussion tenderness is more consistently present with epidural abscess as compared to subdural empyema (Dacey et al., Fraser et al.). Myelography may allow differential diagnosis but regardless, immediate surgical drainage should be accomplished.

Treatment

An acute spinal epidural abscess should be considered to be a surgical emergency requiring laminectomy and drainage at the earliest possible moment. It is a potentially curable lesion, with the degree of recovery depending on the extent and duration of neurologic impairment at the time the diagnosis is made and the surgical procedure accomplished. Heusner found that among 20 patients with this lesion, total recovery occurred in all who had no paralysis at the time of operation or who had weakness of less than 36 hours' duration. In contrast, no patient in whom paralysis had been present longer than 48 hours made a complete neurologic recovery. Prior to the development of surgical and antibiotic therapy, spinal epidural abscess was almost uniformly fatal, with cause of death usually being secondary to the development of generalized septicemia and pulmonary complications.

The suspicion of an epidural abscess preoperatively warrants the initiation of intravenous antibiotics, with the assumption that the causative organism is probably *Staphylococcus* species. A semisynthetic penicillinase-resistant penicillin preparation should be administered, either alone or in combination with penicillin. Purulent material obtained at surgery should be cultured both aerobically and anaerobically, with alterations in the antibiotic regimen being made on the basis of culture and sensitivity results. Antibiotic therapy should be continued for at least ten to 14 days postoperatively. Four weeks of antibiotic therapy is indicated if vertebral osteomyelitis is demonstrated roentgenographically.

An indwelling urinary catheter may be required to prevent overdistention of the bladder in those with neurogenic bladder dysfunction. Postoperatively, certain patients will require an active physical therapy program, which should be started as soon as possible to prevent contractures and joint stiffness.

INFLAMMATORY INTERVERTEBRAL DISC LESIONS IN CHILDREN (SPONDYLARTHRITIS, ACUTE DISC SPACE INFECTION, DISKITIS)

There are now a number of reports that describe an acute or subacute painful syndrome of the low back in children that is usually benign and with characteristic clinical and roentgenographic manifestations (Bremner and Neligan; Doyle, Jamison, Lascari et al.; Milone et al.; Moes, Saenger, Smith and Taylor). The precise cause of the disorder remains speculative, although most investigators regard it to be an acute inflammatory process, and biopsy studies have indicated its staphylococcal origin in several cases (Moes, Milone et al., Smith and Taylor). Despite the isolation of this organism from biopsy of the disc in some patients, considerable speculation remains regarding the cause-and-effect relationship. In a few reported cases, organisms other than *Staphylococcus aureus* have been isolated from disc biopsy (Fischer et al., Spiegel et al., Wong et al.). The lumbar spine is the preferred site of this disease although there are a few reports in which the low thoracic region was affected. In most cases, only one or two disc spaces reveal roentgenographic abnormalities. Although the disorder can occur at any age in childhood, the greatest incidence is between one and four years. Among 20 cases reported by Moes, 14 occurred in children less than four years of age.

Clinical Findings

The onset of symptoms referable to the low back may be preceded by a mild systemic febrile illness or blunt trauma to the back. In other children, the first manifestation of illness is in the form of excessive crying and irritability secondary to low back pain, and low-grade fever. Occasionally, the initial pain seems referred to the hip region on one side and is associated with a limp when walking is attempted. The lumbar pain can vary in intensity from day to day and often persists for several days before stiffness of the back and paravertebral muscle spasm ensues. Eventually, the child refuses to walk at all and subsequently even the sitting position is avoided because of the severity of the discomfort. The parents may observe at this stage that the infant or young child appears reasonably comfortable while lying but screams in pain when pulled to a sitting position, when placed upright with weight-bearing on the feet, or when the trunk is flexed.

An occasional child will never develop the intense pain that is usually considered characteristic of this disorder. The more mildly affected child will complain of some back pain along with stiffness of the low back which inhibits forward bending. Limitation of ambulation may occur only in the first hour or so in the morning after wakening, followed by a lesser degree of discomfort through the rest of the day. Localized spinal percussion tenderness in such cases is often difficult to identify, leading to diagnostic delay until spine x-rays reveal progressive narrowing of the involved disc space.

The signs on examination vary somewhat, depending on the stage of illness and the age of the child. Irritability and screaming evoked from the infant may be so intense that identification and interpretation of other signs on examination is difficult. Spinal rigidity is associated with loss of the normal lumbar lordosis, pain on straight leg raising, and resistance to flexion of the neck. Tenderness is usually marked on blunt percussion over the involved area of the lower spinal column. Of particular importance in differentiating this illness from a spinal epidural abscess is the presence of normal strength, sensation, and deep tendon reflexes in the lower extremities. However, one's ability to demonstrate normal neurologic function in the legs in the young child with this disorder is often limited because of the severity of pain and the resistance to examination.

Fever of low to moderate degree is common in children with spondylarthritis but the white blood cell count is usually either normal or only modestly elevated. Elevation of the erythrocyte sedimentation rate to 40 to 80 millimeters per hour is the most consistent laboratory abnormality and is a valuable diagnostic test. Spinal fluid examination reveals normal findings in most instances. In cases where the diagnosis is suspected from the clinical findings and is supported by characteristic x-ray abnormalities and elevated sedimentation rate, lumbar puncture need not be considered necessary. Other studies of value from the differential diagnostic standpoint include the negative tuberculin skin test and negative brucellosis agglutination test.

Differential diagnostic considerations include several disorders with clinical or roentgenographic features that can resemble this illness. Of greatest importance to exclude quickly is a pyogenic epidural abscess. This process is usually characterized by a more striking febrile response and a greater degree of leukocytosis than occurs with inflammatory disc space lesions, and is more rapidly progressive with associated signs of spinal cord or cauda equina compression. X-ray findings are helpful to differentiate the two only if narrowing of the disc space on the lateral projection has developed. Tuberculous spondylitis usually occurs at vertebral levels higher than the customary site of involvement with acute disc space infection in children, although any region of the vertebral column can be affected with tuberculosis. The absence of evidence of tuberculous disease elsewhere and a negative skin test are important differentiating features. Osteoid osteoma of the lower part of the vertebral spine is a rare lesion but can result in severe local pain with paravertebral muscle spasm. It is identified by x-ray techniques but can be elusive in certain instances. Low back pain with spinal rigidity will occur in some children with primary intraspinal lumbar neoplasms, thus resembling inflammatory disc space lesions. The longer duration of symptoms, the presence of neurologic signs in the lower extremities, and the roentgenographic findings usually allow diagnostic separation of the two conditions. Malignant intraspinal lesions, such as epidural sarcomas or neuroblastomas, also enter the differential diagnosis but usually are rapidly productive of signs of neurologic dysfunction, indicating the need for lumbar myelography.

Roentgenographic Findings

The diagnostic hallmarks of the disease are the roentgenographic abnormalities, which,

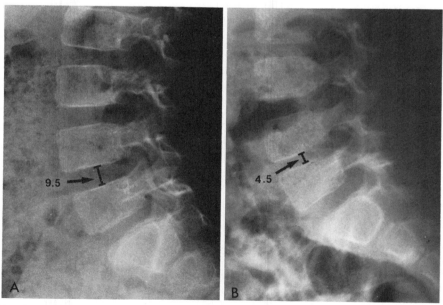

Figure 8–24. Acute intervertebral disc space infection. Photographs demonstrate normal findings in the early stages of the illness with progressive changes during the course of the disease. Five-year-old girl with the abrupt onset of low back pain followed soon thereafter by stiffness of the back and limitation of forward flexion at the hips. *A,* Lateral spine x-ray 2 weeks after onset of back pain. There are no definite roentgenographic abnormalities and the L4–5 disc space measures 9.5 mm. *B,* Repeat lateral spine x-ray 4 weeks later. In the interval, the child has remained symptomatic but with only mild worsening of symptoms. The erythrocyte sedimentation rate at this time was 75 mm. per hour. The L4–5 disc space is now markedly reduced in height and measures only 4.5 mm. Early erosive changes of the posterior aspect of the body of L4 are present. The child subsequently recovered with treatment and the spine x-ray abnormalities reverted to normal.

however, lag in their development behind the clinical symptoms and signs (Fig. 8–24). Two to four weeks may elapse from the onset of back pain until narrowing of the involved lumbar disc space (or spaces) becomes evident. Approximately one to two weeks after disc space narrowing occurs, demineralization with erosion and irregularity of the adjacent vertebral body margins can be visualized (Fig. 8–25). During the next two or three months, the disc space becomes progressively more narrow and the vertebral margins become more distinct as remineralization occurs. Reactive sclerosis of the margins of the involved vertebral bodies may become apparent during the reparative stage. In certain cases, the disc space remains permanently narrow while others return almost to normal width after several months. An occasional patient will develop interbody fusion with body ankylosis as a permanent roentgenographic abnormality.

Radioactive bone scanning is an additional useful diagnostic procedure, and will usually exhibit distinctive abnormalities even before x-ray changes have developed (Wenger et al.). In the series of nine cases of Fischer et al., nuclear imaging with technetium or gallium was abnormal in all, and in seven of the nine was abnormal before changes were observed on standard x-rays of the spine. The typical pattern is increased uptake of the isotope in the vertebral bodies above and below the involved disc space.

Treatment

Management of the child with this condition is usually conservative, with considerable dispute in regard to the need for either antibiotics or immobilization. Several authors have indicated that eventual recovery is to be expected regardless of the therapeutic ap-

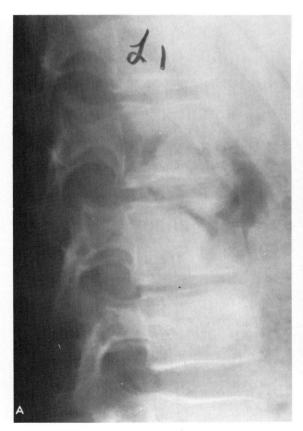

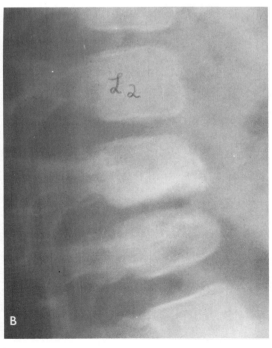

Figure 8–25.   Acute intervertebral disc space infection. *A,* Early changes involving the L3–4 disc space in an 11-year-old girl. The disc is narrowed with minimal apparent changes of the adjacent vertebral bodies. *B,* More advanced abnormalities in a 3-year-old boy. The L3–4 disc space is narrowed. There is demineralization of the vertebral bodies and irregularity of the inferior margin of L3 and superior margin of the L4 vertebral body.

proach. The evidence of staphylococcal infection, at least in some cases, would support the use of a penicillinase-resistant penicillin preparation for a period of three to four weeks after the diagnosis is established. In the acutely ill child with some degree of fever, intravenous methicillin is given for the first 10 to 14 days. In those with mild involvement, dicloxacillin can be given orally in a dosage of 20 to 40 mg. per kilogram per day. Immobilization, either with a body cast or Bradford frame, is helpful for relief of symptoms during the early stages of the illness. Spiegel et al. have recommended that younger children be treated on a Bradford frame followed by plaster immobilization for a period of six weeks to three months. The older child can be immobilized in a brace until pain on activity has ceased. What effect immobilization has on the ultimate outcome remains unestablished, although the prognosis is generally regarded to be favorable in the majority of patients.

The indications for biopsy of the involved disc space by one means or another are unclear, although past experience indicates that the majority of children with this disorder do well with the treatment regimen outlined above. Most authors favor initiation of therapy with a penicillinase-resistant penicillin given intravenously combined with some type of immobilization but without invasive procedures. Persistence of fever or lack of improvement of clinical signs following the initiation of treatment would warrant consideration of biopsy of the disc.

REFERENCES

Abbott, M., and Stern, W. E.: Intracerebral hemorrhage associated with brain abscess. A complication of inappropriate anticoagulation. J.A.M.A. 207:1111–1114, 1969.

Aicardi, J., and Lepintre, J.: Spinal epidural abscess in a one-month-old child. Am. J. Dis. Child. 114:665–667, 1967.

Allen, J. H., Jr., and Cobb, C. A., Jr.: Petrositis: Case reports and review. Am. J. Roentgenol. 84:488–491, 1960.

Altrocchi, P. H.: Acute spinal epidural abscess vs. acute transverse myelopathy. Arch. Neurol. 9:17–25, 1963.

Baker, C. J.: Primary spinal epidural abscess. Am. J. Dis. Child. 121:337–339, 1971.

Batson, O. V.: The function of vertebral veins and their role in the spread of metastasis. Ann. Surg. 112:138, 1940.

Beaty, H. N., Turck, M., and Petersdorf, R. G.: Ampicillin in the treatment of enterococcal endocarditis. Ann. Intern. Med. 65:701–707, 1966.

Bell, W. E., and Butler, C.: Cerebral mycotic aneurysms in children. Neurology 18:81–86, 1968.

Bell, W. E., and Myers, M. G.: *Allescheria (Petriellidum) boydii* brain abscess in a child with leukemia. Arch. Neurol. 35:386–388, 1978.

Beller, A. J., Sahar, A., and Praiss, I.: Brain abscess. Review of 89 cases over a period of 30 years. J. Neurol. Neurosurg. Psychiat. 36:757–768, 1973.

Berg, B., Franklin, G., Cuneo, R., Boldrey, E., and Strimling, B.: Nonsurgical cure of brain abscess: Early diagnosis and follow-up with computerized tomography. Ann. Neurol. 3:474–478, 1978.

Bhandari, Y. W., and Sarkari, N. B. S.: Subdural empyema. A review of 37 cases. J. Neurosurg. 32:35–39, 1970.

Bohmfalk, G. L., Story, J. L., Wissinger, J. P., and Brown, W. E., Jr.: Bacterial intracranial aneurysm. J. Neurosurg. 48:369–382, 1978.

Bremner, A. E., and Neligan, G. A.: Benign form of acute osteitis of the spine in young children. Brit. Med. J. 1:856–860, 1953.

Brodi, E., Adler, J. L., and Daly, A. K.: Bacterial endocarditis due to an unusual species of encapsulated Neisseria. Am. J. Dis. Child. 122:433–437, 1971.

Browder, J., and Meyers, R.: Infections of the spinal epidural space: An aspect of vertebral osteomyelitis. Am. J. Surg. 37:4–26, 1937.

Brown, P.: Septic cavernous sinus thrombosis. Johns Hopkins Med. J. 109:68–75, 1961.

Brunner, H.: Intracranial Complications of Ear, Nose, and Throat Infections. Year Book Publishers, Chicago, 1946.

Buchner, L. H., and Schneierson, S. S.: Clinical and laboratory aspects of Listeria monocytogenes infections. With a report of ten cases. Am. J. Med. 45:904–921, 1968.

Burnard, E. D.: Proptosis as the first sign of orbital sepsis in the newborn. Brit. J. Ophthal. 43:9–12, 1959.

Butler, N. R., Barrie, H., and Paine, K. W. E.: Cerebral abscess as a complication of neonatal sepsis. Arch. Dis. Childh. 32:461–465, 1957.

Calkins, R. A., and Bell, W. E.: Cerebral abscess and cyanotic congenital heart disease. J. Lancet 87:403–410, 1967.

Carey, M. E., Chou, S. N., and French, L. A.: Long-term neurological residue in patients surviving brain abscess with surgery. J. Neurosurg. 34:652–656, 1971.

Chandler, J. R.: Malignant external otitis. Laryngoscope. 78:1257–1294, 1968.

Chandler, J. R.: Pathogenesis and treatment of facial paralysis due to malignant external otitis. Ann. Otol. 81:648–658, 1972.

Cherubin, C. E., and Neu, H. C.: Infective endocarditis at the Presbyterian Hospital in New York City from 1938–1967. Am. J. Med. 51:83–96, 1971.

Clark, D. B., and Clarke, E. S.: Brain abscess as complication of congenital cardiac malformation. Trans. Am. Neurol. Assoc. 77:73–76, 1952.

Clune, J. P.: Septic thrombosis within the cavernous chamber. Review of the literature with recent advances in diagnosis and treatment. Am. J. Ophthal. 56:33–39, 1963.

Collier, J.: Discussion on ocular palsies. Proc. Roy. Soc. Med. 14:10–11, 1921.

Coonrod, J. D., and Dans, P. E.: Subdural empyema. Am. J. Med. 53:85–91, 1972.

Courville, C. B.: Intracranial complications of otitis media and mastoiditis in the antibiotic era. Trans. Am. Laryng. Rhin. Otol. Soc. 59:151–166, 1955.

Courville, C. B., and Nielsen, J. M.: Fatal complications of otitis media, with particular reference to the intracranial lesions in a series of 10,000 autopsies. Arch. Otolaryng. 19:451–501, 1934.

Crocker, E. F., and Leicester, J.: Cerebral abscess due to Listeria monocytogenes. Med. J. Aust. 1:90–92, 1976.

Crocker, E. F., McLaughlin, A. F., Morris, J. G., Benn, R., McLeod, J. D., and Allsop, J. L.: Technetium brain scanning in the diagnosis and management of cerebral abscess. Am. J. Med. 56:192–201, 1974.

Dacey, R. G., Winn, H. R., Jane, J. A., and Butler, A. B.: Spinal subdural empyema: Report of two cases. Neurosurgery 3:400–402, 1978.

Dandy, W. E.: Abscesses and inflammatory tumors in the spinal epidural space (so-called pachymeningitis externa). Arch. Surg. 13:477–494, 1926.

Dinapoli, R. P., and Thomas, J. E.: Neurologic aspects of malignant external otitis: Report of three cases. Mayo Clin. Proc. 46:339–344, 1971.

Domingue, J. N., and Wilson, C. B.: Pituitary abscesses. Report of seven cases and review of the literature. J. Neurosurg. 46:601–608, 1977.

Doyle, J. R.: Narrowing of the intervertebral-disc space in children. Presumably an infectious lesion of the disc. J. Bone Joint Surg. 42-A:1191–1200, 1960.

Duffner, P. K., and Cohen, M. E.: Cystic fibrosis with brain abscess. Arch. Neurol. 36:27–28, 1979.

Duffy, P. E., Sassin, J. F., Summers, D. S., and Lourie, H.: Rhomboencephalitis due to Listeria monocytogenes. Neurology 14:1067–1072, 1964.

Dyer, N. H.: Cerebral abscess in hereditary hemorrhagic telangiectasia: Report of 2 cases in a family. J. Neurol. Neurosurg. Psychiat. 30:563–567, 1967.

Enzmann, D. R., Britt, R. H., and Yeager, A. S.: Experimental brain abscess evolution: Computed tomographic and neuropathic correlation. Radiology 133:113–122, 1979.

Farmer, T. W., and Wise, G. R.: Subdural empyema in infants, children and adults. Neurology 23:254–261, 1973.

Fearnsides, E. G.: Intracranial aneurysms. Brain 39:224–296, 1916.

Felner, J. M., and Dowell, V. R., Jr.: Anaerobic bacterial endocarditis. New Eng. J. Med. 283:1188–1192, 1970.

Ferris, E. J., and Ciembroniewicz, J.: Subdural empyema. Report of a case demonstrating the unusual angiographic triad. Am. J. Roentgenol. 92:838–843, 1964.

Fischbein, C. A., Beckett, K. M., and Rosenthal, A.: Hemophilus aphrophilus brain abscess associated with congenital heart disease. J. Pediat. 83:631–633, 1973.

Fischer, E. G., Shwachman, H., and Wepsic, J. G.: Brain abscess and cystic fibrosis. J. Pediat. 95:385–388, 1979.

Fischer, G. W., Popich, G. A., Sullivan, D. E., Mayfield, G., Mazat, B. A., and Patterson, P. H.: Diskitis: A prospective diagnostic analysis. Pediatrics 62:543–547, 1978.

Forno, L. S., and Billingham, M. E.: Allescheria boydii infection of the brain. J. Pathol. 106:195–198, 1972.

Fraser, R. A. R., Ratzan, K., Wolpert, S. M., and Weinstein, L.: Spinal subdural empyema. Arch. Neurol. 28:235–238, 1973.

Friberg, T. R., and Sogg, R. L.: Ischemic optic neuropathy in cavernous sinus thrombosis. Arch. Ophthal. 96:453–456, 1978.

Gamble, R. C.: Acute inflammations of the orbit in children. Arch. Ophthal. 10:483–497, 1933.

Gardner, W. J.: Otitic sinus thrombosis causing intracranial hypertension. Arch. Otolaryng. 30:253, 1939.

Gellady, A. M., Shulman, S. T., and Ayoub, E. M.: Periorbital and orbital cellulitis in children. Pediatrics 61:272–277, 1978.

Gilroy, J., Andaya, L., and Thomas, V. J.: Intracranial mycotic aneurysms and subacute bacterial endocarditis in heroin addiction. Neurology 23:1193–1198, 1973.

Goldberg, F., Berne, A. S., and Oski, F. A.: Differentiation of orbital cellulitis from preseptal cellulitis by computed tomography. Pediatrics 62:1000–1005, 1978.

Goldman, J. A., Fleischer, A. S., Leifer, W., Parent, A., Schwarzman, S. W., and Raggio, J.: *Candida albicans* mycotic aneurysm associated with systemic lupus erythematosus. Neurosurgery 4:325–328, 1979.

Gradenigo, G.: Über circumscripte leptomeningitis mit spinalen symptomen and über paralyse des N. abducens ototischen ursprungs. Arch. Ohrenh. 51:255–270, 1904.

Greer, M., and Berk, M. S.: Lateral sinus obstruction and mastoiditis. Pediatrics 31:840–844, 1963.

Groff, R. A.: Experimental production of abscess of the brain of cats. Arch. Neurol. Psychiat. 31:199–204, 1934.

Handel, S. F., Klein, W. C., and Kim, Y. W.: Intracranial epidural abscess. Radiology 111:117–120, 1974.

Hara, H. J.: Otogenic meningitis in infancy and childhood in the antibiotic era. Arch. Otolaryng. 70:315–320, 1959.

Haynes, R. E., and Cramblett, H. G.: Acute ethmoiditis. Its relationship to orbital cellulitis. Am. J. Dis. Child. 114:261–267, 1967.

Heidelberger, K. P., Layton, W. M., Jr. and Fisher, R. G.: Multiple cerebral mycotic aneurysms complicating posttraumatic pseudomonas meningitis. J. Neurosurg. 29:631–635, 1968.

Heineman, H. S., and Braude, A. I.: Anaerobic infection of the brain. Am. J. Med. 35:682–697, 1963.

Heineman, H. S., Braude, A. I., and Osterholm, J. L.: Intracranial suppurative disease. Early presumptive diagnosis and successful treatment without surgery. J.A.M.A. 218:1542–1547, 1971.

Hepner, R., and Hager, D.: Staphylococcal orbital sepsis in newborn infants. Southern Med. J. 53:922–925, 1960.

Heusner, A. P.: Nontuberculous spinal epidural infections. New Eng. J. Med. 239:845–854, 1948.

Hitchcock, E., and Andreadis, A.: Subdural empyema: A review of 29 cases. J. Neurol. Neurosurg. Psychiat. 27:422–434, 1964.

Hoefnagel, D., and Joseph, J. B.: Oculosympathetic paralysis in otitis media. New Eng. J. Med. 265:475–477, 1961.

Hoffman, H. J., Hendrick, E. B., and Hiscox, J. L.: Cerebral abscesses in early infancy. J. Neurosurg. 33:172–177, 1970.

Holt, L. E.: A report of five cases of abscess of the brain in infants, together with a summary of 27 collected cases in infants and very young children. Arch. Pediat. 15:81–106, 1898.

Horner, F. A., Berry, R. G., and Frantz, M.: Broken pencil points as a cause of brain abscess. New Eng. J. Med. 271:342–345, 1964.

Horten, B. C., Abbott, G. F., and Porro, R. S.: Fungal aneurysms of intracranial vessels. Arch. Neurol. 33:577–579, 1976.

Hubert, L.: Horner's syndrome with chronic purulent otitis media. Demonstration of a diagnostic test. Laryngoscope. 53:46–49, 1943.

Hughes, W. T.: Generalized aspergillosis. Am. J. Dis. Child. 112:262–265, 1966.

Hulme, A., and Dott, N. M.: Spinal epidural abscess. Brit. Med. J. 1:64–68, 1954.

Hunt, W. E., Meagher, J. N., LaFever, H. E., and Zeman, W.: Painful ophthalmoplegia. Its relation to indolent inflammation of the cavernous sinus. Neurology 11:56–62, 1961.

Jamison, R. C., Heimlich, E. M., Miethke, J. C., and O'Loughlin, B. J.: Non-specific spondylitis of infants and children. Radiology 77:355–367, 1961.

Jarrett, W. H., and Gutman, F. A.: Ocular complications of infection in the paranasal sinuses. Arch. Ophthal. 81:683–688, 1969.

Joachims, H. Z.: Malignant external otitis in children, Arch. Otolaryngol. 22:236–237, 1976.

Joubert, M. J., and Stephanov, M. D.: Computerized tomography and surgical treatment in intracranial suppuration. Report of 30 consecutive unselected cases of brain abscess and subdural empyema. J. Neurosurg. 47:73–78, 1977.

Kalbag, R. M., and Woolf, A. L.: Cerebral venous thrombosis. Oxford University Press, London, 1967, p. 137.

Kaplan, A. M., Itabashi, H. H., Yoshimori, R., and Weil, M. L.: Cerebral abscesses complicating neonatal Citrobacter freundii meningitis. West. J. Med. 127:418–422, 1977.

Kaufman, D. M., and Leeds, N. E.: Computed tomography (CT) in the diagnosis of intracranial abscesses. Brain abscess, subdural empyema, and epidural empyema. Neurology 27:1069–1073, 1977.

Kaufman, D. M., Miller, M. H., and Steigbigel, N. H.: Subdural empyema: Analysis of 17 recent cases and review of the literature. Medicine 54:485–498, 1975.

Keith, W. S.: Subdural empyema. J. Neurosurg. 6:127–139, 1949.

Kim, K. S., Weinberg, P. E., and Magidson, M.: Angiographic features of subdural empyema. Radiology 188:621–625, 1976.

Kinnaird, P. M., Jr., Acker, J. D., and Snead, O. C.: Cavernous sinus thrombosis with vascular steal syndrome. J. Pediat. 94:410–413, 1979.

Klein, D. M., and Cohen, M. E.: Pasteurella multocida brain abscess following perforating cranial dog bite. J. Pediat. 92:588–589, 1978.

Knox, D. L., Clark, D. B., and Schuster, F. F.: Benign VI nerve palsies in children. Pediatrics 40:560–564, 1967.

Kolmer, J. W., Wallenborn, P. A., Jr., and Crowgey, J. E.: Cavernous sinus thrombosis complicating sinusitis and orbital cellulitis. Virginia Med. Monthly 92:134–139, 1966.

Larsen, T. E., Harris, L., and Holden, F. A.: Isolation of Pasteurella multocida from an otogenic cerebellar abscess. Canad. Med. Assoc. J. 101:114–115, 1969.

Lascari, A. D., Graham, M. H., and MacQueen, J. C.: Intervertebral disk infection in children. J. Pediat. 70:751–757, 1967.

Law, J. D., Lehman, R. A. W., Kirsch, W. M., and Ehni, G.: Diagnosis and treatment of abscess of the central ganglia. J. Neurosurg. 44:226–232, 1976.

Leers, W-D., Russell, N. A., and Laroye, G.: Cerebellar abscess due to Blastomyces dermatitidis. Canad. Med. Assoc. J. 107:657–660, 1972.

Legg, N. J., Gupta, P. C., and Scott, D. F.: Epilepsy following cerebral abscess. Brain 96:259–268, 1973.

Lerner, P. I., and Weinstein, L.: Infective endocarditis in the antibiotic era. New Eng. J. Med. 274:199–206, 259–266, 323–331, 388–393, 1966.

Lerner, P. I., Golden, P. F., and Jane, J. A.: Salmonella-infected subdural hematoma. Pediatrics 49:127–128, 1972.

List, C. F.: Diagnosis and treatment of acute subdural empyema. Neurology 5:663–670, 1955.

Lombardo, L., Alonso, P., Arroyo, L. S., Brandt, H., and Mateos, J. H.: Cerebral amebiasis. Report of 17 cases. J. Neurosurg. 21:704–709, 1964.

Londer, L., and Nelson, D. L.: Orbital cellulitis due to Haemophilus influenzae. Arch. Ophthal. 91:89–91, 1974.

Mahony, J. F., Tambyah, J. A., Dalton, V. C., and Wolfenden, W. H.: Pontomedullary listerosis in renal allograft recipient. Brit. Med. J. 2:705, 1974.

Mathew, N. T., Abraham, J., Taori, G. M., and Tyer, G. V.: Internal carotid artery occlusion in cavernous sinus thrombosis. Arch. Neurol. 24:11–16, 1971.

Matson, D. D., and Salam, M.: Brain abscess in congenital heart disease. Pediatrics 27:772–789, 1961.

McDonald, C. A., and Korb, M.: Intracranial aneurysms. Arch. Neurol. Psychiat. 42:298–328, 1939.

McDowell, D. E., Ulmer, J. L., Velo, A. G., Ekren, W. S., and Kriz, J. R.: Cerebral abscess due to Actinomyces israeli. Southern Med. J. 58:227–230, 1965.

McLeod, R., Berry, P. F., Marshall, W. H., Jr., Hunt, S. A., Ryning, F. W., and Remington, J. S.: Toxoplasmosis presenting as brain abscesses. Diagnosis by computerized tomography and cytology of aspirated purulent material. Am. J. Med. 67:711–714, 1979.

Mendelsohn, G., and Hutchins, G. M.: Infective endocarditis during the first decade of life. An autopsy review of 33 cases. Am. J. Dis. Child. 133:619–622, 1979.

Merzbach, D., Freundlich, E., Metzker, A., and Falk, W.: Bacterial endocarditis due to corynebacterium. J. Pediat. 67:792–796, 1965.

Middleton, F. G., Jurgenson, P. F., Utz, J. P., Shadomy, S., and Shadomy, H. J.: Brain abscess caused by Cladosporium trichoides. Arch. Intern. Med. 136:444–448, 1976.

Miller, W. H., and Hesch, J. A.: Nontuberculous spinal epidural abscess. Am. J. Dis. Child. 104:269–275, 1962.

Milone, F. P., Bianco, A. J., Jr., and Ivins, J. C.: Infections of intervertebral disk in children. J.A.M.A. 181:1029–1033, 1962.

Moes, C. A. F.: Spondylarthritis in childhood. Am. J. Roentgenol. 91:578–587, 1964.

Molinari, G. F., Smith, L., Goldstein, M. N., and Satran, R.: Brain abscess from septic cerebral embolism: An experimental model. Neurology 23:1205–1210, 1973.

Morgan, H., Wood, M. W., and Murphy, F.: Experience with 88 consecutive cases of brain abscess. J. Neurosurg. 38:698–704, 1973.

Morriss, F. H., Jr., and Spock, A.: Intracranial aneurysm secondary to mycotic orbital and sinus infection. Report of a case implicating Penicillium as an opportunistic fungus. Am. J. Dis. Child. 119:357–362, 1970.

Munslow, R. A., Stovall, V. S., Price, R. D., and Kohler, C. M.: Brain abscess in infants. J. Pediat. 51:74–79, 1957.

New, P. F. J., Davis, K. R., and Ballantine, H. T., Jr.: Computed tomography in cerebral abscess. Radiology 121:641–646, 1976.

Noonan, J. A., Wilson, C. B., Spencer, F. C., and Talbert, W. M., Jr.: Cerebral and cardiac complications from bacterial complications. Am. J. Dis. Child 116:666–674, 1968.

Norrell, H., and Howieson, J.: Gas-containing brain abscesses. Am. J. Roentgenol. 109:273–276, 1970.

Ojemann, R. G., New, P. F. J., and Fleming, T. C.: Intracranial aneurysms associated with bacterial meningitis. Neurology 16:1222–1226, 1966.

Osler, W.: The Gulstonian lectures on malignant endocarditis. Lancet 1:467–470, 1885.

Palmer, J. J., and Kelly, W. A.: Epidural abscess in a 3-week-old infant: Case report. Pediatrics 50:817–820, 1972.

Panky, G. A.: Acute bacterial endocarditis at the University of Minnesota Hospitals, 1939–1959. Am. Heart J. 64:583–591, 1962.

Panky, G. A.: Subacute bacterial endocarditis at the University of Minnesota Hospital, 1939 through 1959. Ann. Intern. Med. 55:550–561, 1961.

Poncher, H. G., and Blayney, J. R.: Osteomyelitis of the maxilla in nurslings and in infants. Am. J. Dis. Child. 48:730–738, 1934.

Posnikoff, J.: Spontaneous spinal epidural hematoma of childhood. J. Pediat. 73:178–183, 1968.

Pruitt, A. A., Rubin, R. H., Karchmer, A. W., and Duncan, G. W.: Neurologic complications of bacterial endocarditis. Medicine 57:329–343, 1978.

Rahal, J. J., Jr., Meyer, B. R., and Weinstein, L.: Treatment of bacterial endocarditis with cephalothin. New Eng. J. Med. 279:1305–1309, 1968.

Raimondi, A. J., Matsumoto, S., and Miller, R. A.: Brain abscess in children with congenital heart disease. I. J. Neurosurg. 23:588–595, 1965.

Rangell, L., and Glassman, F.: Acute spinal epidural abscess as a complication of lumbar puncture. J. Nerv. Ment. Dis. 102:8–18, 1945.

Rankin, J., and Javid, M.: Nocardiosis of the central nervous system. Neurology 5:815–820, 1955.

Ray, B. S., and Parsons, H.: Subdural abscess complicating frontal sinusitis. Arch. Otolaryng. 37:536–551, 1943.

Ray, H., and Wahal, K. M.: Subarachnoid hemorrhage in subacute bacterial endocarditis. Neurology 7:265–269, 1957.

Roach, M. R., and Drake, C. G.: Ruptured cerebral aneurysms caused by micro-organisms. New Eng. J. Med. 273:240–244, 1965.

Roessman, U., and Friede, R. L.: Candidal infection of the brain. Arch. Path. 84:495–498, 1967.

Rosamond, E.: Epidural abscess complicated by staphylococcus meningitis. J. Pediat. 1:230–232, 1932.

Rosen, F., Deck, J. H. N., and Rewcastle, N. B.: Allescheria boydii—unique systemic dissemination to thyroid and brain. Canad. Med. Assoc. J. 93:1125–1127, 1965.

Rushworth, R. G., and Martin, P. B.: Acute spinal epidural abscess: A case in an infant with recovery. Arch. Dis. Childh. 33:261–264, 1958.

Saenger, E. L.: Spondylarthritis in children. Am. J. Roentgenol. 64:20–31, 1950.

Salibi, B. S.: Bacteroides infection of the brain. Arch. Neurol. 10:629–634, 1964.

Samson, D. S., and Clark, K.: A current review of brain abscess. Am. J. Med. 54:201–210, 1973.

Sanders, D. Y., and Stevenson, J.: Bacteroides infections in children. J. Pediat. 72:673–677, 1968.

Sanford, H. N.: Abscess of the brain in infants under twelve months of age. Am. J. Dis. Child. 35:256–261, 1928.

Schurr, P.: Brain abscess in childhood. Develop. Med. Child. Neurol. 7:433–435, 1965.

Schwarz, G. A., Blumenkrantz, M. J., and Sundmaker, W. L. H.: Neurologic complications of malignant external otitis. Neurology 21:1077–1084, 1971.

Scott, R. M.: Bacterial endocarditis due to Neisseria flava. J. Pediat. 78:673–675, 1971.

Selker, R. G.: Intracranial abscess: Treatment by continuous catheter drainage. Child's Brain 1:368–375, 1975.

Shuster, M., Klein, M. M., Pribor, H. C., and Kozub, W.: Brain abscess due to Nocardia. Arch. Intern. Med. 120:610–614, 1967.

Siber, G. R., Alpert, S., Smith, A. L., Lin, J-S., and McCormack, W. M.: Neonatal central nervous system infection due to Mycoplasma hominis. J. Pediat. 90:625–627, 1977.

Smith, R. F., and Taylor, T. K. R.: Inflammatory lesions of the intervertebral discs in children. J. Bone Joint Surg. 49-A:1508–1520, 1967.

Smith, T. F., O'Day, D., and Wright, P. F.: Clinical implications of preseptal (periorbital) cellulitis in childhood. Pediatrics 62:1006–1009, 1978.

Smith, W. E., McCall, R. E., and Blake, T. J.: *Bacteroides* infections of the central nervous system. Ann. Intern. Med. 20:920–932, 1944.

Solomon, O. D., Moses, L., and Volk, M.: Steroid therapy in cavernous sinus thrombosis. Am. J. Ophthal. 54:1122–1124, 1962.

Sondheimer, F. K., and Knapp, J.: Angiographic findings in the Tolosa-Hunt syndrome: Painful ophthalmoplegia. Radiology 106:105–112, 1973.

Spiegel, P. G., Kengla, K. W., Isaacson, A. S., and Wilson, J. C., Jr.: Intervertebral disc-space inflammation in children. J. Bone Joint Surg. 54-A:284–296, 1972.

Stanton, R. E., Lindesmith, G. G., and Meyer, B. W.: *Escherichia coli* endocarditis after repair of ventricular septal defects. New Eng. J. Med. 279:737–742, 1968.

Stephanov, S.: Experience with multiloculated brain abscesses. J. Neurosurg. 49:199–203, 1978.

Stern, W. E., and Naffziger, H. C.: Brain abscess associated with pulmonary angiomatous malformation. Ann. Surg. 138:521–531, 1953.

Symonds, C.: Intracranial thrombophlebitis. Ann. Roy. Coll. Surg. Eng. 10:347–356, 1952.

Symonds, C.: Otitic hydrocephalus. Neurology 6:681–685, 1956.

Symonds, C. P.: Hydrocephalic and focal cerebral symptoms in relation to thrombophlebitis of dural sinuses and cerebral veins. Brain 60:531–550, 1937.

Symonds, C. P.: Otitis hydrocephalus. Brain 54:55–71, 1931.

Takeoka, T., Gotoh, F., Fukuuchi, Y., and Inagaki, Y.: Tolosa-Hunt syndrome. Arteriographic evidence of improvement in carotid narrowing. Arch. Neurol. 35:219–223, 1978.

Tarkkanen, J. V.: Otogenic brain abscesses. A study of 99 cases including 24 follow-up examined. Acta Otolaryng. Suppl. 185, 1963.

Terrence, C. F., and Samaha, F. J.: The Tolosa-Hunt syndrome (painful ophthalmoplegia) in children. Develop. Med. Child. Neurol. 15:506–509, 1973.

Théron, J., and Djindjian, R.: Comparison of the venous phase of carotid arteriography with direct intracranial venography in the evaluation of lesions at the base of the skull. Neuroradiology 5:43–48, 1973.

Tobey, G. L., and Ayer, J. B.: Dynamic studies of the cerebrospinal fluid in the differential diagnosis of lateral sinus thrombosis. Arch. Otolaryng. 2:50, 1925.

Tolosa, E. J.: Periarteritic lesions of the carotid siphon with the clinical features of a carotid infraclinoidal aneurysm. J. Neurol. Neurosurg. Psychiat. 17:300–302, 1954.

Van Gilder, J. C., Allen, W. E., III, and Lesser, R. A.: Pontine abscess: survival following surgical drainage. J. Neurosurg. 40:386–390, 1974.

Vogel, L. C., Ferguson, L., and Gotoff, S. P.: Citrobacter

infections of the central nervous system in early infancy. J. Pediat. 93:86–88, 1978.

Waage, R.: Bacterium anitratum (B₅W) isolated from cerebral abscesses. Acta Pathol. Microbiol. Scand. 33:268–270, 1953.

Walsh, F. B.: Ocular signs of thrombosis of the intracranial venous sinuses. Arch. Ophthal. 17:46–65, 1937.

Walsh, F. B., and Hoyt, W. F.: Clinical Neuro-ophthalmology. The Williams and Wilkins Company, Baltimore, 1969. Vol. 2, p. 1892.

Warner, J. F., Perkins, R. L., and Cordero, L.: Metronidazole therapy of anaerobic bacteremia, meningitis, and brain abscess. Arch. Intern. Med. 139;167–169, 1979.

Watson, G. W., Fuller, T. J., Elms, J., and Kluge, R. M.: *Listeria* cerebritis. Relapse of infection in renal transplant patients. Arch. Intern. Med. 138:83–87, 1978.

Weickhardt, G. D., and Davis, R. L.: Solitary abscess of the brain-stem. Neurology 14:918–925, 1964.

Weisberg, L. A.: Cerebral computerized tomography in intracranial inflammatory disorders. Arch. Neurol. 37:137–142, 1980.

Wenger, D. R., Bobechko, W. P., and Gilday, D. L.: The spectrum of intervertebral disc-space infection in children. J. Bone Joint Surg. 60-A:100–108, 1978.

Whitener, D. R.: Tuberculous brain abscess. Report of a case and review of the literature. Arch. Neurol. 35:148–155, 1978.

Wise, G. R., and Farmer, T. W.: Bacterial cerebral vasculitis. Neurology 21:195–200, 1971.

Wishingrad, L., Rosenthal, I. M., and Cascino, J. P.: Brain abscess seven years after a Potts anastomosis in case of tetralogy of Fallot. J.A.M.A. 164:1465–1466, 1957.

Wong, A. S., Dyke, J., Perry, D., and Anderson, D. C.: Paraspinal mass associated with intervertebral disk infection secondary to Morazella kingii. J. Pediat. 92:86–88, 1978.

Wright, R. L., and Ballantine, H. T., Jr.: Management of brain abscesses in children and adolescents. Am. J. Dis. Child. 114:113–122, 1967.

Zakrzewski, T., and Keith, J. D.: Bacterial endocarditis in infants and children. J. Pediat. 67:1179–1193, 1965.

Zaky, D. A., Bentley, D. W., Lowy, K., Betts, R. F., and Douglas, R. G., Jr.: Malignant external otitis: A severe form of otitis in diabetic patients. Am. J. Med. 61:298–302, 1976.

Zimmerman, R. A., Bilaniuk, L. T., Shipkin, P. M., Gilden, D. H., and Murtagh, F.: Evolution of cerebral abscess: Correlation of clinical features with computed tomography. A case report. Neurology 27:14–19, 1977.

Chapter Nine

TETANUS

Tetanus, or lockjaw, has been known to affect people since antiquity. The word tetanus first appeared in the works of Hippocrates and was derived from a verb meaning to stretch (Chalian), descriptive of the most dramatic feature of the illness. Tetanus occupies a special position among human bacterial diseases because of its persistently high mortality rate, its agonizing symptoms, and its needless occurrence. It is a disease that is virtually entirely preventable by the judicious use of a safe, inexpensive, and easily administered immunizing agent. It spares no age group and throughout the world has its peak incidence and greatest mortality in the newborn infant and the elderly. Although the incidence of tetanus in this country has declined since 1950, the case-fatality ratio of approximately 65 percent has remained constant for many years (LaForce et al.) (Fig. 9–1).

Tetanus is caused by the exotoxin of *Clostridium tetani,* a gram-positive anaerobic rod with terminal, rounded spores. The exotoxin is notable for its affinity to become fixed to nervous tissue (the Wasserman-Takaki phenomenon) and accounts for the clinical features characteristic of the disease. The tetanus bacillus has its natural habitat in soil and animal feces. The spores are markedly resistant to physical agents and may survive in dirt or dust for many months.

The classic example of the type of injury producing tetanus in childhood is the puncture wound on the plantar surface of the foot which is contaminated by dirt or manure containing tetanus spores. Devitalized, necrotic tissue within the wound supports growth of the anaerobic tetanus bacilli that elaborate

exotoxin, which subsequently results in clinical disease. Although injuries of this type are obviously hazardous in the unimmunized child, it must be emphasized that tetanus is an unpredictable disease and may strike after even trivial or superficial wounds sustained on any part of the body. Furthermore, the occurrence of tetanus in the absence of a previously recognized injury is not uncommon. Even the site of an intramuscular injection or vaccination may become contaminated with tetanus spores and result in tetanus (Patel et al.). The chronically infected middle ear or mastoid antrum can provide an adequate environment for survival of clostridium organisms and give rise to the condition referred to as "otogenic" tetanus. This form of tetanus is not common and appears to be a less severe form of the disease compared to that secondary to acquired wounds (Fischer et al.). Additional causes include automobile injuries, war wounds, and criminal abortions performed under non-sterile conditions. In adults in this country at the present time, the single most common type of wound leading to tetanus is the unsterile one, self-inflicted by the drug addict (Cherubin), in whom the disease is characteristically severe.

Regardless of the circumstances, the requirements for the development of tetanus include the occurrence of a wound or lesion with devitalized or necrotic tissue which will support growth of the anaerobic organism, the presence of toxin-producing tetanus bacilli, and the lack of adequate immunity of the host. On rare occasion, tetanus has been described in persons with greater than the minimal protective level of antibody in the

257

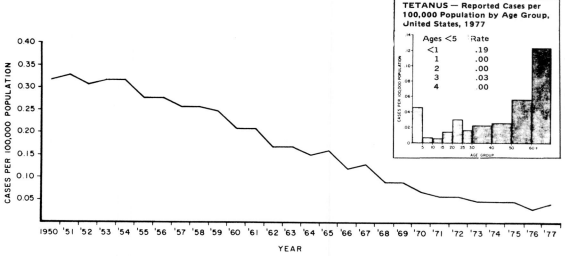

Figure 9–1.   Tetanus. Reported cases per 100,000 population by year, United States, 1950–1977. (From: Morbidity and Mortality Weekly Report, Annual Summary, 1977. Vol. 26, No. 53, Sept. 1978.)

serum. The illness in these patients has generally been mild and sometimes localized (Berger et al.).

Pathogenesis

While it is generally agreed that the harmful effects of *Clostridium tetani* infections result entirely from the neurotoxin produced by the organism, the mechanism by which the toxin gets from the wound to its site of action has been controversial for many years. Most authorities have favored the concept that tetanus toxin absorbed at the site of the wound spreads by centripetal migration along motor nerve trunks to reach the central nervous system, a theory first proposed in 1903 (Morax and Marie, Meyer and Ransom). The precise manner and the anatomic structures responsible for such peripheral neural conveyance of toxin, however, have not been demonstrated. Other authors (Abel et al., Zacks and Sheff) have favored the concept of hematogenous dissemination of the toxin, one which more readily explains the high frequency of trismus as an early symptom regardless of the location of the infected wound. One of the principal objections to the theory of hematogenous spread of toxin has been the restriction of signs to a localized region of the body in patients with local tetanus. Evidence that tetanus toxin has an effect on skeletal muscle (Prabhu and Oester, Zacks and Sheff) has led

to the postulate that toxin spread by the blood stream may result in abnormal discharges from spinal neurons affecting only those skeletal muscles injured by the toxin (Zacks and Sheff). On this basis, local tetanus occurring in one with partial or incomplete immunity might also be explained on the basis of hematogenous spread of toxin from the site of injury.

Once tetanus toxin reaches the spinal cord or brain stem, its primary site of action, resulting in muscle rigidity and spasm, is at the level of inhibitory synapses (Brooks et al., Eccles). Although morphologic changes within the nervous system have often been denied, Illis and Mitchell studied experimental tetanus in rabbits with special staining techniques and demonstrated a progressive distention of dendritic boutons terminaux. Other workers have not been able to reproduce this morphologic abnormality but have described chromatolysis of spinal ventral horn neurons in animals with experimental local tetanus (Tarlov et al.).

Clinical Manifestations

The usual incubation period extending from the injury to the onset of symptoms of tetanus is five to ten days. Variations are well known, however, with some cases having incubation periods as short as two or three days and others as long as several weeks. When the interval between injury and onset of symptoms is prolonged, it is probable that tetanus bacilli have remained dormant within tissue with minimal elaboration of toxin. In many cases, the period of incubation cannot be calculated since an offending wound was not recognized. When it can be determined, the incubation period in tetanus is of prognostic value because those of less than one week's duration are usually followed by severe manifestations and those of longer duration are apt to be associated with milder illnesses.

The initial symptoms of tetanus are variable but most often include low back pain, stiffness of the legs while walking, dysphagia, or restriction of the child's ability to open the mouth. Fever is not usually present at this stage and frequently is minimal throughout the course of the disease. Either trismus or rigidity of the paraspinus or abdominal musculature represents the usual early sign which alerts the physician to the probable diagnosis (Fig. 9–2). Trismus is the symptomatic hallmark of tetanus, although it is by no means specific for this disorder. It is due to spasm of the masseter muscles, and at first causes only mild difficulty with chewing. As worsening occurs, the mouth can barely be opened, and subsequently the teeth cannot be separated at all. With the jaws tightly closed, contraction of facial muscles draws the angles of the mouth up and out resulting in the fixed facial expression referred to as risus sardonicus.

With the passage of hours thereafter, muscle rigidity becomes more generalized and more severe, culminating in recurrent muscle spasms. Spasms may be brief and mild or can be so intense that the back becomes violently arched, projecting the child into a posture of opisthotonus. Recurrent spasmodic episodes occur spontaneously but are also precipitated by a variety of external sensory stimuli. Compression vertebral fractures may occur secondary to violent spasm of the trunk musculature. Multiple consecutive vertebrae are usually involved, with the fourth to the eighth thoracic vertebrae being the most commonly affected sites (Bohrer). Such fractures do not cause spinal cord compression and are usually asymptomatic except for the possible association with back pain. In severe cases, spasmodic "convulsions" seriously interfere with respiratory function because of involvement of the intercostal muscles and diaphragm in addition to the added burden of laryngo-

spasm. Deep cyanosis accompanies such attacks, which may terminate in death unless interrupted by appropriate therapeutic measures.

One of the most striking features of the child with tetanus is the retention of mental alertness and clarity despite the presence of rigidity and muscle spasms. This aspect of the disease is an important differential diagnostic point separating tetanus from several other conditions which resemble it. The preservation of alertness, however, subjects the child to the agonizing pain that accompanies the intense hypertonus and recurrent spasmodic crises. Headache is usually not present in patients with tetanus. The optic discs remain normal and extraocular movements are generally unaffected. Constipation is a common feature of the disease, while urinary retention has been described but is infrequent (Athavale and Pai).

Sympathetic Involvement. Certain patients with severe tetanus exhibit a variety of clinical abnormalities that are believed to be due to overactivity of the sympathetic nervous system (Kerr et al.). Tachycardia, fluctuating hypertension, profuse perspiration, and peripheral vasoconstriction are autonomic disturbances that can complicate the clinical course of this illness. Kerr et al. suggested that glucosuria and hyperglycemia occasionally observed in such patients can also be explained on the basis of increased serum catecholamines. The sympathetic disturbances do not usually create significant management problems, although cardiac arrhythmias and hypertension become dangerous in certain cases. Prys-Roberts et al. have recommended a combination of propranolol and bethanidine to block adrenergic mechanisms and thus alleviate sympathetic overactivity in selected cases. Episodes of profound arterial hypotension have also been observed in patients with tetanus, although the cause is unclear. Corbett et al. studied several such patients and ascribed hypotensive episodes to impairment of baroreceptor reflexes.

Local Tetanus

Local tetanus is an unusual variation of the more generalized disorder and is believed to occur in persons who possess partial immunity to the infection or who sustain minor wounds with only minimal contamination with tetanus bacilli. The patient with local tet-

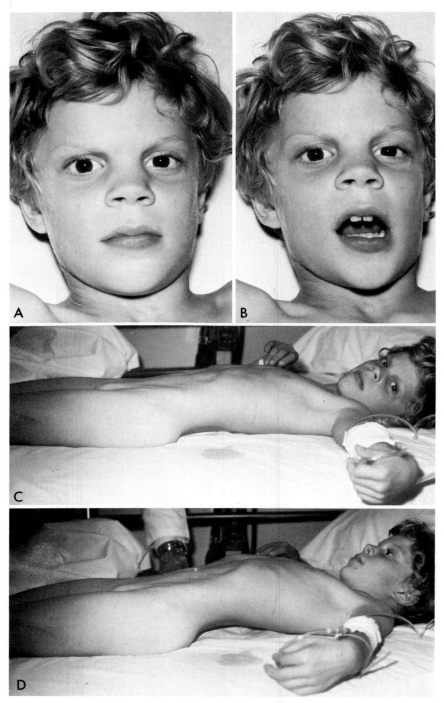

Figure 9–2. Tetanus. Six-year-old unimmunized girl who suffered a puncture wound of the foot 8 days before onset of symptoms. The illness began with back pain, followed by rigidity of the low back and abdomen. Inability to open the mouth normally and difficulty in swallowing were then observed. *A,* Anxious-appearing child who is alert and normally responsive. *B,* Masseter spasm markedly restricts the degree to which the child can open her mouth. *C,* When unstimulated, she lies with her back almost flat on the surface of the bed. Note the apparent spasm of the abdominal muscles. *D,* Tactile stimulation results in immediate paraspinous muscle spasm, producing a concave appearance to her low back.

anus usually first describes muscle stiffness or intermittent twitching of muscle groups in the vicinity of the preceding wound. Brief recurrent localized spasm is soon followed by a persisting state of localized rigidity on which are superimposed more intense spasms precipitated spontaneously, by voluntary use of the extremity, or by external stimulation in the region. Struppler et al. emphasized the provocation of localized spasms by repetitive voluntary muscle contraction, such as opening and closing of the hand, when the process affects one upper limb. The gradual spread of the spasm from its site of origin to neighboring muscles, and, in some cases, involvement of the entire extremity, was referred to by these authors as "recruitment spasm."

The natural course of localized tetanus is variable in that it may remain entirely re-stricted to one area of the body in some cases or evolve to generalized disease in others. The distal portion of one upper limb may be affected in certain patients, with the only additional evidence of involvement elsewhere being in the form of mild trismus. Muscle rigidity and recurrent spasms in local tetanus may persist for weeks or even months before spontaneous resolution gradually leads to complete recovery. In some cases, the illness beginning locally progressively involves the limb and truncal musculature in mild to moderate degree and becomes protracted, with rigidity and spasms persisting for several months, a condition called chronic tetanus (Fig. 9–3).

A type of localized tetanus in which symptoms are limited to dysfunction of certain cranial nerves is referred to as "cephalic tetanus" (Vakil et al.). Persisting rigid contraction of the facial muscles on one side may superficially resemble a peripheral facial palsy, although the superimposed episodic spasms serve to distinguish the two. In the bulbar form of cephalic tetanus, restriction of motion of the tongue and pharyngeal muscles gives rise to dysarthria and dysphagia, which are associated with postural deviation of the head if one sternocleidomastoid muscle is implicated.

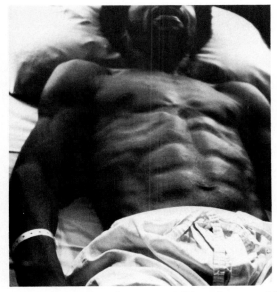

Figure 9–3. Chronic tetanus. Thirty-nine-year-old man with no prior immunizations. Eight weeks before hospital admission, he fell and lacerated the skin in the region of his right knee. Approximately 10 days later he began to have recurrent spasms of the right leg, initially believed to be myoclonic seizures. Over the following days, his right leg became "stiff" and soon thereafter his left leg also was similarly affected. Three weeks after onset, he noticed trismus and persistent spasm of the abdominal muscles. On one occasion he developed laryngospasm on attempting to swallow. Tactile, auditory, or bright light stimuli provoked sudden muscle spasms of his face and trunk musculature. Note the intense, sustained muscle spasm of the pectoralis, abdominal, and biceps muscles. There is persistent retraction of the angles of the mouth. He experienced moderate improvement with five mg. doses of diazepam and eventually recovered after several weeks.

Neonatal Tetanus

Tetanus in the newborn infant is primarily a disease of underdeveloped countries in which prenatal obstetrical care is limited, home deliveries are usual, and custom or convenience dictates the method of cutting and care of the umbilical cord. The two main prerequisites for the occurrence of this illness at the present time are absence of immunity of the mother and the contamination of the umbilical cord with tetanus bacilli. Neonatal tetanus is not unknown in affluent societies but has become much less common as hospital births have increased. In the United States in 1965 and 1966, 54 cases of neonatal tetanus were reported, with a mortality rate of 77 percent (LaForce et al.). The importance of maternal immunity in protecting against this disease is apparent from this series in that only three of the 54 mothers had received any form of tetanus toxoid immunization.

The astonishing statistics in economically deprived countries regarding the incidence of neonatal tetanus have been summarized by Marshall. Her series of 2,198 cases observed in Haiti from 1957 to 1966 exemplifies the magnitude of the problem in a country where neonatal tetanus affects approximately 14 percent of all live births. A similar incidence has been reported from parts of South Africa (Wright) and a figure only slightly lower has been recorded from areas of New Guinea (Schofield et al.). In all these regions, similar factors pertain to newborn care that predispose the child to this disease. Birth of the child generally occurs in unsanitary surroundings and the umbilical cord is severed by unclean scissors, a knife, or whatever instrument is available. The umbilical stump is often completely neglected and becomes contaminated by dirt, or may, by ritual, be coated with various substances such as charcoal, grease, or even cow dung, believed to have antiseptic properties (Athavale and Pai). As the umbilical stump becomes dry and necrotic, it provides an ideal environment for growth of tetanus bacilli and other bacterial pathogens introduced from the dirty utensil used for its severance or from foreign material or dirt applied to its cut surface.

The incubation period in neonatal tetanus is less variable than that in older age groups, although symptoms may appear as early as two days or as late as thirty days. The incubation period usually corresponds to the age of the child since umbilical contamination occurs in the immediate neonatal period. The average time of onset of symptoms is on the fifth to the seventh day after birth. Irritability, incessant crying, and decline in ability to suck are the usual initial symptoms, followed by fever, trismus, and generalized stiffness. Within 12 to 24 hours after the onset, recurrent spasms with flexion of the arms and clenching of the fists are superimposed upon the already present rigid state. Cyanosis and tachycardia accompany the spasms, which become progressively more frequent and severe as hours pass. Fever, dehydration, and acidosis rapidly develop unless prevented by therapeutic measures. Mildly affected infants reveal enhanced deep tendon reflexes, but more severely involved neonates in opisthotonus are so intensely rigid that stretch reflexes may not be elicitable. Unless death occurs owing to respiratory failure or from a complicating bacterial infection such as pneumonia or gastroenteritis, spasms continue for one to three weeks before improvement ensues.

Differential Diagnosis

The diagnosis of tetanus is made on the basis of the historical sequence of development of symptoms, in addition to the physical signs such as trismus, muscle rigidity, and recurrent spasms. Retained mental clarity, rigid abdominal musculature, and the ability to elicit muscle spasms by tactile or painful stimulation are characteristic features and are important diagnostic points for the clinician. The lack of previous active immunization enhances the probability but an immunization history obtained from parents is not always reliable, especially when there are several children in the family. The diagnosis of tetanus cannot be categorically excluded when adequate immunization was said to have been administered, but is significantly reduced if, in fact, such immunization was accomplished. Among 535 patients with tetanus, LaForce et al. found that only eight had reportedly received a full primary course of immunization within ten years before injury.

Laboratory investigations are of little positive help in view of the nonspecific findings. The white blood cell count and erythrocyte sedimentation rate are normal unless altered by complications of the disease, such as aspiration pneumonitis. The cerebrospinal fluid examination also is non-revealing but may be indicated in certain cases when neck rigidity suggests the possibility of septic or aseptic meningitis. Wounds that are identified should be cultured for pathogens, including *Clostridium tetani*, but negative results do not exclude the diagnosis.

Strychnine poisoning bears similarities to tetanus in that postsynaptic inhibition within the spinal cord results in recurrent extensor thrusts and clonic convulsions without loss of consciousness (Maron et al.). The distinguishing feature between these two disorders is the absence of muscle rigidity and trismus in the interval between convulsions in patients intoxicated with strychnine. The history of ingestion of strychnine in pill form or in a rodenticide is of obvious diagnostic importance.

Adverse reactions to certain phenothiazine preparations may also produce dystonic and other postural disturbances that resemble tetanus (Angle and McIntire, Cottom and Newman, Gailitis et al.). Although trismus and muscle rigidity are common in such patients, other movement disorders that enable clinical identification of the problem are usually present. Oculogyric crisis, torticollis, rhythmic protrusion of the tongue, puckering movements of the lips, or facial grimacing are examples of associated signs that are not present in tetanus. Drug-induced dystonic reactions are not dose-related and may occur after a single dose of certain phenothiazines. Prompt improvement after intravenous injection of diphenhydramine serves as both treatment and a diagnostic test.

Status epilepticus may be considered in differential diagnosis, especially when trismus and persistent extensor rigidity are more pronounced than clonic contractions. The loss of consciousness and lack of response to external stimulation in status epilepticus are in contrast to the findings noted in tetanus.

Trismus is often observed in children with meningitis and encephalitis. These central nervous system infections, however, usually disturb the state of awareness, are associated with fever, and are characterized by abnormal CSF findings. It is only the exceptional case in which tetanus is a diagnostic consideration.

The stiff-man syndrome was described in 1956 by Moersch and Woltman. It has remained a disorder of unknown etiology characterized by the adult onset in either sex of progressive muscle stiffness, especially of the truncal musculature, with painful muscle cramps that last for several minutes and are often provoked by movement, noise, or cutaneous stimulation. Although trismus is not usually seen in patients with the so-called stiff-man syndrome, similarities of the clinical features of this disorder to those of subacute or chronic tetanus have been pointed out (Layzer and Rowland). McQuillen et al. described an elderly patient believed to have protracted tetanus with manifestations like those of the stiff-man syndrome and suggested that some cases of previously described stiff-man syndrome may have been examples of unrecognized tetanus.

In the early stages of tetanus, conversion hysteria may be entertained in the differential diagnosis. Hysterical reactions can resemble certain aspects of tetanus but trismus would be unusual, and hysterical "spasmodic" episodes or convulsions are not usually superimposed on a state of persistent muscular rigidity.

Mortality and Sequelae

Tetanus is a serious disease with a high mortality rate; however, even children severely affected may recover completely and show no obvious residual deficits. The fatality rate of tetanus currently varies from 40 to 60 percent in different series when neonatal cases are excluded. Neonatal tetanus creates a greater threat to survival, with mortality rates between 55 and 80 percent in most of the recent reports (Marshall). Death resulting from tetanus in the newborn is more frequent when the disease affects the premature infant and when symptoms begin before the sixth day after birth. In any age group, the shorter the interval between the onset of symptoms and the appearance of muscle spasms, the higher is the fatality rate. Hypothermia often heralds the occurrence of fatal respiratory complications in the neonate, the most common being pneumonitis and acute pulmonary hemorrhage (Salimpour).

It has often been stated that tetanus itself results in no sequelae in patients who survive but that residual deficits may result from cerebral hypoxia or ischemia if the illness is complicated by respiratory insufficiency, cardiac arrest, or compromise of cardiac output. These complicating factors are possible in any age group but have been observed more often when tetanus occurs in the newborn period. Follow-up studies by Illis and Taylor have cast doubt on the previous concepts of total lack of residual effects of tetanus toxin on the nervous system in survivors. Sequelae observed in some patients included irritability, sleep disturbances, myoclonus, postural hypotension, and electroencephalographic abnormalities. While the cause of these residual deficits remains speculative, the authors postulated that some might be autonomic in origin and secondary to sympathetic dysfunction during the acute stage of the illness.

Prevention

There is no natural immunity to tetanus, although the newborn infant receives passive, transplacental protection if the antibody titer of the mother is adequate from preceding active immunization. In addition, the disease itself does not immunize the patient. The reason for the lack of immunity resulting from the disease is unclear but it has been suggested that because of the extreme potency of the toxin, only those persons exposed to a small quantity can survive, and that such minute amounts of the toxin are insufficient to result in antigenic stimulation.

Active Immunization. The most effective method of preventing tetanus is by active immunization of infants and children, which is customarily accomplished using a preparation containing diphtheria and tetanus toxoids and pertussis vaccine. Tetanus toxoid was produced in 1924 by Descombey by formalin detoxification of toxin. Its value and safety as an immunizing agent gradually became evident, and it is now recognized to be one of the most effective prophylactic preparations available to the physician. The remarkable record of tetanus toxoid was illustrated by the military experience in World War II, during which United States forces were generously exposed to this organism. Only 12 cases of tetanus were identified in the troops and at least one-half of these individuals had successfully avoided previous immunization.

The basic immunization series includes injections at ages two, three, and four months plus a reinforcing fourth dose at age fifteen to eighteen months. An additional dose of DPT vaccine at age five to six years is advised, while tetanus boosters thereafter should be given only at ten-year intervals. Studies from Denmark have shown that up to 12 years after the basic immunizing series given in infancy, 96 percent of children still have tetanus antitoxin titers above 0.01 unit per ml. of plasma, the accepted protective level of circulating tetanus antitoxin (Scheibel et al.). The practice in past years of giving tetanus toxoid boosters in the previously immunized child every year or following every wound led to the paradox of hyperimmunization in certain population groups (Peebles et al., Steigman). Adverse reactions from toxoid injection in such hyperimmune persons have generally been mild but can be minimized by a more conservative schedule regarding frequency of booster injections.

Immunization with tetanus toxoid of women during pregnancy also has a role in countries where neonatal tetanus remains a serious threat to the newborn (Athavale and Pai, Schofield et al.). While this would largely eliminate tetanus in the newborn infant, the obvious problem is that those countries with a high incidence of neonatal tetanus are the same countries in which prenatal care either is not sought or is not readily available.

Passive Immunization. Passive immunization may be administered in the form of tetanus antitoxin (T.A.T., A.T.S.) at the time of injury to one not known to have been actively immunized beforehand. Its efficacy was demonstrated in World War I when the incidence of tetanus among injured British forces declined from eight per 1,000 to one per 1,000 following the utilization of prophylactic tetanus antitoxin (Christie). Equine tetanus antitoxin for prophylaxis is usually given by intramuscular injection in a dose of 1,500 units but carries a significant risk of anaphylaxis, serum sickness, or, less commonly, peripheral neuropathy. It is estimated that the administration of equine serum is associated with an incidence of serum sickness in approximately 10 percent and fatal anaphylaxis in one in 100,000 instances (Stiehm). Disseminated encephalomyelitis has also been described as a complication of equine tetanus antitoxin but appears to be rare (Miller and Ramsden, Williams and Chafee).

Tetanus antitoxin of human origin (tetanus immune globulin–human) is now available and is a more acceptable agent for passive immunization against this disease (Shirkey). The primary objection to this material is the higher price as compared with equine antitoxin, but its advantages more than compensate. In addition to a far lesser number of adverse reactions, the protective levels in serum after a single dose of homologous serum is several weeks, thus being considerably longer than with antitoxin of equine origin. Tetanus immune globulin (human) is administered in a dose of 250 to 500 units intramuscularly, the larger dose being selected for more extensive wounds in the adult or older child. Immunization with tetanus toxoid can be initiated simultaneously, but the two agents should be given at different sites using separate syringes (Red Book, 1970).

Other Preventive Measures. Proper management of the wound, including removal of foreign material and excision of devitalized tissue, reduces the possibility that *Clostridium tetani* can flourish and elaborate toxin. Surgical wound management, however, does not totally eliminate the possibility of tetanus and does not compare with the protection provided by previous adequate active immunization. Deep puncture wounds which contain necrotic tissue and harbor dirt and other debris should be treated with antibiotics. *Clostridium tetani* is usually sensitive to penicillin, although the susceptibility of the organism cloistered in avascular, devitalized tissue is questionable.

Prevention and subsequent eradication of neonatal tetanus must largely be based on education of populations in which the disease prevails. Development of prenatal obstetrical care and encouragement of hospital deliveries will have a great impact on this variety of tetanus, as will the more widespread use of active immunization.

Treatment

Decline of the incidence of an infectious disease is evidence of success of medical measures; however, the decreasing occurrence of tetanus has increased the problems of management in one respect. Treatment of the child with tetanus requires expert judgment that depends heavily upon prior experience with the disease. Few practicing physicians see more than an infrequent case of tetanus and thus have little opportunity to develop expertise in its recognition as well as in the complexities of its management. The dilution of clinical experience on this basis is best circumvented by the utilization of regional treatment centers for the multi-specialty care required for patients with this illness. Treatment of the severely affected patient is best accomplished in an intensive care unit staffed by nurses and physicians well versed in respiratory physiology, use of ventilators, and drug therapy. Constant and skilled nursing attention, often for three to six weeks, is an absolute prerequisite for successful treatment. A quiet, darkened room with a minimum of external stimulation has often been recommended. These restrictions have merit but should not be carried to the point that observation is difficult or the necessary examinations are avoided.

General Measures

Wound debridement should be thorough and preferably is done as early as possible in the course of the disease. The precise timing of surgical attention to the wound, however, depends on the status of the patient in other respects. Airway or respiratory problems that might have developed or severe spasms take precedence and must be managed either simultaneously or before the wound is cleansed. Penicillin therapy is initiated by intravenous administration and is continued for a 10-day period. Tetracycline can be used as an alternative in patients allergic to penicillin. Repeated intramuscular injections should be avoided, as they provide an unnecessary painful stimulus which provokes spasms. More seriously affected patients will require a nasogastric tube to decompress the stomach and a urethral catheter to prevent bladder distention. The quantity and quality of intravenous fluids depend on the results of periodic electrolyte and blood gas determinations. When it is apparent that prolonged sedation or possibly even respirator care will be necessary, parenteral hyperalimentation through a superior vena cava catheter will forestall nutritional deficiencies.

Tetanus Antitoxin and Toxoid

The value of serotherapy of any type, once signs of tetanus have appeared, has been debated for years. It is generally agreed that antitoxin has no effect on toxin that is fixed to neural tissue, but it is assumed that it might neutralize toxin that has not yet reached the central nervous system. Most authors (Altemeier and Hummel, Athavale and Pai, Bernhardt and Hickey) continue to advise its use if human tetanus immune globulin is not available, even though the beneficial effects remain questionable.

Tetanus immune globulin (human) is now preferred, primarily because of the greater safety of this preparation when compared to that of equine origin. While claims for greater effectiveness have been made for tetanus immune globulin (human), McCracken et al. found no significant difference when compared to equine antitoxin in a series of newborn infants with tetanus. Tetanus immune globulin (human) is given intramuscularly in the older child or adult in a dose of 3,000 to 6,000 units. The volume of this amount is sufficiently great that two or more injection sites are usually required. It is not recommended for intravenous use.

When tetanus immune globulin (human) is not available, equine antitoxin is used in an intravenous dose of 50,000 units for children, after sensitivity tests are done. This amount should be diluted in a quantity of intravenous fluid so that its administration is accomplished over a 30- to 60-minute period. An additional 5,000 units of equine antitoxin may be infiltrated in and around a wound if one is identified.

In view of the lack of immunity conveyed by the disease, active immunization with tetanus toxoid should be initiated during the recovery phase. The parents of the child must then be encouraged to have the series completed in its usual fashion. In addition, siblings of the patient have also probably not been adequately immunized and this, too, deserves attention.

Sedation and Ventilation

While the above measures are important and should not be underemphasized, it is one's ability to control spasms and maintain adequate ventilation that will determine the outcome of the child more than mildly affected by this illness. Numerous drugs have been used in an effort to produce sedation and control spasms. Barbiturates, phenothiazines, and meprobamate have been the most popular drugs and often have been used in combination at different dosage levels (Crandell and Whitcher, Perlstein et al.). In recent years, diazepam (Valium) has become increasingly popular (Femi-Pearse) and is now considered by many to be the drug of choice. Sedation and reduction in muscle spasms can frequently be accomplished without significant respiratory suppression or other adverse effects. The frequency of intravenous administration and the total daily dosage must be individualized according to the severity of symptoms and the child's response to the drug. Reasonable dosage ranges of diazepam are, for a mild case, 2 to 4 mg. per kilogram per day, for moderate cases 4 to 6 mg. per kilogram per day, and for severe cases 6 to 10 mg. per kilogram per day. Repeated intravenous injections of diazepam are sometimes required at hourly intervals in certain patients or every four hours in others.

Tracheostomy must be considered in every case and should be performed without hesitation in those patients with severe spasms or with laryngospasm. It is vital to anticipate the need for this procedure and to have it accomplished before it is required under emergency circumstances. It facilitates airway management and will be necessary if prolonged respirator care is required. Intermittent oropharyngeal suction will suffice in mild cases but will not be adequate in others and may precipitate muscle spasms as well as laryngospasm.

In extraordinarily severe cases of tetanus, even heavy sedation fails to control muscle spasms, rigidity, or laryngospasm. In others, the spasmodic component is adequately checked but at the expense of suppressing respiratory function to a dangerous level. Such events are an indication for the use of controlled ventilation, usually with muscle paralysis induced by d-tubocurarine or pancuronium bromide. While it is possible to maintain muscle paralysis in the respirator patient without sedation (Ramsey), this experience would probably frighten the child to such a degree that it should be avoided. Attendants must remember that the curarized patient on a respirator looks comatose to observers but is quite aware of his surroundings if not sedated. Discussions about the illness or prognosis should not take place at the bedside or within hearing distance of the patient.

The child with tetanus severe enough to require respirator care will probably need ventilatory assistance and sedation for one to three weeks. Discontinuation of d-tubocurare therapy is determined by intermittent trials with reduction of the dose to ascertain if spasms or rigidity will recur. When spasms do not recur, curare is stopped and spontaneous respirations resume. Sedation therapy is gradually decreased and is finally terminated.

Curare therapy with controlled ventilation and diazepam sedation requires the continued attendance of a skilled anesthesiologist, continuous nursing care, and constant search for complications of the management, as well as of the disease. Periodic chest x-rays are indicated to identify pulmonary complications such as atelectasis, pneumothorax, or pneumonia. Hyperventilation can be recognized and corrected by periodic blood gas analysis. Urine and serum osmolarities and serum electrolytes are also necessary at daily intervals during respirator management.

Neonatal Tetanus—Treatment

The general principles of management of the neonate with tetanus do not differ from those above. Tetanus immune globulin (human) is given intramuscularly in a dose of 500 units, and if not available, tetanus antitoxin of equine origin is used instead. The dose of equine tetanus antitoxin has not been standardized, with recommendations varying from 80,000 units IM (Marshall) to 1,500 units (Patel and Goodluck) but with 10,000 units for the neonate being the most commonly quoted dosage. Penicillin, intravenous fluids, and methods to control temperature elevation are indicated, much as in older children.

Sedation is required and diazepam in dosage described above represents the agent of choice. The advisability of tracheostomy in newborns with tetanus has varied with different authors (Holloway, Thambiran). Tracheostomy is plagued by many serious potential complications in young infants, with the inability to achieve extubation and the development of tracheal stenosis being the most outstanding. When spasms and extensor rigidity cannot be controlled with sedation alone, the current approach is endotracheal intubation and controlled ventilation with the aid of paralysis induced by pancuronium bromide (Adams et al.). Nutrition during the course of treatment can be maintained by nasogastric tube feeding. Following recovery, the infant will require the primary series of immunizations including tetanus vaccine, but this should not be initiated until at least six weeks after the child has received tetanus immune globulin.

REFERENCES

Abel, J. J., Firor, W. M., and Chalian, W.: Researches on tetanus. IX. Further evidence to show that tetanus toxin is not carried to central neurons by way of axis cylinders of motor nerves. Bull. Johns Hopkins Hosp. 63:373, 1938.

Adams, J. M., Kenny, J. D., and Rudolph, A. J.: Modern management of tetanus neonatorum. Pediatrics 64:472–477, 1979.

Altemeier, W. A., and Hummel, R. P.: Treatment of tetanus. Surgery 60:495–505, 1966.

Angle, C. R., and McIntire, M. S.: Persistent dystonia in a brain-damaged child after ingestion of phenothiazine. J. Pediat. 73:124–126, 1968.

Athavale, V. B., and Pai, P. N.: Tetanus—clinical manifestations in children. J. Pediat. 65:590–598, 1964.

Athavale, V. B., and Pai, P. N.: Tetanus neonatorum—clinical manifestations. J. Pediat. 67:649–657, 1965.

Athavale, V. B., and Pai, P. N.: Role of tetanus antitoxin in the treatment of tetanus in children. J. Pediat. 68:289–293, 1966.

Berger, S. A., Cherubin, C. E., Nelson, S., and Levine, L.: Tetanus despite pre-existing antitetanus antibody. J.A.M.A. 240:769–770, 1978.

Bernhardt, L. C., and Hickey, R. C.: Tetanus. Its prophylaxis and treatment. Am. J. Surg. 112:23–27, 1966.

Bohrer, S. P.: Spinal fractures in tetanus. Radiology 85:1111–1116, 1965.

Brooks, V. B., Curtis, D. R., and Eccles, J. C.: The action of tetanus toxin on the inhibition of motoneurons. J. Physiol. 135:655–672, 1957.

Chalian, W.: An essay on the history of lockjaw. Bull. Hist. Med. 8:171–201, 1940.

Cherubin, C. E.: Clinical severity of tetanus in narcotic addicts in New York City. Arch. Intern. Med. 121:156–158, 1968.

Christie, A. B.: Infectious Diseases: Epidemiology and Clinical practice. E. S. Livingstone, Ltd., Edinburgh and London, 1969, p. 742.

Corbett, J. L., Spalding, J. M. K., and Harris, P. J.: Hypotension in tetanus. Brit. Med. J. 3:423–428, 1973.

Cottom, D. G., and Newman, C. G. H.: Dystonic reactions to phenothiazine derivatives. Arch. Dis. Childh. 41:551–553, 1966.

Crandell, D. L., and Whitcher, C. E.: Control of neuromuscular manifestations of severe systemic tetanus. J.A.M.A. 172:15–19, 1960.

Descombey, P.: L'Anatoxine tétanique. Compt. Rend. Soc. Biol. 91:239–241, 1924.

Eccles, J. C.: Pharmacology of central inhibitory synapses. Brit. Med. Bull. 21:19–25, 1965.

Femi-Pearse, D.: Experience with diazepam in tetanus. Brit. Med. J. 2:862–865, 1966.

Fischer, G. W., Sunakorn, P., and Duangman, C.: Otogenous tetanus. A sequela of chronic ear infections. Am. J. Dis. Child. 131:445–446, 1977.

Gailitis, J., Knowles, R. R., and Longobardi, A.: Alarming neuromuscular reactions due to prochlorperazine. Ann. Intern. Med. 52:538–543, 1960.

Holloway, R.: The place of tracheostomy in tetanus neonatorum. Arch. Dis. Childh. 42:546–548, 1967.

Illis, L. S., and Mitchell, J.: The effect of tetanus toxin on boutons terminaux. Brain Res. 18:283–295, 1970.

Illis, L. S., and Taylor, F. M.: Neurological and electroencephalographic sequelae of tetanus. Lancet 1:826–830, 1971.

Kerr, J. H., Corbett, J. L., Prys-Roberts, C., Smith, A. C., and Spalding, J. M. K: Involvement of the sympathetic nervous system in tetanus. Studies on 82 cases. Lancet 2:236–241, 1968.

LaForce, F. M., Young, L. S., and Bennett, J. V.: Tetanus in the United States (1965–1966). Epidemiologic and clinical features. New Eng. J. Med. 280:569–574, 1969.

Layzer, R. B., and Rowland, L. P.: Cramps. New Eng. J. Med. 285:31–40, 1971.

Maron, B. J., Krupp, J. R., and Tune, B.: Strychnine poisoning successfully treated with diazepam. J. Pediat. 78:697–699, 1971.

Marshall, F. N.: Tetanus of the newborn. With special reference to experiences in Haiti, W.I. Adv. Pediat. 15:65–110, 1968.

McCracken, G. H., Jr., Dowell, D. L., and Marshall, F. N.: Double-blind trial of equine antitoxin and human immune globulin in tetanus neonatorum. Lancet 1:1146–1149, 1971.

McQuillen, M. P., Tucker, K., and Pellegrino, E. D.: Syndrome of subacute generalized muscular stiffness and spasm. Arch. Neurol. 16:165–174, 1967.

Meyer, H., and Ransom, F.: Untersuchungen ueber den tetanus. Arch. Exp. Path. Pharmakol. 49:369–416, 1903.

Miller, A. A., and Ramsden, F.: Acute disseminating encephalomyelitis with massive necrosis of spinal cord, probably due to antitetanus serum. J. Clin. Path. 15:314–323, 1962.

Moersch, F. P., and Woltman, H. W.: Progressive fluctuating muscular rigidity and spasm ("stiff-man" syndrome): Report of a case and some observations in 13 other cases. Mayo Clin. Proc. 31:421–427, 1956.

Morax, V., and Marie, A.: Recherches sur l'absorption de la toxine tétanique. Ann. de l'Inst. Pasteur. 17:33, 1903.

Patel, J. C., and Goodluck, P. L.: Serum therapy in neonatal tetanus. Am J. Dis. Child. 114:131–134, 1967.

Patel, J. C., Dhirawani, M. D., Mehta, B. C., and Agarwal, K. K.: Tetanus following intramuscular injection. J. Indian Med. Assoc. 35:505, 1960.

Patel, J. C., Dhirawani, M. D., Mehta, B. C., Agarwall, K. K., and Verdachari, N. S.: Tetanus following vaccination against small pox. Indian J. Pediat. 27:251, 1960.

Peebles, T. C., Levine, L., Eldred, M. C., and Edsall, G.: Tetanus-toxoid emergency boosters. A reappraisal. New Eng. J. Med. 280:575–581, 1969.

Perlstein, M. A., Stein, M. D., and Elam, H.: Routine treatment of tetanus. J.A.M.A. 173:1536–1541, 1960.

Prabhu, V. G., and Oester, Y. T.: Electromyographic changes in skeletal muscle due to tetanus toxin. J. Pharm. Exp. Ther. 138:241, 1962.

Prys-Roberts, C., Corbett, J. L., Kerr, J. H., Smith, A. C., and Spalding, J. M. K.: Treatment of sympathetic overactivity in tetanus. Lancet 1:542–545, 1969.

Ramsey, F. C.: Total paralysis without sedation in the treatment of severe tetanus. Dev. Med. Child. Neurol. 7:56–60, 1965.

Salimpour, R.: Cause of death in tetanus neonatorum. Study of 233 cases with 54 necropsies. Arch. Dis. Childh. 52:587–589, 1977.

Scheibel, I., Bentzon, M. W., Christensen, P. E., and Biering, A.: Duration of immunity to diphtheria and tetanus after active immunization. Arch. Path. Microbiol. Scand. 67:380, 1966.

Schofield, F. D., Tucker, V. M., and Westbrook, G. R.: Neonatal tetanus in New Guinea. Effect of active immunization in pregnancy. Brit. Med. J. 2:785–789, 1961.

Shirkey, H. C.: Tetanus immune globulin (human) in prophylaxis against tetanus. J. Pediat. 67:643–646, 1965.

Steigman, A. J.: Abuse of tetanus toxoid. J. Pediat. 72:753–754, 1968.

Stiehm, E. R.: Standard and special human immune serum globulins as therapeutic agents. Pediatrics 63:301–319, 1979.

Struppler, A., Struppler, E., and Adams, R. D.: Local tetanus in man. Its clinical and neurophysiological characteristics. Arch. Neurol. 8:162–178, 1963.

Tarlov, I. M., Ling, H., and Yamada, H.: Neuronal pathology in experimental local tetanus. Clinical implications. Neurology 23:580–591, 1973.

Thambiran, A. K.: Assisted respiration in the treatment of neonatal tetanus. Arch. Dis. Childh. 43:182–186, 1968.

Vakil, B. J., Singhal, B. S., Pandya, S. S., and Irani, P. F.: Cephalic tetanus. Neurology 23:1091–1096, 1973.

Williams, H. H., and Chafee, F. H.: Demyelinating encephalomyelitis in a case of tetanus treated with antitoxin. New Eng. J. Med. 264:489–491, 1961.

Wright, R.: Tetanus neonatorum. S. Afr. Med. J. 34:111, 1960.

Zacks, S. I., and Sheff, M. F.: Studies on tetanus toxin. J. Neuropath. Exp. Neurol. 23:306–323, 194.

Chapter Ten

BOTULISM

Botulism is a disorder in which the clinical manifestations result from the effects on the neuromuscular junction of a toxin produced by *Clostridium botulinum.* The illness is now recognized to occur in three forms, each with different epidemiologic features and pathogenesis (Black and Arnon). The best known and classic type of botulism is the food-borne variety, which follows ingestion of improperly prepared foods containing preformed *Clostridium botulinum* toxin as well as organisms. The second is an unusual form referred to as wound botulism, which results from wound contamination by the toxin-producing organism. The third variety is infantile botulism, a condition recognized since 1976 in which infants less than six months of age acquire gastrointestinal colonization with *Clostridium botulinum.* Toxin formed within the intestinal tract of the infant is absorbed therefrom, leading to a syndrome manifested by constipation, ocular and bulbar signs, hypotonia, and, in some cases, severe respiratory compromise secondary to muscle weakness.

The term botulism evolved from the Latin term "botulus" (which means sausage) following outbreaks of the clinical illness in Germany in the late 1700's (Tyler). In the years that followed, it became known that a paralyzing and often fatal illness could result from eating smoked or inadequately cooked meat of many kinds, including sausage, uncooked fish, and, rarely, even cheese. In 1894, thirty-four persons in Belgium attended a banquet following a concert and consumed a meal which included preserved ham. Twenty-three people became ill and three died of botulism. From the contaminated ham, Van Ermengem isolated an anaerobic, gram-positive organism, which he named *Bacillus botulinus,*

and subsequently demonstrated that the clinical illness was the result of a toxin produced by the microorganism. In 1956, Meyer reviewed the status of botulism as a world health problem and stated that during the preceding fifty years, approximately 5,635 persons throughout the world had been afflicted by this disease, of whom 1,714 had died of the condition.

In the United States, cases of botulism were identified in the early part of this century and outbreaks continued to appear sporadically. Home-canned vegetables and fruits were the most common offenders, but improperly prepared meat and fish also were recognized to be potential dangers. In 1961, 14 cases were identified in this country and in 1962, ten cases were recognized. In 1963, however, 47 cases of human botulism with 15 deaths were reported in the United States, more than in any single year since 1939. The sharp increase in 1963 was largely attributable to intoxication by type E toxin, traced to contaminated smoked whitefish chub, which originated in the Great Lakes area. Twenty-three cases of botulism were recorded in 1964 in this country and less than 20 cases per year were identified in each of the subsequent six years. In 1976, there were 58 cases of botulism identified in the United States, including 40 that were food-borne, 3 cases of wound botulism, and 15 cases of infant botulism (Black and Arnon) (Fig. 10–1). Since 1943 when wound botulism was first identified, there has been a total of 21 such cases reported in the United States as of January, 1980 (Morbidity and Mortality Weekly Report, Vol. 29, Jan. 25, 1980). Although botulism remains rare, the experiences in 1963 and 1976 make it clear that outbreaks of sig-

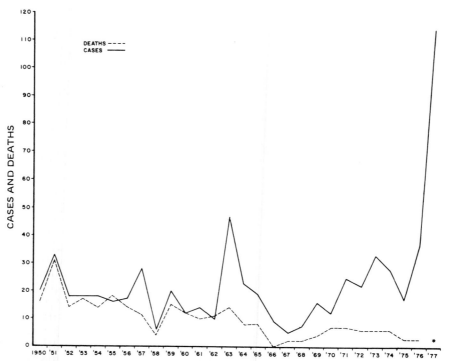

Figure 10–1. Botulism. Reported cases and deaths by year in the United States, 1950–1977. (From: Morbidity and Mortality Weekly Report, Annual Summary, 1977, Volume 26, No. 53, Sept. 1978.)

nificant magnitude can still occur unless food products are properly handled before consumption.

The Organism and Its Toxin

Clostridium botulinum is a gram-positive, anaerobic, spore-forming bacillus whose natural habitat is the soil. It is divided into types A, B, C, D, E, and F on the basis of the immunologic properties of the toxin that is elaborated. The toxin is believed to be formed within the organism and is released on autolysis. It is regarded to be one of the most potent of the biological toxins, and, according to Guyton and MacDonald, as little as 0.25 micrograms of the pure toxin can be lethal in adults. Human beings have been affected by types A and B toxins in most recorded outbreaks, although type E intoxication from fish was prominent in 1963. Human beings appear to be more susceptible to type A toxin, which has been associated with a higher fatality rate than has been the case with toxins of types B or E. Types C, D, and F have only rarely been identified as causes of human disease. Toxins of the various types produce similar symptoms and signs, although gas-

trointestinal features have seemingly been more outstanding in the recent cases due to type E. Although botulinus spores are markedly resistant to physical and chemical agents, the toxin is thermolabile and can be rapidly destroyed by heat. Clostridial spores may withstand boiling for up to 24 hours but can be destroyed by heat under pressure within 20 minutes (Meyers). Both the spores and the toxins survive low temperatures indefinitely and are not destroyed by freezing for many months. The toxins appear to be resistant to gastric and intestinal substances and type E toxin may even be enhanced by trypsin (Duff et al.).

Pathogenesis

Food-borne botulism is caused by the consumption of inadequately cooked food containing *Clostridium botulinum* and its toxin. In addition, the disease can be contracted from wounds contaminated with *Clostridium botulinum* from the soil; however, this has been described only on rare occasions (de Jesus et al., Merson and Dowell). After ingestion, the toxin is absorbed from the gastrointestinal tract and enters the blood stream, where it is carried to its site of action in the vicinity of the neuromuscular junction. Some investigators have suggested the possibility of continued formation of toxin from germination of ingested spores and multiplication of organisms within the intestinal tract of the affected patient. This "toxi-infection" theory presupposes continued growth of *Clostridium botulinum* within the bowel and is a postulate that might be supported by the long duration of neuromuscular block observed in certain patients. Although the possibility of intestinal colonization and subsequent continued elaboration of toxin is a justifiable consideration, it is not generally considered an important factor in human disease except in the syndrome of infantile botulism described later.

In the United States, most outbreaks have resulted from consumption of home-canned or home-jarred vegetables and fruits, including stringbeans, corn, spinach, tomatoes, beets, and peaches. These home-prepared canned foods were often allowed to stand for long periods of time and subsequently eaten without further cooking. The relatively high incidence of botulism in Colorado is believed by Cherington to be the result of the low boiling temperature of water at high altitudes, which is insufficient to destroy spores. Commercially canned foods have only rarely been the source of the disease in this country, but in 1963 commercially prepared fish resulted in several cases of botulism. The source of the organism in fish is not clear, but bottom-feeding fish may ingest spores transmitted to their environment from water drainage from soil. Thus, bacterial contamination of fish may occur before they are obtained from the water and may result in accumulation of lethal amounts of toxin if smoked or pickled and not adequately cooked.

Pathophysiology

Muscle weakness in patients with botulism has been recognized for many years to result from the effects of toxin acting peripherally to interfere with transmission at the neuromuscular junction (Dickson and Shevsky). Transmission along the nerve trunk and contractibility of muscle have not generally been found to be affected (Bishop and Bronfenbrenner, Guttmann and Pratt), although studies by Oh did demonstrate some mild and probably insignificant distal peripheral

nerve dysfunction in botulism. Unlike the block in myasthenia gravis, that present in botulism cannot be overcome with neostigmine (Guyton and MacDonald).

The precise location of the effect of botulinus toxin on the peripheral neuromuscular junction was long debated until the studies by Brooks in 1953 and 1954. He demonstrated that type A toxin caused neuromuscular paralysis by interfering with conduction in the terminal twigs of motor nerves, close to the site of acetylcholine release. Brooks found that the release mechanism of acetylcholine is not inactivated by any direct effect upon it, but merely because impulses from the nerve trunk cannot reach it. Further support for the lack of effect of botulinus toxin on the formation and potential release of acetylcholine is provided by evidence of clinical improvement from guanidine, a drug whose action is the stimulation of acetylcholine release at the cholinergic neuromuscular junction (Cherington and Ryan).

While the vast majority of the clinical manifestations in botulism are secondary to the effects of the toxin on the neuromuscular junction, certain studies have supported a possible central nervous system effect. Polley et al. found marked but transient electroencephalographic changes in animals following the intravenous injection of type A toxin. The presence of prominent "H" reflexes during electrophysiologic study of an adult with botulism also led Tyler to suggest a possible central effect of toxin on spinal neurons.

Clinical Manifestations

The symptoms and signs of food-borne botulism result from ingestion of the toxin elaborated within the organism. The onset of symptoms can occur as early as three hours or as late as five days after ingestion of the toxin, although the usual incubation period is eight to 36 hours. In some outbreaks, patients have noted a peculiar odor or taste, or an abnormal appearance of the food at the time it was consumed. Whittaker et al. observed that type E *Clostridium botulinum* is less proteolytic than type A or B and, therefore, results in little food spoilage which might forewarn the patient of the impending danger.

Approximately one-third of affected patients have gastrointestinal symptoms within a few hours after eating the contaminated food, and in the remainder, either a feeling of weakness or more specific neurologic complaints constitute the initial manifestations. Abdominal symptoms include epigastric pain, nausea, vomiting, constipation, and diarrhea. The gastrointestinal symptoms usually last 12 to 36 hours and probably result from local irritation from the spoiled food rather than from the botulinus toxin within the food. Headache, dizziness, excessive sweating, and malaise may coexist with abdominal symptoms, which can lead one to suspect an infectious gastroenteritis or staphylococcal food poisoning until other signs become evident. An acute surgical abdomen with intestinal obstruction may also be considered when abdominal distention is associated with cramping pain and constipation.

Patients who do not experience abdominal distress sometimes have general feelings of light-headedness or visual abnormalities as the initial manifestation. Diplopia or blurred vision are common early symptoms and frequently represent the very first alteration the patient is aware of. Corresponding findings on examination include ptosis, dilated pupils which respond sluggishly to light, and a variable degree of extraocular muscle paresis or complete external ophthalmoplegia. Lateral rectus paresis was the most common ocular abnormality found among 45 patients examined by Terranova et al. Nystagmus may occur but is less common than pupillary dilatation. Although fixed, dilated pupils are stressed as the ocular hallmark of this condition, Ryan and Cherington have indicated that these findings are not invariably present and that the pupils may occasionally be unaffected even though weakness elsewhere is severe. The optic discs remain normal throughout the course of the disease. Differential diagnostic considerations at this stage include myasthenia gravis, which can be excluded when pupillary abnormalities are present. Guillain-Barré disease, Fisher's syndrome, and acute demyelinating disorders of the brain stem also bear similarities to the neurologic findings in botulism and enter into the differential diagnosis.

With progression of the disease over the next few hours, difficulty in swallowing causing nasal regurgitation of liquids along with slowing and poor articulation of speech becomes evident. The patient loses the ability to protrude the tongue and develops bilateral facial weakness. During this period, generalization of the process results in weakness of the extremities and especially of the neck

musculature. In severe cases, the respiratory muscles may be affected to such an extent that some form of artificial ventilation will be required. Despite the severity of the motor deficits, sensory modalities remain intact and fasciculations are not observed. The weakness is of the hypotonic or flaccid type although deep tendon reflexes either can remain normal or become somewhat diminished. Unless influenced by hypoxia secondary to a respiratory or cardiac arrest, the state of alertness and mentation is not affected. A relatively benign variation of botulism has been described by Jenzer et al. in which the clinical features consist mainly of transient autonomic dysfunction. Affected patients were found to have type B toxin and their symptoms included blurred vision, dryness of the mouth, constipation, and impairment of salivary and lacrimal secretions but no significant bulbar or skeletal muscle weakness. While the illness remained mild in these individuals, a number of their complaints were quite protracted, lasting for several months.

A notable clinical feature in patients with botulism is the absence of fever and the nonspecificity of the basic laboratory tests. Body temperature is usually normal, although several authors have commented on the subnormal temperature observed in some patients. The pulse rate may be slower than average in the early stages of the illness but becomes abnormally rapid as progression occurs. Not more than a modest blood leukocytosis is expected and the urine examination is unrevealing except for the possible finding of proteinuria. Lumbar puncture, likewise, is of help only in a negative fashion. Cells are not expected in the CSF, and other chemical studies are usually normal.

The severely affected patient progresses through the above stages rather rapidly and may expire within 24 hours after the onset of symptoms, usually from a respiratory or cardiac arrest. As expected, the severity of the illness represents a broad spectrum which probably is explained on the basis of the quantity and type of toxin that is ingested. Mildly affected patients have less extensive weakness or only partial deficits of function of certain cranial nerves. Recovery in such persons is often complete one to four days after the beginning of symptoms. More severely affected patients who survive sometimes will have ocular abnormalities that persist for six to eight months, although recovery is usually eventually complete.

Infantile Botulism

Botulism in early infancy was first recognized in this country in California in 1976 (Pickett et al., Midura and Arnon). Prior to that time it was assumed that the disease did not occur in the first year of life because the infant is not exposed to the types of foods that ordinarily represent the vehicle for the organism and its preformed toxin. It is now known, however, that in the infantile form of botulism, preformed toxin is not ingested but that toxin is liberated from *Clostridium botulinum* spores that colonize the intestinal tract. Although an identical illness had been described before (Grover et al.), it was the observation by Pickett and colleagues of two previously normal infants who developed hypotonic weakness, ocular deficits, and bulbar signs which first aroused awareness of this condition. The affected patients were found to have *Clostridium botulinum* and toxin in the stools but not in the serum, and each recovered with conservative management. Thereafter, further examples of the illness were described in California and in other states (Clay et al., McKee et al.) and also in England (Turner et al.).

The clinical manifestations of infantile botulism have been similar in most reports although there is a wide range in the severity of the disorder. Affected infants are between three and 26 weeks of age and have generally been well until the first sign of illness, which in most cases is constipation. This is followed in days or a week or so by poor feeding, weakening of the cry, pooling of oral secretions, and ocular signs. Ptosis, sluggishly reacting dilated pupils, ophthalmoparesis, facial paresis, and dysphagia are common cranial nerve signs, which precede or are found simultaneous to poor head control due to cervical muscle weakness, and generalized hypotonia, hyporeflexia, and weakness. Mildly affected infants continue to breathe adequately but others proceed to respiratory arrest, requiring ventilator therapy. Signs resulting from blockade of the neuromuscular junction persist for a number of days up to several weeks but then gradually recede, to be followed by eventual recovery. The great majority of hospitalized infants identified with this disorder thus far have survived (Arnon et al. 1979), although it has been postulated that infantile botulism is one cause of the sudden, unexpected infant death syndrome. Arnon et al. (1978) found evidence on stool examination to indicate that nine of 211 cases of sudden infant death syndrome could be explained by intestinal colonization with *Clostridium botulinum,* suggesting that more fulminating examples of this disease may be manifested by precipitous respiratory failure.

Diagnosis of infantile botulism is on the basis of the characteristic clinical pattern with laboratory confirmation by the demonstration of *Clostridium botulinum* and botulinum toxin in the stools. Organisms and toxin may persist in stools many weeks after recovery from the illness, allowing retrospective diagnosis in some instances (Arnon et al. 1977). Unlike the adult form of the disease, toxin has not usually been identified in serum in the infantile variety of botulism. Electrodiagnostic tests are important in the recognition of this illness in that motor nerve conduction velocities are normal, but electromyography reveals a characteristic pattern with brief, small amplitude-abundant motor unit potentials (BSAPs), and in some cases, small numbers of fibrillation potentials and positive waves (Clay et al., McKee et al.). Muscle enzymes are normal, as are the findings of cerebrospinal fluid examination.

The source from which the infant with botulism acquires *Clostridium botulinum* has largely been unclear, although it is known that the organism is widely distributed in dust, soil, and a number of agricultural products. Honey is sometimes contaminated with botulinum spores and Arnon et al. (1979) have shown a definite association between exposure to honey and the occurrence of infantile botulism in some of the documented cases. For this reason, it has been recommended that honey should not be used as a sweetener of foods or placed on pacifiers for infants less than 12 months of age.

Treatment of infantile botulism is largely conservative, with the most important aspect being maintenance of adequate ventilation, by respirator support if necessary. Oral feeding should be discontinued until recovery of the swallowing mechanism has occurred. The role of antitoxin is not yet known, and, to this date, has not been used in the majority of identified cases. Since the great majority of infants hospitalized and identified as having this disease have recovered without antitoxin therapy (Johnson et al.), its use in the infant age group should be withheld in view of the potential adverse effects of the preparation. The same is true of oral antibiotics for the purpose of eradication of the organism from the intestinal tract. Since the toxin is released from the bacterium upon bacterial cell lysis, it is theoretically possible that antibiotic therapy might temporarily result in a large amount of toxin suddenly being made available to the circulation, provoking acute respiratory compromise. Worsening of muscle weakness and acute respiratory decompensation in infants with botulism has been attributed to the use of aminoglycoside antibiotics, agents known to interfere with neuromuscular transmission under certain circumstances (L'Hommedieu et al.). Drugs in this category should be avoided in patients with this illness until full recovery of muscle strength has occurred.

Diagnosis

Because of the rare occurrence of this disease, an isolated case or the first case in a cluster is difficult to recognize clinically. Diagnosis is facilitated when a suspected contaminated food that was consumed is mentioned in the history. The possibility of botulism is also more likely to be considered if gastrointestinal symptoms precede neurologic signs, or if more than one person in a group is involved in similar fashion.

Laboratory confirmation of the diagnosis of botulism depends upon the identification of the toxin either in blood from the patient or in the suspected food substance. The usual laboratory technique is the intraperitoneal injection of blood from the patient into mice, some of which are protected by antitoxin of the various types. Toxin-containing blood causes an illness in unprotected mice characterized by progressive muscular and respiratory paralysis and followed by death within a few days after injection. The protection in mice by type-specific antitoxin adds further evidence of the diagnosis and identifies the offending type. It is not clear how long after onset of symptoms toxin can be demonstrated in sera of patients with botulism. Whittaker et al. demonstrated the presence of toxin up to ten days and Christie has suggested that it may be present up to 30 days after the onset of the illness. Saline extracts of food may be studied in similar fashion in an effort to identify the toxin. In addition, the suspected food plus gastric washings and stools from the affected patient should be cultured in an effort to isolate *Clostridium botulinum.*

Examination of the stools for *Clostridium botulinum* and toxin has not been emphasized in the past but has been shown by Dowell et al. (1977) to be an important diagnostic adjunct to serum examination. This is especially true in cases of infantile botulism in which toxin is not usually detected in serum but organisms and toxin are identified in the stools during the acute stage of the illness and often for long periods of time thereafter. In a series of 60 adult patients with food-borne botulism, Dowell and colleagues found that the diagnosis could be confirmed in only 33.3 percent on the basis of identification of toxin in serum but that the confirmation rate was increased to 72.9 percent by analyzing serum for toxin and stools for toxin and organisms.

Treatment

Type-specific antitoxin is recommended for the treatment of botulism although its value has been questioned by certain authorities, especially if it is given after the onset of neurologic signs. Because of the urgency of early initiation of antitoxin treatment, it must be started on the basis of a clinical diagnosis and before there is laboratory confirmation of the presence of the toxin. Bivalent botulism antitoxin of equine origin containing types A and B antitoxin is available from Lederle laboratories, while type E is obtained from the Public Health Service. Prior to its administration, a skin test should be done by the intradermal injection of 0.1 ml. of a 1:10 saline dilution of the material and the reaction read ten to 30 minutes later. A positive test indicating horse serum sensitivity includes the formation of wheals and erythema surrounding the area of injection. The adult dose of bivalent antitoxin is 10,000 units (one vial) given intravenously, which may be repeated every four hours to a total of five vials. The antitoxin for intravenous injection should be diluted 1:10 with 5 percent glucose and the initial 10 ml. should be administered slowly over a five-minute period. It is advisable to have available a syringe containing 1 ml. of 1:1,000 epinephrine hydrochloride when the antitoxin is injected. Use of epinephrine is indicated should the patient develop respiratory distress or anaphylaxis. It is generally believed that the earlier in the course of the illness that the antitoxin is given, the more beneficial it will be. In addition to its use in the patient exhibiting symptoms, antitoxin should be given to others who shared the probable contaminated meal even though symptoms haven't yet appeared.

In those whose illness progresses to the stage of bulbar paresis and respiratory muscle paralysis, artificial ventilation and methods to support blood pressure are necessary. This requires constant and expert surveillance and, in most centers, is best accomplished in an intensive care unit with skilled nurse attendants. Patients needing respirator care require tracheostomy because of the length of the illness.

Guanidine hydrochloride has recently been shown to improve the neuromuscular block in patients with botulism and may provide a means to sustain respiration in some cases without ventilatory assistance (Cherington and Ryan, Scaer et al.). While guanidine frequently brings about improvement of ocular muscle dysfunction, the effect on respiratory function is not constant and is often not beneficial (Puggiari and Cherington). The effect of guanidine is believed to result from its ability to stimulate the release of acetylcholine at the neuromuscular junction. Cherington and Ryan recommended that it be given orally in a dose of 15 to 35 mg. per kilogram per day in divided doses. Other methods of treatment that have been recommended include gastric lavage with 2 percent sodium bicarbonate to neutralize toxin within the stomach, enemas in patients with constipation to accelerate elimination of toxin, and antibiotics to eradicate *Clostridium botulinum* from the intestinal tract (Petty). While such procedures may be of some help in selected cases, the most critical aspects of management remain early identification of the illness and prompt administration of type-specific antitoxin, in addition to the prevention of hypoxia by close attention to the airway and respiratory function.

Mortality from this disease varies, depending on the amount and type of toxin present in the food and the quantity of the contaminated food that is consumed. Mortality rates recorded from series in the past have relatively little meaning, since they vary from 1 to 100 percent. At least it can be said that botulism is a potentially serious disease with a significant mortality rate in persons with generalized involvement that includes respiratory insufficiency.

REFERENCES

Arnon, S. S., Midura, T. F., Clay, S. A., Wood, R. M., and Chin, J.: Infant botulism. Epidemiological, clinical, and laboratory aspects. J.A.M.A. 237:1946–1951, 1977.

Arnon, S. S., Midura, T. F., Damus, K., Wood, R. M., and Chin, J.: Intestinal infection and toxin production by Clostridium botulinum as one cause of sudden infant death syndrome. Lancet 1:1273–1276, 1978.

Arnon, S. S., Midura, T. F., Damus, K., Thompson, B., Wood, R. M., and Chin, J.: Honey and other environmental risk factors for infant botulism. J. Pediat. 94:331–336, 1979.

Bishop, G. H., and Bronfenbrenner, J. J.: The site of action of botulinus toxin. Am. J. Physiol. 117:393–404, 1936.

Black, R. E., and Arnon, S. S.: Botulism in the United States, 1976. J. Infect. Dis. 136:829–832, 1977.

Brooks, V. B.: Motor nerve filament block produced by botulinum toxin. Science 117:334–335, 1953.

Brooks, V. B.: The action of botulinum toxin on motor-nerve filaments. J. Physiol. 123:501–515, 1954.

Cherington, M.: Botulism. Ten-year experience. Arch. Neurol. 30:432–437, 1974.

Cherington, M., and Ryan, D. W.: Botulism and guanidine. New Eng. J. Med. 278:931–933, 1968.

Cherington, M., and Ryan, D. W.: Treatment of botulism with guanidine. Early neurophysiologic studies. New Eng. J. Med. 282:195–197, 1970.

Christie, A. B.: Infectious diseases: Epidemiology and clinical practice. E. S. Livingstone, Ltd., Edinburgh and London, 1969, p. 180.

Clay, S. A., Ramseyer, J. C., Fishman, L. S., and Sedgwick, R. P.: Acute infantile motor unit disorder. Infantile botulism? Arch. Neurol. 34:236–243, 1977.

de Jesus, P. V., Jr., Slater, R., Spitz, L. K., and Penn, A. S.: Neuromuscular physiology of wound botulism. Arch. Neurol. 29:425–431, 1973.

Dickson, E. C., and Shevsky, E.: Studies on the manner in which the toxin of Clostridium botulin acts on the body. J. Exp. Med. 37:711–731, 1923.

Dowell, V. R., Jr., McCroskey, L. M., Hatheway, C. L., Lombard, G. L., Hughes, J. M., and Merson, M. H.: Coproexamination for botulinal toxin and *Clostridium botulinum*. A new procedure for laboratory diagnosis of botulism. J.A.M.A. 238:1829–1832, 1977.

Duff, J. T., Wright, O. C., and Yarinkoky, A.: Activation of Clostridium botulinus type E toxin by trypsin. J. Bact. 72:455–460, 1956.

Grover, W. D., Peckham, G. J., and Berman, P. H.: Recovery following cranial nerve dysfunction and muscle weakness in infancy. Dev. Med. Child. Neurol. 16:163–171, 1974.

Guttmann, L., and Pratt, L.: Pathophysiologic aspects of human botulism. Arch. Neurol. 33:175–179, 1976.

Guyton, A. C., and MacDonald, M. A.: Physiology of botulinus toxin. Arch. Neurol. Psychiat. 57:578–592, 1947.

Jenzer, G., Mumenthaler, M., Ludin, H. P., and Robert, F.: Autonomic dysfunction in botulism B: A clinical report. Neurology 25:150–153, 1975.

Johnson, R. O., Clay, S. A., and Arnon, S. S.: Diagnosis and management of infant botulism. Am. J. Dis. Child. 133:586–593, 1979.

L'Hommedieu, C., Stough, R., Brown, L., Kettrick, R., and Polin, R.: Potentiation of neuromuscular weakness in infant botulism by aminoglycosides. J. Pediat. 95:1065–1070, 1979.

McKee, K. R., Jr., Kilroy, A. W., Harrison, W. W., and Schaffner, W.: Botulism in infancy. Report of a case. Am. J. Dis. Child. 131:857–859, 1977.

Merson, M. H., and Dowell, V. R., Jr.: Epidemiologic

clinical and laboratory aspects of wound botulism. New Eng. J. Med. 289:1005–1010, 1973.

Meyer, K. F.: The status of botulism as a world health problem. Bull. WHO 15:281–298, 1956.

Midura, T. F., and Arnon, S. S.: Infant botulism. Identification of Clostridium botulinum and its toxin in faeces. Lancet 2:934–935, 1976.

Oh, S.: Botulism: Electrophysiologic studies. Ann. Neurol. 1:481–485, 1977.

Petty, C. S.: Botulism: The disease and the toxin. Am. J. Med. Sci. 249:345–359, 1965.

Pickett, J., Berg, B., Chaplin, E., and Brunstetter-Shafer, M-A.: Syndrome of botulism in infancy: Clinical and electrophysiologic study. New Eng. J. Med. 295:770–772, 1976.

Polley, E. H., Vick, J. A., Ciuchta, H. P., Fischetti, D. A., Macchitelli, F. J., and Montanarelli, N.: Botulinum toxin, type A: Effects on central nervous system. Science 147:1036–1037, 1965.

Puggiari, M., and Cherington, M.: Botulism and guanidine. Ten years later. J.A.M.A. 240:2276–2277, 1978.

Ryan, D. W., and Cherington, M.: Human type A botulism. J.A.M.A. 216:513–514, 1971.

Scaer, R. C., Tooker, J., and Cherington, M.: Effect of guanidine on the neuromuscular block of botulism. Neurology 19:1107–1110, 1969.

Terranova, W., Palumbo, J. N., and Breman, J. G.: Ocular findings in botulism type B. J.A.M.A. 241:475–477, 1979.

Turner, H. D., Brett, E. M., Gilbert, R. J., Ghosh, A. C., and Liebeschuetz, H. J.: Infant botulism in England. Lancet 1:1277–1278, 1978.

Tyler, H. R.: Botulism. Arch. Neurol. 9:652–660, 1963.

Tyler, H. R.: Physiologic observations in human botulism. Arch. Neurol. 9:661–670, 1963.

Van Ermengem, E.: Recherches sur des cas d'accidents alimentaires. Rev. Hyg. 18:761–819, 1896.

Van Ermengem, E.: Untersuchungen uber falle van fleischver giftung mit symptomen von botulismus. Zbl. Bakt. 19:442, 1896.

Whittaker, R. L., Gilbertson, R. B., and Garrett, A. S., Jr.: Botulism, type E. Report of eight simultaneous cases. Ann. Intern. Med. 61:448–454, 1964.

Chapter Eleven

MYCOPLASMA INFECTIONS AND THE NERVOUS SYSTEM

Mycoplasma species have biological properties different from both viruses and bacteria and are classified under the Order *Mycoplasmatales*. They are filterable agents with the reproductive unit having a diameter of 125 to 250 millimicrons, thus being similar in size to certain of the myxoviruses. Unlike viruses, mycoplasmas are capable of reproduction in a cell-free medium and thus represent the smallest free-living organisms. They lack a rigid cell wall characteristic of bacteria and, for this reason, are entirely resistant to membrane-active antibiotics, including the penicillins. While bacterial L forms and mycoplasmas have a number of similar properties, they are not considered to be related. The biological properties and characteristics of the *Mycoplasma* species have been reviewed by Hayflick and Chanock.

In 1898, Nocard and Roux isolated in cell-free medium the etiologic agent causing bovine pleuropneumonia, which subsequently was named *Mycoplasma mycoides*. Thereafter, organisms with similar properties were isolated and were referred to as pleuropneumonia-like organisms, and in 1929 the term mycoplasma was proposed by Nowak. In 1938, Reimann coined the term primary atypical pneumonia to describe pneumonia with features atypical in comparison to those caused by the common bacterial offenders. Eaton and colleagues in 1944 reported the isolation of a "filterable" agent from patients with atypical pneumonia which could be propagated in embryonated eggs and which

produced pneumonia in laboratory animals. Many cases of so-called atypical pneumonia were discovered to be associated with the development of cold agglutinins in the serum (Peterson et al.), a finding which suggested that at least a certain number of cases of atypical pneumonia might have an etiologic origin in common. In 1957, it was demonstrated that the Eaton agent could be observed by immunofluorescence in the chick embryo lung (Liu), and in 1962, Chanock et al. identified the pleuropneumonia-like organism causing primary atypical pneumonia to be a mycoplasma, and subsequently the name *Mycoplasma pneumoniae* was assigned.

In addition to *Mycoplasma pneumoniae*, human species of mycoplasma include *Mycoplasma salivarium, Mycoplasma orale,* and the so-called genital strains, including *Mycoplasma hominis, Mycoplasma fermentans,* and T-strains of mycoplasma *(Ureaplasma urealyticum),* with the T-designation assigned because of their property of producing very tiny colonies on agar (Shepard). *Mycoplasma salivarium* and *Mycoplasma orale* are sometimes found in oropharyngeal secretions of healthy persons and are not considered to be significant pathogens.

Among the human mycoplasmas, *Mycoplasma pneumoniae* is by far the most important cause of clinical illness in children. It is now known to be a significant pathogen, producing acute upper and lower respiratory tract infection in humans. The characteristic pattern of lower respiratory infection with

277

Mycoplasma pneumoniae is an insidious onset of cough, fever, and headache in an older child or young adult who is found to have minimally to moderately abnormal physical signs, a normal or near normal total white blood cell count, and pulmonary infiltration of variable degree on chest x-ray (Clyde and Denny, Cordero et al.). In most instances, the roentgenographic abnormalities are patchy and segmental, although lobar consolidation identical to that with pneumococcal pneumonia can occur (Stevens et al.). The average duration of illness is two to three weeks, and it is generally believed that the illness can be somewhat abbreviated by tetracycline or erythromycin therapy. Less common manifestations of infection include hemolytic anemia, gastroenteritis, polyarthritis, pericarditis, and cutaneous lesions of various types. Involvement of the central or peripheral nervous system is believed to be a rare expression of infection with *Mycoplasma pneumoniae*.

Mucocutaneous lesions have been said to occur in 15 to 25 percent of patients with other manifestations of *Mycoplasma pneumoniae* infection. Erythema multiforme of the minor variety and of the Stevens-Johnson type has received greatest attention (Fleming et al., Ludlam et al.), although morbilliform and vesicular rashes have also been described (Lascari et al., Teisch et al.). In most instances, rashes attributed to *Mycoplasma pneumoniae* have occurred in conjunction with respiratory infection; however, erythema multiforme has been described as the sole manifestation of infection (Lyell et al.).

Respiratory infection due to *Mycoplasma pneumoniae* has been recognized most frequently in individuals of from five to 20 years of age. It was previously assumed that infection with this organism rarely occurred in children under five years of age. Recent studies have shown that infection below age five years is probably quite common, although in the majority of instances it remains asymptomatic or produces only minor clinical illness (Brunner et al., Fernald et al.). The immunosuppressed patient does not appear to be at special risk for *Mycoplasma pneumoniae* infections. The illness has been observed in a small number of patients with antibody-deficient syndromes and, while symptoms were more severe than usual, cessation of excretion of the organism and eventual recovery indicated that cell-mediated immunity plays some role in natural resistance (Foy et al.). The lack of development of pulmonary infiltrates in these patients has been used as one bit of evidence that infection of the bronchial mucosa is primary with this organism and that pulmonary infiltration represents a host immune response. Pneumonia caused by *Mycoplasma pneumoniae* has also been said to be more severe than customary in children with sickle-cell disease, although the explanation for this is uncertain (Shulman et al.).

Mycoplasma hominis is frequently found to be present on the genital mucosa of women during pregnancy and often results in colonization of the newborn infant (Klein et al.). Despite this, it rarely gives rise to invasive disease in the neonate or young infant.

Diagnostic Methods

Diagnosis of *Mycoplasma pneumoniae* infection is accomplished by demonstration of an appropriate serum rise in specific antibody titer or by isolation of the organism from body fluids or tissue specimens. Isolation of the organism from blood is rare and has been unsuccessful from CSF specimens in patients with central nervous system involvement. Growth of *Mycoplasma pneumoniae* requires the use of the proper laboratory media and usually requires a period of 10 days or more. Among the serologic techniques, indirect immunofluorescence was originally the standard method; however, it is laborious and has largely been replaced by the complement fixation test and the growth inhibition antibody test. The complement fixation method is most widely available and uses an antigen prepared from lipid extracts of the organism. The complement fixation titer begins to rise in the second week after infection and usually peaks in three to four weeks. Titers remain significantly elevated for several months and fall to minimal levels by two years. A fourfold or greater rise in titer is diagnostic of infection with *Mycoplasma pneumoniae*. A single titer of 1 to 64 or higher in the convalescent period strongly suggests recent infection with this organism.

There is a significant relationship between infection with *Mycoplasma pneumoniae* and a cold agglutinin titer rise; however, the test is nonspecific, since cold agglutinins can be found with other viral infections and do not always develop with *Mycoplasma pneumoniae* infections. Seventy-two to 92 percent of patients with pneumonia who developed cold agglutinins were found to have a titer rise that was indicative of infection with *Mycoplasma pneumoniae* (Chanock et al. 1963); however, it is not uncommon that patients known to have such infections will not develop cold agglutinins (Chanock et al. 1961). The cold agglutinin titer usually becomes positive approximately seven days after onset of infection and peaks in four to six weeks. Agglutinins for the MG strain of streptococci also develop in some persons with *Mycoplasma pneumoniae* infections, although this occurs less often than the development of cold agglutinins.

Mycoplasma pneumoniae *Infections*

Even before the discovery of *Mycoplasma pneumoniae* as the pleuropneumonia-like organism commonly causing acute respiratory infection in young persons, cases were described of aseptic meningitis and acute encephalitis in association with atypical pneumonia or cold-agglutinin-positive respiratory infection (Skoldenberg, Yesnick). With the development of serologic techniques which document the occurrence of infection with *Mycoplasma pneumoniae*, it was found that a variety of neurologic syndromes might occur in association with this infection on rare occasion. The neurologic complications that have been recognized include acute aseptic meningitis and meningoencephalitis, transverse myelitis, acute cerebellar ataxia, and cranial and peripheral neuropathy. The majority of reported cases have occurred in older children and young adults, corresponding to the age group in which symptomatic *Mycoplasma pneumoniae* respiratory infections most commonly occur. In a literature review of 48 patients with central nervous system complications attributed to infection with *Mycoplasma pneumoniae*, Lerer and Kalavsky found that 21 percent had no evidence of respiratory infection, while 58 percent had bronchitis or pneumonia and 21 percent had otitis or upper respiratory signs preceding the neurologic disorder.

Reported examples of aseptic meningitis related to *Mycoplasma pneumoniae* have been mild, transient illnesses followed by rapid recovery (Sterner and Biberfeld). Acute meningoencephalitis associated with *Mycoplasma pneumoniae* infection is usually a rather severe illness manifested by fever, meningeal signs, disturbance in state of consciousness ranging from lethargy to deep coma, and a variety of multifocal or focal signs of cerebral or brain stem dysfunction (Hodges et al., Lerer and Kalavsky). A common pattern characteristic of many of the reported examples has been the rapid development of deep coma associated with seizures and other neurologic signs, followed by prompt and complete recovery over the course of the ensuing days. Although the prognosis is assumed to be favorable in most cases despite the severity of the acute illness, death has been described on rare occasion and permanent sequelae have been observed in some (Dorff and Lind, Lerer and Kalavsky, Taylor et al.).

The CSF in patients with acute meningoencephalitis associated with *Mycoplasma pneumoniae* infection is quite variable. Cells may be absent in the CSF, but in most cases the cellular response varies from 10 to 300 per cu. mm. and occasionally even higher. Lymphocytes usually are the predominant cell type, although in some cases there is initially a polymorphonuclear cell response. The protein content is normal or slightly elevated and the glucose content is expected to be normal. A reduced CSF glucose content has been reported in this disorder (Klimek et al.), but this is an unusual exception. Mycoplasma has not been isolated from the CSF despite repeated attempts. There is little available information to date about the neuropathology of acute meningoencephalitis associated with *Mycoplasma pneumoniae* infection. Cerebral biopsy in one patient reported by Taylor et al. showed softening and edema of the brain and only nonspecific cellular changes. Autopsy cases described by Dorff and Lind revealed cerebral swelling, leptomeningeal infiltration with lymphocytes, granulocytes and macrophages, and thrombi within leptomeningeal vessels. Neuronal degeneration and some perivascular infiltration with mononuclear cells were seen within the brain.

Acute transverse myelitis manifested by long tract signs in concert with a sensory level (Klimek et al.) and a spinal cord syndrome initially resembling poliomyelitis (Warren et al.) have also been identified as rare manifestations of *Mycoplasma pneumoniae* infection. Acute cerebellar ataxia has been attributed to infection with this organism, although the few recorded cases have usually had other features indicative of meningoencephalitis (Steele et al.). Peripheral neuropathy of the Guillain-Barré type and cranial neuropathies are additional conditions that have been associated with infection with *Mycoplasma pneumoniae* (Hodges and Perkins, Steele et al.). In a study of 100 patients with the Guillain-Barré syndrome, Goldschmidt et al. identified serologic evidence of recent infection with *Mycoplasma pneumoniae* in 5 percent.

Combinations of the above types of neurologic insult can also occur, as exemplified by the adult patient described by Rothstein and Kenny who exhibited cranial neuropathy, spinal radiculopathy, myelopathy, and myositis. Arthur and Margolis reported two adults with granulomatous angiitis of the brain in which electron microscopy revealed mycoplasma-like structures within the granulomatous lesions of the vessel walls. The authors suggested a possible causative role of *Mycoplasma* species in this disorder, although additional studies in similar cases will be needed to clarify a possible relationship. The possibility of a disorder in humans characterized by necrotizing arteritis is especially intriguing in view of the cerebral vasculitis which has been shown to occur in turkeys following the intravenous injection of *Mycoplasma gallisepticum* (Clyde and Thomas, Thomas et al.). In at least one instance, *Mycoplasma pneumoniae* has been incriminated as a cause of intrauterine infection, giving rise to a newborn infant with hydrocephalus and other congenital defects (Bray and Hackett).

Although there is little doubt that *Mycoplasma pneumoniae* can provoke most of the previously-described central and peripheral nervous system complications, the mechanism by which tissue injury occurs is entirely unclear. Relative to respiratory infection with this organism, concepts have been proposed that the primary site of attack is upon the bronchial mucosa and that pneumonitis is, perhaps, a manifestation of the host immune response rather than a direct inflammatory reaction secondary to tissue invasion with mycoplasmas (Fernald et al.). The inability to isolate *Mycoplasma pneumoniae* from the CSF, the occasional absence of cells in CSF, and the lack of apparent response to tetracycline in cases of acute meningoencephalitis associated with *Mycoplasma pneumoniae* infection might suggest that tissue immune response plays an important role in the pathogenesis of neurologic signs.

Mycoplasma hominis *Infections*

Mycoplasma hominis and the T-strains are referred to as genital mycoplasmas and are commonly found in the genitourinary tract of healthy women of reproductive age. Genital mycoplasmas are infrequently isolated from prepubertal girls, but, after puberty, genital colonization occurs primarily through sexual contact. While the incidence with which genital colonization occurs varies in different social groups in women of reproductive age, positive isolates have been found in 50 to 70 percent (McCormack et al., Shurin et al.). Thus, it is not surprising that colonization of the newborn infant is a frequent event. Klein and colleagues were able to isolate genital mycoplasmas, most often those of T-strains, from the throat in 22 percent of newborn infants less than 2,500 grams and in 12 percent of neonates over 2,500 grams at birth. Despite their frequent colonization of normal newborn infants, these organisms are uncommonly associated with invasive disease in the neonate. They have been incriminated as a cause of spontaneous abortion (Caspi et al., Jones), of congenital pneumonia (Tafari et al.), of neonatal conjunctivitis (Jones and Tobin), and of suppurative adenopathy in the newborn infant (Powell et al.), but colonization is generally regarded to be common and of little consequence.

Examples of neonatal *Mycoplasma hominis* meningitis have been described in recent years, most often in low-birth-weight infants born of mothers with symptomatic perinatal infection or perinatal complications of other types (Boe et al., Gewitz et al.). Onset of illness in reported cases has been between five and 15 days after birth. Unlike *Mycoplasma pneumoniae* intracranial infections in older persons, in these cases in newborn infants *Mycoplasma hominis* has been recovered from the CSF. In addition, the CSF findings were usually more characteristic of suppurative meningitis in the newborn period, with high cell counts composed mainly of granulocytes and striking elevation of the protein content. Clinical signs indicated severe cerebral injury and the outcome was not favorable in these cases. A further example described by Siber et al. was a premature infant born of a mother with amnionitis. Signs of meningitis appeared at eight days of age, and several days later a frontal abscess was drained, from which *Mycoplasma hominis* was recovered. *Mycoplasma hominis* has also been found to be a cause of meningitis in infants with meningomyeloceles (Wealthall). Neonatal *Mycoplasma hominis* meningitis is a rare disorder but one in which mycoplasmas invade the CSF, resulting in an intense inflammatory response with potential serious cerebral injury. Tetracycline therapy would be indicated in such instances.

REFERENCES

Arthur, G., and Margolis, G.: Mycoplasma-like structures in granulomatous angiitis of the central nervous system. Case reports with light and electron microscopic studies. Arch. Path. Lab. Med. 101:382–387, 1977.

Boe, O., Diderichsen, J., and Matre, R.: Isolation of Mycoplasma hominis from cerebrospinal fluid. Scand. J. Infect. Dis. 5:285–288, 1973.

Bray, P. F., and Hackett, T. N.: Multiple birth defects in a newborn exposed to Mycoplasma pneumoniae in utero. Am. J. Dis. Child. 130:312–314, 1976.

Brunner, H., Prescott, B., Greenberg, H., James, W. D., Horswood, R. L., and Chanock, R. M.: Unexpectedly high frequency of antibody of Mycoplasma pneumoniae in human sera as measured by sensitive techniques. J. Infect. Dis. 135:524–530, 1977.

Caspi, E., Solomon, F., and Sompolinsky, D.: Early abortion and mycoplasma infection. Isr. J. Med. Sci. 8:122–127, 1972.

Chanock, R. M., Hayflick, L., and Barile, M. F.: Growth on artificial medium of an agent associated with atypical pneumonia and its identification as a PPLO. Proc. Natl. Acad. Sci. U.S.A. 48:41–49, 1962.

Chanock, R. M., Mufson, M. A., Bloom, H. H., James, W. D., Fox, H. H., and Kingston, J. R.: Eaton agent pneumonia. J.A.M.A. 175:213–220, 1961.

Chanock, R. M., Mufson, M. A., Somerson, N. L., and Couch, R. B.: Role of mycoplasma (PPLO) in human respiratory disease. Am. Rev. Respir. Dis. 88:218–231, 1963.

Clyde, W. A., Jr., and Denny, F. W.: Mycoplasma infections in childhood. Pediatrics 40:669–684, 1967.

Clyde, W. A., Jr., and Thomas, L.: Pathogenesis studies in experimental Mycoplasma disease: Mycoplasma gallisepticum infections of turkeys. Ann. N. Y. Acad. Sci. 225:413–424, 1973.

Cordero, L., Cuadrado, R., Hall, C. B., and Horstmann, D. M.: Primary atypical pneumonia: An epidemic caused by Mycoplasma pneumoniae. J. Pediat. 71:1–12, 1967.

Dorff, B., and Lind, K.: Two fatal cases of meningoencephalitis associated with Mycoplasma pneumoniae infection. Scand. J. Infect. Dis. 8:49–51, 1976.

Eaton, M. D., Meiklejohn, G., and van Herick, W.: Studies on the etiology of primary atypical pneumonia. A filterable agent transmissible to cotton rats, hamsters, and chick embryos. J. Exp. Med. 79:649–668, 1944.

Fernald, G. W., Collier, A. M., and Clyde, W. A., Jr.: Respiratory infections due to Mycoplasma pneumoniae in infants and children. Pediatrics 55:327–335, 1975.

Fleming, P. C., Krieger, E., Turner, J. A. P., Watty, E. I., Quinn, P. A., and Bannatyne, R. M.: Febrile mucocutaneous syndrome with respiratory involvement associated with isolation of Mycoplasma pneumoniae. Canad. Med. Assoc. J. 97:1458–1459, 1967.

Foy, H. M., Ochs, H., Davis, S. D., Kenny, G. E., and Luce, R. R.: Mycoplasma pneumoniae infections in patients with immunodeficiency syndromes: Report of four cases. J. Infect. Dis. 127:388–393, 1973.

Gewitz, M., Dinwiddie, R., Rees, L., Volikas, O., Yuille, T., O'Connell, B., and Marshall, W. C.: Mycoplasma hominis. A cause of neonatal meningitis. Arch. Dis. Childh. 54:231–239, 1979.

Goldschmidt, B., Menonna, J., Fortunato, J., Dowling, P., and Cook, S.: Mycoplasma antibody in Guillain-Barré syndrome and other neurological disorders. Ann. Neurol. 7:108–112, 1980.

Hayflick, L., and Chanock, R. M.: Mycoplasma species in man. Bact. Rev. 29:185–221, 1965.

Hodges, G. R., and Perkins, R. L.: Landry-Guillain-Barré syndrome associated with Mycoplasma pneumoniae infection. J.A.M.A. 210:2088–2090, 1969.

Hodges, G. R., Fass, R. J., and Saslaw, S.: Central nervous system disease associated with Mycoplasma pneumoniae infection. Arch. Intern. Med. 130:277–282, 1972.

Jones, D. M.: Mycoplasma hominis in abortion. Brit. Med. J. 1:338–340, 1967.

Jones, D. M., and Tobin, B.: Neonatal eye infections due to Mycoplasma hominis. Brit. Med. J. 3:467–468, 1968.

Klein, J. O., Buckland, D., and Finland, M.: Colonization of newborn infants by Mycoplasmas. New Eng. J. Med. 280:1025–1030, 1969.

Klimek, J. J., Russman, B. S., and Quintiliani, R.: Mycoplasma pneumoniae meningoencephalitis and transverse myelitis in association with low cerebrospinal fluid glucose. Pediatrics 58:133–135, 1976.

Lascari, A. D., Garfunkel, J. M., and Mauro, D. J.: Varicella-like rash associated with Mycoplasma infection. Am. J. Dis. Child. 128:254–255, 1974.

Lerer, R. J., and Kalavsky, S. M.: Central nervous system disease associated with Mycoplasma pneumoniae infection: Report of five cases and review of the literature. Pediatrics 52:658–668, 1973.

Liu, C.: Studies on primary atypical pneumonia. I. Localization, isolation, and cultivation of a virus in chick embryos. J. Exp. Med. 106:455–467, 1957.

Ludlam, G. B., Bridges, J. B., and Benn, E. C.: Association of Stevens-Johnson syndrome with antibody for Mycoplasma pneumoniae. Lancet 1:958–959, 1964.

Lyell, A., Gordon, A. M., Dick, H. M., and Sommerville, R. G.: Mycoplasmas and erythema multiforme. Lancet 2:1116–1118, 1967.

McCormack, W. M., Braun, P., Lee, Y-H, Klein, J. O., and Kass, E. H.: The genital mycoplasmas. New Eng. J. Med. 288:78–89, 1973.

Nocard, E., and Roux, E. R.: Le microbe de la peripneumonie. Ann. Inst. Pasteur. 12:240–262, 1898.

Nowak, J.: Morphologie, nature et cycle evolutif du microbe de la peripneumonie des bovides. Ann. Inst. Pasteur (Paris). 43:1330–1352, 1929.

Peterson, O. L., Ham, T. H., and Finland, M.: Cold agglutinins (autohemagglutinins) in primary atypical pneumonias. Science 98:167–168, 1943.

Powell, D. A., Miller, K., and Clyde, W. A., Jr.: Suppurative adenitis in a newborn caused by Mycoplasma hominis. Pediatrics 63:798–799, 1979.

Reimann, H. A.: An acute infection of the respiratory tract with atypical pneumonia. J.A.M.A. 111:2377–2384, 1938.

Rothstein, T. L., and Kenny, G. E.: Cranial neuropathy, myeloradiculopathy, and myositis. Complications of Mycoplasma pneumoniae infection. Arch. Neurol. 36:476–477, 1979.

Shepard, M. C.: T-form colonies of pleuropneumonia-like organisms. J. Bact. 71:362–369, 1956.

Shulman, S. T., Bartlett, J., Clyde, W. A., Jr., and Ayoub, E. M.: The unusual severity of mycoplasmal pneumonia in children with sickle-cell disease. New Eng. J. Med. 287:164–167, 1972.

Shurin, P. A., Alpert, S., Rosner, B., Driscoll, S. G., Lee, Y-H., McCormack, W. M., Santamarina, B. A. G., and Kass, E. H.: Chorioamnionitis and colonization of the newborn infant with genital mycoplasmas. New Eng. J. Med. 293:5–7, 1975.

Siber, G. R., Alpert, S., Smith, A. L., Lin, J-S. L., and McCormack, W. M.: Neonatal central nervous system infection due to Mycoplasma hominis. J. Pediat. 90:625–627, 1977.

Skoldenberg, B.: Aseptic meningitis and meningoencephalitis in cold-agglutinin-positive infections. Brit. Med. J. 1:100–102, 1965.

Steele, J. C., Gladstone, R. M., Thanasophon, S., and Fleming, P. C.: Mycoplasma pneumoniae as a determinant of the Guillain-Barré syndrome. Lancet 2:710–714, 1969.

Steele, J. C., Gladstone, R. M., Thanasophon, S., and Fleming, P. C.: Acute cerebellar ataxia and concomitant infection with Mycoplasma pneumoniae. J. Pediat. 80:467–469, 1972.

Sterner, G., and Biberfeld, G.: Central nervous system complications of Mycoplasma pneumoniae infection. Scand. J. Infect. Dis. 1:203–208, 1969.

Stevens, D., Swift, P. G. F., Johnston, P. G. B., Kearney, P. J., Corner, B. D., and Burman, D.: Mycoplasma pneumoniae infections in children. Arch. Dis. Childh. 53:38–42, 1978.

Tafari, N., Ross, S., Naeye, R. L., Judge, D. M., and Marboe, C.: Mycoplasma T strains and perinatal death. Lancet 1:108–109, 1976.

Taylor, M. J., Burrow, G. N., Strauch, B., and Horstmann, D. M.: Meningoencephalitis associated with pneumonitis due to *Mycoplasma pneumoniae.* J.A.M.A. 199:813–816, 1967.

Teisch, J. A., Shapiro, L., and Walzer, R. A.: Vesiculopustular eruption with Mycoplasma infection. J.A.M.A. 211:1694–1697, 1970.

Thomas, L., Davidson, M., and McClusky, R. T.: Studies of PPLO infection: I. The production of cerebral arteritis by *Mycoplasma gallisepticum* in turkeys: The neurotoxic property of the mycoplasma. J. Exp. Med. 123:897–912, 1966.

Warren, P., Fischbein, C., Mascoli, N., Rudolph, J., and Hodder, D. H.: Poliomyelitis-like syndrome caused by Mycoplasma pneumoniae. J. Pediat. 93:451–452, 1978.

Wealthall, S. R.: Mycoplasma meningitis in infants with spina bifida. Dev. Med. Child Neurol. 17 (Suppl. 35):117–122, 1975.

Yesnick, L.: Central nervous system complications of primary atypical pneumonia. Arch. Intern. Med. 97:93–98, 1956.

PART
II

Viral Infections of the Nervous System

Chapter Twelve

INTRODUCTION— VIRUSES AND THE NERVOUS SYSTEM

Viruses have long been known to be the cause of a multiplicity of human diseases, but the entire spectrum continues to unfold with new observations. The word "virus" is derived from Latin meaning poison or venom; its use in reference to an infecting agent too small to be seen by the conventional microscope dates to the latter part of the nineteenth century. The techniques and advances of modern medicine have developed the means to conquer certain devastating viral infections, but at the same time have led to the development of sophisticated new methods of treatment such as organ transplantation and immunosuppressive therapy, which have added an entirely new dimension to the pathogenic effects of certain viruses.

Knowledge of the chemical and structural properties of viruses and of their mode of reproduction has perplexed investigators for many years and has been clarified only in the recent past. Viruses, unlike bacteria, lack enzymes. Their reproduction is dependent upon living cells that provide the enzyme systems necessary for their replication. The mature virus particle, referred to as the virion, is an obligatory intracellular parasite, dependent upon a living cell for its reproduction. Virions vary in size, from the poliovirus with a diameter of approximately 30 nanometers up to certain poxviruses which are 300 nanometers in diameter. By comparison, a human erythrocyte has a diameter of 7,500 nanometers. The virion is composed of a nucleic acid, either deoxyribonucleic acid (DNA) or

ribonucleic acid (RNA), which is surrounded by a protein shell called the capsid. The morphologic units of the capsid are termed capsomeres. With certain "small" viruses, such as the picornaviruses, the nucleic acid and its surrounding capsid form the nucleocapsid. More complex viruses have, in addition, an envelope which encases the capsid.

Mechanisms of viral infection at the cellular level include the initial step of contact and attachment of the virus to the cell surface, a process called absorption. Penetration is followed by uncoating, which is the liberation of the infectious nucleic acid from its protective coat. The host cell is then directed to synthesize viral protein and assemble new viral particles (Johnson and Johnson). Newly assembled virions are next released from the cell by one of several methods. When the mechanism is by direct cell-to-cell transfer as occurs with herpes viruses, the extracellular fluid is not entered and the virus is thereby not exposed to type-specific humoral antibody.

Classification

Classification of viruses has gradually changed over the years as new methods of analysis of virus characteristics have been developed. Current classification is largely on the basis of features such as type of nucleic acid contained by the virus, capsid symmetry, site of capsid assembly, nucleocapsid envelopment, number of capsomeres, and ether-sensitivity (Melnick) (Table 12–1). The notable exceptions are the members of the arbovirus group, which are classified together on an ecological basis rather than on the basis of physical or biochemical properties. With continued investigation of their characteristics, most of the arboviruses of groups A and B have been classified among the togaviruses, along with the rubella virus.

Classified among the herpesvirus group are several viruses of neurologic importance in man, including *Herpesvirus hominis* types 1 and 2, varicella-zoster virus, cytomegalovirus, and the Epstein-Barr virus. They have been subdivided into two groups on the basis of rapidity of release of virions from infected cells. Viruses in group A are readily released and include *Herpesvirus hominis* types 1 and 2, and *Herpes simiae* of monkeys. Within group B are the varicella-zoster virus, the cytomegaloviruses, and the Epstein-Barr virus, which are more strongly cell-associated and released more slowly. *Herpesvirus hominis* is the most common DNA-containing virus causing acute encephalitis in man, while the cytomegaloviruses are the prevalent viral cause of intra-uterine-acquired fetal infection. The herpes viruses are characterized by a DNA core with a lipid-containing envelope which surrounds the viral capsid.

Among the RNA-containing viruses, the members of greatest importance producing neurologic disease in man are included within the myxoviruses, the picornaviruses, and the togaviruses. As mentioned, the latter includes most, but not all, of the human arboviruses as well as the rubella virus. Of the myxoviruses, the human influenza viruses are classified within the orthomyxovirus group, while the paramyxovirus group includes the mumps, measles, and parainfluenza viruses. The picornaviruses are small RNA viruses, subdivided into at least 65 serotypes of human enteroviruses and 90 rhinovirus serotypes. The name picornavirus is descriptive of its members, with *pico* being derived from small and *rna* indicating the type of contained nucleic acid. Within the enterovirus subgroups, the three serotypes of poliovirus have been recognized for decades with no recent additions, but the number of serotypes of the ECHO viruses and Coxsackie viruses has gradually increased with new discoveries. In recent years, newly identified serotypes have been assigned *enterovirus* type numbers rather than adding additional serotypes to

Table 12–1. Viruses of Neurologic Importance in Man

A. DNA Viruses
Herpesviruses
  Group A
    Herpesvirus hominis, types 1, 2
    Herpes simiae (B virus)
  Group B
    Varicella-zoster virus
    Cytomegalovirus
    Epstein-Barr virus
Adenoviruses
Poxviruses
  Variola virus
  Vaccinia virus
Papovaviruses
B. RNA Viruses
Myxoviruses
  Influenza viruses
  Parainfluenza viruses
  Mumps virus
  Rubeola (measles) virus
Arboviruses (grouping on an ecological basis)
  Mosquito-borne
    California encephalitis virus
    St. Louis encephalitis virus
    Eastern equine encephalitis virus
    Western equine encephalitis virus
    Venezuelan equine encephalitis virus
    Japanese B encephalitis virus (Australian X)
    Yellow fever virus
    Dengue
    West Nile virus
  Tick-borne
    Colorado tick fever virus
    Powassan virus
    Russian spring-summer encephalitis virus
    Louping-ill virus
Picornaviruses
  Enteroviruses
    Polioviruses, types 1, 2, 3
    Coxsackie A virus, type 1–24
    Coxsackie B virus, type 1–6
    Echovirus, type 1–34
  Rhinoviruses (many serotypes)
Togaviruses
  Rubella virus
  Most arboviruses, groups A and B
Arenaviruses
  Lymphocytic choriomeningitis virus
Rhabdoviruses
  Rabies virus

the ECHO or Coxsackie subgroups (Melnick).

Additional RNA-containing viruses of human importance are the rabies virus and lymphocytic choriomeningitis virus. The rabies virus is a representative of a relatively newly classified group referred to as the rhabdovirus group. Other members include the Marburg virus, which is pathogenic for man, and a number of others found in lower species. Lymphocytic choriomeningitis virus is the prototype of the arenaviruses, so-named because of the sandy granules characteristic of the virions.

Neurologic Disorders Associated with Viral Infection

The viral etiology of certain neurologic conditions, such as acute encephalitis, aseptic meningitis, or infection of motor neurons of the spinal cord and brain stem, has been undoubted for many years. This is a group of illnesses about which a great deal of epidemiologic and clinical knowledge has been compiled. For example, certain viruses, such as the arboviruses, cause human disease with well-established seasonal and geographic patterns and, in some instances, even with distinct predilections for attacking patients in certain age groups. *Herpesvirus hominis* type 1 is well-known for its ability to produce a common type of non-seasonal, acute, severe encephalitis, while mumps, Coxsackie, and ECHO viruses characteristically result in aseptic meningitis when they invade the nervous system. Selective involvement of motor neurons in the spinal cord and brain stem has been recognized historically with poliovirus infection; however, in recent years, other enteroviruses and the mumps virus also have

Table 12–2. Neurologic Disorders Associated with Viral Infection

A. Acute illness
 Aseptic meningitis
 Encephalitis, encephalomyelitis
 Post-infectious, post-vaccinal encephalomyelitis
 Acute transverse myelitis
 Poliomyelitis, polio-like myelitis
 Immune brain reaction (acute hemorrhagic
  leukoencephalitis)
B. Chronic illness (chronic progressive viral infections
  of the brain)
 Kuru
 Creutzfeldt-Jakob disease
 Progressive multifocal leukoencephalopathy
 Subacute sclerosing panencephalitis
 Progressive rubella panencephalitis
C. Intrauterine-neonatal illnesses
 Teratogenic disorders (rubella, varicella)
 Chronic viral infection (rubella, cytomegalovirus)
 Neonatal acute infection (Herpesvirus hominis,
  Coxsackie B, ECHO virus)
D. Viral-related disorders
 Reye's syndrome
 Acute cerebellar ataxia
 Guillain-Barré syndrome
 Opsoclonus-polymyoclonus
 Bell's palsy
 Benign sixth nerve palsy of childhood

demonstrated their ability to cause "polio-like" infections.

The relationship of certain viral infections, such as measles and smallpox, to an acute perivenous demyelinating type of encephalitis characteristic of the so-called "post-infectious" encephalitides has also been well established, although the pathogenesis is less clear than with many other types of acute encephalitis. The spectrum of neurologic infection caused by the measles virus, especially, has been expanded by continued observations in recent years. Encephalitis complicating the acute stage of primary measles infection was recognized in the latter part of the last century but is was not until 1965 that the chronic, progressive encephalitis referred to as subacute sclerosing panencephalitis was recognized to be caused by the measles virus (Bouteille et al.). More recently, the measles virus has been incriminated as a cause of a subacute type of encephalitis with distinctive clinical features in immunosuppressed patients (Murphy and Yunis, Wolinsky et al.).

The discovery that viruses can cause chronic infection of the central nervous system in man, producing progressive deteriorative brain disease, was a striking departure from previously held concepts and opened new avenues of research for a number of neurologic disorders. Kuru was the first such human brain disease identified to be a chronic encephalitic disorder. Creutzfeldt-Jakob disease, progressive multifocal leukoencephalopathy, and subacute sclerosing panencephalitis have subsequently been placed in the same category. Chronic progressive panencephalitis caused by the rubella virus is the most recent addition to this list of conditions (Cremer et al., Townsend et al.). Multiple sclerosis and certain other progressive neurologic conditions may also have a viral etiology and are now the subject of intensive investigation in many laboratories.

Viral infection is now known to have some sort of cause-and-effect association with most cases of Guillain-Barré disease, Reye's syndrome, and acute cerebellar ataxia of childhood. The pathogenesis of these viral, or post-viral, syndromes is still quite unclear and probably involves immune mechanisms, and in some instances may require a pre-existent susceptibility or predisposition. The latter seems especially applicable to Reye's syndrome, in view of certain epidemiologic features of the disease. The rare disorder referred to as myoclonic encephalopathy of infancy, or polymyoclonia-opsoclonus, is in the same general category, in that the disease often follows a viral infection or immunization but is not believed to be explained by direct viral invasion of neural tissue. Bell's palsy and a similar condition referred to as benign sixth nerve palsy in childhood (Knox et al.) are also believed to have a viral etiology, largely on the basis of guilt by association. Mononeuropathies of this type are commonly preceded by viral respiratory infections, although a cause-and-effect relationship has rarely been proved. One of the most recent discoveries relating a disorder to a viral etiology is the occurrence of aqueductal stenosis as an aftermath of mumps virus infection. Supported somewhat by clinical observations, the concept was first developed as a result of animal experiments in which the virus-induced aqueductal lesions were found to be similar histologically to those previously assumed to be a congenital anomaly in humans (Johnson and Johnson).

Since the discovery in 1941 of fetal infection by the rubella virus, the significance of viral attack on the immature or developing nervous system has gradually unfolded. We now possess a vast storehouse of knowledge concerning the chronic encephalitis that occurs with intrauterine-acquired cytomegalovirus and rubella virus infections but still have relatively little understanding of the role played by many other viruses. Varicella, *Herpesvirus hominis,* measles, and influenza viruses have all been held suspect as possible causes of intrauterine-acquired encephalitis, and perhaps with teratogenic effects, but with insufficient evidence to be certain to this date. Viral infection can damage the immature nervous system indirectly, either by disturbing the health of the mother or by its effect on the placenta, or, by direct attack on the fetus, causing inflammatory lesions within the brain, chromosomal damage, or alteration of the normal sequence of embryogenesis. Teratogenic effects of intrauterine viral infection, except for those associated with the rubella virus, are more speculative than factual in the human. Studies in animals, however, indicate that congenital anomalies of the nervous system can be induced by fetal virus infection and may be an important factor in certain instances in the human. Neural tube defects have been produced in chick embryos by influenza A infection (Johnson et al., Hamburger and Habel), and aqueductal stenosis resembling the human counterpart has resulted from mumps virus infection in the

hamster (Johnson and Johnson). The blue-tongue virus of sheep also can cause cerebral anomalies in fetal lambs (Shultz and DeLay). There is little doubt that viral infection of the immature nervous system is an underrated factor in the production of a multitude of neurologic abnormalities among infants and children. Defects of neural tube closure, certain cases of epilepsy or mental retardation, and many cases of microcephaly or hydrocephalus may well be the end result of infection early in pregnancy by viruses not generally recognized to be the cause of such defects.

From this brief discussion, it is apparent that viruses can affect the nervous system in a wide variety of ways, giving rise to a remarkable spectrum of neurologic disease. Ingenious laboratory investigations and astute clinical observations by authors mentioned in these chapters have brought together a great deal of comprehension of the many ways that viral infections result in neurologic dysfunction.

REFERENCES

Bouteille, M., Fontaine, C., Bedrenne, C., and Delarue, J.: Sur un cas d' encephalite subaique a inclusions: Etude anatomoclinique et ultrastructurale. Rev. Neurol. 113:454–458, 1965.

Cremer, N. E., Oshiro, L. S., Weil, M. L., Lennette, E. H., Itabashi, H. H., and Carnay, L.: Isolation of rubella virus from brain in chronic progressive panencephalitis. J. Gen. Virol. 29:143–153, 1975.

Hamburger, V., and Habel, K.: Teratogenic and lethal effects of influenza A and mumps viruses on early chick embryos. Proc. Soc. Exp. Biol. Med. 66:608–617, 1947.

Johnson, K. P., Klasnja, R., and Johnson, R. T.: Neural tube defects of chick embryos: An indirect result of influenza A virus infection. J. Neuropath. Exp. Neurol. 30:68–74, 1971.

Johnson, R. T., and Johnson, K. P.: Hydrocephalus following viral infection: The pathology of aqueductal stenosis developing after experimental mumps virus infection. J. Neuropath. Exp. Neurol. 27:591–606, 1968.

Johnson, R. T., and Johnson, K. P.: Slow and chronic virus infections of the nervous system. *In:* Plum, F.: Recent Advances in Neurology. F. A. Davis Company, Philadelphia, 1969.

Knox, D. L., Clark, D. B., and Schuster, F. F.: Benign VI nerve palsies in children. Pediatrics 40:560–564, 1967.

Melnick, J. L.: Classification and nomenclature of animal viruses, 1971. Progr. Med. Virol. 13:462–484, 1971.

Melnick, J. L.: Taxonomy of viruses, 1976. Prog. Med. Virol. 22:211–221, 1976.

Murphy, J. V., and Yunis, E. J.: Encephalopathy following measles infection in children with chronic illness. J. Pediat. 88:937–942, 1976.

Shultz, G., and DeLay, P. D.: Losses in newborn lambs associated with bluetongue vaccination of pregnant ewes. J. Am. Vet. Med. Assoc. 127:224–226, 1955.

Townsend, J. J., Wolinsky, J. S., and Baringer, J. R.: The neuropathology of progressive rubella panencephalitis of late onset. Brain 99:81–90, 1976.

Wolinsky, J. S., Swoveland, P., Johnson, K. P., and Baringer, J. R.: Subacute measles encephalitis complicating Hodgkin's disease in an adult. Ann. Neurol. 1:452–457, 1977.

Chapter Thirteen

VIRAL ENCEPHALITIS AND ASEPTIC MENINGITIS

Viral infections of the central nervous system include a variety of different conditions that can occur in any age group in all degrees of severity. The designations used for such illnesses during life are largely determined by the primary anatomic site of involvement judged clinically. Aseptic meningitis, encephalitis, meningoencephalitis, encephalomyelitis, and myelitis are descriptive terms that are appropriate, depending on whether the main impact of the infection is upon the meninges, the brain, the spinal cord, or combinations of these structures. Such designations are of some predictive importance from the etiologic standpoint, because certain viruses have a propensity to result in one type of neurologic infection more often than another type. For example, mumps, Coxsackie, and ECHO viruses are common causes of aseptic meningitis and, only much less often, result in signs of cerebral parenchymal involvement. Herpesvirus hominis, the arboviruses, and rubeola virus characteristically result in severe encephalitis when they invade the nervous system, and only infrequently provoke aseptic meningitis. Thus, the descriptive diagnosis, in addition to the geographic location and the time of year when the patient acquires the illness, provides a clue to the most likely offending agents.

The clinical manifestations of aseptic meningitis are primarily those of fever, headache, vomiting, and stiffness of the neck along with other signs of meningeal irritation. Irritabil-

ity is common in infants and young children, and a mild degree of lethargy or drowsiness occurs in some. Viral encephalitis is associated with similar findings in many patients but alterations in the state of awareness or behavioral abnormalities represent the symptomatic hallmark of the illness. Agitation or excitement can precede coma in some patients, while others exhibit varying grades of decreased consciousness from the beginning. Papilledema is occasionally observed during the course of viral encephalitis but it is usually mild and without retinal hemorrhages. High-grade papilledema with hemorrhages is sufficiently unusual that its presence should cast doubt on the accuracy of the diagnosis.

The type of neurologic abnormalities that occur in the encephalitic patient depends on the degree of increased intracranial pressure and the areas of the brain most severely affected. Cerebral hemisphere involvement leads to confusion, disorientation, convulsions and variable long tract signs. Movement disorders of many types can result from the effects of the inflammatory process on the basal ganglia and cerebellum. Signs of brain stem dysfunction are often intermixed with above-mentioned signs. Focal neurologic signs can occur with encephalitis regardless of the viral cause, but localizing signs indicative of temporal lobe or orbito-frontal dysfunction are most typical of Herpes simplex encephalitis.

Brain stem encephalitis is an unusual form

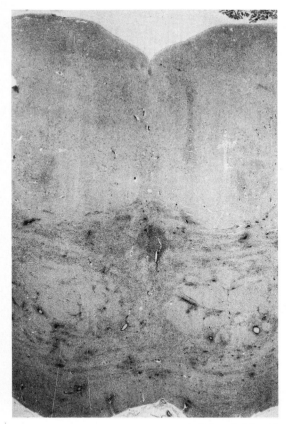

Figure 13–1. Brain stem encephalitis. Child with acute encephalitis manifested primarily by signs of midbrain and pontine involvement. Section through the pons shows heavy perivascular cuffing and vascular distention.

of the disease in which the clinical features are predominantly those of infection within the midbrain, pons, and medulla (Yalaz and Tinaztope, Schain and Wilson, Dayan et al.) (Fig. 13–1). Multiple cranial nerve signs, ataxia, and long tract signs characterize the illness, thus bearing certain features in common with gliomas in the same region. The two illnesses can readily be confused in some instances, especially since posterior displacement of the fourth ventricle on pneumoencephalography can occur with either. Rabies is one type of human encephalitis in which the brain stem is particularly heavily affected, and involvement here probably accounts for the characteristic pharyngeal and laryngeal spasms seen in the early stages of the illness.

Spinal cord involvement with viral neurologic infection usually occurs in association with cerebral dysfunction but can represent the only manifestation of the infectious pro-

cess. It is recognized by the presence of flaccid paraplegia, alteration of deep tendon reflexes, and neurogenic bladder dysfunction.

With any type of viral infection of the central nervous system, the mode of entry of virus, and the mechanism of cell damage therefrom have been only partly clarified. The role of the immune response of the host to a variety of different viral-induced neurologic infections remains unclear and is a subject of continued experimental investigation. There is experimental evidence to indicate that the host immune response is an important factor determining outcome of viral encephalitis (Nathanson and Cole). However, such an immune response can be either detrimental or protective, and both components may be operative in natural infections (Camenga and Nathanson). Spread of virus into the brain by the neural route has been considered important in certain instances but hematogenous dissemination is probably the method by which most viral neurologic infections are brought about (Johnson and Mims). With rabies encephalitis, the human is inoculated at the time of an animal bite in the great majority of cases, and transmission to the brain is by retrograde axoplasmic flow along peripheral nerves. Craig and Nahmias have postulated that Herpes simplex type 1 encephalitis may result from transmission of the virus from the nasopharynx via the olfactory nerves to the frontal and temporal lobes, while type 2 disseminated infection in the newborn or aseptic meningitis in the adult is on a hematogenous basis. The fact that type 1 Herpes simplex virus is rarely isolated from blood or cerebrospinal fluid while type 2 can be in some cases is support for this concept.

With most types of encephalitis, pathologic changes are the end result of invasion of the brain by the offending virus. The pathogenesis of so-called post-infectious or post-vaccinal encephalitis must somehow implicate other factors to account for the striking perivenous demyelination that is characteristic of these disorders. Allergic or immune mechanisms have been implicated in this group, although in certain instances, entry of virus into the brain has been demonstrated. With acute rubeola encephalitis, it is postulated that virus invasion and replication in brain tissue leads to tissue damage, which initiates a host immune response directed against host tissue, leading to the characteristic pathologic changes in the perivenous distribution (ter Meulen et al.).

Viral infections of the central nervous system are reasonably common but when one considers the high frequency of respiratory and systemic viral illness that occurs in children, it is apparent that encephalitis and aseptic meningitis are very infrequent complications of most. It is currently estimated that an etiologic agent can be identified in 50 to 70 percent of viral neurologic infections in laboratories with adequate facilities when a diligent search is made (Klemola et al., Cramblett et al.). The possibility of discovery of a specific cause is greater in cases with aseptic meningitis than in those with encephalitis.

Many viruses can cause acute encephalitis or aseptic meningitis, but most cases result from common viruses, including the enteroviruses, members of the herpesvirus group, the mumps virus, and the arboviruses. Arbovirus and enteroviral infections are generally seasonal illnesses and frequently occur in clusters or epidemics, while Herpes simplex encephalitis is sporadic, occurs at any time of the year, and is regarded to be the most common type of severe, non-seasonal encephalitis. Polio and measles virus infections have now been sharply curtailed in this country by the use of effective immunizing agents but neither is yet eliminated. Less frequent causes are the lymphocytic choriomeningitis virus, the adenoviruses, rabies virus, Epstein-Barr virus, and the presumed virus which causes cat scratch disease. Cytomegalovirus is a notable opportunistic invader of the immunosuppressed host but is a rare cause of primary, acute encephalitis in the immunologically normal older child or adult (Phillips et al.). *Mycoplasma pneumoniae* is an uncommon non-viral cause of encephalitis or aseptic meningitis, clinically identical to infections caused by a host of viral agents (Lerner and Kalavsky, Hodges et al., Sterner and Biberfeld, Taylor et al.). The same is true of various serotypes of leptospira. Viral invasion of the fetal brain is most often due to the rubella virus or the cytomegalovirus, while acute viral infection in the newborn infant is most frequently caused by Herpesvirus hominis type II, ECHO viruses, and Coxsackie group B viruses (Table 13–1). The complete spectrum of the effects of viral infection on the fetal brain remains unknown although studies with animal models indicate that the scope is far broader than is currently recognized (Johnson, Kristensson et al.). What role such fetal infections play in the pathogenesis of defects of neural tube closure, hydrocephalus, and other cerebral malformations remains to be clarified.

Table 13–1. Agents that Cause Congenital and Neonatal Infections with Neurologic Involvement

Rubella
Cytomegaloviruses
Herpesvirus hominis
Varicella
Coxsackie B viruses
ECHO viruses
Polioviruses
Western equine encephalitis virus
Toxoplasma gondii
Treponema pallidum
Bacterial agents
Fungal (Candida, Coccidioides)

Certain other viral or presumed viral disorders are considered to be rare or even doubtful causes of neurologic infection. Roseola is a very common illness in children under two years of age and is known to be a common precipitant of "febrile" seizures. A bulging fontanel syndrome has been described with this illness (Oski) but encephalitis has not been well documented. A few cases of acute hemiplegia have been recorded with roseola (Posson, Rosenblum); however, these are better explained on the basis of a vasculitis with tissue infarction than secondary to encephalitis. Erythema infectiosum ("fifth disease") is another childhood exanthem in which encephalitis is rarely recognized. Balfour et al. described a single case with encephalitic symptoms followed by recovery. Hall and Horner reported a nine-month-old infant with erythema infectiosum complicated by a severe encephalitic-like syndrome, although a cellular response in the cerebrospinal fluid was not found. Rhinoviruses are important etiologic agents of upper respiratory infections in adults and children but only rarely have been implicated as a cause of encephalitis (Holzel). The reoviruses are considered to be rare causes of human disease of any type with the exception of the Colorado tick fever virus, which produces an acute febrile illness with leukopenia and is rarely accompanied by encephalitis. Certain reoviruses are known to be pathogenic in infant mice, in which they produce disseminated disease including hepatitis, encephalitis, and myocarditis. Human neurologic disease due to reovirus infection has been postulated on rare occasion although the etiologic role of the agent has remained uncertain (Joske et al., Krainer and Aronson).

Parainfluenza viruses are common offenders producing croup as well as other respiratory infections in children, and have been implicated as a cause of "febrile" convulsions (Downham et al.) and of Guillain-Barré syndrome (Román et al.). They are not generally recognized to be common causes of encephalitis or viral aseptic meningitis. Parainfluenza virus is one of a number of viruses that have been of interest to investigators as a possible causative factor of multiple sclerosis (ter Meulen et al.).

The role of the influenza viruses in the production of neurologic infection is more complex and has been debated for decades. They are regarded by most to be infrequent causes of neurologic disease, except for the association of influenza B with Reye's syndrome, but have been implicated during certain epidemics in the past (Mellman). In 1919–1920, influenza virus was postulated to be associated with von Economo's encephalitis lethargica in this country. A relationship was never proved and has subsequently been doubted. Numerous cases of encephalitis were attributed to the Asian influenza virus in the epidemic of 1957 but most were not well documented (Anderson and Jares, Bell et al., Friedman et al., Mellman). Illnesses designated acute encephalopathy without hepatic involvement have been described in children in association with influenza A infections but are poorly understood from the standpoint of pathogenesis (Delorme and Middleton). Acute transverse myelopathy, polyneuropathy, and localized mononeuropathy have also been described secondary to influenza virus infection (Wells). A disorder associated with influenza virus infection which is probably considerably more common is referred to as acute, benign myositis (Antony et al., Dietzman et al.). Most cases occur in children between four and 12 years of age. Following the initial illness with fever, malaise, vomiting, and mild respiratory symptoms, the child has the abrupt onset of intense pain and tenderness, especially of the musculature of the lower extremities. Except for an abnormal gait which is markedly restricted because of pain, the neurologic examination reveals few striking abnormalities. The muscle enzymes in serum are found to be elevated and the illness spontaneously resolves after three to five days in most instances. Myoglobulinuria can occur but has been observed more often in adults with acute influenza myositis than in children (Gamboa et al.).

Pathologic examinations in patients with cerebral complications of influenza have been sparse. Identification of perivenous demyeli-nation has led some authors to assume that encephalitis complicating influenza may be of the "post-infectious" type (Hoult and Flewett, Flewett and Hoult). An acute encephalopathy has also occurred following the administration of influenza vaccine in rare instances (Yahr and Lobo-Antunes, Woods and Ellison). Influenza virus infections during pregnancy have been considered to be a possible cause of congenital cerebral malformations by some authors (Coffey and Jessop, Hakosalo and Saxen) and doubted by others (Leck et al.). In an extensive review of the information compiled to 1974, Mackenzie and Houghton were unable to find sufficient evidence to support an association between maternal influenza infection and congenital malformations.

The disorders considered to this point have mainly been of the acute type. It is now known that certain viral encephalitic conditions can follow a subacute or chronic course, especially when the immune state of the patient is other than normal. Progressive multifocal leukoencephalopathy is a chronic, progressive, viral-induced illness seen most often in patients with hematologic malignancies. Subacute or chronic progressive neurologic disorders in the immunosuppressed patient have recently been identified which are caused by the measles virus (Murphy and Yunis, Wolinsky et al.), ECHO virus (Bardelas et al.), adenovirus (Chou et al.), and poliovirus (Davis et al.). Cytomegaloviruses, likewise, are well known for their ability to invade the immunodeficient patient, resulting in prolonged and progressive symptoms, although the clinical features are generally ill-defined (Dorfman). Herpesvirus hominis (simplex) is a common cause of infection in the immunocompromised patient but most cases occur in the form of mucocutaneous disease (Muller et al.). Subacute, progressive encephalitis in atypical form for Herpes simplex virus has also been described in patients with immunosuppressed conditions (Price et al., Linnemann et al.). Examples of disorders with chronic progressive encephalitis in the otherwise healthy individual include Creutzfeldt-Jakob disease and subacute sclerosing panencephalitis, the latter now accepted to be caused by the measles virus.

In addition to the above well-established conditions, it is believed that viral infections of the brain can be manifested in atypical fashion in some instances, resulting in prolonged neurologic dysfunction not easily recognized to be inflammatory in origin.

Chronic localized encephalitis has been proposed to account for certain cases of recurrent seizures in children. Support for this concept is on the basis of histologic evidence of "viral-like" encephalitic changes in surgically obtained brain tissue (Rasmussen et al., Aguilar and Rasmussen). A syndrome of young children characterized by acquired and progressive aphasia associated with temporal lobe spike activity on electroencephalography or overt seizures has also been postulated to be caused by a subacute or chronic viral infection (Gascon et al.). In one reported case of this type, cerebral biopsy revealed meningeal inflammation and cortical changes consistent with a chronic encephalitic process (Lou et al.). There are similar reports of adults with protracted neurologic dysfunction in the form of mental confusion, memory disturbances, behavioral abnormalities, and speech defects, in which brain biopsy has revealed evidence of subacute or chronic encephalitis, but without proof of a viral origin (Brierley et al.).

Benign Myalgic Encephalomyelitis (Iceland Disease)

A curious and poorly understood condition believed but not proved to be of viral origin has been variously called benign myalgic encephalomyelitis, Iceland disease, and epidemic neuromyasthenia. None of these designations is entirely accurate since it is not always epidemic, was described before the outbreak in Iceland, and usually is not associated with definite or objective evidence of either encephalitis or myelitis. Because the illness is benign, although protracted, deaths have not occurred and tissue for examination has not been available. The first known outbreak was observed in Los Angeles in 1938 (Gilliam). The illness appeared in epidemic fashion again in Iceland in 1948 (Sigurdsson et al.) and subsequently in New York State (White and Burtch), in London (Pool et al.), Australia (Pellew), and elsewhere. Acheson reviewed the available literature regarding the disease up to 1969 and noted that of 14 different outbreaks, seven had occurred among hospital staff members.

Young adults have been primarily affected, with an unexplained predisposition for females. The illness has often been confused with polio because of certain clinical similarities and because most cases have occurred in the summer and fall months. The onset is usually abrupt with influenza-like symptoms associated with headache, neck and shoulder girdle pain, vertigo, and myalgia. Upper respiratory infection with malaise often precedes the onset with headache and muscle discomfort by several days.

Persistent muscle aching is considered the hallmark of the syndrome, being present in the great majority of patients. Distal paresthesias are common, and, in the severe cases, a peculiar type of muscle weakness is described. Muscle weakness can be either localized or generalized but rarely is of a severe degree. Slowness in initiation of muscle contraction and jerkiness or inconsistency of maintenance of contraction have been emphasized by some authors (Holt). Deep stretch reflexes are unaffected and atrophy of affected muscle groups does not usually occur. Lethargy, ease of fatigue, and a host of different mental and other neurologic symptoms add to the complexity of the disease. Complaints frequently persist for weeks or even months, sometimes associated with periods of improvement followed by relapse, and often associated with emotional instability. Unequivocal signs of cerebral or spinal cord dysfunction are infrequent, although nystagmus, ataxia, and extensor toe signs have been seen in some cases (Graybill et al.).

Laboratory findings are not distinctive, including cerebrospinal fluid examination, which is normal in most instances. In a few cases, a mild lymphocytic pleocytosis has been found. Most investigators have assumed that the illness is an inflammatory one, although specific causative factors have remained elusive. Innes found evidence of enteroviral infection in four patients with symptoms like those of benign myalgic encephalomyelitis. In two of the four cases, virus was isolated from cerebrospinal fluid.

Encephalitis Lethargica

Of historical interest is the condition referred to as encephalitis lethargica, or von Economo's disease, first described by Constantin von Economo in 1917 following a small outbreak of the disease in Vienna during the winter of 1916–1917. It was the first type of epidemic encephalitis to be recognized, and for a number of years, the terms encephalitis lethargica and epidemic encephalitis were used synonymously. Isolated examples of the same illness had almost certainly been described before, but whether previous epidemics had occurred is uncertain (Hall).

An outbreak of the disease occurred in France in 1917 coincident to that described by von Economo in Austria. In subsequent winters it spread to Italy and thereafter became widespread in Europe and Asia. The most severe epidemic in Europe was recorded in the winter of 1919–1920, and the largest outbreak in Great Britain occurred in 1920–1921. By 1920, it was estimated that at least 10,000 cases had been identified in France since the onset of the recurrent epidemics in 1917. In 1920–1921, 2,360 cases were reported in England and Wales (Hall). The first cases in the United States were recognized in 1918 (Neal), and during the winter of 1918–1919, over 200 cases in this country were identified. The illness recurred annually in many parts of the world, but after approximately eight years its occurrence in epidemic proportions disappeared. The disease did not vanish entirely, however, as isolated examples of what was believed to be encephalitis lethargica continued to be described for years thereafter. In 1956, Espir and Spalding described three cases of encephalitis with features entirely compatible with the diagnosis.

Although encephalitis lethargica was generally assumed to be a viral disorder, no specific cause was ever identified and no definitive laboratory diagnostic test was discovered. Thus, its diagnosis rested on clinical and epidemiological grounds. Since the majority of cases in Europe and in the United States occurred in the cool or winter months it was not believed to be transmitted by mosquito or tick vectors. Some considered the disease to be an altered expression of poliovirus infection but there was little documented support for this concept and much evidence to the contrary. Others postulated an association of epidemics of encephalitis to the world-wide pandemics of influenza. This was especially considered to be likely in this country because many patients with encephalitis lethargica had experienced a preceding influenza-like illness (Neal). The initial outbreaks in Austria and France, however, had preceded the onset of the European epidemics of influenza.

Encephalitis lethargica spared no age group, with cases described from the newborn period to the very elderly. The highest percentage affected with the disease were young and middle-aged adults. Approxi-

mately 25 percent were estimated to be patients under 20 years of age (Blattner). The clinical aspects of the acute stage of the illness were quite variable, but the most typical signs observed in many patients included somnolence or coma and the presence of abnormal ocular signs, often in association with other cranial nerve deficits (Main, Hall). The onset of symptoms was usually abrupt, with fever, malaise, headache, and mental confusion. Lethargy, a sleep-like state, or deep coma was a feature described in a large percentage of cases, and it lasted for variable periods of time. Some patients could be readily aroused by stimulation from the sleep-like appearance, only to exhibit agitation or delirium until sleep again ensued. The prominence of the altered state of awareness led von Economo to refer to the condition in his initial publication in 1917 as "sleeping sickness." Myoclonus was often observed in the later epidemics of encephalitis lethargica, although it was infrequently described in the initial outbreaks.

One of the most remarkable features of this form of encephalitis, from the experience in Europe and Great Britain, was the high percentage of cases in which the cerebrospinal fluid contained no cells or only a slight increase in mononuclear cells. The findings in this country were somewhat different in that a mild cellular response in cerebrospinal fluid was more often found, although this was not invariable (Neal). The illness was widely recognized for its potentially poor outcome, with a mortality rate claimed to be approximately 25 percent. Higher mortality rates were described when select age groups were considered, such as infancy and the elderly.

Perhaps the most lasting memory of von Economo's disease has been the complication of the disorder in the form of postencephalitic Parkinsonism. Early follow-up studies suggested a relatively low incidence of basal ganglia complications following recovery from the illness, but, with the passage of time, it became evident that a high percentage of survivors were afflicted in this fashion. When survivors were re-evaluated up to 10 years after the acute illness, between 50 and 80 percent were found to have manifestations of Parkinsonism (Grossman, Duvoisin and Yahr). In some patients, rigidity and tremor were already evident as the acute phase of the illness was subsiding. The latent period in most before the onset of Parkinsonism was not more than three to five years, but in a few cases many years elapsed before Parkinsonism became manifest (Nielsen). There was no obvious association between the degree of the acute encephalitic illness and the development of Parkinsonism, and, in some, characteristic postencephalitic Parkinsonism was observed in the absence of a past history of acute encephalitis (Duvoisin and Yahr).

The Parkinsonian state that followed acute encephalitis lethargica was distinctive because of its unexplained progressive course, often years after the acute illness, and because of the customary association of other neurologic abnormalities. Hemiparesis, spastic quadriparesis, and cranial nerve palsies were frequently present in surviving patients. Another associated abnormality was oculogyric crises, a painful episodic ocular disorder which was widely held to be pathognomonic of the previous occurrence of encephalitis lethargica. An additional common complication, often associated with tremor, rigidity, and masked facies, was bizarre oral-facial dyskinesias. Parkinsonism complicating this type of encephalitis has been of particular interest because a similar condition has rarely been seen as a sequel to other types of encephalitis. The frequent occurrence of extraocular muscle and pupillary disturbances during the acute stage, as well as the high frequency of Parkinsonism in survivors, is evidence of the predisposition for damage of the substantia nigra and other parts of the upper brain stem in this disease.

Other types of sequelae often noted in survivors of the acute stage included evidence of hypothalamic dysfunction manifested by hyperphagia and obesity, chronic sleep disturbances, and profound personality and emotional abnormalities. Children were especially susceptible to many and varied types of behavioral deviations, which sometimes slowly improved and in other instances remained as a permanent disability (Holt, Main).

Pathologic changes in the brain in the acute stages of encephalitis lethargica were somewhat variable from case to case regarding the severity of the inflammatory infiltrates (Buzzard and Greenfield, Neal). The gross findings usually included generalized cerebral swelling, extensive vascular congestion, and petechial hemorrhages in some cases. Microscopically, there was a mild degree of mononuclear cell infiltration within the meninges, and a heavier perivascular round cell infiltrate in brain. This was often most striking in the midbrain and especially in the periaqueductal gray matter. Cerebral cortical neuronal involvement was usually rather sparse and patchy in distribution in comparison to gray matter injury elsewhere.

The neuropathology in the chronic stage in patients with sequelae revealed variable degrees of diffuse cerebral atrophy. Severe atrophy and gliosis of the corpus striatum was often observed. The most characteristic finding was shrinkage and depigmentation of the substantia nigra. Microscopic examination of this region showed neuronal depletion and glial scarring.

Aseptic Meningitis

Aseptic meningitis (serous or lymphocytic meningitis) is a common syndrome of multiple causes, the most frequent being one of many viral agents. When undesignated etiologically, aseptic meningitis refers to an illness with signs of meningeal irritation, a cellular response without bacterial or fungal pathogens in the cerebrospinal fluid, and a benign and transient clinical course in the majority of cases.

Non-viral causes of the syndrome include the introduction of certain chemotherapeutic agents, Pantopaque, detergents, or alcohol into the cerebrospinal fluid. Starch granules from surgical glove powder introduced at the time of operation can be irritative to meningeal tissues, resulting in aseptic meningitis (Dunkley and Lewis). The intrathecal administration of radioiodinated human serum albumin for isotope cisternography can also give rise to a symptomatic meningeal response (Barnos and Fish, Messert and Rieder).

The disorder referred to as the mucocutaneous lymph node syndrome of infants and young children is associated with aseptic meningitis in some cases (Melish et al.). This recently identified condition is an acute illness of uncertain etiology seen mainly among Japanese children, and is believed by some to be related to, or perhaps identical to, infantile periarteritis nodosa (Landing and Larson).

The tick-borne disorder called Lyme disease, characterized by erythema chronicum migrans and relapsing arthritis, can also be complicated by aseptic meningitis or meningoencephalitis (Reik et al.). The illness is believed to be infectious in origin; however, a causative agent has not yet been identified.

Systemic lupus erythematosus can be associated with aseptic meningitis in acute, chronic, or relapsing fashion (Canoso and

Cohen). In most instances, the meningeal inflammatory disorder has occurred in patients with prior evidence of lupus, and often has gradually merged into or was soon followed by more typical brain involvement with this disease (Sergent et al.). The identification of DNA–anti-DNA complexes in cerebrospinal fluid in these patients has suggested that lupus-induced aseptic meningitis is an immune-mediated disorder (Keeffe et al.).

On rare occasion, spontaneous leakage of cyst contents of a craniopharyngioma can lead to an acute, transient illness with aseptic meningeal irritation, but affected children usually have preceding abnormalities ascribed to the primary illness. A syndrome with meningeal irritation can occur in children following posterior fossa craniectomy for neoplasms (Carmel et al.). An acute, sterile meningeal syndrome has also been described in adults with cerebral glioblastoma multiforme (Bernat). The similarity of this unusual condition to viral aseptic meningitis can lead to considerable diagnostic confusion, especially when it occurs as one of the early manifestations of the neoplastic process. The cause of the meningeal inflammatory process is unclear, but it is believed to be the result of spillage into the cerebrospinal fluid of lipid-containing necrotic tissue from the neoplasm.

Many viruses have been shown to be capable of provoking aseptic meningitis in children and adults, but a relatively small number of viruses account for most of the cases in which an etiologic agent is identified. Members of the Coxsackie B group, several serotypes of the ECHO viruses, and the mumps virus are currently the most common offenders producing aseptic meningitis (Meyer et al., Lepow et al.). Cases of aseptic meningitis caused by the enteroviruses have a definite seasonal occurrence and are especially prone to appear in epidemic fashion, with children and young adults most heavily affected. Polioviruses ranked with those above prior to 1955, when decline in the prevalence of polio infections was achieved by active immunization. The lymphocytic choriomeningitis virus has a predisposition to produce meningeal inflammation when it attacks the human nervous system but is not a common cause when all cases of aseptic meningitis are considered collectively. Herpesvirus hominis on rare occasion will give rise to a benign neurologic infection in the form of aseptic meningitis but is much more often a cause of severe, necrotizing encephalitis.

When aseptic meningitis is caused by Herpesvirus hominis, it is most commonly the result of the type 2 strain, and usually occurs in association with herpes genitalis in the young adult (Jarratt and Hubler, Terni et al.). Meningitis provoked by either type 1 or type 2 Herpesvirus hominis has also been reported in patients with acute leukemia (Cappel and Klastersky, Harford et al.). The arthropod-borne viruses, likewise, usually result in encephalitic signs when a clinically manifested illness occurs, although a mild inflammatory meningeal syndrome has been observed with infection with the St. Louis encephalitis virus (Williams et al.), California virus (Johnson et al.), and Colorado tick fever virus. Aseptic meningitis can also occur as an infrequent manifestation of infectious mononucleosis (Gautier-Smith). Viral aseptic meningitis occurs at any time of the year, but the frequency is highest in the summer and fall months, partly because of the prevalence of enterovirus infections at this time.

Among infectious but non-viral causes of aseptic meningitis are the leptospira and *Mycoplasma pneumoniae*. Leptospirosis characteristically is a biphasic illness, with the initial, or septicemic, phase lasting several days and manifested by chills, fever, headache, myalgia, and often conjunctivitis. Either renal or hepatic involvement may become evident at this time but they are frequently absent. Systemic complaints subside but one or two weeks later the illness in some patients will recur, with headache, vomiting, neck stiffness, and cells in the cerebrospinal fluid. Paradoxically, leptospira can sometimes be isolated from the spinal fluid during the first stage of the infection but not usually during the second phase when meningeal symptoms are present. *Mycoplasma pneumoniae* is well known as a cause of upper and lower respiratory tract infections in children and young adults and is now recognized to be capable of producing various types of neurologic dysfunction, including aseptic meningitis (Sterner and Biberfeld, Hodges et al., Lerer and Kalavsky). Meningeal inflammation with *Mycoplasma pneumoniae* is not clinically different from that caused by other infectious agents except for a higher incidence of associated respiratory infection. Diagnosis, therefore, depends on cold agglutinin and complement fixation antibody titer rises.

The criteria for the diagnosis of aseptic meningitis have been altered somewhat from those outlined by Wallgren in 1925, but it is still generally agreed that the illness is of abrupt onset and of relatively short duration, is manifested by signs of meningeal irritation, and is associated with cells in the cerebrospinal fluid. The neurologic aspects are similar regardless of the infectious cause and consist of fever, headache, vomiting, and stiffness of the neck. Irritability and lethargy are conspicuous in infants and young children and convulsions can occur on a "febrile" basis in this age group. Distinct and unequivocal signs of involvement of the parenchyma of the brain not explained otherwise are not part of the syndrome and indicate the encephalitic character of the disorder. Despite the lack of clinical evidence of significant cerebral involvement in children with aseptic meningitis, diffuse slowing on electroencephalography during the acute stage is not uncommon (Gibbs et al.). Non-neurologic symptoms occasionally accompany the neurologic complaints and sometimes provide a hint of the organism involved. For example, parotitis in a child with aseptic meningitis suggests mumps virus infection but can also rarely occur with Coxsackie infections. Rash is seen with ECHO virus infections more often than with other causes of aseptic meningitis, while severe myalgia raises the consideration of one of the Coxsackie viruses.

Symptoms with viral meningitis last from a few days up to two weeks in most patients, followed by gradual recovery. An occasional child will have subsidence of fever and other general manifestations of the infectious illness but continue to have headache, sometimes with the development of papilledema, for several days or even weeks. The cause of this temporary increased intracranial pressure syndrome is not clear, but it may respond promptly to a brief course of corticosteroid therapy. Much less frequent as an aftermath of aseptic meningitis is the development of progressive communicating hydrocephalus requiring shunting therapy. Still other patients will recover from the acute illness in large part but continue to have a variety of subjective complaints, such as dizziness, malaise, ease of fatigue, or intermittent headaches, for weeks or months thereafter (Lepow et al.).

The cerebrospinal fluid in aseptic meningitis of infectious origin reveals a cellular response which varies from 10 to over 1,000 per cu. mm. Lymphocytes are the predominant cell type in most cases but in the first day or so after onset many cases will show a significant percentage of polymorphonuclear leukocytes. The protein content is raised to between 50 and 100 mg. per 100 ml. and the glucose value is normal in most. A mild reduction in the spinal fluid glucose can occur with certain viral infections, such as mumps and lymphocytic choriomeningitis. The absence of bacteria and fungi by the appropriate methods of examination is one of the laboratory prerequisites of the syndrome.

Recurrent or multiple attacks of aseptic meningitis are not frequent and, in reported cases, have not been explained on the basis of local, anatomic factors or immunologic abnormalities (Klemola and Lapinleimu, Nakao and Miura). An unusual and poorly understood type of recurrent aseptic meningitis is referred to as Mollaret's meningitis. The disorder was first recognized in 1944 by Mollaret and has been observed primarily in European countries. Most cases have been in adults, although a few reports of the illness in children have been published (Georg, Franche et al.). The course of the disease is characterized by repeated attacks of fever associated with signs of meningeal irritation (Bruyn et al.). Onset of each episode is usually abrupt and is manifested by elevation of temperature, headache, malaise, and stiffness of the neck. The first day or so is the most intense from the standpoint of severity of symptoms, after which the attack gradually resolves, disappearing by four to five days after onset. Weeks or months later, the illness recurs in the same fashion, only to again promptly abate, leaving no trace of neurologic deficits. Recurrences may continue over the course of a year or so or over a period of many years in some patients. The average duration over which recurrences occur is three to four years. Nordbring and Gertzen described an adult female with this condition in whom at least 37 attacks of benign aseptic meningitis occurred over a period of 10 years. The illness has largely been unrecognized in this country except for the recent, well-documented cases of Hermans et al. and those of Haynes et al.

The cerebrospinal fluid in the first 24 hours of an attack of Mollaret's meningitis reveals a cellular response of considerable magnitude, predominantly of polymorphonuclear leukocytes. The hallmark of the disease is the presence of large "endothelial" cells in the cerebrospinal fluid which show an irregular and poorly distinct outline of their nuclear and cytoplasmic membranes. These peculiar cells are rapidly lysed in the counting chamber and are easily overlooked for this reason. In addition, they are present in the cerebrospinal fluid only during the first hours of the attack, after which they disappear. By the second day of the episode, lymphocytes are the predominant cell type in the cerebrospinal fluid and remain so until symptoms vanish. The protein content is slightly to moderately increased and the glucose is normal in most cases. Between recurrences, the cerebrospinal fluid reverts to normal.

The etiologic origin of Mollaret's meningitis remains unestablished. It has been considered by some to be related to either Behcet's disease or the Vogt-Koyanagi-Harada syndrome but shows only superficial resemblance to these disorders. Others have placed it in the group referred to as "periodic disease" but this does little to clarify its etiology. No particular therapeutic approach has proved beneficial to the present time.

Acute Transverse Myelitis

Acute transverse myelitis (myelopathy) is a reasonably common but poorly understood disorder which results from many different types of insults to the spinal cord. When the cause is infectious, the illness is appropriately termed myelitis; otherwise it is best designated as a myelopathy. In most cases, an etiologic diagnosis is never established, although pathogenesis in many instances is most likely related to cell-mediated autoimmune mechanisms (Abramsky and Teitelbaum).

The onset is abrupt in most cases, and maximal neurologic deficit is very frequently reached within 24 to 48 hours after the first symptoms. Weakness of the legs or numbness or tingling of the feet represents the initial complaint, often associated with either radicular pain or localized back pain. As the process advances, the legs become progressively weaker and a sensory level is established, indicating the upper level of spinal cord involvement. Whether or not the upper limbs are involved depends on the upper level of the spinal cord insult. Evidence of neurogenic bladder dysfunction usually becomes apparent during the first day after onset. The motor deficit in the extremities can vary in severity and is initially of the flaccid type, often with absent deep tendon reflexes in the involved areas. Within days to weeks, spastic signs ensue, manifested by increased tone, hyperreflexia, and extensor toe signs. Sensory dissociation is seen in some cases, in which there is marked diminution of pain and temperature perception but relative sparing of posterior column function with intact or partially intact position, vibratory, and light touch sensations. This pattern, classically seen in adults with anterior spinal artery occlusion producing infarction of the ventral portion of the spinal cord, can also occur in children on an inflammatory basis. Still other patients have virtual total loss of all sensory modalities below a given level. Any part of the spinal cord can be affected in patients with acute transverse myelopathy but the most common site is the upper to mid-thoracic region.

The outcome of this condition ranges from total recovery within weeks after onset to permanent and nearly complete paralysis of the involved limbs. In patients with poor functional recovery, the persistence of neurogenic bladder dysfunction becomes one of the major problems of management. Of 67 adult and childhood cases of acute transverse myelopathy reviewed by Altrocchi, approximately one-third made a good recovery, one-third experienced fair recovery, and one-third had poor return of function. The outcome was more favorable in the 25 childhood cases described by Paine and Byers, in which 15 improved to a good functional state and only four failed to obtain some useful function.

There are numerous non-infectious conditions known to be causes of acute transverse myelopathy. The symptoms and neurologic signs are similar regardless of the cause, and thus etiologic diagnosis depends on other aspects of the total medical background or laboratory analysis. Ischemic myelopathy is more common in adults than in children and can be associated with atherosclerosis, embolization, systemic lupus erythematosus, or syphilis. A vascular malformation of the spinal cord can cause an acute intramedullary insult of sudden onset but is usually associated with subarachnoid bleeding. Spontaneous spinal epidural hemorrhage is rare in otherwise normal children but can closely resemble acute transverse myelopathy (Packer and Cummins). Time from onset of symptoms to maximum neurologic deficit is usually measured in hours and the correct diagnosis is not likely to be considered until myelography is done. Multiple sclerosis is included in the differential diagnostic list but has been found to be a rare cause of acute transverse myelopathy in a previously well individual (Altrocchi, Lipton and Teasdall).

Ropper and Poskanzer summarized three reported series comprising 149 patients with acute or subacute transverse myelopathy in whom there was follow-up information. Multiple sclerosis developed in only 7 percent of the total group. A more likely possibility in a child with an acute intramedullary spinal cord insult is Devic's syndrome, a demyelinating disease in which spinal cord involvement is associated with acute optic or retrobulbar neuritis manifested as sudden onset of visual loss.

The most important disease to consider and exclude in a child believed to have an acute transverse myelopathy is acute spinal epidural abscess. High fever and exquisite percussion tenderness over one or two spinous processes favor acute spinal epidural abscess while rapid progression of neurologic deficits leading to paraplegia within 24 hours after onset is more suggestive of acute transverse myelopathy. However, symptoms and signs may be remarkably similar, requiring myelography and spinal fluid analysis to differentiate the two illnesses. Myelograms are usually normal in patients with acute transverse myelopathy but, on occasion, focal cord swelling will be sufficiently great to result in a myelographic appearance like that with an intramedullary spinal cord neoplasm, or even cause a complete intraspinal block (Parker and Anderson).

Upper respiratory infection not uncommonly precedes the neurologic symptoms and signs in patients with acute transverse spinal cord insults but their significance remains unknown. Acute myelitis, in the absence of encephalitic signs, has been described in association with mumps (Benady et al.), measles (Senseman), varicella (Johnson and Milbourn, McCarthy and Amer), infectious mononucleosis (Cotton and Webb-Peploe, Silverstein et al.), ECHO virus (Johnson and Eger), poliovirus (Foley and Beresford), Herpes simplex (Klastersky et al.), and Herpes zoster (Hogan and Krigman). Transverse myelitis has also been seen in brucellosis (Abramsky), with rabies (Knutti), following rabies vaccination (Appelbaum et al., Harrington and Olin) and smallpox vaccination (Broadbank). In such cases, the spinal cord syndrome is etiologically associated with the viral illness or immunization, primarily because of their simultaneous or close temporal occurrence.

Virus isolation from the cerebrospinal fluid can also be used as diagnostic evidence from an etiologic standpoint but is rarely successful. Cerebrospinal fluid analysis, otherwise, is not usually helpful although the presence of a large number of cells, especially if associated with fever, is suggestive of an inflammatory disorder. Many of the non-infectious causes of acute transverse myelopathy are also associated with a mild lymphocytic pleocytosis in the cerebrospinal fluid. Corticosteroids are commonly used in treatment of acute transverse myelopathy but their value has not been proved.

Acute Hemorrhagic Leukoencephalitis

Acute hemorrhagic leukoencephalitis is a rare disease of abrupt onset and rapid progession which is manifested by signs of increased intracranial pressure in concert with signs indicative of both focal and multifocal neurologic involvement. Descriptions of the pathology had appeared previously, but it was Hurst in 1941 who first popularized the disease as a pathologic entity. The disorder is one with a high mortality rate and to this date is of uncertain etiology. A high percentage of identified cases have followed nonspecific viral illnesses (Rankin and Dance) or identified infections, such as varicella (Lander), rubeola (Tyler), or scarlet fever (Toomey et al.). It is generally considered to be an immune response of brain tissue to a foreign antigen, although this concept remains speculative. Analogies have been made between this condition and acute disseminated encephalomyelitis and experimental allergic encephalomyelitis (Russell).

Acute hemorrhagic leukoencephalitis most often occurs in older children and young adults; however, cases have been reported as early as two years of age (Byers). The usual sequence of events is the occurrence of a mild viral or respiratory illness followed days or a week or so later by the sudden onset of cerebral involvement. Neurologic manifestations appear abruptly in the form of headache, vomiting, confusion, stiffness of the neck, and lethargy. Progressive deterioration follows and includes the emergence of various signs, which often are seizures, dysphasia, motor deficits, and cranial nerve palsies. Motor disturbances often assume highly localizing features consisting of hemiparesis or focal convulsions, leading one to the erroneous consideration of a cerebral neoplasm, brain abscess, or Herpes simplex encephalitis. Papilledema will develop in some, indicating marked intracranial hypertension. Unless the process can be interrupted by therapy, lethargy and disorientation lead to coma, with eventual internal herniation causing respiratory failure and death. The illness can proceed from onset to deep coma and death as rapidly as 12 to 24 hours.

Fever is not always present but reaches impressively high levels in certain patients. Because of the acuteness of onset of the illness in addition to the frequent presence of fever, neck stiffness, and lethargy, either meningitis or encephalitis is likely to be the initial diagnostic consideration. The peripheral white blood cell count is usually significantly elevated and often contains a preponderance of polymorphonuclear leukocytes. The erythrocyte sedimentation rate is elevated to levels between 50 and 100 mm. per hour in some cases but falls within the normal range in others (Byers, Kristiansen et al.). The cerebrospinal fluid examination likewise shows wide variability but is abnormal in some fashion in the majority of instances. The opening pressure is usually elevated. The glucose content is expected to be normal while the protein value is commonly somewhat elevated. Cells are often present in the cerebrospinal fluid, and in many cases are predominantly polymorphonuclear in type. Numerous red blood cells may also be observed. The cellular response in the cerebrospinal fluid can be sufficiently great to render the fluid cloudy on gross inspection. Because of the confusing and sometimes localizing nature of the neurologic signs, carotid angiography has been performed in a number of cases of acute hemorrhagic leukoencephalitis. Vessel displacement suggestive of a mass lesion has been occasionally observed on angiography, adding further difficulty to the diagnostic analysis (Kristiansen et al., Coxe and Luse).

The pathology of acute hemorrhagic leukoencephalitis includes parenchymal edema of various degree, often strikingly asymmetrical in location. Gross observation of the cerebral cortex reveals no abnormalities, while the white matter shows areas of softening and multiple areas of hemorrhage of variable diameter. Hemorrhagic lesions are confined to one hemisphere in some cases and are bilateral and extensive in others. On microscopic examination, there is a necrotizing angiitis of capillaries and venules in the cerebral white matter or brain stem, with extravasation of polymorphonuclear leukocytes in vessel walls and surrounding tissue. Ring hemorrhages are seen in the region of affected vessels, sometimes sufficiently large to coalesce with adjacent lesions.

The disorder was originally believed to be uniformly fatal and recognizable only on postmortem examination. Biopsy confirma-

tion and intensive therapy have now demonstrated that survival is possible in certain instances (Coxe and Luse, Byers). Treatment includes vigorous methods to control intracranial hypertension and seizures combined with aggressive use of corticosteroids in high dosages.

Differential Diagnosis and Diagnostic Methods

The clinical diagnosis of viral encephalitis in some cases is reasonably sound, but in many others is worrisome and places the clinician in a position of less than complete confidence. It is a diagnosis that rarely should be accepted until consideration has been given to the many other neurologic and systemic conditions which can result in similar findings. Almost any disorder associated with an abrupt onset of headache, disturbances of mentation, or coma can be confused with encephalitis, whether it be other types of infection, metabolic or toxic conditions, or a wide variety of primary diseases of the brain.

The most common differential diagnostic problem is the separation of viral neurologic disease from bacterial meningitis that has already been partially treated or is in the very early stages without previous treatment. Neutrophils predominate in the cerebrospinal fluid in untreated bacterial meningitis but likewise often do so in the initial phases of encephalitis. In addition, the glucose content can be initially normal in meningitis and can even be mildly reduced in certain cases of viral encephalitis or aseptic meningitis. Hypoglycorrhachia, although not typical, has been seen in certain cases with mumps, lymphocytic choriomeningitis, and Herpes simplex infections (Green et al., Sarubbi et al., Wilfert).

Determination of the cerebrospinal fluid lactic acid content can be an important aid in the differentiation of viral from bacterial infection of the central nervous system. Recent studies have shown that the CSF lactic acid level is consistently elevated in the early stages of bacterial meningitis but is usually normal or minimally increased in patients with viral infection of the nervous system (Brook et al., Ferguson and Tearle). The latter is true, assuming that extensive necrotizing cerebral changes have not occurred.

When the cerebrospinal fluid findings are not entirely distinctive and antibiotics have not been given, if the illness is consistent with encephalitis and the Gram stain of the cerebrospinal fluid reveals no bacteria, one can safely withhold antibiotic therapy but repeat the lumbar puncture eight to 12 hours later. Shift of the cell type from neutrophilic to mononuclear, stability or increase in the glucose value, and absence of organisms on the second tap enhance the probability of viral disease (Feigin and Shackelford). The problem is considerably more difficult, however, when the child has received antibiotic therapy before hospital admission or performance of the initial lumbar puncture. Such preliminary therapy does not usually alter the spinal fluid with bacterial meningitis to the point that the diagnosis cannot be established but can do so in certain cases. When this occurs and one cannot be certain whether the illness is a viral or a bacterial one, it is mandatory to treat with the appropriate antibiotics, at least until blood and spinal fluid cultures prove to be negative.

Tuberculous meningitis and cryptococcal meningoencephalitis can resemble viral disease of the nervous system in certain patients. Both illnesses are usually more prolonged and are more likely to be associated with significant reductions of the cerebrospinal fluid glucose. The cerebrospinal fluid protein content is generally higher in any form of granulomatous meningitis than with encephalitis. Rocky Mountain spotted fever is commonly misdiagnosed as viral encephalitis, especially when the characteristic rash is erroneously attributed to previously administered antibiotics. Its occurrence in the spring and early summer, the history of exposure to ticks, associated thrombocytopenia and hyponatremia, and distribution of the rash, allow early diagnosis by the informed clinician. Diagnosis of this rickettsial disease is more likely to be overlooked in the black child, in whom the rash is less easily recognized.

Brain abscess is another infectious condition that enters differential diagnosis in select instances, especially in cases of encephalitis caused by Herpes simplex. The child with Herpesvirus hominis (simplex) encephalitis often has localized temporal or frontotemporal lobe involvement associated with signs of increased pressure and a lymphocytic pleocytosis in the cerebrospinal fluid. The shorter history and other evidence of more widespread cerebral disease clinically and electroencephalographically usually separate this necrotizing infection from focal suppuration, but in some cases angiography or even surgery is required. Radioactive brain scan is a helpful diagnostic tool for localization of a cerebral abscess but can also demonstrate a localized lesion in patients with Herpesvirus hominis encephalitis. With most other types of viral encephalitis, the brain scan is either normal or reveals a diffuse increase of isotope uptake throughout the cerebral hemispheres (Gilday). Computed tomography has now proved to be an exceedingly valuable diagnostic measure to differentiate focal suppurative lesions from Herpes simplex encephalitis, since the findings in patients with brain abscesses are highly specific, especially with the use of contrast enhancement.

Neurologic disorders of abrupt onset which can resemble acute viral encephalitis include the initial generalized convulsion in an epileptic child, the acute encephalopathy of obscure origin complicating certain systemic infections (Lyon et al.), and the encephalopathy associated with Reye's syndrome. Cells are usually not present in the cerebrospinal fluid in these conditions and neck stiffness is rather uncommon. Reye's syndrome is rapidly distinguished in most cases on the basis of the customary metabolic abnormalities, indicated by elevated serum glutamic oxaloacetic transaminase and ammonia levels. Acute hemorrhagic leukoencephalitis is another disorder with many clinical features in common with acute viral encephalitis. Abrupt onset of illness, fever, cells in the cerebrospinal fluid, and signs of diffuse cerebral dysfunction are frequently present in both conditions. Most cases of acute hemorrhagic leukoencephalitis are neither suspected nor recognized until postmortem examination, although diagnosis during life is possible in some cases by brain biopsy (Byers).

Acute drug ingestion frequently is manifested by rapid onset of coma, sometimes raising the question of acute viral infection of the brain. Physical signs, absence of fever, lack of cerebrospinal fluid evidence of infection, and history of drug intake secures the diagnosis in most cases. Fever, coma, and a rapid, labored respiratory pattern, characteristic of salicylate intoxication, can be duplicated by an unusual variety of viral encephalitis in which the insult is primarily localized to the brain stem. Lead encephalopathy can have a precipitous onset in some cases, with seizures followed by deep coma, neck rigidity, and a lymphocytic pleocytosis in the cerebrospinal fluid, thus simulating acute viral encephalitis. Important diagnostic features suggesting an acute encephalopathy secondary to lead ingestion include anemia, proteinuria, lead lines in long bones or lead in the intestinal tract on x-ray examination. Sudden onset of coma and stiff neck are the presenting features in some children with spontaneous intracranial hemorrhage from arteriovenous malformations, thus resembling acute neurologic infection. Grossly bloody cerebrospinal fluid and the results of angiographic studies confirm the diagnosis and eliminate infectious causes from consideration.

In rare cases, certain intracranial neoplasms can masquerade as an acute encephalitic disorder. Symptoms can be of abrupt onset secondary to precipitous obstruction within the posterior fossa. Cerebellar tonsillar herniation accounts for neck stiffness, and cells mistakenly assumed to be of inflammatory origin may be found in the cerebrospinal fluid. Illnesses of this type have been observed with medulloblastoma or ependymoma in the posterior fossa but are more often confused with granulomatous infections than with viral ones. Demonstration of ventricular enlargement and a posterior fossa mass by the appropriate diagnostic studies leads to the correct therapeutic approach. Cerebral reticulum cell sarcoma, or microglioma, is sometimes associated with signs suggestive of inflammatory disease but the course is more prolonged and gradually progressive. Brain stem encephalitis and gliomas

of the brain stem can present in similar fashion, although in most cases neoplasms in this region have a more chronic and gradually progressive clinical pattern. The characteristic pneumoencephalographic appearance of brain stem tumors of posterior displacement of the fourth ventricle has also been described in brain stem encephalitis (Schain and Wilson).

Unusual conditions that may simulate acute viral encephalitis include metabolic disturbances such as hypoglycemia, acute adrenal insufficiency, and hyponatremia of many causes. Multiple cerebral emboli secondary to subacute bacterial endocarditis or left atrial myxoma likewise can resemble viral infection of the brain.

Clinical diagnosis of acute viral encephalitis or aseptic meningitis is predicated on the presence of a compatible history and neurologic findings, the results of cerebrospinal fluid examination, and the accomplishment of sufficient laboratory and ancillary studies to exclude other reasonable considerations (Table 13–2). Cerebrospinal fluid examination is the laboratory study most strongly relied upon for diagnosis of viral infection of the central nervous system, although the results can vary considerably with different types of encephalitis. The spinal fluid is usually clear and colorless to gross inspection in

Table 13–2. Check List of Studies Indicated or to Be Considered in a Child with Acute Viral Encephalitis

A. Studies usually indicated

    Complete blood count
    Urinalysis
    Platelet count
    Tuberculin skin test
    Serum electrolytes
    Blood glucose
    Blood urea nitrogen and creatinine
    Blood culture
    Heterophile agglutination test
    Acute-convalescent phase sera for appropriate infectious agents
    Lumbar puncture and cerebrospinal fluid examination. Includes gram stain for bacteria, India ink
        preparation, culture for bacteria and fungi
    Specimens for viral isolation (stool, CSF, oropharyngeal)
    Skull and chest x-ray
    Electroencephalogram

B. Studies to be considered

    Serum salicylate level
    Serum glutamic oxaloacetic transaminase
    Serum ammonia
    Radioactive brain scan
    Computed cranial tomography
    Electrocardiogram

viral encephalitis but is xanthochromic in some cases caused by Herpesvirus hominis. The cellular response in many cases of encephalitis initially consists of a combination of polymorphonuclear and mononuclear cells, followed in hours or a day or so by a lymphocytic reaction. In Eastern equine encephalitis, polymorphonuclear cells often predominate throughout the illness, while lymphocytes make up the great majority of cells from onset until recovery in acute lymphocytic choriomeningitis. Diagnosis of acute viral encephalitis is not incompatible with an absence of a significant cerebrospinal fluid cellular response, although the frequency with which this occurs is unknown. It is not unusual for the initial lumbar puncture soon after onset of symptoms to yield negative findings, and for the second examination hours or a day or so later to reveal a marked pleocytosis.

Electroencephalography has its greatest value in this group of disorders in demonstrating the diffuseness of the inflammatory process, thus facilitating the exclusion of a focal cerebral lesion. Diffuse, bilateral slow activity, sometimes with intermixed sharp or spike activity, represents the customary abnormality in cases with acute encephalitis. A more distinctive type of abnormality is seen in some cases of Herpes simplex encephalitis, consisting of periodic, focal or lateralized spike or spike–slow wave discharges.

Etiologic diagnosis can sometimes be postulated from the clinical picture but can be confirmed only by a variety of specialized laboratory techniques. Probabilities in regard to the offending virus are predicted on the basis of the age of the child, the epidemiologic aspects of the illness, and the associated nonneurologic symptoms and signs. Aseptic meningitis in the child with parotitis obviously suggests a mumps virus infection, while aseptic meningitis in late summer occurring after a few days of diarrhea raises suspicion of a possible enteroviral infection. Acute encephalitis following several days of pharyngitis in the older child who is found to have splenomegaly and elevated liver enzymes directs one's attention to the consideration of the Epstein-Barr virus as the possible offender. The rapid development of marked impairment of consciousness followed shortly by progressive improvement in the patient with minimal or no CSF cellular response is a rather common pattern associated with encephalitis, or encephalopathy, with *Mycoplasma pneumoniae,* Epstein-Barr virus, or with

cat scratch disease. History of an unprovoked animal bite 30 to 60 days before the onset of numbness or pain at the site of the injury followed by signs of encephalitis is presumptive evidence of rabies encephalitis.

Other important factors relative to the possible etiologic considerations include whether the disease occurs in sporadic or epidemic fashion, the time of the year, and the geographic region the patient is in when the infection is acquired. For example, viral encephalitis in a child in the upper Midwest in late summer is most likely to be the result of infection with the California encephalitis virus, an enterovirus, or the mumps virus. Severe encephalitis in the same region in the winter is more likely to be due to Herpesvirus hominis than other agents. Each section of the country has its own leading probabilities in regard to viral cause of neurologic infection and should be known by physicians in the various regions.

There are three general laboratory approaches to the determination of an etiologic diagnosis. These include serologic methods, viral isolation, and microscopic techniques (Gershow, Lennette, Schmidt). Chance of success with these procedures depends on many factors but the initial one under control of the practitioner is the adequacy of specimens submitted for analysis. Materials collected must be appropriate for the most likely viral pathogens, and should be properly obtained and transported to the virology diagnostic laboratory. Specimens should be accompanied by a concise summary of the clinical information that allows the virologist to employ the procedures appropriate to the situation.

Serologic tests are valuable but have the disadvantage of the time required for antibody rise to occur after onset of the illness and the large number of antigens needed if extensive screening is done (Table 13–3). Complement fixation, neutralization, and hemagglutination inhibition tests are the methods most frequently used, but all require serial specimens to demonstrate a four-fold or greater titer rise. Fluorescent antibody tests have acquired increased importance in viral diagnosis but demand technical expertise and are of limited availability. They are methods used both for the demonstration of viral antigen in brain tissue after death and on certain types of specimens obtained during life. Immunofluorescent demonstration of viral antigen within cells in cerebrospinal fluid has recently been added to the diagnos-

Table 13–3. Serologic Tests To Be Considered in a Child with Symptoms and Signs Suggestive of Aseptic Meningitis or Viral Meningoencephalitis (Depending on Season and Geographic Location)

Mumps
Herpesvirus hominis (H. simplex)
Coxsackie A, B
ECHO virus, types 1–34
Poliovirus, I, II, III
Arthropod-borne viruses
    California virus
    Eastern equine
    Western equine
    St. Louis encephalitis virus
    Venezuelan equine
    Colorado tick fever virus
    Powassan virus
Rubella
Rubeola
Adenovirus
Cytomegalovirus
Lymphocytic choriomeningitis
Influenza and parainfluenza
Varicella-Zoster
Heterophile agglutination, Epstein-Barr virus
Mycoplasma pneumoniae
Rocky Mountain spotted fever
Leptospirosis
Brucellosis

tic capability in certain laboratories (Lindeman et al., Dayan and Stokes).

Microscopic methods for etiologic viral diagnosis have not been widely used because of their lack of specificity and, in part, because of the difficulty in obtaining tissue during life in patients with neurologic infections. Imprint preparations have been useful in rabies, and the presence of intranuclear inclusions in brain is suggestive but not diagnostic in the child suspected clinically to have Herpes simplex encephalitis. Inclusion bodies are also seen in encephalitis caused by other members of the herpes group and in rubeola (measles) encephalitis. Morphologic examination is of greater practical value when applied to cutaneous lesions caused by one of the herpes viruses. In the preeruptive stage of measles, microscopic examination of stained scrapings from the conjunctival or pharyngeal regions will reveal multinucleated giant cells, so-called Warthin-Finkeldey cells. The presence of these cells can be of diagnostic importance in isolated cases, although measles is not likely to be suspected until the rash appears, unless exposure has occurred.

Virus isolation has become an important diagnostic tool, especially when used in conjunction with other laboratory techniques.

Viral isolation from cerebrospinal fluid is almost never successful in cases of arthropod-borne encephalitis, is uncommon in Herpesvirus hominis encephalitis, but is relatively frequent when encephalitis is caused by mumps, ECHO, or Coxsackie viruses. Recovery of a virus from the patient does not necessarily mean an illness can be attributed to that particular virus. When the virus isolated is from brain or cerebrospinal fluid, the probability is very high that a neurologic infection can be attributed to the isolated agent.

Being intracellular parasites, viruses multiply only within a living host and thus isolation for diagnostic purposes requires inoculation of infected material into embryonated eggs, animals, and, especially, tissue cell cultures. Viral growth is identified indirectly on the basis of cell death or changes in the cell morphology, referred to as the cytopathogenic effect. Some cytopathic alterations are virtually specific for certain viral groups. Absolute identification of the isolated virus in most instances is accomplished by the use of chemical procedures and specific immune sera.

Pathology

There are several histologic alterations in the central nervous system that are common to most types of acute viral encephalitis, but a few varieties have characteristic changes which, while not diagnostic of the offending virus, are often suggestive of it. Brain swelling and vascular congestion seen on gross observation and a cellular exudate microscopically are conspicuous abnormalities in most cases of encephalitis. When death occurs in the early stages, the cellular infiltrate within brain tissue or meninges is made up partly or even largely of polymorphonuclear leukocytes. In later stages, the exudate is predominantly mononuclear in type, in addition to plasma cells and large phagocytes. Perivascular mononuclear infiltration is one of the commonest findings in encephalitis but is also seen in certain non-infectious conditions. Microglial proliferation is found to a variable extent in most cases of viral encephalitis, often in the immediate vicinity of degenerating nerve cells. The presence of numerous small cells surrounding a neuron undergoing regressive changes is called neuronophagia and is also commonly seen in viral infections of the brain. Neuronal changes vary from mild chromatolysis to total disintegration.

The arbovirus encephalitides occurring in the United States have no distinctive pathologic changes which consistently set them apart from other types of encephalitis. Neuronal damage is usually fairly severe, and alterations of blood vessel walls occur more frequently than is usual with most other viral infections. In Eastern equine encephalitis, polymorphonuclear leukocytes are more pronounced in the cortical and meningeal exudate than in other arthropod-borne infections. The neuropathology of California virus encephalitis has not been well described because of the limited number of identified fatalities. The pathology of St. Louis encephalitis and Japanese B encephalitis shows striking similarities, with hallmarks of both types being widespread neuronal destruction in the cerebral cortex, the basal ganglia, and the brain stem, in addition to meningeal infiltration and perivascular cuffing with mononuclear cells (Zimmerman, McCordock et al.).

Herpesvirus hominis encephalitis in the older infant or child is associated with typical morphologic changes in the majority of cases. It is an acute, necrotizing, and sometimes hemorrhagic process in which there is a predisposition for severe involvement of one or both orbital surfaces of the frontal lobe or fronto-temporal lobes. Softening, necrosis, or hemorrhagic necrosis of these regions, often with internal herniation, is characteristic of this infection. Microscopically, there is the customary meningeal and perivascular inflammatory cellular infiltration, glial nodules, and variable degrees of neuronal degeneration. Perivascular cuffing with polymorphonuclear leukocytes is one of the characteristic histologic features of this illness. Eosinophilic intranuclear inclusions of Cowdry type A in oligodendroglia and to a lesser extent in other glial cells and neurons represent one of the hallmarks of the disease although they are seen in certain other viral infections as well (Table 13–4). The cerebral pathology of Herpesvirus hominis encephalitis in the newborn infant is similar although the spectrum regarding severity is perhaps greater because early death can result from other organ system involvement.

Encephalitis caused by Herpes zoster likewise is associated with similar pathologic changes, although the inflammatory reaction is usually less intense and the tendency for fronto-temporal localization is less striking. The cytomegalovirus is the other member of the herpes group which attacks the brain, usually in the form of an intrauterine infec-

Table 13–4. Classification of Inclusion Bodies Found Within Brain Tissue

Intranuclear:

Type A—(Single and large; often surrounded by a clear halo)
    Herpes simplex encephalitis
    B virus encephalitis (monkey virus, Herpesvirus simiae)
    Cytomegalic inclusion disease (Cytomegalovirus disease)
    Progressive multifocal leukoencephalopathy
    Measles encephalitis
    Subacute sclerosing panencephalitis

Type B—(Multiple and small)
    Poliomyelitis
    Several types of brain tumors (cytoplasmic "inclusions")
    Marinesco bodies (normal findings, non-viral)

Intracytoplasmic:

Viral:
    Rabies (Negri and Lyssa bodies)
    Poliomyelitis
    Measles encephalitis
    Cytomegalic inclusion disease

Non-Viral:
    Lafora bodies
    Pick's bodies
    Lewy bodies

tion or as a complication of immunosuppression in an older individual. The diffuse meningeal and parenchymal inflammatory response is most often less than with other types of herpetic encephalitis. Cytomegalovirus encephalitis in the newborn child or young infant has a decided predisposition for involvement of the periventricular subependymal matrix, especially in the lateral ventricular regions. In this region, one sees glial cells and, less often, neurons which are abnormally enlarged and contain intranuclear or intracytoplasmic Cowdry type A inclusions. Ependymal damage, periventricular necrosis, and calcium deposition adjacent to the ventricular wall are additional common findings.

Rubella encephalitis in the neonate is an infection acquired by transplacental transmission in which there is a chronic leptomeningitis in addition to degenerative cerebral vascular lesions that lead to areas of focal ischemic necrosis of the parenchyma of the brain. Rabies is a severe, diffuse encephalitis with features in common with many other types but with a notable predilection to attack cortical gray matter and the brain stem. The cytoplasmic inclusions of rabies are called Negri bodies and are found in neurons which otherwise reveal few if any structural alterations. These inclusions are distinct, rounded, eosinophilic bodies most readily identified in the hippocampus of the temporal lobe and Purkinje cells of the cerebellum.

The greatest departure from the conventional findings of acute viral encephalitis is seen in the group referred to as post-infectious or post-vaccinal encephalomyelitis. This acute neurologic disturbance has been associated with several viral infections such as measles, mumps, and varicella. It has also followed smallpox and rabies vaccination, and has been described as a complication of typhoid fever (Ramachandran et al.). Extensive white matter damage with perivenous demyelination with only minimal or mild cortical abnormality is the pathologic hallmark of this condition (Fig. 13–2). Petechial hemorrhages are often found in the white matter, and in some cases, hemorrhage is diffuse and extensive. Although the pathogenesis of the histopathology of this group of disorders remains unclear, it is assumed that tissue injury by an invading antigen provokes a host immune response, with resulting attack on host tissue.

Management and Control

Treatment of the child with viral aseptic meningitis or acute encephalitis is largely conservative and includes measures dictated by the needs of the individual patient. Mild infections require little more than close observation and methods to relieve headache, while severe illnesses may demand intensive treatment to support the life of the child. Fluid and electrolyte therapy, methods to control hyperthermia, skin care, and attention to bladder function are all vital aspects of the management of the encephalitic patient. When intravenous fluids are required, mild restriction of the total daily volume, perhaps to 75 to 80 percent of the maintenance requirements, is appropriate because of the common occurrence of cerebral swelling associated with encephalitis. Marked and persistent hyperthermia is undesirable in the en-

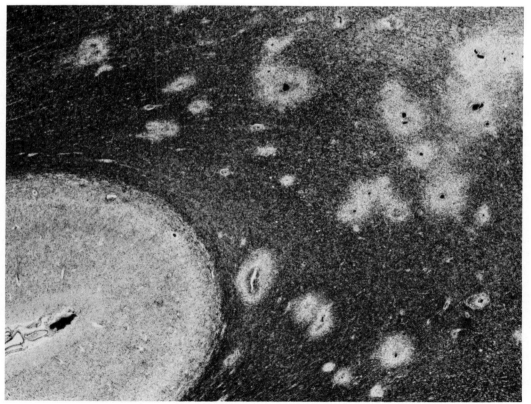

Figure 13–2. Perivenous demyelinating encephalomyelitis. Multiple zones of perivenous demyelination (trichrome stain).

cephalitic patient with increased intracranial pressure. Sponging may suffice for some while cooling blankets will be needed for others to bring the body temperature down to acceptable levels.

Agitation or hyperkinesis can usually be controlled by the use of proper restraints combined with sedative drugs such as diazepam or chlorpromazine. Recurrent convulsions or status epilepticus require both diligent nursing care and judicious administration of anticonvulsant medications. Intravenous diazepam or short-acting barbiturates are used for prolonged or severe seizures. Once the initial convulsion is controlled, a maintenance regimen with phenobarbital given every six or eight hours is advisable.

Airway obstruction or ventilatory failure becomes a threat to the convulsing child as well as to others with markedly depressed state of consciousness. Airway suction, intubation, tracheotomy, and the use of a mechanical ventilator are steps determined by the needs of the child. The advisability of measures to reduce increased intracranial pressure in the child with encephalitis is a controversial matter about which there is little to base judgment. Corticosteroids, glycerol, or mannitol are agents commonly used for this purpose but should be withheld unless reasonably clear-cut indications develop. They are not indicated in the patient who is mildly or moderately ill, without papilledema, who is showing a stable or improving clinical course. Consideration of the use of such drugs is warranted when there is progressive deterioration, episodes of decerebration, signs consistent with internal herniation, or the presence of significant papilledema in the child with depressed consciousness. In severe cases, it is usually very difficult to judge from clinical signs the presence of, or degree of, increase in intracranial pressure. When one cannot be certain and concern exists over the possible adverse effects of intracranial hypertension, the use of an indwelling intracranial bolt for continuous pressure monitoring can be of great value. This allows the appropriate administration of antiedema osmotic agents or the use of controlled ventilation to keep the intracranial pressure at a safe level. Corticosteroids are commonly used to reduce cerebral edema in many conditions but experience indicates that they are often of limited value for this purpose in patients with acute viral encephalitis. Because of postulated concern of their potential ability to enhance dissemination of Herpesvirus hominis, measles, and varicella viruses, corticosteroids should probably not be used as antiedema agents in encephalitis caused by these viruses.

Specific antiviral treatment for the various forms of viral encephalitis remains in the investigative stage but is a field showing a glimmer of promise for future development (Hirschman, Weinstein and Chang). Except for possible beneficial effects of adenine arabinoside in Herpesvirus hominis encephalitis, specific chemotherapy has had little influence on viral neurologic infections to this time.

Control measures have achieved remarkable results in regard to the prevalence of certain viruses, most notable being the effects of vaccines against the polio and measles viruses. Human rabies can be largely curtailed by the enforcement of available public health principles. Mosquito control measures likewise can significantly influence outbreaks of arbovirus encephalitis even though complete eradication of these diseases is still beyond our means.

ENTEROVIRUS INFECTIONS

The picornaviruses are small RNA viruses which include the many serotypes of the enteroviruses and the rhinoviruses. The viruses of the polio, Coxsackie, and ECHO groups constitute the enteroviruses, which share a number of common biological properties, their frequent habitation of the intestinal tract of man, and certain similarities in regard to clinical and epidemiologic aspects of the illnesses they produce. Members of all three groups cause both sporadic and epidemic disease, which, in temperate climates, occur more commonly in summer and early fall. The polioviruses were in the past by far the most common of the enteroviruses causing serious neurologic disease or death, but they can now be controlled by active immunization given in early infancy.

Paralytic disease due to involvement of motor neurons in the brain stem or spinal cord was for many years recognized to be the cardinal neurologic manifestation of the poliovirus, even though it was known that asymptomatic or mild infections were much more common. Even before the decline in the occurrence of poliomyelitis with the use of the vaccine, similar illnesses with muscle weakness were identified with Coxsackie or ECHO virus infection and, in other countries, by the Russian spring-summer virus. A polio-like clinical illness has also been recognized with infection caused by the louping ill virus, a member of the Russian spring-summer virus complex (Likar and Dane), and by the West Nile virus, a virus related to Japanese B and St. Louis encephalitis viruses (Godoth et al.). Limb weakness is generally milder when caused by non-polio enteroviruses, and bulbar involvement has been observed only on rare occasion. A "polio-like" syndrome complicating acute, severe asthmatic attacks has been described by several authors, although a causative virus has not been identified (Danta, Hopkins, Ilett et al., Wheeler and Ochoa). These cases have been characterized by sudden onset of flaccid weakness of one extremity immediately following an acute and severe asthmatic attack and have generally been followed by subtotal recovery. Clinical and electrophysiologic studies have been compatible with anterior horn cell involvement but no pathologic documentation has been available. The best explanation for such cases, although yet to be proved, is that a viral illness provokes the acute asthmatic episode and at the same time gives rise to a localized anterior horn cell inflammatory process resulting in flaccid limb paresis (Shapiro et al.).

The most frequent neurologic condition associated with certain serotypes of the Coxsackie and ECHO viruses is aseptic meningitis, which occurs most often in children and is usually a benign, self-limited illness. Certain members of all three enteroviruses have been associated with acute cerebellar ataxia and also with Reye's syndrome. On rare occasion, Coxsackie and ECHO viruses have been believed responsible for the occurrence of the Guillain-Barré syndrome. Although viral infections are not generally considered to represent a serious threat to the child with deficient antibody-mediated immunity, vaccine-associated poliomyelitis in children with agammaglobulinemia is now well-known (Wyatt, Wright et al.). In addition, a dermatomyositis-like syndrome associated with persistent central nervous system infection with ECHO virus has recently been described in children with antibody-deficiency states (Bardelas et al., Wilfert et al.).

Diagnosis of neurologic conditions due to the enteroviruses can sometimes be suspected from clinical and epidemiologic data. Serologic methods are valuable for confirmation of diagnosis but are frequently impractical because of the large number of serotypes that are potential offenders. Virus isolation from stool or oropharynx is often successful but alone does not necessarily mean the isolated virus is the cause of a neurologic infection. Isolation of virus from cerebrospinal fluid establishes the diagnosis and can frequently be achieved with Coxsackie or ECHO infections. Recovery of the poliovirus from cerebrospinal fluid, however, is rare.

Poliovirus Infections

Polio (poliomyelitis, "infantile paralysis," Heine-Medin disease) was for many years one of the most feared of all infectious diseases because of its devastating and often permanent effect on motor neurons of the spinal cord and brain stem. Historically, the disease dates back to ancient times but was first clearly defined as a clinical entity in a monograph in 1840 written by a German orthopedist named Jacob Heine. Karl Medin of Sweden in 1890 contributed further to the knowledge of the illness and made clear its predisposition to occur in epidemic fashion. The contributions of these two men led Wickman in 1907 to propose the eponym "Heine-Medin disease," a term that became popular for a decade or so thereafter but eventually was replaced by the previously used designation of poliomyelitis.

The illness had been recognized in this country for many years before the turn of the century but the first recorded large-scale outbreak occurred in Vermont in 1894 in which 132 cases were identified (Caverly). The illness thereafter appeared to gradually increase in this country until 1907 when an epidemic of major proportions occurred in New York City, with estimates of the number of affected persons ranging from several hundred up to 2,500 (Lovett). Two years later, in 1909, Landsteiner and Popper working in Vienna, postulated the viral etiology of the disease after producing flaccid paralysis in a monkey by the intraperitoneal injection of an emulsion of spinal cord tissue obtained from a human fatal case. Histologic examination of the monkey spinal cord revealed changes very similar to those which by then had become known to occur in fatal human cases of poliomyelitis.

In the years that followed, the impact of poliovirus infections in this country became progressively evident and an enormous research effort to understand and combat the disease gradually unfolded. Outbreaks of variable magnitude occurred each summer and fall, some with crippling results on hundreds of patients. Large epidemics occurred in the Northeast in 1911 and again in 1916, and on the West Coast in 1934. A landmark in the historical sequences surrounding the disease occurred in the late 1920's with the invention of the tank respirator by Dr. Philip Drinker of Boston, a device soon named the "iron lung." The name of Sister Elizabeth Kenny emerged on the medical scene in the early 1940's following her denouncements of the previously held passive attitudes of treatment with complete rest and total immobilization of painful or paralyzed extremities. Her methods of treatment quickly received wide publicity around the world and provoked widely divergent responses from members of the medical profession, some being supportive while others expressed vehement opposition. The end-result was the generation of new attitudes about the management of both the acute and the chronic stages of poliomyelitis, but at the price of considerable ill will among professionals involved with the disease. The potential ability to eradicate the infection came a step closer in 1949 when Enders, Weller, and Robbins isolated and cultivated polioviruses

in vitro in non-neural tissue. Inactivated polio vaccine (Salk) was introduced in 1955 and live attenuated vaccine (Sabin) became widely used in 1962 in the United States and elsewhere. Trivalent oral polio vaccine was introduced in 1963 and is the preparation in current use. A review of the history of poliomyelitis from ancient times through the eventual conquest of the disease has been eloquently written by Dr. John Paul and published in 1971.

The impact of active immunization was dramatic, proving that the disease is potentially preventable (Fig. 13–3). In 1954, there were 18,308 reported cases of paralytic polio in this country, and in 1965, the reported number had fallen to 61 (Morbidity and Mortality Weekly Report, 1967). From 1969 through 1976, there were a total of 132 cases of paralytic poliomyelitis reported in this country, of which 44 were classified as vaccine-associated (Nightingale). This dramatic decline in the incidence of this disease illustrates the remarkable effectiveness of the vaccine, but, at the same time, the existence of the virus indicates the potential danger of future epidemics should the immunity in the population not be sustained.

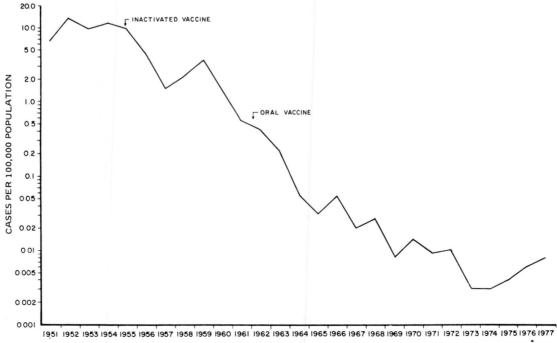

Figure 13–3. Paralytic poliomyelitis. Reported cases per 100,000 population by year, United States, 1951–1977. (From: Morbidity and Mortality Weekly Report, Annual Summary, 1977, Volume 26, No. 53, Sept. 1978).

Clinical Aspects

The route by which the poliovirus reaches the central nervous system has been debated for years and remains a controversial issue. As early as 1914, Flexner and Amoss demonstrated experimentally the definite affinity of the virus for neural tissue but showed that blood-borne virus did not enter the brain or spinal cord unless there was preexistent injury to the choroid plexus. Their studies confirmed the concept of the ability of the virus to be transmitted along peripheral or cranial nerves to gain entrance into the brain and spinal cord. Flexner and Amoss proposed that the route of entrance of the virus causing human neurologic disease was via the respiratory mucosa, with transmission along olfactory nerves into the brain stem and spinal cord. Subsequent authors postulated invasion by hematogenous spread through the region of the area postrema (Nathanson and Bodian), and entrance through the mucosa of the oropharynx and intestinal tract, with virus transmission along nerve fibers (Sabin, 1956).

Of the three poliovirus serotypes, type 1 has been the most frequent cause of endemic and epidemic paralytic disease and type 2 is the least paralytogenic strain. The incubation period of poliovirus infection varies from six to 20 days and perhaps can be somewhat shorter or more prolonged in certain cases. Most epidemics in temperate regions have occurred in summer and early fall, although sporadic cases can occur throughout the year. Infections caused by the polioviruses have been classified as asymptomatic, abortive, nonparalytic, and paralytic. Types of paralytic polio include spinal, bulbar, and bulbospinal. Primary cerebral involvement with diffuse encephalitic signs therefrom is a doubtful manifestation of poliovirus infection. The condition referred to as polioencephalitis, associated clinically with confusion, disorientation, stupor, or coma, has been attributed to a severe inflammatory reaction within the brain stem reticular formation and the hypothalamus rather than to higher cerebral involvement (Bodian). It is now known that, in the majority of cases, infection with the poliovirus is asymptomatic or occurs in the form of a transient, minor illness. Paralytic disease is, or was in the past, the unusual expression of poliovirus infection.

Abortive polio is a brief illness manifested by fever, malaise, and other non-specific symptoms followed by recovery in two to four days. Non-paralytic polio in essence is aseptic meningitis without parenchymal signs of involvement and is clinically similar to meningeal infections produced by other enteroviruses. The illness of greatest consequence is paralytic polio, or poliomyelitis, which classically begins with fever, sore throat, and other non-specific signs lasting one or two days, followed by a few days of apparent well-being when fever recurs in association with headache, vomiting, and signs of meningeal irritation. In some cases the brief prodromal stage is absent or unrecognized and the initial symptoms are those of a febrile illness with meningeal signs. Limb pain or painful muscle spasms may be the first evidence of parenchymal neurologic involvement, but more often the rapid evolution of flaccid muscle weakness is observed within one or two days after onset of the meningeal signs. Weakness or paralysis develops quickly, and, once begun, it achieves its maximal severity within 48 hours in most cases. The cause of muscle spasm occurring in the early stages in some cases of poliomyelitis has never been adequately explained. Theories proposed include the possibility of a direct attack of the virus on muscle or an irritative effect from inflamed anterior horn cells. The most attractive postulate is that muscle spasm represents a "release from inhibition" of functional anterior horn cells secondary to damage of inhibitory internuncial neurons in the spinal cord (Kabat and Knapp).

The pattern of muscle weakness in paralytic polio varies a great deal from patient to patient but asymmetry of limb involvement is a notable but not invariable feature. Certain muscle groups of one arm or one leg are selectively affected in some cases, but in others flaccid paraplegia or quadriplegia will occur. Anterior horn cells of the cervical and lumbar spinal cord enlargement areas seem especially vulnerable, although any area of the spinal cord can be affected. Upper cervical or thoracic cord involvement results in diaphragm and intercostal muscle weakness manifested by a shallow, rapid, but regular respiratory pattern.

Bulbar polio may occur with or without spinal cord disease and is manifested by dysfunction of lower cranial nerves, often in asymmetrical fashion. The most life-threatening aspect of bulbar polio results from inflammation of certain nuclear groups of the medullary reticular formation, the so-called vasomotor "centers." The respiratory pattern in such cases is characterized by its irregularity punctuated by episodes of apnea, in addition to hypertension and abnormalities of the rate and rhythm of the pulse. Peripheral vascular collapse or the sudden appearance of pulmonary edema (Baker) are the common terminal events in such cases. Facial paralysis is observed in some patients with other signs of bulbar polio, and, rarely, has been stated to be the only paralytic sign of the disease (Sherman and Kimelblot, Winter). Nystagmus is seen occasionally, while external ophthalmoplegia is quite infrequent. The relative sparing of extraocular muscle function in polio is, according to Murray and Walsh, partly explained by the anatomic difference of innervation of these muscles as compared to other somatic musculature. The ratio of nerve to muscle fibers in the extraocular muscles is in the range of one to five, and thus, a large percentage of the motor nuclei must be damaged to create functional disturbances.

Polioencephalitis is much less common than either the spinal or the medullary form of the disease. Disturbances of consciousness, convulsions, variable brain stem signs, and either flaccid or spastic deficits of the extremities are found in this unusual form of poliovirus infection, which carries a high mortality rate. Of the different neurologic syndromes that can occur in polio, approximately 45 to 50 percent of cases are predominantly spinal, 10 to 15 percent are bulbar, 15 percent are bulbospinal, and 1 to 5 percent have "encephalitic" features reflecting extensive damage within the brain stem and diencephalon. Non-paralytic polio has been estimated to account for 25 to 28 percent of the cases (Smith et al., Weinstein et al.). Mortality from poliovirus infections is higher in adults than in children, and when all types are included, ranges from 5 to 10 percent. Bulbar, bulbospinal, and bulboencephalitic cases are the most threatening and have been fatal in 25 to 35 percent.

In any of the neurologic forms of poliovirus infection, the cerebrospinal fluid usually reveals a pleocytosis which initially may be largely polymorphonuclear but rapidly becomes lymphocytic in type. The cell count ranges from 50 to 200 per cu. mm. in most but can be greater or less in some cases. As early as 1912, Draper and Peabody showed that in the initial days after onset of the illness, polymorphonuclear leukocytes often account for 80 to 90 percent of the cells in the cerebrospinal fluid. Thereafter, lymphocytes come to predominate, but, by two to three weeks after onset, the cell count decreases to normal or near normal. The authors also demonstrated that the protein content of cerebrospinal fluid in poliomyelitis reveals a modest increase, which may persist to some degree for approximately two months.

Paralytic polio spares no age group, is more common in males than females, and occurs during pregnancy at a frequency greater than expected (Weinstein et al., Aycock). The peak age incidence of the disease in the nineteenth century and prior to 1930 was in infants and children less than five years of age. Thereafter, the most susceptible age shifted to the five- to nine-year-old age group and, correspondingly, more cases were observed in adults (Dehn, Weinstein et al.). The infant is relatively protected for the first four to six months after birth because of transplacental antibody transfer from the mother (Aycock and Kramer); however, numerous cases have been described in early infancy and even in the newborn period (Abramson and Greenberg, Abramson et al., Mouton et al.). Transplacental passage of the virus from mother to fetus has been postulated (Shelokov and Weinstein), but in the vast majority of hundreds of cases of polio complicating pregnancy, the newborn infant remained unaffected.

A number of factors have been proposed in past years which have been assumed to be related to susceptibility to polio or to severity and localization of inflammatory lesions once they occurred. Of the many such considerations, relatively few have been of proven importance, and in the overwhelming majority of cases there is no explanation why a given child is afflicted with paralyzing disease while many others experience only transient and insignificant poliovirus illnesses. Exposure to the virus and lack of preceding immunity remain the primary factors which determine whether infection will be acquired.

Previous tonsillectomy was recognized years ago to have an effect on the localization of poliovirus infection of the nervous system (Eley and Flake, Top). It was never proved that the incidence of polio was higher in tonsillectomized patients, but studies have shown that when polio did occur, the frequency of bulbar involvement was higher in tonsillectomized patients than in persons otherwise. The explanation for this was never established despite many postulates.

Administration of the vaccine itself has, on rare occasion, been the determining factor resulting in paralytic disease (Cesario et al.,

Balduzzi and Glasgow, Haneberg and Ør-stavik). Only a limited number of cases of vaccine-associated paralytic polio in otherwise healthy persons have been reported and these have occurred in recipients of the vaccine as well as in contacts of vaccinees (Schonberger et al.). All three types of the polio virus have been incriminated. A number of cases of paralytic involvement from polio vaccine have been observed in children with immunodeficient syndromes. This has occurred in patients with defects of either cellular or humoral immunity as well as in those with combined immunodeficiency syndromes (Chang et al., Lopez et al., Feigin et al., Riker et al., Saulsbury et al.). Characteristic features of poliovirus neurologic infection in the immunodeficient host include a prolonged incubation period of one to three months, a severe and often subacute illness, and prolonged viral shedding (Wright et al.). Davis et al. have described an infant with immunodeficiency associated with dwarfism with cartilage-hair hypoplasia who developed a slowly progressive neurologic disorder with onset three months after receiving her last oral polio vaccination. The clinical findings were atypical for poliomyelitis but the pathologic findings were consistent with this diagnosis, and poliovirus was isolated from brain tissue.

It is now accepted that patients with immune deficiency diseases of virtually any type, or those with immunosuppression from drug treatment or radiation therapy, should not be given oral polio vaccine. In addition, to the degree possible, such patients should avoid close contact with recipients of this vaccine for a three-week period after vaccination.

Unusual Neurologic Manifestations

Several unusual neurologic manifestations of poliovirus infection have been described, such as acute cerebellar ataxia (Mendez-Cashion et al., Curnen and Chamberlin) and an association with Reye's syndrome (Brunberg and Bell). Sensory loss is generally assumed not to accompany the flaccid, areflexic paresis or paralysis of polio, but, in rare cases, disturbances of sensation are found as a result of lesions in dorsal horns of the spinal cord or as part of the picture of an acute transverse myelitis (Plum, Foley and Beresford). Still another observation antagonistic to the usual concepts of the natural course of the disease is the onset of progressive anterior horn cell degeneration many years after the acute illness. Late progression has been noted in adults who had experienced paralytic polio in childhood. It is characterized by an insidious onset and predisposition to involve muscle groups previously affected in the acute stage (Campbell et al., Mulder et al., Anderson et al.). Several postulates have been developed to explain this finding, the most plausible being that of Mulder et al., who suggested that neurons partially damaged during the acute illness become more vulnerable to the aging process than are otherwise normal cells.

Diagnosis and Pathology

Diagnosis of poliovirus infection can sometimes be suspected from the clinical and epidemiologic findings, especially when the illness is of the paralytic type in a patient without prior polio immunization. Poliomyelitis can usually be distinguished from the Guillain-Barré syndrome because of the differences in the clinical pattern but also on the basis of the differences in the cerebrospinal fluid findings in the two disorders. Acute bulbar polio with lower cranial nerve dysfunction can resemble botulism, although pupillary dilatation and extraocular muscle paresis is customary in botulism and uncommon with polio. In addition, epidemiologic features and CSF findings help differentiate the two disorders.

Neutralization and complement fixation tests on serial serum specimens are the most valuable laboratory diagnostic aids for poliovirus infections, in addition to techniques to isolate and type the virus from stool and nasopharyngeal specimens. Poliovirus can often be recovered from stools for two to three weeks after onset of the illness, and sometimes longer. Unlike other enteroviruses, the poliovirus can rarely be isolated from the cerebrospinal fluid in patients with neurologic infection (Wright and Ward).

One of the striking features of the pathology of this disease is the selectivity of distribution of the lesions and the almost consistent sparing of other parts of the central nervous system. In the spinal cord, the most severe gray matter lesions are in the anterior columns. The degree of damage varies from one level to another but often is most intense at the cervical or lumbar enlargements of the cord. Lesions are usually bilateral at any one segment but can be conspicuously asymmetrical. The inflammatory reaction can also involve the intermediate and posterior horns, but not to the extent of the involvement of the anterior horns. The spinal cord may be the only site of disease, or can be affected in concert with lesions in the brain stem and elsewhere. Within the brain stem, cellular infiltration can be seen in many of the cranial nerve motor nuclei, but is most apparent in the region of the vestibular nuclei and the reticular formation. Other sites affected in severe cases include the tectal nuclei, the roof nuclei of the cerebellum, the hypothalamus, and the thalamus. Unlike most other types of viral encephalitis, the cerebral cortex is characteristically spared with poliovirus infection, except for the precentral gyrus, where lesions

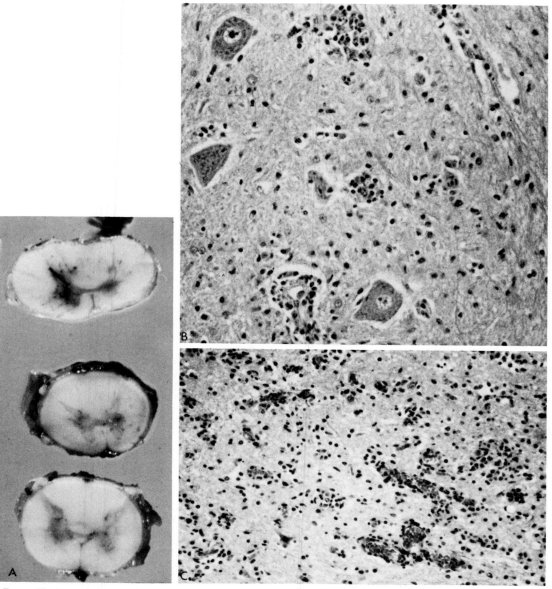

Figure 13–4. Poliomyelitis, acute stage. *A,* Severe congestion and petechial hemorrhages within the gray matter of the spinal cord. *B,* Various stages of neuronal damage and neuronophagia of anterior horn cells of the spinal cord. *C,* Extensive inflammatory reaction within the anterior gray matter of the spinal cord 7 days after onset of muscle weakness.

may be found but are usually mild in degree (Bodian). Likewise, the corpus striatum is generally unaffected, although there is occasionally mild involvement of the globus pallidum. White matter involvement in the spinal cord is far less extensive than that of the gray matter, and, if present at all, it is in the form of perivascular infiltration with lymphocytes and phagocytic cells (Feigin).

The microscopic pathology of paralytic polio varies, depending on the duration of the illness at the time of death. The earliest visible changes in the spinal cord in the acute stage consist of infiltration with lymphocytes and polymorphonuclear leukocytes in the ventral horns, in addition to chromatolysis of nerve cells in the region (Fig. 13–4). Congestion of vessels and petechial hemorrhages may also be observed when the inflammatory reaction is intense. Collections of inflammatory cells are sparse in some areas and sufficiently dense in other regions to obscure early neuronal changes. The spinal meninges commonly exhibit inflammatory cell infiltration of variable degee, while the cerebral meninges may be entirely spared.

With the passage of time beyond the acute insult, the cellular infiltration becomes less dense, but neurons that are irreversibly damaged undergo necrosis and neuronophagia. This is followed by atrophy of the ventral roots due to loss of myelinated nerve fibers, and denervation atrophy of the involved muscles. In the chronic stages, severely damaged ventral horns contain few or no viable neuronal elements, and may assume a cavitary or cystic appearance to gross observation (Fig. 13–5). Similar degenerative changes are seen in certain areas of gray matter in the brain stem when this region is affected.

Coxsackie Virus Infections

The first strains of the Coxsackie viruses were isolated in 1947 by Dalldorf and Sickles and were so named after the town in New York State where they were recovered. They were separated into two groups on the basis of the pathologic changes produced in suckling mice. There are now 23 types in group A and 6 types in group B, identifiable by neutralization and complement fixation tests, using specific immune serum prepared in animals. Like other enteroviruses, the Coxsackie viruses can cause a variety of clinical illnesses in all age groups, but do so especially in children, and occur in all parts of the world. Most Coxsackie virus infections are mild and self-limited, but their spectrum ranges from asymptomatic disease to conditions with a fatal outcome. The incubation period is usually three to five days but can be as long as ten to 14 days.

Coxsackie viruses have been etiologically associated with a number of clinical syndromes, some of which are primarily caused by members of one of the two groups, while others can result from several types of either group (Table 13–5). A given serotype can cause different illnesses in different patients; for example, Coxsackie A16 is the usual isolate in children with hand, foot, and mouth disease but on rare occasion it has been recovered from spinal fluid in patients with aseptic meningitis. Herpangina is an acute febrile illness in which small, discrete vesicles are formed on the soft palate and adjacent oral mucosa, caused by several types of group A Coxsackie viruses and considerably less often by group B viruses. Acute lymphonodular pharyngitis is a similar transient pharyngitis due to group A type 10 virus, and is characterized by small, raised, nodular lesions on the oral and pharyngeal mucosa (Steigman et al.). Hand, foot, and mouth disease is one of the few Coxsackie infections in which the clinical features are themselves suggestive of a specific etiologic serotype. The majority of the cases result from Coxsackie A16, although A10 and A5 have less often been associated with this illness (Froeschle et al., Meadow, Adler et al.). Features of the illness include stomatitis, a maculopapular rash, vesicles on the hands and feet, and a strong predisposition to affect children in outbreaks in the summer and fall. Epidemic myalgia (Bornholm disease) has occasionally been associated with group A viruses but is mainly due to members of Coxsackie group B viruses. Like most enteroviral infections, it has its highest incidence in the summer and fall and occurs in outbreaks as well as sporadically. Fever is usual but severe muscle pain and tenderness, especially of the chest and abdomen, is the symptomatic hallmark of the disease. Myocarditis, pericarditis, and disseminated disease of the newborn infant are manifestations of the various types of group B Coxsackie viruses and are examples of illnesses that may depart from the usual benign nature of Coxsackie-induced disease.

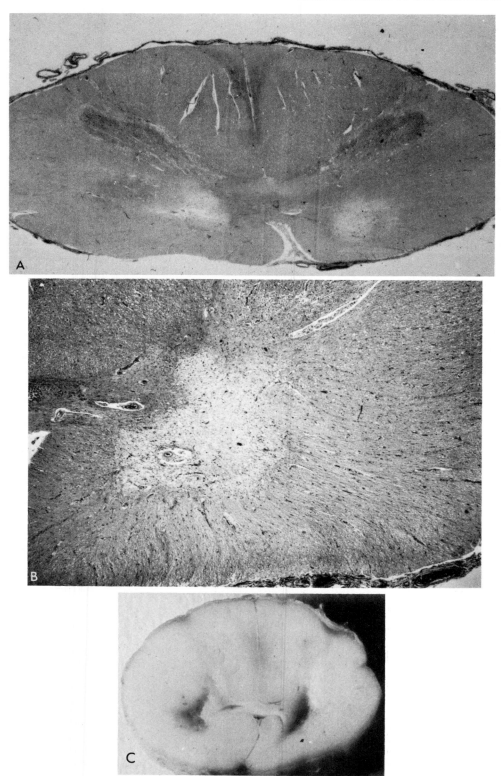

Figure 13–5. Poliomyelitis, chronic stage. *A,* Rarefaction of the anterior horns bilaterally, associated with virtually total neuronal loss and extensive gliosis. *B,* Higher-power view of the damaged ventral horn which assumes a microcystic appearance. *C,* Cross section of the spinal cord in the chronic stage of the disease. The anterior horn regions bilaterally have a cavitary appearance as the result of necrotic changes.

Table 13–5. Conditions Etiologically Associated with Coxsackie Viruses

Herpangina
Epidemic myalgia (Bornholm disease)
Hand, foot, and mouth disease
Acute lymphonodular pharyngitis
Febrile illness with exanthem
Acute respiratory infection
Hepatitis
Myocarditis
Pericarditis
Disseminated neonatal disease (encephalomyocarditis)
Neurologic disease
    Aseptic meningitis
    Encephalitis
    Polio-like paralytic disease
    Acute cerebellar ataxia (rare)
    Guillain-Barré syndrome (rare)
    Acute hemiplegia of infancy-childhood

Neurologic Manifestations

In keeping with the enteroviruses generally, certain Coxsackie viruses are important causes of neurologic disease of different types and severity. Aseptic meningitis is by far the most common neurologic disorder provoked by the Coxsackie viruses. Encephalitis and paralytic disease resembling that caused by the poliovirus are much less frequent but more threatening. Acute cerebellar ataxia (Berg and Jelke) and Guillain-Barré disease (Jackson) on rare occasion have also been associated with Coxsackie viruses of certain strains. Acute hemiplegia of infancy or childhood is an ill-defined but not infrequent disorder which is characterized by the sudden onset of localizing neurologic signs, including hemiparesis and, often, focal seizures. The condition is usually assumed to be the result of a cerebral vascular occlusive episode, although a specific cause is not found in most instances. An inflammatory or infectious arterial lesion has been proposed to account for some examples of this stroke-like disorder (Shillito, Harwood-Nash et al.). Acute hemiplegia believed to be secondary to focal vasculitis due to Coxsackie A9 infection has been described by Roden et al. A similar clinical syndrome in a three-month-old child was reported by Chalhub et al. who favored focal encephalitis caused by Coxsackie A9 to be the underlying pathology. The virus was isolated from cerebrospinal fluid in both cases.

The Coxsackie viruses have been found to represent the most frequent viral cause of aseptic meningitis in recent years (Lennett et al., Meyer et al.), and cases are predomi-

nantly, but not entirely, the result of infection by the members of group B. Coxsackie B5 has been the most prevalent offender (Cramblett et al., Syverton et al., Heathfield et al.), while several different types of group A viruses have also been incriminated. Coxsackie virus aseptic meningitis in most cases is manifested by fever in addition to symptoms and signs of meningeal inflammation, but in some the neurologic aspects are accompanied by myocarditis (Price et al.) or other features of Coxsackie infection such as severe myalgia. Exanthems are not usually seen in children with Coxsackie virus aseptic meningitis but have been described in certain instances (Cherry). In children and young adults, aseptic meningitis is a transient illness followed by recovery without sequelae in the majority of instances. In an occasional patient, following subsidence of the acute phase of the illness, there is persistence of headaches and other signs of increased intracranial pressure, sometimes with the development of papilledema (Wooley). The pathogenesis of this increased pressure syndrome is not clear and perhaps varies in different patients, but some recover promptly with corticosteroid therapy.

Encephalitis is a much less frequent manifestation of Coxsackie infection but has been described in all degrees of severity, including some with a fatal outcome (Jarcho et al., Walters, Heathfield et al.). Parenchymal nervous system involvement in the form of acute paralytic disease caused by non-poliovirus enteroviruses became increasingly evident with the decline of polio infections secondary to immunization programs (Lennett et al., Magoffin et al., Ranzenhofer et al., Steigman). Coxsackie A4, 7, 9, and B2, 3, 4, and 5 have been associated with lower motor neuron involvement within the spinal cord. Like polio infections, flaccid limb weakness due to Coxsackie viruses is usually asymmetrical and associated with fever, meningeal signs, and cells in the cerebrospinal fluid. Spinal cord damage from Coxsackie infection is rarely as severe as it sometimes is with paralytic disease due to the poliovirus. Most Coxsackie-induced paralytic cases are fairly mild and are followed by eventual improvement or complete recovery. With any type of neurologic infection caused by the Coxsackie viruses, the cerebrospinal fluid usually shows a lymphocytic pleocytosis, although neutrophils may predominate in the early stages. In some cases, the initial spinal tap done soon after onset of symptoms will be without cells but a second examination two or three days later will reveal 50 to 500 cells per cu. mm. The glucose content remains normal but the protein value is usually elevated.

Infection of the newborn and young infant with Coxsackie group B viruses carries a greater potential hazard than infection in older patients. Myocarditis is the primary manifestation in some young infants (Hosier and Newton, Robino et al.), and in others the central nervous system is the organ mainly affected (Brightman et al., Swender et al., Rantakallio et al.). In some cases, the illness is mild and transient but a more widely recognized pattern is severe, disseminated neonatal infection manifested by myocarditis, encephalitis, and hepatitis, and sometimes associated with pulmonary and adrenal involvement (Kibrick and Benirschke). The newborn child with widespread Coxsackie group B infection exhibits features similar to those of bacterial sepsis or other types of neonatal viral infection. The clinical manifestations vary, depending on the type and extent of organ system involvement, but can include tachypnea, bradycardia, poor feeding, lethargy, irritability, jaundice, hepatomegaly, and fever in some cases. Severe bleeding can occur when liver involvement is extensive. When cardiorespiratory disturbances are severe, the signs of encephalitis can be submerged among the more generalized signs, and neurologic involvement can be unrecognized unless cerebrospinal fluid abnormalities are found. Disseminated neonatal disease caused by Coxsackie viruses is a serious condition with a significant mortality rate. Infants with more localized infection may show only mild signs and recover completely. Coxsackie infection in the neonate is sometimes acquired in utero (Kibrick and Benirschke) but more often is contracted from perinatal transmission from the mother or from exposure after birth to other infants or adults harboring the virus.

Diagnosis

Diagnosis of Coxsackie virus infection is sometimes suggestive on the basis of clinical and epidemiologic findings but can only be confirmed by serologic and virologic techniques. Four-fold complement fixation and neutralization antibody titer rises on serial serum specimens, or isolation of the virus, are the usual methods of diagnosis of Coxsackie virus disease. Like other enteroviral infections, those caused by the Coxsackie viruses

are most common in the summer and fall months of the year.

ECHO Virus Infections

Following the discovery of the Coxsackie viruses, another group of enteroviruses was recognized which also were occasionally found in the intestinal tract of man. They were initially called "orphan" viruses because they were not then known to cause disease in animals or man, but later received the designation, ECHO (enteric cytopathogenic human orphan) viruses. Although the term has survived and now is in common usage, the viruses were not "orphans" for long. They were soon found to be associated with a wide array of human illnesses and within a short time after discovery were recognized to be a common cause of epidemic and sporadic aseptic meningitis. ECHO 6 was the first type to be unequivocally associated with meningeal infection (Davis and Melnick), but numerous other serotypes were soon implicated. At least 34 serotypes are now known (Wenner and Behbehani), although certain of those originally included among the ECHO viruses have been reclassified in other groups.

In general, ECHO virus infections are usually mild and self-limited, occur in any age group but especially in children five to 12 years of age, and, in temperate climates, have their highest incidence in the summer and early fall. The incubation period of ECHO virus infections, like that of the other enteroviruses, is usually three to five days but may range up to ten days. Clinical syndromes that have been identified due to different types of the ECHO viruses include a transient febrile illness with rash of several possible types, mild upper respiratory infection, gastroenteritis, pericarditis, and neonatal disease with widespread involvement. Some outbreaks received a special designation because of certain unusual characteristics of the clinical illness. For example, "Boston exanthem" was the name given to an illness originally observed in Boston and subsequently in Pittsburgh which consists of fever and other nonspecific symptoms of a few days' duration. With defervescence, a rubelliform rash appears, first on the face and chest, lasting one to five days. The illness thus resembles roseola but has been found to be caused by ECHO virus 16 (Neva et al., Neva). Infections produced by ECHO virus 16 were infrequently observed for a number of years following the initial outbreaks, but recently have again occurred with clinical features similar to the original descriptions (Hall et al.).

Neurologic Manifestations

Neurologic infections are one of the most important manifestations of ECHO virus disease and are usually in the form of aseptic meningitis. Meningoencephalitis can also occur and, less commonly, paralytic disease which resembles that caused by the poliovirus is produced by the ECHO virus. Reye's syndrome (Haynes et al.), acute cerebellar ataxia (McAllister et al.), and Guillain-Barré disease (Urano et al.) have been attributed to the ECHO viruses on rare occasion.

Aseptic meningitis has resulted from almost all serotypes of the ECHO virus, in this country and in many others. They have been found to be the cause of approximately 10 to 20 percent of all cases of aseptic meningitis in which the etiology is identified (Lennette et al., Lepow et al.). ECHO virus type 9 has been one of the more prevalent causes of this syndrome, both in epidemic (Oren et al., Sabin et al., Soloman et al., Portnoy et al., Haynes et al., Levitt et al.) and in sporadic fashion (Saslaw et al.). Outbreaks of ECHO 9 aseptic meningitis, like those caused by other types, have occurred predominantly in the warmer months of the year and have shown a male-to-female preference of between two and four to one.

The symptoms are usually of abrupt onset with fever, headache, and signs of meningeal irritation representing the usual early manifestations of the illness. Photophobia, dizziness, sore throat, mild diarrhea, and muscular pains are additional complaints described by some patients. Infrequently, the illness assumes a biphasic pattern, with one or two days of fever and malaise followed by one to three days without symptoms. Fever then recurs, in addition to other features of meningeal irritation. Rash has been described in 10 to 12 percent of patients with ECHO virus type 9 aseptic meningitis (Portnoy et al., Haynes et al.). The exanthem is usually erythematous and maculopapular in appearance, but can have a petechial quality which simulates meningococcemia (Frothingham). Of 18 patients with ECHO 4 aseptic meningitis reported by Spudis and Cramblett, five were observed to have a macular rash. Rash and neurologic manifestations have also been described in some cases with ECHO virus 16 infection (Hall et al.). In certain ECHO virus epidemics, the presence of rash has been age-determined, being much more common among infants and young children, and less frequent in older patients (Sabin et al.).

Large outbreaks of aseptic meningitis caused by other serotypes have appeared from time to time. A total of 130 cases due to ECHO type 6 occurred in the western part of New York State in 1955 (Karzon et al.). Eighty-two percent of all patients were between four and 15 years of age. Rash was observed in only two cases of the entire group, but muscle stiffness or muscle spasm was notable in the great majority of affected children. ECHO virus type 3 was isolated by Haynes and co-workers from 29 children in Columbus, Ohio between August and November, 1970. Twenty-four patients were classified as having aseptic meningitis while one child had meningeal infection, pericarditis, and myocarditis. Encephalitic manifestations occurred in one other child. ECHO virus 17, previously known to be a cause of sporadic aseptic meningitis, made its appearance in large scale in certain communities in Great Britain in 1969. Over a two-year period, the virus was isolated from 152 patients, 89 of whom exhibited neurologic symptoms (Hart and Miller). Approximately 75 percent of cases were children and almost one-half were less than five years of age. A very similar outbreak again occurred in England in the summer and fall of 1974, this one caused by ECHO virus 19 (Codd et al.). Fifty percent of the cases were in children under eight years of age and 8 percent were in infants less than six months of age. The illness was described as "serious" in magnitude in only eight patients of the total of 268 cases, seven of the eight being under six months of age. An epidemic of ECHO virus 18 aseptic meningitis occurred in Australia in 1969 (Kennett et al.) and reappeared in Durham, North Carolina, in 1972 (Wilfert et al.). Of the 103 cases of aseptic meningitis observed between June and the end of August, most were patients from the Durham area, 80 percent were under 25 years of age, and the majority were caused by ECHO virus 18. Virus was isolated from 73 percent of the cerebrospinal fluid specimens that were cultured. ECHO virus 18 had been recognized previously as a sporadic cause of aseptic meningitis (Eckert et al.), but the Durham epidemic was the first recorded large outbreak in this country due to this serotype.

Although ECHO virus epidemics have primarily attacked school-age children, young infants and even neonates can also be affected in either epidemic or sporadic fashion. An outbreak of ECHO virus type 3 in Virginia in 1970 had its highest attack rate for children under six months of age (Peters et al.). A similar localized epidemic in New Haven in 1965 was caused by ECHO 11 and in more than one-half of all the identified cases the infants were less than six months of age (Miller et al.). Young infants were also predominantly involved in the series published by Linnemann et al. in which the offending organism was ECHO 4.

In the neonatal period, ECHO virus infection has not received the notoriety that has been bestowed on the disseminated form of Coxsackie B infection but is considerably more common. Similarly to ECHO virus infections in general, those in newborn and young infants usually are seen in summer or fall months of the year (Lake et al.). ECHO virus infection in the newborn has resulted from several different types, often with severe neurologic involvement (McDonald et al., Philip and Larson, Nogen and Lepow, Krous et al., Cramblett et al.). The source of the virus producing neonatal disease has not been clearly established in most instances but it is assumed that infection can be acquired in utero, during the birth process, or by contamination in the nursery after delivery. The clinical manifestations in reported cases have resembled those of viral or bacterial neonatal infection generally, and have included fever, apneic spells, poor feeding, lethargy, jaundice, petechiae, and hepatosplenomegaly. In some instances, the occurrence of convulsions, sudden peripheral vascular collapse, thrombocytopenia, and polymorphonuclear pleocytosis in cerebrospinal fluid make clinical differentiation from bacterial sepsis or meningitis impossible until the results of cultures clarify the diagnosis (Bacon and Sims, Lake et al.). Neurologic involvement has been quite variable but can be severe. In some neonates, evidence of central nervous system involvement has been present despite minimal or no cerebrospinal fluid abnormalities (McDonald et al., Philip and Larson). Massive hepatic necrosis and disseminated intravascular coagulation have been found in certain fatal cases (Philip and Larson, Krous et al.).

Neurologic disease produced by ECHO viruses is generally mild and followed by recovery without sequelae, although chronic neurologic impairment can result, especially when the newborn or young infant is involved (Sells et al.). An occasional child with enteroviral aseptic meningitis will seemingly recover from the acute infectious part of the illness but will have persistent headaches for days or even weeks thereafter. Papilledema can develop in such patients secondary to increased intracranial pressure, and response to corticosteroids is sometimes dramatic. Members of the ECHO group can cause severe or even fatal encephalitis although this is considerably less common than an acute meningeal syndrome and has been described with only a few ECHO serotypes. Peters et al. reported an unusual type of neurologic involvement caused by ECHO 25 in a child with acute onset of hemichorea and hemiparesis with a mild cellular reaction in the CSF. The illness was associated with a focal low-density lesion in the basal ganglia on the opposite side on the cranial computed tomogram.

ECHO virus has also been implicated as a cause of myelitis (Johnson and Eger) and has been added to the list of viruses somehow associated with Reye's syndrome (Haynes et al.). In addition, several ECHO virus serotypes, like certain of the Coxsackie viruses, have been found to cause flaccid limb paresis or paralysis without sensory loss, identical to that with poliovirus infection. Fatal cases with bulbar and spinal cord involvement have been associated with ECHO type 2 and 11 infection (Steigman, Steigman and Lipton). Illnesses less severe but typical of paralytic poliomyelitis have also been caused by ECHO type 3 (Williams et al., Stevenson and Hambling), type 4 (Kopel et al.), and types 6, 9, 16, and 30 (Hammon et al., Ashkenazi and Melnick, Kleinman et al.). Some reports of ECHO virus-induced focal limb paralysis have suggested that prognosis for recovery is more favorable when caused by this virus compared to paralytic disease due to the poliovirus. Of the series of 130 cases of ECHO 6 aseptic meningitis described by Karzon et al., mild or minor neuromuscular abnormalities were frequently observed during the acute stage of the illness. Reflex loss was noted in 16 percent and mild muscle weakness in 39 percent, but recovery occurred in the great majority.

None of the members of the enterovirus group have been considered to be significant causes of disease in the immunosuppressed patient or in patients with disturbances in antibody-mediated immunity. Bardelas et al., however, have described a child with hypogammaglobulinemia who developed a progressive disorder ending fatally which was caused by disseminated infection with ECHO virus 24. The illness was associated with a dermatomyositis-like syndrome and the cerebrospinal fluid revealed a lymphocytic pleocytosis present over the course of a number of months. ECHO virus was isolated from the cerebrospinal fluid, and at autopsy there was lymphocytic infiltration within the meninges and in a perivascular distribution in the brain. Two similar children with primary hypogammaglobulinemia complicated by subacute and progressive ECHO virus encephalitis were described by Webster et al. In one of the cases, dermatomyositis-like features improved after treatment with infusions of plasma containing virus-specific antibody, although the child subsequently died of encephalitis. Immune plasma was also tried in the patient reported by Bodensteiner et al. but the illness ended in death five years after the onset of the neurologic disorder. Five additional patients with agammaglobulinemia were reported by Wilfert et al., three of whom also had a dermatomyositis-like syndrome. Although the neurologic complaints of these children varied considerably, all had a cerebrospinal fluid pleocytosis on repeated examinations and all had ECHO viruses of various serotypes isolated from the cerebrospinal fluid. Persistent neurologic infection in these cases led the authors to suggest that intact B-cell function is essential for termination of central nervous system enterovirus infection.

Diagnosis

Diagnosis of neurologic infections due to the ECHO viruses depends on serologic and virologic methods because of the nonspecificity of the clinical syndrome. An enterovirus is suspected when aseptic meningitis or encephalitis occurs in association with rash, myocarditis, or focal, flaccid limb paresis. Diagnosis, however, must be established by demonstration of an antibody titer rise or isolation of the offending virus. The peripheral white blood cell count is subject to considerable variation, being normal in some cases but elevated to levels as high as 25,000 per cu. mm. in others. The cerebrospinal fluid usually shows a lymphocytic pleocytosis, although in the first day or so of the illness polymorphonuclear leukocytes may be predominant. In some cases, the cerebrospinal fluid cellular response is minimal, but in most, 50 to 500 cells per cu. mm. are present. Over 2,000 cells per cu. mm. can be found in exceptional instances. Cases have been described in which enterovirus was isolated from cerebrospinal fluid in the absence of a significant cellular response (Yeager et al., Wilfert et al.).

Occasionally, the combination of peripheral blood leukocytosis and a neutrophilic response in the cerebrospinal fluid is sufficiently marked that bacterial meningitis is suspected until cultures prove negative (Haynes et al., Miller et al.). The cerebrospinal fluid glucose content is normal while the protein content is often increased to levels between 50 and 150 mg. per 100 ml. Fourfold or greater rises of type specific serum neutralization, complement fixation, or hemagglutination inhibition antibodies are diagnostic of ECHO virus infection. Feces, oropharyngeal secretions, and cerebrospinal fluid are specimens from which ECHO viruses can sometimes be recovered from children with aseptic meningitis or encephalitis. Isolation of the virus only from stools is of suggestive diagnostic value but is not proof that the neurologic infection is caused by the virus that is isolated. ECHO virus is isolated with relative ease from cerebrospinal fluid in children with aseptic meningitis. It is successful with infections caused by the ECHO virus group more often than many other viruses and is more likely to be accomplished when the specimen is obtained early in the course of the illness.

MEASLES ENCEPHALITIS (ENCEPHALOMYELITIS)

The disease referred to as measles (rubeola) had been recognized for centuries but was clearly separated from other exanthematous conditions by Thomas Sydenham in the seventeenth century. Thereafter, it became known as a highly contagious disease transmitted from person to person by droplet spread of virus-containing respiratory secretions. The measles virus is an RNA-containing myxovirus in the paramyxovirus group and, along with the distemper and rinderpest viruses, is placed in the medipest subgroup (Melnick).

The significance and broad spectrum of measles virus infections have come to be recognized only in recent years and gradually continue to unfold as new observations are made. The hazard of this virus to the immunosuppressed child and the occurrence of a chronic, progressive encephalitis in the form of subacute sclerosing panencephalitis are relatively recent additions to our knowledge of the effects of the measles virus. Its possible role as a cause of fetal defects is an additional topic of concern in the past few years, and is one that remains to be clarified (Jespersen et al.).

An incubation period of ten to 14 days precedes the initial symptoms of measles of fever, coryza, and conjunctivitis. The first distinctive features of the illness are the Koplik spots, which are observed on the buccal mucosa two to three days after onset of symptoms and two to three days before onset of the cutaneous rash. The diagnostic importance of these lesions was emphasized by Henry Koplik of New York in 1896. In his description in the *Archives of Pediatrics,* Koplik stated that "on the buccal mucous membrane and inside the lips, we invariably see a distinct eruption. It consists of small, irregular spots, of a bright red color. In the center of each spot, there is noted, in strong daylight, a minute bluish white speck. These red spots, with accompanying specks of a bluish white color, are absolutely pathognomonic of beginning measles, and when seen can be relied upon as a forerunner of the skin eruption."

The second distinctive feature of measles is the erythematous maculopapular rash, which makes its debut behind the ears and along the hairline of the forehead before spreading over the face and eventually comes to involve the trunk and limbs (Fig. 13–6). With spread of the rash, the constitutional symptoms worsen and fever is accentuated. After two to four days, the rash begins to fade, and does so in the same order that it had appeared. A characteristic feature of measles which can be of diagnostic importance in some cases is the presence of multinucleated giant cells, referred to as Warthin-Finkeldey giant cells. They can be demonstrated by histologic examination of conjunctival or pharyngeal scrapings and are present even before the appearance of the exanthem and for a few days after its onset. Antibodies make their appearance in the serum soon after the appearance of the rash and persist for many years, providing a reliable indication of immunity. Measles virus is present in blood, urine, and respiratory secretions during the prodromal stage of the illness but is isolated by laboratory means only with considerable difficulty.

Measles is a disease of considerable significance when one considers the intensity of symptoms of the acute illness as well as the threat of several possible serious complications. Bronchopneumonia caused by secondary invading bacteria is one of the most common serious complications, while acute encephalitis is perhaps the one most feared. Purulent otitis media can develop in severe cases, and in past years, sometimes led to suppurative mastoiditis. Another observation made in the past was the occurrence of measles as an immediate antecedent of childhood pulmonary tuberculosis (Lincoln et al.). Whether it was an actual causative precipitant of tuberculosis in such cases has been a subject of debate and remains unsettled (Christie). The mortality rate from measles in this

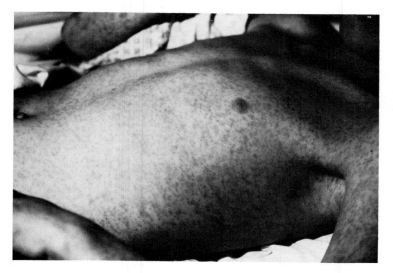

Figure 13–6. Characteristic erythematous maculopapular eruption with measles. Eleven-year-old boy with onset of rash 4 days previously, first noticed on the forehead. One day prior to admission, he became confused and developed neck stiffness, diffuse hyperreflexia, and neurogenic bladder dysfunction, indicative of acute measles encephalomyelitis. CSF contained 42 white blood cells per cu. mm., 54 percent neutrophils. Complete recovery eventually followed.

country has been quite low, but this is not true in other parts of the world. In many underdeveloped countries with widespread malnutrition and a high incidence of a variety of chronic infections, measles represents a serious disease and is among the major causes of childhood death (Ogbeide, Morley, Teneja et al.).

The danger of infection with measles virus is enhanced considerably in the child with an immunocompromised condition. Death from giant cell pneumonia is well known in children with leukemia (Breitfeld et al., Siegel et al.), and has also occurred in other disorders with immune disturbances, such as combined immunodeficiency syndrome (Mihatsch et al.) and with cyclophosphamide-treated nephrotic syndrome (Meadow et al.). The onset of pulmonary involvement in immunosuppressed patients occurs at variable periods of time after the acute measles infection and may be as long as a year thereafter. In addition, the acute, systemic measles infection in such children can occur in the absence of a rash or the absence of a measles antibody response. A more recent discovery is another type of process which can be caused by the measles virus in the immunosuppressed patient in the form of a subacute, progressive encephalitis (Murphy and Yunis, Wolinsky et al.). The identification of this condition expands the spectrum of neurologic dysfunction produced by this virus and is discussed in the subsequent section.

Following the isolation of the measles virus by Enders and Peebles in 1954 and its subsequent attenuation by Katz et al., the way was paved for the eventual licensure of two measles vaccines in 1963. These included a live attenuated measles virus vaccine and a formalin-inactivated vaccine. Before licensure of the live attenuated vaccine in 1963, there were approximately 500,000 cases of measles and between 300 and 400 cases of measles encephalitis reported per year in the United States. By 1968, the use of the vaccine had reduced the number of reported measles cases to 25,000, a decreased incidence of 95 percent (Krugman). The incidence of measles encephalitis, estimated to occur in approximately one per 1,000 cases, correspondingly declined in dramatic fashion.

The major step toward control of natural measles did not, however, remove the measles virus from medical interest or importance. Outbreaks of considerable magnitude have continued to occur (Weiner et al., Shasby et al.), generally with a shift in the age

groups involved, from the younger child in past years, to the older child and adolescent group currently. Most cases have been in unimmunized children, although some have occurred in children who were immunized before one year of age or who received live measles vaccine that had lost its potency because of improper handling (Krugman et al.). Soon after the initial reduction in the occurrence of the natural disease, measles virus or a measles-like virus was incriminated as a causative factor in the production of subacute sclerosing panencephalitis. Unexpected but usually insignificant complications, such as thrombocytopenia, were observed following the use of the live vaccine (Bachand et al., Alter et al., Oski and Naiman), while measles post-vaccinal encephalitis has occurred only rarely (Nader and Warren), and certainly with a much lower incidence than encephalitis following natural measles. The Guillain-Barré syndrome has also been reported following administration of live measles vaccine but also appears to be exceedingly unusual (Grose and Spigland).

Another remarkable change of character of infection produced by the measles virus was observed in recipients of killed vaccine when they were exposed to live measles virus months or years later. This "atypical measles" infection was characterized by high fever, tachypnea, myalgia, peripheral edema, and a macular, vesicular, or purpuric rash, which began distally on the lower limbs and progressed cephalad (Cherry et al., Nader et al., Fulginiti et al.). Koplik spots were usually absent and, unlike natural measles, pneumonia, sometimes associated with pleural effusion, was present in most cases (Young et al.). The resolution of pulmonary infiltrates in the acute stage is sometimes followed by the chronic persistence of pulmonary nodules roentgenographically (Laptook et al.). An adverse reaction to live measles vaccine administration to children previously inoculated with killed virus vaccine also was observed (Scott and Bonanno), adding evidence that the killed virus somehow acted as a sensitizing agent. As a result of these altered host responses, inactivated measles vaccine was removed from availability.

Neurologic Complications of Measles

Acute Neurologic Complications. Our understanding of the types of acute nervous system involvement, the frequency of occurrence, and the pathogenesis of any form of neurologic involvement by the measles virus has never been clear. In part, this is explained by the complexity of the problem but is also the result of the tendency in the past to label almost any central nervous system disorder which occurred during the course of measles as "encephalitis." Statistics dealing with complications or sequelae were sometimes compiled from hospitalized patients without sufficient regard to the concept that only the more severe or complicated cases needed hospital admission whereas in the mild or "average" case the patient remained at home and frequently was never evaluated medically at all. The current availability of a method which can potentially eliminate natural measles, it is hoped, will limit the resources for the future study of the acute neurologic complications to the experimental arena.

Neurologic disturbances associated with measles only rarely mentioned in the literature include acute blindness, probably due to bilateral retrobulbar neuritis (Strom, Schlossberg and Prizer, Tyler), acute transient cerebellar ataxia (Tyler, Griffith), and peripheral polyneuropathy (Berkovich and Schneck, Peterman et al., Roseman and Aring), sometimes with characteristics of the Guillain-Barré syndrome. So-called "febrile" seizures unaccompanied by other clinical or cerebrospinal fluid evidence of encephalitis can occur in young children with measles but are not common.

An additional non-encephalitic complication of measles is the abrupt onset of hemiplegia, usually preceded by or developing simultaneously with repetitive focal convulsions. The cerebrospinal fluid is usually unremarkable in such patients and the hemiparesis is often permanent. Hemiplegia and other associated unilateral focal signs are most likely the result of cerebral arterial occlusion secondary to an inflammatory process affecting the vessel wall.

An acute encephalopathy manifested by symptoms and signs of increased intracranial pressure which rapidly leads to coma, decerebrate rigidity, and death has also been observed during the course of measles (Tyler). The cerebrospinal fluid in this disorder is unremarkable except for increased pressure, and the neuropathology is that of profound brain swelling and internal herniations but without features of encephalitis or perivenous demyelination. This disorder, sometimes referred to as "toxic" encephalopathy

or "acute encephalopathy of obscure origin" (Lyon et al.), has been described following a variety of childhood infections and has many similarities with Reye's syndrome. Neurologic complications of measles, such as acute hemiplegia and acute, fulminating encephalopathy, remain unclear in regard to pathogenesis but should be considered separate from measles encephalomyelitis, which is more common and has different pathologic and prognostic characteristics.

The most common acute adverse neurologic reaction in children with measles has been variously referred to as measles encephalitis or encephalomyelitis, post-infectious encephalomyelitis, para-infectious encephalomyelitis, measles perivascular myelinoclasis, and measles hyperergic encephalomyelitis. The term, post-infectious encephalomyelitis, is somewhat misleading in that symptoms or signs of the cerebral process occur in the early stages of the systemic illness in some cases and, rarely, will even precede the appearance of the rash (Holliday). Because the disorder is now believed to be associated with cerebral invasion by the measles virus and since both the brain and spinal cord are usually affected, the term acute measles encephalomyelitis would appear to be appropriate. In addition to the well-known symptomatic forms of measles encephalomyelitis, studies have suggested that the measles virus commonly involves the brain, even in the absence of clinical neurologic dysfunction. Gibbs et al. found significant slow electroencephalographic abnormalities in 51 percent of 680 patients with measles without signs of encephalitis. Cerebrospinal fluid abnormalities in some patients with uncomplicated measles also suggest that subclinical cerebral involvement is relatively common in this disease (Adams et al.).

The frequency of encephalomyelitis in measles has varied greatly in different reports, but the most widely accepted figures have been approximately one case in 600 (Hoyne and Slotkowski) to one in 1,000 (La Boccetta and Tornay). The occurrence of neurologic involvement appears unrelated to the intensity of the rash or the severity of the systemic illness. In most cases, the onset of neurologic symptoms is between the second and fifth day after the appearance of the rash, but the illness can even precede the first symptoms of measles or occur anytime in the first two weeks thereafter. Recurrence of temperature along with headache, confusion, convulsions, lethargy, or coma are the usual early signs. Monoparesis, paraplegia, and neurogenic bladder or bowel dysfunction sometimes are found, indicative of spinal cord involvement. Cerebellar ataxia is seen in some or may become evident as gradual recovery allows ambulation, but is rarely a prominent feature of the illness. The neurologic signs in measles encephalomyelitis usually reflect both diffuse and multifocal abnormalities of the cerebrum, brain stem, and spinal cord, and thus are complex and variable from case to case. Isolated myelitis with minimal or no evidence of intracranial pathology is one of the least common forms of the disease. The mortality rate of acute measles encephalomyelitis is in the range of 10 to 15 percent and neurologic sequelae compromise function in approximately 20 percent of survivors (Tyler, Hoyne and Slotkowski).

In the great majority of cases of measles encephalomyelitis, the cerebrospinal fluid reveals abnormalities, which include a lymphocytic pleocytosis, a mild to moderate increase in the protein content, and a variable opening pressure which may be either normal or elevated (Peterman and Fox). The glucose content is normal or mildly elevated.

The pathogenesis of measles encephalomyelitis has been a subject of debate and dispute since the complication was first recognized many years ago. Proposed theories included direct invasion of the brain by the measles virus, activation of a latent neurotrophic virus by the systemic disease, and a cerebral reaction to a foreign substance, which is referred to as "allergic" or "immunologic" in nature. Such considerations arose because of the inability to isolate virus from the brain of affected patients and because of the characteristic perivenous demyelination observed in the brain in fatal cases. Virtually identical pathologic changes are seen in encephalomyelitis associated with measles, some cases due to mumps and varicella, smallpox, and following vaccination for smallpox and rabies (Ferraro and Roizin 1957, Adams and Kubik). The microscopic alterations in these conditions differ considerably from those classically described in viral encephalitis but show striking similarity to the cerebral lesions in experimental allergic encephalomyelitis (Ferraro et al. 1950). The concept was therefore developed that the "post-infectious" and "post-vaccinal" encephalomyelitides must have certain common pathogenic factors, presumably somehow related to an "allergic" or "hypersensitivity" reaction of the host tissue to the multiplying virus, or to products of damage inflicted by the virus on tissue (Koprowski).

Recent studies have provided definite evidence that the measles virus does invade the brain in measles encephalomyelitis. Laboratory findings supporting this concept were published as early as 1942 when Shaffer et al. produced a measles-like clinical illness in monkeys following injection into the animals of a suspension made from postmortem-obtained brain tissue of a child with acute measles encephalitis. In 1966, Adams and colleagues demonstrated the presence of cytoplasmic and nuclear inclusion bodies in 15 of 20 fatal cases, and also found multinucleated giant cells in the brain in five cases of measles encephalitis, findings suggestive of viral invasion of brain tissue. Ter Meulen et al. succeeded in isolation of measles virus from the brain in a fatal case of encephalomyelitis by the method of co-cultivation of cells of the infected brain with those of African green monkey kidney tissue. Although these observations and findings strongly support the concept of direct involvement of the brain by the measles virus, ter Meulen et al. pointed out that such infection is not a simple one since, in their case, the virus could not be isolated directly but required co-cultivation techniques.

The precise explanation for the pathologic alterations in measles encephalomyelitis remains unclear but it seems probable that the process is in some way induced by virus invasion of the brain. Individual predisposition may be required for the resulting cerebral reaction, which appears to be a host immune response to the virus or to products of tissue damage induced by the virus, leading to the morphologic changes which include perivenous edema and cellular infiltration, followed by perivenous demyelination.

The cerebral pathology in the early stages of measles encephalomyelitis reveals a meningeal cellular infiltrate of variable degree, as well as cerebral swelling with venous congestion, petechial hemorrhages in white matter in some cases, and perivenous infiltration with mononuclear cells followed by perivenous edema. Myelin destruction with relative sparing of axons is subsequently established in the perivenous distribution. Demyelination also occurs in subpial and subependymal regions in the brain and spinal cord (Adams and Kubik). Glial and neuronal cytoplasmic and nuclear inclusion bodies resembling Cowdry type A inclusions, along with small multinucleated giant cells, represent the hallmark of measles infection in the acute stage (Adams et al., Adams, ter Meulen). Neuronal degenerative changes are usually minimal to mild in the acute stage. Changes in the cerebral cortex consist of an increase in microglia and the presence of swollen astrocytes. In general, the pathologic alterations are most prominent in the white matter of the cerebrum, brain stem, and spinal cord, although the gray matter is not entirely spared.

Treatment of the child with encephalomyelitis complicating measles is fundamentally conservative, with measures to prevent marked hyperthermia, to control seizures, and to maintain fluid and electrolyte balance. Increased intracranial pressure should be managed by the prevention of hyperthermia, use of intravenous mannitol as indicated, and controlled ventilation as necessary. As is the case with any type of severe encephalitis, respiratory compromise enhances the degree of intracranial hypertension and increases the risk of internal herniation. Corticosteroids have been recommended by some in view of the postulates regarding pathogenesis, but the value of this form of therapy has not been proved (Karelitz and Eisenberg).

Subacute and Chronic Neurologic Complications. The discovery of an association of the measles virus with a chronic, progressive encephalitis in the form of subacute sclerosing panencephalitis added a new dimension to the spectrum of neurologic disease provoked by this virus. Dawson, in 1933, described a type of chronic encephalitis in previously normal children which was believed to be of viral origin and which was then called Dawson's subacute inclusion body encephalitis. It was not until 1965, however, that the measles virus was incriminated, when Bouteille et al. demonstrated paramyxovirus nucleocapsids in the brain of children with the disease, by this time referred to as subacute sclerosing panencephalitis. Subsequent studies revealed that measles antibody titers were elevated in serum and cerebrospinal fluid in such patients, and that measles virus could be cultivated from brain tissue.

Following the introduction of measles vaccine, the disease decreased considerably in frequency. Concern then arose over the possibility of its occurrence following vaccine administration (Modlin et al.), although the risk has been shown to be much less than

after natural measles (Krugman, 1977). The precise role played by the measles virus in producing this type of chronic encephalitis has remained a subject of speculation to the present date. The disease affects previously normal children, although in a few cases a preceding viral infection with a different virus has raised suspicion of virus-associated immunosuppression which somehow allows activation of a latent myxovirus infection (Feorino et al., Hochberg et al.). Most cases, however, occur without such an association, and little is known as to predisposing factors accounting for this illness.

A subacute and moderately rapid progressive form of encephalitis in the immunosuppressed patient is the most recently identified expression of neurologic disease caused by the measles virus. In 1973, Breitfeld and colleagues described two children with leukemia in remission who developed a progressive fatal encephalitis caused by the measles virus. One child had coexistent Hecht's giant-cell pneumonia, and in both the neurologic process became evident within a few months of the primary measles infection, with death occurring within six months of the primary illness. Thereafter, there appeared several reports establishing the existence of a type of subacute progressive encephalitis caused by the measles virus in the immunosuppressed patient (Murphy and Yunis, Pullan et al., Smyth et al., Aicardi et al., Haltia et al., Wolinsky et al.). This illness differs from acute measles encephalitis by the longer time interval between the primary infection with measles and the onset of cerebral signs, by its occurrence in the immunosuppressed patient, and by features more of a progressive, degenerative character and less of an inflammatory process. It departs from the usual pattern of subacute sclerosing panencephalitis by its onset in closer proximity to the primary measles infection, the more rapid course, and again, its occurrence in the patient with a previously identified underlying systemic disease. The electroencephalographic findings in the subacute form of immunosuppressive measles encephalitis include a variety of diffuse or focal abnormalities which are unlike the characteristic "suppression burst" pattern seen with SSPE. In addition, there has not been a consistent elevation of the CSF measles antibody titer in the subacute form in the immunosuppressed patient, as occurs with SSPE.

Most cases thus far described of subacute measles encephalitis have been leukemic children in remission, although the illness has occurred in an adult with Hodgkin's disease (Wolinsky et al.) and in a 21-year-old man following renal transplantation (Agamanolis et al.). The primary measles infection has usually occurred two to six months before onset of the neurologic disorder, but in rare instances no definite preceding infection with the measles virus had been recognized (Agamanolis et al.). Recurrent seizures, often with gradual deterioration of the state of mentation and alertness, are the usual initial signs of the disorder. Seizures are frequently focal in type, and in several cases have been in the form of epilepsia partialis continua or segmental myoclonus. Other neurologic signs are variable but commonly suggest the presence of a diffuse but multifocal cerebral process. The child with rhabdomyosarcoma complicated by subacute measles encephalitis described by Haltia et al. was found to have a retinopathy during life similar to that described with subacute sclerosing panencephalitis. In most reported instances, gradual deterioration is followed by death a few weeks after onset of the neurologic manifestations. Cerebrospinal fluid examination during the course of the illness is usually non-revealing and, notably, contains either no cells or an insignificant number of white blood cells.

On neuropathologic examination in such cases, the gross appearance of the brain may be normal, but microscopic examination reveals prominent findings, including eosinophilic inclusions in glial cells and neurons, and giant cells in some instances. Microglial nodules and perivascular round cell infiltration are seen in variable degree, and can be entirely absent. The extensive degree of neuronal loss and fibrillary astrocytosis characteristic of subacute sclerosing panencephalitis is not found with this disorder. Electron micrographs of formalin-fixed tissue show tubular aggregates consistent with those of myxovirus infection, confirmed by immunofluorescent methods (Pullan et al., Wolinsky et al.).

Thus, the neurologic complications of infection with the measles virus are legion and represent a broad spectrum of disorders which occur in different settings. Acute measles encephalitis, a perivenous demyelinating form of encephalitis, was the first to be identified and will continue to be a serious health hazard unless measles can be entirely curtailed by immunization. Subacute sclerosing panencephalitis, classified among the chronic encephalitides, was next identified, and, finally, a subacute measles encephalitis in the immunosuppressed patient has been recognized. Cases of the latter have shown a rather characteristic clinical pattern which allows suspicion of the etiologic source but which is progressive and is not amenable to currently available therapy.

MUMPS ASEPTIC MENINGITIS AND ENCEPHALITIS

Mumps, or epidemic parotitis, is a common and usually benign viral disease, most often seen in children between four and ten years of age, with an incubation period of 14 to 18 days, and which affects males more often than females. The illness rarely occurs in the first year of life. Inapparent infections with this virus are frequent, estimated to be in the range of 30 to 40 percent. The common symptomatic manifestation of the illness is inflammation of the salivary glands characterized by tender swelling of the parotid glands and usually associated with fever and malaise. Certain cases have associated symptomatic orchitis, pancreatitis, aseptic meningitis, or encephalitis. Still others are manifested only by neurologic symptoms and signs with no apparent salivary gland involvement, and diagnosed only by serologic and virologic methods.

The mumps virus, classified among the paramyxovirus group of the myxoviruses (Melnick), is widely recognized to be one of the most common causes of acute aseptic meningitis, but recently, investigators have suggested another possible role of this virus in the production of neurologic disease. Experiments in suckling hamsters by Johnson and Johnson in 1968 demonstrated that intracerebral inoculation of mumps virus produced an infection of ependymal cells associated with a temporary, marked perivascular inflammatory response. Eventual loss of ependyma resulted in stenotic changes of the aqueduct of Sylvius, subsequently leading to pronounced hydrocephalus. Fluorescent antibody staining for virus antigen revealed that virus growth was almost entirely confined to the ependymal cells.

Other investigators later showed that inoculation of the mumps virus into the amniotic sac could also induce destructive ependymitis followed by hydrocephalus in newborn hamsters (Kilham and Margolis). Mumps virus inoculated into the cerebrum of fetal rhesus monkeys also results in virus replication within the fetal tissues leading to hydrocephalus, although the pathologic changes are different in the monkey as compared to the hamster (London et al.). In the monkey, the ventricular enlargement is most striking in the posterior horns and when obstructive lesions are found, they are at a variety of levels within the ventricular system and not confined to the periaqueductal region. Following these observations, Timmons and Johnson and, later, Bray described children who developed hydrocephalus secondary to aqueductal obstruction, 27 and 30 months, respectively, after having naturally acquired mumps, with neurologic symptoms transiently present during the acute illness. A cause-and-effect relationship was only suggestive and not proved in these cases.

Additional evidence supporting the concept of mumps virus infection causing ependymal damage has come from electron microscopic studies of cerebrospinal fluid of children with mumps aseptic meningitis. Herndon et al. demonstrated the presence of ependymal cells and cytoplasmic inclusions of viral nucleocapsid-like material in the cerebrospinal fluid of several children with this illness, findings not identified in control subjects with other viral neurologic infections. Further studies will be required to determine if the mumps virus is a cause of acquired hydrocephalus in older children or of congenital hydrocephalus secondary to transplacentally transmitted intrauterine infection. Little is known to date of the possible damaging effects of the mumps virus when acquired by the fetus early in pregnancy. The majority of pregnancies complicated by mumps follow an uneventful course, although there are reports of fetal abnormalities resulting (Greenberg and Beilly, Holowach et al.).

The mumps virus is one of the most common viral causes of neurologic infection encountered in clinical practice. Any level of the nervous system can be affected during the course of this illness, either preceding or following symptoms of parotid gland involvement. In some children, the mumps virus gives rise to neurologic infection in the absence of parotitis. Aseptic meningitis is by far the most common central nervous system complication of mumps. Encephalitis is much less common but is prognostically less favorable, while transverse myelitis and polyneuritis have been described rather infrequently

(Scheid, Benady et al.). Aseptic meningitis accounted for 81 percent of the 42 cases of central nervous system mumps virus infection in the series of Lennette et al. and for 74 percent of 91 cases of Meyer et al. Of 137 patients with neurologic involvement described by Johnstone et al., only six had encephalitic signs and the remaining 131 were classified as aseptic meningitis.

The incidence with which aseptic meningitis or encephalitis complicates infection with the mumps virus is not known. Previous estimates have varied from less than 1 percent to better than one-half of all cases, and thus are of limited value. The remarkable variations in the estimates are due to many factors, one being the different diagnostic criteria that have been used. Compilation of a hospital-oriented series is obviously misleading since most cases of mumps are mild and many are never seen medically. Considering all cases of mumps in children, the incidence of significant clinical neurologic involvement associated with a cerebrospinal fluid pleocytosis must be quite low. Conversely, it is probable that during the viremic stage, the virus frequently invades the central nervous system. In one series, a cerebrospinal fluid cellular response was observed in over 60 percent of all clinically apparent mumps infections (Bang and Bang).

Mumps aseptic meningitis or encephalitis affects males more than females in a ratio of approximately two to one. It occurs at any time of year but the peak incidence is during spring and early fall. The diagnosis is established most readily when neurologic symptoms are preceded by parotitis. Clinical evidence of parotitis occurred in only 37 percent of cases of mumps aseptic meningitis-encephalitis reported by Johnstone et al., in 53 percent of cases described by Levitt et al., in 43 percent of those in the series of Ritter, and in 47 percent in the group collected by Azimi et al. Thus, in 50 percent or more of cases with neurologic involvement by the mumps virus, serologic or virologic tests provide the only indicators of the etiologic diagnosis. In cases in which parotitis does occur, the onset of neurologic symptoms may precede the first evidence of parotid swelling by several days, but more often will develop three to ten days afterward. Several authors have noted that mumps aseptic meningitis most often develops two to three days after the onset of parotitis, while those with encephalitic manifestations more often have the appearance of neurologic symptoms seven to nine days following parotitis.

Symptoms and signs in the child with mumps aseptic meningitis include fever, which often spikes to high levels the day of onset of the neurologic complaints. Headache and vomiting are usual, in association with neck stiffness and other signs of meningeal irritation. A certain degree of malaise and lethargy are acceptable with this syndrome, which usually lasts three to seven days, when recovery occurs. Mumps encephalitis is a more severe illness that may begin with fever and meningeal signs but is promptly complicated by mental confusion, disorientation, drowsiness, convulsions, or a variety of other cerebral, brain stem or spinal cord signs. This illness is likely to be a more protracted one, can be followed by lasting sequelae, and, rarely, can be fatal (Bistrian et al., Donohue et al., Schwarz et al., Taylor and Toreson).

The peripheral white blood cell count varies from normal to over 25,000 per cu. mm. in children with central nervous system mumps infection and cannot be used as a differentiation of viral from bacterial disease. Serum amylase is elevated in most children with mumps parotitis but has been found to be normal in most patients with mumps meningitis or encephalitis without parotid gland involvement (Azimi et al.). Cerebrospinal fluid findings in children with mumps aseptic meningitis or encephalitis include a pleocytosis ranging from 10 to 2,000 cells per cu. mm. Lymphocytes are the predominant cell type in most but polymorphonuclear leukocytes can be more prevalent, especially on the first or second day of the illness. The protein content is usually normal or only mildly increased. The cerebrospinal fluid glucose value is normal in the majority of cases, although reduction to levels between 20 and 40 mg. per 100 ml. is seen in some cases (Wilfert, Levitt et al., Azimi et al.).

Diagnosis of mumps meningitis or encephalitis is reasonably obvious in those in whom parotitis precedes the neurologic complaints, but depends on serologic and virologic methods otherwise. Serologic diagnosis can sometimes be established in the first week of the illness on a single serum specimen by measuring complement-fixing antibodies against both the "S" or soluble antigen, and the "V" or viral antigen, but is more reliably accomplished by the demonstration of an antibody

titer rise during the course of the illness. In the acute stage of mumps infection of any form, the serum contains antibodies against the "S" antigen and negligible or low titers against "V" antigen. Both rise during convalescence, and subsequently the anti-"S" antibody declines more rapidly than does the anti-"V" antibody titer. Diagnosis can also be confirmed in some cases by isolation of the mumps virus in cell culture from the cerebrospinal fluid obtained in the early stages of the illness. Another possible diagnostic technique recently described is the detection of mumps antigen in cerebrospinal fluid cells by fluorescent antibody staining (Boyd and Vince-Ribaric).

Mumps virus infection of the central nervous system is usually a benign disease, from which complete recovery occurs. No significant sequelae were observed in the series of 33 patients of Azimi et al. or among 137 cases described by Johnstone et al. Of 30 cases, Ritter found no residual deficits except for one child who developed seizures two years after the illness. Although sequelae have been described (Oldfelt, Kilham, Miller et al.), they are infrequent in children following mumps aseptic meningitis but may occur secondary to encephalitis.

Death from mumps encephalitis has been infrequently reported and thus, only limited descriptions of the neuropathology are available. Bistrian et al. in 1973 claimed that to that date only approximately 70 fatal cases had been described, many of them poorly documented. Donohue and colleagues in 1955 gave a detailed report of the central nervous system pathology in two fatal cases and stated that, to that time, there were only three or perhaps four adequate descriptions of the pathology of mumps encephalitis. The more detailed reports (Donohue et al., Taylor and Toreson, Schwarz et al.) have almost consistently revealed acute perivascular demyelination and necrosis of cerebral and brain stem white matter, similar to that described with the so-called "post-infectious" encephalitides associated with smallpox or rabies vaccination or rubeola. Additional changes include perivascular infiltrations with lymphocytes and plasma cells, and variable degrees of microglial proliferation. Cerebral cortical changes are usually minimal. The meningeal infiltration is only slight to moderate in most cases. It is generally assumed that mumps aseptic meningitis or encephalitis is associated with direct invasion of the nervous system by the mumps virus. It is not clear how this brings about perivenous myelin destruction, which perhaps is the result of a poorly understood immunologic reaction of brain tissue to the presence of the virus antigen (Robbins) or to a product of tissue damage induced by the virus.

LYMPHOCYTIC CHORIOMENINGITIS

Lymphocytic choriomeningitis is an uncommon human illness caused by a virus which recently has been classified among the arenaviruses (Rowe et al.). As the first recognized member, it is considered the prototype of the group. Other members of the arenaviruses that produce human disease include the Lassa virus, and viruses that cause Argentinian hemorrhagic fever and Bolivian hemorrhagic fever (Casals). The name arenavirus, derived from the word for "sandy," emphasizes the characteristic fine granules observed in the virion in ultrathin sections. Members of this group are ribonucleic acid–containing viruses which produce a typical cytopathogenic effect in the Vero tissue culture cell line of African green monkey kidney. The best known carrier of the lymphocytic choriomeningitis virus is the mouse, although hamsters have also been implicated as a source of human infection (Hirsch et al.).

The lymphocytic choriomeningitis virus was first discovered by Armstrong and Lillie in 1933 in monkeys and mice that were being used to study the St. Louis encephalitis virus. The term lymphocytic choriomeningitis was chosen for the virus because of the marked cellular response that it produces within the choroid plexus and meninges of the monkey. The virus was first isolated from the cerebrospinal fluid of humans with aseptic meningitis by Rivers and Scott in 1935 and for a period of time thereafter was considered to be the main cause of aseptic meningitis, a concept dispelled by later studies (Adair et al.).

Lymphocytic choriomeningitis is usually a benign disease which most often affects young adults or older children (Green et al.). The virus is a common inhabitant of rodents and most human cases result from inhalation of virus-containing dried excreta of mice. Laboratory workers dealing with hamsters or mice can contract the illness from infected animals (Baum et al., Hinman et al.). Human infection sometimes results in asymptomatic disease or in a transient influenza-like illness

following an incubation period believed to be approximately eight days in length. The systemic illness is characterized by fever, malaise, headache, and myalgia which last from a few days to one or two weeks. Arthralgia and orchitis are occasionally described during this phase of the disease. Leukopenia and thrombocytopenia are commonly identified laboratory abnormalities in the initial phases of the systemic stage of the illness (Vanzee et al.).

In some cases, the illness subsides with the resolution of the systemic symptoms, but in others it assumes a biphasic quality, with the second stage being manifested by neurologic symptoms and signs. In the majority of instances, this is in the form of an acute aseptic meningitis associated with fever, headache, vomiting, and meningeal signs which persist for a week or so before recovery ensues. Less often, encephalitic signs prevail in variable degrees of severity. Still another pattern the disorder may assume is the appearance of aseptic meningitis or meningoencephalitis as the primary symptomatic phase, without a preceding stage with systemic complaints. On rare occasion, signs of aseptic meningitis will persist for several weeks prior to spontaneous resolution (Chesney et al.).

Cerebrospinal fluid in patients with neurologic involvement with lymphocytic choriomeningitis virus shows a cellular response, usually in the range of 500 to 2,000 cells per cu. mm., 90 to 100 percent being lymphocytes. The protein content is raised in most cases to levels between 50 and 150 mg. per 100 ml. and the glucose value is normal or, occasionally, somewhat reduced (Green et al.). An unusual variation in the CSF findings was described by Chesney et al. in a child with protracted meningitis caused by the lymphocytic choriomeningitis virus in which a significant eosinophilic pleocytosis was present.

Aseptic meningitis caused by the lymphocytic choriomeningitis virus is usually an acute, transient illness from which almost all affected patients recover without apparent sequelae. Hydrocephalus has been described as a residual deficit but is unusual (Tindall and Gladstone). Prognosis is more guarded in those with encephalitic manifestations, but recovery is also the rule in this group (Meyer et al.). Death can occur from this illness but is distinctly infrequent (Warkel et al.).

Diagnosis of lymphocytic choriomeningitis depends on serologic and virologic techniques since the aseptic meningitis or meningoencephalitis caused by this virus is entirely non-specific. Complement-fixing antibodies rise slowly, usually requiring three to four weeks to develop, and subsequently disappear by five to six months. Neutralizing antibodies achieve diagnostic levels even more slowly, taking up to eight weeks to develop. The neutralizing antibody titer declines at a less rapid rate and persists to some degree long after the infection subsides. Specific antibodies in serum can also be demonstrated by indirect fluorescent antibody testing. Virus isolation from blood and cerebrospinal fluid is sometimes successful during the acute stage of the illness.

The pathogenesis of human neurologic infections with the lymphocytic choriomeningitis virus remains unclear. Several interesting observations, however, have been made by Cole et al. and Monjan et al. following inoculation of the rodent brain with this virus. These investigators demonstrated that inoculation of virus into the brain of the adult mouse produces extensive involvement of the meninges, choroid plexus, and ependyma. If the inoculation is followed by an immunosuppressive dose of cyclophosphamide, the mouse is protected against the lethal effects of the virus but develops a state of chronic carrier infection, with the virus present in brain but without tissue pathology. Likewise, intracerebral challenge of untreated newborn mice results in a chronic viral carrier state, with high levels of the lymphocytic choriomeningitis virus in blood and brain without tissue damage, thus representing a state of immunologic tolerance. As opposed to these effects in either adult or newborn mice, experimental infection in rats or mice at four days of age gives rise to a severe CNS parenchymal infection and subsequent cerebellar necrosis. These experiments suggested to Cole et al. that lesions in the nervous system induced by this virus are immune-mediated, and thus are influenced by factors that regulate immunologic mechanisms. It is probable that this concept is partially applicable to human infection as well.

The pathology of human neurologic infection with the lymphocytic choriomeningitis virus is little known since the disease is rarely fatal. In the case described by Warkel and colleagues, the most obvious findings included a meningeal perivascular inflammatory response consisting mainly of lymphocytes and mononuclear cells, in addition to similar infiltrates in distended Virchow-Robin spaces of the cerebral cortex. Mild to moderate neuronal changes were present in wide areas of the brain, including the brain stem. Lymphocytic infiltration was also observed in the spinal cord and nerve roots.

ADENOVIRUS ENCEPHALITIS

The adenoviruses were discovered in 1953 and, from the beginning, were recognized to be a cause of upper respiratory infection in children and adults and epidemic influenza-like illness in military recruits (Rowe et al., Hilleman and Werner). Seventy-seven distinct species of this DNA-containing virus group have been identified, over 30 of which come from humans (Ginsberg). Various designations were initially applied to these agents until 1956 when it was proposed that they be called the adenoviruses (Enders et al.). The adenovirus group are medium-sized, ether-resistant viruses, which possess 252 capsomeres.

Diseases produced by the adenoviruses involve the respiratory tract predominantly and, to a less degree, the eye. Most of the respiratory infections of children provoked by these viruses affect the upper respiratory tract but bronchiolitis occurs and also pneumonia, sometimes in severe form or even with a fatal outcome (Benyesh-Melnick, Gold et al.). In military recruits the influenza-like illness with associated respiratory symptoms is usually caused by type 4 adenovirus, a strain that is rarely recovered from children. Rash is uncommon with any adenovirus infection but has been described in a pattern resembling that of meningococcemia (Sahler and Wilfert). Conjunctivitis, pharyngoconjunctivitis, and keratoconjunctivitis are other manifestations of adenovirus infection, especially due to type 8. An association of adenoviruses with pertussis has been made, with some reports suggesting an independent causative role of a certain serotype of adenovirus (Connor). In other reports, mixed infection with adenovirus and *Bordetella pertussis* has been identified in children with the pertussis syndrome (Klenk et al., Nelson et al.), with the presence of adenovirus probably representing reactivation of latent viral infection rather than being a primary causative factor in the production of the illness (Baraff et al.).

Relatively few well-documented cases of encephalitis or meningoencephalitis caused by the adenoviruses have been reported. In addition, certain reported cases of adenovirus encephalitis, indeed, had some form of neurologic complication, but the absence of cells and the normal protein content in the cerebrospinal fluid, the elevated pressure, plus the finding of cerebral edema as the predominant autopsy finding (Similä et al. 1970) raises questions in regard to the pathogenesis of the neurologic abnormality. Although there is no doubt that encephalitis can be caused by this group of viruses, certain cases with neurologic symptoms and signs may have represented an acute encephalopathy with brain swelling in the absence of actual viral invasion of brain tissue. Ladisch et al. described three children with adenovirus pneumonia complicated by severe cerebral injury with coma, convulsions, and death. There was no evidence of encephalitis pathologically; however, widespread extrapulmonary endothelial damage suggested a toxic or immunopathologic process. Among the cases of adenovirus type 7 infection in children reported by Sutton et al., one developed acute cerebellar ataxia two weeks after upper respiratory infection. Improvement followed but complete recovery of cerebellar function did not occur.

Adenovirus encephalitis was first described by LeLong et al., who isolated type 7 adenovirus from the cerebrospinal fluid and brain of a child with fatal encephalitis. Among subsequently reported cases of encephalitis in which the adenovirus strain was identified, type 7 has been the most common but types 1, 2, 3, 5, 6, and 12 have also been isolated (Similä et al. 1970, Faulkner and Rooyen, Kelsey). In most cases, encephalitis has coexisted with other manifestations of severe, generalized adenovirus disease, most often occurring in infants and children less than four years of age. Similä and colleagues described 29 children with severe infections due to adenoviruses, eight of whom had encephalitic manifestations. These patients were quite ill, because of both pulmonary and extrapulmonary infectious involvement. The apparent greater susceptibility of the younger child to widespread infection, including encephalitis, is also reflected by the reports of Gabrielson et al. and Huttunen. The severity of neurologic signs varies, but in most cases encephalitic manifestations have been fairly intense, including stupor or coma, neck rigidity, and convulsions. Among the eight cases described by Similä et al., death occurred in three. A more benign illness with aseptic meningitis can occur with adenovirus infection but is unusual.

Adenovirus has recently been found to be a cause of progressive subacute encephalitis in an adult with lymphoma, thus acting in opportunistic fashion in a setting of host immunosuppression (Chou et al.). The cerebral pathology in this case included perivascular cuffing, astrocytic and microglial proliferation, and large, basophilic nuclear inclusions. Adenovirus encephalitis has also been described in a child with acute leukemia during leukemic relapse (Kelsey). As mentioned, the cerebrospinal fluid findings are quite variable in children with central nervous system involvement with adenovirus. Pleocytosis may or may not be present and the protein content is normal in some and elevated in others. The cellular response in the cerebrospinal fluid in the initial stages of the illness can be predominantly polymorphonuclear or mononuclear in type.

Adenovirus infection is diagnosed by the demonstration of a fourfold or greater antibody titer rise in acute and convalescent sera. Because encephalitis usually occurs with pulmonary and other organ system disease, efforts should be made to isolate the virus from respiratory secretions and stools as well as from the cerebrospinal fluid. Characteristic cytopathogenic effects in tissue culture appear from two days to two weeks after inoculation. The virus is identified definitively as an adenovirus by complement-fixation titrations with hyperimmune rabbit serum.

ARBOVIRUS (ARTHROPOD-BORNE) ENCEPHALITIDES

More than 300 distinct arboviruses have been recognized, of which approximately 60 infect man (Casals). Relatively few cause serious neurologic disease, especially in the United States. The arbovirus group is a heterogeneous one from the standpoint of biochemical and physical properties, and its members are classified together primarily on an ecological basis (Melnick). The commonly referred to subgroups, including group A and group B, are established on the basis of common antigenic characteristics (Table 13–6). With progressive characterization of these RNA viruses, many have been assigned to established virus groups. For example, most of the group A and B arboviruses are now placed within the togavirus group, while the Colorado tick fever virus has been classified among the reovirus group. The vectors of these viruses accounting for human disease are the mosquito and the tick. Mosquito-borne viruses include California encephalitis

Table 13–6. Classification of the Arboviruses That Cause Human Disease*

Group A
  Eastern equine encephalitis
  Western equine encephalitis
  Venezuelan equine encephalitis
  Semliki forest

Group B
  St. Louis encephalitis
  Japanese B encephalitis
  Murray Valley encephalitis
  Dengue
  Yellow fever
  West Nile fever
  Russian spring-summer encephalitis complex
    Russian spring-summer encephalitis
    Central European encephalitis
    Far Eastern spring-summer encephalitis
    Louping ill
    Powassan
    Kyasanur forest disease
    Omsk hemorrhagic fever
    Kumlinge disease of Finland

California group

Arboviruses in the reovirus group
  Colorado tick fever
  Bluetongue

*Modified from Melnick.

virus, St. Louis encephalitis virus, the equine encephalitis viruses, Japanese B encephalitis virus, Murray Valley virus, and West Nile virus. The tick-borne group is composed of Colorado tick fever virus, Powassan virus, Russian spring-summer encephalitis virus, and the louping ill virus.

Arthropod-borne encephalitides in the United States are characterized by their seasonal incidence, their predominance in certain geographic regions of the country, and the tendency of certain of them to cause disease in epidemic fashion. California virus encephalitis is the most common arbovirus encephalitis in many of the upper midwestern states and in Ohio. It is almost exclusively a disease of children but infrequently affects the infant under one year of age. The encephalitic illness is usually severe, although death is most infrequent, and only a minority of infected children are left with residual deficits.

St. Louis encephalitis occurs over broad areas west of the Mississippi River, as well as in certain eastern states to a lesser degree. The disease carries a mortality rate that has varied from 5 to 20 percent in different epidemics and is particularly severe in the elderly age group. Unlike California virus en-

cephalitis, this illness is much more common in adults than in children.

Eastern equine encephalitis is an uncommon disease which in past years has been observed in epidemic fashion along the eastern seaboard, in Louisiana, and in Texas. Wild birds are the reservoir, while horses and man are the principal hosts. Children, and especially infants, are particularly susceptible to this illness which has a mortality rate of almost 70 percent and a high incidence of sequelae among survivors.

Western equine encephalitis virus also shows a predisposition to attack the infant but the clinical illness is generally less intense than with the Eastern variety. Western equine encephalitis occurs epidemically and sporadically west of the Mississippi River, with most cases arising in California and Texas. The mortality rate overall is approximately 10 percent.

Venezuelan equine encephalitis virus has only recently produced clinical disease in humans in the United States. Only a few cases with symptomatic illness have been described in Florida, Texas, and California, and most of these have been mild.

Colorado tick fever is only rarely associated with encephalitis and Powassan virus infections of humans are extremely limited in frequency.

A curious disorder of either children or adults which occurs in Connecticut, Rhode Island, and on Cape Cod is referred to as Lyme disease. It has been established to be a tick-borne illness but is not yet known to be viral in origin since the causative organism has not been isolated. Lyme disease has variable clinical manifestations, the most common including cutaneous and articular involvement. In one series, 11 percent were found to have neurologic manifestations in combination with other symptoms (Reik et al.). The usual first sign of the illness is the development of a cutaneous red macule, which then expands to form a red ring with central clearing, a lesion termed erythema chronicum migrans. Some patients will subsequently develop recurrent attacks of monarticular arthritis or migratory polyarthritis, and, less often, the illness is complicated by neurologic signs. The latter occur in the form of aseptic meningitis or meningoencephalitis, with a CSF lymphocytic pleocytosis and a normal protein content. Chorea, localized neuropathy, and polyneuropathy have also been described, either alone or in association with meningoencephalitis (Reik et al.). The frequent occurrence of serum cryoglobulins has been used as evidence suggesting that circulating immune complexes may be important in the production of tissue injury accounting for neurologic disease in these patients. While aseptic meningitis or encephalitis often follows a protracted or relapsing course for weeks or months, the ultimate outcome is usually favorable, although sequelae can occur.

Murray Valley encephalitis is now recognized to be identical to what in past years was called Australian X disease. The virus is a member of the Japanese B group and, like the latter, is engaged in a bird-mosquito cycle (Miles). Man becomes infected by the bite of virus-laden Culex mosquitoes. Large outbreaks occurred in Australia in 1917 and 1918, and again in 1951. Human cases were then not observed until 1956 when a few instances of encephalitis occurred (Anderson et al.), and cases subsequently have been sporadic. Epidemics have occurred in the months of February, March, and April. The clinically manifested illness is usually severe, although inapparent infections far outnumber the cases with overt encephalitis. In a large serologic survey by Anderson et al., there was one case of severe encephalitis for every 700 infections with the Murray Valley encephalitis virus. Of the series of 40 cases of Murray Valley encephalitis reported by Anderson in the 1951 epidemic, 23 were children under 12 years of age and 17 of the 40 cases were fatal. The neuropathology of Murray Valley encephalitis is similar to that of Japanese B encephalitis (Robertson). In the acute stage, there is meningeal infiltration with inflammatory cells and diffuse and multifocal cortical damage, as well as involvement of thalamic neurons, and severe injury to Purkinje cells. Inflammatory perivascular cuffing in white matter is variable in degree.

West Nile fever virus is a group B arbovirus related to the viruses of Murray Valley encephalitis and St. Louis encephalitis. Infection by this virus is seen primarily in Africa, Egypt, Israel, and India, where birds serve as the reservoir and the Culex mosquito is the principal vector. West Nile fever in children is usually a benign illness manifested by fever, headache, myalgia, lymphadenopathy, and rash. The incubation period is two to six days, and neurologic involvement in this age group is unusual. In adults, and especially in elderly persons, West Nile fever is often a more severe illness. Fever and lymphadenopathy are usual symptoms, and acute meningoenceph-

alitis is not rare in this age group (Pruzanski and Altman). Death from the illness is much more frequent in the elderly than in younger persons. Godoth et al. described a 22-year-old man with West Nile fever manifested by a polio-like illness with acute onset of an asymmetrical flaccid paresis of one leg and a mixed cellular pleocytosis in the CSF. Improvement followed but the patient was left with residual weakness of the affected limb. Diagnosis of infection caused by the West Nile fever virus is on the basis of the clinical picture, the epidemiology of the illness, adequate rise in complement-fixing or neutralizing antibodies, and recovery of the virus from blood or CSF.

The Russian spring-summer encephalitis complex represents a group of antigenically related, tick-borne viruses of wide geographic distribution and with variable clinical manifestations (Work). Included among the disorders caused by various strains of this virus complex are encephalitic disorders, such as Russian spring-summer encephalitis, Central European encephalitis, louping ill, and Powassan virus encephalitis. Among the non-encephalitic illnesses are Kyasanur forest disease and Omsk hemorrhagic fever, conditions with striking clinical similarities.

Russian spring-summer virus encephalitis is a severe, seasonal, tick-borne disease occurring in Siberia and other parts of Russia as well as in central Europe, with a mortality rate estimated to be 20 to 30 percent. Outbreaks usually occur in the summer months of May and June, and most cases are seen in communities where people have close access to forested areas. The illness differs from its Central European counterpart in that it is more severe with a higher mortality rate, and without the diphasic character of the latter condition. The onset of the illness is acute, with rapid development of high fever, meningeal signs, and signs of cerebral dysfunction. Bulbar muscle weakness is seen in some severely affected cases. In a certain proportion of patients, the illness is complicated by flaccid weakness and atrophy of muscles of the cervical region, around the shoulder girdle, and of the proximal part of the upper extremities. Complete recovery of the "paralytic" aspects of tick-borne encephalitis occurs in some, while others have persistent focal muscle weakness and atrophy, identical to that caused by the poliovirus (Smorodintsev). In a recent publication, Ogawa and colleagues have described a patient who developed a slowly progressive dementing process with long tract and cerebellar signs 13 years after acute Russian spring-summer encephalitis. Pathologic and immunologic studies implicated the Russian spring-summer virus, suggesting that it may be another cause of chronic panencephalitis analogous to the measles virus.

Central European tick-borne encephalitis occurs in epidemics in central and eastern Europe. Like louping ill, it is usually a biphasic illness with an initial stage with influenza-like symptoms followed by a second phase with severe encephalitis. Shoulder girdle paralysis may accompany the symptoms of encephalitis. In addition to its transmission by tick bite, the biphasic form of tick-borne encephalitis in Europe can be acquired by man by drinking milk from goats infected by tick bite (Shtilbance). The mortality rate from Central European encephalitis is relatively low. Russian investigators have reported favorable results in the treatment of Eurasian acute tick-borne encephalitis with pancreatic ribonuclease (Glukhov et al.).

Kyasanur forest disease of India is an acute systemic disease of humans and monkeys that closely resembles Omsk hemorrhagic fever, both of which are caused by a virus of the Russian spring-summer complex (Work). Symptoms of Kyasanur forest disease are of abrupt onset, with fever, headache, prostration, ocular inflammation, and, in some cases, with bleeding from the nose, mouth, or abdominal viscera. Encephalitic features are not usually recognized, and cerebrospinal fluid examination is normal. Leukopenia is a constant feature of the illness during the acute stage.

Louping ill is a tick-borne disease of sheep of Scotland and North Ireland that is manifested primarily by cerebellar ataxia. The illness occurs mainly between the months of March and June, corresponding to the period of maximal activity of the Ixodes tick vector. The virus causing this illness is also serologically closely related to the virus of Russian spring-summer encephalitis. Accidental laboratory infection in humans has occurred several times with this virus (Rivers and Schwentker), and a few naturally occurring cases have also been observed. The illness in man is usually a diphasic one, with the initial phase consisting of fever, sore throat, malaise, and leukopenia. Improvement follows, but three to four weeks after onset, symptoms and signs of aseptic meningitis or meningoencephalitis emerge. The neurologic aspects of the illness persist for one to four weeks when gradual recovery ensues. The louping ill virus can also result in an acute illness in man in a fashion resembling poliomyelitis (Likar and Dane). Weakness or paralysis of the lower motor neuron type follows signs of meningeal irritation and is usually followed by functional recovery. Webb et al. found louping-ill antibody in the cerebrospinal fluid of patients with laboratory-acquired disease and postulated that antibody is partially derived locally from neural tissue. Because of the possibility of neuronal damage secondary to virus-antibody interactions, they used corticosteroids therapeutically with apparent good results.

Inapparent infections far outnumber clinical illness with the arthropod-borne viruses with the exception of Eastern equine encephalitis, in which the ratio of symptomatic to inapparent infection is believed to be in the range of 1 to 10 to 50. When symptomatic neurologic infection does occur, it tends to be more severe, considering the group collectively, than occurs with many of the other viral causes of encephalitis. Diagnosis can frequently be suspected by the epidemiologic aspects of the illness, including the time of year of occurrence, the geographic region involved, and especially the recent previous recognition of arbovirus encephalitis in the community. Efforts should be made to isolate the offending virus from blood, stool, and cerebrospinal fluid in life but this is rarely successful with this group of illnesses. For this reason, confirmation of the diagnosis in most cases must be on the basis of the demonstration of a serial rise in antibody titer in the blood during the course of the infection. There is no specific treatment for most of these types of viral encephalitis, although survival in many cases depends on conservative measures such as control of hyperthermia, termination and prevention of convulsions, and management of other secondary complicating factors. Preventive measures include vector control by one of several methods, diminution of exposure to vectors of persons in certain age groups to the degree possible, and the development of vaccines, which has met with limited success to the present time.

California Virus Encephalitis

California virus encephalitis is an arthropod-borne, seasonal infection which almost exclusively affects children. The disease was first recognized in California but subsequently has been shown to be more prevalent in certain forested, midwestern states. The California virus was first isolated in 1943 from pools of mosquitoes from Kern County, California (Hammon and Reeves). The first reports of encephalitis in humans caused by this virus appeared in 1952 from California, and included studies which revealed that inapparent infections in man were quite common (Hammon and Reeves). Among several hundred persons tested from Kern County, approximately 11 percent showed antibody evidence of previous infection with this virus.

Absolute documentation of human California virus encephalitis resulted from a fatal case in a four-year-old girl who died in La Crosse, Wisconsin, in September, 1960. The virus, now referred to as the La Crosse strain, was recovered from brain tissue of the child and was subsequently reported by Thompson et al. in 1965. During this time period, surveys demonstrated that many adults in Wisconsin had serologic evidence of past infection with California encephalitis virus, indicating a high incidence of inapparent or subclinical illness in this region (Thompson et al.). The investigations also revealed a relationship between frequency of positive serologic response and duration of outdoor exposure. Reports of cases of California encephalitis in children thereafter became prevalent. From 1963 to 1969, 352 cases were diagnosed in this country, almost 50 percent being identified in Ohio (Hilty et al.) and a significant number of the others from Wisconsin and Minnesota (Johnson et al., Balfour et al., Chun et al., Cramblett et al.). The disease has also occurred in California, Florida (Quick et al.), and other midwestern states.

Most cases of California virus encephalitis in the midwestern region have been caused by the La Crosse strain, the principal vector for which is the Aedes mosquito. The mechanism by which winter survival of the virus occurs was not clear until investigators demonstrated transovarial passage of the virus in *Aedes triseriatus* (Watts et al., Balfour et al.). Small woodland mammals, including chipmunks, squirrels, and rabbits, are hosts of the La Crosse strain of California virus and account for summer amplification of virus transmission (Gauld et al.). Viremia in these animals, however, is of relatively short duration and does not account for overwintering of the virus. The Aedes species which transmits this virus is found in wooded areas, breeding within small pores near the base of

hardwood trees, and with a limited flying range from the breeding sites (Balfour et al.). These characteristics explain the much higher incidence of symptomatic infection among children from rural areas and probably also the predisposition of boys more than girls to acquire the illness. Almost all reported cases of California virus encephalitis have been in children, but relatively few cases have been observed among infants less than one year of age, in contrast to the Western and Eastern equine viruses, which show a striking predisposition to attack the infant. Four to 10 years is the most susceptible age range, and males are considerably more often affected than females.

Adults are remarkably resistant to encephalitis caused by this virus, although Copps and Elston mentioned a single case which occurred in a man in his mid-twenties. Serologic surveys have shown that adults acquire California virus infection but do so asymptomatically, somehow being capable of preventing hematogenous spread of the virus to the brain. Johnson and Johnson found that experimental California virus infection in mice is similar to human infection in that resistance to encephalitis following extraneural inoculation increases with the age of the animal. When suckling mice were inoculated subcutaneously, initial viral growth occurred locally, followed by viremia and eventual invasion of the brain by growth of the virus in endothelial cells of small cerebral vessels. A similar experiment in adult mice with the California virus was not followed by virus proliferation, even at the inoculated site. Thus, viremia and cerebral invasion could not occur, even though the adult mouse brain remained susceptible to the infection by direct intracerebral inoculation. Unlike the experimental adult model, which did not react to the extraneural inoculation with an antibody response, the adult human does show an antibody response to extraneural infection, suggesting that some extraneural growth of virus does take place (Johnson and Johnson).

California virus encephalitis is a seasonal disease, with its frequency of occurrence being dependent on the activity of its mosquito vector. First cases are recognized in the month of June, and the illness peaks in August and early September, only to vanish in early October until the following season. The incubation period is not well documented but is believed to be short, perhaps in the range of three to seven days. The clinical illness varies in severity, with a minority of cases manifested by mild symptoms such as malaise, fever, headache, and gastrointestinal complaints. A benign aseptic meningitis syndrome characterized by fever, headache, nuchal rigidity, and a lymphocytic pleocytosis in the cerebrospinal fluid can be caused by the California virus but represents an unusual manifestation (Johnson et al.).

Most cases follow a fairly constant pattern in which a two- or three-day prodrome of fever and systemic signs is followed by a severe illness lasting seven to ten days, from which recovery occurs and sequelae are relatively few. Fever and headache are nearly always present, often with vomiting, complicated 24 to 48 hours later by a rapid decline in consciousness or the abrupt development of generalized or focal convulsions. Seizures are a common feature of this type of encephalitis, having been described in over 50 percent of cases in most large series (Cramblett et al., Chun et al.). The decided tendency for the occurrence of convulsions in children with California virus encephalitis is a point aiding clinical differentiation of this illness from enteroviral meningoencephalitis in which seizures are much less frequent. At the peak of the illness, the febrile child is either lethargic and disoriented, or unresponsive to most forms of external stimulation except perhaps deep pain. Tremulousness, rigidity of neck and limbs, and hyperreflexia are common signs, while approximately 20 percent exhibit focal neurologic abnormalities. Anything more than minimal papilledema is not anticipated with this condition. The presence of significant papilledema with hemorrhages would be so unusual that it would raise serious doubt as to the correctness of the diagnosis. Diminution of fever and gradual improvement of responsiveness and other neurologic signs ordinarily evolve between three and seven days after onset.

Laboratory studies during the acute stage include a peripheral white blood cell count which sometimes is normal but more often is elevated up to 25,000 per cu. mm. The cerebrospinal fluid cellular response varies from an absence of leukocytes up to more than 600 per cu. mm., but in the majority, 50 to 200 cells per cu. mm. are present. Initially, the cerebrospinal fluid pleocytosis may be made up of both neutrophils and lymphocytes, but the latter soon predominate. The cerebrospinal fluid glucose content is normal or mildly elevated, and the protein value is normal in most cases and increased only in the minority.

The electroencephalogram during the acute stage has its greatest value as an indicator of the diffuse nature of the inflammatory process. Tracings usually show generalized medium to high-voltage delta slow activity, sometimes with some localizing aspects but not with the conspicuous focal disturbances seen with a cerebral abscess or with Herpes simplex encephalitis.

Diagnosis of California virus encephalitis is suspected in the child with signs of a diffuse, nonsuppurative neurologic infection in a known endemic region between the months of July and October. The virus is not recovered from blood or cerebrospinal fluid, and thus confirmation of the diagnosis is on the basis of a four-fold or greater rise in antibody titers. The hemagglutination inhibition and neutralization antibody titers rise rapidly from one week after onset of the illness to peak by three weeks and then persist at relatively high levels for as long as two years. The complement-fixation antibody titer rises more slowly, usually reaching its highest level about five weeks after onset. It then falls fairly rapidly and persists thereafter at low levels. Serologic diagnosis of California encephalitis by immunofluorescence has recently been developed (Kalis et al.).

Despite the common severity of the acute encephalitic manifestations, the majority of children with California virus encephalitis survive the illness. Fatalities have been extremely rare, with the best known being the case described by Thompson et al. from whom the virus was first isolated. The two-month-old infant described by Hammon and Reeves in 1952 managed to survive the acute phase of the disease, but with sequelae that culminated in death at age 11 months. Hilty et al. mentioned a single fatal case among their series of 50 children with California virus encephalitis. Following recovery, most children are free of major neurologic sequelae (Rie et al.) although behavior or learning disturbances have occasionally been noted (Matthews et al., Sabatino and Cramblett). A small percentage suffer recurrent convulsions as a complication of the illness (Grabow et al.). Chun and colleagues described persistent left hemiparesis in one child and Balfour et al. noted lasting mild weakness of one upper extremity in a single youngster after this illness.

Little is known of the pathology of California encephalitis since the great majority of identified patients have survived. In the fatal case described by Thompson et al., the brain was swollen and microscopic abnormalities were largely confined to the cerebral cortex and basal ganglia. Perivascular cuffing and neuronal degenerative changes were the most conspicuous findings. Inclusion bodies were not present. Tissue obtained by temporal lobe biopsy in one patient revealed pale foci and some degree of cortical vacuolization (Balfour et al.).

St. Louis Encephalitis

St. Louis encephalitis virus is among the group B arboviruses and is a cause of seasonal encephalitis in epidemic or sporadic fashion in many areas in this country. The name of the virus is derived from the first recorded epidemic of the disease which occurred in St. Louis, Missouri, in 1933. Outbreaks as well as sporadic cases (Blattner and Heys) have since been observed in many states, but the illness has been most prevalent in Texas, California, and other western and southwestern regions. Clusters of cases have appeared in Florida and New Jersey, indicating the potential widespread nature of this viral illness. St. Louis encephalitis virus is believed to be harbored by birds, with humans becoming infected through the bite of mosquitos that acquired their infection by feeding on viremic birds. Studies during certain outbreaks of St. Louis encephalitis have shown that inapparent infections far exceed symptomatic ones.

The encephalitis epidemic in and around St. Louis in 1933 occurred in the late summer months and resulted in 1,097 identified cases, an estimated attack rate of approximately 100 cases per 100,000 population (Leake et al., Hempelmann, Jones, Muckenfuss et al.). The overall mortality rate was 20 percent, a mortality rate considerably higher than has occurred in more recent epidemics. Children were affected much less often than adults and, generally, there was a definite increase in the incidence of the infection with increasing age. The case fatality rate followed a similar pattern. Among patients less than 20 years of age, the mortality rate was only 6 percent but, in those over 70 years, death occurred in approximately 70 percent. A much smaller but clinically similar outbreak of encephalitis had occurred one year previously, in 1932, in Paris, Illinois. The attack rate there was estimated to be 433 cases per 100,000 population, over four times that of

the St. Louis epidemic the following year (Leake et al.). St. Louis was struck with another epidemic in 1937 in which 750 encephalitis cases occurred. A virus isolated from brain tissue at autopsy was found to be immunologically identical to the one previously recovered in 1933.

St. Louis encephalitis subsequently became recognized as a mosquito-borne infection occurring in late summer and early fall mainly in the western and southwestern parts of this country. However, in 1959, a limited epidemic of St. Louis encephalitis was identified in Florida with clinical characteristics very similar to those of the St. Louis experience of 1933 (Skinner). Adults were affected more often than children and the mortality rate was higher in the older age groups. Houston, Texas, was the site of another major epidemic in 1964 during which more than 700 clinical cases and 32 deaths resulted (Phillips and Melnick, Barrett et al., Riggs et al.). As in previous outbreaks, adults were more often involved than children and males more than females. The youngest childhood case was an infant five weeks of age, and no deaths were observed among affected children. House sparrows and pigeons were believed to be the important avian hosts accounting for the spread of the infection by mosquitoes in the Houston epidemic (Lord et al.). Smaller outbreaks developed again in Corpus Christi, Texas, in the summer of 1965 and in Corpus Christi and Dallas in 1966. There were 76 confirmed cases in Corpus Christi in 1966, an attack rate of 41 cases per 100,000 (Williams et al.). The severity of the infection in this epidemic was relatively mild in that only two deaths occurred among the 76 confirmed cases. The Dallas outbreak included 145 confirmed cases with an attack rate of 15 per 100,000 (Hopkins et al.). 1975 was a banner year for St. Louis encephalitis in the United States, during which there was a record number of 2,131 laboratory-documented human cases with a case-fatality ratio of 8 percent (Creech). Several eastern states reported the occurrence of the illness for the first time, and the metropolitan Chicago area experienced its first outbreak with 269 known cases.

As an arthropod-borne infection, St. Louis encephalitis is a seasonal disease which occurs between the months of July and early October. Like most types of encephalitis, the spectrum of the clinical illness ranges from very mild, with almost imperceptible neurologic signs or signs only of aseptic meningitis, to an extremely severe illness which can lead to death within days after onset. The usual child with the disease experiences an abrupt onset with fever, headache, and vomiting. Alteration of sensorium is usual, including drowsiness, confusion, delirium, or coma, while neck rigidity and seizures are much less constant. Strikingly focal neurologic signs are uncommon. Tremulousness and hyperreflexia are frequently observed but are not invariable. Electromyographic abnormalities indicative of lower motor neuron involvement during the acute stage was a frequent finding in the patients examined by Southern et al. Fever persists for several days and usually abates before overall improvement begins to occur. The usual duration of the illness is one to two weeks. Death from St. Louis encephalitis in children is unusual but severely affected patients may retain persistent neurologic sequelae. Lasting deficits following this infection are lower in frequency than occurs with Eastern or Western equine encephalitis. In part, this is because of the lower incidence of St. Louis encephalitis in the infant age group compared to the equine encephalitides.

The white blood cell count during the first week of the illness may be normal but more often is elevated to levels between 10,000 and 20,000 per cu. mm. Hyponatremia caused by inappropriate antidiuretic hormone secretion is not infrequent in moderately or severely ill patients (Brinker et al.). The cerebrospinal fluid is clear or slightly opalescent, and in the majority of cases reveals a lymphocytic pleocytosis of 50 to 500 cells per cu. mm. The glucose content is normal or elevated and the protein value in most is between 50 and 100 mg. per 100 ml. The virus has only rarely been isolated from cerebrospinal fluid or blood (Blattner and Heys). Diagnosis is established by the demonstration of a four-fold or greater rise in complement fixation and hemagglutination inhibition antibody titers between acute and convalescent phase sera.

The pathology of St. Louis encephalitis is a nonsuppurative inflammatory reaction of the brain and meninges, which includes vascular congestion, perivascular mononuclear cell infiltrates, microglial proliferation, and neuronal degeneration with some degree of neuronophagia (McCordock et al., Shinner). Inflammation occurs throughout the central nervous system, including the spinal cord, and is often most severe in the substantia nigra, where changes resemble those previously seen in the von Economo type of epidemic encephalitis (Suzuki and Phillips).

Eastern Equine Encephalitis

Eastern equine encephalitis is a relatively rare disease compared to the other arthropod-borne encephalitides that occur within the United States. Outbreaks of limited size occurred in Massachusetts in 1938 when 34 cases were identified (Farber et al., Getting), in Louisiana in 1947 in which there were ten human cases (Hauser), and again in Massachusetts in 1956 with 12 cases (Feemster). Up to 1956, Feemster claimed that a total of 50 Eastern equine encephalitis cases had been identified in Massachusetts and 25 in all other states. Human disease with this virus has remained infrequent, although the disease periodically has recurred in various geographic areas. From 1955 to 1973, there were 23 confirmed human cases of Eastern equine encephalitis in Florida, representing approximately 19 percent of all cases reported in the United States during this period (Bigler et al.). No cases were identified in Massachusetts from 1957 until 1970 when a five-month-old child experienced a non-fatal infection with this virus (Levitt et al.). Despite this relatively low attack rate upon humans, the virus continues to be isolated periodically from horses in eastern seaboard states and Texas (Morbidity and Mortality Weekly Reports, 11 Aug. 1973, Morris et al.). Previous human epidemics have usually occurred in conjunction with epidemics in horses. Wild birds are believed to serve as reservoirs of the virus, which is transmitted to man and horses by several different mosquito vectors (Kissling et al.).

The Eastern equine encephalitis virus was first isolated in 1933 from horses in Virginia, Delaware, and Maryland by Ten Broeck and Merrill. In southeastern Massachusetts in the late summer of 1938, an encephalitis epidemic spread among horses until almost 300 equines had been affected, of which more than 90 percent died. Approximately three weeks after the onset of the epidemic in horses, a type of epidemic encephalitis that had not previously been seen began to appear in humans. The illness was characterized by abrupt onset, high fever, profound and diffuse cerebral involvement, and a strikingly high mortality rate. Of a total of 34 identified human cases, death occurred in 65 percent (Farber et al.) and, of the survivors, only one was believed to have recovered free of sequelae (Ayers and Feemster). There was a remarkable predisposition for the virus to attack children in this epidemic. Seventy percent of all cases were in children less than 10 years of age and 25 percent occurred in infants under one year of age. During the outbreak, Eastern encephalitis virus was isolated from the brain of a pigeon and from pheasants (Fothergill and Dingle, Tyzzer et al.). For the first time, the virus also was recovered from the brain in fatal human cases (Fothergill et al.). The 1938 epidemic established the Eastern equine encephalitis virus as a potential serious seasonal threat to the health and welfare of young children but, fortunately, the following 40 years demonstrated the magnitude of the danger to be less than might have been suspected at that time. Despite the relative infrequency of the disease, the proportion of inapparent infections to clinical cases is considered to be low compared to other arthropod-borne encephalitides, perhaps in the range of 10 to one to 50 to one.

The most notable clinical characteristic of Eastern equine encephalitis is its intense severity. The onset of the illness in infants is usually abrupt, with fever and encephalitic signs present from almost the beginning of the illness. Older children and adults may experience one or two days with more generalized symptoms such as nausea, malaise, and headache before drowsiness, confusion, neck stiffness or convulsions supervene. Once neurologic signs become evident, they advance rapidly within 24 to 48 hours to reach their maximal degree of severity. Temperature promptly rises to 103° F to 106° F, and diffuse rigidity or hypertonicity is accompanied by coma. Nonpitting edema of the face and distal part of the limbs has frequently been described in infants during the second or third day of the illness. In fatal cases, death is not uncommon within one to three days after onset. In survivors, the first week tends to be the most severe, followed by gradual resolution but with variable degrees of eventual recovery. As already noted, the mortality rate is high and most who survive the acute illness are left with lasting neurologic deficits. Complete recovery without sequelae has been described (Webster) and is more likely to occur in the adult than in the child.

Blood leukocytosis with an increase of immature forms is present in the acute stage of the disease. The cerebrospinal fluid is under increased pressure in most cases and contains cells which number from 200 to 2,000 per cu. mm. Polymorphonuclear leukocytes constitute over 50 percent of the cerebrospinal fluid cellular response. Unlike most types of viral encephalitis, this neurophilic predomi-

nance can persist into the second week of the illness. The virus is not usually isolated from blood or cerebrospinal fluid, and diagnosis depends on a four-fold or greater rise in complement fixation and neutralizing antibody titers between paired sera. Antibody response is usually rapid, sometimes showing rise early in the second week of the disease. Clinical diagnosis can be suspected when acute, severe encephalitis occurs in late summer in proximity to a previously recognized outbreak in horses.

The pathology of this condition includes expected findings such as diffuse brain swelling, vascular congestion, areas of softening, and perivascular cuffing. One of the most distinctive features of the pathology of Eastern equine encephalitis is the presence of polymorphonuclear leukocytes in the meningeal and cerebral infiltrates. Neuronal damage within the cerebral cortex and deep nuclear gray matter is severe but often patchy. In some cases, the most severe neuronal damage is found in the basal ganglia and the brain stem. Extensively damaged nerve cells are phagocytized by neutrophils, unlike the conspicuous neuronophagia observed in Japanese B encephalitis. In a fatal case studied by electron microscopy by Bastian and colleagues, togavirus particles were found within the cytoplasm of oligodendroglial cells and in the extracellular spaces.

Western Equine Encephalitis

Periodic epizootics among horses had occurred in the western part of the United States for many years preceding the isolation of the Western equine encephalitis virus by Meyer et al. in 1930. Although human infections were suspected, it was not until 1938 that Howitt first recovered the virus from the brain of a child who had died of acute encephalitis in California. In the same year, human and equine cases of encephalitis caused by this virus were observed in North Dakota and Saskatchewan (Breslich et al.). A major human epidemic of Western equine encephalitis broke out in 1941 in Minnesota, North Dakota, and adjacent provinces of Canada. Over 3,000 cases occurred, with a mortality rate of about 10 percent. The largest percentage of the identified cases were among the elderly and the very young. During this outbreak, the susceptibility of infants to this infection and the severity of the disease when it occurred in this age group became evident.

Of 509 cases seen in Manitoba, 27 were under one year of age (Medovy). The attack rate in infants less than one year of age was estimated to be 200 per 100,000 compared to an attack rate of 44 per 100,000 in the population generally (Donovan and Bowman). A similar tendency was later demonstrated in epidemics in California. In 174 confirmed cases seen from 1945 to 1950, Lennette and Longshore found that approximately 20 percent were among infants less than one year of age. More recent studies have indicated that between 20 and 30 percent of all cases of Western equine encephalitis occur in infants less than one year of age (Finley et al., Herzon et al.). Even fetal involvement can be produced by this virus, which is able to cross the placenta during the viremic stage in the pregnant mother. In reported cases of transplacentally transmitted Western equine encephalitis, the maternal illness had occurred near term and the neonate exhibited encephalitic signs in the first week after birth (Copps and Giddings, Shinefield and Townsend).

Western equine encephalitis occurs in horses and humans in many areas west of the Mississippi River but the greatest concentration of cases has been in California and Texas. It is mosquito-borne and thus is generally observed in late summer and early fall in either sporadic or epidemic form. The method of survival of the virus from one epidemic season to another has been debated but it is believed that birds serve as the reservoir host from which the mosquito vectors acquire the virus (Kissling et al.). Inapparent infections far outnumber cases with clinical illness, probably in the range of 60 to one in young children and 1,000 to one in adults. The illness in the infant is usually abrupt in onset and is characterized by irritability and fever, rapidly leading to stiffness of the neck, rigidity, convulsions, coma, and a bulging fontanel. The older child or adult in most instances experiences fever, chills, headache, and myalgia for one to three days before more clear-cut encephalitic signs emerge. The severity is more variable in older persons than in infants and may extend from only mild lethargy to a state of deep coma with intense rigidity. In survivors, the usual duration of the illness is five to 10 days, with gradual subsidence of the symptoms. Cerebrospinal fluid shows a cellular response which initially includes both neutrophils and lymphocytes but later becomes a lymphocytic pleocytosis. The protein content is mildly elevated. The virus has been recovered from cerebrospinal fluid only rarely (Sciple et al.), and thus diagnosis depends on the demonstration of a four-fold or greater antibody rise by complement fixation, neutralization, or hemagglutination inhibition tests.

The overall mortality rate of Western equine encephalitis is usually placed at approximately 10 percent but is somewhat higher in the infant age group. Sequelae from this infection have been extensively studied, especially by Finley. In a follow-up series of over 600 cases, there was a strong correlation between the age of the patient at the time of the illness and the incidence and severity of neurologic sequelae. According to Finley, over 50 percent of surviving patients who sustained the illness in the first year of life retained major neurologic deficits. In contrast, significant residual deficits were found in only 5 percent of adult patients. A similar trend was found in the studies by Earnest and colleagues. In neither of these studies was Parkinson's syndrome found to complicate preceding Western equine encephalitis. The commonly identified sequelae include mental retardation, behavioral abnormalities, convulsions, and spastic deficits.

The pathological features of Western equine encephalitis include swelling and hyperemia of the brain on gross examination. Microscopically, there is meningeal and perivascular round cell infiltration of variable degree. The inflammatory reaction can usually be observed throughout the brain but generally is of maximal intensity in the basal ganglia and the upper portion of the brain stem. Glial nodules are readily found but neuronophagia within the cerebral cortex is usually minimal (Haymaker). Foci of tissue necrosis in a perivascular distribution in cerebral white matter are seen in some cases (Weil and Breslich). Noran and Baker emphasized the vascular involvement observed in certain instances, consisting of endothelial hyperplasia of small vessels, sometimes leading to complete vessel occlusion. Among those in whom death occurs in the subacute or chronic stages, the inflammatory vascular process can result in wide zones of tissue infarction with extensive cystic degeneration.

Venezuelan Equine Encephalitis

With the viruses of Eastern and Western equine encephalitis already having been discovered, epidemics among horses appeared in 1935 in Colombia and in 1938 in Venezuela. This led to the recognition of still another arthropod-borne equine virus, first isolated by Beck and Wyckoff in 1938 and Kubes and Rios in 1939. It was subsequently called Venezuelan equine encephalitis virus. It was not then known whether man could be infected with this virus, but, in 1943, mild febrile illnesses of an influenza type were described in laboratory workers who handled the virus (Casals et al., Lennette and Koprowski). The possibility of serious human disease became documented in 1944 when two deaths occurred in Trinidad, British West Indies (Randall and Mills, Gilyard). Venezuelan equine encephalitis virus was isolated from the brain in these cases, one of which preceded and one of which occurred coincident to an epidemic among horses in the same region.

Koprowski and Cox described four additional human laboratory-acquired cases in 1947. These illnesses in adults varied from mild symptoms with fever, headache, and myalgia of short duration to more alarming complaints, which included chills, lethargy, and delirium. All recovered without sequelae. Thereafter, Venezuelan equine encephalitis continued to occur in South and Central America, primarily affecting horses but also with some identified cases in humans. In 1960, Work found Venezuelan equine encephalitis antibodies in Seminole Indians in Florida, and soon thereafter Chamberlain et al. isolated the virus from Culex mosquitoes in the Everglades National Park. Clinical disease was not observed in man in the United States until 1968 when a 53-year-old woman in Florida experienced a transient but fairly severe febrile illness with chills, vomiting, and headache (Ehrenkranz et al.). Cerebrospinal fluid examination revealed a mixed pleocytosis and an elevated protein content while serologic studies demonstrated a serial rise in Venezuelan equine virus antibodies. A similar case in an elderly man subsequently was identified, also in Florida (Morbidity and Mortality Weekly Reports, 13 Nov. 1971). In 1971, the disease spread from Mexico into southern Texas, resulting in a major epidemic in horses with many equine deaths and a number of human infections but without human fatalities (Sudia et al.). As a result of this outbreak, a large-scale program of vaccination of equines with Venezuelan equine encephalitis vaccine has been promoted in an effort to interrupt the natural transmission chain of the virus (Sudia and Newhouse).

It is now known that there are several different antigenic strains of the Venezuelan equine encephalitis virus and that the pathogenic capabilities for horses varies greatly among the different viral strains (Walton et al.). The principal vertebrate host is the horse but, during epizootic spread, the virus may spill over to man, rodents, and birds. Mosquitoes serve as the vector, transmitting the virus. The incubation period of the disease in man is relatively short, judging from laboratory-acquired infections where exposure is known (Koprowski and Cox) and is probably in the range of three to four days. Most human cases have been mild, manifested by fever, myalgia, and vomiting. Headache and lethargy have represented the primary evidence of neurologic involvement in such patients. Severe encephalitis, sometimes terminating fatally, can occur with this disease but is uncommon (Randall and Mills). Diagnosis is confirmed by rise in titer of complement fixation and hemagglutination inhibition antibodies in serum.

Japanese B Encephalitis

Japanese B encephalitis is a disease of Asian countries which is caused by a member of the group B arboviruses and is transmitted to man by the bite of various species of Culex and Aedes mosquitoes. The disease received its name to differentiate it from type A encephalitis, the designation originally assigned to encephalitis lethargica (Kaneko and Aoki). Wild birds are the main hosts but swine, horses, goats, and rats have also been found to harbor Japanese B encephalitis virus. Human disease occurs both sporadically and epidemically and is seen in Japan, Korea, Okinawa, China, the Philippines, Vietnam, and in eastern parts of Russia. The only acute cases seen in the United States are acquired in the Far East in persons traveling therefrom. The virus is believed to be quite prevalent in endemic regions. In Japan, studies have shown that approximately 10 percent of nonimmune children contract the infection each year and that 500 to 1,000 inapparent infections occur for each case with clinically apparent disease (Southam).

Although Japanese B encephalitis virus was not isolated until 1936, previous epidemics in Japan in 1924 and 1935 are believed to have been caused by this organism (Hashimoto et al.). Outbreaks occurred in Okinawa in 1945 (Sabin), and in Korea in 1946 (Sabin et al.)

and 1949 (Hullinghorst et al.). Over 5,000 cases were reported among Koreans in the 1949 epidemic. In 1950, approximately 300 American soldiers contracted Japanese B encephalitis in Korea between the months of August and October (Lincoln and Sivertson). Cases have continued to occur virtually every season in the Far East and, more recently, American troops were again affected in Vietnam (Ketel and Ognibene).

Japanese B encephalitis has the usual range of severity from mild to fulminating but, in general, the disease is considered to be one of the more severe forms of viral encephalitis, associated with significant morbidity and mortality rates. Among persons indigenous to the endemic areas, the highest attack rate is in those over 65 years of age and under 15 years of age (Richter and Shimojyo). During the Korean epidemic in 1949, 63 percent of identified cases were in children between two and 12 years of age (Hullinghorst et al.). Infections in the first year of life with this virus are unusual. The disease can occur at any time of year in certain tropical Asian regions, but most cases occur in summer and early fall when conditions are favorable for the arthropod vectors.

Symptoms are usually rapid but not sudden in onset. Many patients experience fever, malaise, and headache for two or three days before the more specific signs indicative of a meningoencephalitis become evident. Less often, the first observed manifestations are mental confusion or convulsions. Fever quickly reaches levels of 104° F or higher and is associated with chills and headache in a high percentage of afflicted patients. Neck rigidity, mental confusion, disorientation, delirium, and combativeness are variable in degree but present to some extent in most. Photophobia is common and generalized muscle weakness in the second or third week of the illness has been mentioned by several authors (Dickerson et al., Ketel and Ognibene). Diffuse, severe weakness sometimes requires continued bed confinement even after most other symptoms have abated. An infrequent finding in the acute stage is localized limb paresis associated with other signs of anterior horn cell involvement such as atrophy and reflex loss. Other common signs during the acute stage of Japanese B encephalitis are tremor of the head and extremities, rigidity, hyperreflexia, and weight loss. Dickerson et al. observed that most patients during the acute illness developed a mask-like, expressionless face and also ocular tremulousness,

suggestive of basal ganglia or brain stem dysfunction.

Laboratory studies in most patients with Japanese B encephalitis include a leukocytosis and elevation of the sedimentation rate. The cerebrospinal fluid is clear to opalescent, depending on the number of white cells present. The cerebrospinal fluid pleocytosis varies from 20 to 500 cells per cu. mm. In the first few days, both neutrophils and lymphocytes may be present, but thereafter lymphocytes predominate. The glucose content is normal or raised and the protein value is usually between 50 and 100 mg. per 100 ml. Japanese B encephalitis virus is infrequently recovered from the cerebrospinal fluid or blood, and therefore diagnosis depends on demonstration of a four-fold or greater antibody titer rise on paired sera specimens. Complement-fixing antibodies often rise slowly in this disease and up to six weeks may be required for diagnostic titer elevation to occur.

The reported mortality rate of Japanese B encephalitis has varied in different publications but generally can be regarded to be high in populations indigenous to the endemic zones. Among Japanese people from 1948 to 1959, over 36,000 cases were reported and the outcome was fatal in more than 15,000, a mortality rate of approximately 40 percent (Richter and Shimojyo). In the civilian epidemic in Korea in 1949, there were 5,548 reported encephalitis cases with death occurring in 2,429, a mortality of 43 percent (Hullinghorst et al.).

In contrast to these figures, however, are much lower mortality statistics of Japanese B encephalitis among U.S. troops in the Far East. In 1950, there was a death rate of only 8.5 percent among 201 men with the illness (Lincoln and Sivertson). More recently in Vietnam, only one fatality occurred among 57 identified cases (Ketel and Ognibene). The discrepancy between such figures has been partially explained by the difference in medical and nursing management, including maintenance of fluid and electrolyte requirements and control of seizures. Age factors may also be an important determinant because the young and the aged are more often affected in those indigenous to the endemic areas, while the majority of the encephalitis cases in military persons are necessarily among young adults. Lasting sequelae following Japanese B encephalitis usually are in the category of disturbances of higher cortical function or motor deficits. Dickerson et al. found 12 percent of survivors to have disabling residual defects, and other authors have found sequelae to occur in up to 20 percent (Richter and Shimojyo, Weaver et al.).

The pathology of Japanese B encephalitis in the acute stage includes vascular congestion within the meninges and the brain, and widespread perivascular lymphocytic infiltration and cuffing (Zimmerman). Neuronal degenerative changes and conspicuous neuronophagia are characteristic of the disease. Microglial proliferation and petechial hemorrhages are commonly observed. Inflammatory changes in the brain, brain stem, and spinal cord are extensive and widespread, but in certain cases, the greatest impact is within the thalamus and substantia nigra. Areas of necrosis can be seen in these regions as well as within the cerebral cortex. The neuropathology in the chronic stages of the disease has been studied by Ishii et al. who examined tissue in patients in whom death occurred 12 to 67 years after the acute illness. Symmetrical lesions most intense in the thalamus, substantia nigra, and Ammon's horn were found. The thalamic and nigral lesions consisted of multiple small oval areas of decreased cellularity adjacent to areas with glial scarring. Focal lesions in the cerebral cortex were generally less striking than those in the thalamus and substantia nigra.

Colorado Tick Fever Encephalitis

Colorado tick fever is usually a benign acute viral disease which occurs throughout much of the western part of the United States. The virus causing this illness has been classified among the reovirus group. With the exception of the rare Powassan virus infections, Colorado tick fever is probably the only tick-borne virus infection of man in this country. The vast majority of cases are manifested in the form of an acute, transient, febrile illness from which complete recovery follows. Neurologic complications such as aseptic meningitis or meningoencephalitis are rare. Colorado tick fever is transmitted to man by the wood tick, *Dermacentor andersoni,* and thus the disease occurs within the environmental range of this insect vector. Most cases are seen in the spring and early summer months in Colorado, Wyoming, Utah, Idaho, and Nevada, but the illness can occur elsewhere in persons who recently traveled in these regions. The disease affects children as well as adults, with the highest incidence in males between 15 and 40 years of age.

History of exposure to ticks or the discovery of a tick on the body of the ill patient is usually found in the patient with this disease. The incubation period is three to six days, followed by the abrupt onset of the febrile illness, which lasts seven to ten days in most instances. Fever, headache, and myalgia are the usual first symptoms, in some cases associated with vomiting and abdominal pain. The febrile reaction is characteristically diphasic with the first period of temperature elevation lasting two to three days, followed by remission of approximately equal length. Fever then recurs and persists for an additional two or three days at which time symptoms gradually resolve. Tachycardia, conjunctival injection, and pharyngeal erythema are observed during the course of the illness, and splenomegaly is found in some cases. Rash is infrequent and was seen in 12 percent of the 115 cases compiled by Spruance and Bailey and in only 5 percent of 228 cases reported by Goodpasture et al. The low incidence of rash and its macular or maculopapular quality when it does occur are important points of difference between Colorado tick fever and Rocky Mountain spotted fever, the condition it is most often confused with.

Leukopenia is a common, although not constant, laboratory feature of Colorado tick fever, with white blood counts found in most cases to be lower than 4,000 per cu. mm. (Silver et al.). Leukopenia generally is most marked during the second febrile phase. Diagnosis is established by isolation of the virus from blood obtained during the acute stage of the illness or by demonstration of complement fixation or neutralization antibody titer rises between the acute and convalescent stages of the disease. Viremia usually persists throughout the acute phase of the illness and in some for several weeks thereafter (Goodpasture et al.). For this reason, laboratory confirmation is possible in most cases by utilization of the appropriate tissue culture methods. Significant antibody titer rises occur more slowly than with many viral infections and may not reach diagnostic levels for three to five weeks after the onset of symptoms.

Aseptic meningitis or meningoencephalitis are infrequent complications of Colorado tick fever, having occurred in only three of 115 cases in the series of Spruance and Bailey. In reported cases, encephalitis has been fairly severe but with a good prognosis in most instances (Fraser and Schiff, Draughn et al.). The cerebrospinal fluid usually shows a lymphocytic pleocytosis in those with neurologic manifestations, although neutrophils may predominate in the initial stages. The glucose is normal and the protein content is elevated, sometimes up to 300 mg. per 100 ml. The virus has been recovered from the cerebrospinal fluid in certain cases. Of interest are the findings of Florio et al., in which the virus was recovered from the cerebrospinal fluid in patients with Colorado tick fever without clinical evidence of encephalitis or cells in the cerebrospinal fluid.

Powassan Virus Encephalitis

Powassan virus is a tick-borne, group B arbovirus that is a member of the Russian spring-summer encephalitis virus complex and which is a rare cause of human infection in this country. In the United States, the virus has been isolated from ticks in Colorado and South Dakota, and from ticks, woodchucks, and foxes in New York State (Whitney and Jamnback). The few reported cases of encephalitis caused by this virus have been from the state of New York and from Canada.

The first and only isolation until recently of the Powassan virus from human brain tissue was reported by McLean and Donohue in 1959. The affected patient was a five-year-old child who lived in Powassan, Ontario, Canada, thus accounting for the name of the virus. His illness occurred in September, 1958 and consisted of an acute encephalitis with headache, fever, neck stiffness, and hemiplegia. Coma supervened and the child died six days after onset of symptoms. The brain revealed perivascular and parenchymal infiltration with mononuclear cells and microglial nodules. An additional isolate of the virus from brain tissue was obtained from a fatal case in 1975 (Morbidity and Mortality Weekly Reports, Vol. 24, 1975). The patient was an 82-year-old farmer in New York State who died eight days after the onset of encephalitis.

Only a few additional cases of Powassan virus encephalitis have been reported, mostly in children and virtually all from New York State or Canada (Smith et al.). The disease usually occurs in late summer or early fall, consistent with the activity of the tick vector. It is characterized by fairly severe encephalitic signs, including headache, fever, convulsions, disturbance in consciousness, and focal deficits in some. Recovery usually follows but lasting deficits can occur. Antibody response is rapid and diagnosis depends on the demonstration of a four-fold or greater rise in complement fixation or hemagglutination-inhibiting antibody titer.

REFERENCES

Abramsky, O.: Neurological features as presenting manifestations of brucellosis. Eur. Neurol. 15:281–284, 1977.

Abramsky, O., and Teitelbaum, D.: The autoimmune features of acute transverse myelopathy. Ann. Neurol. 2:36–40, 1977.

Abramson, H., and Greenberg, M.: Acute poliomyelitis in infants under one year of age: Epidemiological and clinical features. Pediatrics 16:478–487, 1955.

Abramson, H., Greenberg, M., and Magee, M. C.: Poliomyelitis in the newborn infant. J. Pediat. 43:167–173, 1953.

Acheson, E. D.: The clinical syndrome variously called benign myalgic encephalomyelitis, Iceland disease and epidemic neuromyasthenia. Am. J. Med. 26:569–595, 1969.

Adair, C. V., Gauld, R. L., and Smadel, J. E.: Aseptic meningitis, a disease of diverse etiology: clinical and etiologic studies on 854 cases. Ann. Intern. Med. 39:675–704, 1953.

Adams, J. M.: Clinical pathology of measles encephalitis and sequelae. Neurology 18: Part 2:52–56, 1968.

Adams, J. M., Baird, C., and Filloy, L.: Inclusion bodies in measles encephalitis. J.A.M.A. 195:290–298, 1966.

Adams, R. D., and Kubik, C. S.: The morbid anatomy of the demyelinative diseases. Am. J. Med. 12:510–546, 1952.

Adler, J. L., Mostow, S. R., Mellin, H., Janney, J. H., and Joseph, J. M.: Epidemiologic investigation of hand, foot, and mouth disease. Am. J. Dis. Child. 120:309–313, 1970.

Agamanolis, D. P., Tan, J. S., and Parker, D. L.: Immunosuppressive measles encephalitis in a patient with a renal transplant. Arch. Neurol. 36:686–690, 1979.

Aguilar, M. J., and Rasmussen, T.: Role of encephalitis in pathogenesis of epilepsy. Arch. Neurol. 2:663–676, 1960.

Aicardi, J., Goutieres, F., Arsenio-Nunes, M-L., and Lebon, P.: Acute measles encephalitis in children with leukemia. Pediatrics 59:232–239, 1977.

Alter, H. J., Scanlon, R. T., and Schechter, G. P.: Thrombocytopenic purpura following vaccination with attenuated measles virus. Am. J. Dis. Child. 115:111–112, 1968.

Altrocchi, P. H.: Acute transverse myelopathy. Arch. Neurol. 9:111–119, 1963.

Anderson, A. D., Levine, S. A., and Gellert, H.: Loss of ambulatory ability in patients with old anterior poliomyelitis. Lancet 2:1061–1063, 1972.

Anderson, S. G.: Murray Valley encephalitis: Epidemiological aspects. Med. J. Aust. 1:97–100, 1952.

Anderson, S. G., Dobrotworsky, N. V., and Stevenson, W. J.: Murray Valley encephalitis in the Murray Valley, 1956 and 1957. Med. J. Aust. 2:15–17, 1958.

Anderson, S. G., Donnelley, M., Stevenson, W. J., Caldwell, N. J., and Eagle, M.: Murray Valley encephalitis: Surveys of human and animal sera. Med. J. Aust. 1:110–114, 1952.

Anderson, W. W., and Jaros, R. M.: Neurologic complications of Asian influenza. Neurology 8:568–570, 1958.

Antony, J. H., Procopis, P. G., and Ouvrier, R. A.: Benign acute childhood myositis. Neurology 29:1068–1071, 1979.

Appelbaum, E., Greenberg, M., and Nelson, J.: Neurological complications following antirabies vaccination. J.A.M.A. 151:188–191, 1953.

Armstrong, C., and Lillie, R. D.: Experimental lymphocytic choriomeningitis of monkeys and mice produced by a virus encountered in studies of the 1933 St. Louis encephalitis epidemic. Pub. Health Rep. 49:1019–1027, 1934.

Ashkenazi, A., and Melnick, J. L.: Topics in microbiology. Enteroviruses—A review of their properties, and associated disease. Am. J. Clin. Path. 38:209–229, 1962.

Aycock, W. L.: Frequency of poliomyelitis in pregnancy. New Eng. J. Med. 225:405–408, 1941.

Aycock, W. L., and Kramer, S. D.: Immunity to poliomyelitis in mothers and the newborn as shown by the neutralization test. J. Exp. Med. 52:457, 1930.

Ayres, J. C., and Feemster, R. F.: The sequelae of Eastern equine encephalomyelitis. New. Eng. J. Med. 240:960–962, 1949.

Azimi, P. H., Cramblett, H. G., and Haynes, R. E.: Mumps meningoencephalitis in children. J.A.M.A. 207:509–512, 1969.

Bachand, A. J., Rubenstein, J., and Morrison, A. N.: Thrombocytopenic purpura following live measles vaccine. Am. J. Dis. Child. 113:283–285, 1967.

Bacon, C. J., and Sims, D. G.: Echovirus 19 infection in infants under six months. Arch. Dis. Childh. 51:631–633, 1976.

Baker, A. B.: Poliomyelitis. 16. A study of pulmonary edema. Neurology 7:743–751, 1957.

Balduzzi, P., and Glasgow, L. A.: Paralytic poliomyelitis in a contact of a vaccinated child. New Eng. J. Med. 276:796–797, 1967.

Balfour, H. H., Jr., Schiff, G. M., and Bloom, J. E.: Encephalitis associated with erythema infectiosum. J. Pediat. 77:133–136, 1970.

Balfour, H. H., Jr., Edelman, C. K., Bauer, H., and Siem, R. A.: California arbovirus (La Crosse) infections. III. Epidemiology of California encephalitis in Minnesota. J. Infect. Dis. 133:293–301, 1976.

Balfour, H. H., Jr., Siem, R. A., Bauer, H., and Quie, P. G.: California arbovirus (La Crosse) infections. I. Clinical and laboratory findings in 66 children with meningoencephalitis. Pediatrics 52:680–691, 1973.

Balfour, H. H., Jr., Edelman, C. K., Cook, F. E., Barton, W. I., Buzicky, A. W., Siem, R. A., and Bauer, H.: Isolates of California encephalitis (La Crosse) virus from field-collected eggs and larvae of *Aedes triseriatus:* Identification of the overwintering site of California encephalitis. J. Infect. Dis. 131:712–716, 1975.

Bang, H. O., and Bang, J.: Involvement of the central nervous system in mumps. Acta Med. Scand. 113:487–505, 1943.

Baraff, L. J., Wilkins, J., and Wehrle, P. F.: The role of antibiotics, immunizations, and adenoviruses in pertussis. Pediatrics 61:224–230, 1978.

Bardelas, J. A., Winkelstein, J. A., Seto, D. S. Y., Tsai, T., and Rogol, A. D.: Fatal ECHO 24 infection in patient with hypogammaglobulinemia: Relationship to dermatomyositis-like syndrome. J. Pediat. 90:396–399, 1977.

Barnes, B., and Fish, M.: Chemical meningitis as a complication of isotope cisternography. Neurology 22:83–91, 1972.

Barrett, F. F., Yow, M. D., and Phillips, C. A.: St. Louis encephalitis in children during the 1964 epidemic. J.A.M.A. 193:381–385, 1965.

Bastian, F. O., Wende, R. D., Singer, D. B., and Zeller, R. S.: Eastern equine encephalomyelitis. Histopathologic and ultrastructural changes with isolation of the virus in a human case. Am. J. Clin. Path. 64:10–13, 1975.

Baum, S. G., Lewis, A. M., Jr., Rowe, W. P., and Huebner, R. J.: Epidemic nonmeningitic lymphocytic-choriomeningitis-virus infection. An outbreak in a population of laboratory personnel. New Eng. J. Med. 274:934–936, 1966.

Beck, C. E., and Wyckoff, R. W. G.: Venezuelan equine encephalomyelitis. Science 88:530, 1938.

Bell, W. E., McKee, A. P., and Utterback, R. A.: Asian influenza virus as a cause of acute encephalitis. Neurology 8:500–502, 1958.

Benady, S., Zvi, A. B., and Szabo, G.: Transverse myelitis following mumps. Acta Paediat. Scand. 62:205–206, 1973.

Benyesh-Melnick, M., and Rosenberg, H. S.: The isolation of adenovirus type 7 from a fatal case of pneumonia and disseminated disease. J. Pediat. 64:83–87, 1964.

Berg, R., and Jelke, H.: Acute cerebellar ataxia in children associated with Coxsackie viruses group B. Acta Paediat. Scand. 54:497–502, 1965.

Berkovich, S., and Schneck, L.: Ascending paralysis associated with measles. J. Pediat. 64:88–93, 1964.

Bernat, J. L.: Glioblastoma multiforme and the meningeal syndrome. Neurology 26:1071–1074, 1976.

Bigler, W. J., Lassing, E. B., Buff, E. E., Prather, E. C., Beck, E. C., and Hoff, G. L.: Endemic eastern equine encephalitis in Florida: A twenty-year analysis, 1955–1974. Am. J. Trop. Med. 25:884–890, 1976.

Bistrian, B., Phillips, C. A., and Kaye, I. S.: Fatal mumps meningoencephalitis. Isolation of virus premortem and postmortem. J.A.M.A. 222:478–479, 1972.

Blattner, R. J.: Encephalitis lethargica type A encephalitis, von Economo's disease. J. Pediat. 49:370–372, 1956.

Blattner, R. J., and Heys, F. M.: Isolation of St. Louis encephalitis virus from the peripheral blood of a human subject. J. Pediat. 28:401–406, 1946.

Blattner, R. J., and Heys, F. M.: St. Louis encephalitis. Occurrence in children in the St. Louis area during nonepidemic years 1939–1944. J.A.M.A. 129:854–857, 1945.

Bodensteiner, J. B., Morris, H. H., Howell, J. T., and Schochet, S. S.: Chronic ECHO type 5 virus meningoencephalitis in x-linked hypogammaglobulinemia: Treatment with immune plasma. Neurology 29:815–819, 1979.

Bodian, D.: Histopathologic basis of clinical findings in poliomyelitis. Am. J. Med. 6:563–578, 1949.

Bouteille, M., Fontaine, C., Bedrenne, C., and Delarue, J.: Sur un cas d'encephalite subaigue avec inclusions: Etude anatomoclinique et ultrastructurale. Rev. Neurol. 113:454–458, 1965.

Boyd, J. F., and Vince-Ribaric, V.: The examination of cerebrospinal fluid cells by fluorescent antibody staining to detect mumps antigen. Scand. J. Infect. Dis. 5:7–15, 1973.

Bray, P. F.: Mumps—a cause of hydrocephalus? Pediatrics 49:446–449, 1972.

Breitfeld, V., Hashida, Y., Sherman, F. E., Odagiri, K., and Yunis, E. J.: Fatal measles infection in children with leukemia. Lab. Invest. 28:279–291, 1973.

Breslich, P. J., Rowe, P. H., and Lehman, W. L.: Epidemic encephalitis in North Dakota. J.A.M.A. 113:1722–1724, 1939.

Brierley, J. B., Corsellis, J. A. N., Hierons, R., and Nevin, S.: Subacute encephalitis of later adult life. Mainly affecting the limbic areas. Brain 83:357–368, 1960.

Brightman, V. J., Scott, T. F. M., Westphal, M., and Boggs, T. R.: An outbreak of Coxsackie B-5 virus infection in a newborn nursery. J. Pediat. 69:179–192, 1966.

Brinker, K. R., Paulson, G., Monath, T. P., Wise, G., and Fass, R. J.: St. Louis encephalitis in Ohio, September 1975. Clinical and EEG studies in 16 cases. Arch. Intern. Med. 139:561–566, 1979.

Broadbank, T. W.: Postvaccinal myelitis. J.A.M.A. 97:227–228, 1931.

Brook, I., Bricknell, K. S., Overturf, G. D., and Finegold, S. M.: Measurement of lactic acid in cerebrospinal fluid of patients with infections of the central nervous system. J. Infect. Dis. 137:384–390, 1978.

Brunberg, J. A., and Bell, W. E.: Reye syndrome. An association with type 1 vaccine-like poliovirus. Arch. Neurol. 30:304–306, 1974.

Bruyn, G. W., Straathof, L. J. A., and Raymakers, G. M. J.: Mollaret's meningitis. Neurology 12:745–753, 1962.

Buzzard, E. F., and Greenfield, J. G.: Lethargic encephalitis: Its sequelae and morbid anatomy. Brain 13:305–338, 1919.

Byers, R. K.: Acute hemorrhagic leukoencephalitis: Report of three cases and review of the literature. Pediatrics 56:727–735, 1975.

Camenga, D. L., and Nathanson, N.: An immunopathologic component in experimental togavirus encephalitis. J. Neuropath. Exp. Neurol. 34:492–500, 1975.

Campbell, A. M. G., Williams, E. R., and Pearce, J.: Late motor neuron degeneration following poliomyelitis. Neurology 19:1101–1106, 1969.

Canoso, J. J., and Cohen, A. S.: Aseptic meningitis in systemic lupus erythematosus. Report of three cases. Arthritis Rheum. 18:369–374, 1975.

Cappel, R., and Klastersky, J.: Herpetic meningitis (type 1) in a case of acute leukemia. Arch. Neurol. 28:415–416, 1973.

Carmel, P. W., Fraser, R. A. R., and Stein, B. M.: Aseptic meningitis following posterior fossa surgery in children. J. Neurosurg. 41:44–48, 1974.

Casals, J.: Arboviruses. Am. J. Clin. Path. 57:762–770, 1972.

Casals, J.: Arenaviruses. Yale J. Biol. Med. 48:115–140, 1975.

Casals, J., Curnen, E. C., and Thomas, L.: Venezuelan equine encephalomyelitis in man. J. Exp. Med. 77:521–530, 1943.

Caverly, C. S.: Notes of an epidemic of acute anterior poliomyelitis. J.A.M.A. 26:1–5, 1896.

Cesario, T. C., Nakano, J. H., Caldwell, G. G., and Youmans, R. A.: Paralytic poliomyelitis in an unimmunized child. Am. J. Dis. Child. 118:895–898, 1969.

Chalhub, E. G., De Vivo, D. C., Siegel, B. A., Gado, M. H., and Feigin, R. D.: Coxsackie A9 focal encephalitis associated with acute infantile hemiplegia and porencephaly. Neurology 27:574–579, 1977.

Chamberlain, R. W., Sudia, W. D., Coleman, P. H., and Work, T. H.: Venezuelan equine encephalitis virus from south Florida. Science 145:272–274, 1964.

Chang, T. W., Weinstein, L., and MacMahon, H. E.: Paralytic poliomyelitis in a child with hypogammaglobulinemia: Probable implication of type 1 vaccine strain. Pediatrics 37:630–636, 1966.

Cherry, J. D.: Newer viral exanthems. Adv. Pediat. 16:233–286, 1969.

Cherry, J. D., Feigin, R. D., Lobes, L. A., Jr., and Shackelford, P. G.: Atypical measles in children previously immunized with attenuated measles virus vaccines. Pediatrics 50:712–717, 1972.

Chesney, P. J., Katcher, M. L., Nelson, D. B., and Horowitz, S. D.: CSF eosinophilia and chronic lymphocytic choriomeningitis virus meningitis. J. Pediat. 94:750–752, 1979.

Chou, S. M., Roos, R., Burrell, R., Gutmann, L., and Harley, J. B.: Subacute focal adenovirus encephalitis. J. Neuropath. Exp. Neurol. 32:34–50, 1973.

Christie, A. B.: Infectious Diseases: Epidemiology and Clinical Practice. E. S. Livingstone, Ltd. Edinburgh, 1969.

Chun, R. W. M., Thompson, W. H., Grabow, J. D., and Matthews, C. G.: California arbovirus encephalitis in children. Neurology 18:369–375, 1968.

Codd, A. A., Hale, J. H., Bell, T. M., Sims, D. G., Bacon, C. J., and Gardner, P. S.: Epidemic of echovirus 19 in the north-east of England. J. Hyg. Camb. 76:307–317, 1976.

Coffey, V. P., and Jessop, W. J. E.: Maternal influenza and congenital deformities. A prospective study. Lancet 2:935–938, 1959.

Coffey, V. P., and Jessop, W. J. E.: Maternal influenza and congenital deformities. A follow-up study. Lancet 1:748–751, 1963.

Cole, G. A., Gilden, D. H., Monjan, A. A., and Nathanson, N.: Lymphocytic choriomeningitis virus: pathogenesis of acute central nervous system disease. Fed. Proc. 30:1831–1841, 1971.

Conner, J. D.: Evidence for an etiologic role of adenoviral infection in pertussis syndrome. New Eng. J. Med. 283:390–394, 1970.

Copps, S. C., and Elston, A. C. V.: California virus (La Crosse strain) encephalitis. Wisc. Med. J. 68:329–331, 1969.

Copps, S. C., and Giddings, L. E.: Transplacental transmission of Western equine encephalitis. Pediatrics 24:31–33, 1959.

Costillo, C. E.: Informe sobre una reciente epidemia de encefalitis equina Venezelana en la zona norte del estado Zulia. Rev. Venez. Sanid. Asist. Soc. 29:325–348, 1964.

Cotton, P. B., and Webb-Peplee, M. M.: Acute transverse myelitis as a complication of glandular fever. Brit. Med. J. 1:654–655, 1966.

Coxe, W. S., and Luse, S. A.: Acute hemorrhagic leukoencephalitis. A clinical and electron-microscope report of 2 patients treated with surgical decompression. J. Neurosurg. 20:584–596, 1963.

Craig, C. P., and Nahmias, A. J.: Different patterns of neurologic involvement with Herpes simplex virus types 1 and 2: Isolation of Herpes simplex virus type 2 from the buffy coat of two adults with meningitis. J. Infect. Dis. 127:365–372, 1973.

Cramblett, H. G., Stegmiller, H., and Spencer, C.: California encephalitis virus infections in children. J.A.M.A. 198:108–112, 1966.

Cramblett, H. G., Haynes, R. E., Azimi, P. H., Hilty, M. D., and Wilder, M. H.: Nosocomial infection with Echovirus type II in handicapped and premature infants. Pediatrics 51:603–607, 1973.

Cramblett, H. G., Moffet, H. L., Black, J. P., Shulenberger, H., Smith, A., and Colonna, C. T.: Coxsackie virus infections. Clinical and laboratory studies. J. Pediat. 64:406–414, 1964.

Creech, W. B.: St. Louis encephalitis in the United States, 1975. J. Infect. Dis. 135:1014–1016, 1977.

Curnen, E. C., and Chamberlin, H. R.: Acute cerebellar ataxia associated with poliovirus infection. Yale J. Biol. Med. 34:219–233, 1962.

Dalldorf, G., and Sickles, G. M.: An unidentified, filterable agent isolated from feces of children with paralysis. Science 108:61, 1948.

Danta, G.: Electrophysiological study of amyotrophy associated with acute asthma (asthmatic amyotrophy). J. Neurol. Neurosurg. Psychiat. 38:1016–1021, 1975.

Davis, D. C., and Melnick, J. L.: Association of ECHO virus type 6 with aseptic meningitis. Proc. Soc. Exp. Biol. Med. 92:839–843, 1956.

Davis, L. E., Bodian, D., Price, D., Butler, I. J., and Vickers, J. H.: Chronic progressive poliomyelitis secondary to vaccination of an immunodeficient child. New Eng. J. Med. 297:241–245, 1977.

Dawson, J. R., Jr.: Cellular inclusions in cerebral lesions of lethargic encephalitis. Am. J. Path. 9:7–15, 1933.

Dayan, A. D., and Stokes, M. I.: Rapid diagnosis of encephalitis by immunofluorescent examination of cerebrospinal fluid cells. Lancet 1:177–179, 1973.

Dayan, A. D., Gooddy, W., Harrison, M. J. G., and Rudge, P.: Brain stem encephalitis caused by Herpesvirus hominis. Brit. Med. J. 4:405–406, 1972.

Dehn, H. M.: The age incidence of poliomyelitis in Cleveland. Pediatrics 1:83–89, 1948.

Delorme, L., and Middleton, P. J.: Influenza A virus associated with acute encephalopathy. Am. J. Dis. Child. 133:822–824, 1979.

Dickerson, R. B., Newton, J. R., and Hansen, J. E.: Diagnosis and immediate prognosis of Japanese B encephalitis. Observations based on more than 200 patients with detailed analysis of 65 serologically confirmed cases. Am. J. Med. 12:277–288, 1952.

Dietzman, D. E., Schaller, J. G., Ray, C. G., and Reed, M. E.: Acute myositis associated with influenza B infection. Pediatrics 57:255–258, 1976.

Donohue, W. L., Playfair, F. D., and Whitaker, L.: Mumps encephalitis. Pathology and pathogenesis. J. Pediat. 47:395–412, 1955.

Donovan, C. R., and Bowman, M.: Some epidemiological features of poliomyelitis and encephalitis, Manitoba, 1941. Canad. J. Publ. Health 33:246, 1942.

Dorfman, L. J.: Cytomegalovirus encephalitis in adults. Neurology 23:136–144, 1973.

Downham, M. A. P. S., McQuillin, J., and Gardner, P. S.: Diagnosis and clinical significance of parainfluenza virus infections in children. Arch. Dis. Childh. 49:8–15, 1974.

Draper, G., and Peabody, F. W.: A study of the cerebrospinal fluid and blood in acute poliomyelitis. Am. J. Dis. Child. 3:153–169, 1912.

Draughn, D. E., Sieber, O. F., and Umlauf, H. J., Jr.: Colorado tick fever encephalitis. Clin. Pediat. 4:626–628, 1965.

Drinker, P., and McKhann, C. F.: The use of a new apparatus for the prolonged administration of artificial respiration; a fatal case of poliomyelitis. J.A.M.A. 92:1658–1660, 1929.

Dunkley, B., and Lewis, T. T.: Meningeal reaction to starch powder in the cerebrospinal fluid. Brit. Med. J. 2:1391–1392, 1977.

Duvoisin, R. C., and Yahr, M. D.: Encephalitis and parkinsonism. Arch. Neurol. 12:227–239, 1965.

Earnest, M. P., Goolishian, H. A., Calverley, J. R., Hayes, R. O., and Hill, H. R.: Neurologic, intellectual, and psychologic sequelae following western encephalitis.

A follow-up study of 35 cases. Neurology 21:969–974, 1971.

Eckert, G. L., Barron, A. L., and Karzon, D. T.: Aseptic meningitis due to ECHO virus type 18. Am. J. Dis. Child. 99:1–3, 1960.

Ehrenkranz, N. I., Sinclair, M. C., Buff, E., and Lyman, D. O.: The natural occurrence of Venezuelan equine encephalitis in the United States. First case and epidemiologic investigations. New Eng. J. Med. 282:298–302, 1970.

Eley, R. C., and Flake, C. G.: Acute anterior poliomyelitis following tonsillectomy and adenoidectomy. J. Pediat. 13:63–70, 1938.

Enders, J., Bell, J., Dingle, J., Francis, J., Jr., Hilleman, M., and Huebner, R.: "Adenoviruses": Group name proposed for new respiratory-tract diseases. Science 124:119, 1956.

Enders, J. F., Weller, T. H., and Robbins, F. C.: Cultivation of the Lansing strain of poliomyelitis virus in cultures of various human embryonic tissues. Science 109:85, 1949.

Enders, J. P., and Peebles, T. C.: Propagation in tissue cultures of cytopathogenic agents from patients with measles. Proc. Soc. Exp. Biol. Med. 86:277–286, 1954.

Espir, M. L. E., and Spalding, J. M. K.: Three recent cases of encephalitis lethargica. Brit. Med. J. 1:1141–1144, 1956.

Farber, S., Hill, A., Connerly, M. L., and Dingle, J. H.: Encephalitis in infants and children caused by the virus of the Eastern variety of equine encephalitis. J.A.M.A. 114:1725–1731, 1940.

Faulkner, R., and van Rooyen, C. E.: Adenovirus types 3 and 5 isolated from the cerebrospinal fluid of children. Canad. Med. Assoc. J. 87:1123–1125, 1962.

Feemster, R. F.: Equine encephalitis in Massachusetts. New Eng. J. Med. 257:701–704, 1957.

Feigin, I.: Lesions in the white matter in acute poliomyelitis. Neurology 7:399–403, 1957.

Feigin, R. D., and Shackelford, P. G.: Value of repeat lumbar puncture in the differential diagnosis of meningitis. New Eng. J. Med. 289:571–574, 1973.

Feigin, R. D., Guggenheim, M. A., and Johnsen, S. D.: Vaccine-related paralytic poliomyelitis in an immunodeficient child. J. Pediat. 79:642–647, 1971.

Feorino, P. M., Humphrey, D., Hochberg, F., and Chilicote, R.: Mononucleosis-associated subacute sclerosing panencephalitis. Lancet 2:530–532, 1975.

Ferguson, I. R., and Tearle, P. V.: Gas liquid chromatography in the rapid diagnosis of meningitis. J. Clin. Path. 30:1163–1167, 1977.

Ferraro, A., and Roizin, L.: Hyperergic encephalomyelitides following exanthematic diseases, infectious diseases, and vaccination. J. Neuropath. Exp. Neurol. 16:423–445, 1957.

Ferraro, A., Roizin, L., and Cazzullo, C. L.: Experimental studies in allergic encephalomyelitis. J. Neuropath. Exp. Neurol. 9:18–28, 1950.

Finkeldey, W.: Riesenzellbefunde, bei akuter wurmfortsatzentzündung. Ein beitrag zur histopathologie der veränderungen des wurmfortsatzes im masserninkubationsstadium. Virchows Arch. 284:518, 1932.

Finley, K. H.: Postencephalitis manifestations of viral encephalitides. In: Fields, W. S., and Blattner, R. J.: Viral Encephalitis. Springfield, Ill., Charles C Thomas, 1958.

Finley, K. M., Fitzgerald, L. H., Richter, R. W., Riggs, N., and Shelton, J. T.: Western encephalitis and cerebral ontogenesis. Arch. Neurol. 16:140–164, 1967.

Flewett, T. H., and Hoult, J. G.: Influenzal encephalopathy and postinfluenzal encephalitis. Lancet 2:11–15, 1958.

Flexner, S., and Amoss, H. L.: Localization of the virus and pathogenesis of epidemic poliomyelitis. J. Exp. Med. 20:249–268, 1914.

Florio, L., Miller, M. S., and Mugrage, E. R.: Colorado tick fever. Recovery of virus from human cerebrospinal fluid. J. Infect. Dis. 90:285–289, 1952.

Foley, K. M., and Beresford, H. R.: Acute poliomyelitis beginning as transverse myelopathy. Arch. Neurol. 30:182–183, 1974.

Fothergill, L. D., and Dingle, J. H.: Fatal disease of pigeons caused by virus of Eastern variety of equine encephalomyelitis. Science 88:549, 1938.

Fothergill, L. D., Dingle, J. H., Farber, S., and Connerley, M. L.: Human encephalitis caused by the virus of the Eastern variety of equine encephalomyelitis. New Eng. J. Med. 219:411, 1938.

Franche, M., Brauner, E., Cuciureanu, G., Baltiev, A., Petrovanu, I., and Grigoriu, A.: La meningite leucocytaire multirecurrente (consideration au sujet d'un cas). Presse Med. 75:1839, 1967.

Fraser, C. H., and Schiff, D. W.: Colorado tick fever encephalitis. Pediatrics 29:187–190, 1962.

Friedman, J. H., and Cancellieri, R.: Central nervous system complications of Asian influenza. New York J. Med. 58:859–862, 1958.

Froesche, J. E., Nahmias, A. J., Feorino, P. M., McCord, G., and Naib, Z.: Hand, foot, and mouth disease (Coxsackievirus A16) in Atlanta. Am. J. Dis. Child. 114:278–283, 1967.

Frothingham, T. E.: ECHO virus type 9 associated with three cases simulating meningococcemia. New Eng. J. Med. 259:484–485, 1958.

Fulginiti, V. A., Eller, J. J., Downie, A. W., and Kempe, C. H.: Altered reactivity to measles virus. Atypical measles in children previously immunized with inactivated measles virus vaccines. J.A.M.A. 202:1075–1080, 1967.

Gabrielson, M. O., Joseph, C., and Hsiung, G. D.: Encephalitis associated with adenovirus type 7 occurring in a family outbreak. J. Pediat. 68:142–144, 1966.

Gamboa, E. T., Eastwood, A. B., Hays, A. P., Maxwell, J., and Penn, A. S.: Isolation of influenza virus from muscle in myoglobinuric polymyositis. Neurology 29:1323–1335, 1979.

Gascon, G., Victor, D., Lombroso, C. T., and Goodglass, H.: Language disorder, convulsive disorder, and electroencephalographic abnormalities. Acquired syndrome in children. Arch. Neurol. 28:156–162, 1973.

Gauld, L. W., Hanson, R. P., Thompson, W. H., and Sinha, S. K.: Observations on a natural cycle of La Crosse virus (California group) in southwestern Wisconsin. Am J. Trop. Med. 23:983–992, 1974.

Gautier-Smith, P. C.: Neurological complications of glandular fever (infectious mononucleosis). Brain 88:323–334, 1965.

Georg, A. J.: Recidiverende meningitis. Nord. Med. 47:556, 1952.

Gershon, A. A.: Diagnostic virology. Pediat. Clin. N. Amer. 18:73–86, 1971.

Getting, V. A.: Equine encephalomyelitis in Massachusetts. An analysis of the 1938 outbreak, a follow-up of cases and a report of a mosquito survey. New Eng. J. Med. 224:999–1006, 1941.

Gibbs, F. A., Gibbs, E. L., Carpenter, P. R., and Spies, H. W.: Electroencephalographic abnormality in "uncomplicated" childhood diseases. J.A.M.A. 171:1050–1055, 1959.

Gibbs, F. A., Gibbs, E. L., Carpenter, P. R., and Spies, H. W.: Electroencephalographic study of patients with acute aseptic meningitis. Pediatrics 29:181–186, 1962.

Gilday, D. L.: Various radionuclide patterns of cerebral inflammation of infants and children. Am. J. Roentgenol. 120:247–253, 1974.

Gilliam, A. G.: Epidemiological study of an epidemic diagnosed as poliomyelitis occurring among the personnel of the Los Angeles County General Hospital during the summer of 1934. Public Health Bulletin, U.S. Treasury Dept. No. 240, 1938.

Gilyard, R. T.: Clinical study of Venezuelan virus equine encephalomyelitis in Trinidad, B. W. I. J. Am. Vet. M. A. 106:267–277, 1945.

Ginsberg, H. S.: Adenoviruses. Am. J. Clin. Path. 57:771–776, 1972.

Glukhov, B. N., Jerusalimsky, A. P., Canter, V. M., and Salganik, R. I.: Ribonuclease treatment of tick-borne encephalitis. Arch. Neurol. 33:598–603, 1976.

Godoth, N., Weitzman, S., and Lehmann, E E.: Acute anterior myelitis complicating West Nile Fever. Arch. Neurol. 36:172–173, 1979.

Gold, R., Wilt, J. C., Adhikari, P. K., and Macpherson, R. I.: Adenoviral pneumonia and its complications in infancy and childhood. J. Canad. Assoc. Radiol. 20:218–224, 1969.

Goodpasture, H. C., Poland, J. D., Francy, D. B., Bowen, G. S., and Horn, K. A.: Colorado tick fever: Clinical, epidemiologic, and laboratory aspects of 228 cases in Colorado in 1973–1974. Ann. Intern. Med. 88:303–310, 1978.

Grabow, J. D., Matthews, G. G., Chun, R. W. M., and Thompson, W. H.: The electroencephalogram and clinical sequelae of California arbovirus encephalitis. Neurology 19:394–404, 1969.

Graybill, J. R., Silva, J., Jr., O'Brien, M. S., and Reinarz, J. A.: Epidemic neuromyasthenia. A syndrome or disease? J.A.M.A. 219:1440–1443, 1972.

Green, W. R., Sweet, L. K., and Prichard, R. W.: Acute lymphocytic choriomeningitis. A study of twenty-one cases. J. Pediat. 35:688–701, 1949.

Greenberg, M. W., and Beilly, J. S.: Congenital defects in the infant following mumps during pregnancy. Am. J. Obstet. Gynecol. 57:805–806, 1949.

Griffith, J.: "Acute cerebellar encephalitis." Am. J. Med. Sci. 162:781, 1921.

Grose, C., and Spigland, I.: Guillain-Barré syndrome following administration of live measles vaccine. Am. J. Med. 60:441–443, 1976.

Grossman, M.: Sequels of acute epidemic encephalitis. J.A.M.A. 78:959–962, 1922.

Hakosalo, J., and Saxen, L.: Influenza epidemic and congenital defects. Lancet 2:1346–1347, 1971.

Hall, A. J.: Encephalitis lethargica (epidemic encephalitis). Lancet 1:731–740, 1923.

Hall, C. B., and Horner, F. A.: Encephalopathy with erythema infectiosum. Am. J. Dis. Child. 131:65–67, 1977.

Hall, C. B., Cherry, J. D., Hatch, M. H., Nelson, D. B., and Winter, H. S.: The return of Boston exanthem. Echovirus 16 infections in 1974. Am. J. Dis. Child. 131:323–326, 1977.

Haltia, M., Paetau, A., Vaheri, A., Erkkilä, H., Donner, M., Kaakinen, K., and Holmström, T.: Fatal measles encephalopathy with retinopathy during cytotoxic chemotherapy. J. Neurol. Sci. 32:323–330, 1977.

Hammon, W. M., and Reeves, W. C.: Recent advances in the epidemiology of the arthropod-borne encephalitides. Am. J. Pub. Health 35:994–1004, 1945.

Hammon, W. M., and Reeves, W. C.: California encephalitis virus. A newly described agent. Calif. Med. 77:303–309, 1952.

Hammon, W. M., Yohn, D. S., Ludwig, E. H., Pavia, R. A., Sather, G. E., and McCloskey, L. W.: A study of certain non-poliomyelitis and poliomyelitis enterovirus infections. J.A.M.A. 167:727–735, 1958.

Haneberg, B., and Ørstavik, I.: Poliomyelitis associated with oral poliovaccine. Report on two cases. Acta Paediat. Scand. 61:105–108, 1972.

Harford, C. G., Wellinghoff, W., and Weinstein, R. A.: Isolation of herpes simplex virus from the cerebrospinal fluid in viral meningitis. Neurology 25:198–200, 1975.

Harrington, R. B., and Olin, R.: Incomplete transverse myelitis following rabies duck embryo vaccination. J.A.M.A. 217:2137–2138, 1971.

Hart, R. J. C., and Miller, D. L.: Echovirus-17 infections in Britain 1969–71. Lancet 2:661–664, 1973.

Harwood-Nash, D. C., McDonald, P., and Argent, W.: Cerebral arterial disease in children. An angiographic study of 40 cases. Am. J. Roentgenol. 111:672–686, 1971.

Hashimoto, H., Kudo, M., and Uraguchi, K.: Experiences in the summer epidemics of acute encephalitis in Tokyo. J.A.M.A. 106:1266–1268, 1936.

Hauser, G. H.: Human equine encephalomyelitis, Eastern type, in Louisiana. New Orleans Med. Surg. J. 100:551–558, 1948.

Haymaker, W.: Mosquito-borne encephalitides. *In*: van Bogaert et al.: Encephalitides. Elsevier, Amsterdam, 1961.

Haynes, B. F., Wright, R., and McCracken, J. P.: Mollaret meningitis. A report of three cases. J.A.M.A. 236:1967–1969, 1976.

Haynes, R. E., Cramblett, H. G., and Kronfol, H. J.: Echovirus 9 meningoencephalitis in infants and children. J.A.M.A. 208:1657–1660, 1969.

Haynes, R. E., Cramblett, H. G., Hilty, M. D., Azimi, P. H., and Crews, J.: ECHO virus type 3 infections in children: Clinical and laboratory studies. J. Pediat. 80:589–595, 1972.

Heathfield, K. W. G., Pilsworth, R., Wall, B. J., and Corsellis, J. A. N.: Coxsackie B5 infections in Essex, 1965, with particular reference to the nervous system. Quart. J. Med. 36:579–595, 1967.

Heine, J.: Beobachtungen uber lahmungszustande der untern extremitaten und deren behandlung. Stuttgart, Köhler, 1840.

Hempelmann, T. C.: The symptoms and diagnosis of encephalitis (1933 St. Louis epidemic). J.A.M.A. 103:733–735, 1934.

Hermans, P. E., Goldstein, N. P., and Wellman, W. E.: Mollaret's meningitis and differential diagnosis of recurrent meningitis. Report of case, with review of the literature. Am. J. Med. 52:128–140, 1972.

Herndon, R. M., Johnson, R. T., Davis, L. E., and Descalzi, L. R.: Ependymitis in mumps virus meningitis. Arch. Neurol. 30:475–479, 1974.

Herzon, H., Shelton, J. T., and Bruyn, H. B.: Sequelae of Western equine and other arthropod-borne encephalitides. Neurology 7:535–548, 1957.

Hilleman, M. R., and Wener, J. R.: Recovery of new agent from patients with acute respiratory illness. Proc. Soc. Exp. Biol. Med. 85:183–188, 1954.

Hilty, M. D., Haynes, R. E., Azimi, P. H., and Cramblett, H. G.: California encephalitis in children. Am. J. Dis. Child. 124:530–533, 1972.

Hinman, A. R., Fraser, D. W., Douglas, R. G., Bowen, G. S., Kraus, A. L., Winkler, W. G., and Rhodes, W. W.: Outbreak of lymphocytic choriomeningitis virus infections in medical center personnel. Am. J. Epidemiol. 101:103–110, 1975.

Hirsch, M. S., Moellering, R. C., Jr., Pope, H. G., and Poskanzer, D. C.: Lymphocytic-choriomeningitis-virus infection traced to a pet hamster. New Eng. J. Med. 291:610–612, 1974.

Hirschman, S. A.: Approaches to antiviral chemotherapy. Am. J. Med. 51:699–703, 1971.

Hochberg, F. H., Lehrich, J. R., Richardson, E. P., Jr., Feorino, P., and Astrom, K. E.: Mononucleosis-associated subacute sclerosing panencephalitis. Acta Neuropath. 34:33–40, 1976.

Hodges, G. R., Fass, R. J., and Saslaw, S.: Central nervous system disease associated with *Mycoplasma pneumoniae* infection. Arch. Intern. Med. 130:277–282, 1972.

Hogan, E. L., and Krigman, M. R.: Herpes zoster myelitis. Evidence of viral invasion of spinal cord. Arch. Neurol. 29:309–313, 1973.

Holliday, P. B.: Pre-eruptive neurological complications of the common contagious diseases—rubella, rubeola, roseola, and varicella. J. Pediat. 36:185–198, 1950.

Holowach, J., Thurston, D. L., and Becker, B.: Congenital defects in infants following mumps during pregnancy. a review of the literature and a report of chorioretinitis due to fetal infection. J. Pediat. 50:689–694, 1957.

Holt, G. W.: Epidemic neuromyasthenia. The sporadic form. Am. J. Med. Sci. 249:98–112, 1965.

Holt, W. L.: Epidemic encephalitis. A follow-up study of two-hundred and sixty-six cases. Arch. Neurol. Psychiat. 38:1135–1144, 1937.

Holzel, A., Smith, P. A., and Tobin, J. O'H.: A new type of meningoencephalitis associated with a rhinovirus. Acta Paediat. Scand. 54:168–174, 1965.

Hopkins, C. C., Hollinger, F. B., Johnson, R. F., Dewlett, H. J., Newhouse, V. F., and Chamberlain, R. W.: The epidemiology of St. Louis encephalitis in Dallas, Texas, 1966. Am. J. Epidemiol. 102:1–15, 1975.

Hopkins, I. J.: A new syndrome: Poliomyelitis-like illness associated with acute asthma in childhood. Austral. Pediat. J. 10:273–276, 1974.

Hosier, D. M., and Newton, W. A., Jr.: Serious Coxsackie infection in infants and children. Am. J. Dis. Child. 96:251–267, 1958.

Hoult, J. G., and Flewett, T. H.: Influenzal encephalopathy and postinfluenzal encephalitis. Histological and other observations. Brit. Med. J. 1:1847–1850, 1960.

Howitt, B.: Recovery of the virus of equine encephalomyelitis from the brain of a child. Science 88:455–456, 1938.

Hoyne, A. L., and Slotkowski, E. L.: Frequency of encephalitis as a complication of measles. Report of twenty cases. Am. J. Dis. Child. 73:554–558, 1947.

Hullinghorst, R. L., Burns, K. F., Choi, Y. T., and Whatley, L. L.: Japanese B encephalitis in Korea. The epidemic of 1949. J.A.M.A. 145:460–466, 1951.

Hurst, E. W.: Acute hemorrhagic leukoencephalitis: a previously undefined entity. Med. J. Aust. 2:1–6, 1941.

Huttunen, L.: Adenovirus type 7–associated encephalitis. Scand. J. Infect. Dis. 2:151–153, 1970.

Ilett, S. J., Pugh, R. J., and Smithells, R. W.: Poliomyelitis-like illness after acute asthma. Arch. Dis. Childh. 52:738–740, 1977.

Innes, S. G. B.: Encephalomyelitis resembling benign myalgic encephalomyelitis. Lancet 1:969–971, 1970.

Ishii, T., Matsushita, M., and Hamada, S.: Characteristic residual neuropathological features of Japanese B encephalitis. Acta Neuropath. 38:181–186, 1977.

Jackson, A. L.: A clinical study of the Landry-Guillain-Barré syndrome with reference to aetiology, including the role of Coxsackie virus infections. South African J. Lab. Clin. Med. 7:121–137, 1961.

Jarco, L. W., Fred, H. L., and Castle, C. H.: Encephalitis and poliomyelitis in the adult due to Coxsackie virus group B, type 5. New Eng. J. Med. 268:235–238, 1963.

Jarratt, M., and Hubler, W. R., Jr.: Herpes genitalis and aseptic meningitis. Arch. Dermatol. 110:771–772, 1974.

Jespersen, C. S., Littauer, J., and Sagild, V.: Measles as a cause of fetal defects. A retrospective study of ten measles epidemics in Greenland. Acta Paediat. Scand. 66:367–372, 1977.

Johnson, D. A., and Eger, A. W.: Myelitis associated with an Echo-virus. J.A.M.A. 201:637–638, 1967.

Johnson, K. P., and Johnson, R. T.: California encephalitis. II. Studies of experimental infection in the mouse. J. Neuropath. Exp. Neurol. 27:390–400, 1968.

Johnson, K. P., Lepow, M. L., and Johnson, R. T.: California encephalitis. I. Clinical and epidemiological studies. Neurology 18:250–254, 1968.

Johnson, R., and Milbourn, P. E.: Central nervous system manifestations of chickenpox. Canad. Med. Assoc. J. 102:831–834, 1970.

Johnson, R. T.: Effects of viral infection on the developing nervous system. New Eng. J. Med. 287:599–604, 1972.

Johnson, R. T., and Johnson, K. J.: Hydrocephalus following viral infection: The pathology of aqueductal stenosis developing after experimental mumps virus infection. J. Neuropath. Exp. Neurol. 27:591–606, 1968.

Johnson, R. T., and Mims, C. A.: Pathogenesis of viral infections of the nervous system. New Eng. J. Med. 278:23–30, 1968.

Johnstone, J. A., Ross, C. A. C., and Dunn, M.: Meningitis and encephalitis associated with mumps infection. Arch. Dis. Childh. 47:647–651, 1972.

Jones, A. B.: The encephalitis epidemic in St. Louis city and county, 1933. Prognosis. J.A.M.A. 103:825, 1934.

Joske, R. A., Keall, D. D., Leak, P. J., Stanley, N. F., and Walters, M. N. I.: Hepatitis-encephalitis in humans with reovirus infection. Arch. Intern. Med. 113:811–816, 1964.

Kabat, H., and Knapp, M. E.: The mechanism of muscle spasm in poliomyelitis. J. Pediat. 24:408–416, 1944.

Kalis, J. M., Burgess, A. C., and Balfour, H. H., Jr.: Serologic diagnosis of California (La Crosse) encephalitis by immunofluorescence. J. Clin. Microbiol. 1:448–450, 1975.

Kaneko, R., and Aoki, Y.: Über die encephalitis epidemica in Japan. Ergebn. d. inn. Med. u. Kinderh. 34:342–456, 1928.

Karelitz, S., and Eisenberg, M.: Measles encephalitis. Evaluation of treatment with adrenocorticotropin and adrenal corticosteroids. Pediatrics 27:811–818, 1961.

Karson, D. T., Hayner, N. S., Winkelstein, W., Jr., and Barron, A. L.: An epidemic of aseptic meningitis syndrome due to ECHO virus type 6. Pediatrics 29:418–431, 1962.

Katz, S. L., Milovanovic, M. V., and Enders, J. F.: Propagation of measles virus in cultures of chick embryo cells. Proc. Soc. Exp. Biol. Med. 97:23–29, 1958.

Keeffe, E. B., Bardana, E. J., Jr., Harbeck, R. J., Pirofsky, B., and Carr, R. I.: Lupus meningitis. Antibody to deoxyribonucleic acid (DNA) and DNA: anti-DNA complexes in cerebrospinal fluid. Ann. Intern. Med. 80:58–60, 1974.

Kelsey, D. S.: Adenovirus meningoencephalitis. Pediatrics 61:291–293, 1978.

Kennett, M. L., Ellis, A. W., Lewis, F. A., and Gust, I. D.: An epidemic associated with echovirus type 18. J. Hyg. 70:325–334, 1972.

Ketel, W. B., and Ognibene, A. J.: Japanese B encephalitis in Vietnam. Am. J. Med. Sci. 261:271–279, 1971.

Kibrick, S., and Benirschke, K.: Acute aseptic myocarditis and meningoencephalitis in the newborn child infected with Coxsackie virus group B, type 3. New Eng. J. Med. 255:883–889, 1956.

Kibrick, S., and Benirschke, K.: Severe generalized disease (encephalohepatomyocarditis) occurring in the newborn period and due to infection with Coxsackie virus, group B. Evidence of intrauterine infection with this agent. Pediatrics 22:857–874, 1958.

Kilham, L.: Mumps meningoencephalitis with and without parotitis. Am. J. Dis. Child. 78:324–333, 1949.

Kilham, L., and Margolis, G.: Induction of congenital hydrocephalus in hamsters with attenuated and natural strains of mumps virus. J. Infect. Dis. 132:462–466, 1975.

Kissling, R. E., Chamberlain, R. W., Nelson, D. B., and Stamm, D. D.: Studies on the North American arthropod-borne encephalitides. VIII. Equine encephalitis studies in Louisiana. Am. J. Hyg. 62:233–254, 1955.

Klastersky, J., Cappel, R., Snoeck, J. B., Flament, J., and Thiry, L.: Ascending myelitis in association with Herpes-simplex virus. New Eng. J. Med. 287:182–184, 1972.

Kleinman, H., Cooney, M. K., Nelson, C. B., Owen, R. R., Boyd, L., and Swanda, G.: Aseptic meningitis and paralytic disease due to newly recognized enterovirus. J.A.M.A. 187:90–95, 1964.

Klemola, E., and Lapinleimu, K.: Multiple attacks of aseptic meningitis in the same individual. Brit. Med. J. 1:1087–1090, 1964.

Klemola, E., Weckman, N., Haltia, K., and Kääriäinen, L.: The Guillain-Barré syndrome associated with acquired cytomegalovirus infection. Acta Med. Scand. 181:603–607, 1969.

Klenk, E. L., Gaultney, J. V., and Bass, J. W.: Bacteriologically proved pertussis and adenovirus infection. Possible association. Am. J. Dis. Child. 124:203–207, 1972.

Knutti, R. E.: Acute ascending paralysis and myelitis due to the virus of rabies. J.A.M.A. 93:754–758, 1929.

Kopel, F. B., Shore, B., and Hodes, H. L.: Nonfatal bulbospinal paralysis due to ECHO 4 virus. J. Pediat. 67:588–593, 1965.

Koplik, H.: The diagnosis of the invasion of measles from a study of the exanthema as it appears on the buccal mucous membrane. Arch. Pediat. 13:918–922, 1896.

Koprowski, H.: The role of hyperergy in measles encephalitis. Am. J. Dis. Child. 103:273–278, 1962.

Koprowski, H., and Cox, H. R.: Human laboratory infection with Venezuelan equine encephalomyelitis virus. Report of four cases. New Eng. J. Med. 236:647–654, 1947.

Krainer, L., and Aronson, B. E.: Disseminated encephalomyelitis in human with recovery of hepato-encephalitis virus (HEV). J. Neuropath. Exp. Neurol. 18:339–342, 1959.

Kristensson, K., Olsson, Y., and Sourander, P.: Viral encephalitis: Pathogenesis in the immature brain. Dev. Med. Child. Neurol. 16:382–394, 1974.

Kristiansen, K., Harkmark, W., and Cohen, M. M.: Acute hemorrhagic encephalitis. Neurology 6:503–509, 1956.

Krous, H. F., Dietzman, D., and Ray, C. G.: Fatal infections with Echovirus type 6 and 11 in early infancy. Am. J. Dis. Child. 126:842–846, 1973.

Krugman, R. D., Meyer, B. C., Enterline, J C., Parkman, P. D., Witte, J. J., and Meyer, H. M., Jr.: Impotency of live-virus vaccines as a result of improper handling in clinical practice. J. Pediat. 85:512–514, 1974.

Krugman, S.: Present status of measles and rubella immunization in the United States: A medical progress report. J. Pediat. 78:1–16, 1971.

Krugman, S.: Present status of measles and rubella immunization in the United States: A medical progress report. J. Pediat. 90:1–12, 1977.

Kubes, V., and Rios, F. A.: Causative agent of infectious equine encephalomyelitis in Venezuela. Science 90:20, 1939.

LaBoccetta, A. C., and Tornay, A. S.: Measles encephalitis. Report of 61 cases. Am. J. Dis. Child. 107:247–255, 1964.

Ladisch, S., Lovejoy, F. H., Hierholzer, J. C., Oxman, M. N., Strieder, D., Vawter, G. F., Finer, N., and Moore, M.: Extrapulmonary manifestations of adenovirus type 7 pneumonia simulating Reye syndrome and the possible role of an adenovirus toxin. J. Pediat. 95:348–355, 1979.

Lake, A. M., Lauer, B. A., Clark, J. C., Wesenberg, R. L., and McIntosh, K.: Enteroviral infections in neonates. J. Pediat. 89:787–791, 1976.

Lander, H.: A case of acute hemorrhagic leucoencephalitis (Hurst) complicating varicella. J. Path. Bact. 70:157–165, 1955.

Landing, B. H., and Larson, E. J.: Are infantile periarteritis nodosa with coronary artery involvement and fatal mucocutaneous lymph node syndrome the same? Comparison of 20 patients from North America with patients from Hawaii and Japan. Pediatrics 59:651–662, 1977.

Landsteiner, K., and Popper, E.: Uebertragung der poliomyelitis acuta auf affen. Ztschr. f. Immunitatsforch u. Exper. Ther. 2:377–390, 1909.

Laptook, A., Wind, E., Nussbaum, M., and Shenker, I. R.: Pulmonary lesions in atypical measles. Pediatrics 62:42–46, 1978.

Leake, J. P., Musson, E. K., and Chope, H. D.: Epidemiology of epidemic encephalitis, St. Louis type. J.A.M.A. 103:728–731, 1934.

Leck, I., Hay, S., Witte, J. J., and Greene, J. C.: Malformations recorded on birth certificates following A2 influenza epidemics. Pub. Health Rep. 84:971–979, 1969.

LeLong, M., Lepine, P., Alison, F., LeTan-Vinh Stage, P., and Chany, C.: La pneumonie a virus du group A.P.C. chez le nourrison; isolement du virus. Les lesions anatomohistologiques. Arch. Franc. Pediat. 13:1092–1095, 1956.

Lennette, E. H.: Laboratory diagnosis of viral infections: general principles. Am. J. Clin. Path. 57:737–750, 1972.

Lennette, E. H., and Koprowski, H.: Human infection with Venezuelan equine encephalomyelitis virus: report on eight cases of infection acquired in the laboratory. J.A.M.A. 123:1088–1095, 1943.

Lennette, E. H., and Longshore, W. A.: Western equine and St. Louis encephalitis in man, California, 1945–1950. Calif. Med. J. 75:189, 1951.

Lennette, E. H., Magoffin, R. L., and Knouf, E. G.: Viral central nervous system disease. J.A.M.A. 179:687–695, 1962.

Lepow, M. L., Carver, D. H., Wright, H. T., Jr., Woods, W. A., and Robbins, F. C.: A clinical, epidemiologic and laboratory investigation of aseptic meningitis during a four-year period, 1955–1958. I. Observations concerning etiology and epidemiology. New Eng. J. Med. 266:1181–1187, 1962.

Lepow, M. L., Coyne, N., Thompson, L. B., Carver, D. H., and Robbins, F. C.: A clinical, epidemiologic and laboratory investigation of aseptic meningitis during the four-year period, 1955–1958. II. The clinical disease and its sequelae. New Eng. J. Med. 266:1188–1193, 1962.

Lerer, R. J., and Kalavsky, S. M.: Central nervous system disease associated with *Mycoplasma pneumoniae* infection. Report of five cases and review of the literature. Pediatrics 52:658–668, 1973.

Levitt, L. P., Lovejoy, F H., Jr., and Daniels, J. B.: Eastern equine encephalitis in Massachusetts—First human case in 14 years. New Eng. J. Med. 284:540, 1971.

Levitt, L. P., Rich, T. A., Kinde, S. W., Lewis, A. L., Gates, E. H., and Bond, J. O.: Central nervous system mumps. A review of 64 cases. Neurology 20:829–834, 1970.

Levitt, L. P., Bond, J. O., Hall, I. E., Jr., Dame, G. M., Buff, E. E., Marston, C., and Prather, E. C.: Meningococcal and ECHO-9 meningitis. Report of an outbreak. Neurology 20:45–51, 1970.

Likar, M., and Dane, D. S.: An illness resembling acute poliomyelitis caused by a virus of the Russian spring-summer encephalitis/louping ill group in northern Ireland. Lancet 1:456–458, 1958.

Lincoln, A. F., and Silvertson, S. E.: Acute phase of Japanese B encephalitis. Two hundred and one cases in American soldiers, Korea, 1950. J.A.M.A. 150:268–283, 1952.

Lincoln, E. M., Sordillo, S. V. R., and Davies, P. A.: Tuberculous meningitis in children. J. Pediat. 57:807–823, 1960.

Lindeman, J., Muller, W. K., Versteeg, J., Bots, G. T., and Peters, A. C. B.: Rapid diagnosis of meningo-encephalitis, encephalitis. Immunofluorescent examination of fresh and in vitro cultured cerebrospinal fluid cells. Neurology 24:143–148, 1974.

Linnemann, C. C., Jr., Steichen, J., Sherman, W. G., and Schiff, G. M.: Febrile illness in early infancy associated with ECHO virus infection. J. Pediat. 84:49–54, 1974.

Linnemann, C. C., Jr., First, M. R., Alvira, M. M., Alexander, J. W., and Schiff, G. M.: Herpesvirus hominis type 2 meningoencephalitis following renal transplantation. Am. J. Med. 61:703–708, 1976.

Lipton, H. L., and Teasdall, R. D.: Acute transverse myelopathy in adults. Arch. Neurol. 28:252–257, 1973.

London, W. T., Kent, S. G., Palmer, A. E., Fucillo, D. A., Houff, S. A., Saini, N., and Sever, J. L.: Induction of congenital hydrocephalus with mumps virus in rhesus monkeys. J. Infect. Dis. 139:324–328, 1979.

Lopez, C., Biggar, W. D., Park, B. H., and Good, R. A.: Nonparalytic poliovirus infections in patients with severe combined immuno-deficiency disease. J. Pediat. 84:497–502, 1974.

Lord, R. D., Calisher, C. H., and Doughty, W. P.: Assessment of bird involvement in three urban St. Louis encephalitis epidemics. Am. J. Epidemiol. 99:364–367, 1974.

Lord, R. D., Calisher, C. H., Chappell, W. A., Metzger,

W. R., and Fischer, G. W.: Urban St. Louis encephalitis surveillance through wild birds. Am. J. Epidemiol. 99:360–363, 1974.

Lou, H. C., Brandt, S., and Bruhn, P.: Progressive aphasia and epilepsy with a self-limited course. *In*: Penry, J. K.: Epilepsy, The Eighth International Symposium. Raven Press, New York, 1977.

Lovett, R. W.: The occurrence of infantile paralysis in the United States and Canada in 1910. Am. J. Dis. Child. 2:65–74, 1911.

Lyon, G., Dodge, P. R., and Adams, R. D.: The acute encephalopathies of obscure origin in infants and children. Brain 83:680–706, 1961.

MacKenzie, J. S., and Houghton, M.: Influenza infections during pregnancy: Association with congenital malformations and with subsequent neoplasms in children, and potential hazards of live virus vaccines. Bact. Rev. 38:356–370, 1974.

Magoffin, R. L., Lennette, E. H., Hollister, A. C., Jr., and Schmidt, N. J.: An etiologic study of clinical paralytic poliomyelitis. J.A.M.A. 175:269–278, 1961.

Main, A.: Lethargic encephalitis: The Glasgow epidemic of 1923. J. Hyg. 31:162–188, 1931.

Matthews, C. G., Chun, R. W. M., Grabow, J. D., and Thompson, W. H.: Psychological sequelae in children following California arbovirus encephalitis. Neurology 18:1023–1030, 1968.

McAllister, R., Hummeler, K., and Coriell, L.: Acute cerebellar ataxia. Report of a case with isolation of type 9 ECHO virus from the cerebrospinal fluid. New Eng. J. Med. 261:1159–1162, 1959.

McCarthy, J. T., and Amer, J.: Postvaricella acute transverse myelitis: A case presentation and review of the literature. Pediatrics 62:202–204, 1978.

McCordock, H. A., Collier, W., and Gray, S. H.: The pathologic changes of the St. Louis type of acute encephalitis. J.A.M.A. 103:822–825, 1934.

McDonald, L. L., St. Geme, J. W., Jr., and Arnold, B. H.: Nosocomial infection with ECHO virus type 31 in a neonatal intensive care unit. Pediatrics 47:995–999, 1971.

McLean, D. M., and Donohue, W. L.: Powassan virus: Isolation of virus from a fatal case of encephalitis. Canad. Med. Assoc. J. 80:708–711, 1959.

Meadow, S. R.: Hand, foot, and mouth diseases. Arch. Dis. Childh. 40:560–564, 1965.

Meadow, S. R., Weller, R. O., and Archibald, R. W. R.: Fatal systemic measles in a child receiving cyclophosphamide for nephrotic syndrome. Lancet 2:876–878, 1969.

Medin, O.: Ueber eine epidemie von spinaler kinderlahmung. Verhandl. d. 10 Int. Med. Kongr., 1890. 2:6, 37, 47, 1891.

Medovy, H.: Western equine encephalomyelitis in infants. J. Pediat. 22:308–318, 1943.

Melish, M. E., Hicks, R. M., and Larson, E. J.: Mucocutaneous lymph node syndrome in the United States. Am. J. Dis. Child. 130:599–607, 1976.

Mellman, W. J.: Influenza meningitis. J. Pediat. 53:292–297, 1958.

Melnick, J. L.: Classification and nomenclature of animal viruses, 1971. Progr. Med. Virol. 13:462–484, 1971.

Mendez-Cashion, D., Sanchez-Longo, L. P., Valcarel, M., and Rosen, L.: Acute cerebellar ataxia in children associated with infection by poliovirus 1. Pediatrics 29:808–815, 1962.

Messert, B., and Rieder, M. J.: RISA cisternography. Study of spinal fluid changes associated with intrathecal RISA injection. Neurology 22:789–792, 1972.

Meyer, H. M., Jr., Johnson, R. T., Crawford, I. P., Dascomb, H. E., and Rogers, N. G.: Central nervous system syndromes of "viral" etiology. A study of 713 cases. Am. J. Med. 29:334–347, 1960.

Meyer, K. F., Haring, C. M., and Howitt, B.: Etiology of epizootic encephalomyelitis of horses in San Joaquin Valley. Science 74:227, 1931.

Mithatsch, M. J., Ohnacker, H., Just, M., and Nars, P-W.: Lethal measles giant cell pneumonia after live measles vaccination in a case of thymic alymphoplasia Gitlin. Helv. Paediat. Acta 27:143–146, 1972.

Miles, J. A. R.: Epidemiology of the arthropod-borne encephalitides. Bull. W.H.O. 22:339–371, 1960.

Miller, D. G., Gabrielson, M. O., Bart, K. J., Opton, E. M., and Horstman, D. M.: An epidemic of aseptic meningitis, primarily among infants, caused by Echovirus 11-prime. Pediatrics 41:77–90, 1968.

Miller, H. G., Stanton, J. B., and Gibbons, J. L.: Parainfectious encephalitis and related syndromes: A critical review of the neurological complications of certain specific fevers. Quart. J. Med. 25:427–505, 1956.

Modlin, J. F., Jabbour, J. T., Witte, J. J., and Halsey, N. A.: Epidemiologic studies of measles, measles vaccine, and subacute sclerosing panencephalitis. Pediatrics 59:505–512, 1977.

Mollaret, M. P.: La meningite endothélio-leucocytaire multi-recurrente benigne. Syndrome nouveau ou maladie nouvelle? Rev. Neurol. 76:57–76, 1944.

Monjan, A. A., Cole, G. A., Gilden, D. H., and Nathanson, N.: Pathogenesis of cerebellar hypoplasia produced by lymphocytic choriomeningitis virus infection of neonatal rats. J. Neuropath. Exp. Neurol. 32:110–124, 1973.

Morbidity and Mortality Weekly Reports. Vol. 16, 19 Aug., 1967.

Morbidity and Mortality Weekly Reports. Vol. 20, 13 Nov., 1971.

Morbidity and Mortality Weekly Reports. Vol. 22, 11 Aug., 1973.

Morbidity and Mortality Weekly Reports. Vol. 24, 1975, p. 379.

Morley, D. C.: Measles in Nigeria. Am. J. Dis. Child. 103:230–233, 1962.

Morris, C. D., Caines, A. R., Woodall, J. P., and Bast, T. F.: Eastern equine encephalomyelitis in upstate New York, 1972–1974. Am. J. Trop. Med. 24:986–991, 1975.

Mouton, C. M., Smillie, J. G., and Bower, A. G.: Report of ten cases of poliomyelitis in infants under six months of age. J. Pediat. 36:482–492, 1950.

Muckenfuss, R. S., Armstrong, C., and Webster, L. T.: Etiology of the 1933 epidemic of encephalitis. J.A.M.A. 103:731–733, 1934.

Mulder, D. W., Rosenbaum, R. A., and Layton, D. D., Jr.: Late progression of poliomyelitis or forme fruste amyotrophic lateral sclerosis? Mayo Clin. Proc. 47:756–761, 1972.

Muller, S. A., Herrmann, E. C., Jr., and Winkelmann, R. K.: Herpes simplex infections in hematologic malignancies. Am. J. Med. 52:102–114, 1972.

Murphy, J. V., and Yunis, E. J.: Encephalopathy following measles infection in children with chronic illness. J. Pediat. 88:937–942, 1976.

Murray, R. G., and Walsh, F. B.: Ocular abnormalities in poliomyelitis and their pathogenesis. Canad. Med. Assoc. J. 70:141–147, 1954.

Nader, P. R., and Warren, R. J.: Reported neurologic disorders following live measles vaccine. Pediatrics 41:997–1001, 1968.

Nader, P. R., Horwitz, M. S., and Rousseau, J.: Atypical exanthem following exposure to natural measles: Eleven cases in children previously inoculated with killed vaccine. J. Pediat. 72:22–28, 1968.

Nakao, T., and Miura, R.: Recurrent virus meningitis. Pediatrics 47:773–776, 1971.

Nathanson, N., and Bodian, D.: Experimental poliomyelitis following intramuscular virus injection. III. The effect of passive antibody on paralysis and viremia. Bull. Johns Hopkins Hosp. 111:198–220, 1962.

Nathanson, N., and Cole, G. A.: Immunosuppression and experimental virus infection of the nervous system. Adv. Virus Res. 16:397–448, 1970.

Neal, J. B.: Lethargic encephalitis. Arch. Neurol. Psychiat. 2:271–290, 1919.

Nelson, K. E., Gavitt, F., Batt, M. D., Kallick, C. A., Reddi, K. T., and Levin, S.: The role of adenoviruses in the pertussis syndrome. J. Pediat. 86:335–341, 1975.

Neva, F. A.: A second outbreak of Boston exanthem disease in Pittsburgh during 1954. New Eng. J. Med. 254:838–843, 1956.

Neva, F. A., Feemster, R. F., and Gorback, I. J.: Clinical and epidemiological features of an unusual epidemic exanthem. J.A.M.A. 155:544–548, 1954.

Nielsen, J. M.: Complications of encephalitis of the von Economo type. Bull. Los Angeles Neurol. Assoc. 18:84–90, 1953.

Nightingale, E. O.: Recommendations for a national policy on poliomyelitis vaccination. New Eng. J. Med. 297:249–253, 1977.

Nogen, A. G., and Lepow, M. L.: Enteroviral meningitis in very young infants. Pediatrics 40:617–626, 1969.

Noran, H. H., and Baker, A. B.: Western equine encephalitis: The pathogenesis of the pathological lesions. J. Neuropath. Exp. Neurol. 4:269–276, 1945.

Nordbring, F., and Gertzen, O.: Benign recurrent aseptic meningitis (Mollaret's meningitis). Scand. J. Infect. Dis. 3:75–78, 1971.

Ogawa, M., Okubo, H., Tsuji, Y., Yasui, N., and Someda, K.: Chronic progressive encephalitis occurring 13 years after Russian spring-summer encephalitis. J. Neurol. Sci. 19:363–373, 1973.

Ogbeide, M. I.: Measles in Nigerian children. J. Pediat. 71:737–741, 1967.

Oldfelt, V.: Sequelae of mumps meningoencephalitis. Acta Med. Scand. 134:405–414, 1949.

Oren, J., Schiff, G. M., Foder, A. R., and Mohr, D. V.: Aseptic meningitis on an Indian reservation. Am. J. Dis. Child. 102:843–852, 1961.

Oski, F. A.: Roseola infantum. Another cause of bulging fontanel. Am. J. Dis. Child. 101:376–378, 1961.

Oski, F. A., and Naiman, J. L.: Effect of live measles vaccine on the platelet count. New Eng. J. Med. 275:352–356, 1966.

Packer, N. P., and Cummins, B. H.: Spontaneous epidural haemorrhage: A surgical emergency. Lancet 1:356–358, 1978.

Paine, R. S., and Byers, R. K.: Transverse myelopathy in childhood. Am. J. Dis. Child. 85:151–163, 1953.

Parker, J. J., and Anderson, W. B.: Myelitis simulating spinal cord tumor. Am. J. Roentgenol. 95:942–946, 1965.

Paul, J. R.: A History of Poliomyelitis. Yale University Press, New Haven, 1971.

Pellew, R. A. A.: Clinical description of disease resembling poliomyelitis. Med. J. Aust. 1:944, 1951.

Peterman, A. F., Daly, D. D., Dion, F. R., and Keith, H. M.: Infectious neuronitis (Guillain-Barré syndrome) in children. Neurology 9:533–539, 1959.

Peterman, M. G., and Fox, M. J.: Encephalitis as a complication of measles. A report of thirteen cases. Am. J. Dis. Child. 46:512–517, 1933.

Peters, A. C. B., Vielvoye, G. J., Versteeg, J., Bots, G. T. A. M., and Lindeman, J.: ECHO 25 focal encephalitis and subacute hemichorea. Neurology 29:676–681, 1979.

Peters, A. H., O'Grady, J. E., and Milanovich, R. A.: Aseptic meningitis associated with Echovirus type 3 in very young children. Am. J. Dis. Child. 123:452–456, 1972.

Philip, A. G. S., and Larson, E. J.: Overwhelming neonatal infection with ECHO 19 virus. J. Pediat. 82:391–397, 1973.

Phillips, C. A., and Melnick, J. L.: Community infection with St. Louis encephalitis virus. Serologic study of the 1964 epidemic in Houston. J.A.M.A. 193:207–211, 1965.

Phillips, C. A., Fanning, W. L., Gump, D. W., and Phillips, C. F.: Cytomegalovirus encephalitis in immunologically normal adults. Successful treatment with vidarabine. J.A.M.A. 238:2299–2300, 1977.

Plum, F.: Sensory loss with poliomyelitis. Neurology 6:166–172, 1956.

Pool, J. H., Walton, J. N., Brewis, E. G., Uldall, P. R., Wright, A. E., and Gardner, P. S.: Benign myalgic encephalomyelitis in Newcastle Upon Tyne. Lancet 1:733–737, 1961.

Portnoy, B., Hanes, B., Pierce, N. F., Leedom, J. M., Kunzman, E. E., and Wehrle, P. F.: Aseptic meningitis associated with ECHO virus type 9 infection. Calif. Med. 102:262–267, 1965.

Posson, D. D.: Exanthem subitum (roseola infantum) complicated by prolonged convulsions and hemiplegia. J. Pediat. 35:235–236, 1949.

Price, R., Chernik, N. L., Horta-Barbosa, L., and Posner, J. B.: Herpes simplex encephalitis in an anergic patient. Am. J. Med. 54:222–228, 1973.

Price, R. A., Garcia, J. H., and Rightsel, W. A.: Choriomeningitis and myocarditis in an adolescent with isolation of Coxsackie B-5 virus. Am. J. Clin. Path. 53:825–831, 1970.

Pruzanski, W., and Altman, R.: Encephalitis due to West Nile fever virus. World Neurol. 3:525–528, 1962.

Pullan, C. R., Noble, T. C., Scott, D. J., Wisniewski, K., and Gardner, P. S.: Atypical measles infections in leukemic children on immunosuppressive treatment. Brit. Med. J. 1:1562–1565, 1976.

Quick, D. T., Smith, A. G., Lewis, A. L., and Sather, C. E.: California virus infection. A case report. Am. J. Trop. Med. 14:456, 1965.

Ramachandran, S., Wickremesinghe, H. R., and Perera, M. V. F.: Acute disseminated encephalomyelitis in typhoid fever. Brit. Med. J. 1:494–495, 1975.

Randall, R., and Mills, J. W.: Fatal encephalitis in man due to Venezuelan virus of equine encephalomyelitis in Trinidad. Science 99:225, 1944.

Rankin, N. E., and Dance, J.: Case of acute hemorrhagic leucoencephalitis. Brit. Med. J. 2:808–809, 1956.

Rantakallio, P., Lapinleimu, K., and Mantyjarvi, R.: Coxsackie B5 outbreak in a newborn nursery with 17 cases of serous meningitis. Scand. J. Infect. Dis. 2:17–23, 1970.

Rantakallio, P., Saukkonen, A. L., Krause, U., and Lapinleimu, K.: Follow-up study of 17 cases of neonatal Coxsackie B5 meningitis and one with suspected myocarditis. Scand. J. Infect. Dis. 2:25–28, 1970.

Ranzenhofer, E. R., Dizon, F. C., Lipton, M. M., and Steigman, A. J.: Clinical paralytic poliomyelitis due to Coxsackie virus group A, type 7. New Eng. J. Med. 259:182, 1958.

Rasmussen, T., Olszewski, J., and Lloyd-Smith, D.: Focal seizures due to chronic localized encephalitis. Neurology 8:435–445, 1958.

Reik, L., Steere, A. C., Bartenhagen, N. H., Shope, R. E., and Malawista, S. E.: Neurologic abnormalities of Lyme disease. Medicine 58:281–294, 1979.

Richter, R., and Shimojyo, S.: Neurologic sequelae of Japanese B encephalitis. Neurology 11:553–559, 1961.

Rie, H. E, Hilty, M. D., and Cramblett, H. F.: Intelligence and coordination following California encephalitis. Am. J. Dis. Child. 125:824–827, 1973.

Riggs, S., Smith, D. L., and Phillips, C. A.: St. Louis encephalitis in adults during the 1964 Houston epidemic. J.A.M.A. 193:284–288, 1965.

Riker, J. B., Brandt, C. D., Chandrou, R., Arrobio, J. O., and Nakano, J. H.: Vaccine-associated poliomyelitis in a child with thymic abnormality. Pediatrics 48:923–929, 1971.

Ritter, B. S.: Mumps meningoencephalitis in children. J. Pediat. 52:424–433, 1958.

Rivers, T. M., and Schwentker, F. F.: Louping ill in man. J. Exp. Med. 59:669–685, 1934.

Rivers, T. M., and Scott, T F. M.: Meningitis in man caused by a filterable virus. Science 81:439–440, 1935.

Robbins, F. C.: Evidence for and against the immunologic nature of experimental "allergic" and post-infectious encephalomyelitis. In: Kies and Alvord: Allergic Encephalomyelitis. Charles C Thomas, Springfield, Illinois, 1959.

Robertson, E. G.: Murray Valley encephalitis: Pathological aspects. Med. J. Aust. 1:107–110, 1952.

Robino, G., Perlman, A., Togo, Y., and Reback, J.: Fatal neonatal infection due to Coxsackie B2 virus. Report of generalized infection and myocarditis in the newborn. J. Pediat. 61:911–918, 1962.

Roden, V. J., Cantor, H. E., O'Connor, D. M., Schmidt, R. R., and Cherry, J. D.: Acute hemiplegia of childhood associated with Coxsackie A9 viral infection. J. Pediat. 86:56–58, 1975.

Román, G., Phillips, C. A., and Poser, C. M.: Parainfluenza virus type 3. Isolation from CSF of a patient with Guillain-Barré syndrome. J.A.M.A. 240:1613–1615, 1978.

Ropper, A. H., and Poskanzer, D. C.: The prognosis of acute and subacute transverse myelopathy based on early signs and symptoms. Ann. Neurol. 4:51–59, 1978.

Roseman, E., and Aring, C. D.: Infectious polyneuritis. Medicine 20:463–494, 1941.

Rosenblum, J.: Roseola infantum (exanthema subitum) complicated by hemiplegia. Am. J. Dis. Child. 69:234–236, 1945.

Rowe, W. P., Heubner, R., Gilmore, L., Parrott, R., and Ward, T.: Isolation of a cytopathogenic agent from human adenoids undergoing spontaneous degeneration in tissue culture. Proc. Soc. Exp. Biol. Med. 84:570–573, 1953.

Rowe, W. P., Murphy, F. A., Bergold, G. H., Casals, J., Hutchin, J., Johnson, K. M., Lehmann-Grube, F., Mims, C. A., Traub, E., and Webb, P. A.: Arenaviruses: Proposed name for a newly defined virus group. J. Virol. 5:651–652, 1970.

Russell, D. S.: The nosological unity of acute hemorrhagic leukoencephalitis and acute disseminated encephalomyelitis. Brain 78:369–376, 1955.

Sabatino, D. A., and Cramblett, H. G.: Behavioral sequelae of California encephalitis virus infection in children. Dev. Med. Child Neurol. 10:331–337, 1968.

Sabin, A. B.: Epidemic encephalitis in military personnel. Isolation of Japanese B virus on Okinawa in 1945, serologic diagnosis, clinical manifestations, epidemiologic aspects and use of mouse brain vaccine. J.A.M.A. 133:281–293, 1947.

Sabin, A. B.: Pathogenesis of poliomyelitis: Reappraisal in the light of new data. Science 123:1151–1157, 1956.

Sabin, A. B., Krumiegel, E. R., and Wigand, R.: Echo 9 virus disease. Am. J. Dis. Child. 96:197–219, 1958.

Sabin, A. B., Schlesinger, R. W., Ginder, D. R., and Matumoto, M.: Japanese B encephalitis in American soldiers in Korea. Am. J. Hyg. 46:356–375, 1947.

Sahler, O. J. Z., and Wilfert, C. M.: Fever and petechiae with adenovirus type 7 infection. Pediatrics 53:233–235, 1974.

Sarubbi, F. A., Jr., Sparling, P. F., and Glezen, W. P.: Herpesvirus hominis encephalitis. Virus isolation from brain biopsy in seven patients and results of therapy. Arch. Neurol. 29:268–273, 1973.

Saslaw, S., Wooley, C. F., and Anderson, G. R.: Aseptic meningitis syndrome. Report of eleven cases with cerebrospinal fluid isolation of enteroviruses. Arch. Intern. Med. 105:69–75, 1960.

Schain, R. J., and Wilson, G.: Brainstem encephalitis with radiographic evidence of medullary enlargement. Neurology 21:537–539, 1971.

Scheid, W.: Mumps virus and the central nervous system. World Neurology 2:117–130, 1961.

Schlossberg, F. R., and Prizer, M.: Retinal changes with marked impairment of vision in measles. Am. J. Ophthal. 23:998–1000, 1940.

Schmidt, N. J.: Tissue culture in the laboratory diagnosis of viral infections. Am. J. Clin. Path. 57:820–828, 1972.

Schonberger, L. B., McGowan, J. E., Jr., and Gregg, M. B.: Vaccine-associated poliomyelitis in the United States, 1961–1972. Am. J. Epidemiol. 104:202–211, 1976.

Schwarz, G. A., Yang, D. C., and Noone, E. L.: Meningoencephalomyelitis with epidemic parotitis. Arch. Neurol. 11:453–462, 1964.

Sciple, G. W., Ray, G., LaMotte, L. C., Holden, P., Gardner, P., Crane, G., and Bublis, M. D.: Western encephalitis with recovery of virus from cerebrospinal fluid. Neurology 17:169–171, 1967.

Scott, T. F. M., and Bonanno, D. E.: Reactions to live-measles-virus vaccine in children previously inoculated with killed-virus vaccine. New Eng. J. Med. 277:248–250, 1967.

Sells, C. J., Carpenter, R. L., and Ray, C. G.: Sequelae of central-nervous-system enterovirus infections. New Eng. J. Med. 293:1–4, 1975.

Senseman, L. A.: Myelitis complicating measles. Arch. Neurol. Psychiat. 53:309–310, 1945.

Sergent, J. S., Lockshin, M. D., Klempner, M. S., and Lipsky, B. A.: Central nervous system disease in systemic lupus erythematosus. Therapy and prognosis. Am. J. Med. 58:644–654, 1975.

Shaffer, M. F., Rake, G., and Hodes, H. L.: Isolation of virus from a patient with fatal encephalitis complicating measles. Am. J. Dis. Child. 64:815–819, 1942.

Shapiro, G. G., Chapman, J. T., Pierson, W. E., and Bierman, C. W.: Poliomyelitis-like illness after acute asthma. J. Pediat. 94:767–768, 1979.

Shasby, D. M., Shope, T. C., Downs, H., Herrmann, K. L., and Polkowski, J.: Epidemic measles in a highly vaccinated population. New Eng. J. Med. 296:585–589, 1977.

Shelokov, A., and Weinstein, L.: Poliomyelitis in the early neonatal period: Report of a case of possible intrauterine infection. J. Pediat. 38:80–84, 1951.

Sherman, I. C., and Kimelblot, S. J.: Facial paralysis in poliomyelitis. Report of 3 patients with unusual delayed paralysis. Neurology 9:282–287, 1959.

Shillito, J., Jr.: Carotid arteritis: A cause of hemiplegia in childhood. J. Neurosurg. 21:540–551, 1964.

Shinefield, M. R., and Townsend, T. E.: Transplacental transmission of western equine encephalitis. J. Pediat. 43:21–25, 1953.

Shinner, J. J.: St. Louis virus encephalomyelitis. Arch. Path. 75:309–322, 1963.

Shtilbance, I. I.: Possibility of natural infection in men with tick-borne encephalitis without tick's bite. Neuropath. Psychiat. 52:33–38, 1952.

Siegel, M. M., Walter, T. K., and Ablin, A. R.: Measles pneumonia in childhood leukemia. Pediatrics 60:38–40, 1977.

Sigurdsson, B., Sigurjonsson, J., Sigurdsson, J., Thorbelsson, J., and Gudmundsson, K. R.: Disease epidemic in Iceland simulating poliomyelitis. Am. J. Hyg. 52:222–238, 1950.

Silver, H. K., Meiklejohn, G., and Kempe, C. H.: Colorado tick fever. Am. J. Dis. Child. 101:30–36, 1961.

Silverstein, A., Steinberg, G., and Nathanson, M.: Nervous system involvement in infectious mononucleosis. Arch. Neurol. 26:353–358, 1972.

Similä, S., Ylikorkala, O., and Wasz-Hocket, O.: Type 7 adenovirus pneumonia. J. Pediat. 79:605–611, 1971.

Similä, S., Jouppila, R., Salmi, A., and Pohjonen, R.: Encephalomeningitis in children associated with an adenovirus type 7 epidemic. Acta Paediat. Scand. 59:310–316, 1970.

Smith, E., Harris, I. L., and Rosenblatt, P.: Acute poliomyelitis. A clinical and statistical study of 263 cases. J. Pediat. 43:9–20, 1953.

Smith, R., Woodall, J. P., Whitney, E., Diebel, R., Gross, M. A., Smith, V., and Bast, T. F.: Powassan virus infection. A report of three human cases of encephalitis. Am. J. Dis. Child. 127:691–693, 1974.

Smorodintsev, A. A.: Tick-borne spring-summer encephalitis. Progr. Med. Virol. 1:210–247, 1958.

Smyth, D., Tripp, J. H., Brett, E. M., Marshall, W. C., Almeida, J., Dayan, A. D., Coleman, J. C., and Dayton, R.: Atypical measles encephalitis in leukaemic children in remission. Lancet 2:574, 1976.

Solomon, P., Weinstein, L., Chang, T., Artenstein, M. S., and Ambrose, C. T.: Epidemiologic, clinical and laboratory features of an epidemic of type 9 ECHO virus meningitis. J. Pediat. 55:609–619, 1959.

Southam, C. M.: Serological studies of encephalitis in Japan. II. Inapparent infections by Japanese B encephalitis virus. J. Infect. Dis. 99:163–169, 1956.

Southern, P. M., Jr., Smith, J. W., Luby, J. P., Barnett, J. A., and Sanford, J. P.: Clinical and laboratory features of epidemic St. Louis encephalitis. Ann. Intern. Med. 71:681–689, 1969.

Spruance, S. L., and Bailey, A.: Colorado tick fever. A review of 115 laboratory confirmed cases. Arch. Intern. Med. 131:288–293, 1973.

Spudis, E. V., and Cramblett, H. G.: ECHO 4 meningoencephalitis. Arch. Neurol. 12:404–409, 1965.

Steigman, A. J.: Poliomyelitic properties of certain non-polio viruses. Enteroviruses and Heine-Medin disease. J. Mount Sinai Hosp. 25:391–404, 1958.

Steigman, A. J., and Lipton, M. M.: Fatal bulbospinal paralytic poliomyelitis due to ECHO 11 virus. J.A.M.A. 174:178–179, 1960.

Steigman, A. J., Lipton, M. M., and Braspennickx, H.: Acute lymphonodular pharyngitis: A newly described condition due to Coxsackie A virus. J. Pediat. 61:331–336, 1962.

Sterner, G., and Biberfeld, G.: Central nervous system complications of Mycoplasma pneumoniae infection. Scand. J. Infect. Dis. 1:203–208, 1969.

Stevenson, J., and Hambling, M. H.: Paralysis in Echovirus-3 infection. Lancet 1:525–526, 1968.

Strom, T.: Acute blindness as post-measles complication. Acta Paediat. 42:60–65, 1953.

Swender, P. T., Shott, R. J., and Williams, M. L.: A community and intensive care nursery outbreak of Coxsackievirus B5 meningitis. Am. J. Dis. Child. 127:42–45, 1974.

Sudia, W. D., and Newhouse, V. F.: Epidemic Venezuelan equine encephalitis in North America: A summary of virus-vector-host relationships. Am. J. Epidemiol. 101:1–13, 1975.

Sudia, W. D., McLean, R. G., Newhouse, V. F., Johnston, J. G., Jr., Miller, D. L., Trevino, H., Bowen, G. S., and Sather, G.: Epidemic Venezuelan equine encephalitis in North America in 1971: Vertebrate field studies. Am. J. Epidemiol. 101:36–50, 1975.

Sudia, W. D., Newhouse, V. F., Beadle, L. D., Miller, D. L., Johnston, J. G., Jr., Young, R., Calisher, C. H., and Maness, K.: Epidemic Venezuelan equine encephalitis in North America in 1971: Vector studies. Am. J. Epidemiol. 101:17–35, 1975.

Sutton, R. N. P., Pullen, H. J. M., Blackledge, P., Brown, E. H., Sinclair, L., and Swift, P. N.: Adenovirus type 7; 1971–1974. Lancet 2:987–991, 1976.

Suzuki, M., and Phillips, C. A.: St. Louis encephalitis. A histopathologic study of the fatal cases from the Houston epidemic in 1964. Arch. Path. 81:47–54, 1966.

Syverton, J. T., McLean, D. M., daSilva, M. M., Doany, H. B., Cooney, M., Kleinman, H., and Bauer, H.: Outbreak of Coxsackie B5 virus. J.A.M.A. 164:2015–2019, 1957.

Taneja, P. N., Ghai, O. P., and Bhakoo, O. N.: Importance of measles to India. Am. J. Dis. Child. 102:226–229, 1962.

Taylor, F. B., Jr., and Toreson, W. E.: Primary mumps meningoencephalitis. Arch. Intern. Med. 112:216–221, 1963.

Taylor, M. J., Burrow, G. N., Strauch, B., and Horstmann, D. M.: Meningoencephalitis associated with pneumonitis due to Mycoplasma pneumoniae. J.A.M.A. 199:813–816, 1967.

Ten Broeck, C., and Merrill, M. H.: Serological difference between eastern and western equine encephalomyelitis virus. Proc. Soc. Exp. Biol. Med. 21:217–220, 1933.

ter Meulen, V., Koprowski, H., Iwasaki, Y., Käckell, Y. M., and Müller, D.: Fusion of cultured multiple-sclerosis brain cells with indicator cells: Presence of nucleocapsids and virions and isolation of parainfluenza-type virus. Lancet 2:1–5, 1972.

ter Meulen, V., Müller, D., Käckell, Y., Katz, M., and Meyermann, R.: Isolation of infectious measles virus in measles encephalitis. Lancet 2:1172–1175, 1972.

Terni, M., Caccialanza, P., Cassai, E., and Kieff, E.: Aseptic meningitis in association with herpes progenitalis. New Eng. J. Med. 285:503–504, 1971.

Thompson, W. H., Kalfayan, B., and Anslow, R. O.: Isolation of California encephalitis group virus from a fatal human illness. Am. J. Epidemiol. 81:245–253, 1965.

Thompson, W. H., Trainer, D. O., Allen, V., and Hale, J. B.: The exposure of wildlife workers in Wisconsin to ten zoonotic diseases. Trans. N. Amer. Wildlife Nat. Res. Conf. 28:215, 1963.

Timmons, G. D., and Johnson, K. P.: Aqueductal stenosis and hydrocephalus after mumps encephalitis. New Eng. J. Med. 283:1505–1507, 1970.

Tindall, G. T., and Gladstone, L. A.: Hydrocephalus as a sequel to lymphocytic choriomeningitis. Neurology 7:516–518, 1957.

Toomey, J. A., Dembo, L. H., and McConnell, G.: Acute hemorrhagic encephalitis. Report of a case following scarlet fever. Am. J. Dis. Child. 25:98–106, 1923.

Top, F. H.: Incidence of cranial nerve paralysis in poliomyelitis in relation to presence or absence of tonsils. I. In a metropolitan area. Pediatrics 21:94–105, 1958.

Top, F. H.: Incidence of cranial nerve paralysis in poliomyelitis in relation to presence or absence of tonsils. II. In a largely rural area. Pediatrics 21:106–111, 1958.

Tyler, H. R.: Neurological complications of rubeola (measles). Medicine 36:147–167, 1957.

Tyzzer, E. E., Sellards, A. W., and Bennett, B. L.: Occurrence in nature of "equine encephalomyelitis" in ring-necked pheasant. Science 88:505, 1938.

Urano, T., Kawase, T., Kodaira, K., Takeuchi, Y., Kikuchi, T., and Kimura, M.: Guillain-Barré syndrome associated with ECHO virus type 7 infections. Pediatrics 45:294–295, 1970.

Vanzee, B. E., Douglas, R. G., Jr., Betts, R. F., Bauman, A. W., Fraser, D. W., and Hinman, A. R.: Lymphocytic choriomeningitis in university hospital personnel. Clinical features. Am. J. Med. 58:803–809, 1975.

von Economo, C.: Encephalitis lethargica. Wien Klin. Wschr. 30:581–585, 1917.

Wallgren, A.: Une nouvelle maladie infectieuse du systeme nerveux central? (Meningite aseptique aigue.) Acta Paediat. 4:158–182, 1925.

Walters, J. H.: Postencephalitic Parkinson syndrome after meningoencephalitis due to Coxsackie virus Group B, Type 2. New Eng. J. Med. 263:744–747, 1960.

Walton, T. E., Alvarez, O., Jr., Buckwalter, R. M., and Johnson, K. M.: Experimental infection of horses with enzootic and epizootic strains of Venezuelan equine encephalomyelitis virus. J. Infect. Dis. 128:271–282, 1973.

Warkel, R. L., Rinaldi, C. F., Bancroft, W. H., Cardiff, R. D., Holmes, G. E., and Wilsnack, R. E.: Fatal acute meningoencephalitis due to lymphocytic choriomeningitis virus. Neurology 23:198–203, 1973.

Warthin, A. S.: Occurrence of numerous large giant cells in the tonsils and pharyngeal mucosa in the prodromal stage of measles. Report of four cases. Arch. Path. 11:864–874, 1931.

Watts, D. M., Pantuwatana, S., De Foliart, D., Yuill, T. M., and Thompson, W. H.: Transovarial transmission of La Crosse virus (California encephalitis group) in the mosquito, *Aedes triseriatus.* Science 182:1140–1141, 1973.

Weaver, O. M., Pieper, S., and Kurland, R.: Epidemiology of arthropod-borne encephalitis. V. Japanese B encephalitis. Sequelae. Neurology 8:887–889, 1958.

Webb, H. E., Connolly, J. H., Kane, F. F., O'Reilly, K. J., and Simpson, D. I. H.: Laboratory infections with louping-ill with associated encephalitis. Lancet 2:255–258, 1968.

Webster, A. D. B., Tripp, J. H., Hayward, A. R., Dayan, A. D., Doshi, R., MacIntyre, E. H., and Tyrrell, D.

A. J.: Echovirus encephalitis and myositis in primary immunoglobulin deficiency. Arch. Dis. Childh. 53:33–37, 1978.

Webster, H. F.: Eastern equine encephalomyelitis in Massachusetts. Report of two cases, diagnosed serologically, with complete clinical recovery. New Eng. J. Med. 255:267–270, 1956.

Weil, A., and Breslich, P. J.: Histopathology of the central nervous system in the North Dakota epidemic encephalitis. J. Neuropath. Exp. Neurol. 1:49–58, 1942.

Weiner, L. B., Corwin, R. M., Nieburg, P. I., and Feldman, H. A.: A measles outbreak among adolescents. J. Pediat. 90:17–20, 1977.

Weinstein, L., and Chang, T. W.: The chemotherapy of viral infections. New Eng. J. Med. 289:725–730, 1973.

Weinstein, L., Aycock, W. L., and Feemster, R. F.: Relation of sex, pregnancy and menstruation to susceptibility in poliomyelitis. New Eng. J. Med. 245:54–58, 1951.

Weinstein, L., Selokov, A., Seltser, R., and Winchell, G. D.: A comparison of the clinical features of poliomyelitis in adults and in children. New Eng. J. Med. 246:296–302, 1952.

Wells, C. E. C.: Neurological complications of so-called "influenza." A winter study in Southeast Wales. Brit. Med. J. 1:369–373, 1971.

Wenner, H. A., and Behbehani, A. M.: ECHO viruses. Monogr. Virol. 1:1–72, 1968.

Wheeler, S. D., and Ochoa, J.: Poliomyelitis-like syndrome associated with asthma. A case report and review of the literature. Arch. Neurol. 37:52–53, 1980.

White, D. N., and Burtch, R. B.: Iceland disease. A new infection simulating acute anterior poliomyelitis. Neurology 4:506–516, 1954.

Whitney, E., and Jamnback, H.: The first isolations of Powassan virus in New York State. Proc. Soc. Exp. Biol. Med. 119:432–439, 1965.

Wickman, I.: Beiträge zur Konntnis der Heine-Medinschen Krankheit (poliomyelitis acuta und verwandter erkrankungen). Karger, Berlin, 1907.

Wilfert, C. M.: Mumps meningoencephalitis with low cerebrospinal-fluid glucose, prolonged pleocytosis and elevation of protein. New Eng. J. Med. 280:855–859, 1969.

Wilfert, C. M., Lauer, B. A., Cohen, M., Costenbader, L., and Myers, E.: An epidemic of echovirus 18 meningitis. J. Infect. Dis. 131:75–78, 1975.

Wilfert, C. M., Buckley, R. H., Mohanakumar, T., Griffith, J. F., Katz, S. L., Whisnant, J. K., Eggleston, P. A., Moore, M., Treadwell, E., Oxman, M. N., and Rosen, F. S.: Persistent and fatal central-nervous-system echovirus infections in patients with agammaglobulinemia. New Eng. J. Med. 296:1485–1489, 1977.

Williams, H., MacArthur, P., Bell, E. J., and Lamb, R.: Paralysis in echovirus-3 infection. Lancet 1:425, 1968.

Williams, K. H., Hollinger, F. B., Metzger, W. R., Hopkins, C. C., and Chamberlain, R. W.: The epidemiology of St. Louis encephalitis in Corpus Christi, Texas, 1966. Am. J. Epidemiol. 102:16–24, 1975.

Winter, S. T.: Facial paralysis in poliomyelitis. A follow-up of 58 patients. Pediatrics 59:876–880, 1957.

Wolinsky, J. S., Swoveland, P., Johnson, K. P., and Baringer, J. R.: Subacute measles encephalitis complicating Hodgkin's disease in an adult. Ann. Neurol. 1:452–457, 1977.

Woods, C. A., and Ellison, G. W.: Encephalopathy following influenza immunization. J. Pediat. 65:745–748, 1964.

Wooley, C. F.: Intracranial hypertension associated with recovery of a Coxsackie virus from the cerebrospinal fluid. Neurology 10:572–574, 1960.

Work, T. H.: Russian spring-summer virus in India. Kyasanur forest disease. Progr. Med. Virol. 1:248–277, 1958.

Work, T. H.: Serological evidence of arbovirus infection in the Seminole Indians of Southern Florida. Science 145:270–272, 1964.

Work, T. H.: Tick-borne viruses. A review of an arthropod-borne virus problem of growing importance in the tropics. Bull. W.H.O. 29:59–74, 1973.

Wright, H. T., Jr., and Ward, R.: Detection of poliovirus type 1 in human cerebrospinal fluid. J. Pediat. 66:489–494, 1965.

Wright, P. F., Hatch, M. H., Kasselberg, A. G., Lowry, S. P., Wadlington, W. B., and Karzon, D. T.: Vaccine-associated poliomyelitis in a child with sex-linked agammaglobulinemia. J. Pediat. 91:408–412, 1977.

Wyatt, H. V.: Poliomyelitis in hypogammaglobulinemics. J. Infect. Dis. 128:802–806, 1973.

Yahr, M. D., and Lobo-Antunes, J.: Relapsing encephalomyelitis following the use of influenza vaccine. Arch. Neurol. 27:182–183, 1972.

Yalaz, K., and Tinaztepe, K.: Brain stem encephalitis. Acta Paediat. Scand. 63:235–240, 1974.

Yeager, A. S., Bruhn, F. W., and Clark, J.: Cerebrospinal fluid: Presence of virus unaccompanied by pleocytosis. J. Pediat. 85:578–580, 1974.

Young, L. W., Smith, D. I., and Glasgow, L. A.: Pneumonia of atypical measles. Am. J. Roentgenol. 110:439–448, 1970.

Zimmerman, H. M.: The pathology of Japanese B encephalitis. Am. J. Path. 22:965–991, 1946.

Chapter Fourteen

HERPES VIRUS INFECTIONS OF THE NERVOUS SYSTEM

The members of the herpes group of viruses which cause neurologic disease in man include Herpesvirus hominis (Herpes simplex), varicella-zoster virus, the cytomegaloviruses, and the Epstein-Barr virus (Table 14–1). The latter is the most recent addition to the group as a cause of human disease. The E-B herpesvirus is now accepted to be etiologically associated with infectious mononucleosis, which in rare instances is complicated by neurologic dysfunction. The virus can also give rise to acute encephalitis or the Guillain-Barré syndrome in the absence of clinical evidence of infectious mononucleosis (Grose et al.). Worthy of mention, also, is the Herpes simiae (Herpes B) virus which can accidentally infect man, leading to a severe and often fatal encephalomyelitis. Such cases have only rarely been described and result from exposure in the laboratory to monkeys or monkey tissues harboring the virus (Fierer et al., Bryan et al.).

Herpes simplex virus, varicella-zoster virus, and the cytomegaloviruses all share certain biologic and morphologic similarities,

but there are a number of notable differences in regard to their clinical implications and neuropathologic features. For example, each is capable of producing severe, disseminated disease in the newborn, and intranuclear inclusion bodies represent the pathologic hallmark of all. The neonatal diseases associated with cytomegalovirus and Herpes simplex, however, are quite different; the latter usually appears in the form of an acute illness and the virus is acquired during labor or delivery and often manifested by a vesicular rash in addition to visceral involvement. Neonatal cytomegalovirus infection is usually a transplacentally transmitted condition; the infant at birth either is asymptomatic or exhibits evidence of chronic viral infection of one or more organ systems. Neonatal varicella is an unusual infection which occurs when the mother acquires the disease immediately before or at the time of birth of the child. In most cases, it is a benign illness in the newborn infant manifested primarily by a cutaneous rash, although dissemination with pulmonary and other visceral involvement can occur. Acute encephalitis in the otherwise normal older child or adult is a relatively common expression of Herpes simplex virus but is unusual with the other two viruses. Acute encephalitis caused by the cytomegalovirus or varicella-zoster virus has come to be more frequently recognized with lymphoreticular malignancies or secondary to immunosuppressive drug therapy.

Table 14–1. Herpesviruses of Neurologic Importance

Herpesvirus hominis, types I, II
Varicella-Zoster virus
Cytomegaloviruses
Epstein-Barr virus
Herpes simiae (B virus)

HERPESVIRUS HOMINIS (SIMPLEX) INFECTIONS OF THE NERVOUS SYSTEM

Herpesvirus hominis has been characterized as having a diameter ranging from 1,800 to 2,500 angstroms and consists of a capsid composed of 162 subunits called capsomeres which surround the viral core containing deoxyribonucleic acid (Kaplan). Herpesvirus hominis (simplex) is now known to exist as two antigenic types, each with different biological characteristics. Differentiation of the two types is accomplished by laboratory techniques, which include the microneutralization method, the microindirect hemagglutination test, and the direct immunofluorescent method (Nahmias et al., Fuccillo et al.). Type 1 Herpesvirus hominis, the "oral" strain, causes most cases of herpetic gingivostomatitis (Fig. 14–1), recurrent herpetic labialis, and herpes encephalitis in the child or the adult. Type 2, the "genital" strain, is implicated as the cause of vulvovaginitis, cervicitis, and disseminated disease in the newborn. The type 2 virus has also been shown to be capable of producing benign aseptic meningitis in adults, usually associated with herpes genitalis (Jarratt and Hubler, Terni et al.), and rarely, an acute meningoencephalitis in adults (Morrison et al.). An unusual syndrome has been described in adults with ano-genital herpes infection characterized by acute urinary retention and sensory disturbances in the sacral dermatomes (Oates and Greenhouse). It is believed that this transient disorder is the result of a herpetic lumbosacral meningomyelitis.

The reason for the different forms of neurologic involvement induced by the two types of Herpesvirus hominis is not yet clear. Mode of transmission of the virus may be one important factor, and it has been proposed by Craig and Nahmias that type 2 strains spread to the central nervous system by the hematogenous route while type 1 strains usually reach the brain by direct neural spread. Although this postulate remains conjectural, support for the concept includes the infrequency with which the type 1 virus can be isolated from blood or cerebrospinal fluid compared to the higher rate of successful isolation of the type 2 virus (Craig and Nahmias, Stalder et al.). Transmission of type 1 virus into brain along the olfactory nerves or trigeminal nerve and subsequently via tentorial nerves is also suggested by the striking predisposition of encephalitic involvement of anatomically associated structures, such as the medial portion of the temporal lobe and the orbitofrontal region of the frontal lobe (Davis and Johnson). Animal experiments with inoculation of the cornea with type 1 Herpes simplex, likewise, have shown rapid transmission of the virus into the brain along sensory nerves, most likely within axon cylinders, followed by slower cell-to-cell extension within the central nervous system (Knotts et al.).

Herpes simplex infections in childhood cover a wide spectrum of clinical conditions which are divided into primary and recurrent infections. Primary infection occurs in the susceptible host without antibody and in many cases results in an inapparent illness. Symptomatic primary illnesses may be in the form of an acute gingivostomatitis, vulvovaginitis, or keratoconjunctivitis. Herpetic whitlow is a cutaneous infection caused by Herpes simplex which is unusual in children but has been reported as an occupational hazard of nurses, dentists, and others who have heavy exposure to the virus by virtue of prolonged hand contact within the oral cavity of patients (Stern et al.). More recently, herpetic lesions of the fingers or hands caused by type 2 virus have been recognized in adults with genital infection, presumably secondary to direct contact with the genital lesion (Glogau et al.). The lesion presents as a painful vesicle on the

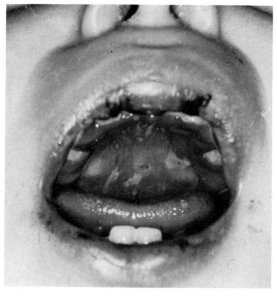

Figure 14–1. Herpes gingivostomatitis. Two-year-old child with fever and painful ulcerative lesions on the lips and buccal mucosa, caused by Herpes simplex, type I.

terminal segment of the finger or on the hand followed by the eruption of other vesicles, which soon coalesce producing a honeycombed appearance. Local pain is often intense, while fever or generalized symptoms are mild or absent. Spontaneous healing follows in 10 to 14 days. Eczema herpeticum refers to a severe cutaneous herpetic infection superimposed on atopic eczema. Herpes encephalitis in infants and young children is the result of primary infection in most, but in older children and adults may represent either a primary or a reactivation process.

The most common form of recurrent infection due to Herpes simplex is herpes labialis, the well-known "fever blister" or cold sore. Herpes simplex virus is the best known among viruses with a latent state punctuated by symptomatic recurrences (Docherty and Chopan). The site of persistence of the virus has been uncertain but observations accumulated over a number of years have indicated that it is most likely within trigeminal and other sensory ganglia. Cushing, in 1904, described the occurrence of herpetic cutaneous lesions following posterior rootlet section. The development of Herpes simplex facial lesions following trigeminal sensory root section thereafter was commonly recognized and was described in detail in publications by Carton and Kilbourne, and by Carton in 1952 and 1953. These authors demonstrated that 28 of 30 patients developed herpetic lesions in the distribution of the second and third divisions of the trigeminal nerve after posterior root section and that such lesions did not occur following peripheral interruption of the trigeminal nerve or after section of the intramedullary portion of its sensory root. These observations did not clarify the site of residence of the virus during the latent stage but did demonstrate the effect of manipulation of sensory neural structures on its reactivation.

The probability that the virus is harbored during the period of latency in sensory ganglia has been advanced by recent success in recovery of Herpes simplex virus from human trigeminal ganglia (Bastian et al., Baringer and Swoveland) and from other sensory ganglia (Baringer). This, now, seems reasonably certain although the factors that provoke reactivation of the virus with its movement down the axon to result in recurrent herpes infection at the skin or mucosal site subserved by the appropriate sensory ganglion remains unclear. Pazin and colleagues have made the interesting observation that even the minimal degree of manipulation or trauma to the trigeminal sensory root associated with microsurgical decompression of the root can be sufficient to result in reactivation of herpes infection. In their series of 56 patients undergoing this procedure for trigeminal neuralgia, 21 (38 percent) developed facial herpetic lesions within ten days following surgery. Davis and Johnson have postulated that localization of acute Herpes simplex encephalitis to the orbitofrontal and temporal lobe is perhaps determined by direct spread of virus from the trigeminal ganglion along the tentorial nerves to the anterior and middle fossa structures.

In addition to the above well-established conditions, the implications of the Herpes simplex virus have gradually been broadened. It is recognized to be a rare cause of erythema multiforme (MacDonald and Feiwel) and has been incriminated by some as a cause of incontinentia pigmenti (Palmgren). Type 2 herpesvirus antibodies have been found to be higher in a series of multiple sclerosis patients than in controls (Catalano); however, the significance remains unestablished. Herpes simplex has also been suggested to be the offender in some cases of Bell's palsy (McCormick) and other types of recurrent neuropathy (Constantine et al., Krohel et al.). Considerable attention has been focused on the possible oncogenic properties of the herpesvirus (Allen and Cole), and especially on Herpesvirus hominis type 2 as a cause of carcinoma of the cervix (Rawls et al., Catalano and Johnson). Herpesvirus has been isolated from the brain of an adult with a malignant glioma but the cause-and-effect relationship remains speculative (Benjamin et al.).

Herpes simplex virus has not been as widely recognized as a hazard to the patient with malignant disease or other conditions with immunosuppression as varicella-zoster or the cytomegaloviruses. Most infections with Herpes simplex in such patients are of the cutaneous or mucocutaneous type and are usually self-limited and of little consequence. In some cases with hematologic malignancies or following renal transplantation, mucocutaneous lesions become widespread or chronic, and may lead to ulcerative involvement of the trachea or esophagus (Logan et al., Montgomerie et al., Muller et al., Stone et al.). Disseminated Herpes simplex infection with multiple organ involvement, sometimes including the brain, has been described in a variety of conditions, including leukemia (Faden et al., Ruiz-Palacios et al.), thymic dysplasia (Sutton et al.), Wiskott-Aldrich syndrome (St. Geme et al.), and with eczema herpeticum (Monif et al.). Disseminated infection has also been seen in patients with widespread burns (Foley et al.), secondary to corticosteroid therapy in a patient with acute drug overdose (Abraham and Manko), and very rarely in an otherwise normal person without underlying disease or immunosuppression (Joseph and Vogt).

Involvement of the central nervous system with Herpes simplex virus without widespread dissemination elsewhere in the immunosuppressed patient has been infrequently reported and is believed to be a rare event. Cappel and Klastersky described a 23-year-old man with leukemia with acute aseptic meningitis caused by type 1 Herpes simplex. Fatal encephalitis from Herpes simplex virus has occurred in children with sex-linked hypogammaglobulinemia (Linnemann et al., 1973), and has also been observed in an adult following renal transplantation (Linnemann et al., 1976). In the latter instance, the illness was an acute one caused by type 2 virus, and provoked a severe cerebral vasculitis. The adult with Hodgkin's disease described by Price and colleagues departs strikingly from the usual cerebral response to this virus in that the encephalitic illness was subacute in type, being gradually progressive over seven weeks with minimal febrile response or meningeal signs. There were Cowdry type A inclusion bodies in oligodendroglia at autopsy, in addition to neuronal and glial degenerative changes. Findings typical of acute Herpes simplex encephalitis, such as localized hemorrhagic necrosis and perivascular inflammatory cell infiltrates, however, were not present. The absence of these pathologic features led the authors to postulate that in this immunosuppressed individual, the cerebral injury resulted primarily from the cytotoxic effect of the virus, giving rise to neuropathology different from that of the usual case of acute Herpes simplex encephalitis in the otherwise normal person, in whom cerebral changes result from both the direct cytotoxic effects of the virus and the host immune response to the foreign antigen.

Herpesvirus Hominis (Simplex) Encephalitis

Herpesvirus hominis (simplex) has been known to be the cause of an acute sporadic,

necrotizing and hemorrhagic encephalitis with intranuclear inclusion bodies since 1941 when Smith and colleagues first isolated the virus from the brain of an afflicted patient. It is an illness that has stimulated a great deal of interest in recent years because of the frequent diagnostic importance of certain radiologic procedures, distinctive neuropathologic features, and the increasing possibility of beneficial response to certain therapeutic modalities.

The precise incidence of acute Herpes simplex encephalitis is unknown but it is often claimed to be the most frequent severe or fatal nonseasonal encephalitis in this country (Johnson et al., 1968). The sporadic form of encephalitis is now recognized to be due in the majority of cases to the type 1 strain, which can occur in any age group ranging from infancy to the elderly. Earlier authors considered Herpes simplex encephalitis to be a primary infection in most cases. This is probably true when the disease occurs in infancy or in the early childhood years, but in older persons encephalitis may represent either a primary or a reactivation infection. Several reports are now available in which Herpes simplex encephalitis developed in persons with recurrent herpes labialis (Leider et al., Nolan et al.) and, in one instance, several months following herpes keratitis (Balfour and Lockman).

The vast majority of childhood or adult cases of acute necrotizing encephalitis due to this virus have been in previously normal persons without predisposing causes for severe infectious disease. As mentioned earlier, encephalitis has been observed on infrequent occasion as part of widespread dissemination in persons with underlying disorders associated with immunosuppression (Faden et al., Sutton et al.). Only a few reports exist of Herpes simplex encephalitis without widespread visceral involvement in the immunocompromised patient (Linnemann et al., 1976; Price et al.). That described by Price et al. was especially remarkable in that the disorder manifested itself in the form of subacute encephalitis with atypical clinical and pathologic findings.

Clinical Manifestations

Central nervous system infection with Herpesvirus hominis is usually in the form of an acute severe encephalitis which occurs in either sex of any age and at any time of the year. It is generally regarded to be more prevalent during the colder months, corresponding to the higher incidence of upper respiratory infections (McKee et al.). Benign aseptic meningitis (Terni et al., Leider et al., Olson et al.) can be caused by this virus but is infrequent, especially in childhood. The occasional observation of aseptic meningitis associated with genital Herpes simplex infection suggested to earlier workers that the benign meningeal infection is more commonly caused by herpesvirus type 2 than type 1. Craig and Nahmias and Stalder et al. have recently added support to this concept by isolation of type 2 Herpes simplex virus from cerebrospinal fluid in adults with aseptic meningitis. Such patients exhibit meningeal signs and headache in association with a febrile illness with a cerebrospinal fluid lymphocytic pleocytosis. The illness is usually less than a week in duration, and is followed by gradual recovery. Still another unusual type of neurologic infection due to Herpes simplex is an acute myelitis without evidence of significant cerebral involvement (Klastersky et al., Craig and Nahmias).

Similarly to other types of viral encephalitis, that due to Herpes simplex shows variable symptoms and signs from patient to patient. In infancy and early childhood, the clinical features usually include fever, vomiting, lethargy, and convulsions, which may be either focal or generalized or both (Bellanti et al., Brunell and Dodd, Kent and Nicholson, Wenzl and Rubio). There is little from the history or physical findings to suggest a herpetic cause in this age group, but on rare occasion vesicular skin lesions (Bellanti et al.) or gingivostomatitis (Brunell and Dodd) coexist, suggesting the probable viral offender.

In the older child, as in the adult, the manifestations are often more complex but may include combinations of symptoms and signs which prove to be etiologically suggestive. Approximately 30 percent of patients report preceding symptoms of an upper respiratory infection several days before onset of the encephalitic manifestations (Olson et al.). Fever, intense headache, vomiting, lethargy, and mental confusion are usual early complaints, which may persist for hours or even several days before progression of the illness occurs. Drachman and Adams emphasized the frequency with which psychological disturbances have been observed in the initial stages of the illness, before lethargy or coma supervene. Restlessness, irritability, hyperkinesis, disorientation, or hallucinations may coexist with headache and fever or even precede such features. Uncinate seizures are occasion-

ally described in the initial stages of the illness, representing the first sign which later will indicate severe temporal lobe disease. Progressive decline in awareness is frequently associated with neck rigidity and the subsequent occurrence of repetitive convulsions, often focal motor in type. The optic fundi are usually normal during the early stages of this illness although low-grade papilledema may ultimately develop in some. Unlike patients with the disseminated neonatal form of the disease, the older patient with acute Herpes simplex encephalitis only rarely exhibits coexisting inflammatory involvement of the ocular structures (Minckler et al.).

At variable periods of time after the onset of the illness, a significant feature of Herpesvirus hominis encephalitis in some patients is the emergence of signs of focal cerebral dysfunction. Localizing neurologic signs include focal seizures, hemiparesis, lateralizing deep reflex alterations, homonymous field defects, and dysphasia. Among 36 patients with herpes encephalitis described by Olson et al., 28 were noted to have localizing signs at some point during the illness. The localizing neurologic signs frequently reflect the predisposition for medial temporal lobe or orbital-frontal lobe involvement by this virus. In some patients, the signs indicative of unilateral fronto-temporal lobe disease are so outstanding that brain tumor or abscess is the primary diagnostic consideration (Bennett et al., Carmon et al., Pierce et al.). The possibility of a focal mass lesion is further supported in certain cases by the results of special studies such as electroencephalography, computed cranial tomography, and angiography. Craniotomy and biopsy is required in cases of this sort in order to exclude a surgically treatable lesion and to establish the diagnosis of Herpes simplex encephalitis.

As the illness progresses and lethargy proceeds to a state of coma, evidence of increased intracranial pressure is superimposed upon the already-present signs of diffuse and focal cerebral involvement. Various brain stem signs may be observed at different stages of the illness, including nystagmus, anisocoria, extraocular muscle palsies, and facial paresis. In unusual cases, the major site of the inflammatory process is confined to the brain stem, with relatively few coexisting signs of supratentorial involvement (Dayan et al., Ellison and Hanson). The presence of deep coma, marked hyperpyrexia, significant papilledema, or frequently recurring convulsions all indicate an unfavorable outcome and are usually followed by death.

As the illness progresses, transtentorial herniation leads to oculomotor paralysis with dilated pupils. Episodes of decerebration may result either from midbrain compression secondary to herniation or from inflammatory necrotizing changes within the brain stem. Cardiorespiratory arrest is the end result of either of the latter two components of the illness.

The mortality rate in Herpesvirus hominis encephalitis is unquestionably high but is perhaps somewhat overestimated from the available statistics. Because absolute diagnosis is dependent upon autopsy or cerebral biopsy and since performance of biopsy is biased toward more severely affected cases, collected data may not include cases that are more mildly affected. Thus, the 60 to 70 percent mortality rate often stated for this disease may be misleadingly high (Meyer et al., Olson et al.). Furthermore, the relationship of antiviral drug therapy in regard to its influence on morbidity and mortality remains to be clarified. Among survivors, neurologic sequelae are common and frequently are of an incapacitating magnitude. The severity of acute Herpes simplex encephalitis is reflected from the series of 15 brain-biopsy-proven cases reported by Williams and Lerner. Among the 15, eight died, and of the seven survivors, only one recovered without major neurologic disability. It is possible for a remarkable degree of functional recovery to follow severe herpesvirus encephalitis (Johnson et al., 1972; Rennick et al.), although it appears to be an infrequent occurrence.

Laboratory Findings

The basic laboratory examinations including hemoglobin, white blood cell count and urinalysis are helpful mainly in a negative way and are subject to variations from patient to patient. The white blood cell count may be normal or significantly elevated ·and the differential count may be unremarkable or shifted to the left. Serum electrolytes are usually normal unless altered by recurrent vomiting, although hyponatremia has been described with herpes encephalitis, and is believed due to inappropriate antidiuretic hormone secretion (Rovit et al.).

Cerebrospinal fluid examination is an important diagnostic aid in this disease but does not always reveal the expected abnormalities. The opening pressure may be normal or elevated or may be normal on the first tap but markedly increased on a subsequent examination. The fluid is usually clear and contains a variable number of cells, the type of which depends to some degree on when in the illness the examination is performed. During the first day or so after onset of symptoms, polymorphonuclear neutrophils are often more abundant than lymphocytes, but thereafter mononuclear cells become more prevalent. The number of cells in the usual case varies from 50 up to several hundred per cu. mm. Many red blood cells or even xanthochromia of the spinal fluid specimen is sometimes observed with Herpes simplex encephalitis, a finding emphasized to be of diagnostic importance by Miller et al. This finding in the cerebrospinal fluid is not surprising in view of the frequency with which cerebral hemorrhagic necrosis is observed at autopsy. In exceptional cases, the cerebrospinal fluid cell count is surprisingly and misleadingly normal (Marshall, Kent and Nicholson, Olson et al., Nolan et al., Drachman and Adams), a finding which often is an indication to consider repeating the study at a subsequent time. The cerebrospinal fluid glucose is normal to elevated in most cases, although significantly reduced glucose levels have been observed in some instances (Morrison et al., Sarubbi et al., Johnson et al., 1972). The protein content is usually elevated to levels between 60 and 200 mg. per 100 ml. In addition to the appropriate studies to exclude bacterial and fungal disease, a spinal fluid specimen should be obtained to attempt to isolate the offending virus. This is not usually successful, as spinal fluid is a poor source for viral isolation in patients with acute Herpes simplex encephalitis.

The electroencephalogram is a helpful diagnostic aid in patients with Herpes simplex encephalitis in that it generally adds evidence of diffuse cerebral dysfunction but often also reflects the predilection of the herpes virus for focal frontal or temporal lobe involvement. Among 13 patients studied by Nolan et al., six had focal slow abnormalities in one frontal or temporal lobe. Such focal electrical disturbances with Herpes simplex encephalitis usually consist of periodic delta bursts, at times with intermixed sharp activity arising from the same region (Illis and Taylor). Periodic, lateralized slow and spike discharges do not occur in all patients with acute Herpes simplex encephalitis and in some cases are not observed in the initial symptomatic stages but emerge with progression of the illness (Ch'ien et al., Smith et al., 1975). Their presence is strong supportive evidence of the herpetic etiology in the patient with acute encephalitis, and also facilitates decisions for the optimal site for cerebral biopsy, when indicated. The occurrence of repetitive lateralizing complexes on the electroencephalogram indicates a severe cerebral insult and has been said to represent a poor prognostic sign (Elian). The generalized electroencephalographic abnormalities along with the quality of the focal disturbances usually allow differentiation of this type of acute encephalitis from a brain abscess.

Abnormalities on radioactive brain scan consisting of focal uptake of the isotope have been observed more often with Herpes simplex encephalitis than with other types of viral encephalitis (Balfour et al., Mishkin) (Fig. 14–2). This may be diagnostically helpful when encephalitis is recognized as the probable explanation for the child's illness but can be misleading if a focal mass lesion is the primary consideration. How often scans are abnormal in this disease is unclear from the literature, but among six examinations in the series of Nolan et al., three were normal, two were diffusely abnormal and one showed focal uptake of the isotope. One may assume that those cases associated with focal necrotizing temporal lobe changes are more likely to be associated with focal scan abnormalities. Although the radioactive brain scan may reveal informative data in such patients, it is important not to delay other aspects of diagnostic and therapeutic management if the scan cannot be performed rapidly.

Computed cranial tomography has been shown to be one of the best methods to demonstrate focal edema in the temporal or fronto-temporal region in patients with acute Herpes simplex encephalitis (Fig. 14–3). Swelling is apparent in the form of an area of variable size of decreased density compared to other areas of brain tissue, and is sometimes observed even when there are no clinical signs indicative of localized cerebral involvement. In cases with focal hemorrhagic necrosis, the unenhanced computed tomogram demonstrates areas of increased density intermixed within the broader zone of low density (Enzmann et al.). When no abnormalities are found on the initial scan in the early stages of the illness, the development of focal swelling may be seen on subsequent scans three to six days later. In some cases, contrast enhancement demonstrates a gyral configuration in the abnormal area of low density on the non-enhanced scan (Davis et al.). The procedure also provides evidence of the degree of ventricular shift, if present, and is useful to exclude the possibility of cerebral abscess, which can be a diagnostic consideration in the patient with Herpes simplex encephalitis.

Carotid angiography was frequently utilized in the past in patients suspected to have Herpes simplex encephalitis, primarily to exclude a focal mass lesion but also to illustrate

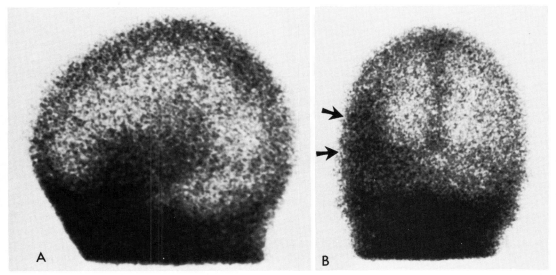

Figure 14–2. Abnormal radionuclide brain scan in acute Herpes simplex encephalitis. Seventeen-year-old girl in the fourth day of the illness. *A,* Lateral view demonstrates dense isotope uptake in the left temporal region extending into the parietal area. *B,* PA view shows the uptake of the isotope in the left temporal lobe (arrows).

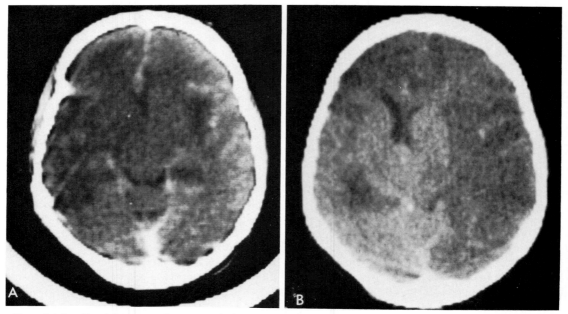

Figure 14–3.   Cranial computed tomography in acute Herpes simplex encephalitis illustrating change over 6 days' duration. *A,* Computed tomogram with contrast infusion done approximately 5 days after onset of illness. There are faint areas of decreased density in both temporal areas in addition to diffuse enhancement in the right parieto-temporal cortical areas. *B,* Computed tomogram with contrast infusion 6 days after the first scan. There are now patchy areas of decreased density in the left temporal region but much more extensive involvement over a wide area of the right cerebral hemisphere resulting in a very marked shift of the lateral ventricles to the left.

unilateral frontal or temporal lobe swelling (Radcliffe et al.). With the advent of computed tomography, angiographic study has become less popular as a diagnostic aid with this disease, but can still provide valuable information in select instances when clinical findings are somewhat atypical.

Pathology

Herpesvirus hominis encephalitis is associated with distinctive neuropathologic changes although isolation of the virus or demonstration of Herpes simplex antigen within brain by immunofluorescence is required for absolute diagnosis. The brain is usually swollen and congested, sometimes asymmetrically so. Swelling and hemorrhagic necrosis is commonly observed in one or both temporal regions, at times resulting in considerable shift of the ventricular system and transtentorial herniation (Fig. 14–4). In common with other forms of acute viral encephalitis are lymphocytic infiltration of the meninges, perivascular collections of lymphocytes and histiocytes in the cortex and adjacent white matter, and microglial proliferation. The inflammatory

exudate in Herpes simplex encephalitis frequently contains more polymorphonuclear leukocytes and the degree of cerebral vasculitis is greater than occurs with encephalitis caused by other herpesviruses, such as the cytomegaloviruses and varicella-zoster virus. Neuronal degenerative changes accompany the inflammatory process, but the most notable microscopic feature of the disease is the presence of eosinophilic intranuclear inclusion bodies of various sizes and shapes within oligodendroglia and, more rarely, within neurons or other glial cells (Itabashi et al.) (Fig. 14–5). Intranuclear inclusions are not diagnostic of Herpesvirus hominis encephalitis, since they occur in other conditions, including varicella-zoster encephalitis, cytomegalovirus disease, and some cases of acute measles encephalitis. In addition, inclusions are not always found in patients with Herpes simplex encephalitis. They may be absent or sparse in those with a rapid course who expire within two or three days after onset of symptoms. Although Cowdry type A inclusions have been considered to represent fixation artifacts by some observers (Swanson et al.), they are now generally believed to be alterations in the nucleoplasm specifically related to viral replication (Baringer and Griffith, Chou and Cherry).

An unusual form of pathology has been described by Koenig et al. in a young adult with acute Herpes simplex encephalitis who showed an initial favorable response to adenine arabinoside therapy. Soon after near total recovery, the patient exhibited relapse of encephalopathic signs and, on brain biopsy, was then found to have changes compatible with immune-mediated perivenous demyelinating encephalitis. The significance of this finding is uncertain but perhaps suggests that residual deficits seen in survivors of acute Herpes simplex encephalitis are secondary to the host immune response in addition to the cerebral cytotoxic effect of the virus.

Diagnosis

Diagnosis of Herpesvirus hominis encephalitis is dependent upon recognition of the possibility from the clinical findings and neurologic studies, the exclusion of bacterial and fungal disease by the appropriate laboratory procedures, and confirmation of the herpetic etiology by a combination of serologic, morphologic, and virologic techniques (Table 14–2). The disease is a consideration in any

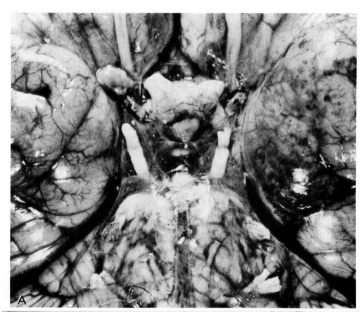

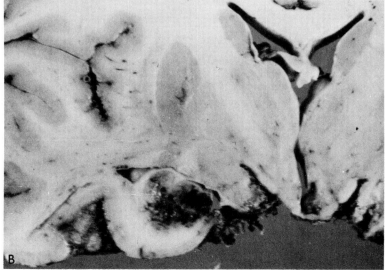

Figure 14–4. Acute Herpes simplex encephalitis. *A,* Severe swelling, softening, and hemorrhagic necrosis of the medial aspect of the left temporal lobe. *B,* Coronal section of the brain, demonstrating temporal lobe hemorrhage and necrosis.

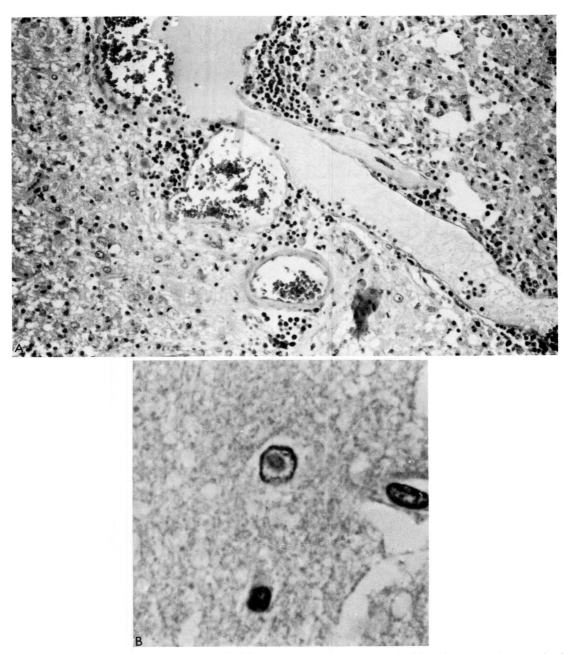

Figure 14–5. Acute Herpes simplex encephalitis. *A,* Severe necrotizing encephalitis with perivascular round cell infiltration (H&E, 100×). *B,* Typical Cowdry type A intranuclear inclusion within a glial cell.

Illustration continued on opposite page.

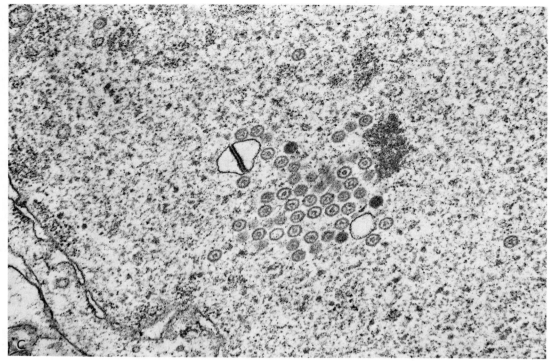

Figure 14–5. Continued. C, Electron microscopy showing Herpesvirus hominis virions within the nucleus of an oligodendroglial cell.

child with acute encephalitis, the cause of which is not readily apparent, but becomes a primary concern when the illness is severe, appears to be steadily progressive, and becomes associated with focal neurologic signs pointing to temporal lobe involvement. Severe encephalitis in the winter months is also

Table 14–2. Diagnostic Methods—Herpes Simplex Encephalitis

Clinical features
Neurologic studies
  Cerebrospinal fluid examination
  Electroencephalogram
  Radioactive brain scan
  Computed cranial tomography
Serologic methods
  Complement-fixation, neutralization antibody titer rise
  Serum to CSF antibody ratio
Morphologic techniques (brain biopsy or autopsy)
  Necrotizing, hemorrhagic encephalitis
  Cowdry type A inclusion bodies
  Typical Herpesvirus virions on electron microscopy
Virologic methods
  Viral isolation (cytopathogenic effect in tissue culture)
  Immunofluorescence (specific antigen in brain tissue, CSF cells)

suggestive of the possibility of Herpesvirus hominis encephalitis because of the absence of arthropod-borne encephalitic disorders at this time. Erythocytes plus mononuclear cells in the spinal fluid is an additional diagnostic hint but is not consistently present. Localizing as well as diffuse abnormalities on the electroencephalogram, a focal uptake of isotope on the radioactive brain scan, or a localized area of decreased density in the frontal or temporal region on computed tomography, and evidence of temporal lobe swelling on angiography in the encephalitic patient are all supportive evidence of Herpes simplex as the offender but, like other diagnostic features, are not always present in patients with this disease.

Laboratory diagnosis includes serologic and morphologic examinations but absolute confirmation requires isolation and identification of the virus from brain tissue since recovery of the virus from cerebrospinal fluid is unusual in previously normal persons with acute encephalitis. During life, this can be accomplished only by brain biopsy, a procedure with certain technical complexities and hazards, especially when increased intracranial pressure is marked. The primary reason for establishing a herpetic etiology of encephalitis in life is the consideration of antiviral treatment, which should be initiated early in the course of the illness if such therapy is to be used. For this reason, the decision to proceed with cerebral biopsy requires considerable judgment and experience so that the proper candidates are selected for brain biopsy and the initiation of drug treatment.

When cerebral biopsy is judged to be indicated, it is important to select the most appropriate side and site from which tissue is to be obtained. One hopes to biopsy an area involved in the acute inflammatory process, but not one which is frankly necrotic. Deciding on the optimal site for biopsy is aided somewhat by clinical findings, but in most cases, is determined more by the localization of abnormalities on electroencephalography and computed tomography. Biopsy of less affected areas of brain is less likely to yield diagnostically positive information. Tissue obtained by biopsy should include specimens for light and electron microscopy, immunofluorescent study, and viral, bacterial, and fungal cultures. If continuous intracranial pressure monitoring is to be done to assist management of intracranial hypertension, placement of the monitoring device can be accomplished at the time the biopsy is performed.

Serologic Techniques. A four-fold or greater rise in complement-fixing or neutralizing antibodies to Herpes simplex in acute and convalescent specimens of serum is supportive evidence but cannot be used as proof of the diagnosis of Herpes simplex encephalitis. Serologic methods are the basis for diagnosis of central nervous system infections caused by arthropod-borne viruses and certain other viruses; however, these are associated with consistent serologic responses and are not viruses with a latency state in man with periodic recurrences. A significant increase in antibody titer can occur with activation of latent Herpes simplex virus with or without mucocutaneous lesions. Activation of latent herpes infection may be provoked by a variety of systemic or febrile illnesses which are unrelated to the herpesvirus but which lead to antibody titer rises to this virus. Thus, for example, the child with meningococcal disease may exhibit a significant rise in antibody titer to Herpes simplex even though the virus has no causative relationship to his neurologic signs. Furthermore, the traditional concept that primary and reactivation herpetic infections can be differentiated by the

presence or absence of antibodies at the onset of the illness and the rate of titer rise likewise is in error (Johnson et al., 1968).

The other limiting aspect of the serologic method of diagnosis for Herpes simplex encephalitis is the time required for the titer rise to occur between the paired sera specimens. The decision to use specific antiviral treatment must be made rapidly and preferably early in the course of the illness. In addition, many patients will have expired before the convalescent specimen is drawn. The measurement of Herpes simplex antibodies in cerebrospinal fluid may become an important diagnostic tool with this disease although the test is associated with certain problems (Lerner et al., MacCallum et al.). Unless the initial titer proves to be significantly elevated, a rising titer may be necessary for diagnostic purposes since Herpes simplex antibodies have been found in cerebrospinal fluid of normal persons, especially in those subject to recurrent oral herpetic infection (Russell and Saertre). Studies by Levine et al. have shown that CSF antibody titers can be of greater value by determining the serum-to-CSF ratio; however, the usefulness of the procedure for rapid diagnosis may still be limited by the time required for significant titer rise to develop.

Morphologic Techniques. The presence of Cowdry type A intranuclear inclusion bodies in the older infant or child with encephalitis provides strong evidence for a Herpes simplex etiologic origin but does not entirely establish the diagnosis. Inclusion bodies are not always seen in brain tissue with this disease and are present in certain other conditions. However, the main drawback of this method on brain biopsy material when rapid diagnosis is required is that several days are needed to properly prepare and examine the tissue. For this reason and because of the lack of total specificity, light microscopic examination of brain biopsy material for inclusion bodies is not usually relied upon for decisions of whether or not to treat. A pathologic method which is useful for rapid diagnosis is electron microscopic examination of biopsy material. This procedure can provide a presumptive diagnosis within 24 to 36 hours after tissue is obtained by the demonstration of herpesvirus particles within cells. Although the various herpesviruses share similar morphologic features on electron microscopy, one can be confident the offender is Herpes simplex when acute encephalitis occurs in the previously normal person and is associated with necrotizing, hemorrhagic changes with cerebral vasculitis seen on light microscopic examination.

Virologic Methods. Absolute confirmation of Herpesvirus hominis encephalitis is accomplished by isolation of the virus from the brain in tissue culture or by the demonstration of specific viral antigen within brain tissue by immunofluorescence (Liu and Llanes-Rodas). The typical cytopathogenic effect produced by this virus in tissue culture usually appears within a period of two to four days. Immunofluorescence performed on frozen material can establish the diagnosis within three hours after receipt of tissue in the laboratory but is highly technical and is available only in a limited number of centers. A somewhat less complex means to demonstrate Herpes simplex antigen in brain tissue is the indirect immunoperoxidase method, as described by Benjamin and Ray. It also provides results rapidly, utilizes cell suspensions rather than frozen sections, and requires reagents that can be prepared relatively easily. Immunofluorescent examination of cerebrospinal fluid cells for herpes antigen has recently been developed, with some success to date, and shows promise as an important diagnostic method in the future (Dayan and Stokes, Sommerville, Taber et al.).

Treatment

General principles of management of the child with Herpes simplex encephalitis are similar to those with other types of encephalitis although the performance of brain biopsy and the administration of antiviral therapy provide a number of special considerations in regard to treatment of this infection. Maintenance of fluid and electrolyte balance, methods of prevention or correction of marked hyperthermia, and control of seizures require constant attention by the physician in charge. Disturbances of fluid and electrolyte metabolism can result from the disease itself but are especially troublesome when adenine arabinoside is used therapeutically because the fluid volume required to administer the drug can lead to fluid overload and marked serum hyponatremia.

Increased intracranial pressure secondary to brain swelling creates a serious threat to life in some patients and warrants use of one of several methods of treatment when it develops (Bell and McCormick). One of the main problems in its management is awareness of its presence and its degree, factors that can be alleviated in seriously ill patients by the use of one of the methods of continuous intracranial pressure monitoring. With a minute-to-minute estimate of the level of intracranial pressure, one can combat pressure elevations by controlling ventilation to lower the arterial pCO_2, the use of intravenous mannitol periodically as indicated, and systemic fluid restriction to the degree possible. When high-grade intracranial hypertension does not respond to these measures, the next step would include high-dose barbiturate therapy in conjunction with the above modalities.

Because of the complexities of these therapeutic endeavors, the severely affected child is best managed in an intensive care unit with facilities for such care. Measurements of central venous pressure or pulmonary wedge pressure add important information helpful in the regulation of intravenous fluid administration.

Corticosteroids have been recommended by a number of authors as a means of controlling intracranial hypertension in Herpes simplex encephalitis. In some reports, beneficial effects have been attributed to corticosteroid therapy (Habel and Brown, Upton et al.), while other authors advise caution in their use with infections caused by this virus (Baringer, 1974). The immunosuppressive effects of corticosteroids, including the depression of interferon production, could possibly enhance replication of the virus and its dissemination within brain tissue. In addition, the occurrence of disseminated herpes infection in a young adult has been partially attributed to corticosteroid therapy in a recently published case (Abraham and Manko). Although the literature does not clearly reflect adverse effects from corticosteroid treatment in Herpes simplex encephalitis, its use should be avoided on theoretical grounds and other measures should be selected to control cerebral swelling with this disease.

Antiviral Drug Therapy. A number of experimental drugs have been used for treatment of Herpes simplex encephalitis in the past two decades. The antiviral effects of these investigational drugs in the clinical setting have been variably interpreted by different workers, but the limiting factor with certain of the preparations has been their associated toxic properties. Synthetic agents to stimulate interferon production in vivo were investigated but continued interest waned because of their side effects and when it was demonstrated that herpesvirus infection results in increased interferon levels (Bellanti et al.). Further investigations with interferon have included the intrathecal administration in newborn infants with generalized Herpes simplex infection (De Clercq et al.) and experimental study of antiherpes effects of interferon combined with adenine arabinoside (Bryson and Kronenberg). The antiviral drugs that have received most attention for treatment of this infection have included idoxuridine (5-iodo-2-deoxyuridine), cytosine arabinoside (1-B-D-arabinofuranosylcytosine, Ara-C), and adenine arabinoside (9-B-D-arabinofuranosyladenine, Ara-A, Vidarabine). The latter is currently the sole survivor as far as continuation with clinical trials and shows promise as an important treatment modality.

Idoxuridine, a halogenated pyrimidine which resembles thymidine, was shown to inhibit growth of Herpes simplex virus in vitro and was suggested for clinical use as an antiherpes drug by Calabresi in 1963. Clinical trials with the preparation were begun by Breeden et al. in 1966, and thereafter there were a number of favorable reports of its effect in patients with Herpes simplex encephalitis (Evans et al., Marshall, Meyer et al., Nolan et al.). Less optimistic publications were to appear (Fishman et al., Haynes et al.), and soon the severity of the drug's adverse effects, including stomatitis, leukopenia, and thrombocytopenia, became evident. Experimental studies with animals demonstrated the lack of effectiveness of idoxuridine in decreasing virus content in brain tissue and also revealed the possibility of severe developmental lesions of the cerebellum, retina, and kidney when used in the newborn period (Percy, Hatch). A double-blind study published in 1975 resulted in the termination of clinical trials with idoxuridine because of its lack of effectiveness as well as the unacceptable degree of myelosuppression (Boston Interhospital Virus Study Group).

Cytosine arabinoside was synthesized in 1959, and after achieving importance in cancer chemotherapy it was shown to possess antiviral activity in vitro owing to its DNA-inhibiting qualities (Buthala). The drug showed promise as one useful in the treatment of Herpes simplex encephalitis because of its water solubility, its lesser degree of toxicity than idoxuridine, and initial favorable reports following its clinical use (Farris and Blaw, Juel-Jensen, Hryniuk et al.). Myelotox-

icity was subsequently shown to be a problem in some instances, and results of experimental studies did not support beneficial effects of the drug (Griffiths et al.). The immunosuppressive properties of the preparation raised concern regarding its possible effect on the host response to infection (Mitchell et al.), while other studies revealed damage to the external granular cell layer of the cerebellum when newborn mice were treated with cytosine arabinoside (Shimada et al.). As a result of the many potential problems as well as the lack of proof of effectiveness, Ara-C has largely been abandoned as a drug for treatment of Herpes simplex encephalitis (Alford and Whitley).

Adenine arabinoside (Ara-A) is the latest purine nucleoside to receive attention for treatment of Herpes simplex encephalitis and shows considerable promise thus far in both experimental and clinical studies. It disturbs normal cellular metabolism less than other purine and pyrimidine derivatives (Steele et al., 1975), is metabolized relatively slowly to arabinosyl hypoxanthine, which itself has antiviral properties, and penetrates the blood-brain barrier (Whitley et al., 1975). In doses of 10 to 20 mg. per kilogram per day intravenously, toxic effects have been mild and not usually of serious consequence but can include leukopenia, thrombocytopenia, hypokalemia, vomiting, and tremulousness (Ross et al., Whitley et al., 1977). Inappropriate release of antidiuretic hormone resulting in hyponatremia has also been attributed to adenine arabinoside (Ramos et al.). One problem with the drug in its present form is the large fluid volume required for its administration because of its relative insolubility. This complicates management of the commonly present intracranial hypertension and requires careful monitoring of the intracranial pressure as well as the central venous pressure. The initial reports of Ara-A treatment of acute Herpes simplex encephalitis have been favorable in cases when the drug has been administered early in the illness (Taber et al.), although future refinements of the drug and its utilization are to be anticipated. In the first reasonably large series to be published comparing patients with Herpes simplex encephalitis treated with Ara-A against untreated controls, the mortality rate among 18 treated cases was 28 percent while mortality in patients not receiving the drug was 70 percent (Whitley et al., 1977).

A major practical problem with the use of

the drug is the high desirability of confirmation of the diagnosis before initiation of therapy and the need for brain biopsy to establish the diagnosis. This requires an invasive procedure in the early stages of the illness when the patient is still reasonably alert, an approach reluctantly agreed to by many clinicians when the subsequent course of the illness cannot be predicted. To perform a brain biopsy which proves negative for Herpes simplex is undesirable, while withholding potentially effective therapy until coma supervenes in the patient subsequently proved to have Herpes simplex encephalitis is equally dissatisfying. This dilemma will not be satisfactorily resolved until a less invasive but reliable method of confirming the diagnosis of acute Herpes simplex encephalitis is achieved.

Neonatal Disseminated Herpesvirus Hominis Infection

Herpesvirus hominis infection in the newborn infant differs from that in the older child or adult in many important aspects. It is caused by a different antigenic strain in most cases. It is much more likely to be a disseminated illness with multiple organ system involvement, and, in those with encephalitis, vesicular lesions are present on the skin in more than 50 percent, which provide an excellent available source for isolation of the virus. Like other types of infection in the newborn, there is a predilection for Herpesvirus hominis to affect the premature infant. The remarkable tendency for this virus to produce widespread, disseminated disease in the neonate is a curious phenomenon not entirely explained by immunologic differences compared to his older counterpart. Disseminated disease appearing after the first few weeks of life is decidedly infrequent and, when it does occur, is usually associated with some underlying process, such as severe burns (Foley et al.), herpetic infection complicating eczema (Monif et al.), severe malnutrition (Becker et al.), following renal transplantation (Montgomerie et al.) and other immune disorders (Sutton et al.), or with debilitating conditions for which corticosteroids are administered (Abraham and Manko).

The virus is usually acquired by the infant from the mother's infected birth canal either soon before delivery or during the birth process. The mother is often entirely asymptomatic and the herpetic lesions are identified on the cervix or vaginal wall only by careful examination. The maternal lesions are initially vesicular but usually rupture soon after formation, resulting in shallow erosions, which may be painful. Less often, maternal genital herpes is associated with fever, local discomfort, vaginal discharge and obvious ulcerative lesions in the perineal region (White). Lesions may last only a few days or can persist for several weeks in association with a variety of symptoms. Over 95 percent of genital herpes infections and more than 80 percent of neonatal Herpesvirus hominis infections are caused by the type 2 strain (Nahmias et al.), a virus presumably acquired by adults mainly by venereal transmission.

Since the first report of disseminated infection in the newborn by Hass in 1935, many subsequent studies and publications have enlarged our understanding of the disease. It is now recognized that the disseminated form is not invariably fatal (Torphy et al.) and that the degree and extent of involvement represents a spectrum with considerable variation (Fig. 14–6). The infection can be limited to the eye or the skin (Berkovich and Ressel), or, in unusual cases, can affect only one major internal organ, such as the brain or the liver. Localized skin lesions due to Herpes simplex in the infant without other organ system disease can even assume the segmental distribution characteristic of Herpes zoster and thus be misdiagnosed unless viral isolation studies are performed (Music et al.) (Fig. 14–7). The available information also suggests that the Herpes simplex virus can be transplacentally transmitted to the fetus in utero (Mitchell and McCall, Sieber et al.) and can have teratogenic effects when transmitted to the fetus early in pregnancy, resulting in congenital malformations in the newborn infant (South et al.).

The frequency with which neonatal Herpesvirus hominis infections occur is not known. Using previous conservative estimates, Hanshaw (1973) suggested that if neonatal Herpesvirus hominis infection occurred once in every 20,000 deliveries, there would be expected approximately 160 such cases per year in this country. While it has not been well documented statistically, it is generally believed that either the incidence or the recognition of genital Herpes simplex infection has significantly increased in the past two decades (Amstey).

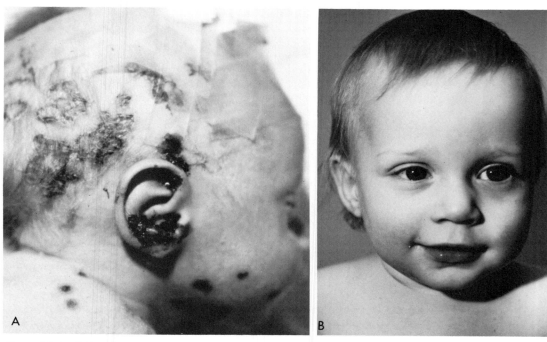

Figure 14–6. Disseminated neonatal Herpes simplex infection with a favorable outcome. *A,* Ten-day-old infant with birth weight of 2020 grams. He was born by cesarean section because of arrest of labor. During labor, a clamp was attached to the scalp transvaginally for fetal monitoring. The child did well until 5 days after birth when vesicles were observed on the scalp at the site of the previously attached clamp. Herpesvirus hominis, type II, was isolated from the vesicle fluid. By 10 days of age, vesicles which ruptured and crusted had spread over the scalp, external ear, and face. He was febrile, irritable, had vomiting, was listless, and exhibited a bulging fontanel. Hepatospleno-megaly was present by this time. CSF examination revealed 400 white blood cells per cu. mm., 95 percent neutrophils. The CSF protein content was 264 and the glucose was 25 mg. per 100 ml. Cytopathogenic effect in tissue culture consistent with Herpesvirus hominis appeared from the CSF in 2 days. The child's condition stabilized and was then followed by gradual improvement. *B,* At 11 months of age, the child was developmentally and neurologically normal. Head circumference was 46 cm.; retinae and optic discs were normal. The child babbled, took a few steps alone, and pulled up to a standing position. He was subsequently seen at 4 years of age and was normal.

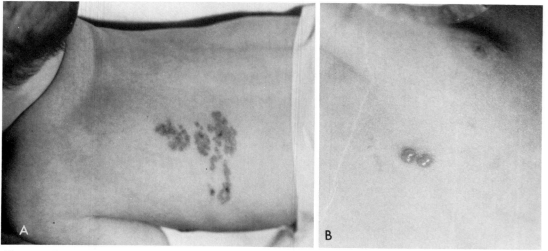

Figure 14–7. Cutaneous lesions caused by Herpes simplex in a 16-day-old infant. *A,* Lesions on the posterior thorax assume a radicular pattern resembling that usually associated with Herpes zoster. *B,* Vesicles on the skin in the anterior axillary line in the same child. Herpes simplex was isolated from these vesicular lesions.

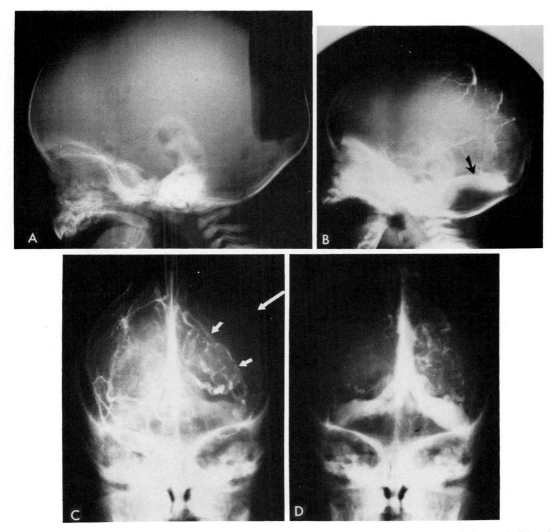

Figure 14–8. Probable intrauterine-acquired Herpes simplex infection resulting in congenital encephalitis with severe cerebral injury. Child's mother was believed to have had genital herpes infection in early pregnancy but diagnosis was never proved. At birth, the infant weighed 2600 grams and was hypotonic and poorly responsive. At 5 days of age, a rash was described and Herpes simplex was subsequently isolated from vesicular lesions. She was found to have chorioretinitis and metaphyseal lesions in long bones, consistent with an intrauterine viral infection. There was bilateral abnormal cranial transillumination. At 2 weeks of age, the child was hypothermic, poorly responsive, hypotonic but hyperreflexic, and had a diminished Moro reflex. CSF obtained by lumbar puncture demonstrated 410 white blood cells per cu. mm. all of which were lymphocytes, protein of 835 and glucose of 0 mg. per 100 ml. Virus was not obtained from the CSF. *A,* Lateral skull x-ray with air placed in the subdural space after subdural taps had revealed massive subdural fluid collections. Subdural fluid contained a protein content of 411 mg. per 100 ml. and 21 white blood cells per cu. mm. *B,* Angiogram, late venous phase, lateral view, shows striking distention of the transverse sinuses with tortuosity of cortical veins indicative of venous obstruction. *C,* Angiogram, venous phase, AP view. The short arrows indicate the surface of the cerebrum containing cortical veins, which is compressed medially by the overlying subdural effusion of massive proportion. The longer white arrow points to the edge of the skull, indicating the size of the subdural fluid collection. Note again the distention and tortuosity of the venous channels. *D,* Angiogram, late venous phase, AP view, demonstrates the gross distention of the transverse sinuses bilaterally but more striking on the left than the right. In this instance, the transplacentally transmitted infection, which was most likely Herpes simplex, resulted in a severe diffuse cerebral injury and produced obstruction of the venous outflow from the brain, giving rise to increased intracranial venous pressure and bilateral subdural effusions. (Courtesy of Dr. JoAnna Seibert, Little Rock, Arkansas.)

Clinical Manifestations

Because most neonatal infections with Herpes simplex virus result from acquisition by the infant of the virus from the birth canal during delivery, and since the incubation period is two to 12 days, the onset of symptoms in the infected newborn ranges from two to 12 days after birth. The most common time for the appearance of the initial manifestations of the illness is on the fifth or sixth postnatal day. A much less common source of newborn infection is nosocomial spread from one infected infant to another or from mother, nurses, or other hospital attendants (Francis et al.). Acquisition of the virus from infected maternal breast milk has also been described but is assumed to be rare (Dunkle et al.). The presence of herpetic vesicular skin lesions at birth (Sieber et al.) or their appearance within one day after birth indicates that the infection was either transplacentally transmitted from mother to child late in pregnancy or that ascending infection from the mother's birth canal has occurred. The latter is more likely if premature rupture of membranes has complicated the pregnancy near term.

Still another unusual form of neonatal involvement with Herpesvirus hominis is the result of transplacental transmission of the virus early in pregnancy leading to abortion or congenital anomalies at birth (Fig. 14–8). South et al. described a prematurely born infant with microcephaly, microphthalmia, intracranial calcification, and cutaneous lesions at birth from which Herpesvirus hominis was isolated. A similar case was described by Florman et al. in which the infant was small for gestational age, had neonatal pneumonitis, thrombocytopenia and hepatomegaly, and subsequently exhibited microcephaly and intracranial calcifications in a periventricular distribution. Herpes simplex type 1 was isolated from the child's urine and cerebrospinal fluid.

In a report by Montgomery et al., the teratogenic effects attributed to Herpes simplex type 2 infection early in pregnancy included a congenital cardiac defect and deformed digits. The infant was of low birth weight and had chorioretinitis and recurrent crops of cutaneous vesicles, from which the virus was isolated. Growth retardation and developmental delay characterized the postnatal clinical course. Chalhub et al. described a newborn infant believed to have transplacentally acquired Herpes simplex infection in the first trimester of pregnancy. Abnormalities included microcephaly with foci of cerebral calcification seen pathologically, hepatosplenomegaly with extensive hepatic calcification on x-ray and Cowdry type A inclusions microscopically, bilateral cataracts and chorioretinitis, and lesions in the distal femurs and proximal tibias similar to those seen with congenital rubella. Two additional examples of intrauterine-acquired Herpes simplex infection resulting in severe cerebral damage, microphthalmia, and cutaneous lesions present at birth have been described by Komorous et al. Cibis and Burde reported a child in whom Herpesvirus hominis was isolated from a congenital cataract removed at age 18 months and speculated that it may have resulted from fetal infection early in pregnancy.

The initial clinical manifestations in the neonate with Herpesvirus hominis infection are variable, depending on whether the illness is localized to the skin or the ocular structures, or is of the disseminated type. The infant with only herpetic vesicles on the skin or with conjunctivitis may otherwise appear entirely well or may exhibit only mild fever and irritability. Such localized lesions can be transient, followed by complete recovery, or may subsequently evolve into the more common and more serious disseminated form. Although the cutaneous or the ocular localized type of neonatal herpes infection is generally regarded to be benign, a certain number of such infants will subsequently show persisting neurologic deficits, developmental retardation, or chorioretinitis with visual loss (Hovig et al.). Unexpected sequelae of this sort indicate that the infection was more widespread than recognized and that cerebral involvement may be manifested only by irritability and a certain degree of lethargy during the acute stage. Cases of this type point out the desirability of cerebrospinal fluid examination whenever the infant exhibits any form of herpesvirus infection in the first few days of life.

The frequency with which neonatal herpes infection occurs in either localized or disseminated fashion is difficult to judge from the available literature. Of 14 cases presented by Pettay et al., nine had widespread disease, four had predominantly cutaneous involvement, and one infant had only neurologic manifestations but subsequently developed vesicles on the skin. Nahmias and colleagues reviewed 148 cases from the literature of which 98 were of the disseminated type. Of the 98 cases, neurologic involvement was identified in 40. Forty-eight patients were placed in the localized category but this included 25 in which the primary site of infection was the brain. Considering all the available information, it appears that disseminated neonatal herpes infection is far more common than disease localized to one organ system and that the brain is affected to some degree in a significant percentage of those with widespread disease.

The initial signs of illness in the newborn infant with disseminated Herpes simplex infection are usually non-specific, including poor feeding, vomiting, lethargy, respiratory distress, and fever. Within hours or a few days after onset, many affected infants will develop cutaneous manifestations or ocular signs, which represent the most common early diagnostic clue regarding the etiology of the condition. The usual skin lesions are vesicular in type and may be either single or clustered (Fig. 14–9). The forehead or scalp is the customary site of the first lesions but

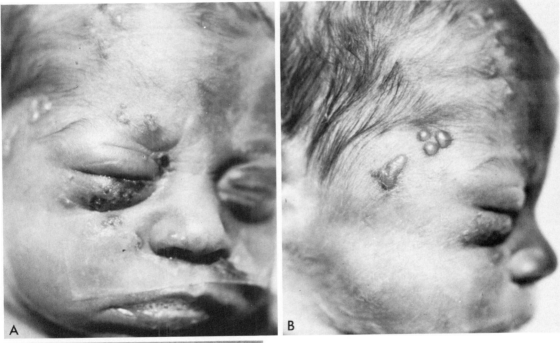

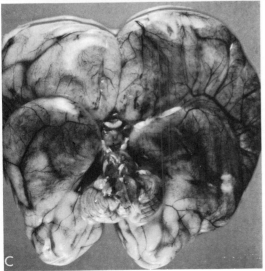

Figure 14–9. Disseminated neonatal Herpes simplex infection. *A* and *B*, Nine-day-old female infant with a birth weight of 1420 grams. The mother was not ill at the time of delivery and was not known to have genital herpes. Except for mild respiratory distress, child did well until 5 days after birth when she developed conjunctivitis on the right. Eyelid swelling and scalp vesicles appeared on the seventh day. By the ninth day after birth, the vesicular lesions had spread and the child was lethargic. CSF examination revealed no cells, a glucose of 56 and protein content of 172 mg. per 100 ml. At 14 days of age, she was more lethargic and had recurrent convulsions. CSF at this time contained 50 white blood cells per cu. mm. and a protein content of 260 mg. per 100 ml. Herpesvirus hominis was isolated from a cutaneous vesicle and from the second CSF specimen. Death occurred 3 weeks after birth. *C*, The brain is severely swollen and congested. Although the brain is diffusely affected, the greatest damage is to the frontal and temporal lobes bilaterally.

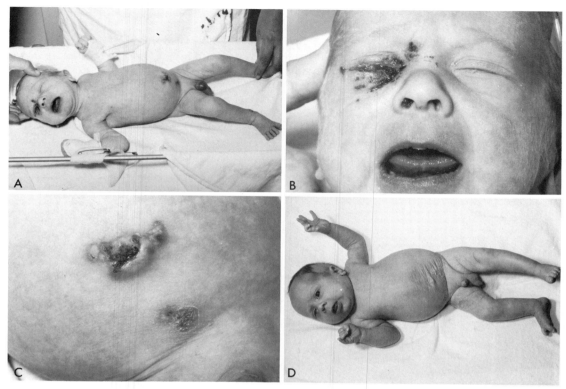

Figure 14–10. Disseminated neonatal Herpes simplex infection, type II. *A,* Sixteen-day-old infant with birth weight of 3240 grams. Child's mother had cervical herpetic lesions at the time of delivery. The child was normal at birth but on the fourth postnatal day had a total serum bilirubin of 16.8 mg. per 100 ml. He became febrile on the sixth day after birth and was considered to have bacterial sepsis for the next few days. CSF was unremarkable and cultures of blood and CSF remained negative. Conjunctivitis developed on the eleventh day after birth. Vesicles appeared on the skin around the right eye and on the abdomen the following day. At 16 days of age, the child had seizures, became lethargic, and developed hepatosplenomegaly. *B* and *C,* Cutaneous lesions on the sixteenth day after birth are crusted and necrotic. *D,* The child survived the illness and at age 6 weeks has right microphthalmia and is mildly hypertonic and hyperreflexic.

they can be located anywhere on the body. In some, the first lesions observed are erythematous macules, which later become vesicular and eventually are converted to ulcerative or crusted areas that may become confluent (Hovig) (Fig. 14–10). Secondary bacterial infection of the skin lesions can lead the unwary to the mistaken diagnosis of impetigo. Unilateral or bilateral conjunctivitis in the infant with vesicular skin lesions is an additional diagnostic signal suggesting herpetic infection. The extent of ocular disease varies from a mild conjunctivitis or keratoconjunctivitis to a severe necrotizing chorioretinitis or panuveitis which will leave the survivor with profound visual deficits (Hagler et al.).

Visceral organs most profoundly affected in disseminated neonatal Herpesvirus hominis infection are the liver, adrenal glands, and the brain, although many other structures may also be implicated. Hepatomegaly,

excessive bleeding due to prolongation of the prothrombin time, and elevation of serum liver enzymes indicate hepatic invasion by the virus. In some, serious liver disease will be evident clinically several days before significant liver or spleen enlargement can be detected. Jaundice can be the presenting abnormality in infants with this disease but is less common than the signs described above. The early manifestations of encephalitis may be only lethargy and vomiting, with evidence that the brain is involved coming largely from abnormalities found in the cerebrospinal fluid. More often, lethargy progresses to coma and is associated with convulsions, rigidity or flaccidity, nystagmus, or a tense fontanel. The cerebrospinal fluid is clear in appearance, unless the child is jaundiced, and often contains red blood cells and lymphocytes, which vary in number from a few up to several hundred per cu. mm. The glucose

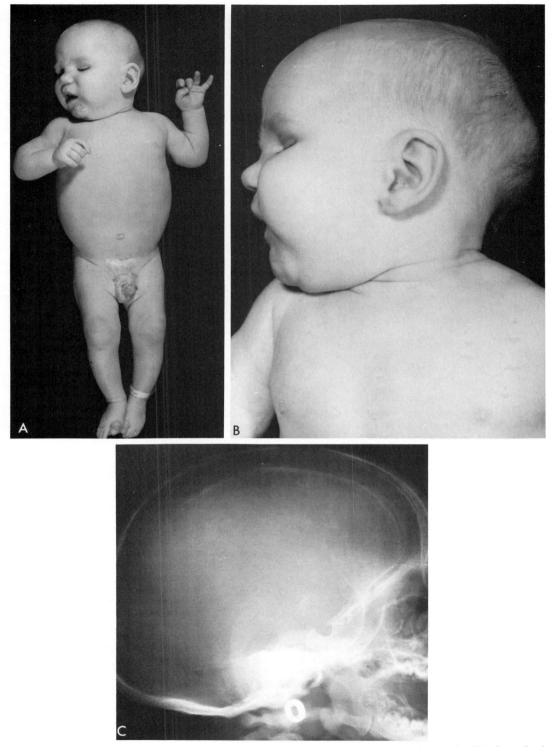

Figure 14–11. Late sequelae of neonatal Herpes simplex encephalitis. *A* and *B,* Six-month-old infant who had severe disseminated infection with onset 5 days after birth. At age 6 months, he is microcephalic, blind with bilateral microphthalmia, and has spastic limbs. *C,* Skull x-ray shows calcification within damaged brain, outlining a markedly distended ventricular system.

content is not reduced unless the child is hypoglycemic, while the protein content is elevated in most cases, with levels ranging from 80 to 600 mg. per 100 ml.

During the illness, it is not unusual for the infant to develop abnormal bleeding from puncture wounds, from the umbilicus or the gastrointestinal tract, or from other sites. Excessive bleeding results either from severe hepatic injury or from disseminated intravascular coagulation (Miller et al., Catalona et al., Shershow et al.). Hemorrhagic tendencies usually are seen in infants with other obvious evidence of diffuse herpetic disease. On rare occasion, the first and virtually only clinical evidence of the disease is the sudden onset of massive bleeding, which rapidly leads to death of the child. Such infants are likely to be considered to have vitamin K deficiency hemorrhagic disease of the newborn until necropsy reveals the characteristic morphologic changes of Herpesvirus hominis infection of the liver and other organs, from which the virus is isolated.

Disseminated Herpesvirus hominis infection in the newborn must be regarded to be a life-threatening illness with a high mortality rate. Nahmias et al. found that previously published cases reflected a 96 percent death rate. The course of the disease is very rapid in some cases, with death occurring only hours after the first signs of illness. More often, the duration between onset and death is five to 10 days. The degree of major organ system involvement differs from case to case, however, and survival can occur, even in those severely affected by the illness (Pettay et al., Torphy et al.). Frentz et al. described a 2,800-gram newborn infant with type 2 Herpesvirus hominis infection in whom the virus was recovered from the cerebrospinal fluid. The child recovered and, at age 18 months, exhibited no obvious developmental or other abnormalities.

Of infants who do recover, sequelae are common and are frequently severe, especially in those with cerebral involvement during the acute stage. Clinical residual deficits may include microcephaly, spasticity, convulsions, mental retardation, and blindness (Fig. 14–11). Pathologic correlates in survivors who expired at a later date have included diffuse cystic encephalomalacia (Mirra, Smith et al.) or hydranencephaly (Young et al.). Diffuse calcification in the brain is sometimes observed on skull x-ray months after the acute illness (Fig. 14–12). Adrenal cortical insufficiency has also been described as a resid-

ual of the acute process (Bahrani et al.). An interesting course that has been observed in a small number of infants who recovered from the acute illness is the periodic recurrence of crops of cutaneous vesicles without other signs of viral dissemination (Frentz et al., Gershon et al., Hovig et al., Smith et al.). In the child described by Torphy et al., recurrent vesicles continued to appear on the skin up to 26 months of age, and Herpesvirus hominis type 2 was isolated therefrom.

Diagnosis

Diagnostic principles in the neonate with Herpesvirus hominis infection are similar to those in the older child described above. One must suspect the possibility from the clinical findings, exclude a bacterial cause by appropriate studies, and confirm the diagnosis by a combination of serologic, morphologic, and virologic laboratory examinations.

Because of certain differences in the newborn form of this disease as compared to the older child with herpesvirus encephalitis, brain biopsy is rarely indicated or required in this age group to establish the diagnosis during life. Since most infants with the illness acquire the virus from the mother, the presence of maternal genital herpes infection adds support to the herpetic etiology when the infant develops signs of infection. If maternal lesions weren't observed earlier, the pelvic examination should be repeated when the child becomes ill with skin vesicles or encephalitis in the first two weeks after birth. The presence of cutaneous vesicles or conjunctivitis in association with cerebral or hepatic involvement greatly facilitates rapid diagnosis because it makes available an external source from which the virus can be isolated. Fluid containing the virus can be aspirated from the vesicular lesions and, in tissue culture, may reveal the characteristic herpetic cytopathogenic effect within one to three days. Herpetic virions within exfoliated cells in the vesicle fluid are identifiable with the electron microscope in approximately the same period of time. When facilities are available, cells in vesicle fluid or from conjunctival scrapings can be shown to contain herpesvirus antigen by immunofluorescence even more rapidly (Pettay et al., Taber et al., 1976). It is important to recognize that skin vesicles due to this viral disease may become pustular with staphylococci cultured from aspirated material. This does not exclude Herpesvirus hominis as a possible cause and means only that secondary infection of the lesion has occurred.

External lesions also provide a readily available source of material for morphologic examination. Scrapings or biopsy from the margin or bed of skin vesicles (Tzanck smear) or from inflamed conjunctivae reveal multinucleated giant cells or inclusion-bearing cells consistent with infection by a member of the herpes group of viruses. In addition to vesicle fluid or the conjunctivae as sources, herpesvirus in the neonatal type of infection can sometimes be isolated from urine (Chang et al.), stool, nasopharynx, or rarely even blood. The cerebrospinal fluid is generally regarded to be a poor source for viral isolation in the older child with Herpesvirus hominis encephalitis but is more often positive in the newborn infant with the disseminated form of the disease.

Serologic methods of diagnosis are less helpful in neonatal herpes than either morphologic or virologic techniques. If the mother has had no previous illnesses with types 1 or 2 herpesvirus prior to developing genital herpes near term, the infant will probably have undetectable antibody levels at the onset of the illness. If the mother has had previous infection with type 1 Herpesvirus hominis, the newborn baby may have a significant passively transferred antibody titer but is not necessarily protected against type 2 disease. The development of a four-fold or greater antibody titer rise in the infant's serum will require two to four weeks in most cases and thus has limited immediate diagnostic value during the acute stage of the illness. Within a week after onset of the neonatal disease, specific IgM herpetic antibody can be detected in the infant's serum by indirect fluorescent antibody methods and provides presumptive evidence of Herpes simplex infection (Nahmias et al.).

Because of the severity, the rapid rate of progression in certain cases, and the peculiar clinical variations that sometimes occur, diagnosis often remains unsuspected until the necropsy is performed and histologic examination accomplished. The brain reveals variable findings, including swelling, softening, and lymphocytic infiltration as well as intranuclear inclusion bodies in oligodendroglia and, less often, in other cells. As compared to Herpesvirus hominis encephalitis in the older child, that occurring in the neonate tends to be a more uniform process with less of the selectivity for the temporal lobe or orbital frontal lobes. Hepatitis may be mild, with intranuclear inclusion bodies in addition to other inflammatory cell infiltrates, but in some cases the process is characterized by massive and widespread hepatic necrosis (Fig. 14–13). Similar findings may be present in the adrenal glands and other structures, and virus can usually be isolated from various organs if the material is properly handled. Mirra has recently pointed out vascular changes in neonatal disseminated Herpes simplex infection, which include intimal fibrosis and severe granulomatous inflammation of the medial wall of the aorta.

Prevention and Treatment

The most important method of prevention of neonatal Herpes simplex infection is the detection of maternal genital herpes during pregnancy, and delivery by Cesarean section if the maternal lesions are evident at term. Hanshaw has estimated that the risk of neonatal infection is approximately 10 percent in women with cytologic or clinical evidence of genital Herpesvirus hominis infection after 32 weeks' gestation. The risk increases to approximately 40 percent if the virus is present at the time of delivery, unless the infant is delivered abdominally. Delivery by section does not always prevent viral contamination of the infant, particularly if premature rupture of membranes has occurred (Zavoral et al.). Recognition of genital herpetic infection in the mother can easily be overlooked, especially in those cases where the primary site of the infection is the uterine cervix.

A problem over which there is considerable dispute is the most appropriate isolation techniques in the newborn nursery relative to the Herpes simplex virus. All agree that the child with clinical illness caused by this virus should be strictly isolated and that the asymptomatic newborn infant born to a mother with active genital herpes should be separated from other infants in the nursery. The infant should be isolated until discharge from the hospital or for 21 days if he remains in hospital for that period of time. Visintine et al. also recommend that the infant born vaginally of a mother with a genital herpes infection should have topical idoxuridine or Ara-A ointment applied to the eyes in addition to periodic viral cultures of the mouth, eyes, CSF, and other specimens. The extent and duration of separation of the well infant from the mother with genital infection is a point of

Text continued on page 386

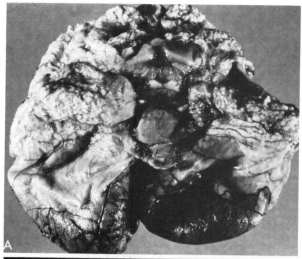

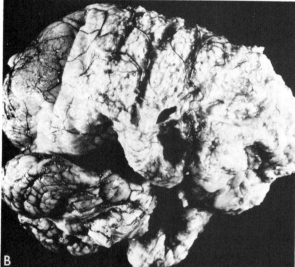

Figure 14–12. Late effects of neonatal Herpes simplex encephalitis. Necropsy findings at age 18 months of the infant shown in Figure 14–11. *A* and *B*, Diffuse and extensive damage to the brain with nodular calcification of the cerebral cortex. *C*, Widespread calcification in necrotic cortical tissue is demonstrated in the postmortem radiograph with the brain removed from the skull.

Illustration continued on opposite page

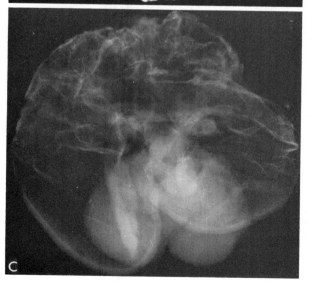

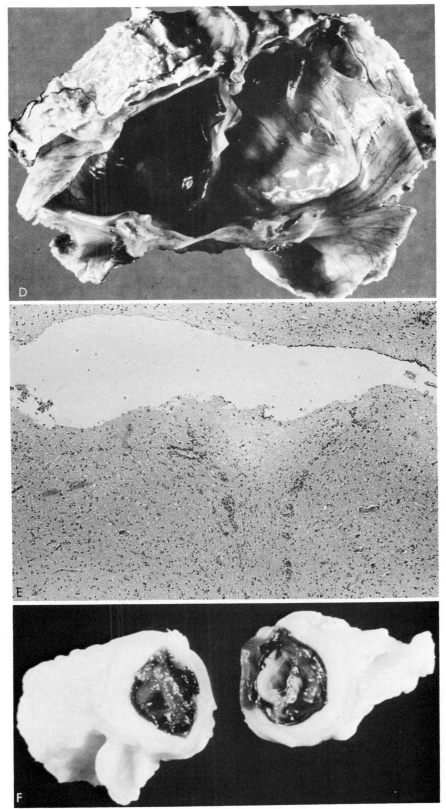

Figure 14–12 Continued. *D* and *E*, Hydrocephalus and thinned cerebral mantle secondary to aqueductal gliosis. *F*, Remnants of destroyed ocular structures encased in bone.

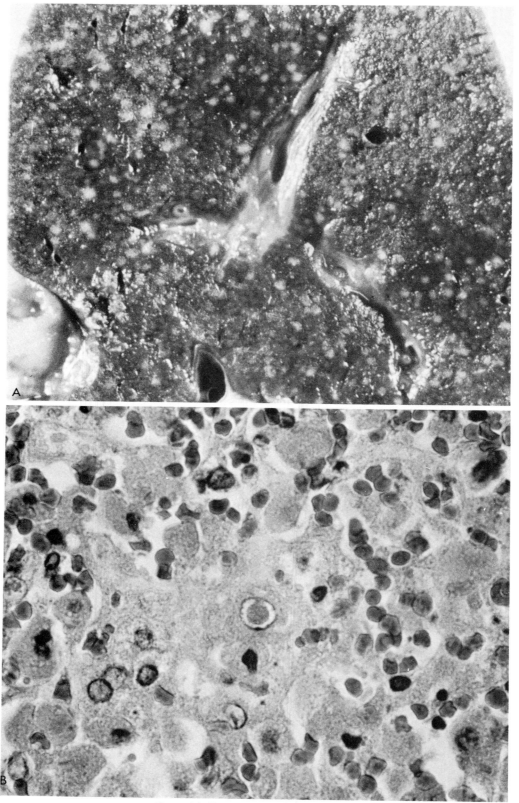

Figure 14–13.   See legend on opposite page

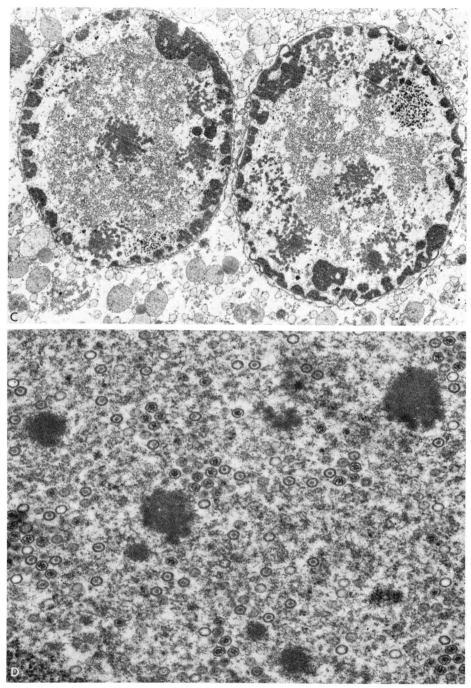

Figure 14–13.   Liver pathology in disseminated neonatal Herpes simplex infection. *A,* Gross appearance of the liver showing multiple, small (2 to 4 mm.) necrotic foci. *B,* Typical Cowdry type A inclusion body near the center of the photograph. *C,* Electron micrograph showing large number of target-like Herpesvirus hominis virions in the nuclei of two hepatocytes. *D,* Electron micrograph, higher power, revealing numerous virions, many with target-like appearance.

dispute, although the safest approach from the infant's standpoint is to discourage intimate contact of the baby with the mother until the maternal lesions have cleared (Light, Visintine et al.). Oral herpetic lesions in nursery personnel are probably rare sources of infection of the newborn infant. In addition, since oral lesions in adults are often asymptomatic, a policy designed to prevent infant contamination can be only partially successful. Nevertheless, nursery attendants with active oral lesions or herpetic whitlows should be reassigned to other duties that do not include contact with infants less than one month of age until the active infection has subsided (Haynes et al.).

Treatment of the infant who exhibits evidence of disseminated disease with Herpes simplex remains in the speculative stage except for conservative measures such as control of seizures, local ocular therapy, and the provision of adequate fluids and electrolytes. Bleeding secondary to hepatic dysfunction is managed by administration of vitamin K and, at times, the use of fresh whole blood. If bleeding is due to intravascular coagulation, heparin therapy deserves consideration but is fraught with difficulties in the newborn.

The history of antiviral drug therapy in the newborn infant with Herpes simplex infection is similar to that of the older child and adult outlined earlier. Idoxuridine (5-iodo-2-deoxyuridine) achieved popularity for a time following apparent beneficial results when used in uncontrolled fashion (Charnock and Cramblett, Duffli and Nahmias, Golden et al., Partridge and Millis, Pettay et al.). The use of the drug in the newborn period was of concern because of the possibility that it might disturb normal cellular metabolism, leading to maturational disturbances within the brain. The subsequent demonstration of its degree of toxicity and relative ineffectiveness as an antiviral drug terminated its clinical use for this illness.

Cytosine arabinoside was the next preparation to receive attention for treatment of systemic neonatal Herpes simplex infection, but it likewise was shown to have serious limitations. Experimental studies revealed that it could produce defective development of the cerebellum and retina when administered in the newborn period (Percy and Hatch, Shimada et al.).

The preliminary studies with adenine arabinoside (Ara-A) for treatment of neonatal systemic Herpes simplex infections show promise but will require continued investi-

gation (Ch'ien et al., 1975; Steele et al.). The drug has advantages over those previously investigated, including a lesser degree of toxicity, less degree of suppression of the host immune response, and less inhibition of normal cellular metabolism. The current treatment regimen is a dose of 15 mg. per kilogram per day, given by continuous intravenous drip for 12 hours daily for 10 days. Laboratory studies for monitoring of possible myelosuppression or hepatotoxicity are performed periodically during the course of treatment.

VARICELLA-ZOSTER INFECTIONS

The relationship between varicella (chickenpox) and herpes zoster has intrigued investigators for years and has acquired great importance in this era of organ transplantation, prolonged survival from hematologic malignancies, and immunosuppressive and corticosteroid therapy. As early as 1888 and again in 1909, von Bokay suggested that the two illnesses were related after observing several cases of chickenpox developing in children following exposure to adults with herpes zoster. The occurrence of varicella subsequent to contact with an adult with zoster has since been recorded many times, while the reverse is recognized to occur less often. The virus causing the two conditions is now known to be the same, with the immune state of the host representing the variable which accounts for the differences in clinical expression of the illness. Rake and colleagues demonstrated by electron microscopy that virions from vesicles in the two diseases were morphologically identical and that zoster virus particles were agglutinated when exposed to serum from patients recovering from varicella. Weller and Coons examined viruses from varicella and zoster vesicles using the fluorescent antibody method. They found no antigenic differences between the viral agents from the two illnesses, adding further evidence that the viruses are identical.

Since one virus, now referred to as the varicella-zoster virus (or Herpesvirus varicellae), has been shown to be the cause of both varicella and herpes zoster, it is recognized that varicella is the primary infection, occurring mainly in children without prior immunity, and that zoster is a secondary, usually reactivation, infection in one only partially immune. It is presumed that following the primary varicella infection, the virus remains latent within dorsal root ganglia. With decline in protective antibody years later, the virus migrates along the sensory nerves, eventually reaching the cutaneous nerve endings where it is released to produce the characteristic vesicles of herpes zoster aligned in radicular distribution. The process of reactivation of the dormant virus occurs for no apparent reason in most afflicted patients, but in others is provoked by another febrile illness, by irradiation therapy, with malignancy, or secondary to immunosuppressive drug therapy. Infection in children with varicella-zoster virus is generally regarded to be benign; however, in the newborn period the illness carries greater risk, and in patients who are immunosuppressed the danger of visceral dissemination is strikingly increased.

Varicella (Chickenpox)

Varicella is widely known as a highly contagious disease of children which occurs primarily in late winter or early spring and which is mild in the majority of cases, with neurologic or other serious complications being infrequent. While the degree of severity of the illness varies considerably in chil-

dren, the infection is symptomatic in most, with subclinical infection being quite infrequent. The incubation period ranges from 10 to 21 days, with an average of 16 days. Fever or malaise may be the initial symptom but the vesicular eruption is the most characteristic feature of the illness in most children. Vesicles are first noticed on the trunk and promptly extend to the face and scalp. The rash spreads rapidly, and, within two to four days after onset, lesions in different stages are present over the trunk, face and proximal portions of the extremities (Fig. 14–14). Most have reached the crusted stage within six days after onset, by which time systemic manifestations of the illness have usually subsided. Virus can be isolated from vesicle fluid during the first three days after onset of the rash but rarely thereafter (Gold). Thus, by the time the skin lesions have all reached the crusted stage, the child is no longer considered contagious. Rise in complement-fixing antibodies can confirm the recent occurrence of infection with varicella-zoster virus but is not a reliable method of determining the immune status of persons otherwise. The recently developed fluorescent antibody to membrane antigen technique is a more sen-

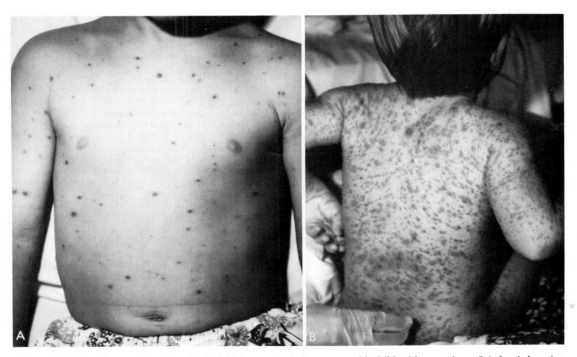

Figure 14–14. Uncomplicated varicella (chickenpox). *A,* Four-year-old child with eruption of 4 days' duration. Illness was very mild with only slight temperature elevation. *B,* Three-year-old child with extensive cutaneous lesions. Fever was 102°F and symptoms included anorexia and irritability. The child had been exposed to a sibling with varicella 2 weeks prior to onset of illness. Complete recovery followed.

sitive method to detect susceptibility or immunity to this virus, and is of particular importance for this purpose in immunocompromised patients (Williams et al., Gershon and Krugman).

Of the various types of complications of varicella, the most common is secondary cutaneous bacterial infection. Rarely in childhood, the illness is associated with varicella pneumonia (Eisenklam), a serious complication which is a recognized threat when the disease occurs in the leukemic child or in the adult (Sargent et al.). Hemorrhagic complications, likewise, are rare with varicella but have been described in the form of purpura fulminans (Becker and Buckley) or consump-

tion coagulopathy. Thrombocytopenia without other coagulation defects can occur with varicella, and at least in one case, has resulted in fatal cerebral hemorrhage (Tobin and ten Bensel). The risk of varicella is increased in the child with a malignant condition, especially during treatment with chemotherapeutic agents. Although most children who acquire the illness while receiving such drugs do recover, the incidence of disseminated infection is increased considerably compared to its infrequent occurrence in otherwise normal children (Fig. 14–15). In the series of Feldman et al. of children receiving anti-cancer treatment who acquired varicella, 32 percent had evidence of visceral dissemi-

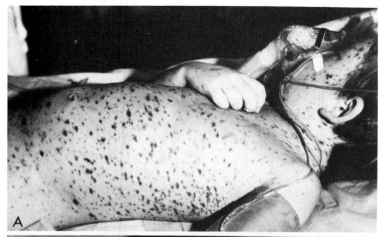

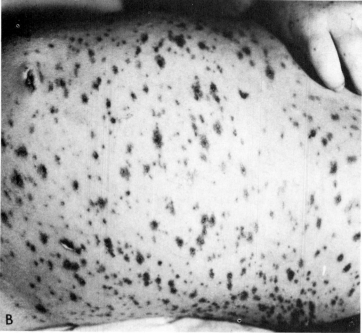

Figure 14–15. Severe varicella with dissemination in a child with leukemia. Seven-year-old boy with bone marrow relapse of leukemia 6 weeks before onset of varicella. He experienced continued elaboration of new vesicles over 10 days at which time the cutaneous lesions became hemorrhagic *(A, B)*. The illness was complicated by varicella pneumonia and, approximately 12 days after the onset of the rash, he developed recurrent grand mal convulsions with coma between seizures. Varicella virus was isolated from the blood but not from the CSF. He survived the illness but was left with severe neurologic sequelae secondary to encephalitis.

nation, and the mortality rate in the entire group was 7 percent.

The danger associated with varicella in a child receiving chronic corticosteroid therapy for another underlying disease is widely discussed but poorly understood. Haggerty and Eley in 1956 emphasized the possibility of a fatal outcome from varicella in certain children treated with corticosteroids. Further observations have indicated that varicella in a steroid-treated child with an underlying disease which disturbs the immune mechanism is indeed hazardous and may result in viral dissemination and death. On the other hand, when the primary disease does not cause immunologic compromise, the danger of varicella in the child on steroids is unproved (Falliers and Ellis). In this latter group of patients, Falliers and Ellis suggested that some of the reported deaths may have been secondary to sudden and total discontinuation of corticosteroid therapy at the onset of the exanthem, thus perhaps resulting in acute adrenal insufficiency.

Varicella occurring during pregnancy is a matter of special concern, not only because of the greater severity of the infection in the adult, but also because of the potential implications to the fetus or the neonate. Maternal varicella, active just before or at the time of birth of the child, may be transplacentally transmitted to the fetus, resulting in neonatal varicella (Hubbard). One can be certain that varicella is transplacentally transmitted only if the illness in the neonate occurs within the first nine days after birth since the incubation period extends from 10 to 21 days. In addition to intrauterine transmission of the virus during the viremic stage, the infant is susceptible to viral contamination during passage through the birth canal if vesicles are present on the mother at this time. Of 15 mothers with varicella within two weeks prior to delivery, infection developed in four of the infants within three weeks after birth (Abler).

Varicella in the newborn child is generally a benign illness but significant complications occur more often than in older children. Dissemination of the infection to the lungs, liver, adrenal glands, and other organs has been observed in certain cases, some with a fatal outcome. Ehrlich et al. suggested from literature review that congenital varicella is fatal in approximately 20 percent of cases. Another remotely possible complication of maternal varicella late in pregnancy is the occurrence of a subclinical infection in the neonate followed by reactivation in the form

of herpes zoster in infancy or childhood. Lewkonia and Jackson reported an 18-month-old child with herpes zoster ophthalmicus whose mother had varicella five weeks before term.

Although reports are few, varicella in the early weeks of pregnancy may result in congenital defects in the baby, and perhaps can result in chronic viral persistence, analogous to that with intrauterine-acquired rubella. What percentage of fetuses will be affected in teratogenic fashion when chickenpox occurs in early pregnancy is unknown but is probably very low (Brunell). Laforet and Lynch described a case of maternal varicella in the eighth week of pregnancy followed by birth of a child with hepatomegaly, hypoplasia of the right lower extremity, and evidence of cerebral atrophy on pneumoencephalography. The child subsequently developed seizures and was found to have nystagmus, optic atrophy, and pigmentary abnormalities of the retina. A report by McKendry and Bailey described maternal varicella in the eleventh week of pregnancy, resulting in a low-birth-weight infant with multiple cutaneous scars and hypoplasia of the right upper limb. The child subsequently grew poorly, developed seizures, and was found to have chorioretinitis and scoliosis. Dilated lateral ventricles were demonstrated on pneumoencephalography. Similar findings were reported by Savage et al. in a newborn infant whose mother had contracted varicella in the ninth week of pregnancy. Low birth weight, hypoplasia of the left upper extremity with depressed cutaneous scars, and a unilateral Horner's syndrome characterized this child's abnormalities. Congenital defects similar to those described above were present in the child reported by Rinvik; the mother had acquired varicella in the fifteenth week of pregnancy. Birth weight was abnormally low, hypoplasia of the right leg and foot were observed, and cutaneous scars in a zigzag pattern extended down the posterior aspect of the right thigh. Chorioretinitis was present and pneumoencephalography demonstrated cerebral atrophy.

More recently, Srabstein et al. described an infant born at 41 weeks' gestation with a birth weight of 2,000 grams whose mother had varicella between the 13th and 15th week of pregnancy. The child had microphthalmia with cataracts, cutaneous scars in the lumbar region, and atrophy of the left lower limb. She remained apathetic, had recurrent myoclonic seizures, and died at six months of age.

The brain revealed marked ventricular dilatation secondary to obstruction of the foramina of Monro. Histologic findings confirmed a severe, necrotizing encephalomyelitis in addition to a destructive ependymitis. Although virus isolation was unsuccessful, serologic tests during life supported the diagnosis of infection with varicella-zoster virus. Thus, the pattern, including low birth weight, microphthalmia and other ocular defects, skin scarring, hypoplastic limbs, and a variety of neurologic defects, seems sufficiently constant in reported cases to indicate that intrauterine-acquired varicella can have teratogenic and injurious effects upon the fetus (Brice, Frey et al., Charles et al.).

Maternal infection with the varicella-zoster virus in the form of herpes zoster has less clearly been related to congenital defects, although Duehr reported two such infants with congenital cataracts. Microphthalmia was also present in one and the other had talipes equinovarus and developmental retardation, in addition to lens opacities.

Neurologic Complications of Varicella

Since the same virus causes chickenpox and herpes zoster, it is somewhat artificial to discuss the neurologic complications separately. From the clinical standpoint, however, certain differences are apparent regarding the neurologic disorders that afflict the child with classic chickenpox as compared to the patient with herpes zoster.

The varicella virus has been implicated as a cause of a variety of neurologic conditions in childhood, some of which remain speculative, and most of which are unusual to rare. Among the most infrequent of such disorders complicating chickenpox are optic neuritis (Hatch) and the Guillain-Barré syndrome (Welch, Boughton), of which only a few examples have been reported. Acute hemorrhagic leukoencephalitis has also been reported as a rare complication of varicella (Lander).

Of greater interest is the association between varicella and Reye's syndrome, the latter being the most common cause of death in children with varicella (Takashima and Becker). This disorder is an acute, severe encephalopathy with fatty infiltration of the viscera, particularly of the liver. The brain is usually swollen but without an inflammatory response. Biochemical alterations include marked elevations in the serum glutamic oxaloacetic transaminase and ammonia levels. In some cases, severe hypoglycemia also occurs. Pathogenesis of this fulminating disorder remains unclear but preceding viral infections of various types have been recognized in most cases (Riley). The association of Reye's syndrome with a preceding infection with the varicella virus has now been made on many occasions (Abruzzi, Brown and Madge, Glick et al., Jenkins et al., Norman), and it is estimated that approximately 8 percent of cases of Reye's syndrome follow varicella.

It is likely that the syndrome of acute encephalopathy with fatty degeneration of the liver is a reaction that may be triggered by a variety of different preceding stimuli. Its relationship to varicella is of particular interest, however, because a number of cases reported as examples of varicella encephalitis have probably been in this category. Furthermore, an acute, severe encephalopathy with no spinal fluid pleocytosis or inflammatory cells in the brain and without the characteristic visceral changes of Reye's syndrome may complicate chickenpox (Johnson and Milbourn). The relationship, if any, of this fulminating illness to Reye's syndrome is unclear.

Varicella Encephalitis. The incidence with which encephalitis complicates chickenpox in childhood is difficult to estimate from the literature, in part because there has been little effort to separate those with encephalitis from patients with an acute encephalopathy, which most likely is pathogenetically different. Even cases of acute cerebellar ataxia associated with varicella have been included with encephalitis in some series. The acute ataxic syndrome in most instances is sufficiently different from cases with encephalitis that it deserves being placed in a special category, recognizing that its cause is undetermined. In addition, in some cases, manifestations of the illness are a blending of different features of these various disorders so that one cannot be certain of the underlying pathology unless brain tissue becomes available for histologic examination. In view of these diagnostic complexities, the often stated figures that encephalitis occurs with chickenpox in approximately one in 1,000 to one in 5,000 cases have relatively little meaning. It is probable that acute varicella encephalitis in the previously normal individual is a very rare disorder (Takashima and Becker).

A rare but usually fatal central nervous system response to varicella infection is an acute encephalopathy in which the brain becomes rapidly and profoundly edematous, leading to tentorial herniation and brain stem compression. Except for cerebral swelling and acute neuronal degeneration of variable degree, little is found in the brain or elsewhere to account for the process. The onset of symptoms is abrupt, with vomiting and irritability, soon to be followed by a rapid decline in awareness leading to deep coma and signs of decerebration. The absence of cells in the cerebrospinal fluid and the lack of an inflammatory response in brain tissue set this disorder apart from the condition better referred to as encephalitis. In our present state of knowledge, this condition is more appropriately called an acute encephalopathy secondary to varicella, the pathogenesis remaining unknown. Its possible relationship to Reye's syndrome is a point of interesting speculation.

In addition to encephalitis, varicella in childhood may be complicated by either a benign aseptic meningitis or an acute transverse myelitis (Johnson and Milbourn, Krabbe, Smith). Of the few reports in the literature of post-varicella acute transverse myelitis, most describe a favorable outcome with complete or nearly complete recovery. Permanent spinal cord dysfunction, however, can result from this illness (McCarthy and Amer).

Encephalitic manifestations most commonly appear on the fourth to sixth posteruptive day, although neurologic signs can occur even before the rash develops (Underwood, Holliday). A generalized convulsion may be the first sign of neurologic involvement, but more often headache, vomiting, and fever followed by decline in consciousness are the initial manifestations. Meningeal signs are usual and, as in other types of viral encephalitis, manifestations of cerebral dysfunction are variable. Stretch reflexes and muscle tone may be either enhanced or decreased and some patients exhibit focal deficits, such as hemiparesis, ataxia, localized seizures, or cranial nerve abnormalities.

Cerebrospinal fluid examination in the usual case of chickenpox encephalitis reveals clear fluid under moderately increased pressure. Pleocytosis varies from 10 to 150 cells per cu. mm. with an occasional case in which the cell count is even higher. At the onset of the disease, polymorphonuclear cells may predominate but are soon replaced by lymphocytes. Like other types of encephalitis, cells can be entirely absent in the spinal fluid (Gibel et al.). The glucose content is normal or increased, as is the cerebrospinal fluid protein value.

The severity of varicella encephalitis is variable, as is the mortality rate reported in different series in the literature. Appelbaum and colleagues found a mortality rate of 5 percent in a series of 59 cases. Boughton reported an 18 percent mortality among 39 patients, and Johnson and Milbourn observed a 35 percent fatality rate in a series of 23 patients with cerebral signs during the illness. In survivors, sequelae may reflect either focal or diffuse neurologic injury of either the cerebrum, cerebellum, or brain stem. Lipsett et al. described a unique neurologic disturbance following varicella complicated by pneumonia in a six-year-old boy. The acute illness was followed by hyperphagia, recurrent hyperthermia, and secondary hypothyroidism. Gliosis and lymphocytic infiltration were found in the hypothalamus at autopsy.

Like other types of exanthematous encephalitis in childhood, that secondary to chickenpox has been attributed to direct viral invasion of the brain by some authors and to an "allergic" or immune cerebral reaction by others. Speculation remains appropriate but accumulating evidence seems more consistent with the concept of direct viral invasion of the brain, especially in light of recent findings (McCormick et al.).

Acute Cerebellar Ataxia. In some children with varicella unassociated with signs of encephalitis, an acute ataxic syndrome appears five to ten days following the development of the eruption or, rarely, even before the rash is noted (Goldston et al.). Truncal ataxia resulting in a markedly incoordinated gait is often the only sign of neurologic dysfunction. In others, the cerebellar signs are preceded by headache or vomiting and are compounded by lethargy, irritability, and evidence of increased intracranial pressure. Ataxia is transient in most, with complete recovery following within a week or so. The cerebrospinal fluid is frequently entirely normal, but a lymphocytic pleocytosis or a mild increase in the protein content may be present (Johnson and Milbourn).

Acute cerebellar ataxia with varicella has been considered by many authors to be an "encephalitic" manifestation in which the inflammatory process affects primarily the cerebellum (Levin, Johnson and Milbourn). The probability of direct viral invasion of the central nervous system in cases of acute cerebellar ataxia has been supported by the demonstration of varicella-zoster antigen in cerebrospinal fluid cells by immunofluorescent staining (Peters et al.). In addition, in some cases with clear-cut and severe encephalitic signs plus spinal fluid pleocytosis, cerebellar ataxia is a prominent part of the illness before lethargy or coma supervenes. In most cases, however, the ataxic syndrome exists without fever, without other symptoms, and with a normal spinal fluid examination, all of which cast some degree of doubt on the encephalitic postulate. In these cases, the disorder is best considered an acute cerebellar response to a varicella infection but the pathogenesis is unclear.

Herpes Zoster

As mentioned earlier, varicella is now considered to be a primary infection in one unimmune while herpes zoster is a secondary, or reactivation, infection in one with partial immunity from previous illness with the virus. Although the virus causing varicella and herpes zoster is the same, there are striking differences in the two conditions. Varicella is mainly a disease of children, with a seasonal distribution of late winter and early spring, and with cutaneous lesions that are diffuse. Herpes zoster occurs throughout the year, is much more common in those in the sixth to the eighth decades of life, and is characterized by an eruption which is usually segmental in distribution. In contrast to the high degree of contagiousness of varicella among unimmune children, herpes zoster is usually a sporadic disease with a much lower degree of person-to-person spread.

Despite its prevalence in late middle-age and the elderly, zoster does occur in children (Fig. 14–16) and has even been reported in the neonate (Bonar and Pearsall, Freud et al.). In most reports of neonatal herpes zoster, the diagnosis has been based on the location and pattern of the vesicular eruption and is, therefore, open to question. This is especially true since zoster-like cutaneous lesions in the young infant have now been described as a result of Herpes simplex infection (Music et al.). When herpes zoster does occur in children, the illness is similar to that in adults except that it is usually milder (Brunell et al.) and without the post-herpetic neuralgia syndrome that sometimes complicates the adult illness.

Herpes zoster is believed to occur when there is reactivation of the virus which has remained latent within the dorsal root gan-

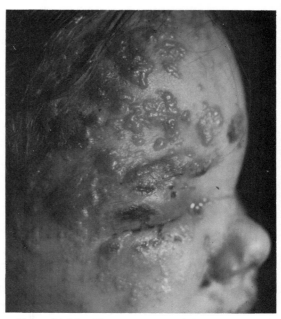

Figure 14–16. Herpes zoster ophthalmicus in a 3-year-old girl with no underlying or predisposing illness, and no prior history of varicella. Symptoms included headache, vomiting, and pain in the face and eye. Temperature was 102°F. CSF examination was normal. Complete spontaneous recovery occurred within 10 to 14 days.

glia. Much less frequently, the illness develops following contact with a child with chickenpox, suggesting direct viral transmission from one patient to another who has waning immunity to the virus. The initial clinical manifestation of the illness is often tingling or pain in the cutaneous region where vesicles subsequently will appear. Within a few days, vesicles develop in the distribution of one to three sensory nerve segments. The cutaneous eruption is unilateral in the majority of cases. The most common site of involvement is the thoracic region, with the distribution of supply of the ophthalmic division of the trigeminal nerve being the second most predisposed area. Some patients are virtually asymptomatic except for the localized eruption, while others have low-grade fever, headache, posterior cervical pain, or malaise. Regardless of the site of the cutaneous lesions, certain patients with herpes zoster are found to have an elevation of the cerebrospinal fluid protein content with a modest lymphocytic pleocytosis (Gold). Approximately 50 percent of patients with uncomplicated herpes zoster have been found to have lymphocytes in the cerebrospinal fluid (Appelbaum et al.).

Herpes zoster of the cutaneous area supplied by the first division of the trigeminal nerve is referred to as herpes zoster ophthalmicus and is of special importance because of the possibility of ocular involvement on the affected side. Whenever the nasociliary branch of the first division is affected, as indicated by extension of the eruption to the tip of the nose, the likelihood of ocular inflammation is high. Conversely, when the nose is spared and the eruption is limited to the forehead, the eye is usually not affected. Corneal ulceration with subsequent visual loss may result, or, the process can be complicated by keratitis, uveitis, or secondary glaucoma (Pierce and Jenkins). A rare complication of herpes zoster ophthalmicus is extraocular muscle weakness, which may involve the third, fourth, and sixth cranial nerves in variable combination (Goldsmith, Carmody). Ultimate recovery of ocular motility has occurred in most such reported cases but the site of the nerve injury has not been clarified. Ophthalmic herpes zoster can also be complicated by the occurrence of a delayed, contralateral hemiparesis (Cope and Jones, Gilbert, Hughes, Laws). Hemiparesis usually develops several weeks after the appearance of the facial lesions, and is of variable severity and duration. Angiographic studies have demonstrated arteritis of intracranial vessels in the form of segmental arterial constrictions in these cases, presumably the result of inflammatory changes of the vessel wall (Pratesi et al., Walker et al.).

Motor weakness of the lower motor neuron type is infrequent with herpes zoster. Although not the most common form of motor zoster, perhaps the best known is that in which the seventh cranial nerve is affected. The association of a unilateral peripheral facial paralysis with herpetic lesions in the external auditory canal and on the external ear has been known as the Ramsay Hunt syndrome since his description in 1907. Hunt postulated herpetic involvement of the geniculate ganglion in such cases; however, the concept was refuted by Denny-Brown et al. Few pathologic studies have been done in patients with so-called "geniculate herpes zoster," although inflammation of the seventh nerve itself seems more likely than primary involvement of the geniculate ganglion (Sachs and House). It is probable that acquired peripheral facial palsy without associated external ear lesions can also occur from varicella-zoster virus infection (Ohsaki et al.).

Motor zoster is unusual at any age, and only a few cases in childhood have been described (Nachman). Among 1,210 cases of herpes zoster, Thomas and Howard found only 61 with segmental zoster paresis. Muscle weakness in such cases usually occurs within two weeks after onset of the rash. It is possible, however, for weakness to precede the rash (Fee and Evarts), resulting in a perplexing diagnostic problem until the characteristic vesicular lesions appear on the skin. Segmental weakness usually corresponds anatomically to the cutaneous eruption but in exceptional cases, the distributions of the two types of involvement are slightly different. Eventual recovery of the motor disturbance is the rule in most cases. In addition to involvement of any of the four limbs or the abdomen or face, the diaphragm can be affected secondary to phrenic nerve dysfunction (Brostoff). The site of the pathology in segmental motor zoster remains speculative. Some authors favor anterior rootlet inflammation while others postulate anterior horn cell involvement. Electromyography of affected muscle groups reveals denervation potentials indicating lower motor neuron dysfunction.

One of the most notable characteristics of herpes zoster is its tendency to occur in patients with malignancy, especially the leukemias and the lymphomas (Keidan and Mainwaring). The increased incidence of zoster with malignancy has been clearly documented by Feldman and colleagues who studied 1,132 children with cancer, of whom 9 percent developed herpes zoster at some point during their illness. Children at greatest risk were those with Hodgkin's disease, in whom 22 percent experienced infection with herpes zoster. Ten percent of patients with acute lymphoblastic leukemia-lymphosarcoma and 5 percent with solid tumors had zoster. Three deaths were attributable to herpes zoster among the total group of 101 children whose neoplastic disease was complicated by this infectious illness. Sokal and Firat found that among 600 patients with Hodgkin's disease, 8 percent had one or more episodes with infection with the varicella-zoster virus. In ten of 49 cases, the cutaneous lesions became disseminated, indicating the decreased resistance of such patients to this viral illness. Factors that have been suggested which predispose the patient with lymphoma to herpes zoster include neoplastic masses in proximity to nerve rootlets, local irradiation therapy, immunosuppressive and corticosteroid therapy, and altered immune conditions secondary to the neoplastic disease itself. An interesting recent observation that might explain the increased risk of zoster dissemination in some cancer patients is the decreased ability of such patients to produce vesicle-fluid interferon (Armstrong et al.).

The usual uncomplicated course of varicella in children with agammaglobulinemia with abnormalities in humoral immunity is evidence of the importance of the cell-mediated immune system in recovery from this illness. The presence of defects in cellular immune function in some patients with malignant disease, such as Hodgkin's disease, is perhaps one of the primary reasons for the high susceptibility of such patients to herpes zoster and for the frequent severity of the illness (Ruckdeschel et al.). Herpes zoster frequently heals more slowly and is more often associated with disseminated skin lesions in the immunosuppressed host than in the otherwise normal person. The illness is rarely life-threatening, however, and eventual recovery occurs in the majority of instances.

An increased incidence of zoster has also been observed in immunosuppressed patients without neoplastic disease. Rifkind found six cases of herpes zoster in a series of 73 patients with renal transplantation who had received immunosuppressive and irradiation therapy. Complement-fixation antibody response to the infection was not inhibited or delayed in these persons. In five of the six patients, the onset of zoster occurred one to three weeks after local irradiation to the implanted kidney.

Diagnosis

Clinical recognition of herpes zoster is usually not difficult because of the characteristic appearance of the rash and its radicular distribution. Diagnostic difficulty is encountered when there is localized pain or sensory complaints before the eruption develops, or in the rare patient with segmental muscle weakness that precedes the cutaneous vesicles. A zoster-like eruption in the newborn infant or young child requires serologic and virologic confirmation, since Herpes simplex can produce similar lesions (Music et al., Mok).

Morphologic evidence that a vesicular eruption is due to a virus of the herpes group can be accomplished by the Tzanck test, performed by examination of cells from the base of a cutaneous vesicle. Scrapings from the floor of the lesion are stained appropriately, with most favoring the Giemsa stain. Multinucleated giant cells with eosinophilic nuclear inclusions is consistent with infection of the herpes group (Fig. 14–17). Where facilities permit, specific immunofluorescent antibody testing of the scraping will confirm the diagnosis of varicella-zoster infection. Cells of the same type have been observed from smallpox lesions (Heydenreich) but the latter is now only a theoretical consideration.

Complement-fixation antibody response to the varicella-zoster virus is a reliable diagnostic method, with the most valuable information resulting from a four-fold or greater antibody titer rise between the acute and convalescent specimens. A single titer of greater than one to 64 is considered significant because it is considerably higher than expected in the normal population. Since herpes zoster represents reactivation subsequent to a previous infection with the same virus, titer rises are often more rapid and much higher than occurs with chickenpox in childhood. Following zoster infection, a significant antibody titer persists for a few months, but by one year detectable antibodies are usually absent.

The most definitive laboratory diagnostic method for varicella-zoster infection is viral isolation and identification. Fluid from zoster vesicles inoculated into appropriate tissue culture will reveal the typical cytopathogenic effect of the herpes group of viruses. Absolute identification of the isolated agent is on the basis of serologic tests. Virus may be isolated from vesicles for several days after their appearance but cannot be obtained once dried lesions have evolved. Gold reported isolation of the virus from the cerebrospinal fluid in two patients with herpes zoster who did not have clinical evidence of encephalitic manifestations.

Meningoencephalitis complicating herpes zoster does not usually create diagnostic problems from the etiologic standpoint, as is the case with Herpes simplex. The presence of encephalitis is evident from the clinical signs in addition to the electroencephalographic findings and the results of the cerebrospinal fluid examination. Herpes zoster can be assumed to be the etiologic agent because of the presence of the vesicular eruption and, thus, brain biopsy is usually neither indicated nor necessary. A note of caution is necessary, however, in cancer patients with herpes zoster who suddenly manifest signs of

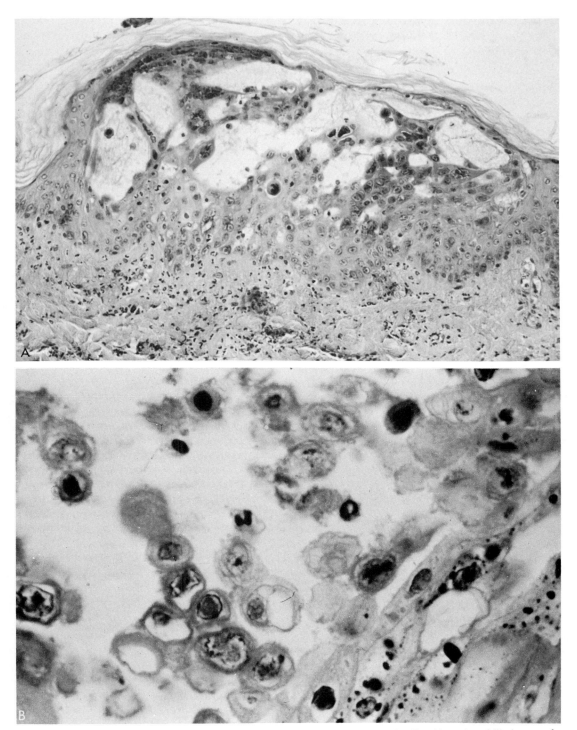

Figure 14–17.   Varicella-zoster skin vesicle. *A,* Multinucleated giant cells and cells with eosinophilic intranuclear inclusions, consistent with infection with a virus of the herpes group. *B,* Higher power with several cells bearing darkly stained intranuclear inclusions.

intracranial infection. Viral and bacterial disease may coexist in the immunologically suppressed patient, and the meningeal signs may be due to suppurative meningitis rather than to the anticipated varicella-zoster virus.

Herpes Zoster Meningoencephalitis

Herpes zoster encephalitis is an unusual disorder in any age group but especially in childhood. Of the few cases reported in children, some are open to question regarding accuracy of diagnosis (McCormick), while others have been in the form of a mild aseptic meningitis (Nachman) rather than encephalitis. Of 14 cases of zoster encephalitis described by Appelbaum and colleagues, three were under the age of 20 years.

Central nervous system complications in patients with herpes zoster include aseptic meningitis, meningoencephalitis, and encephalomyelitis. The symptoms and signs exhibited are determined by the location of the inflammatory reaction. Zoster myelitis is the rarest of these conditions but may be fatal, as in the adult case reported by Rose et al. The majority of cases of encephalitis have the onset of cerebral symptoms two to eight days following the development of the cutaneous eruption. Symptoms are usually of abrupt onset and include headache, fever, vomiting, and change in sensorium. Meningeal signs are present in most, while other manifestations, including long tract signs, pathologic reflexes, or cranial nerve palsies, are variable from case to case. Convulsions have not often been reported and papilledema has been observed only in the minority of described cases. The severity and outcome of zoster encephalitis runs the gamut of possibilities. In some cases, the illness is brief followed by complete recovery, while in others deep coma rapidly proceeds to death. The limited number of proven cases of zoster encephalitis reported to date is insufficient to allow accurate statements about expected frequency of complete recovery, recovery with sequelae, or death. If any conclusions can be drawn, the relatively few autopsy cases thus far reported would suggest that death from this disease is infrequent. From a study of eight cases of Herpes zoster meningoencephalitis, Norris et al. concluded that the illness usually tends to be relatively benign, although severe neurologic involvement can occur.

Cerebrospinal fluid examination in most cases of zoster meningoencephalitis reveals a lymphocytic pleocytosis, with the total number of cells ranging from ten up to several hundred per cu. mm. A cellular response itself does not necessarily indicate encephalitic involvement since cells in the spinal fluid are often present in otherwise uncomplicated cases of cutaneous herpes zoster. Among the 14 cases of encephalitis described by Appelbaum et al., two were notable because of the absence of cells in the spinal fluid. Other usual findings in the cerebrospinal fluid in zoster encephalitis include a normal or elevated glucose content and a protein value in the range of 60 to 200 mg. per 100 ml.

Pathogenesis and Pathology. Several different pathogenetic mechanisms have been postulated because of the variable findings on microscopic examination described by different investigators (Thalhimer, Denny-Brown et al.). Most authors have favored direct viral invasion of brain but others considered the encephalitis to be the result of an "allergic" reaction, or due to activation of another latent virus in the brain. In 1969, McCormick et al. described two cases of varicella-zoster encephalomyelitis associated with reticuloendothelial malignancies. In one case, varicella-zoster virus was isolated from the brain, and in both, virus particles were demonstrated in the brain by electron microscopic examination. In addition to multiple areas of perivenous encephalomalacia and macrophage infiltration, numerous type A intranuclear inclusion bodies were seen. Hogan and Krigman reported an adult with Herpes zoster myelitis which was particularly notable because of the absence of an underlying malignant disease. Viral invasion was proved by the finding of Cowdry type A inclusion bodies in addition to the isolation of the varicella-zoster virus from the spinal cord.

It is probable that direct viral invasion of the brain and spinal cord is the usual cause of the encephalitic manifestations in zoster encephalitis (Fig. 14–18), thus resembling the neuropathology of Herpes simplex encephalitis. Whether visceral dissemination of the virus in patients with Herpes zoster is promoted by cytotoxic or corticosteroid therapy, or is more likely to occur in association with leukemia or lymphoma, remains unclear. A viremic phase has been demonstrated in children with malignancies who develop cutaneous zoster lesions (Feldman et al., 1977).

Treatment

In certain situations, it is important to prevent varicella-zoster virus infection when ex-

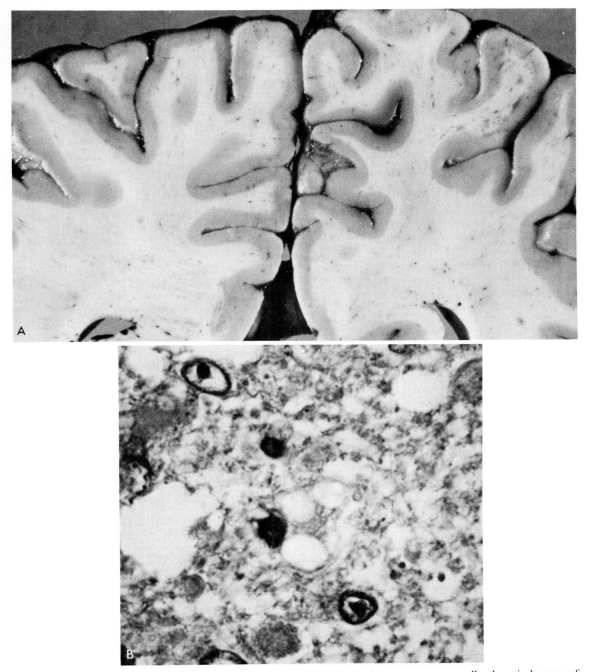

Figure 14–18. Zoster encephalitis. *A,* Coronal section of the brain shows numerous small subcortical zones of necrosis. Pathologically, the changes in zoster meningoencephalitis are generally less necrotizing than in encephalitis caused by Herpes simplex. *B,* Intranuclear inclusion bodies in the spinal cord in zoster encephalomyelitis.

posure to an active case is recognized. This is especially true of children at risk of severe varicella, including those with certain immunodeficiency diseases, leukemia, lymphoma, or patients taking immunosuppressive drug therapy. Zoster immune globulin, prepared from plasma from patients recovering from herpes zoster, has been shown to be an effective preventive agent if given within 72 hours after exposure (Brunell et al., Brunell and Gershon, Gershon et al.). Zoster immune globulin is administered in dosage of 1.25 to

5 ml., depending on body weight of the patient (Morbidity and Mortality Weekly Reports, Feb. 17, 1973). Zoster immune plasma has also been used effectively to prevent varicella in the high-risk patient (Balfour et al.). It has the advantage of greater accessibility compared to zoster immune globulin but the disadvantage of possible transmission of hepatitis. Preliminary experimental trials with a live varicella virus vaccine have shown favorable results regarding both a serologic response to the vaccine and clinical evidence of protection against the development of the illness (Asano et al.). The vaccine has been administered to a limited number of children on corticosteroid therapy and with leukemia in remission without apparent adverse effects and with seroconversion (Izawa et al.).

Principles of management of the patient with varicella-zoster meningoencephalitis are similar to those with encephalitis in general, including fluid and electrolyte therapy, prevention of hyperthermia, and control of seizures. The use of corticosteroids for control of brain swelling is a controversial matter but probably should be avoided because of possible adverse effects on the immune mechanisms. Treatment with cytosine arabinoside was considered for a while but the drug was not shown to be beneficial, has unacceptable toxic effects when given systemically, and was found to prolong the cutaneous eruption in some compromised patients (Stevens et al., Betts et al.). Initial reports of the use of adenine arabinoside (Ara-A) for treatment of cutaneous zoster in immunosuppressed patients have been promising. When given in the early stages of the illness, there has been cessation of new vesicle formation and accelerated clearance of virus from the skin lesions (Whitley et al., 1976, Ch'ien et al., 1976). There is little information regarding the value of adenine arabinoside in patients with visceral dissemination of the varicella-zoster virus, including encephalitis.

CYTOMEGALOVIRUS INFECTIONS

The term cytomegalovirus was proposed by Weller, Hanshaw, and Scott in 1960 for a group of viruses that had long been referred to as the salivary gland viruses. They are classified within the herpes group and, when examined with the electron microscope, are similar to Herpesvirus hominis and the varicella-zoster virus although minor differences have been described (Smith and Rasmussen).

Similar to the latter, the cytomegalovirus consists of a nucleic acid core of deoxyribonucleic acid enveloped by a capsid with 162 capsomeres and surrounded by one or more membranes. A remarkable feature of human infection with this virus is the induction of abnormal cellular enlargement, a response referred to as cytomegalia, and affected cells exhibit characteristic intranuclear or intracytoplasmic inclusion bodies (Fig. 14–19).

Inclusion-containing cells in tissues of stillborn fetuses and newborn infants were observed as early as 1904 (Jesionek and Kiolemenoglou, Ribbert). The generalized nature of the illness and the peculiar cellular morphology suggested an infectious process to examiners but most assumed it to be some form of parasitic infestation. Goodpasture and Talbot (1921) observed such cells in the lungs, liver, and kidney of an infant and proposed the term "cytomegalia" to emphasize the abnormal cellular enlargement that often was associated with intranuclear inclusion bodies. Farber and Wolbach (1932) described the frequent occurrence of inclusion bodies within salivary glands of children with a variety of fatal diseases and also described two childhood cases in which identical inclusion-bearing cells were widely distributed in multiple organs. Evidence gradually accumulated which suggested that the disseminated neonatal and infantile disease which often resembled erythroblastosis and which was characterized by cytomegalia with inclusions was one of viral origin.

In 1947, Cappell and McFarlane described two infants who died of multiple organ system involvement in which characteristic cytomegalic cells were present. The authors postulated that the illness was the result of dissemination of the salivary gland virus, and thereafter the terms "cytomegalic inclusion disease" or "salivary gland virus infection" became popular (Wyatt et al., Smith and Vellios). Fetterman, in 1952, showed that clinical diagnosis of cytomegalic inclusion disease was possible by demonstration of large cells containing inclusion bodies within the urine of affected infants. The procedure was helpful for a period of time but was never entirely reliable, and it is now infrequently used since more accurate diagnostic methods have become available.

Isolation of the cytomegalovirus was accomplished in 1956 and provided the impetus for the subsequent development of reliable diagnostic methods as well as the ability to define more clearly the clinical spectrum of infection due to this group of viruses. In-

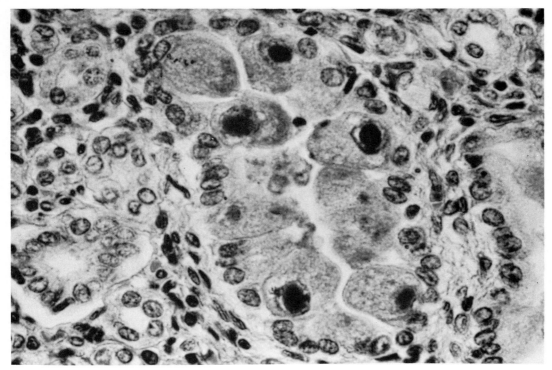

Figure 14–19. Characteristic cellular changes in congenital cytomegalovirus disease. Moderately enlarged renal tubule cells (cytomegalia), and typical type A intranuclear inclusions.

dependently and almost simultaneously, Smith in St. Louis, Rowe and associates in Bethesda, and Weller and colleagues in Boston succeeded in cultivating the cytomegalovirus in vitro, the circumstances of the discovery in each laboratory having been reviewed by Weller (1970).

For several years both before and after isolation of the cytomegaloviruses, they were considered to be of clinical importance primarily because of their ability to cause a disseminated, neonatal condition referred to as cytomegalic inclusion disease. The disorder was then believed to be almost uniformly fatal and was recognized to result from maternal to fetal transmission, which caused in the infant an illness with signs similar to those of congenital infections produced by rubella, toxoplasmosis, and syphilis. Isolation of the cytomegalovirus in 1956 was eventually followed by many observations and investigations which led to a gradual unfolding of the true scope of this viral group in regard to its significance as a cause of human disease. It is now known that more than 1 percent of newborn infants are excreting the virus in the urine and that most such infants are clinically normal, at least in the newborn period. The classic disseminated neonatal disease is, ac-

cordingly, an unusual expression of the infection at one end of a broad spectrum of involvement.

Serologic studies have shown that few humans pass through adult life without contracting the infection. Clinical illness in the healthy adult, however, is unusual, a feature which has made it difficult to document the time during pregnancy when maternal to fetal transmission occurs. In addition to its silent prevalence in the healthy population, the cytomegalovirus has come to be recognized as an important opportunistic invader in the debilitated or immunosuppressed patient in whom tissue damage from the infection can occur regardless of age. Disseminated infection with this virus has also been identified in a child with disturbance in neutrophil motility in whom serum inhibitors of leukotaxis were present (Soriano et al.) and in another with Wiskott-Aldrich syndrome (Root and Speicher).

Clinical Spectrum

The most devastating illness attributable to the cytomegaloviruses is the congenital form acquired in utero from an asymptomatic mother. The severe, disseminated form of this syndrome is, in fact, infrequent and especially so in comparison to the more benign ways the virus affects humans. The manifestations of neonatal cytomegalic inclusion disease are legion, as described below, and include in variable combination hepatosplenomegaly, jaundice, thrombocytopenia, purpura, pneumonitis, and chorioretinitis. The most crippling aspect of the disease results from chronic encephalitis, with a predilection for the virus to affect periventricular tissues. Such cerebral involvement is recognized clinically in the form of microcephaly, abnormalities of muscle tone, and developmental retardation (Haymaker et al.).

With the development of serologic and viral isolation methods for diagnosis of cytomegalovirus infections, it became apparent that most infected newborns did not exhibit the disseminated form, which had become recognized as the classic expression of the illness. Weller and Hanshaw (1962) advised that neonatal hepatitis without other organ system involvement could result from intrauterine transmission of this virus. Chorioretinitis as the only evidence of congenital infection also has been established (Lonn) and it is now known that the brain may be the only organ sufficiently affected to give rise to clinical signs. It is likewise probable that low birth weight without other clinical abnormalities can result from intrauterine infection.

The spectrum of neonatal infection thus extends from severe fetal or neonatal disease incompatible with life to the more common state of asymptomatic infection, evidenced by cytomegaloviruria, which tends to be notably chronic, persisting for months or even years after the infection is acquired. Starr and Gold tested 507 newborn infants and found eight (1.5 percent) to be excreting the virus in the urine. Seven were without signs of illness and one revealed cerebral calcifications on x-ray. Stern identified three of 118 (2.5 percent) apparently healthy newborn infants to be viral excreters, although two were subsequently shown to be mentally retarded. A series of 2,147 infants studied by Starr and colleagues revealed 1.2 percent to be congenitally infected with the cytomegalovirus. The remarkable prevalence of the cytomegalovirus in the neonate, now documented repeatedly in recent years, places it as the most common congenital viral infection (Melish and Hanshaw).

Among infants between two and five months of age, approximately 8 percent have been found to excrete the virus in the urine (Anderson et al.), and up to five years, 10 percent are viral excreters (Stern). Serologic studies in adults have indicated that approximately 80 percent show evidence of prior infection with the cytomegalovirus (Rowe et al.). In comparison to the 1 to 2 percent of newborns who shed the virus in the urine, 3 percent of women during pregnancy were found to have cytomegaloviruria by Feldman, and more than 6 percent in the series of Reynolds and colleagues. The latter authors also found that 11 percent of women at some point during pregnancy had the virus in cervical excretions.

The seemingly high urine and cervical excretion rate of this virus during pregnancy has been interpreted by some investigators to mean that pregnancy provokes reactivation of latent virus. Stagno and colleagues (1975), however, found that the prevalence of cytomegalovirus was low during the first trimester of pregnancy and gradually rose until the third trimester when over 11 percent were excreting the virus. Recovery of virus from the cervix in a nonpregnant control group occurred in 9.4 percent, suggesting to the authors that the early part of pregnancy is associated with a suppressing effect on viral excretion, which late in gestation comes to approximate the rate of viral shedding found in the young adult female population generally. Cytomegalovirus has been identified in semen and has been found to persist therein for 14 months in an immunologically normal, asymptomatic adult male (Lang et al.). This observation has suggested the possibility of venereal transmission of this virus.

The newborn infant, therefore, can acquire the virus in utero, contract it by direct contamination during delivery, or become colonized through ingestion of contaminated breast milk or by exposure to other sources of infection in the postnatal environment. Although the newborn child excreting cytomegalovirus is usually asymptomatic, Hanshaw (1971) has cautioned that inapparent neonatal infection is not always innocuous and that some infants will subsequently exhibit neurologic damage in the form of deafness, hyperactive behavior, or mental retardation. He earlier proposed (1966) that fetal or neonatal cytomegalovirus infection may be an important cause of microcephaly in children who had no prior extraneural manifestations of the infectious process. Reynolds and colleagues have also provided evidence suggesting that inapparent congenital cytomegalovirus infection is an important cause of auditory damage and, perhaps, of mental retardation. Among 51 infants born with subclinical cytomegalovirus infection, Stagno et al. (1977) found seven (13.7 percent) subsequently to be affected with significant sensorineural hearing loss. They calculated therefrom that perhaps as many as 4,000 infants are born per year in this country who will have handicaps of hearing impairment resulting from this infectious illness. Certain cases of infantile myoclonic seizures with hypsarrhythmia on electroencephalography may also represent an unrecognized manifestation of congenital cytomegalovirus infection (Feldman and Schwartz).

Acquired cytomegalovirus infection in the older child or adult is usually inapparent but may result in long-term viral excretion in urine or saliva, as occurs in the infant. The most common form of symptomatic infection with this virus in the otherwise normal older child or adult is an illness resembling infectious mononucleosis with atypical lymphocytes in blood, a negative heterophile antibody titer, and significant liver involvement (Toghill et al., Reller, Lui and Chang). This condition is referred to as cytomegalovirus mononucleosis and is generally a benign disease except for the possibility of persistent hepatic damage. Cytomegalovirus is the most common cause of heterophile-negative mononucleosis, a syndrome that can also be produced by the Epstein-Barr virus, *Toxoplasma gondii,* and the rubella virus (Horwitz et al.). Acute cytomegalovirus encephalitis in immunologically normal older children or adults is acknowledged to be quite rare but has been reported (Duchowny et al., Phillips et al.). Acquired cytomegalovirus infection has also been implicated as a cause of Menetrier disease (Leonidas et al.) and has been linked with the Guillain-Barré syndrome (Klemola et al., Jordan et al.). In one series of 92 patients with Guillain-Barré disease, substantially elevated complement fixation titers were found in 30 (33 percent) and four-fold or greater alterations on serial tests were identified in 21 (Dowling et al.). Among 94 patients with acute polyneuropathy studied by Schmitz and Enders using virus-specific IgM techniques, 10 were shown to have had a preceding and recent cytomegalovirus infection. Acute brachial plexus neuropathy has also been attributed to cytomegalovirus infection (Duchowny et al.).

Cytomegalovirus and Hematologic Malignancy. Of greater importance in the older child or the adult is the role of the cytomegalovirus as an opportunistic pathogen in patients with neoplastic disease such as leukemia or lymphoma (Peach). Infection with cytomegalovirus in such patients is associated with a variable degree of clinical involvement, ranging from asymptomatic viral excretion to severe illness. Cox and Hughes evaluated 36 leukemic children excreting cytomegalovirus in urine or saliva and found that 11 had viremia at some point during the study. Only three of the 11 had significant clinical disease therefrom, two with chorioretinitis and one with a mononucleosis-like syndrome.

Although symptoms caused by viral invasion do occur in some immunosuppressed patients, in most instances evidence of cytomegalovirus infection is unexpectedly found at necropsy or is identified by viral isolation techniques during life. Cytomegalic inclusion-bearing cells may be found in multiple organs, often with little additional inflammatory response. The lungs may be the only organ containing evidence of the disease and is the most consistently involved tissue when the process is disseminated (Gottman and Beatty, Bodey et al.). Pulmonary involvement with cytomegalovirus represents a spectrum ranging from asymptomatic disease to rapidly progressive interstitial pneumonitis leading to death (Abdallah et al.). The gastrointestinal tract, adrenal glands, and liver also frequently reveal histologic evidence of cytomegalovirus infiltration in such cases. Disseminated infection with this virus can play a significant role in the terminal illness in the patient with hematologic malignancy. However, the symptoms and signs in the terminal illness cannot usually be attributed solely to this virus, and other infections are commonly present as well (Armstrong et al.). Such infections are frequently bacterial in origin but in some cases include other opportunistic invaders such as *Toxoplasma gondii* (Luna and Lichtiger) or Aspergillus species (Meyer et al.). Simultaneous pulmonary involvement with cytomegalovirus and *Pneumocystis carinii* has been recorded in many cases (Abdallah et al.).

Cytomegalovirus and Renal Transplantation. Another condition with altered immune mechanisms in which the cytomegaloviruses have achieved prominence is that of renal transplantation (Anderson and Spencer) and, to a lesser degree, cardiac transplantation (Schober and Herman). The cytomegaloviruses are now recognized to be the most common cause of viral infection in patients receiving transplanted kidneys. Recipients of renal transplants are usually chronically debilitated from their underlying disease and, to prevent rejection of the transplanted kidney, require large doses of drugs and radiation therapy that produce immunologic suppression. In many such patients, the infection identified at necropsy cannot be correlated with a well-defined clinical syndrome in life, but in others it gives rise to characteristic cytomegalovirus mononucleosis (Balakrishnan et al.) or to fatal pneumonia (Craighead et al.).

Visual symptoms secondary to cytomegalovirus retinitis have also been recognized in patients following renal transplantation (Aaberg et al.). Retinitis is the first manifestation of systemic infection with this virus in some cases, and generally is associated with distinctive ophthalmoscopic findings. The process can be either unilateral or bilateral, and results in retinal vessel sheathing, retinal edema, and scattered hemorrhages and exudates (Murray et al.). The degree of visual impairment depends on the extensiveness of the retinal inflammatory response but can become severe as the exudative process advances. Dorfman described three post-transplant patients who developed neurologic manifestations prior to death in whom cytomegalovirus pneumonia was associated with a diffuse glial nodule encephalitis but with relatively little inflammatory response in the meninges or in the .cerebral perivascular spaces.

Kanich and Craighead identified evidence of cytomegalovirus infection at necropsy in eight of 25 (32 percent) renal transplant recipients, while Rifkind and colleagues recorded its presence in 27 of 51 (53 percent) post-transplant cases at autopsy. Of 15 patients who died following renal transplantation, 10 (66 percent) were found to have evidence of cytomegalovirus infection by Craighead and associates. Fine et al. performed a clinical study on 21 children who received renal allografts and observed that eight of the 21 (38 percent) had cytomegaloviruria and that clinical symptoms could be attributed to the viral infection in four of the eight cases. Recent studies have indicated an incidence of cytomegalovirus infection of 50 to 90 percent in renal transplant patients (Kanich and Craighead, Fiala et al.), of whom somewhat less than half develop clinical symptoms of illness.

In patients who are seropositive prior to transplantation, it is assumed that transplantation and immunosuppression results in reactivation of latent infection. Studies by Ho and colleagues, however, indicated that when seronegative patients received kidneys from seropositive donors, there was a very high incidence of post-transplant cytomegalovirus infection and that the transplanted kidney was the source of infection. They also demonstrated that infection manifested by clinical illness was considerably higher in previously seronegative patients with primary infection compared to patients who had been seropositive prior to transplantation. The study by Betts et al. yielded similar findings in that among 16 seronegative patients who received a transplant from a seropositive donor, 14 experienced clinical illness, which included fever, pneumonitis, or evidence of hepatic dysfunction. The authors suggested that allograft loss and primary cytomegalovirus infection following transplantation might be reduced by avoiding the use of a seropositive donor for a seronegative recipient. There is also evidence that the immunosuppressive effect of primary cytomegalovirus infection in previously seronegative transplant patients may be an important factor that increases the patient's susceptibility to opportunistic fungal infections (Chatterjee et al.).

Cytomegalovirus and the Post-perfusion Syndrome. The post-perfusion syndrome has been recognized since 1960 (Kreel et al.) as an illness occurring two to six weeks after cardiopulmonary bypass for open-heart surgery, lasting one to four weeks, and manifested by a mononucleosis-like syndrome including fever, splenomegaly, abnormal liver function tests, and atypical lymphocytes in the peripheral blood. It has been estimated to occur in 3 to 7 percent of patients undergoing open-heart surgery (Lang et al.) and since 1966 has been recognized to be related to the cytomegalovirus (Kääriänen et al.). The illness has been mild in most reported cases and is followed by eventual complete recovery. The cytomegalovirus is now believed to be the cause of the disorder and most likely is transmitted to the patient in transfused blood administered at the time of the operative procedure (Embil et al., Lang and Hanshaw, Caul et al.). Recent studies by Prince et al. have supported the concept of cytomegalovirus transmission by blood transfusion in addition to evidence that seroconversion occurs more commonly in immunosuppressed patients receiving multiple blood transfusions as compared to those with normal immune mechanisms.

Congenital Cytomegalic Inclusion Disease

Although neonatal disseminated cytomegalic inclusion disease in its classic form is infrequently seen by practitioners, the congenital form of infection in all of its varied expressions is believed to have considerable medical and social significance. Of the 1 percent or more of newborn infants excreting the virus, Hanshaw (1971) has estimated that approximately 10 percent will exhibit neurologic sequelae, although most will have no abnormal neurologic signs in the neonatal period. Weller (1971) has calculated that as many as 3,700 infants are born each year in this country who will have some degree of cerebral damage induced by cytomegalovirus infection, while Stagno et al. (1977) have estimated that up to 4,000 infants born each year will have a significant degree of auditory impairment from the illness, a large percentage of whom are subclinically infected at birth.

Congenital cytomegalovirus infection manifested by severe symptomatic disease is transplacentally transmitted to the fetus in most instances, although direct contamination during delivery from an infected maternal uterine cervix is the most common cause of perinatally acquired subclinical infection (Reynolds et al., 1973; Granström et al.). Intrauterine blood transfusion or administration of blood products to the infant after birth are other possible sources of infection (Yeager). In addition, the infant may become infected from others in the environment at any time after birth and either remain asymptomatic or develop overt signs of disease. Low-birth-weight infants requiring prolonged intensive care treatment for respiratory distress syndrome may be at particular risk. Ballard et al. identified in sick, pre-term infants a rather distinct syndrome characterized by hepatosplenomegaly, transient deterioration in respiratory status, and lymphocytosis. The illness in these infants occurred several weeks after birth and was usually assumed to be caused by bacterial sepsis until cytomegalovirus was isolated.

When the clinical signs of infection are first noted at two or three months of age, it may be impossible to be certain whether the infection was contracted in utero, during delivery, or postnatally. The time of acquisition of fetal infection has remained obscure in most cases, largely owing to the usual inapparent nature of the illness in the adult. Documentation of the time of maternal infection is also made difficult since cytomegalovirus excretion in the urine may persist for months or up to two years after the infection is acquired. Davis et al. recorded the occurrence of cytomegalovirus mononucleosis in the first trimester of pregnancy, with the virus subsequently being recovered from fetal tissues at 22 weeks' gestation. It is generally assumed that fetal infection can occur at any time during pregnancy and that maternal to fetal transmission most often follows a primary maternal infection during the viremic stage. To support this concept are observations that indicate that a young, primiparous mother is more likely to give birth to a cytomegalovirus-infected infant (Starr et al.). In the series of congenitally infected infants reported by Melish and Hanshaw, the mean maternal age was 19.4 years and 70 percent of the mothers were primigravidas.

Abnormalities of the newborn infant indicative of a teratogenic effect of the cytomegalovirus are distinctly unusual but have been described, especially in regard to cerebral anomalies. Certain authors (Dudgeon) have used the observation that anomalies are rare in infected infants as evidence suggesting that fetal infection with cytomegalovirus more often occurs after the period of organogenesis, as compared to the common first trimester fetal involvement with maternal rubella. Furthermore, maternal cytomegalovirus infection during pregnancy, even with placental involvement, is not invariably followed by transmission of the illness to the child (Hayes and Gibas).

Because fetal involvement has been regarded as the result of primary maternal infection, it has generally been assumed that if one child is infected at birth, subsequent pregnancies will be spared. This has been true in the majority of cases, but examples of congenital cytomegalovirus infection in consecutive pregnancies have been reported (Krech et al., Embil et al.), although the second-born infected infants have not had severe clinical illness. Stagno and colleagues (1973) described two siblings born three years apart, each infected in utero by the same or a closely related strain of cytomegalovirus. Either endogenous reactivation or reinfection was postulated, with the virus being transmitted to the second fetus in spite of maternal immunity. The concept that intrauterine transmission of cytomegalovirus occurs predominantly with primary maternal infection is less certain than was previously suspected. Maternal genital infections with cytomegalovirus are commonly recurrent, and such recurrences no doubt contribute to perinatally acquired infections in the new-born infant. Their role as a factor in intra-uterine transmission of the virus to the fetus is unclear; however, Stagno et al. (1977) have provided evidence that maternal immunity may not provide protection to the fetus against cytomegalovirus infection.

The neonate or young infant with overt signs of cytomegalovirus infection usually has evidence of multiple organ system involve-ment. The signs, however, are variable from case to case, as is their time of appearance and the severity of the disease. The birth weight of infected infants is frequently ab-normally low in comparison to the duration of the pregnancy. In the series of Weller et al. (1962), the average birth weight was 2,279 grams. Among the 20 affected infants de-scribed by McCracken and associates, the birth weight of 14 was less than 2,500 grams. Furthermore, postnatal growth retardation is common in those who survive. The severely affected infant may expire within hours after birth, or may survive for variable periods of time thereafter. Hepatomegaly, splenomeg-aly, jaundice, thrombocytopenia, purpura, hemolytic anemia, pneumonitis, chorioretin-itis, and encephalitis are the most common manifestations of congenital cytomegalic in-clusion disease and may all be present in the infant devastated by the illness (Medearis) (Fig. 14–20). Chorioretinitis is estimated to occur in approximately 25 percent of infants with cytomegalic inclusion disease (Lonn). It may be unilateral or bilateral and can either be of little significance or result in severe vis-ual loss.

Enlargement of the liver with associated biochemical abnormalities of hepatic dys-function represents the most constant feature of the disease and may be present at birth or be first noted days or weeks thereafter (Weller and Hanshaw). In addition, pro-longed hepatosplenomegaly can be the only sign of congenital cytomegalovirus infection (Stern and Tucker). Jaundice is prolonged in some cases, lasting for weeks or months, and hepatosplenomegaly may persist into the sec-ond year of life (Emanuel and Kenny). Chronic hepatitis persisting through the first year will give rise to secondary complications in some, including growth failure due to in-testinal malabsorption, as well as hypocal-cemia and osteomalacia (Kopelman et al.). Thoene et al. described one child with con-

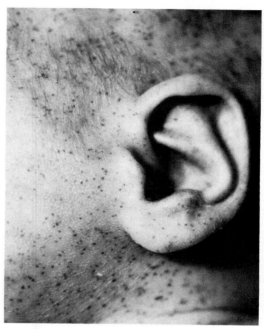

Figure 14–20. Congenital cytomegalovirus infection. Characteristic petechial rash that can be associated with several congenital infections. Infant is 2 hours of age, birth weight 2100 grams. The child has hepatospleno-megaly and a platelet count of 15,000. She developed tachypnea at 6 hours of age due to viral pneumonitis and subsequently developed intractable cardiac failure resulting from myocarditis. Cytomegalovirus was re-covered from the urine. The child expired at 14 days of age.

genital or perinatal cytomegalovirus infection who was found to have tyrosinemia at age three months. The enzymatic disturbance re-sulting in the defect in tyrosine metabolism was believed to have been the result of he-patic dysfunction secondary to the viral ill-ness.

Hemolytic anemia is more common with cytomegalovirus infection in infancy than with other congenital infections and may be present in the newborn period or develop at a later date. Hemolysis usually occurs in con-junction with other aspects of the systemic disease but can be the presenting feature of the illness (Franklin). Hemolytic anemia in combination with hepatitis within 24 hours after birth is easily confused with erythro-blastosis secondary to blood group incompat-ibility and, furthermore, both conditions may exist simultaneously (McEnery and Stern). An additional unusual presenting sign asso-ciated with severe hepatitis in the newborn is marked abdominal distention as the result of massive ascites (Frank et al.).

Indirect inguinal hernia has been observed

in infants with cytomegalic inclusion disease and appears to be more than coincidence. Of 14 male infants with congenital cytomegalovirus disease examined by Lang, 11 had developed inguinal hernia by five months of age. McCracken et al. found two of eight infected infants to have bilateral inguinal hernia. A rare manifestation of the disease in the newborn is the presence of long bone lesions on x-ray consisting of longitudinal bands of lucency in the distal femoral metaphysis, identical to those seen in congenital rubella (Andersen et al. 1979, Graham et al.). An additional rare occurrence is the coexistence of congenital cytomegalic inclusion disease with toxoplasmosis (Demian et al.), aspergillosis (Buttrick and Roberts), or *Pneumocystis carinii* pneumonia (Hamperl). The child with congenital cytomegalovirus infection and pulmonary *Pneumocystis carinii* described by Weinberg and associates was of particular interest because it was the first described to have monoclonal macroglobulinemia.

Regardless of the severity of the disease or whether it is manifested by involvement of a single organ or of multiple organs, the infected newborn who survives is likely to continue to shed the virus in the urine for months or even years. In addition, a prolonged postnatal cytomegaloviremia has also been demonstrated following congenital infection (Lang and Noren). The persistence of the virus in blood despite the presence of circulating antibody is perhaps explained by its intracellular location, which provides protection from destruction by specific antibody. Studies by Lang and Noren have suggested that circulating leukocytes may play an important role in maintaining a state of cytomegalovirus latency.

Neurologic Involvement. The brain may be entirely spared in the infant with congenital cytomegalic inclusion disease but, if affected, it is often the site of the most devastating aspect of the illness. Some infants exhibit manifestations of severe cerebral disease soon after birth in the form of convulsions, hypotonicity or spasticity, and obvious microcephaly. In others, the neurologic signs are initially minimal or absent but become apparent several months later in the form of developmental delay or as the rate of head growth lags behind expectations. Cerebral involvement is most widely recognized as part of the spectrum of multiple organ system disease in this condition, but it is now known that the brain can be selectively affected with no signs of dysfunction of other organ systems (Walker and Tobin). Microcephaly is the single most constant reflection of cerebral disease due to the intrauterine encephalitis, and is often associated with generalized ventricular enlargement due to the encephaloclastic effect of the virus on brain tissue. Of the 17 infants with generalized disease reported by Weller and Hanshaw, 14 had microcephaly at birth or developed it subsequently. In the series of 18 infants with congenital cytomegalic inclusion disease described by McCracken et al., seven were found to be microcephalic during the first few weeks of life.

A distinctive periventricular calcification is observed roentgenographically in some cytomegalovirus-induced microcephalic children (Daurelle et al., Haymaker et al.) (Fig. 14–21). This pattern of calcification lining enlarged ventricles in a baby with an abnormally small head is so infrequently seen in other conditions that it alone is strongly suggestive of the diagnosis of congenital cytomegalovirus infection. Should the infant survive and the ventricles enlarge markedly, the subependymal calcifications may become so dispersed that their periventricular location will no longer be apparent (Fig. 14–22). In this case, the calcification may acquire the disseminated distribution more characteristic of congenital toxoplasmosis. The periventricular location of the calcification seen on x-ray provides a visual marker of the susceptibility of the subependymal matrix of the lateral ventricles to cytomegalovirus encephalitis acquired in utero. Most affected infants with such calcification have it already present in the newborn period, but in some it will develop in the following weeks or months.

Hydrocephalus manifested by progressive ventricular distention and abnormal head enlargement can occur but is far less common than microcephaly. Hanshaw (1971) stated that of more than 100 symptomatic infants with cytomegalic inclusion disease that he had studied, only two developed hydrocephalus. Regardless of the type of cerebral involvement, the infant who manifests neurologic signs of cytomegalovirus infection in the neonatal period can be expected to have lasting deficits, should he survive. Microcephaly and cerebral calcifications are particularly poor prognostic signs, and all infants with these findings will have severe sequelae (Berenberg and Nankervis).

The neuropathology of congenital cytomegalic inclusion disease is that of a chronic encephalitis with characteristic cellular transformation and with certain regional predilec-

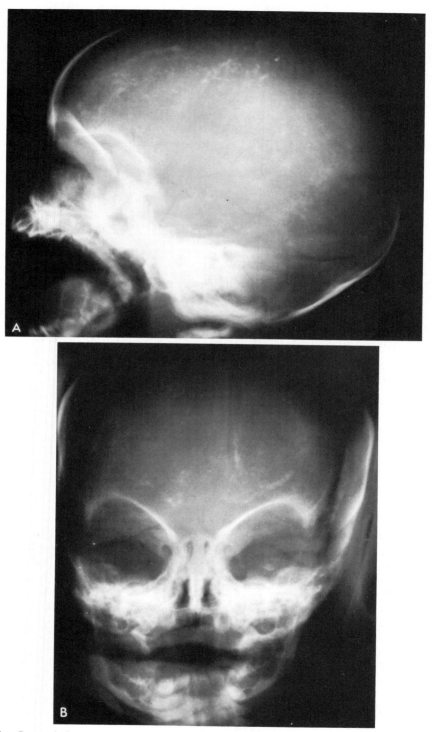

Figure 14–21.   Congenital cytomegalovirus disease. *A,* Lateral skull x-ray of a 5-week-old infant. There is faint intracerebral calcification which lies in a periventricular location and outlines markedly distended lateral ventricles. *B,* AP view of the skull allows more precise localization of the calcium deposition in the periventricular subependymal tissue. (Courtesy of Dr. William McAlister and Dr. Arthur Prensky, St. Louis, Missouri.)

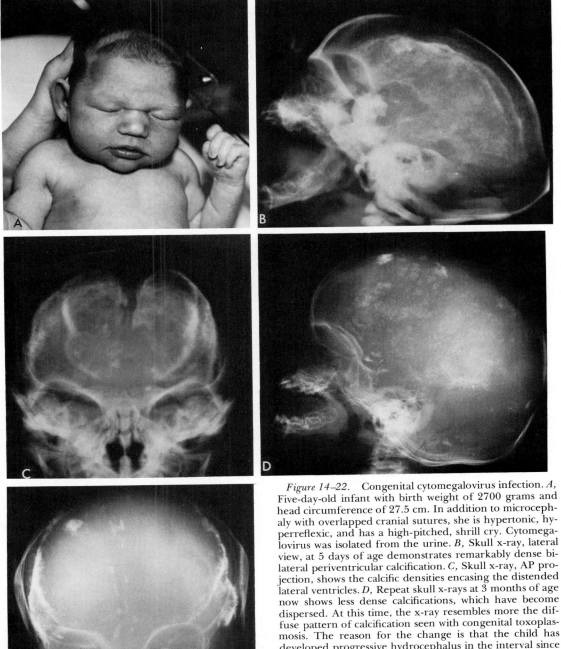

Figure 14–22.   Congenital cytomegalovirus infection. *A,* Five-day-old infant with birth weight of 2700 grams and head circumference of 27.5 cm. In addition to microcephaly with overlapped cranial sutures, she is hypertonic, hyperreflexic, and has a high-pitched, shrill cry. Cytomegalovirus was isolated from the urine. *B,* Skull x-ray, lateral view, at 5 days of age demonstrates remarkably dense bilateral periventricular calcification. *C,* Skull x-ray, AP projection, shows the calcific densities encasing the distended lateral ventricles. *D,* Repeat skull x-rays at 3 months of age now shows less dense calcifications, which have become dispersed. At this time, the x-ray resembles more the diffuse pattern of calcification seen with congenital toxoplasmosis. The reason for the change is that the child has developed progressive hydrocephalus in the interval since the first x-ray at 5 days and the ventricles have now become extremely dilated, displacing the calcification peripherally. *E,* The periventricular location of the calcification can still readily be ascertained on the AP view of the skull. The curvilinear pattern outlines the size of the lateral ventricles. Although this case is an excellent demonstration of periventricular calcification caused by congenital cytomegalovirus infection, it is atypical and unusual because of the extreme density of the calcific deposits.

tions. In general there is less meningeal and parenchymal inflammatory response than occurs with other types of viral encephalitis (Fig. 14–23). The periventricular subependymal matrix, especially of the lateral ventri-

cles and to a lesser degree of the third and fourth ventricles, is most consistently and severely affected. In these regions, one sees glial cells and, less often, abnormally enlarged neurons that contain intranuclear and,

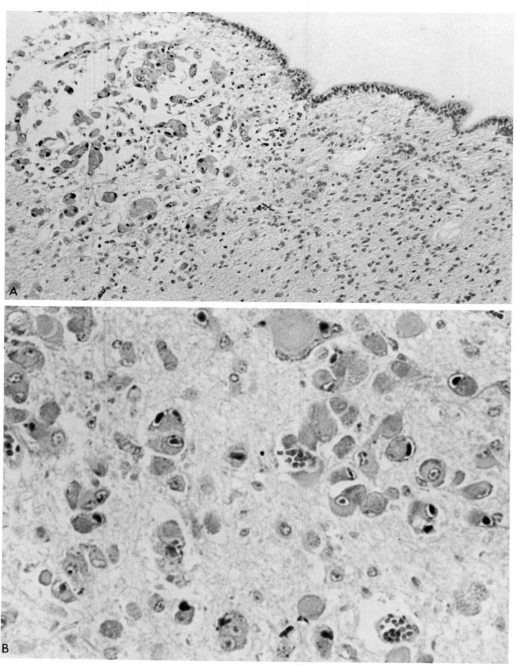

Figure 14–23. Congenital cytomegalovirus infection with encephalitis. Death occurred at 10 weeks of age. *A,* Small area of necrosis in the periventricular subependymal matrix. There is cellular enlargement, with some cells containing intranuclear inclusions. *B,* Higher-power view demonstrating the variable size of enlarged cells and many type A inclusions.

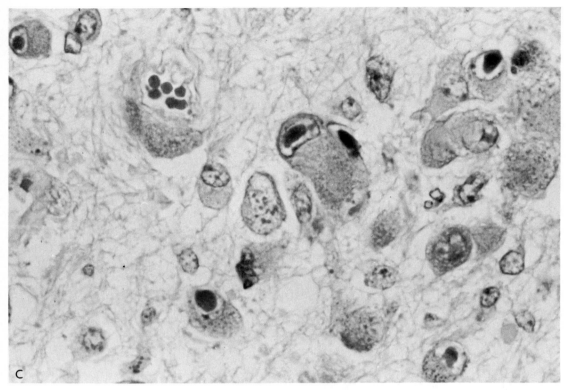

Figure 14–23 Continued. C, Prominent intranuclear inclusions.

occasionally, intracytoplasmic Cowdry type A inclusion bodies. When severely damaged, the regions adjacent to the ventricles appear necrotic and contain various amounts of mineral deposits, which correlate with the roentgenographic findings mentioned above (Elliott and Elliott) (Fig. 14–24). Destruction of the ependymal lining and granular ependymitis is commonly seen adjacent to the more severe periventricular lesions. Microglial nodules and astrocytosis are also found in different regions of the cerebral white matter.

Gross observation of the brain reveals it to be abnormally small in severely affected cases but with mild to moderate lateral ventricular distention. Ventricular enlargement is usually the result of injury and subsequent atrophy of brain tissue and thus is associated with a reduced size of the head in most instances. This is in contrast to the findings in congenital toxoplasmosis, in which hydrocephalus with increased pressure signs and head enlargement commonly results from aqueductal obstruction, an event that generally does not occur with cytomegalic inclusion disease (Wolf and Cowan).

There are several reports in which poly-microgyria vera coexisted with other pathologic evidence of congenital cytomegalovirus infection (Bignami and Appicciutoli, Crome and France, Diezel), suggesting the possibility of a teratogenic effect of the infection when it occurs in early intrauterine life. Porencephaly has also been described (Navin and Angevine), as well as cerebellar hypoplasia combined with cerebral anomalies (Ceballos et al.). Other anomalies, such as congenital cardiac disease, have only rarely been mentioned, but McCracken et al. described abnormalities of the first embryonic arch such as micrognathia and high arched palate in five of 18 infants with congenital cytomegalic inclusion disease.

Diagnosis

Congenital and neonatal infections due to cytomegalovirus, toxoplasma, rubella, Herpesvirus hominis, syphilis, and various bacterial agents all share common clinical findings and thus enter into the differential diagnosis. Coxsackie B virus in the newborn also may produce a disseminated illness with hepatitis, myocarditis, pneumonia, and en-

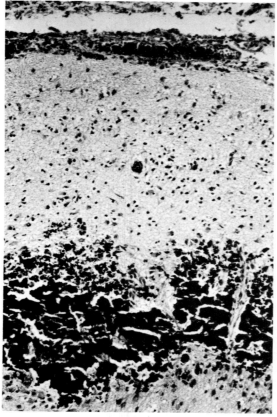

Figure 14–24. Congenital cytomegalovirus disease with encephalitis. Heavy periventricular calcium deposition which corresponds to that observed on skull x-rays.

and young infant is dependent upon the results of the appropriate cultures, serologic studies, and histologic examinations.

Laboratory confirmation of cytomegalovirus infection is based on virologic, serologic, and morphologic methods of examination. Demonstration of inclusion-bearing cells in the urine (Fetterman, Naim) is no longer widely used because of its lack of specificity and the frequency of false-negative examinations. An electron microscopic method for the rapid detection of herpesvirus in the urine has been described and is a procedure with considerable promise despite its technical complexity (Lee et al.). The lack of absolute specificity of this technique for the cytomegalovirus is only a slight distraction because of the infrequency with which other herpesviruses are found in the urine in the newborn age group. Isolation of the virus in urine is now the method of choice for the detection of either symptomatic or inapparent cytomegalovirus infection. The characteristic cytopathogenic effect in tissue culture may be observed as early as two days but, if not, the inoculated cultures should be observed for six weeks before it is assumed that infection is absent. In general, the cytopathogenic effect in tissue culture occurs more slowly with the cytomegaloviruses than with Herpes simplex. Because of the lability of the virus, shipped specimens may be inadequate for diagnostic purposes.

Clinicians should attempt to isolate the virus not only from urine but also from pharyngeal specimens and leukocytes in buffy coat in suspect cases. Because of the prevalence of cytomegaloviruria in infancy and early childhood, it must be recognized that demonstration of the virus in the urine does not necessarily provide proof that the child's illness is caused by this virus. The virus cannot usually be isolated from cerebrospinal fluid in congenitally infected infants, although recovery therefrom has been reported (Jamison and Hathorn).

Serologic methods available include the neutralization and complement fixation tests, with most laboratories using the latter for diagnostic purposes. In addition to being less cumbersome, the complement fixation test has the advantage of detecting antibody against most strains of the cytomegalovirus, using a single antigen (Hanshaw 1969). Complement-fixing antibodies appear a few weeks after the primary infection and reach peak levels four to eight weeks after onset of the disease. Because the complement fixation test

cephalitis. Certain differences are common, but not constant, with the various neonatal infections and thus cannot be used as conclusive evidence to separate the possibilities. For example, hydrocephalus is more often seen with congenital toxoplasmosis, while microcephaly is more common with cytomegalic inclusion disease or congenital rubella. Intracranial calcification, if present, tends to be more diffuse in the neonate with toxoplasmosis and is periventricular in location in cytomegalovirus infection, although a certain degree of overlap does occur. Cataracts and cardiac disease are common expressions of congenital rubella but are not always present. Neonatal Herpesvirus hominis infection is usually manifested as an acute, febrile disorder with vesicular skin lesions or conjunctivitis but also has features that overlap with the previously discussed congenital infections. Although the clinical differences are often diagnostically suggestive, differentiation of the various infections in the newborn depends on IgG immunoglobulins which are transplacentally transferred, the newborn's antibody titer usually corresponds to the antibody titer in the serum of the mother. Absence of antibody at birth can be assumed to nearly exclude congenital cytomegalovirus infection, but a positive complement fixation titer can occur either passively from the mother in an uninfected infant or in the presence of disease. Serial titers are necessary to distinguish passively transferred antibody from the mother, which should diminish or disappear by four months of age. A rising titer or one persisting beyond six months of age is indicative of cytomegalovirus infection acquired before birth or in early infancy. Krech et al. state that the complement fixation test may give negative results after six months of age in the congenitally infected infant, although neutralizing antibodies persist at high titers. This has been attributed to the inability of antibody produced by the infant to fix complement in the presence of the cytomegalovirus antigen.

The fluorescent antibody test (Anderson and Michaels, Hanshaw 1969) for detection of specific IgM antibody is the most reliable serologic test for diagnosis of congenital cytomegalovirus infection in the first year after birth. Since macroglobulins (IgM) of maternal origin are not transmitted to the fetus, the presence of specific IgM antibody in the newborn infant's serum is indicative of congenital infection. After the first year, the production of IgM antibody by the congenitally infected infant may decline and subsequently become undetectable. The other limitation of the test is its relative lack of availability. Counterimmunoelectrophoresis for the detection of precipitating antibodies to cytomegalovirus has been shown to be a useful diagnostic tool for identification of acute infection in adults, but its application in the newborn period remains to be studied (Fortunato et al.).

Treatment

Management of the infant with cytomegalic inclusion disease is essentially conservative, including methods for the control of seizures, if present, and for the prevention of dangerous levels of serum indirect bilirubin. Anemia and hemorrhagic complications may also require attention in the neonatal period. The infected infant shedding cytomegalovirus in saliva or urine must be considered a potential threat to other infants in the hospital nursery. Appropriate isolation precautions should be instituted to prevent contamination of other infants or hospital attendants who are pregnant.

Specific drug therapy for symptomatic congenital cytomegalovirus infection has been unsatisfactory in general and remains a topic of continued investigation. Corticosteroids have been favored by some (Birdsong et al., van Gelderen) but, except for their effect on thrombocytopenia or hemolytic anemia, proof of benefit is lacking. Feigin et al. treated a newborn infant with cytomegalic inclusion disease with floxuridine (5-fluorouracil-2-deoxyriboside), but they observed no beneficial effect and were still able to isolate the virus from saliva and cerebrospinal fluid at the termination of the therapy. The drug is no longer recommended for treatment in this age group, in part because it has been shown to interfere with cellular maturation of the cerebellum in newborn animals (Langman et al.). Cytosine arabinoside has had relatively few trials with cytomegalovirus disease but results likewise have been disappointing (Emodi et al., Kraybill et al., McCracken and Luby). Although the drug is effective against the virus in vitro, it has not been demonstrated to be of clinical value in the infected patient. There is only limited information to date regarding the antiviral effects of adenine arabinoside for cytomegalovirus infections. Clinical trials have not been impressive although reduction in urine excretion of the virus following treatment has been observed in congenitally infected infants (Ch'ien et al., 1974). Adenine arabinoside has not been found to be effective for cytomegalovirus infection in immunosuppressed patients (Ch'ien et al., 1974; Rytel and Kauffman). Investigators have recently developed and tested a live cytomegalovirus vaccine that will stimulate complement fixation and neutralizing antibody production in susceptible persons with minimal side effects (Elek and Stern). It is hoped that further experiments with the vaccine will lead to its wide-scale availability and subsequent elimination of mental retardation caused by this viral disease.

EPSTEIN-BARR VIRUS INFECTIONS

Infectious mononucleosis was long considered to be an infectious disease of viral origin, but it was not until the Epstein-Barr virus was found to be the cause that many aspects of the epidemiology of the disorder and variations of its clinical expression came to be understood. In 1964 in London, Epstein and Barr identified a virus of the herpes group which they had isolated from cell lines from Burkitt's African malignant lymphoma, a virus subsequently named the Epstein-Barr virus. During laboratory investigation with the virus, Gertrude and Werner Henle at the University of Pennsylvania observed that one of their technicians developed antibodies to the virus following infectious mononucleosis. Additional studies led to the publication in 1968 implicating the Epstein-Barr virus as the cause of infectious mononucleosis (Henle et al., 1968).

In the same year, Niederman, McCollum, and the Henles demonstrated by immunofluorescent tests the absence of antibodies against the Epstein-Barr virus in pre-illness sera of 29 persons but their presence in all during and following infectious mononucleosis. They showed these antibodies to be distinctive from the more transient heterophil antibodies and, after reaching peak levels three to four weeks after onset of symptoms, to persist indefinitely thereafter. Also in 1968, Evans and colleagues at Yale confirmed by serologic testing the causative role of the Epstein-Barr virus in infectious mononucleosis and demonstrated that the majority of young adults with this illness will develop positive heterophil-antibody tests. Subsequent investigations have revealed that specific immunoglobulin M type antibodies are detectable early in the illness (Banatvala et al.), that the virus can be recovered from leukocyte cultures from the ill patient (Diehl et al.), and that the Epstein-Barr virus persists in oropharyngeal secretions long after clinical recovery from infectious mononucleosis (Miller et al.).

Infectious mononucleosis in past years was widely regarded as a rare disease in young children because the characteristic clinical syndrome was rarely observed and the heterophil test was generally negative in patients in this age group with ill-defined febrile illnesses. With the development of serologic tests to document the occurrence of Epstein-Barr virus infection, it became evident that primary infection with this virus, conferring life-long immunity, occurs frequently in children under 10 years of age but usually in asymptomatic or atypical fashion and usually without positive heterophil antibody tests (Sumaya, Tamir et al.).

Conversely, the primary infection in the young adult leads to a much higher incidence of clinically manifested infectious mononucleosis, most often associated with a positive heterophil antibody response. In certain underdeveloped countries, the majority of children have experienced primary infection by 10 years of age, resulting in few young adults remaining who are susceptible. Delayed primary infection in societies with more favorable socioeconomic conditions accounts for a greater incidence of the clinical illness in more highly developed countries (Epstein and Achong). Thus, the availability of a serologic tool for diagnosis has brought about considerable enlightening of the epidemiologic features of this infection in recent years.

The virus is now recognized as a very common one, with the highest incidence of primary infection occurring in the first decade. Infection in the young child is usually inapparent or atypical in pattern but conveys permanent immunity. Antibodies against the Epstein-Barr virus can be demonstrated in this age group but the heterophil response has usually been negative, although recent studies have shown that, with highly sensitive assay methods, the heterophil antibody response is greater in young children than was previously suspected (Fleisher et al.). Infection with the Epstein-Barr virus is less frequent in young adults but much more often is expressed in the form of heterophil-positive infectious mononucleosis. In older persons, the illness becomes progressively less common but can occur even in the elderly (Horwitz et al.). Heterophil-negative mononucleosis-like syndromes can be caused by other organisms, the most common being the cytomegaloviruses. The rubella virus and *Toxoplasma gondii* are additional causes of a clinical syndrome with features like those of infectious mononucleosis (Horwitz et al.).

Clinical Aspects

The clinical manifestations and severity of infectious mononucleosis can vary considerably in certain patients, although in most the symptoms and signs are quite stereotyped. The incubation period has not been precisely identified but is believed to range between 30 and 50 days. Sore throat, headache, malaise, and anorexia are the customary initial complaints, followed by intermittent fever, which persists for a week or two. The pharyngeal region is usually erythematous, sometimes with petechial lesions and occasionally with a gray membrane reminiscent of that which occurs in diphtheria. Generalized adenopathy, which is mildly tender in some regions, is a constant feature of the illness, and is associated with splenomegaly in approximately 85 percent of older children with the illness (Baehner and Shuler). Hepatomegaly is much less common, although biochemical evidence of hepatic involvement is present in most. Maculopapular rash occurs only infrequently in patients with infectious mononucleosis unless ampicillin is administered, which, for uncertain reasons, provokes an eruption in a high percentage (Patel, Pullen et al.). Duration of illness is usually one to three weeks, with gradual resolution of symptoms being followed by eventual complete recovery in the great majority. The illness is generally a benign one, although death can occur on rare occasion from splenic rupture, secondary to neurologic complications, from coincident bacterial infections, or from hepatic involvement (Harries and Ferguson).

The white blood cell count is variable from patient to patient and depends somewhat on the stage of the illness. Leukopenia is occasionally observed in the first week but thereafter the total count is usually from 10,000 to 20,000 per cu. mm. and occasionally will be substantially higher. Neutrophils may predominate in the early stages followed by a change to an absolute lymphocytosis, which is one of the hallmarks of the disease. Dow-

ney and McKinley in 1923 first described the atypical lymphocytes which usually constitute 10 to 20 percent of the mononuclear cells and are characterized by their larger than normal size, abundant basophilic cytoplasm, and irregular or ragged margins (Fig. 14–25). Granulation and vacuolation cause the cytoplasm of these cells to appear foamy. The shape of the nucleus is oval or bean-shaped and may be either centrally placed within the cell or located in an eccentric position. The nuclear chromatin of some Downey cells resembles that of a lymphoblast and thereby raises consideration of the possibility of acute leukemia until the bone marrow is examined. Atypical lymphocytes, as well as the development of heterophil antibodies and certain of the clinical manifestations of the illness, are now believed to reflect the host immune response rather than direct viral effects (Miller). Atypical lymphocytes described above are seen not only in infectious mononucleosis but also occur in a variety of viral illnesses, especially in younger children. In most such illnesses, however, they number less than 10 percent, whereas in infectious mononucleosis they usually constitute more than 10 percent of the lymphocytic cell population. Unusual hematologic complications of infectious mononucleosis include thrombocytopenia (Clarke and Davies, Radel and Schorr) and acute hemolytic anemia (Shashaty et al.).

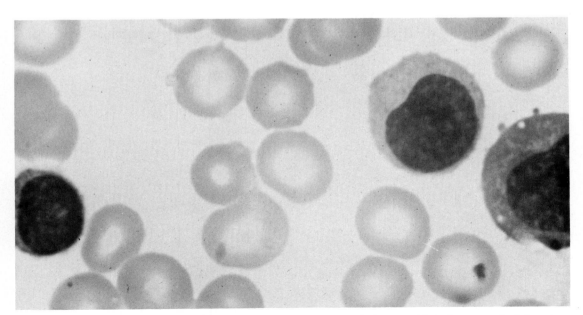

Figure 14–25. Downey cells, infectious mononucleosis. There is a single normal lymphocyte to the left and two atypical lymphocytes (Downey cells) which are enlarged and contain foamy cytoplasm and indented nuclei.

The Paul-Bunnell heterophil agglutination test has been a valuable diagnostic method for identification of this illness since the first description of the procedure in 1932 (Paul and Bunnell). The basis for the test is the presence of heterophil agglutinins for sheep red cells in the serum of patients with infectious mononucleosis. Similar agglutinins may be present in normal individuals or in those who have received horse serum and must be distinguished by absorption tests. Those present in patients with infectious mononucleosis are absorbed by ox cells but not by guinea-pig kidney. The absolute titer after absorption required for diagnosis has not been established, but a single titer of 1:112 is usually considered sufficient. A number of spot or slide tests have become available as screening tests to identify this antibody. They have the advantage of rapidity and simplicity of performance but can yield false positive responses. The heterophil antibody usually appears in serum during the first or second week of the illness and after rising to peak levels will subsequently decline, disappearing in two to six months. Heterophil antibodies appear to be distinct from the variety of antibodies provoked by the Epstein-Barr virus, and, the relationship between them remains unclear. Heterophil antibodies fail to develop during inapparent infection with the virus, and, infrequently, will not develop in young adults with Epstein-Barr virus infectious mononucleosis. Because heterophil antibody is a macroglobulin of the 19S type, it is not usually found in the cerebrospinal fluid of patients with infectious mononucleosis who do not have neurologic involvement (Gutmann). The cerebrospinal fluid heterophil test may be positive, however, in those with neurologic complications.

There are now various immunofluorescent methods for the detection of distinct Epstein-Barr virus antibodies (Henle et al., 1974), although the tests are not widely performed. Antibodies against viral capsid antigen rise rapidly after onset of illness and peak in three to five weeks, thereafter declining but remaining in some measure for life. Antibodies to early antigen also become elevated rapidly but then diminish, disappearing a few months after onset of infection. Because of the rapid elevation of these antibody titers after onset of illness, they have often peaked when the first serum specimen is obtained. Thus, a significant rise between paired serum specimens sometimes cannot be demonstrated, but the absolute value or a significant decline in titer will be sufficient for diagnosis. Specific Epstein-Barr virus antibodies have been demonstrated in cerebrospinal fluid by indirect immunofluorescence in a child with infectious mononucleosis with encephalitis (Joncas et al.). Another recently developed technique which holds promise as a method of documenting recently acquired infection is the demonstration of Epstein-Barr virus-specific IgM, which is consistently present in the acute stage but disappears within two to three months (Schmitz and Scherer, Edwards and McSwiggan).

These specific tests for the Epstein-Barr virus are of particular value for the diagnosis of infections in childhood, which are frequently heterophil-negative. They have also allowed diagnosis of Epstein-Barr virus infections in certain patients in the adult age group with the Guillain-Barré syndrome or acute encephalitis in which other signs of infectious mononucleosis were not distinct and heterophil tests were not diagnostic (Grose et al., 1975).

Neurologic Complications

Central Nervous System Complications

Neurologic complications of infectious mononucleosis have been recognized since 1931 when Johansen described aseptic meningitis and Epstein and Dameshek reported encephalitis in patients with this disease. A variety of different central nervous system complications have subsequently been identified but are not regarded to be common (Table 14–3). The incidence of significant complications involving either the central or peripheral nervous system has been variously

Table 14–3. Neurologic Conditions Associated with the Epstein-Barr Virus

Aseptic meningitis
Acute meningoencephalitis
Transverse myelitis
Reye's syndrome
Cofactor provoking subacute sclerosing panencephalitis
Intracranial hemorrhage secondary to thrombocytopenia
Guillain-Barré syndrome
Brachial plexus neuropathy
Cranial or peripheral mononeuropathy
Acute cerebellar ataxia
Acute papillitis

quoted by different authors. Bergin esti- mated neurologic complications to occur in 1 to 2 percent, while Silverstein and col- leagues found neurologic involvement in more than 5 percent of 144 patients with in- fectious mononucleosis.

When neurologic manifestations do occur, they may appear with the more general symptoms and signs of infectious mononu- cleosis, or they may not develop until the dis- ease has nearly run its course (Gautier- Smith). Neurologic involvement can also pre- cede other features of the systemic illness (Smith, Epstein and Dameshek) or occur in the absence of other signs of infectious mon- onucleosis and without the development of heterophil antibodies (Grose et al., 1975). This is especially true in children in whom encephalitis caused by this virus is more likely to occur without diagnostic elevations of het- erophil antibodies, and in whom other signs of infectious mononucleosis can be easily overlooked (Lange et al.). Such cases are identified only by the performance of specific Epstein-Barr virus antibody tests. In keeping with the peak age of occurrence of infectious mononucleosis, most cases of encephalitis or encephalomyelitis with the illness have been in young adults. The same complications, however, are well known in children (Karpin- ski, Silver et al., Thelander and Shaw, Walsh et al.). A single case of fatal cerebral hemor- rhage secondary to thrombocytopenia in an adult with infectious mononucleosis has been reported (Goldstein and Porter).

The spectrum of central nervous system in- volvement in infectious mononucleosis varies from aseptic meningitis, manifested by head- ache, nuchal rigidity, and cerebrospinal fluid pleocytosis, to severe encephalitis associated with deep coma and other signs of diffuse cerebral dysfunction. Acute cerebellar ataxia can complicate Epstein-Barr virus infection in the absence of other encephalitic signs and, in rare instances, will occur without other physical signs typical of infectious mononu- cleosis (Cleary et al.). The virus of infectious mononucleosis has now been identified as one of several that can provoke Reye's syn- drome with an acute, severe encephalopathy and fatty infiltration of the liver and other viscera (Dorman et al., Rahal and Henle).

Encephalitis may be ushered in by gener- alized convulsions, but more often the child complains of headache and exhibits lethargy, drowsiness, or mental confusion before more florid manifestations such as seizures or un- responsiveness supervene. Focal signs includ- ing hemiplegia or dysphasia accompany clin- ical evidence of more generalized cerebral dysfunction in some cases (Smith). Enceph- alomyelitis refers to clinical evidence of both cerebral and spinal cord disease (Slade, Am- bler et al.) and may be combined with cranial or peripheral nerve deficits in certain pa- tients. In addition to spinal cord involvement present in patients with encephalomyelitis, infectious mononucleosis on rare occasion is complicated by an isolated acute transverse myelitis (Cotton and Webb-Peploe). Bladder or bowel dysfunction, paraplegia or quadri- plegia, and a sensory level characterize this disorder. Signs of cerebellar dysfunction such as ataxia or nystagmus may coexist with or even precede other symptoms of encephalitis (Dowling and Van Slyck, Landes et al., Las- celles et al.). Severe chorea accompanied other signs of meningeal irritation and cere- bral involvement in the case described by Friedland and Yahr.

Cerebrospinal fluid in children with any of the neurologic complications of infectious mononucleosis usually reveals variable abnor- malities, a lymphocytic pleocytosis being the most common. The cellular response is not usually marked and may consist of only a few lymphocytes per cu. mm. or up to 200 cells in certain cases. Detailed inspection of the cel- lular response in the cerebrospinal fluid may identify atypical lymphocytes identical to those in the blood (Finkel). Opening pressure and protein content can be either normal or elevated, while the cerebrospinal fluid glu- cose is normal. Prognosis is good in the ma- jority of patients with encephalitis complicat- ing infectious mononucleosis, and permanent sequelae are unusual but not unknown (Slade, Silverstein et al.).

Neuropathological descriptions have been sparse, since most patients with encephalitis associated with Epstein-Barr virus infection recover. Histologic findings of cases that have been reported have been variable and have not resolved the issue of whether the cerebral process is an encephalopathy secondary to the host immune response to the infection or is best termed an acute encephalitis with viral invasion of brain giving rise to cytotoxic in- jury. In some cases, the predominant abnor- malities in the brain have been degenerative in type, with only minimal evidence of an in- flammatory response (Bergin, Custer and Smith, Dolgopol and Husson). An occipital lobe biopsy in one case revealed perivascular lymphocytic infiltration in the white matter in addition to myelin destruction interpreted to represent an "allergic" encephalopathy (Ambler et al.). In the autopsy described by Sworn and Urich, the brain was swollen and showed a heavy inflammatory response in the cerebral cortex with perivascular lymphocytic cuffing and lymphocytic infiltration within the parenchyma. The white matter revealed some degree of edema but only slight inflammatory changes. The pathology was judged to be consistent with an acute encephalitis by the authors.

An additional point favoring viral invasion of the central nervous system in patients with neurologic signs is the finding of Epstein-Barr virus antibody in cerebrospinal fluid (Joncas et al.). Antibody in cerebrospinal fluid is not anticipated in patients with uncomplicated infectious mononucleosis (Hochberg et al.). In at least one case of encephalitis complicating infectious mononucleosis, the Epstein-Barr virus has been isolated from cerebrospinal fluid (Halsted and Chang). While the pathogenesis of this neurologic complication of Epstein-Barr virus infection remains unclear, perhaps it is somewhat variable from patient to patient, with viral invasion of the brain giving rise to direct cytotoxic effects and host immune response of different intensity in different patients.

The most recent association of the Epstein-Barr virus with central nervous system disease is its possible role in the production of subacute sclerosing panencephalitis. Feorino et al. have described three children with this illness in whom evidence of measles virus was found but was preceded by infectious mononucleosis. In all, the duration of subacute sclerosing panencephalitis was unusually short. In one, there was evidence of measles virus as well as Epstein-Barr virus within brain tissue (Hochberg et al.). The authors proposed that the Epstein-Barr virus is perhaps one of several viruses that can activate a latent measles virus infection by altering immune mechanisms, thus precipitating the clinical syndrome of subacute sclerosing panencephalitis.

Peripheral Nervous System Complications

There are several reports of peripheral or cranial nerve involvement in patients with infectious mononucleosis, but the total number of cases included indicates the infrequency of these complications. Isolated cranial nerve dysfunction has only rarely been observed in

this disease and is usually transient with complete recovery expected. Unilateral oculomotor nerve palsy in a ten-year-old boy with infectious mononucleosis was reported by Nellhaus. Davidson and Salter described an adult with infectious mononucleosis who developed bilateral facial paralysis during the illness in the absence of other evidence of peripheral neuropathy. Despite the localized neurologic involvement in this case, the cerebrospinal fluid contained 30 lymphocytes per cu. mm. Unilateral facial palsy has also been attributed to this infectious illness (Grose et al., 1973). Patients with hypoglossal nerve palsy complicating infectious mononucleosis have been reported by DeSimone and Snyder and by Sibert. In both instances, weakness of the tongue was unilateral and occurred without other cranial nerve involvement. Edema of the optic discs without evidence of increased intracranial pressure has been noted in a few patients (Ashworth and Motto, Piel et al.), presumably as a manifestation of acute optic neuritis secondary to infectious mononucleosis.

Peripheral mononeuropathy also has been observed on rare occasions in patients with infectious mononucleosis, illustrated by the report of Sakena in which long thoracic nerve involvement resulted in serratus anterior paralysis. We have seen a 14-year-old boy with an acute, unilateral brachial neuropathy which developed as the systemic manifestations of infectious mononucleosis were subsiding (Fig. 14–26). Tsairis and colleagues also mentioned the occurrence of acute brachial neuropathy in two patients with infectious mononucleosis. An additional rare variation of neuropathic involvement with infectious mononucleosis is an acute autonomic neuropathy manifested by orthostatic hypotension, abnormalities of sweating, and disturbances of the pupillary reflex mechanisms (Yahr and Frontera).

The most widely recognized peripheral nerve disorder associated with infectious mononucleosis is a symmetrical polyneuropathy of the type referred to as the Guillain-Barré syndrome (Creaturo, Davie et al., Ricker et al.). While this complication has been reported in children (Hiller and Fox), the majority of such patients have been persons in their late teens or early twenties. The onset of this disorder is usually characterized by numbness or weakness of the distal part of the lower extremities, followed by progressive motor dysfunction of the legs in ascending fashion with subsequent weakness of

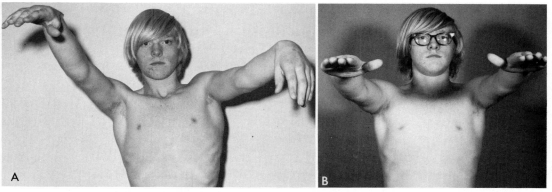

Figure 14–26. Acute left brachial neuropathy associated with infectious mononucleosis in a 14-year-old boy. *A,* During the recovery stage of infectious mononucleosis, the patient first noticed transient pain in the left deltoid region, followed by weakness and decreased reflexes in the left arm. Deltoid, biceps and triceps weakness was moderate in degree, while wrist-drop was complete. *B,* Muscle weakness began to improve 2 to 3 weeks after onset, and recovery was nearly complete 8 weeks after onset.

the arms and hands. Sensory loss may be entirely absent or, at most, is only partially present in the distal regions of the limbs. Bilateral peripheral facial paralysis frequently accompanies generalized weakness, and, less commonly, other cranial nerves are implicated. In severe cases, external ophthalmoplegia and bulbar dysfunction may ensue (Davie et al.), and, if associated with intercostal muscle weakness, creates a threat to life possibly requiring assisted ventilation.

The speed of recovery is usually proportional to the degree and extent of motor weakness at the peak of the illness. Mildly affected patients usually recover completely within three to six weeks after onset. More severely affected persons often require two to six months for restoration of muscle strength and some retain permanent muscle weakness. Reviewing the reported cases up to 1963, Davie et al. found that acute polyneuropathy complicating infectious mononucleosis had been fatal in about 25 percent of the cases. This figure is almost certainly misrepresentative of the seriousness of this type of neurologic complication and perhaps reflects the tendency for fatalities in a usually benign disease to gain entrance into the literature.

A single case of the Fisher syndrome has been described in a child complicating heterophil-positive infectious mononucleosis (Price et al.). This disorder is believed by most to be a variant of the Guillain-Barré syndrome and consists of the sudden onset of external ophthalmoplegia, ataxia, and areflexia.

The cerebrospinal fluid in patients with polyneuropathy secondary to infectious mononucleosis generally contains an increase in protein content and a normal glucose value. Unlike cases of Guillain-Barré disease unassociated with an identifiable infectious illness, a significant number of those secondary to infectious mononucleosis have revealed a lymphocytic pleocytosis (Davie et al.). In certain patients with the Guillain-Barré syndrome, high serum levels of antibodies to the Epstein-Barr virus have been found, even in the absence of clinical evidence of infectious mononucleosis (Grose and Feorino, Grose et al., 1975).

REFERENCES

Aaberg, T. M., Cesarz, T. J., and Rytel, M. W.: Correlation of virology and clinical course of cytomegalovirus retinitis. Am. J. Ophthal. 74:407–415, 1972.

Abdallah, P. S., Mark, J. B. D., and Merigan, T. C.: Diagnosis of cytomegalovirus pneumonia in compromised hosts. Am. J. Med. 61:326–332, 1976.

Abler, C.: Neonatal varicella. Am. J. Dis. Child. 107:492–494, 1964.

Abraham, A. A., and Manko, M. A.: Disseminated Herpesvirus hominis 2 infection following drug overdose. Arch. Intern. Med. 137:1198–1200, 1977.

Abruzzi, W. A.: Varicella encephalitis. N. Y. State J. Med. 61:3912–3915, 1961.

Alford, C. A., Jr., and Whitley, R. J.: Treatment of infections due to Herpesviruses in humans: A critical review of the state of the art. J. Infect. Dis. 133(Suppl.): 101–108, 1976.

Allen, D. W., and Cole, P.: Viruses and human cancer. New Eng. J. Med. 286:70–82, 1972.

Ambler, M., Stoll, J., Tzamaloukas, A., and Albala, M. M.: Focal encephalomyelitis in infectious mononucleosis. Ann. Intern. Med. 75:579–583, 1971.

Amstey, M. S.: Maternal viral infection with adverse results: cytomegalovirus and herpesvirus. Semin. Perinatol. 1:1–10, 1977.

Andersen, H. K., Brostrøm, K., Hansen, B., Leerhøy, J., Pedersen, M., Østerballe, O., Felsager, U., and Mogensen, S.: A prospective study of the incidence and significance of congenital cytomegalovirus infection. Acta Paediat. Scand. 68:329–336, 1979.

Andersen, H. K., Gravesen, J. J., and Iversen, T.: Cytomegalovirus infection among infants admitted to a pediatric department. Acta Paediat. Scand. 61:445–451, 1972.

Andersen, H. K., and Spencer, E. S.: Cytomegalovirus infection among renal allograft recipients. Acta Med. Scand. 186:7–19, 1969.

Anderson, C. H., and Michaels, R. H.: Cytomegalovirus infection: Detection by direct fluorescent-antibody technique. Lancet 2:308–309, 1972.

Appelbaum, E., Kreps, S. I., and Sunshine, A.: Herpes zoster encephalitis. Am. J. Med. 32:25–31, 1962.

Appelbaum, E., Rachelson, M. H., and Dolgopol, V. B.: Varicella encephalitis. Am. J. Med. 15:223–230, 1953.

Armstrong, D., Haghbin, M., Balakrishnan, S. L., and Murphy, M. L.: Asymptomatic cytomegalovirus infection in children with leukemia. Am. J. Dis. Child. 122:404–407, 1971.

Armstrong, R. W., Gurwith, M. J., Waddell, D., and Merigan, T. C.: Cutaneous interferon production in patients with Hodgkin's disease and other cancers infected with varicella or vaccinia. New Eng. J. Med. 283:1182–1187, 1970.

Asano, Y., Nakayama, H., Yazaki, T., Ito, S., Isomura, S., and Takahashi, M.: Protective efficacy of vaccination in children in four episodes of natural varicella and zoster in the ward. Pediatrics 59:8–12, 1977.

Asano, Y., Nakayama, H., Yazaki, T., Kato, R., Hirose, S., Tsuzuki, K., Ito, S., Isomura, S., and Takahashi, M.: Protection against varicella in family contacts by immediate inoculation with live varicella vaccine. Pediatrics 59:3–7, 1977.

Ashworth, J., and Motto, S. A.: Infectious mononucleosis complicated by bilateral papilloretinal edema. New Eng. J. Med. 237:544–545, 1947.

Baehner, R. L., and Shuler, S. E.: Infectious mononucleosis in childhood. Clinical expressions, serologic findings, complications, prognosis. Clin. Pediat. 6:393–399, 1967.

Bahrani, M., Boxerbaum, B., Gilger, A. P., Rosenthal, M. S., and Teree, T. M.: Generalized herpes simplex and hypoadrenocorticism. Am. J. Dis. Child. 111:437–445, 1966.

Balakrishnan, S. L., Armstrong, D., Rubin, A. L., and Stenzel, K. H.: Cytomegalovirus infection after renal transplantation. J.A.M.A. 207:1712–1714, 1969.

Balfour, H. H., Jr., Groth, K. E., McCullough, J., Kalis, J. M., Marker, S. C., Nesbit, M. E., Simmons, R. L., and Najarian, J. S.: Prevention or modification of varicella using zoster immune plasma. Am. J. Dis. Child. 131:693–696, 1977.

Balfour, H. H., Jr., and Lockman, L. A.: Herpesvirus encephalitis following herpes keratitis. Am. J. Dis. Child. 126:357–359, 1973.

Balfour, H. H., Jr., Loken, M. K., and Blaw, M. E.: Brain scan in a patient with herpes simplex encephalitis. J. Pediat. 71:404–407, 1967.

Ballard, R. A., Drew, L., Hufnagle, K. G., and Riedel, P. A.: Acquired cytomegalovirus infection in preterm infants. Am. J. Dis. Child. 133:482–485, 1979.

Banatvala, J. E., Best, J. M., and Waller, D. K.: Epstein-Barr virus-specific IgM in infectious mononucleosis, Burkitt lymphoma, and nasopharyngeal carcinoma. Lancet 1:1205–1208, 1972.

Baringer, J. R.: In: Thompson, R. A., and Green, J. R.: Advances in Neurology, Volume 6. Raven Press, New York, 1974, pp. 41–51.

Baringer, J. R.: Recovery of Herpes simplex virus from human sacral ganglions. New Eng. J. Med. 291:828–830, 1974.

Baringer, J. R., and Griffith, J. F.: Experimental herpes simplex encephalitis: Early neuropathologic changes. J. Neuropath. Exp. Neurol. 29:89–104, 1970.

Baringer, J. R., and Swoveland, P.: Recovery of Herpessimplex virus from human trigeminal ganglions. New Eng. J. Med. 288:648–650, 1973.

Bastian, F. O., Rabson, A. S., Lee, C. L., and Tralka, T. S.: Herpesvirus hominis: isolation from human trigeminal ganglion. Science 178:306–307, 1972.

Becker, F. T., and Buckley, R. P.: Purpura fulminans associated with varicella. Arch. Derm. 94:613–618, 1966.

Becker, W. B., Kipss, A., and McKenzie, D.: Disseminated herpes simplex virus infection. Am. J. Dis. Child. 115:1–8, 1968.

Bell, W. E., and McCormick, W. F.: Increased Intracranial Pressure in Children, 2nd Edition. W. B. Saunders Company, Philadelphia, 1978.

Bellamy, J.: Cytomegalic inclusion body disease occurring in twins. Am. J. Clin. Path. 24:1040, 1954.

Bellanti, J. A., Catalano, L. W., Jr., and Chambers, R. W.: Herpes simplex encephalitis: Virologic and serologic study of a patient treated with an interferon inducer. J. Pediat. 78:136–145, 1971.

Bellanti, J. A., Guin, G. H., Grassi, R. M., and Olson, L. C.: Herpes simplex encephalitis: Brain biopsy and treatment with 5-iodo-2'-deoxyuridine. J. Pediat. 72:266–275, 1968.

Benjamin, D. R., and Ray, C. G.: Use of immunoperoxidase on brain tissue for the rapid diagnosis of herpes encephalitis. Am. J. Clin. Path. 64:472–476, 1975.

Benjamin, S. P., McCormack, L. J., Chatty, M. E., and Dohn, D. F.: Coexistent herpes simplex encephalitis and malignant astrocytoma. Cleveland Clin. Quart. 39:135–143, 1972.

Bennett, D. R., ZuRhein, G. M., and Roberts, T. S.: Acute necrotizing encephalitis. Arch. Neurol. 6:96–113, 1962.

Berenberg, W., and Nankervis, G.: Long-term follow-up of cytomegalic inclusion disease of infancy. Pediatrics 46:403–410, 1970.

Bergin, J. D.: Fatal encephalopathy in glandular fever. J. Neurol. Neurosurg. Psychiat. 23:69–73, 1960.

Berkovich, S., and Ressel, M.: Neonatal herpes keratitis. J. Pediat. 69:652–653, 1966.

Betts, R. F., Freeman, R. B., Douglas, G., and Talley, T. E.: Clinical manifestations of renal allograft derived primary cytomegalovirus infection. Am. J. Dis. Child. 131:759–763, 1977.

Betts, R. F., Zaky, D. A., Douglas, R. G., and Royer, G.: Ineffectiveness of subcutaneous cytosine arabinoside in localized herpes zoster. Ann. Intern. Med. 82:778–783, 1975.

Bignami, A., and Appicciutoli, L.: Micropolygyria and cerebral calcification in cytomegalic inclusion disease. Acta Neuropath. 4:127–137, 1964.

Birdsong, M., Smith, D. E., Mitchell, F. N., and Corey, J. H., Jr.: Generalized cytomegalic inclusion disease in newborn infants. J.A.M.A. 162:1305–1308, 1956.

Bodey, G. P., Wertlake, P. T., Douglas, G., and Levin,

R. H.: Cytomegalic inclusion disease in patients with acute leukemia. Ann. Intern. Med. 62:899–906, 1965.

Bonar, B. E., and Pearsall, C. J.: Herpes zoster in the newborn. Am. J. Dis. Child. 44:398–402, 1932.

Boston Interhospital Virus Study Group and the NIAID-Sponsored Cooperative Antiviral Clinical Study. Failure of high dose 5-iodo-2'-deoxyuridine in the therapy of Herpes simplex virus encephalitis. Evidence of unacceptable toxicity. New Eng. J. Med. 292:600–603, 1975.

Boughton, C. R.: Varicella-zoster in Sydney: II. Neurological complications of varicella. Med. J. Aust. 2:444–447, 1966.

Breeden, C. J., Hall, T. C., and Tyler, H. R.: Herpes simplex encephalitis treated with systemic 5-iodo-2'-deoxyuridine. Ann. Intern. Med. 65:1050–1056, 1966.

Brice, J. E. H.: Congenital varicella resulting from infection during second trimester of pregnancy. Arch. Dis. Childh. 51:474–476, 1976.

Brostoff, J.: Diaphragmatic paralysis after herpes zoster. Brit. Med. J. 2:1571–1572, 1966.

Brown, R. E., and Madge, G. E.: Hepatic degeneration and dysfunction in Reye's syndrome. Am. J. Dig. Dis. 16:1116–1122, 1971.

Brunell, P. A.: Varicella-zoster infections in pregnancy. J.A.M.A. 199:315–317, 1967.

Brunell, P. A., and Dodd, K.: Isolation of herpesvirus hominis from the cerebrospinal fluid of a child with bacterial meningitis and gingivostomatitis. J. Pediat. 65:53–56, 1964.

Brunell, P. A., and Gershon, A. A.: Passive immunization against varicella-zoster infections and other modes of therapy. J. Infect. Dis. 127:415–423, 1973.

Brunell, P. A., Miller, L. H., and Lovejoy, F.: Zoster in children. Am. J. Dis. Child. 115:432–437, 1968.

Brunell, P. A., Ross, A., Miller, L. H., and Kuo, B.: Prevention of varicella by zoster immune globulin. New Eng. J. Med. 280:1191–1194, 1969.

Bryan, B. L., Espana, C. D., Emmons, R. W., Vijayan, N., and Hoeprich, P. D.: Recovery from encephalomyelitis caused by *Herpesvirus simiae*. Report of a case. Arch. Intern. Med. 135:868–870, 1975.

Bryson, Y. J., and Kronenberg, L. H.: Combined antiviral effects of interferon, adenine arabinoside, hypoxanthine arabinoside, and adenine arabinoside-5'-monophosphate in human fibroblast cultures. Antimicrob. Agents Chemother. 11:299–306, 1977.

Buthala, D. A.: Cell culture studies on antiviral agents: I. Action of cytosine arabinoside and some comparisons with 5-iodo-2'-deoxyuridine. Proc. Soc. Exp. Biol. Med. 115:69–77, 1964.

Buttrick, D. D., and Roberts, L.: Generalized cytomegalic inclusion disease. Report of two cases with associated fungal infection, one involving aspergillosis, the second with candidiasis. Am. J. Dis. Child. 110:319–328, 1965.

Calabresi, P.: Current status of clinical investigation with 6-azauridine, 5-iodo-2'-deoxyuridine and related derivatives. Cancer Res. 23:1260–1267, 1963.

Cappel, R., and Klastersky, J.: Herpetic meningitis (type 1) in a case of acute leukemia. Arch. Neurol. 28:415–416, 1973.

Cappell, D. F., and McFarland, M. N.: Inclusion bodies (protozoan-like cells) in the organs of infants. J. Path. Bact. 59:385–398, 1947.

Carmody, R. F.: Herpes zoster ophthalmicus complicated by ophthalmoplegia and exophthalmos. Arch. Ophthal. 18:707–711, 1937.

Carmon, A., Behar, A., and Beller, A. J.: Acute necrotizing haemorrhagic encephalitis presenting clinically as a space occupying lesion. A clinico-pathological study of six cases. J. Neurol. Sci. 2:328–343, 1965.

Carton, C. A.: Effect of previous sensory loss on the appearance of Herpes simplex following trigeminal sensory root section. J. Neurosurg. 10:463–468, 1953.

Carton, C. A., and Kilbourne, E. D.: Activation of latent Herpes simplex by trigeminal sensory-root section. New Eng. J. Med. 246:172–176, 1952.

Catalano, L. W., Jr.: Herpesvirus hominis antibody in multiple sclerosis and amyotrophic lateral sclerosis. Neurology 22:473–478, 1972.

Catalano, L. W., Jr., and Johnson, L. D.: Herpesvirus antibody and carcinoma in situ of the cervix. J.A.M.A. 217:447–450, 1971.

Catalano, L. W., Jr., Safley, G. H., Museles, M., and Jarzynski, D. J.: Disseminated herpesvirus infection in a newborn infant. J. Pediat. 79:393–400, 1971.

Caul, E. O., Clarke, S. K. R., Mott, M. G., Perham, T. G. M., and Wilson, R. S. E.: Cytomegalovirus infections after open heart surgery. Lancet 1:777–781, 1971.

Ceballos, R., Ch'ien, L. T., Whitley, R. J., and Brans, Y. W.: Cerebellar hypoplasia in an infant with congenital cytomegalovirus infection. Pediatrics 57:155–157, 1976.

Chalhub, E. G., Baenziger, J., Feigen, R. D., Middlekamp, J. N., and Shackelford, G. D.: Congenital Herpes simplex type II infection with extensive hepatic calcification, bone lesions and cataracts: Complete postmortem examination. Dev. Med. Child Neurol. 19:527–534, 1977.

Chang, T. W., Solomon, P., and Weinstein, L.: Generalized fatal herpes simplex infection in a newborn infant. J. Pediat. 68:473–475, 1966.

Charles, N. C., Bennett, T. W., and Margolis, S.: Ocular pathology of the congenital varicella syndrome. Arch. Ophthalmol. 95:2034–2037, 1977.

Charnock, E. L., and Cramblett, H. G.: 5-Iodo-2'-deoxyuridine in neonatal herpesvirus hominis encephalitis. J. Pediat. 76:459–463, 1970.

Chatterjee, S. N., Fiala, M., Weiner, J., Stewart, J. A., Stacey, B., and Warner, N.: Primary cytomegalovirus and opportunistic infections. Incidence in renal transplant recipients. J.A.M.A. 240:2446–2449, 1978.

Ch'ien, L. T., Boehm, R. M., Robinson, H., Liu, C., and Frenkel, L. D.: Characteristic early electroencephalographic changes in Herpes simplex encephalitis. Clinical and virologic studies. Arch. Neurol. 34:361–364, 1977.

Ch'ien, L. T., Cannon, N. J., Whitley, R. J., Diethelm, A. G., Dismukes, W. E., Scott, C. W., Buchanan, R. A., and Alford, C. A., Jr.: Effect of adenine arabinoside on cytomegalovirus infections. J. Infect. Dis. 130:32–39, 1974.

Ch'ien, L. T., Whitley, R. J., Alford, C. A., Jr., and Gallasso, G. J.: Adenine arabinoside for therapy of herpes zoster in immunosuppressed patients: Preliminary results of a collaborative study. J. Infect. Dis. 133(Suppl.): A184–191, 1976.

Ch'ien, L. T., Whitley, R. J., Nahmias, A. J., Lewin, E. B., Linnemann, C. C., Jr., Frenkel, L. D., Bellanti, J. A., Buchanan, R. A., and Alford, C. A., Jr.: Antiviral chemotherapy and neonatal Herpes simplex virus infection: A pilot study-experience with adenine arabinoside (Ara-A). Pediatrics 55:678–685, 1975.

Chou, S. M., and Cherry, J. D.: Ultrastructure of Cowdry type A inclusions. I. In human herpes simplex encephalitis. Neurology 17:575–586, 1967.

Cibis, A., and Burde, R. M.: Herpes simplex virus-induced congenital cataracts. Arch. Ophthal. 85:220–223, 1971.

Clarke, B. F., and Davies, S. H.: Severe thrombocytopenia in infectious mononucleosis. Am. J. Med. Sci. 248:703–708, 1964.

Cleary, T. G., Henle, W., and Pickering, L. K.: Acute cerebellar ataxia associated with Epstein-Barr virus infection. J.A.M.A. 243:148–149, 1980.

Constantine, V. S., Francis, R. D., and Montes, L. F.: Association of recurrent herpes simplex with neuralgia. J.A.M.A. 205:131–133, 1968.

Cope, S., and Jones, A. T.: Hemiplegia complicating ophthalmic zoster. Lancet 2:898–899, 1954.

Cotton, P. B., and Webb-Peploe, M. M.: Acute transverse myelitis as a complication of glandular fever. Brit. Med. J. 1:654–655, 1966.

Cox, F., and Hughes, W. T.: Cytomegaloviremia in children with acute lymphatic leukemia. J. Pediat. 87:190–194, 1975.

Craig, C. P., and Nahmias, A. J.: Different patterns of neurologic involvement with Herpes simplex virus types 1 and 2: Isolation of Herpes simplex virus type 2 from the buffy coat of two adults with meningitis. J. Infect. Dis. 127:365–372, 1973.

Craighead, J. E., Hanshaw, J. B., and Carpenter, C. B.: Cytomegalovirus infection after renal allotransplantation. J.A.M.A. 201:725–728, 1967.

Creaturo, N. E.: Infectious mononucleosis and polyneuritis (Guillain-Barré syndrome). Report of a case of facial diplegia treated with 2, 3 dimercaptopropanol (BAL). J.A.M.A. 143:234–236, 1950.

Crome, L., and France, N. E.: Microgyria and cytomegalic inclusion disease in infancy. J. Clin. Path. 12:427–434, 1959.

Cushing, H.: Perineal zoster with notes upon cutaneous segmentation postaxial to the lower limb. Am. J. Med. Sci. 127:375–391, 1904.

Cushing, H.: Surgical aspects of major neuralgia of trigeminal nerve: Report of twenty cases of operation on Gasserian ganglion with anatomic and physiologic notes on consequence of its removal. J.A.M.A. 44:773–779, 860–865, 920–929, 1002–1008, 1088–1093, 1905.

Custer, R. P., and Smith, E. B.: The pathology of infectious mononucleosis. Blood 3:830–857, 1948.

Daurelle, G., Smith, G. F., and Riemer, W.: Periventricular calcification and cytomegalic inclusion disease in newborn infant. J.A.M.A 167:989–991, 1958.

Davidson, R. J. L., and Salter, R. H.: Infectious mononucleosis presenting with facial diplegia. Brit. Med. J. 1:954, 1964.

Davie, J. C., Ceballos, R., and Little, S. C.: Infectious mononucleosis with fatal neuronitis. Arch. Neurol. 9:265–272, 1963.

Davis, J. M., Davis, K. R., Kleinman, G. M., Kirchner, H. S., and Taveras, J. M.: Computed tomography of Herpes simplex encephalitis, with clinicopathological correlation. Radiology 129:409–417, 1978.

Davis, L. E., and Johnson, R. T.: An explanation for the localization of Herpes simplex encephalitis. Ann. Neurol. 5:2–5, 1979.

Davis, L. E., Tweed, G. V., Stewart, J. A., Bernstein, M. T., Miller, G. L., Gravelle, C. R., and Chin, T. D. Y.: Cytomegalovirus mononucleosis in a first trimester pregnant female with transmission to the fetus. Pediatrics 48:200–206, 1971.

Dayan, A. D., Gooddy, W., Harrison, M. J. G., and Rudge, P.: Brain stem encephalitis caused by herpesvirus hominis. Brit. Med. J. 4:405–406, 1972.

Dayan, A. D., and Stokes, M. I.: Rapid diagnosis of encephalitis by immunofluorescent examination of cerebrospinal-fluid cells. Lancet 1:177–179, 1973.

De Clercq, E., Edy, V. G., De Vlieger, H., Eeckels, R., and Desmyter, J.: Intrathecal administration of interferon in neonatal herpes. J. Pediat. 86:736–739, 1975.

Demian, S. D. E., Donnelly, W. H., Jr., and Monif, G. R. G.: Coexistent congenital cytomegalovirus and toxoplasmosis in a stillborn. Am. J. Dis. Child. 125:420–421, 1973.

Denny-Brown, D., Adams, R. D., and Fitzgerald, P. J.: Pathologic features of herpes zoster: A note on "Geniculate Herpes." Arch. Neurol. Psychiat. 51:216–231, 1944.

DeSimone, P. A., and Snyder, D.: Hypoglossal nerve palsy in infectious mononucleosis. Neurology 28:844–847, 1978.

Diehl, V., Henle, G., Henle, W., and Kohn, G.: Demonstration of a herpes group virus in cultures of peripheral leukocytes from patients with infectious mononucleosis. J. Virol. 2:663–669, 1968.

Diezel, P. B.: Mikrogyrie infolge cerebraler speicheldrüsenvirus infektion in rahmen einer generalisierten cytomegalie bei einem saügling zugleich ein beitrag zur theorie der windungsbildung. Virchows Arch. Path. Anat. 325:109, 1954.

Docherty, J. J., and Chopan, M.: The latent Herpes simplex virus. Bact. Rev. 38:337–355, 1974.

Dolgopol, V. B., and Husson, G. S.: Infectious mononucleosis with neurologic complications. Report of a fatal case. Arch. Intern. Med. 83:179–196, 1949.

Dorfman, L. J.: Cytomegalovirus encephalitis in adults. Neurology 23:136–144, 1973.

Dorman, J. M., Glick, T. H., Shannon, D. C., Galdabini, J., and Walker, A.: Complications of infectious mononucleosis. A fatal case in a 2-year-old child. Am. J. Dis. Child. 128:239–242, 1974.

Dowling, M. D., Jr., and Van Slyck, E. J.: Cerebellar disease in infectious mononucleosis. Arch. Neurol. 15:270–274, 1966.

Dowling, P., Menonna, J., and Cook, S.: Cytomegalovirus complement fixation antibody in Guillain-Barré syndrome. Neurology 27:1153–1156, 1977.

Downey, H., and McKinley, L. A.: Acute lymphadenosis compared with acute leukemia. Arch. Intern. Med. 32:82–85, 1923.

Drachman, D. A., and Adams, R. D.: Herpes simplex and acute inclusion-body encephalitis. Arch. Neurol. 7:45–63, 1962.

Duchowny, M., Caplan, L., and Siber, G.: Cytomegalovirus infection of the adult nervous system. Ann. Neurol. 5:458–461, 1979.

Dudgeon, J. A.: Cytomegalovirus infection. Arch. Dis. Childh. 46:581–583, 1971.

Duehr, P. A.: Herpes zoster as a cause of congenital cataract. Am. J. Ophthal. 39:157–161, 1955.

Dunkle, L. M., Schmidt, R. R., and O'Connor, D. M.: Neonatal Herpes simplex infection possibly acquired via maternal breast milk. Pediatrics 63:250–251, 1979.

Edwards, J. M. B., and McSwiggan, D. A.: Studies on the diagnostic value of an immunofluorescence test for EB virus-specific IgM. J. Clin. Path. 27:647–651, 1974.

Ehrlich, R. H., Turner, J. A. P., and Clarke, M.: Neonatal varicella. J. Pediat. 53:139–147, 1958.

Eisenklam, E. J.: Primary varicella pneumonia in a three-year-old girl. J. Pediat. 69:452–454, 1966.

Elek, S. D., and Stern, H.: Development of a vaccine against mental retardation caused by cytomegalovirus infection in utero. Lancet 1:1–5, 1974.

Elian, M.: Herpes simplex encephalitis. Prognosis and long-term follow-up. Arch. Neurol. 32:39–43, 1975.

Elliott, G. B., and Elliott, K. A.: Observations on cerebral cytomegalic inclusion disease of the foetus and newborn. Arch. Dis. Childh. 37:34–39, 1962.

Ellison, P. H., and Hanson, P. A.: Herpes simplex: A possible cause of brain-stem encephalitis. Pediatrics 59:240–243, 1977.

Emanuel, E., and Kenny, G. E.: Cytomegalic inclusion disease of infancy. Pediatrics 38:957–965, 1966.

Embil, J. A., Folkins, D. F., Haldane, E. V., and van Rooyen, C. E.: Cytomegalovirus infection following extracorporeal circulation in children. Lancet 2:1151–1155, 1968.

Embil, J. A., Ozere, R. L., and Haldane, E. V.: Congenital cytomegalovirus infection in two siblings from consecutive pregnancies. J. Pediat. 77:417–421, 1970.

Emodi, G., Sartorius, J., Just, M., Rohner, F., and Buhler, V.: Virus studies in the treatment of congenital cytomegalovirus infections by cytosine arabinoside. Helv. Paediat. Acta 27:557–564, 1972.

Enzmann, D. R., Ranson, B., Norman, D., and Talberth, E.: Computed tomography of Herpes simplex encephalitis. Radiology 129:419–425, 1978.

Epstein, M. A., and Achong, B. G.: Pathogenesis of infectious mononucleosis. Lancet 2:1270–1272, 1977.

Epstein M. A., and Barr, Y. M.: Cultivation in vitro of human lymphocytes from Burkitt malignant lymphoma. Lancet 1:252–253, 1964.

Epstein, S. H., and Dameshek, W.: Involvement of the central nervous system in a case of glandular fever. New Eng. J. Med. 205:1238–1241, 1931.

Evans, A. D., Gray, O. P., Miller, M. H., Jones, E. R. V., Weeks, R. D., and Wells, C. E. C.: Herpes simplex encephalitis treated with intravenous idoxuridine. Brit. Med. J. 2:407–410, 1967.

Evans, A. S., Niederman, J. C., and McCollum, R. W.: Seroepidemiologic studies of infectious mononucleosis with EB virus. New Eng. J. Med. 279:1121–1127, 1968.

Faden, H. S., Bybee, B. L., Overall, J. C., Jr., and Lahey, M. J.: Disseminated Herpesvirus hominis infection in a child with acute leukemia. J. Pediat. 90:951–953, 1977.

Falliers, C. J., and Ellis, E. F.: Corticosteroids and varicella. Six-year experience in an asthmatic population. Arch. Dis. Childh. 40:593–599, 1965.

Farber, S., and Wolbach, S. B.: Intranuclear and cytoplasmic inclusions (Protozoan-like bodies) in the salivary glands and other organs of infants. Am. J. Path. 8:123–135, 1932.

Farris, W. A., and Blaw, M. E.: Cytarabine treatment of herpes simplex encephalitis. Arch. Neurol. 27:99–102, 1972.

Fee, C. F., and Evarts, C. M.: Motor paralysis of the lower extremities in herpes zoster. Cleveland Clin. Quart. 35:169–176, 1968.

Feigin, R. D., Shackelford, P. G., DeVivo, D. C., and Haymond, M. W.: Floxuridine treatment of congenital cytomegalic inclusion disease. Pediatrics 48:318–321, 1971.

Feldman, R. A.: Cytomegalovirus infection during pregnancy. Am. J. Dis. Child. 117:517–521, 1969.

Feldman, R. A., and Schwartz, J. F.: Possible association between cytomegalovirus infection and infantile spasms. Lancet 1:180–181, 1968.

Feldman, S., Chaudary, S., Ossi, M., and Epp, E.: A viremic phase for herpes zoster in children with cancer. J. Pediat. 91:597–600, 1977.

Feldman, S., Hughes, W. T., and Daniel, C. B.: Varicella in children with cancer: Seventy-seven cases. Pediatrics 56:388–397, 1975.

Feldman, S., Hughes, W. T., and Kim, H. Y.: Herpes zoster in children with cancer. Am. J. Dis. Child. 126:178–184, 1973.

Feorino, P. M., Humphrey, D., Hochberg, F., and Chilicote, R.: Mononucleosis-associated subacute sclerosing panencephalitis. Lancet 2:530–532, 1975.

Fetterman, G. H.: A new laboratory aid in the clinical diagnosis of inclusion disease of infancy. Am. J. Clin. Path. 22:424–425, 1952.

Fiala, M., Payne, J. E., Berne, T. V., Moore, T. C., Henle, W., Montgomerie, J. Z., Chatterjee, S. N., and Guze, L. B.: Epidemiology of cytomegalovirus infection after transplantation and immunosuppression. J. Infect. Dis. 132:421–433, 1975.

Fierer, J., Bazeley, P., and Braude, A. I.: Herpes B virus encephalomyelitis presenting as ophthalmic zoster. Ann. Intern. Med. 79:225–228, 1973.

Fine, R. N., Grushkin, C. M., Anand, S., Lieberman, E., and Wright, H. T., Jr.: Cytomegalovirus in children. Postrenal transplantation. Am. J. Dis. Child. 120:197–202, 1970.

Finkel, H. E.: Infectious mononucleosis encephalitis. Am. J. Med. Sci. 249:425–427, 1965.

Fishman, M. A., Haymond, M. W., and Middelkamp, J. N.: Failure of idoxuridine treatment in herpes simplex encephalitis. Am. J. Dis. Child. 122:250–252, 1971.

Fleisher, G., Lennette, E. T., Henle, G., and Henle, W.: Incidence of heterophil antibody responses in children with infectious mononucleosis. J. Pediat. 94:723–728, 1979.

Florman, A. L., Gershon, A. A., Blackett, P. R., and Nahmias, A. J.: Intrauterine infection with Herpes simplex virus. Resultant congenital malformations. J.A.M.A. 225:129–132, 1973.

Foley, F. D., Greenawald, K. A., Nash, G., and Pruitt, B. A., Jr.: Herpesvirus infection in burned patients. New Eng. J. Med. 282:652–656, 1970.

Fortunato, J., Goldschmidt, B., Menonna, J., Dowling, P., and Cook, S.: Rapid detection of antibodies to cytomegalovirus by counterimmunoelectrophoresis. J. Infect. Dis. 135:435–437, 1977.

Francis, D. P., Herrmann, K. L., MacMahon, J. R., Chavigny, K. H., and Sanderlin, K. C.: Nosocomial and maternally acquired Herpesvirus hominis infections. Am. J. Dis. Child. 129:889–893, 1975.

Frank, D. J., DeVaux, W. D., Perkins, J. R., and Perrin, E. V.: Fetal ascites and cytomegalic inclusion disease. Am. J. Dis. Child. 112:604–607, 1966.

Franklin, A. J.: Cytomegalovirus infection presenting as acute haemolytic anaemia in an infant. Arch. Dis. Childh. 47:474–475, 1972.

Frentz, J. M., Gohd, R. S., and Woody, N. C.: Untreated neonatal herpes simplex 2 meningitis without apparent neurologic damage. J. Pediat. 85:77–79, 1974.

Freud, P., Rook, G. D., and Gurian, S.: Herpes zoster in the newborn. Am. J. Dis. Child. 64:895–897, 1942.

Frey, H. M., Bialkin, G., and Gershon, A. A.: Congenital varicella: Case report of a serologically proved long-term survivor. Pediatrics 59:110–112, 1977.

Friedland, R., and Yahr, M. D.: Meningoencephalopathy

secondary to infectious mononucleosis. Unusual presentation with stupor and chorea. Arch. Neurol. 34:186–188, 1977.

Fuccillo, D. A., Moder, F. L., Catalano, L. W., Jr., Vincent, M. M., and Sever, J. L.: Herpesvirus hominis types I and II: A specific microindirect hemagglutination test. Proc. Soc. Exp. Biol. Med. 133:735–739, 1970.

Gautier-Smith, P. C.: Neurological complications of glandular fever (infectious mononucleosis). Brain 88:323–334, 1965.

Gershon, A. A., Fish, I., and Brunell, P. A.: Herpes simplex infection of the newborn. Am. J. Dis. Child. 124:739–741, 1972.

Gershon, A. A., and Krugman, S.: Seroepidemiologic survey of varicella: Value of specific fluorescent antibody test. Pediatrics 56:1005–1008, 1975.

Gershon, A. A., Steinberg, S., and Brunell, P. A.: Zoster immune globulin. A further assessment. New Eng. J. Med. 290:243–245, 1974.

Gibel, H., Kramer, B., and Naji, A. F.: Encephalitis complicating chickenpox. Am. J. Dis. Child. 99:669–679, 1960.

Gilbert, G. J.: Herpes zoster ophthalmicus and delayed contralateral hemiplegia. J.A.M.A. 229:302–304, 1974.

Glick, T. H., Ditchek, N. T., Salitsky, S., and Freimuth, E. J.: Acute encephalopathy and hepatic dysfunction. Association with chickenpox in siblings. Am. J. Dis. Child. 119:68–71, 1970.

Glogau, R., Hanna, L., and Jawetz, E.: Herpetic whitlow as part of genital virus infection. J. Infect. Dis. 136:689–692, 1977.

Gold, E.: Serologic and virus-isolation studies of patients with varicella or herpes-zoster infection. New Eng. J. Med. 274:181–185, 1966.

Golden, B., Bell, W. E., and McKee, A. P.: Disseminated herpes simplex with encephalitis in a neonate. J.A.M.A. 209:1219–1221, 1969.

Goldsmith, M. O.: Herpes zoster ophthalmicus with sixth nerve palsy. Canad. J. Ophthal. 3:279–283, 1968.

Goldstein, E., and Porter, D. Y.: Fatal thrombocytopenia with cerebral hemorrhage in mononucleosis. Arch. Neurol. 20:533–535, 1969.

Goldston, A. S., Millichap, J. G., and Miller, R. H.: Cerebellar ataxia with pre-eruptive varicella. Am. J. Dis. Child. 106:197–200, 1963.

Goodpasture, E. W., and Talbot, F. B.: Concerning the nature of protozoan-like cells in certain lesions of infancy. Am. J. Dis. Child. 21:415–425, 1921.

Gottmann, A. W., and Beatty, E. C., Jr.: Cytomegalic inclusion disease in children with leukemia or lymphosarcoma. Am. J. Dis. Child. 104:180–184, 1962.

Graham, C. B., Thal, A., and Wassum, C. S.: Rubella-like bone changes in congenital cytomegalic inclusion disease. Radiology 94:39–43, 1970.

Granström, M. L., Leinikki, P., Santavuori, P., and Pettay, O.: Perinatal cytomegalovirus infection in man. Arch. Dis. Childh. 52:354–359, 1977.

Griffiths, J. F., Fitzwilliam, J. F., Casagranda, S., and Butler, S. R.: Experimental herpes simplex virus encephalitis. Comparative effects of treatment with cytosine arabinoside and adenine arabinoside. J. Infect. Dis. 132:506–510, 1975.

Grose, C., and Feorino, P. M.: Epstein-Barr virus and Guillain-Barré syndrome. Lancet 2:1285–1287, 1972.

Grose, C., Feorino, P. M., Dye, L. A., and Rand, J.: Bell's palsy and infectious mononucleosis. Lancet 2:231–232, 1973.

Grose, C., Henle, W., Henle, G., and Feorino, P. M.:

Primary Epstein-Barr virus infections in acute neurologic diseases. New Eng. J. Med. 292:392–395, 1975.

Gutmann, L.: The heterophile antibody and cerebrospinal fluid. Neurology 18:269–270, 1968.

Habel, A. H., and Brown, J. K.: Dexamethasone in herpes-simplex encephalitis. Lancet 1:695, 1972.

Haggerty, R. J., and Eley, R. C.: Varicella and cortisone. Pediatrics 18:160–162, 1956.

Hagler, W. S., Walters, P. V., and Nahmias, A. J.: Ocular involvement in neonatal herpes simplex virus infection. Arch. Ophthal. 82:169–176, 1969.

Halsted, C. C., and Chang, R. S.: Infectious mononucleosis and encephalitis: Recovery of EB virus from spinal fluid. Pediatrics 64:257–258, 1979.

Hamperl, H.: Pneumocystis infection and cytomegaly of the lungs in the newborn and adult. Am. J. Path. 32:1–13, 1956.

Hanshaw, J. B.: Cytomegalovirus complement-fixing antibody in microcephaly. New Eng. J. Med. 275:476–479, 1966.

Hanshaw, J. B.: Congenital cytomegalovirus infection: Laboratory methods of detection. J. Pediat. 75:1179–1185, 1969.

Hanshaw, J. B.: Congenital cytomegalovirus infection: A fifteen year perspective. J. Infect. Dis. 123:555–561, 1971.

Hanshaw, J. B.: Herpesvirus hominis infections in the fetus and the newborn. Am. J. Dis. Child. 126:546–555, 1973.

Harries, J. T., and Ferguson, A. W.: Fatal infectious mononucleosis with liver failure in two sisters. Arch. Dis. Childh. 43:480–485, 1968.

Hass, G. M.: Hepato-adrenal necrosis with intranuclear inclusion bodies: Report of a case. Am. J. Path. 11:127–142, 1935.

Hatch, H. A.: Bilateral optic neuritis following chickenpox. Report of case with apparently complete recovery. J. Pediat. 34:758–759, 1949.

Hayes, K., and Gibas, H.: Placental cytomegalovirus infection without fetal involvement following primary infection in pregnancy. J. Pediat. 79:401–405, 1971.

Haymaker, W., Girdany, B. R., Stephens, J., Lillie, R. D., and Fetterman, G. H.: Cerebral involvement with advanced periventricular calcification in generalized cytomegalic inclusion disease in the newborn. J. Neuropath. Exp. Neurol. 13:562–586, 1954.

Haynes, R. E., Azimi, P. H., and Cramblett, H. G.: Fatal herpesvirus hominis (herpes simplex virus) infections in children. J.A.M.A. 206:312–319, 1968.

Haynes, R. E., Sherard, E. S., Cramblett, H. G., Azimi, P. H., and Hilty, M. D.: Treatment of herpesvirus encephalitis with iododeoxyuridine. J. Pediat. 83:102–105, 1973.

Henle, G., Henle, W., and Diehl, V.: Relation of Burkitt's tumor-associated herpes-type virus to infectious mononucleosis. Proc. Natl. Acad. Sci. U.S.A. 59:94–101, 1968.

Henle, W., Henle, G. E., and Horwitz, C. A.: Epstein-Barr virus specific diagnostic tests in infectious mononucleosis. Human Pathology 5:551–565, 1974.

Heydenreich, J. S. S.: An outbreak of smallpox in an urban area. S. Afr. Med. J. 39:463–466, 1965.

Hiller, R. I., and Fox, M. J.: Infectious neuronitis associated with infectious mononucleosis. Marquette M. Rev. 7:152, 1942.

Ho, M., Suwansirikul, S., et al.: The transplanted kidney as a source of cytomegalovirus infection. New Eng. J. Med. 293:1109–1112, 1975.

Hochberg, F. H., Lehrich, J. R., Richardson, E. P., Jr., Feorino, P., and Aström, K. E.: Mononucleosis-associated subacute sclerosing panencephalitis. Acta Neuropath. 34:33–40, 1976.

Hogan, E. L., and Krigman, M. R.: Herpes zoster myelitis. Arch Neurol. 29:309–313, 1973.

Holliday, P. B., Jr.: Pre-eruptive neurological complications of the common contagious diseases—rubella, rubeola, roseola, and varicella. J. Pediat. 36:185–198, 1950.

Horwitz, C. A., Henle, W., Henle, G., Polesky, H., Balfour, H. H., Jr., Siem, R. A., Borken, S., and Ward, P. C. J.: Heterophil-negative infectious mononucleosis and mononucleosis-like illnesses. Laboratory confirmation of 43 cases. Am. J. Med. 63:947–957, 1977.

Horwitz, C. A., Henle, W., Henle, G., Segal, M., Arnold, T., Lewis, F. B., Zanick, D., and Ward, P. C. J.: Clinical and laboratory evaluation of elderly patients with heterophil-antibody positive infectious mononucleosis. Report of seven patients, ages 40 to 78. Am. J. Med. 61:333–339, 1976.

Hovig, D. E., Hodgman, J. E., Mathies, A. W., Jr., Levan, N., and Portnoy, B.: Herpesvirus hominis (simplex) infection with recurrences during infancy. Am. J. Dis. Child. 115:438–444, 1968.

Hryniuk, W., Foerster, J., Shojania, M., and Chow, A.: Cytarabine for herpesvirus infections. J.A.M.A. 219:715–718, 1972.

Hubbard, T. W.: Varicella occurring in an infant twenty-four hours after birth. Brit. Med. J. 1:822, 1878.

Hughes, W. N.: Herpes zoster of the right trigeminal nerve with left hemiplegia. Neurology 1:167–169, 1951.

Hunt, J. R.: On herpetic inflammations of the geniculate ganglion. A new syndrome and its complications. J. Nerv. Ment. Dis. 34:73–96, 1907.

Illis, L. S., and Taylor, F. M.: The electroencephalogram in herpes-simplex encephalitis. Lancet 1:718–721, 1972.

Itabashi, H. H., Bass, D. M., and McCulloch, J. R.: Inclusion body of acute inclusion encephalitis. Arch. Neurol. 14:493–505, 1966.

Izawa, T., Ihara, T., Hattori, A., Iwasa, T., Kamiya, H., Sakurai, M., and Takahashi, M.: Application of a live varicella vaccine in children with acute leukemia or other malignant diseases. Pediatrics 60:805–809, 1977.

Jamison, R. M., and Hathorn, A. W., Jr.: Isolation of cytomegalovirus from cerebrospinal fluid of a congenitally infected infant. Am. J. Dis. Child. 132:63–64, 1978.

Jarratt, M., and Hubler, W. R., Jr.: Herpes genitalis and aseptic meningitis. Arch. Dermatol. 110:771–772, 1974.

Jenkins, R., Dvorak, A., and Patrick, J.: Encephalopathy and fatty degeneration of the viscera associated with chickenpox. Pediatrics 39:769–771, 1967.

Jesionek, A., and Kiolemenoglou, B.: Ueber einen befund von protozoenartigen gibeen in den organen eines hereditarleuetischen fotus. Munchen Med. Wehnschr. 51:1905–1907, 1904.

Johansen, A. H.: Serous meningitis and infectious mononucleosis. Acta Med. Scand. 76:269–272, 1931.

Johnson, K. P., Rosenthal, M. S., and Lerner, P. I.: Herpes simplex encephalitis. The course of five virologically proven cases. Arch. Neurol. 27:103–108, 1972.

Johnson, R., and Milbourn, P. E.: Central nervous system manifestations of chickenpox. Canad. Med. Assoc. J. 102:831–834, 1970.

Johnson, R. T., Olson, L. C., and Buescher, E. L.: Herpes simplex virus infections of the nervous system. Problems in laboratory diagnosis. Arch. Neurol. 18:260–264, 1968.

Joncas, J. H., Chicoine, L., Thivierge, R., and Bertrand, M.: Epstein-Barr virus antibodies in the cerebrospinal fluid. A case of infectious mononucleosis with encephalitis. Am. J. Dis. Child. 127:282–285, 1974.

Jordan, M. C., Rousseau, W. E., Stewart, J. A., Noble, G. R., and Chin, T. D. Y.: Spontaneous cytomegalovirus mononucleosis. Ann. Intern. Med. 79:153–160, 1973.

Joseph, T. J., and Vogt, P. J.: Disseminated herpes with hepatoadrenal necrosis in an adult. Am. J. Med. 56:735–739, 1974.

Juel-Jensen, B. E.: Severe generalized primary herpes treated with cytarabine. Brit. Med. J. 2:154–155, 1970.

Kääriäinen, L., Klemola, E., and Paloheimo, J.: Rise of cytomegalovirus antibodies in infectious mononucleosis-like syndrome after transfusion. Brit. Med. J. 1:1270–1272, 1966.

Kanich, R. E., and Craighead, J. E.: Cytomegalovirus infection and cytomegalic inclusion disease in renal homotransplant recipients. Am. J. Med. 40:874–882, 1966.

Kaplan, A. S.: Recent studies of the herpesviruses. Am. J. Clin. Path. 57:783–793, 1972.

Karpinski, F. E., Jr.: Neurologic manifestations of infectious mononucleosis in childhood. Pediatrics 10:265–270, 1952.

Keidan, S. E., and Mainwaring, D.: Association of herpes zoster with leukemia and lymphoma in children. Clin. Pediat. 4:13–17, 1965.

Kent, T. H., and Nicholson, D. P.: Herpes simplex encephalitis. Am. J. Dis. Child. 108:644–647, 1964.

Klastersky, J., Cappel, R., Snoeck, J. M., Flament, J., and Thiry, L.: Ascending myelitis in association with herpes simplex virus. New Eng. J. Med. 287:182–184, 1972.

Klemola, E., Weckman, N., Haltia, K., and Kääriäinen, L.: The Guillain-Barré syndrome associated with acquired cytomegalovirus infection. Acta Med. Scand. 181:603–607, 1967.

Knotts, F. B., Cook, M. L., and Stevens, J. G.: Pathogenesis of herpetic encephalitis in mice after ophthalmic inoculation. J. Infect. Dis. 130:16–27, 1974.

Koenig, H., Rabinowitz, S. G., Day, E., and Miller, V.: Post-infectious encephalomyelitis after successful treatment of Herpes simplex encephalitis with adenine arabinoside. New Eng. J. Med. 300:1089–1093, 1979.

Komorous, J. M., Wheeler, C. E., Briggaman, R. A., and Caro, I.: Intrauterine Herpes simplex infections. Arch. Dermatol. 113:918–922, 1977.

Kopelman, A. F., Halsted, C. C., and Minnefor, A. B.: Osteomalacia and spontaneous fractures in twins with congenital cytomegalic inclusion disease. J. Pediat. 81:101–105, 1972.

Krabbe, K. H.: Varicella myelitis. Brain 48:535–539, 1925.

Kraybill, E. N., Sever, J. L., Avery, G. B., and Movassaghi, N.: Experimental use of cytosine arabinoside in congenital cytomegalovirus infection. J. Pediat. 80:485–487, 1972.

Krech, U., Knojajev, Z., and Jung, M.: Congenital cytomegalovirus infection in siblings from consecutive pregnancies. Helv. Paediat. Acta 26:355–362, 1971.

Krech, V. H., Jung, M., and Jung, F.: Cytomegalovirus infections in man. S. Karger, Basel, 1971.

Kreel, I., Zaroff, L. I., Canter, J. W., Krasna, I., and Baronofsky, I. D.: Syndrome following total body perfusion. Surg. Gynec. Obst. 111:317–321, 1960.

Krohel, G. B., Richardson, J. R., and Farrell, D. F.: Herpes simplex neuropathy. Neurology 26:596–597, 1976.

Laforet, E. G., and Lynch, C. L., Jr.: Multiple congenital defects following maternal varicella. Report of a case. New Eng. J. Med. 236:534–537, 1947.

Lander, H.: A case of acute haemorrhagic leukoencephalitis (Hurst) complicating varicella. J. Path. Bact. 70:157–165, 1955.

Lange, B. J., Berman, P. H., Bender, J., Henle, W., and Hewetson, J. F.: Encephalitis in infectious mononucleosis: Diagnostic considerations. Pediatrics 58:877–879, 1976.

Laws, H. W.: Herpes zoster ophthalmicus complicated by contralateral hemiplegia. Arch. Ophthalmol. 63:273–280, 1960.

Lee, F. K., Nahmias, A. J., and Stagno, S.: Rapid diagnosis of cytomegalovirus infection in infants by electron microscopy. New Eng. J. Med. 299:1266–1270, 1978.

Leonidas, J. C., Beatty, E. C., and Wenner, H. A.: Ménétrier disease and cytomegalovirus infection in childhood. Am. J. Dis. Child. 126:806–808, 1973.

Lerner, A. M., Lauter, C. B., Nolan, D. C., and Shippey, M. J.: Passive hemagglutinating antibodies in cerebrospinal fluids in Herpesvirus hominis encephalitis. Proc. Soc. Exp. Biol. Med. 140:1460–1466, 1972.

Levin, S.: Cerebellar ataxia following chickenpox. Lancet 1:1222–1223, 1960.

Levine, D. P., Lauter, C. B., and Lerner, A. M.: Simultaneous serum and CSF antibodies in Herpes simplex virus encephalitis. J.A.M.A. 240:356–360, 1978.

Lewkonia, I. K., and Jackson, A. A.: Infantile herpes zoster after intrauterine exposure to varicella. Brit. Med. J. 3:149, 1973.

Light, I. J.: Postnatal acquisition of Herpes simplex virus by the newborn infant: A review of the literature. Pediatrics 63:480–482, 1979.

Linnemann, C. C., Jr., First, M. R., Alvira, M. M., Alexander, J. W., and Schiff, G. M.: Herpesvirus hominis type 2 meningoencephalitis following renal transplantation. Am. J. Med. 61:703–708, 1976.

Linnemann, C. C., Jr., May, D. B., Schubert, W. K., Caraway, C. T., and Schiff, G. M.: Fatal viral encephalitis in children with x-linked hypogammaglobulinemia. Am. J. Dis. Child. 126:100–103, 1973.

Lipsett, M. B., Dreifuss, F. E., and Thomas, L. B.: Hypothalamic syndrome following varicella. Am. J. Med. 32:471–475, 1962.

Liu, C., and Llanes-Rodas, R.: Application of the immunofluorescent technic to the study of pathogenesis and rapid diagnosis of viral infections. Am. J. Clin. Path. 57:829–834, 1972.

Logan, W. S., Tindall, J. P., and Elson, M. L.: Chronic cutaneous herpes simplex. Arch. Derm. 103:606–614, 1971.

Lonn, L. I.: Neonatal cytomegalic inclusion disease chorioretinitis. Arch. Ophthal. 88:434–438, 1972.

Lui, W. Y., and Chang, W. K.: Cytomegalovirus mononucleosis in Chinese infants. Arch. Dis. Childh. 47:643–646, 1972.

Luna, M. A., and Lichtiger, B.: Disseminated toxoplasmosis and cytomegalovirus infection complicating Hodgkin's disease. Am. J. Clin. Path. 55:499–505, 1971.

MacCallum, F. O., Chinn, I. J., and Gostling, J. V. T.: Antibodies to Herpes-simplex virus in the cerebrospinal fluid of patients with herpetic encephalitis. J. Med. Microbiol. 7:325–331, 1974.

MacDonald, A., and Feiwel, M.: Isolation of herpes virus from erythema multiforme. Brit. Med. J. 2:570–571, 1972.

Marshall, W. J. S.: Herpes simplex encephalitis treated with idoxuridine and external decompression. Lancet 2:579–580, 1967.

McAllister, R. M., Wright, H. T., Jr., and Tasem, W. M.: Cytomegalic inclusion disease in newborn twins. J. Pediat. 64:278–281, 1964.

McCarthy, J. T., and Amer, J.: Postvaricella acute transverse myelitis: A case presentation and review of the literature. Pediatrics 62:202–204, 1978.

McCormick, D. P.: Herpes-simplex virus as cause of Bell's palsy. Lancet 1:937–939, 1972.

McCormick, G. W.: Encephalitis associated with herpes zoster. J. Pediat. 30:473–474, 1947.

McCormick, W. F., Rodnitzky, R. L., Schochet, S. S., Jr., and McKee, A. P.: Varicella-zoster encephalomyelitis. Arch. Neurol. 21:559–570, 1969.

McCracken, G. H., Jr., and Luby, J. P.: Cytosine arabinoside in the treatment of congenital cytomegalic inclusion disease. J. Pediat. 80:488–495, 1972.

McCracken, G. H., Jr., Shinefield, H. W., Cobb, K., Rausen, A. R., Dische, M. R., and Eichenwald, H. F.: Congenital cytomegalic inclusion disease. Am. J. Dis. Child. 117:522–539, 1969.

McEnery, G., and Stern, H.: Cytomegalovirus infection in early infancy. Arch. Dis. Childh. 45:669–673, 1970.

McKee, A. P., Hudson, J. D., Kimura, J., and McCormick, W. F.: Herpes simplex infections. Southern Med. J. 61:217–225, 1968.

McKendry, J. B. J., and Bailey, J. D.: Congenital varicella associated with multiple defects. Canad. Med. Assoc. J. 108:66–68, 1973.

Medearis, D. N.: Observations concerning human cytomegalovirus infection and disease. Bull. Johns Hopkins Hosp. 114:181–211, 1964.

Melish, M. E., and Hanshaw, J. B.: Congenital cytomegalovirus infection. Developmental progress of infants detected by routine screening. Am. J. Dis. Child. 126:190–194, 1973.

Meyer, J. S., Bauer, R. B., Rivera-Olmos, V. M., Nolan, D. C., and Lerner, A. M.: Herpesvirus hominis encephalitis. Arch. Neurol. 23:438–450, 1970.

Meyer, R. D., Young, L. S., Armstrong, D., and Yu, B.: Aspergillosis complicating neoplastic disease. Am. J. Med. 54:6–15, 1973.

Miller, D. R., Hanshaw, J. B., O'Leary, D. S., and Hnilicka, J. V.: Fatal disseminated herpes simplex virus infection and hemorrhage in the neonate. J. Pediat. 76:409–415, 1970.

Miller, G.: Epstein-Barr herpesvirus and infectious mononucleosis. Prog. Med. Virol. 20:84–112, 1975.

Miller, G., Niederman, J. C., and Andrews, L.: Prolonged oropharyngeal excretion of Epstein-Barr virus after infectious mononucleosis. New Eng. J. Med. 288:229–232, 1973.

Miller, J. K., Hesser, F., and Tompkins, V. N.: Herpes simplex encephalitis. Ann. Intern. Med. 64:92–103, 1966.

Minckler, D. S., McLean, E. B., Shaw, C. M., and Hendrickson, A.: Herpesvirus hominis encephalitis and retinitis. Arch. Ophthal. 94:89–95, 1976.

Mirra, J. M.: Aortitis and malacoplakia-like lesions of the brain in association with neonatal herpes simplex. Am. J. Clin. Path. 56:104–110, 1971.

Mishkin, F. S.: Radionuclide angiogram and scan findings in case of herpes simplex encephalitis. J. Nuclear Med. 11:608–609, 1970.

Mitchell, J. E., and McCall, F. C.: Transplacental infection by Herpes simplex virus. Am. J. Dis. Child. 106:207–209, 1963.

Mitchell, M. S., Kaplan, S. R., and Calabresi, P.: Alteration of antibody synthesis in the rat by cytosine arabinoside. Cancer Res. 29:896–904, 1969.

Mok, C. H.: Zoster-like disease in infants and young children. New Eng. J. Med. 285:294, 1971.

Monif, G. R. G., Brunell, P. A., and Hsiung, G. D.: Visceral involvement by herpes simplex virus in eczema herpeticum. Am. J. Dis. Child. 116:324–327, 1968.

Montgomerie, J. Z., Becroft, D. M. O., Croxson, M. C., Doak, P. B., and North, J. D. K.: Herpes-simplex-virus infection after renal transplantation. Lancet 2:867–871, 1969.

Montgomery, J. R., Flanders, R. W., and Yow, M. D.: Congenital anomalies and herpesvirus infection. Am. J. Dis. Child. 126:364–366, 1973.

Morbidity and Mortality Weekly Reports. Vol. 22, Feb. 17, 1973.

Morrison, R. E., Miller, M. H., Lyon, L. W., Griffiss, J. M., and Artenstein, M. S.: Adult meningoencephalitis caused by Herpesvirus hominis type 2. Am. J. Med. 56:540–544, 1974.

Muller, S. A., Herrmann, E. C., Jr., and Winkelmann, R. K.: Herpes simplex infections in hematologic malignancies. Am. J. Med. 52:102–114, 1972.

Murray, H. W., Knox, D. L., Green, W. R., and Susel, R. M.: Cytomegalovirus retinitis in adults. A manifestation of disseminated viral infection. Am. J. Med. 63:574–584, 1977.

Music, S. I., Fine, E. M., and Togo, Y.: Zoster-like disease in the newborn due to herpes-simplex virus. New Eng. J. Med. 284:24–26, 1971.

Nachman, A. R.: Neurologic complications of herpes zoster. Pediatrics 7:200–205, 1951.

Nahmias, A. J., Alford, C. A., and Korones, S. B.: Infection of the newborn with herpesvirus hominis. Adv. Pediat. 17:185–226, 1970.

Nahmias, A. J., Chiang, W. T., Del Buono, I., and Duffey, A.: Typing of Herpesvirus hominis strains by a direct immunofluorescent technique. Proc. Soc. Exp. Biol. Med. 132:386–390, 1969.

Nahmias, A. J., Dowdle, W. R., Josey, W. E., Naib, Z. M., Painter, L. M., and Luce, C.: Newborn infection with herpesvirus hominis types 1 and 2. J. Pediat. 75:1194–1203, 1969.

Naib, Z. M.: Cytologic diagnosis of cytomegalic inclusion-body disease. Am. J. Dis. Child. 105:153–159, 1963.

Navin, J. J., and Angevine, J. M.: Congenital cytomegalic inclusion disease with porencephaly. Neurology 18:470–472, 1968.

Nellhaus, G.: Isolated oculomotor nerve palsy in infectious mononucleosis. Neurology 16:221–224, 1966.

Niederman, J. C., McCollum, R. W., Henle, G., and Henle, W.: Infectious mononucleosis. Clinical manifestations in relation to EB virus antibodies. J.A.M.A. 203:205–209, 1968.

Nolan, D. C., Carruthers, M. M., and Lerner, A. M.: Herpesvirus hominis encephalitis in Michigan. New Eng. J. Med. 282:10–13, 1970.

Nolan, D. C., Lauter, C. B., and Lerner, A. M.: Idoxuridine in herpes simplex virus (type 1) encephalitis. Ann. Intern. Med. 78:243–246, 1973.

Norman, M. G.: Encephalopathy and fatty degeneration of the viscera in childhood. Canad. Med. Assoc. J. 99:522–526, 1968.

Norris, F. H., Jr., Leonards, R., Calanchini, P. R., and Calder, C. D.: Herpes-zoster meningoencephalitis. J. Infect. Dis. 122:335–338, 1970.

Oates, J. K., and Greenhouse, P. R. D. H.: Retention of urine in anogenital herpetic infection. Lancet 1:691–692, 1978.

Ohsaki, M., Chiba, S., and Nakao, T.: Bell's palsy in infants associated with varicella-zoster virus infection. J. Pediat. 84:103–104, 1974.

Olson, L. C., Buescher, E. L., Artenstein, M. S., and Parkman, P. D.: Herpesvirus infections of the human central nervous system. New Eng. J. Med. 277:1271–1277, 1967.

Palmgren, B.: The relationship of dermatitis herpetiformis to incontinentia pigmenti in newborn infants. Pediatrics 29:295–302, 1962.

Partridge, J. W., and Millis, R. R.: Systemic herpes simplex infection in a newborn treated with intravenous idoxuridine. Arch. Dis. Childh. 43:377–381, 1968.

Patel, B. M.: Skin rash with infectious mononucleosis and ampicillin. Pediatrics 40:910–911, 1967.

Paul, J. R., and Bunnell, W. W.: The presence of heterophile antibodies in infectious mononucleosis. Am. J. Med. Sci. 183:80–104, 1932.

Pazin, G. J., Ho, M., and Jannetta, P. J.: Reactivation of Herpes simplex virus after decompression of the trigeminal nerve root. J. Infect. Dis. 138:405–409, 1978.

Peace, R. J.: Cytomegalic inclusion disease in adults. Am. J. Med. 24:48–56, 1958.

Percy, D. H., and Hatch, L. A.: Experimental infection with Herpes simplex virus type 2 in newborn rats: Effects of treatment with iododeoxyuridine and cytosine arabinoside. J. Infect. Dis. 132: 256–261, 1975.

Peters, A. C. B., Versteeg, J., Lindeman, J., and Bots, G. T. A. M.: Varicella and acute cerebellar ataxia. Arch. Neurol. 35:769–771, 1978.

Pettay, O., Leinikki, P., Donner, M., and Lapinleimu, K.: Herpes simplex virus infection in the newborn. Arch. Dis. Childh. 47:97–103, 1972.

Phillips, C. A., Fanning, W. L., Gump, D. W., and Phillips, C. F.: Cytomegalovirus encephalitis in immunologically normal adults. Successful treatment with vidarabine. J.A.M.A. 238:2299–2300, 1977.

Piel, J. J., Thelander, H. E., and Shaw, E. B.: Infectious mononucleosis of the central nervous system with bilateral papilledema. J. Pediat. 37:661–665, 1950.

Pierce, N. F., Portnoy, B., Leeds, N. E., Morrison, R. L., and Wehrle, P. F.: Encephalitis associated with herpes simplex infection presenting as a temporal-lobe mass. Neurology 14:708–713, 1964.

Pratesi, R., Freemon, F. R., and Lowry, J. L.: Herpes zoster ophthalmicus with contralateral hemiplegia. Arch. Neurol. 34:640–641, 1977.

Price, R., Chernik, N. L., Horta-Barbosa, L., and Posner, J. B.: Herpes simplex encephalitis in an anergic patient. Am. J. Med. 54:222–228, 1973.

Price, R. L., O'Conner, P. S., and Rothner, A. D.: Acute ophthalmoplegia, ataxia, and areflexia (Fisher syndrome) in childhood. Cleveland Clin. Quart. 45:247–252, 1978.

Prince, A. M., Szmuness, W., Millian, S. J., and David, D. S.: A serologic study of cytomegalovirus infections associated with blood transfusions. New Eng. J. Med. 284:1125–1131, 1971.

Pullen, H., Wright, N., and Murdoch, J. M.: Hypersensitivity reactions to antibacterial drugs in infectious mononucleosis. Lancet 2:1176–1178, 1967.

Radcliffe, W. B., Guinto, F. C., Jr., Adcock, D. F., and Krigman, M. R.: Herpes simplex encephalitis. Arch. Neurol. 10:595–603, 1964.

Radel, E. G., and Schorr, J. B.: Thrombocytopenic purpura with infectious mononucleosis: Report of 2 cases and review of the literature. J. Pediat. 63:46–60, 1963.

Rake, G., Blank, H., Coriell, L. L., Nagler, F. P., and Scott, T. F. M.: The relationship of varicella and herpes zoster. J. Bact. 56:293, 1948.

Rahal, J. J., and Henle, G.: Infectious mononucleosis and Reye's syndrome: A fatal case with studies for Epstein-Barr virus. Pediatrics 46:776–780, 1970.

Ramos, E., Timmons, R. F., and Schimpff, S. C.: Inappropriate antidiuretic hormone following adenine arabinoside administration. Antimicrob. Agents Chemother. 15:142–144, 1979.

Rawls, W. E., Tompkins, W. A. F., Figueroa, M. E., and Melnick, J. L.: Herpesvirus type 2: Association with carcinoma of the cervix. Science 161:1255–1256, 1968.

Reller, L. B.: Granulomatous hepatitis associated with acute cytomegalovirus infection. Lancet 1:20–22, 1973.

Rennick, P. M., Nolan, D. C., Bauer, R. B., and Lerner, A. M.: Neuropsychologic and neurologic follow-up after herpesvirus hominis encephalitis. Neurology 23:42–47, 1973.

Reynolds, D. W., Stagno, S., Hosty, T. S., Tiller, M., and Alford, C. A., Jr.: Maternal cytomegalovirus excretion and perinatal infection. New Eng. J. Med. 289:1–5, 1973.

Reynolds, D. W., Stagno, S., Stubbs, K. G., Dahle, A. J., Livingston, M. M., Saxon, S. S., and Alford, C. A.: Inapparent congenital cytomegalovirus infection with elevated cord IgM levels. Causal relation with auditory and mental deficiency. New Eng. J. Med. 290:291–296, 1974.

Ribbert, H.: Ueber protozoenartigen zellen in der niere eines syphilitischen neugeborenen und in der parotis von kindern. Centralbl. Allg. Path. Path. Anat. 15:945–948, 1904.

Ricker, W., Blumberg, A., Peters, C. H., and Widerman, A.: The association of the Guillain-Barré syndrome with infectious mononucleosis. Blood 2:217–226, 1947.

Rifkind, D.: The activation of varicella-zoster virus infections by immunosuppressive therapy. J. Lab. Clin. Med. 68:463–474, 1966.

Rifkind, D., Goodman, N., and Hill, R. B.: The clinical significance of cytomegalovirus infection in renal transplant recipients. Ann. Intern. Med. 66:1116–1128, 1967.

Riley, H. D., Jr.: Reye's syndrome. J. Infect. Dis. 125:77–81, 1972.

Rinvik, R.: Congenital varicella encephalomyelitis in surviving newborn. Am. J. Dis. Child. 117:231–235, 1969.

Root, A. W., and Speicher, C. E.: The triad of thrombocytopenia, eczema, and recurrent infections (Wiskott-Aldrich syndrome) associated with milk antibodies, giant-cell pneumonia, and cytomegalic inclusion disease. Pediatrics 31:444–454, 1963.

Rose, F. C., Brett, E. M., and Burston, J.: Zoster encephalomyelitis. Arch. Neurol. 11:155–172, 1964.

Ross, A. H., Julia, A., and Balakrishnan, C.: Toxicity of adenine arabinoside in humans. J. Infect. Dis. 133 (Suppl.): 192–198, 1976.

Rovit, R. L., and Sigler, M. H.: Hyponatremia with herpes simplex encephalitis. Arch. Neurol. 10:595–603, 1964.

Rowe, W. P., Hartley, J. W., Waterman, S., Turner, H. C., and Huebner, R. J.: Cytopathogenic agent resembling human salivary gland virus recovered from tissue cultures of human adenoids. Proc. Soc. Exp. Biol. Med. 92:418–424, 1956.

Ruckdeschel, J. S., Schimpff, S. C., Smyth, A. C., and Mardiney, M. R., Jr.: Herpes zoster and impaired cell-associated immunity to the varicella-zoster virus in patients with Hodgkin's disease. Am. J. Med. 62:77–85, 1977.

Ruiz-Palacios, G., Pickering, L. K., van Eys, J., and Conklin, R.: Disseminated herpes simplex with hepatoadrenal necrosis in a child with acute leukemia. J. Pediat. 91:757–759, 1977.

Russell, A. S., and Saertre, A.: Antibodies to Herpes-simplex virus in "normal" cerebrospinal fluid. Lancet 1:64–65, 1976.

Rytel, M. W., and Kauffman, H. M.: Clinical efficacy of adenine arabinoside in therapy of cytomegalovirus infections in renal allograft recipients. J. Infect. Dis. 133:202–205, 1976.

Sachs, E., Jr., and House, R. K.: The Ramsey Hunt syndrome. Neurology 6:262–268, 1956.

Saksena, H. C.: Paralysis of the serratus anterior following glandular fever. Brit. Med. J. 2:267, 1943.

Sargent, E. N., Carson, M. J., and Reilly, E. D.: Roentgenographic manifestations of varicella pneumonia with postmortem correlation. Am. J. Roentgen. 98:305–317, 1966.

Sarubbi, F. A., Jr., Sparling, P. F., and Glezen, W. P.: Herpesvirus hominis encephalitis. Virus isolation from brain biopsy in seven patients and results of therapy. Arch. Neurol. 29:268–273, 1973.

Savage, M. O., Moosa, A., and Gordon, R. R.: Maternal varicella infection as a cause of fetal malformations. Lancet 1:352–354, 1973.

Schmitz, H., and Enders, G.: Cytomegalovirus as a frequent cause of Guillain-Barre syndrome. J. Med. Virol. 1:21–27, 1977.

Schmitz, H., and Scherer, M.: IgM antibodies to Epstein-Barr virus in infectious mononucleosis. Arch. Gesamte Virusforsch. 37:332–339, 1972.

Schober, R., and Herman, M. M.: Neuropathology of cardiac transplantation. Survey of 31 cases. Lancet 1:962–967, 1973.

Shashaty, G. G., and Atamer, M. A.: Hemolytic uremic syndrome associated with infectious mononucleosis. Am. J. Dis. Child. 127:720–722, 1974.

Shearer, W. T., Schreiner, R. L., Marshall, R. E., and Barton, L. L.: Cytomegalovirus infection in a newborn dizygous twin. J. Pediat. 81:1161–1165, 1972.

Shershow, L. W., Ekert, H., Swanson, V. L., Wright, H. T., Jr., and Gilchrist, G. S.: Intravascular coagulation in generalized herpes simplex infection of the newborn. Acta Paediat. Scand. 58:535–539, 1969.

Shimada, M., Wakaizumi, S., Kasubuchi, Y., and Kusonoki, T.: Cytarabine and its effect on cerebellum of suckling mouse. Arch. Neurol. 32:555–559, 1975.

Sibert, J. R.: Hypoglossal nerve palsy complicating a case of infectious mononucleosis. Postgrad. Med. J. 48:691–692, 1972.

Sieber, O. F., Jr., Fulginiti, V. A., Brazie, J., and Umlauf, H. J., Jr.: In utero infection of the fetus by herpes simplex virus. J. Pediat. 69:30–34, 1966.

Silver, H. K., Robertson, W. O., Wray, J. D., and Gruskay, F. L.: Involvement of the central nervous system in infectious mononucleosis in childhood. Am. J. Dis. Child. 91:490–494, 1956.

Silverstein, A., Steinberg, G., and Nathanson, M.: Nervous system involvement in infectious mononucleosis. Arch. Neurol. 26:353–358, 1972.

Slade, J. deR.: Involvement of the central nervous system in infectious mononucleosis. New Eng. J. Med. 234:753–757, 1946.

Smith, D. C.: Acute myelitis following varicella. Am. J. Dis. Child. 10:445, 1915.

Smith, J. B., Groover, R. V., Klass, D. W., and Houser, W.: Multicystic cerebral degeneration in neonatal Herpes simplex virus encephalitis. Am. J. Dis. Child. 131:568–572, 1977.

Smith, J. B., Westmoreland, B. F., Reagan, T. J., and Sandok, B. A.: A distinctive clinical EEG profile in Herpes simplex encephalitis. Mayo Clin. Proc. 50:469–474, 1975.

Smith, J. N., Jr.: Complications of infectious mononucleosis. Ann. Intern. Med. 44:861–873, 1956.

Smith, K. O., and Rasmussen, L. E.: Morphology of cytomegalovirus (salivary gland virus). J. Bact. 95:1319–1325, 1963.

Smith, M. G.: Propagation in tissue cultures of a cytopathogenic virus from human salivary gland virus (SGV) disease. Proc. Soc. Exp. Biol. Med. 92:424–430, 1956.

Smith, M. G., Lennette, E. H., and Reames, H. R.: Isolation of virus of herpes simplex and demonstration of intranuclear inclusions in case of acute encephalitis. Am. J. Path. 17:55–68, 1941.

Smith, M. G., and Vellios, F.: Inclusion disease or generalized salivary gland virus infection. Arch. Path. 50:862–884, 1950.

Sokal, J. E., and Firat, D.: Varicella-zoster infection in Hodgkin's disease. Am. J. Med. 39:452–463, 1965.

Sommerville, R. G.: Rapid identification of neurotropic viruses by an immunofluorescent technique applied to cerebrospinal fluid cellular deposits. Arch. Gesamte Virusforsch. 19:63–69, 1966.

Soriano, R. B., South, M. A., Goldman, A. S., and Smith, C. W.: Defect of neutrophil motility in a child with recurrent bacterial infections and disseminated cytomegalovirus infection. J. Pediat. 83:951–958, 1973.

South, M. A., Tompkins, W. A. F., Morris, C. R., and Rawls, W. E.: Congenital malformation of the central nervous system associated with genital type (type 2) herpesvirus. J. Pediat. 75:13–18, 1969.

Srabstein, J. C., Morris, N., Larke, R. P. B., deSa, D. J., Castelino, B. B., and Sum, E.: Is there a congenital varicella syndrome? J. Pediat. 84:239–243, 1974.

St. Geme, J. W., Jr., Prince, J. T., Burke, B. A., Good, R. A., and Krivit, W.: Impaired cellular resistance to herpes-simplex virus in Wiskott-Aldrich syndrome. New Eng. J. Med. 273:229–234, 1965.

Stagno, S., Reynolds, D. W., Lakeman, A., Charamella, L. J., and Alford, C. A., Jr.: Congenital cytomegalovirus infection: Consecutive occurrence due to viruses with similar antigenic compositions. Pediatrics 52:788–794, 1973.

Stagno, S., Reynolds, D. W., Huang, E. S., Thames, S. D., Smith, R. J., and Alford, C. A., Jr.: Congenital cytomegalovirus infection. Occurrence in an immune population. New Eng. J. Med. 296:1254–1258, 1977.

Stagno, S., Reynolds, D., Dsiantos, A., Fuccillo, D. A., Smith, R., Tiller, M., and Alford, C. A., Jr.: Cervical cytomegalovirus excretion in pregnant and nonpregnant women: Suppression in early gestation. J. Infect. Dis. 131:522–527, 1975.

Stagno, S., Reynolds, D. W., Amos, C. S., Dahle, A. J., McCollister, F. P., Mohindra, I., Ermocilla, R., and Alford, C. A.: Auditory and visual defects resulting from symptomatic subclinical congenital cytomegalovirus and toxoplasma infections. Pediatrics 59:669–678, 1977.

Stalder, H., Oxman, M. N., Dawson, D. M., and Levin, M. J.: Herpes simplex meningitis: Isolation of Herpes simplex virus type 2 from cerebrospinal fluid. New Eng. J. Med. 289:1296–1298, 1973.

Starr, J. G., Bart, R. D., Jr., and Gold, E.: Inapparent congenital cytomegalovirus infection. New Eng. J. Med. 282:1975–1978, 1970.

Starr, J. G., and Gold, E.: Screening of newborn infants for cytomegalovirus infection. J. Pediat. 73:820–824, 1968.

Steele, R. W., Chapa, I. A., Vincent, M. M., Hensen, S. A., and Keeney, R. E.: Effects of adenine arabinoside on cellular immune mechanisms in humans. Antimicrob. Agents Chemother. 7:203–207, 1975.

Steele, R. W., Keeney, R. E., Brown, J., III, and Young, E. J.: Cellular immune responses to herpesviruses during treatment with adenine arabinoside. J. Infect. Dis. 135:593–599, 1977.

Stern, H.: Isolation of cytomegalovirus and clinical manifestations of infection of different ages. Brit. Med. J. 1:665–669, 1968.

Stern, H., Elek, S. D., Millar, D. M., and Anderson, H. F.: Herpetic whitlow. A form of cross-infection in hospitals. Lancet 2:871–874, 1959.

Stern, H., and Tucker, S. M.: Cytomegalovirus infection in the newborn and in early childhood. Lancet 2:1268–1271, 1965.

Stevens, D. A., Jordan, G. W., Waddell, T. F., and Merigan, T. C.: Adverse effect of cytosine arabinoside on disseminated zoster in a controlled trial. New Eng. J. Med. 289:873–878, 1973.

Stone, W. J., Scowden, E. B., Spannuth, C. L., Lowry, S. P., and Alford, R. H.: Atypical Herpesvirus hominis type 2 infection in uremic patients receiving immunosuppressive therapy. Am. J. Med. 63:511–516, 1977.

Sumaya, C. V.: Primary Epstein-Barr virus infections in children. Pediatrics 59:16–21, 1977.

Sutton, A. L., Smithwick, E. M., Seligman, S. J., and Kim, D.-S.: Fatal disseminated Herpesvirus hominis type 2 infection in an adult associated with thymic dysplasia. Am. J. Med. 56:545–553, 1974.

Swanson, J. L., Craighead, J. E., and Reynolds, E. S.: Electron microscopic observations on herpesvirus hominis (herpes simplex virus) encephalitis in man. Lab. Invest. 15:1966–1981, 1966.

Sworn, M. J., and Urich, H.: Acute encephalitis in infectious mononucleosis. J. Path. 100:201–205, 1970.

Taber, L. H., Brasier, F., Couch, R. B., Greenberg, S. B., Jones, D., and Knight, V.: Diagnosis of Herpes simplex virus infection by immunofluorescence. J. Clin. Microbiol. 3:309–312, 1976.

Taber, L. H., Greenberg, S. B., Perez, F. I., and Couch, R. B.: Herpes simplex encephalitis treated with vidarabine (adenine arabinoside). Arch. Neurol. 34:608–610, 1977.

Takashima, S., and Becker, L. E.: Neuropathology of fatal varicella. Arch. Path. Lab. Med. 103:209–213, 1979.

Tamir, D., Benderly, A., Levy, J., Ben-Porath, E., and Vonsover, A.: Infectious mononucleosis and Epstein-Barr virus in children. Pediatrics 53:330–335, 1974.

Terni, M., Caccialanza, P., Cassai, E., and Kieff, E.: Aseptic meningitis in association with herpes progenitalis. New Eng. J. Med. 285:503–504, 1971.

Thalhimer, W.: Herpes zoster: Central nervous system lesions similar to those of epidemic (lethargic) encephalitis. Arch. Neurol. Psychiat. 12:73–79, 1924.

Thelander, H. E., and Shaw, E. B.: Infectious mononucleosis. With special reference to cerebral complications. Am. J. Dis. Child. 61:1131–1145, 1941.

Thoene, J., Sweetman, L., Shafai, T., Kennaway, N., Fellman, J., and Nyhan, W.: Tyrosinemia associated with perinatal infection with cytomegalovirus. J. Pediat. 92:108–112, 1978.

Thomas, J. E., and Howard, F. M., Jr.: Segmental zoster paresis—a disease profile. Neurology 22:459–466, 1972.

Tobin, J. D., Jr., and ten Bensel, R. W.: Varicella with thrombocytopenia causing fatal intracerebral hemorrhage. Am. J. Dis. Child. 124:577–578, 1972.

Toghill, P. J., Bailey, M. E., Williams, R., Zeegen, R., and Bown, R.: Cytomegalovirus hepatitis in the adult. Lancet 1:1351–1354, 1967.

Torphy, D. E., Ray, C. G., McAlister, R., and Du, J. N. H.: Herpes simplex virus infection in infants: A spectrum of disease. J. Pediat. 76:405–408, 1970.

Tsairis, P., Dyck, P. J., and Mulder, D. W.: Natural history of brachial plexus neuropathy. Arch. Neurol. 27:109–117, 1972.

Tuffli, G. A., and Nahmias, A. J.: Neonatal herpetic infection. Am. J. Dis. Child. 118:909–914, 1969.

Underwood, E. A.: The neurological complications of varicella: A clinical and epidemiological study. Brit. J. Child. Dis. 32:83–107, 117–196, 241–263, 1935.

Upton, A. R. M., Barwick, D. D., and Foster, J. B.: Dexamethasone treatment in herpes-simplex encephalitis. Lancet 1:290–291, 1971.

van Gelderen, H. H.: Successfully treated cytomegalic disease in a newborn infant. Acta Pediat. 48:169–174, 1959.

Visintine, A. M., Nahmias, A. J., and Josey, W. E.: Genital herpes. Perinatal Care. 2:32–41, 1978.

von Bokey, J.: Über den ätiologischen zusammenhang der varizellen mit gewissen fällen von herpes zoster. Wien. Klin. Wschr. 22:1323–1326, 1909.

Walker, G. H., and Robin, J. O'H.: Cytomegalovirus infection in the north west of England. Arch. Dis. Childh. 45:513–522, 1970.

Walker, R. J., Gammal, T. E., and Allen, M. G.: Cranial arteritis associated with herpes zoster. Radiology 107:109–110, 1973.

Walsh, F. C., Poser, C. M., and Carter, S.: Infectious mononucleosis encephalitis. Pediatrics 13:536–543, 1954.

Weinberg, A. G., McCracken, G. H., LoSpalluto, J., and Luby, J. P.: Monoclonal macroglobulinemia and cytomegalic inclusion disease. Pediatrics 51:518–524, 1973.

Welch, R. G.: Chickenpox and the Guillain-Barré syndrome. Arch. Dis. Childh. 37:557–559, 1962.

Weller, T. H.: Cytomegaloviruses: The difficult years. J. Infect. Dis. 122:532–539, 1970.

Weller, T. H.: The cytomegaloviruses: Ubiquitous agents with protean clinical manifestations. Part I. New Eng. J. Med. 285:203–214, 1971.

Weller, T. H.: The cytomegaloviruses: Ubiquitous agents with protean clinical manifestations. Part II. New Eng. J. Med. 285:267–274, 1971.

Weller, T. H., and Coons, A. H.: Fluorescent antibody studies with agents of varicella and herpes zoster propagated in vitro. Proc. Soc. Exp. Biol. Med. 86:789–794, 1954.

Weller, T. H., and Hanshaw, J. B.: Virologic and clinical observations on cytomegalic inclusion disease. New Eng. J. Med. 266:1233–1244, 1962.

Weller, T. H., Hanshaw, J. B., and Scott, D. M. E.: Serologic differentiation of viruses responsible for cytomegalic inclusion disease. Virology 12:130–132, 1960.

Weller, T. H., Macaulay, J. C., Craig, J. M., and Wirth, P.: Isolation of intranuclear inclusion producing agents from infants with illnesses resembling cytomegalic inclusion disease. Proc. Soc. Exp. Biol. Med. 94:4–12, 1957.

Wenzl, J. E., and Rubio, T.: Encephalitis due to herpesvirus hominis in an infant: Treatment with idoxuridine. Southern Med. J. 63:457–459, 1970.

White, J. G.: Fulminating infection with herpes-simplex virus in premature and newborn infants. New Eng. J. Med. 269:455–460, 1963.

Whitley, R. J., Ch'ien, L. T., Buchanan, R. A., and Alford, C. A., Jr.: Studies on adenine arabinoside—a model for antiviral chemotherapeutics. In: Pollard, M.: Antiviral Mechanisms: Perspectives in Virology. Vol. 9, pp. 315–336, Academic Press, New York, 1975.

Whitley, R. J., Ch'ien, L. T., Dolin, R., Galasso, G. J., and Alford, C. A., Jr.: Adenine arabinoside therapy of herpes zoster in the immunosuppressed. New Eng. J. Med. 294:1193–1199, 1976.

Whitley, R. J., Soong, S-J., Dolin, R., Galasso, G. J., Ch'ien, L. T., Alford, C. A., and the Collaborative Study Group: Adenine arabinoside therapy of biopsy-proved Herpes simplex encephalitis. New Eng. J. Med. 297:289–294, 1977.

Williams, B. B., and Lerner, A. M.: Some previously unrecognized features of herpes simplex virus encephalitis. Neurology 28:1193–1196, 1978.

Williams, V., Gershon, A. A., and Brunell, P. A.: Serologic response to varicella-zoster membrane antigens measured by indirect immunofluorescence. J. Infect. Dis. 130:669–672, 1974.

Wolf, A., and Cowen, D.: Perinatal infections of the central nervous system. J. Neuropath. Exp. Neurol. 18:191–243, 1959.

Wyatt, J. P., Saxton, J., Lee, R. S., and Pinkerton, H.: Generalized cytomegalic inclusion disease. J. Pediat. 36:271–294, 1950.

Yahr, M. D., and Frontera, A. T.: Acute autonomic neuropathy. Its occurrence in infectious mononucleosis. Arch. Neurol. 32:132–133, 1975.

Yeager, A. S.: Transfusion-acquired cytomegalovirus infection in newborn infants. Am. J. Dis. Child. 128:478–483, 1974.

Young, G. F., Knox, D. L., and Dodge, P. R.: Necrotizing encephalitis and chorioretinitis in a young infant. Arch. Neurol. 13:15–24, 1965.

Zavoral, J. H., Ray, W. L., Kinnard, P. G., and Nahmias, A. J.: Neonatal herpetic infection. J.A.M.A. 213:1492–1493, 1970.

Chapter Fifteen

CAT SCRATCH DISEASE

General Aspects of the Disease

Cat scratch disease is usually a benign, self-limited illness that is transmitted to humans by the scratch or bite of a healthy cat. The illness had been recognized as early as 1932 by Debré and by Foshay (Carithers 1970) but the initial report by Debré and colleagues did not appear until 1950. The large series of cases reported by certain authors (Carithers et al., Margileth) suggests that the disease is not infrequent, and according to Carithers et al., 75 percent of reported cases have occurred in children. Whether the predisposition for the illness to occur in children and young adults is merely related to more intimate exposure to cats or is due to other factors is not apparent.

The incubation period is not always precise unless the patient recalls a specific encounter with a cat which resulted in an abrasion. Often there is a history of continual close contact with one or more cats and repeated cutaneous scratches. Three to 14 days after incurring the inoculation, a primary lesion develops in about 50 percent of the patients according to Job, and in 95 percent in the experience of Carithers (1978). The lesion is in the form of a small papule measuring up to one centimeter in diameter which is located at the site of the original contamination. It is usually on the dorsum of the hand, the fingers, or the foot but can be on any exposed surface that is accessible to the claws of the cat. The primary lesion may resolve within one or two weeks after its appearance or can persist for several weeks before it disappears.

Although a primary lesion at the site of inoculation is sometimes never observed, regional lymphadenitis is consistently present and is the hallmark of the disease. Lymph node enlargement develops two to six weeks after the primary lesion first appears. The location of the enlarged node depends upon the original site of the inoculation. Since the hand is usually the assaulted site, unilateral axillary lymphadenitis is most common. In other patients, the location of the enlarged node or nodes is in the cervical, preauricular, submandibular, epitrochlear, or inguinal region. Lymphadenitis can be symptomless or the involved nodes may become tender as progressive enlargement occurs. Resolution and spontaneous disappearance of the adenopathy usually will occur after a few weeks. In a small number of patients, the involved node or nodes eventually become fluctuant, indicating that suppuration has occurred.

Most patients with cat scratch disease are either asymptomatic except for localized adenopathy or exhibit only mild systemic complaints. Anorexia, generalized aching, malaise, or abdominal discomfort in some cases will be associated with fever, which varies from 101° to 103°. Rash of any variety is unusual but maculopapular eruptions have been described, as has erythema nodosum (Steiner et al., Young). Other unusual clinical manifestations include thrombocytopenic purpura (Jim), osteolytic skeletal lesions (Carithers et al., Rauschkolb), and the neurologic complications discussed below. An infrequent variant of cat scratch disease occurs when the bulbar or palpebral conjunctiva is the site of primary infection. The resulting granulomatous conjunctivitis and preauricular or cervical lymphadenitis is referred to as the oculoglandular syndrome of Parinaud (Carithers 1978, Cassady and Culbertson). Except for the portal of entry and thus the location of the primary lesion, this form of cat scratch disease is similar in regard to clinical course and diagnostic tests to the more common glandular form of the disease.

Etiology

Cat scratch disease is an infectious illness generally believed to be caused by a virus. The causative agent has not been isolated and transmission to animals has generally been unsuccessful (Job). Atypical mycobacteria were once considered to be the possible cause of the illness on the basis of skin test results (Boyd and Craig) but have been excluded by subsequent studies (Warwick). A herpes virus has been implicated by some workers (Kalter et al., Turner et al.) while more importance has been placed on studies that have suggested the virus is in the psittacosis-lymphogranuloma group (Mollaret et al.) or possesses antigens common to these organisms. With the use of antigens of this group, approximately 50 percent of patients with cat scratch disease have been found to have significant complement-fixation titers compared to 3 percent to 6 percent in a control population (Warwick).

Diagnosis

Conventional laboratory studies usually reveal an initial leukopenia followed by a modest leukocytosis coincident with progressive enlargement of the involved lymph nodes. The erythrocyte sedimentation rate may be normal or increased but not usually to high levels. A negative tuberculin skin test aids in the exclusion of tuberculosis, although a positive test does not categorically eliminate the diagnosis of cat scratch disease.

The intradermal skin test using cat scratch antigen was developed by Foshay and is considered to be highly specific for this disease. The antigen is obtained from an aspirate from a lymph node of an infected patient and is administered intradermally in a dose of 0.1 ml. To avoid false negative tests, the skin test antigen should be applied at least one week after the initial development of enlargement of the involved node (Carithers 1978). A positive reaction is an area of induration of 5 mm. or more, with or without surrounding erythema, in 48 to 72 hours. It has been estimated that 94 percent of patients with a clinical course compatible with cat scratch disease will have a positive skin test reaction (Margileth), while false positive reactions occur in only 2 percent of the population in general who do not have contact with cats (Margileth). The incidence of false positive tests is higher in healthy persons who have close and repeated exposure to cats. An increase in the size of the enlarged nodes and a transient febrile reaction may accompany a positive skin test. Biopsy of the skin test site for histologic examination can be of value in certain diagnostically complex cases. The histology of the injection site compatible with cat scratch disease is the presence of a granulomatous infiltrate with lymphocytes, plasma cells, epithelioid cells, and giant cells in some instances (Czarnetzki et al.).

Needle aspiration of a suppurative lymph node may be diagnostically valuable to exclude bacterial infection as well as therapeutically helpful to control fever and tenderness. Lymph node biopsy may be indicated when the diagnosis remains uncertain.

Neurologic Complications

The first report of encephalitis or encephalopathy associated with cat scratch disease was that of Stevens in 1952. Additional reports with neurologic involvement followed, most of which described brief illnesses with complete recovery and with similar clinical manifestations (Brooksaler, Paxson and McKay, Pollen, Smith and Darling, Steiner et al., Thompson and Miller, Weinstein and Meade). According to Lyon, approximately 38 patients with cat scratch disease with neurologic complications had been reported up to 1971. Of 585 cases of cat scratch disease mentioned by Carithers, only two were complicated by encephalitic features. Radicular or cranial nerve involvement can also occur with cat scratch disease but is even less common than cerebral complications (Weinstein and Meade).

Although cerebral complications of cat scratch disease are unusual, they are often dramatic in terms of the symptoms and signs. Headache, confusion, and drowsiness are frequent initial manifestations of neurologic dysfunction and can develop anytime from three days to six weeks after the usual signs of cat scratch disease. A generalized convulsion in some cases is the first sign indicating cerebral involvement, but more often headache and drowsiness are present for hours or a few days before seizures occur. Several authors have commented upon the precipitous deterioration associated with recurrent convulsions, coma, and fever, which is followed within hours or a day or so by rapid improvement and subsequent recovery within a few days (Lyon, Torres et al., Weinstein and Meade). A seven-year-old child reported by Selby and Walker had the sudden onset of hemiplegia and aphasia attributable to an inflammatory arteritis of the left internal carotid and middle cerebral arteries demonstrated angiographically. This observation raises speculation as to the possible role of cerebral vascular involvement in other cases of cat scratch disease complicated by neurologic signs in which the CSF is unremarkable and rapid recovery follows.

Diffuse muscle weakness has been observed in several cases (Paxson and McKay, Steiner et al.), suggesting a myelitic component but without histologic verification. Weinstein and Meade described a patient with evidence of both cerebral and spinal cord involvement in cat scratch disease and stated that the duration required for recovery will perhaps be prolonged when the spinal cord is affected. Although the patient can appear critically ill at the peak of the illness, cessation of convulsions and restoration of alertness lead to full recovery without residual deficits in the vast majority. An exception to the usual benign course of cat scratch encephalitis was reported by Silberman et al. in which a 19-year-old woman died three days after the onset of coma and convulsions. Necropsy demonstrated mononuclear infiltration of meninges, diffuse multiple hemorrhages in cerebral white matter, and perivascular cuffing with lymphocytes and macrophages.

Cerebrospinal fluid examination in patients with encephalitic complications of cat scratch disease is frequently entirely normal. A mild cellular response occurs in some cases and the protein content may be slightly elevated. In several reported cases, the cerebrospinal fluid glucose has been in the range of 60 to 80 mg. per 100 ml., a finding not uncommon with several types of viral encephalitis. The electroencephalogram is almost uni-formly abnormal, with generalized slow activity evident during the acute phase of the encephalitic state. Reversal toward normal lags behind clinical signs of improvement but eventually occurs.

It is unclear whether the neurologic manifestations that may besiege the child with cat scratch disease represent an encephalitis with invasion of the brain by the causative agent, or an encephalopathy in which the brain responds adversely to an unidentified factor without actual infiltration by the organism or secondary to an inflammatory or immune vasculitis. In those patients with marked temperature elevation, nuchal rigidity, and a lymphocytic pleocytosis in cerebrospinal fluid, the process is probably an encephalitic one, although this will remain unproved unless an infectious agent can be isolated from the cerebrospinal fluid or brain tissue. While of scientific interest, the distinction is of little importance from the standpoint of management since therapeutic principles probably remain the same in either situation. Treatment is supportive, including measures to control seizures, to maintain fluid and electrolyte balance, and to prevent hyperthermia. Corticosteroid therapy might be considered if vasculitis could be demonstrated to be present; however, this remains speculative.

REFERENCES

Boyd, G. L., and Craig, G.: Etiology of cat-scratch fever. J. Pediat. 59:313–317, 1961.

Brooksaler, F.: Cat scratch disease with encephalopathy. Am. J. Dis. Child. 107:185–187, 1964.

Carithers, H. A.: Cat-scratch disease. Notes on its history. Am. J. Dis. Child. 119:200–203, 1970.

Carithers, H. A.: Oculoglandular disease of Parinaud. A manifestation of cat-scratch disease. Am. J. Dis. Child. 132:1195–1200, 1978.

Carithers, H. A., Carithers, C. M., and Edwards, R. O., Jr.: Cat-scratch disease. Its natural history. J.A.M.A. 207:312–316, 1969.

Cassady, J. V., and Culbertson, C. S.: Cat-scratch disease and Parinaud's oculoglandular syndrome. Arch. Ophthal. 50:68–74, 1953.

Czarnetzki, B. M., Pomeranz, J. R., Khandekar, P. K., Wolinsky, E., and Belcher, R. W.: Cat-scratch disease skin test. Studies of specificity and histopathologic features. Arch. Dermatol. 111:736–739, 1975.

Debré, R., Lamy, M., Jammet, M. L., Costil, L., and Mozziconacci, P.: La maladie des griffes du chat. Sem. Hop. Paris. 26:1895–1904, 1950.

Jim, R. T. S.: Thrombocytopenic purpura in cat scratch disease. J.A.M.A. 176:146, 1961.

Job, J. C.: Cat-scratch disease. In: Debré, R., and Celers,

J.: Clinical Virology. W. B. Saunders Company, Philadelphia, 1970.

Kalter, S. S., Kim, C. S., and Heberling, R. L.: Herpeslike virus particles associated with cat-scratch disease. Nature 224:190, 1969.

Lyon, L. W.: Neurologic manifestations of cat-scratch disease. Report of a case and review of the literature. Arch. Neurol. 25:23–27, 1971.

Margileth, A. M.: Cat-scratch disease: Nonbacterial regional lymphadenitis. A study of 145 patients and a review of the literature. Pediatrics 42:803–818, 1968.

Mollaret, P., Reilly, J., Bastin, R., and Tournier, P.: La decouverte du virus de la lymphoreticulose benigne d'inoculation. Presse. Méd. 59:681–701, 1951.

Paxson, E. M., and McKay, R. J., Jr.: Neurologic symptoms associated with cat scratch disease. Pediatrics 20:13–21, 1957.

Pollen, R. H.: Cat-scratch encephalitis. Neurology 18:1031–1033, 1968.

Rauschkolb, R. R.: Cat scratch disease. A selective review. Arch. Derm. 79:674, 1959.

Selby, G., and Walker, G. L.: Cerebral arteritis in cat-scratch disease. Neurology 29:1413–1418, 1979.

Silberman, J., Deza, L., and Zaidman, J.: Acute hemorrhagic leukoencephalopathy following cat scratch disease. J. Neuropath. Exp. Neurol. 25:121, 1966.

Smith, R. E., and Darling, R. M.: Encephalopathy of cat-scratch disease. Am. J. Dis. Child. 99:123–124, 1960.

Steiner, M. M., Vuckovitch, D., and Hadawi, S. A.: Cat-scratch disease with encephalopathy. J. Pediat. 62:514–520, 1963.

Stevens, H.: Cat-scratch fever encephalitis. Am. J. Dis. Child. 84:218–222, 1952.

Thompson, T. E., and Miller, K. F.: Cat scratch encephalitis. Ann. Intern. Med. 39:146–151, 1953.

Torres, J. R., Sanders, C. V., Strub, R. L., and Black, F. W.: Cat-scratch disease causing reversible encephalopathy. J.A.M.A. 240:1628–1629, 1978.

Turner, W., Bigley, N. J., Dodd, M. O., and Anderson, G.: Hemagglutinating virus isolated from cat scratch disease. J. Bact. 80:430–435, 1960.

Warwick, W. J.: The cat scratch syndrome, many diseases or one disease? Progr. Med. Virol. 9:256–301, 1967.

Weinstein, L., and Meade, R. H.: The neurologic manifestations of cat scratch disease. Am. J. Med. Sci. 229:500–505, 1955.

Young, D. L.: Cat scratch disease: cause of erythema nodosum and splenomegaly. Texas J. Med. 57:278, 1961.

Chapter Sixteen

RABIES

In many parts of the world, including India, the Philippines, Vietnam, and countries in Latin America, rabies is a serious health problem causing many deaths and necessitating prophylactic immunization of large numbers of persons each year (Miller and Nathanson). In the United States, human rabies has become so rare that most practicing physicians will not encounter a case during their professional lifetimes. The management of the child who has sustained an animal bite, however, is a continual problem which requires the perplexing decision of whether or not to administer prophylactic therapy. The primary purpose of this chapter is to provide the knowledge of the disease and its epidemiology that is essential for judgments regarding prevention.

The rabies virus is an RNA virus which is now classified among the rhadovirus group (Melnick). The term "street virus" has been used in reference to rabies virus occurring in nature in contrast to "fixed virus," which results from laboratory passage from one animal to another. Pasteur and colleagues in 1884 demonstrated that by serial passage of virus from rabbit to rabbit, a modified virus would result which eventually retained little ability to infect dogs when given subcutaneously. This so-called "fixed virus" also differed from that occurring in nature by its inability to produce Negri bodies in tissue, characteristic of the natural infection in animals and humans. In 1885, a small boy severely bitten by a rabid dog was taken to Pasteur who administered his newly developed vaccine to the child without adverse effects. The child remained well and the Pasteur treatment for prevention of rabies was thereby established and soon adopted the world over.

Rabies has been considered a world-wide disease, although recently it has become rare in humans in the United States and is almost absent in England. From 1946 until 1968, only eight fatal cases of rabies were recorded in England, all of which had been acquired by animal bites outside the boundaries of that country (Macrae). In the United States, there were almost 500 human deaths due to rabies from 1940 to 1960, but between 1961 and 1970 only 16 fatal cases were reported (Morbidity and Mortality Weekly Reports, Vol. 19, Aug. 1971). In 1971, just two fatal cases of rabies were identified in the United States, one of which was acquired outside the boundaries of this country (Annual Summary Rabies—1971). The incidence of the human disease in each of the following years in this country has been approximately the same (Fig. 16–1). Ireland, Australia, and New Zealand are additional countries where eradication of the disease has been successful.

Transmission of rabies to man is largely dependent on the existence of the virus in wild and domestic animals. The dog has been the most notable vector in the mind of the public but, with measures to control stray dog populations plus widespread vaccination of domestic pets, this source of rabies has diminished precipitously. In this country, 8000 cases of rabies in dogs were recorded in 1946 compared to 412 in 1966 (Morbidity and Mortality Weekly Reports, Vol. 16, May 13, 1967) and 235 in 1971 (Annual Summary Rabies—1971). In laboratory-confirmed cases of animal rabies in the United States from 1953 through 1977, the dog was the most commonly infected species for the first seven years of this period but has ranked far down the list in the past decade. In the past several years, the skunk has been the most important

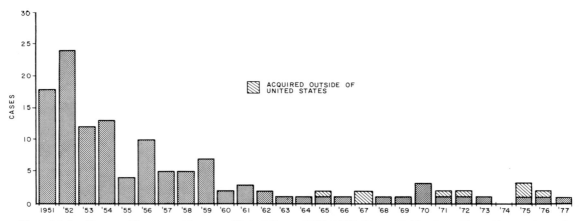

Figure 16–1. Reported human rabies cases, United States, 1951–1977. (From: Rabies Surveillance Report Annual Summary, 1977, U.S. Department of Health, Education and Welfare.)

wildlife reservoir in this country, accounting for almost 50 percent of the total incidence (Table 16–1). Wild rodents, such as mice and chipmunks, and pet rodents, including hamsters and guinea pigs, are not usually considered to be in the rabies cycle. Bites from these small animals are commonplace but generally do not represent a rabies threat. In Africa, the mongoose has been an important source of human rabies, while in Canada and certain European countries, the fox is the largest single reservoir.

Rabies transmitted by bats to cattle and other animals was recognized in the early part of this century. In 1929, the first human cases secondary to bites of vampire bats were recognized in Trinidad when 17 fatal cases occurred (Pawan). Unlike rabies transmitted by the more common wild animal species, these cases secondary to bat bites were nota-

Table 16–1. Reported Rabies Cases in the United States by Type of Animal, 1953–1977. Includes Guam, Puerto Rico, Virgin Islands.*

YEAR	DOGS	CATS	FARM ANIMALS	FOXES	SKUNKS	BATS	OTHER ANIMALS	MAN	TOTAL
1953	5,688	538	1,118	1,033	319	8	119	14	8,837
1954	4,083	462	1,032	1,028	547	4	118	8	7,282
1955	2,657	343	924	1,223	580	14	98	5	5,844
1956	2,592	371	794	1,281	631	41	126	10	5,846
1957	1,758	382	714	1,021	775	31	115	6	4,802
1958	1,643	353	737	845	1,005	68	157	6	4,814
1959	1,119	292	751	920	789	80	126	6	4,083
1960	697	277	645	915	725	88	108	2	3,457
1961	594	217	482	614	1,254	186	120	3	3,470
1962	565	232	614	594	1,449	157	114	2	3,727
1963	573	217	531	622	1,462	303	224	1	3,933
1964	409	220	594	1,061	1,909	352	238	1	4,784
1965	412	289	625	1,038	1,582	484	153	1	4,584
1966	412	252	587	864	1,522	377	183	1	4,198
1967	412	293	691	979	1,568	414	250	2	4,609
1968	296	157	457	801	1,400	291	210	1	3,613
1969	256	165	428	888	1,156	321	307	1	3,522
1970	185	135	399	771	1,235	296	252	3	3,276
1971	235	222	484	677	2,018	465	289	2	4,392
1972	232	184	547	645	2,095	504	218	2	4,427
1973	180	139	448	477	1,851	432	170	1	3,698
1974	232	121	303	302	1,421	537	239	0	3,155
1975	129	104	200	276	1,226	514	223	3	2,675
1976	116	106	198	187	1,468	737	332	2	3,146
1977	120	108	217	122	1,631	637	346	1	3,182

*From: Rabies Surveillance Report Annual Summary 1977, U.S. Department of Health, Education and Welfare.

ble for the high incidence of paralytic signs due to diffuse spinal cord involvement. The vampire bat of Mexico and Central and South America has continued to be a source of the rabies virus to humans and domestic animals. More recently, however, non-vampire bats of the fructivorous and insectivorous types have been shown to be capable of harboring and transmitting rabies virus to humans (Girard et al., Kent and Finegold, Lennette et al.).

Insectivorous bats of either the free-living or colonial type harboring rabies virus have been identified in almost all states in this country and, thus, create a continual potential threat to the human and animal population. As opposed to the high incidence of paralytic symptoms said to have occurred in Trinidad resulting from bites of rabid vampire bats, cases in this country transmitted by insectivorous bats have been manifested mainly by encephalitic features, often preceded by pain and numbness in the region of the bite. Bats infected with rabies virus may appear ill and demonstrate abnormal behavior or, unlike most other rabid animals, can be asymptomatic carriers of the virus but still capable of transmitting the disease.

While animal-to-man transmission of rabies virus is the cause of the human disease in the overwhelming majority of instances, the possibility of man-to-man spread has long been a cause of speculation and concern. The importance of this mode of spread is primarily related to the possible danger to hospital attendants who may become exposed to the virus during attempts to restrain and manage the agitated and irrational victim. There is documented evidence that rabies virus can be present in the saliva of humans with rabies (Duffy et al., Meyer) and, therefore, could conceivably be transmitted to other humans through bites or contamination of wounds by the infected saliva. Meyer has stated that human-to-human transmission of rabies has been infrequently observed because of the usual prompt use of prophylactic therapy in those persons intimately exposed to the saliva of an ill patient.

Houff et al. described a single case in which rabies was transmitted from person to person via a corneal transplant. The donor had no history of an animal bite and experienced an atypical illness characterized by paralytic signs and external ophthalmoparesis. Rabies was not considered because of the unusual clinical features until the recipient died of the disease 50 days after corneal transplantation. A second example of human-to-human transmission of rabies via a corneal transplant has been reported (Morbidity and Mortality Weekly Reports, Vol. 29, Jan. 25, 1980). In this instance, also, the donor had atypical signs characterized by a flaccid quadriparesis which preceded coma.

Pathogenesis

Introduction of the rabies virus into the human is almost always by the bite of an infected animal, transmitting the virus present in its salivary glands and saliva. On very rare occasion, rabies has been acquired by humans by airborne transmission (Conomy et al.). From its site of inoculation, the virus is believed to spread to the central nervous system along peripheral nerves by retrograde axoplasmic flow (Baltazard, Tsiang). The rapidity of migration along neural pathways, and thus the incubation period, is probably related more to the severity of tissue damage plus the richness of innervation of involved tissues than to the linear distance from the site of inoculation to the brain. A temporary viremic phase perhaps exists, although efforts to isolate rabies virus from the blood have usually been unsuccessful (Schindler). How the virus reaches the salivary glands is controversial. Christie suggested that after entrance and replication in nerve cells, the virus may then spread centrifugally along peripheral nerves to salivary and other tissues. Upon arrival within the brain or spinal cord, the virus enters cells and undergoes its multiplication process, eventually resulting in lesions characteristic of encephalitis but with certain features peculiar to infection with this particular virus.

Clinical Features

The incubation period in most cases of human rabies is between 30 and 60 days, although longer incubation periods are well known (Warrell et al.). For the illness to become symptomatic less than 15 days after the inoculating bite is unusual, as are incubation periods reported in the literature of one to two years. Some authors have suggested that the incubation period depends on the site of the inoculation and thus the distance the virus must travel to reach the brain. This relationship has not been proved and is doubted by most investigators (Dupont and

Earle, Johnson). Most authors now favor such factors as the severity of the attack, the degree of tissue damage, and the quantity of virus contaminating tissues to be more closely related to the incubation period.

The initial symptoms of rabies in the human may be either generalized in type, including a feeling of anxiety or depression, malaise, anorexia, headache, and fever, or, more often, in the form of an abnormal sensation or superficial pain in the region of the bite. For example, the child bitten on the hand one to two months previously may first complain of numbness, hyperesthesia, or tingling in the hand, which soon spreads to involve the entire arm and perhaps even the face and chest on the same side. Excessive perspiration is occasionally described in the involved regions. Fever persists or develops if not previously present, and sensitivity to external stimuli such as noises or bright light will often commence.

Within a day or two after onset, apprehension or signs of hyperexcitability develop which lead to mental confusion and disorientation. It is difficult to restrain the child during this period, with his desire for aimless and purposeless walking about resembling compulsive activity. Behavior often becomes intermittently maniacal and makes restraint necessary, but the person applying restraint risks being bitten or scratched by the disoriented patient. Stretch reflexes and muscle tone are generally enhanced at this stage and are joined by signs of autonomic dysfunction. Pupillary dilatation, tachycardia, excessive perspiration, and increased lacrimation and salivation are seen in variable degrees. Neck stiffness usually develops but is not always marked.

Painful, spasmodic contraction of the muscles of the swallowing mechanism result in the symptom best known in rabies, which is referred to as hydrophobia, or "fear of water." Violent spasm of the deglutition muscles is provoked by every attempt to swallow, and in some, by even the sight or thought of water. As a result, saliva pools in the patient's oral cavity and is allowed to drool from the mouth. Laryngeal spasms usually accompany the spasmodic contractions of the pharyngeal musculature, possibly causing airway obstruction sufficient to produce convulsions or a posture of opisthotonus. Occasionally, cardiac arrest and death will ensue during such a hypoxic episode. In some cases, the irritability of the throat musculature is less intense and causes only mild dysphagia with a feeling of tightness or constriction in the pharyngeal region. It is presumed that the recurrent pharyngeal and laryngeal spasms so characteristic of rabies is explained by the striking predilection for brain stem inflammatory involvement before the cerebrum is affected to the degree that disturbance of consciousness occurs. The intermittent episodes of alteration of the respiratory pattern associated with recurrent pharyngeal spasms in the early stage of the illness gradually merge into various types of respiratory irregularities as the patient becomes progressively more unresponsive (Warrell et al.).

Death frequently occurs during the excitement phase, with the total duration of the disease usually being three to eight days. With intensive management of the metabolic abnormalities, airway, and respiratory failure, survival for several weeks after onset of the disease is possible but is infrequent (Bhatt et al.). On rare occasions, the illness assumes a fulminating course with death occurring less than 24 hours after the initiation of symptoms. In some, hyperexcitability, tremulousness, and motor restlessness are followed by a paralytic phase before death ensues. Weakness in such patients may be either symmetrical or asymmetrical, is associated with loss of stretch reflexes, and can include various cranial nerve deficits. Generalized paralytic signs are followed by progressive decline in the patient's state of responsiveness, proceeding to deep coma. The pulse rate increases, hypotension and circulatory insufficiency develop, and fever becomes progressively higher. Eventual cardiorespiratory arrest leads to death. Prolongation of life beyond eight or ten days after the onset of clinical rabies is sufficiently unusual that it raises doubt about the correctness of the diagnosis, assuming that ventilatory assistance is not resorted to. More chronic illnesses in patients at risk to develop rabies on the basis of a preceding animal bite are more likely to be due to an adverse neurologic reaction to previously administered rabies vaccine or antirabies serum than to rabies itself.

A less common mode of presentation of rabies is with paretic or paralytic features before the occurrence of the more usual signs of encephalitic involvement. Motor weakness may first appear in the limb that was bitten and is usually preceded by local pain or paresthesias. Spasms of the muscles of deglutition may not develop until near the terminal stages of the disease in such patients. In these atypical cases, the initial brunt of the infection is within the spinal cord, resulting in a necrotizing inflammatory myelopathy (Knutti et al.). Unless a history of an animal bite is volunteered, the presentation of the illness with flaccid paresis of the limbs followed by bulbar paresis and bilateral facial weakness is likely to be confused with the Guillain-Barré syndrome (Houff et al.).

Animal Rabies

Clinical rabies in the animal, for example, the dog, bears similarity to the illness in the human in many respects. It is important to note, however, that there is considerable variation in the manifestations of rabies in different animal species. For example, cats infected with the rabies virus are notable for the vicious behavior they exhibit, while rabid cattle remain docile while dying of the disease. After sustaining a bite from a rabid animal, the dog is asymptomatic for 20 to 40 days, at which time restlessness, irritability, and fever develop. Within a day or so, recurrent pharyngeal spasms occur, associated with periods of hyperirritability and excitement intermixed with phases of depression and lassitude.

Rabies in the dog has been categorized as either the "furious" or the "dumb" type depending on the prominence of the clinical features. The former variety is characterized by the signs of excitement and irritability while the "dumb" type refers to paralytic and depressive features. As noted above, the infected dog commonly exhibits features of both types in various degrees during the illness. Unprovoked biting or vicious attack may occur at any time. Even during the depressive or quiet periods, the animal is dangerous and may snap or bite unpredictably. The child trying to soothe his dog who is obviously ill but lying quietly with saliva issuing from the mouth is especially vulnerable at this time. Muscle weakness or paralysis eventually supervenes as the dog becomes more emaciated and develops a sinister, "wild-eyed" appearance. Spasms become more frequent, interspersed by attempts to bite anything or anyone in reach. Death usually occurs within eight to ten days after onset.

Laboratory Findings

The conventional laboratory studies are of little diagnostic help in rabies and reveal no specific changes. The white blood cell count can be either normal or somewhat elevated, with a modest increase in immature leukocytes. Glucosuria is occasionally found, as is a mild degree of proteinuria during the febrile phase of the illness. The cerebrospinal fluid pressure is normal or elevated but is rarely increased markedly. The CSF is usually clear and colorless and may be without cells. More often, there is a cellular response of 10 to 100 cells per cu. mm., most or all of which are lymphocytes. Both the CSF glucose and protein contents are frequently mildly elevated but not usually to a marked degree. Near the terminal stages of the illness, profound hyperthermia commonly occurs, as well as serum hyponatremia and hypochloremia, possibly secondary to hypothalamic dysfunction with inappropriate antidiuretic hormone secretion.

Pathology

The histopathology of human rabies is that of a severe encephalitis similar to that caused by certain other viruses. It is most notable for the predilection for involvement of gray matter more than white matter and for its predisposition to involve the brain stem. Cerebral, cerebellar, and spinal cord inflammatory changes are present in variable degrees. Inflammatory and degenerative lesions of sensory ganglia and peripheral nerves are also well known (Tangchai and Vejjajiva).

The inflammatory response in rabies is rather nonspecific and consists of perivascular cuffs of lymphocytes and plasma cells in addition to a microglial response and a certain degree of neuronophagia. Brain stem structures, including the pontine tegmentum and the cranial nerve nuclei in the floor of the fourth ventricle, commonly show a heavy inflammatory cell infiltrate associated with neuronal destruction. Meningeal infiltration is usually slight and sometimes is more marked over the spinal cord than over the surface of the brain.

Negri bodies have been recognized to be the pathologic hallmark of rabies encephalitis since their discovery by Negri in 1903. These cytoplasmic inclusions are usually most numerous within neurons in the hippocampus of the temporal lobe and in Purkinje cells of the cerebellum (Fig. 16–2). Paradoxically, regions most abundant in Negri bodies often reveal few other inflammatory changes. Conversely, areas showing the most severe inflammatory exudate may contain no cyto-

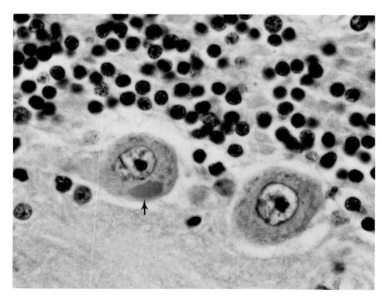

Figure 16–2. Rabies. Negri body within the cytoplasm of a Purkinje cell of the cerebellum.

plasmic inclusions of the Negri type. Neurons containing Negri bodies usually appear otherwise normal or at most reveal only mild chromatolytic changes. Furthermore, Negri bodies cannot invariably be found in rabies encephalitis, and in the series studied by Dupont and Earle they were identified in only 71 percent of the cases.

Negri bodies are well-defined, round or oval eosinophilic cytoplasmic inclusions which vary in size from 5 to 25 microns. The inner structure of the Negri body is essential for positive identification and consists of numerous basophilic granules 0.2 to 0.5 micron in diameter, sometimes arranged in rosette fashion (Tierkel). A peculiar characteristic of this cytoplasmic inclusion is its occurrence with infection by the so-called "street" virus but its absence with the "fixed" virus obtained by laboratory passage from animal to animal. They tend to be larger and more abundant in patients with a longer clinical course before death and are more often absent in those who die following a short illness. This is true in animal rabies also and is one reason why premature sacrifice of a biting animal suspected of being rabid is ill-advised. The precise nature of the Negri body has remained controversial, as have the factors stimulating its formation. Examination with the electron microscope has revealed the Negri body to contain a large number of viral particles (Gonzalez-Angulo et al., Leech), a finding previously identified by fluorescent antibody staining methods (Goldwasser and Kissling).

Negri bodies are specific for rabies and their presence indicates the presence of this virus, making this the only type of acute viral encephalitis in humans for which an etiologic diagnosis can be confirmed by light microscopy. Negri bodies must, however, be distinguished from other types of neuronal inclusions which bear certain resemblances (Derakhshan). Inclusion bodies of canine distemper, for example, can be observed in the brain of dogs and foxes but can be distinguished by their lack of internal structure and their more homogeneous matrix.

Structures similar to Negri bodies in rabies but lacking an inner structure with special staining are referred to as lyssa bodies. These cytoplasmic inclusions are frequently more numerous than Negri bodies but are less specific because identical structures sometimes occur in other conditions. Sung and colleagues studied the ultrastructure of inclusions in the brain in rabies and found that typical Negri bodies did not always exhibit the basophilic inner bodies, a finding, they postulate, that depends on the degree of virus replication. These authors have suggested that lyssa bodies in the brain of a human or animal with rabies may actually be nothing more than Negri bodies without recognizable inner structures. Bàbes nodules were once considered characteristic of rabies but are now recognized to represent clusters of microglial cells similar to those occurring in many types of viral encephalitis and referred to as glial nodules.

Diagnosis

The Attacking Animal

Whenever possible, an animal that bites a human should be captured and confined for a minimum of ten days. Signs indicating that the animal is rabid during the observation period should be reported immediately to the person who was bitten and to his attending physician. The lack of development of symptoms or signs during this period can be assumed to indicate that the animal is not rabid. The premature killing of such animals will complicate laboratory confirmation of rabies, since the formation of Negri bodies in the brain is related to the length of the clinical illness. Should death occur or clinical symptoms of rabies develop requiring that the animal be killed, the head should be removed and shipped under refrigeration to a facility capable of performing the appropriate examinations to establish the presence of rabies. Shipment should be prompt and by messenger whenever possible. The head is best transported in a watertight metal container which is placed in a second, larger metal container with ice packed inside the larger, outer tin. Freezing of the head with dry ice is not desirable because microscopic examination will be delayed until thawing occurs.

Laboratory detection of rabies in the deceased animal is on the basis of identification of Negri bodies by staining of impression smears of brain, fluorescent antibody preparations to demonstrate the viral antigen within brain tissue, and intracerebral inoculation of mice for histologic evidence of the development of Negri bodies and for subsequent viral identification by neuralization tests. The details of laboratory diagnosis by these methods can be found in World Health Organization Monograph Series Number 23, 1966.

The Attacked Human

A person sustaining a bite is considered as *being exposed* to the rabies virus if the attacking animal is shown to be rabid. The person is *assumed* to have been exposed if bitten by a bat or if the animal that inflicted the bite escapes. This is especially true when the attacking animal is of a type known in the geographic area to be occasionally infected with the rabies virus or when the attack was vicious

and unprovoked. For reasons that probably vary from case to case, untreated humans bitten by a rabid animal do not always develop the disease. Precise figures in this regard do not exist but it has been stated that only about 15 percent of humans attacked by a rabid animal will succumb from rabies, even without post-exposure treatment (Tierkel). This figure may be misleadingly low and should not deter one from the established guidelines regarding treatment when possible exposure to the rabies virus has occurred.

Once symptoms or signs in the human have developed, diagnosis during life is largely dependent upon the history of exposure to the virus by animal attack and the features of the encephalitic illness characteristic of the disease. The absence of a history of an animal bite renders the possibility of rabies less likely in the symptomatic patient but by no means excludes the diagnosis. In the series of 49 cases reported by Dupont and Earle, no evidence of a preceding bite was found in 34.7 percent. Antibody titer rises are of value but have their limitations, in part because of the prior administration of serum or vaccine in most cases and also because of the usual abbreviated duration of the illness. In patients who survive over two weeks from onset of symptoms, significant titer rises in blood and CSF are expected and achieve levels considerably higher than those expected from immunization alone.

Reports exist of isolation of the virus from saliva obtained from the patient during life, but this source is not consistently positive (Bhatt et al., Duffy et al.). Virus also has been recovered from cerebrospinal fluid obtained during life (Kent and Finegold). The value of cerebrospinal fluid as a source of rabies virus identification by fluorescent antibody techniques remains unclear in view of the infrequency with which such attempts have been made. Corneal impression smears stained by the direct fluorescent antibody method to detect rabies antigen in corneal epithelial cells have been found to be a useful method for early diagnosis, although performance of the test requires a high degree of technical skill (Koch et al.).

Proof that human encephalitis is due to the rabies virus depends largely on examination of brain tissue after death. The most rapid and easiest procedure is the detection of Negri bodies in the appropriate areas of the brain. In addition to the impression method which may establish a positive diagnosis within one hour after the specimen is received, conventional paraffin-embedded preparations allow detailed examination of the encephalitic lesions. The impression method for detection of Negri bodies is done by obtaining sections approximately 3 mm. in thickness from Ammon's horn, the cerebellum, and the cerebral cortex. The thin slices are placed on a clean wooden spatula and a clean glass slide is gently pressed against the cut surface of the tissue. Several impressions can be made on each slide and several slides from the different anatomic regions are prepared. The slide is flooded with Sellers' stain immediately after the impression is made. The stain is allowed to remain for several seconds and is then gently removed by flooding with water. The slide is air-dried, the tissue covered with a cover-slip, and examination under oil can then be done. With the Sellers' stain, neurons assume a blue coloration while the Negri body is stained purplish-red to bright red with basophilic internal granular bodies. While Negri bodies have an intracytoplasmic location in permanent sections, the inclusions may be seen in an extracellular location on impression smears owing to tissue disruption during the preparation.

When Negri bodies are not detected, the fluorescent antibody test assumes greater importance. This procedure also can be rapidly performed and is highly accurate but requires expert technical skill by one trained in the method and its interpretation. The procedure consists of labeling antibody with fluorescent dye, permitting the antibody to react with specific antigen if present, and examining the results of the reaction with the fluorescent microscope. When examining tissue for the rabies virus, most laboratories tag antibodies with fluorescein isothiocyanate. Antigen reacting with antibody thus tagged will appear under ultraviolet light as brightly colored, greenish-yellow objects against a bluish background (Dean). Although there is a high correlation between the results of the fluorescent antibody test and mouse inoculation studies, it is possible to have fluorescent-positive but mouse-negative results, since the fluorescent antibody test identifies killed antigen as well as live virus.

Mouse inoculation of brain and salivary gland tissue is necessary when Negri bodies are not found. Mice of all ages are susceptible to intracerebrally injected rabies virus but those 21 to 35 days old are preferable (Koprowski). Following the preparation and injection of the suspension into the brain of liv-

ing mice, a single animal is sacrificed each day, beginning on about the fifth day. Examination of the mouse brain for Negri bodies and for rabies antigen by fluorescent antibody staining is then accomplished. Rabies virus rarely causes signs of illness in mice sooner than five days after intracerebral inoculation. When clinical signs of illness in the laboratory mice do appear, this can be assumed to be suggestive of but not proof of rabies. Confirmation must be on the basis of histologic and immunofluorescent examinations. Absolute identification of the virus is obtained by the serum-virus neutralization test (Johnson).

Preventive Measures

Control measures to reduce the occurrence of rabies depend upon wide-scale and enforced vaccination of domestic dogs and cats, the elimination of stray dogs, and, to the degree possible, the reduction of wild-life vector populations. Pre-exposure immunization followed by periodic booster doses is advised for persons in certain high-risk occupations. Those who receive pre-exposure immunization should have their serum tested for neutralizing antibody approximately four weeks after the last injection. If subsequently exposed to rabies, the individual who had demonstrated a significant antibody titer would require only a reduced treatment regimen, while one who showed no titer rise would require complete post-exposure treatment.

Treatment of the local wound resulting from an animal bite should be accomplished as soon as possible. Thorough and repeated cleansing of the area with generous amounts of soap and water or with quaternary ammonium compounds (1:1000 benzalkonium chloride) is the most effective method of eliminating saliva possibly containing the virus. Puncture wounds are difficult to clean adequately but can be managed by exposing the depths of the wound to jets delivered from a syringe. Either soap and water or a variety of antiseptic solutions may be used for wound cleansing. Corrosive substances that injure normal tissue add little to elimination of the virus and should be avoided. Devitalized tissue should be excised and bite wounds should not be closed immediately by suturing. Infiltration of the wound with antirabies serum is indicated with severe lesions when there is a reasonable probability that the biting animal is rabid. The total dose of hyperimmune serum to be administered to the patient is calculated and a fraction (perhaps 500 units) of the total is injected into the area of the wound, with the rest being given intramuscularly. Tetanus prophylaxis is administered at the same time.

Rabies Vaccine (Active Immunization)

While human rabies has decreased appreciably in recent years, the practitioner continues to be challenged by the frequent and difficult decision of whether or not to administer the vaccine to one sustaining an animal bite. Each case must be individualized before a plan of action can be arrived at. One weighs the discomfort and potential complications of the treatment against the possibility that rabies will develop. These factors are judged in conjunction with established guidelines outlined in Table 16–2. Several factors must be considered, including the type of animal that inflicted the wound and whether it has been captured and confined, the circumstances that resulted in the biting incident, the severity and location of the wound, the vaccination status of the animal, and the presence of rabies in the geographic region. Facial wounds are generally considered to be more dangerous than extremity bites. Unprovoked attacks, especially by an animal that appeared ill or acted in an abnormal fashion, are also more indicative of the need for prophylactic treatment.

The rabies vaccine most widely used in past years was one of two types. The Semple vaccine is of nervous tissue origin in which fixed rabies virus is grown in rabbit brain and is inactivated with phenol. Duck embryo vaccine was licensed in the United States in 1957 and is prepared by the injection of embryonated duck eggs with fixed virus which is inactivated with beta-propiolactone. The latter preparation has been the recommended one until recently, largely because of the lesser frequency of adverse neurologic reactions, although the antigenic responses following its administration are rather poor. Greenberg and Childress compared antibody responses of the two vaccines and found that duck embryo vaccine stimulated an earlier production of antibodies than the Semple vaccine but, by 15 days after administration, the antibody titers were approximately the same. Local reactions to the vaccines were similar.

Prophylactic treatment with rabies vaccine is not invariably successful. Subsequent death due to rabies in patients thus treated is well known (Anderson et al.) but not entirely understood. Between 1957 and 1967, there were six rabies deaths among 117,700 persons given vaccine of nervous tissue origin and seven deaths in 172,000 persons who received duck embryo vaccine (Morbidity and Mortality Weekly Reports, Volume 16, May 13, 1967). The percentage of those receiving the vaccines who were actually exposed to rabies is not known. Possible factors explaining failure of the vaccine in the prevention of rabies include interference from hyperimmune rabies serum, insufficient quantity of vaccine, or impotency of the vaccine preparation.

Rabies duck embryo vaccine treatment consists of not less than 14 daily injections given subcutaneously in a dose recommended by the manufacturer. For severe exposures, especially those about the face, 21 daily doses are advised, with rotation of the sites of in-

Table 16–2. Guide for Post-Exposure Antirabies Prophylaxis*

The following recommendations are intended only as a guide. They may be modified according to knowledge of the species of biting animal and circumstances surrounding the biting incident.

WILD ANIMAL	CONDITION OF ANIMAL AT TIME OF ATTACK	TREATMENT OF EXPOSED HUMAN
Skunk Fox Coyote Raccoon Bat	Regard as Rabid	RIG + HDCV[1]

DOMESTIC ANIMAL	CONDITION OF ANIMAL AT TIME OF ATTACK	TREATMENT OF EXPOSED HUMAN
Cat and dog	Healthy Unknown (Escaped) Rabid or Suspected Rabid	None[2] RIG + HDCV RIG + HDCV[1]

Code: RIG—Rabies Immune Globulin, Human
HDCV—Human Diploid Cell Rabies Vaccine
DEV—Duck Embryo Vaccine
[1]Discontinue vaccine if fluorescent antibody tests of animal killed at time of attack are negative. If HDCV is not available, use DEV.
[2]Begin RIG + HDCV at first sign of rabies in biting dog or cat during holding period (10 days).
*From: Morbidity and Mortality Weekly Reports, Vol. 13, No. 23, June 13, 1980.

jection. Two booster doses are recommended, one at ten days and the second at 20 days after completion of the primary course. The administration of antirabies serum prior to the initiation of vaccine therapy may interfere with the antigenic properties of the vaccine (Corey et al.). Because of this, it is recommended that 21 daily doses of vaccine be given whenever hyperimmune rabies serum is used at the onset of treatment.

A rabies vaccine derived from growth of rabies virus in human diploid cells is the most recent development for rabies post-exposure prophylaxis and is now the recommended preparation. The vaccine is believed to be far safer than any of the previously available vaccines, is highly immunogenic, resulting in higher levels of serum neutralizing antibodies than other vaccines, and results in high antibody titers after only four or five doses (Aoki et al., Bahmanyar et al., Plotkin and Wiktor, Wiktor et al.). Human cell vaccine is now available in many parts of the world but has the disadvantage for underdeveloped countries of a high cost of production.

Neurologic Complications from Rabies Vaccine

Rabies vaccine of nervous tissue origin has long been known for its potential ability to produce neurologic complications in human recipients (Shiraki et al.). Such adverse reactions are believed to occur in one in 4000 to 8000 persons receiving the vaccine but different series in the past showed marked variation in this regard. Among one group, neurologic complications occurred in one in 600 patients, while in another, only one in 9073 were affected (Appelbaum et al.).

The most common rabies post-vaccinal neurologic complication following administration of the Semple vaccine was an acute encephalomyelitis. Transverse myelitis and peripheral neuropathy have also been described but are much less common. With the suckling mouse brain vaccine, Toro et al. in Colombia found that of 21 patients who experienced neurologic vaccine reactions, 16 (76 percent) had an acute polyneuropathy identical to the Guillain-Barré syndrome except for its unusual severity. Six of the 16 cases ended fatally. The onset of symptoms of post-vaccinal encephalomyelitis is usually eight to 21 days after the first injection of rabies vaccine. Clinical findings vary but include a combination of encephalitic, myelitic,

and meningeal signs in addition to fever early in the course of the illness. A lymphocytic pleocytosis in the cerebrospinal fluid is present in most cases, with the cell count usually between 10 and 200 per cu. mm. The illness is usually brief with recovery occurring in the majority. Corticosteroid therapy has been recommended although its value remains speculative.

With the introduction of duck embryo vaccine, it was hoped that active immunity against this virus could be induced with complete safety. This has not been totally achieved, although neurologic complications have been significantly reduced. In addition to frequent minor local reactions (Cereghino et al.), neurologic complications have been noted in approximately one in every 25,000 persons receiving rabies duck embryo vaccine (Morbidity and Mortality Weekly Reports, Vol. 16, May 13, 1967). Of two patients with acute transverse myelitis secondary to duck embryo vaccine reported by Harrington and Olin, both recovered completely. Rubin et al. estimated that approximately 424,000 persons received duck embryo rabies vaccine between 1958 and 1971. Serious reactions among recipients included 22 cases of anaphylaxis, five cases with cranial or peripheral neuropathy, four with transverse myelitis, and four with acute encephalopathy. Two of the latter patients died but it is unclear whether death occurred from the vaccine or from rabies. The available data indicate that neurologic complications from this preparation are infrequent and that death therefrom is decidedly unusual.

Hyperimmune Rabies Serum (Passive Immunization)

Hyperimmune serum in combination with rabies vaccine is believed to be the most effective method of post-exposure prophylaxis. Since one of the currently available serum preparation is of equine origin, the frequent occurrence of serum sickness or anaphylactic shock requires that its use be restricted to absolute indications. History of horse serum allergy should be sought and intradermal sensitivity tests performed before serum is administered. Indications for use of hyperimmune serum noted in Table 16–2 include most severe exposures and all bites by animals believed to be or known to be rabid. Because repeated doses of hyperimmune serum producing persistence of passive antibody will interfere with vaccine antigenicity, only a single dose is recommended, to be followed immediately by initiation of vaccine treatment. The advised dose is 1000 units (one vial) per 40 pounds of body weight (Morbidity and Mortality Weekly Reports, Vol. 16, May 13, 1967). A fraction of this total amount may be infiltrated around the local wound if desired.

In an attempt to minimize the high incidence of allergic reactions to equine serum, investigators have developed and studied rabies immune globulin of human origin (Loofbourow et al., Winkler et al.). This preparation is made from plasma from donors who had received rabies vaccine. Loofbourow et al. state that dosage of the human-prepared material must be critically calculated so that interference with active immunity will not occur. Human serum is preferable to that of equine origin because of the lesser risk of serum reactions and because of its longer half-life in the circulation.

Treatment

Once symptoms of rabies encephalitis in the human have developed, it has been assumed that a fatal outcome will inevitably result. Description of cases with survival from illnesses which were most likely rabies has raised questions regarding the previously considered uniformly fatal outcome of this disease (Hattwick et al., Porras et al.). The first surviving patient was a six-year-old boy in Ohio who was bitten by a rabid bat on October 10, 1970 (Hattwick et al.). Four days after the attack, the child was started on a 14-day course of duck embryo vaccine but on October 30, 1970, he experienced lethargy and anorexia. He subsequently developed fever and other signs of encephalitis, in addition to a lymphocytic pleocytosis in the cerebrospinal fluid. Although rabies virus could not be isolated and brain biopsy was not conclusive, his serum neutralization titer rose to a level of 1:63,000 by three months after onset of the illness, a titer far exceeding that expected from vaccine treatment. With conservative measures to maintain adequate ventilation, prevent hypoxia, and reduce intracranial hypertension, the child survived and subsequently was said to show only mild neurologic deficits.

Another reported survival was a 45-year-old woman in Argentina who was bitten by a dog that died four days later (Porras et al.).

Twenty-one days after being bitten, the patient developed paresthesias at the site of the injury, followed by motor deficits, ataxia, seizures, and other encephalitic signs. Diagnosis was on the basis of epidemiologic features of the illness and serum and CSF rabies neutralizing titers which reached levels of 1:640,000 and 1:160,000, respectively. Her recovery was said to be complete 13 months after onset.

The above descriptions of cases of human rabies with recovery would suggest the advisability of measures to support respiration and prevent cerebral injury from hypoxia until evidence of brain death is demonstrated by the customary methods. In this regard, the therapeutic approach for rabies is analogous to that for tetanus. The patient should be isolated and hospital attendants warned of the danger of bites or the contamination by saliva. Examiners and nurses should wear gowns and rubber gloves. Attendants accidentally bitten or otherwise intimately exposed to oral secretions of the patient may require a course of vaccine therapy. Experimental evidence of the ability of adrenocorticotrophic hormones to reactivate rabies virus infection would suggest that corticosteroids be avoided as a means to control increased intracranial pressure in the human disease (Soave et al.).

Restraint of the excited patient is necessary and often requires physical methods in addition to large quantities of sedative drugs. The drugs of choice are a matter of personal preference but one may be astonished at the relative lack of effect unless very large doses are used. Diazepam is a reasonable choice to achieve sedation in view of its safety in addition to its potential anticonvulsant effects. Phenobarbital may be added if seizures become frequent.

REFERENCES

Anderson, J. A., Daly, F. T., Jr., and Kidd, J. C.: Human rabies after antiserum and vaccine postexposure treatment. Case report and review. Ann. Intern. Med. 64:1297–1302, 1966.

Annual Summary Rabies —1971. Department of Health, Education, and Welfare Publication No. (HSM) 72–8126. May, 1972.

Aoki, F. Y., Tyrell, D. A. J., Hill, L. E., and Turner, G. S.: Immunogenicity and acceptability of a human diploid-cell culture rabies vaccine in volunteers. Lancet 1:660–662, 1975.

Appelbaum, E., Greenberg, M., and Nelson, J.: Neurological complications following antirabies vaccination. J.A.M.A. 151:188–191, 1953.

Bahmanyar, M., Fayaz, A., Nour-Salehi, S., Mohammadi,

M., and Koprowski, H.: Successful protection of humans exposed to rabies infection. Post-exposure treatment with the new human diploid cell rabies vaccine and antirabies serum. J.A.M.A. 236:2751–2754, 1976.

Baltazard, M.: Rabies, *In:* Debré and Celers, R. J.: Clinical Virology. W. B. Saunders Co., Philadelphia, 1970.

Bhatt, D. R., Hattwick, M. A. W., Gerdsen, R., Emmons, R. W., and Johnson, H. N.: Human rabies. Diagnosis, complications, and management. Am. J. Dis. Child. 127:862–869, 1974.

Cereghino, J. J., Osterud, H. T., Pinnas, J. L., and Holmes, M. A.: Rabies: A rare disease but a serious pediatric problem. Pediatrics 45:839–844, 1970.

Christie, A. B.: Infectious Diseases: Epidemiology and Clinical Practice. E. & S. Livingstone, Ltd., Edinburgh, 1969.

Conomy, J. P., Leibovitz, A., McCombs, W., and Stinson, J.: Airborne rabies encephalitis: Demonstration of rabies virus in the human central nervous system. Neurology 27:67–69, 1977.

Corey, L., Hattwick, M. A. W., Baer, G. M., and Smith, J. S.: Serum neutralizing antibody after rabies post-exposure prophylaxis. Ann. Intern. Med. 85:170–176, 1976.

Dean, D. J.: The fluorescent antibody test. *In:* World Health Organization. Monograph Series, Number 23, 1966.

Derakhshan, I.: Is the Negri body specific for rabies? A light and electron microscopical study. Arch. Neurol. 32:75–79, 1975.

Duffy, C. E., Woolley, P. V., Jr., and Nolting, W. S.: Rabies. A case report with notes on the isolation of the virus from saliva. J. Pediat. 31:440–447, 1947.

Dupont, J. R., and Earle, K. M.: Human rabies encephalitis. A study of forty-nine fatal cases with a review of the literature. Neurology 15:1023–1034, 1965.

Girard, K. F., Hitchcock, H. B., Edsall, G., and MacCready, R. A.: Rabies in bats in southern New England. New Eng. J. Med. 272:75–80, 1965.

Goldwasser, R. A., and Kissling, R. E.: Fluorescent antibody staining of street and fixed rabies virus antigen. Proc. Soc. Exp. Biol. Med. 98:219, 1958.

González-Angulo, A., Márquez-Monter, H., Feria-Velasco, A., and Zavala, B. J.: The ultrastructure of Negri bodies in Purkinje neurons in human rabies. Neurology 20:323–328, 1970.

Greenberg, M., and Childress, J.: Vaccination against rabies with duck-embryo and Semple vaccines. J.A.M.A. 173:333–337, 1960.

Harrington, R. B., and Olin, R.: Incomplete transverse myelitis following rabies duck embryo vaccination. J.A.M.A. 216:2137–2138, 1971.

Hattwick, M. A. W., Weis, T. T., Stechschulte, C. J., Baer, G. M., and Gregg, M. B.: Recovery from rabies. A case report. Ann. Intern. Med. 76:931–942, 1972.

Houff, S. A., Burton, R. C., Wilson, R. W., Henson, T. E., London, W. T., Baer, G. M., Anderson, L. J., Winkler, W. G., Madden, D. L., and Sever, J. L.: Human-to-human transmission of rabies virus by corneal transplant. New Eng. J. Med. 300:603–604, 1979.

Johnson, H. N.: The serum-virus neutralization test. *In:* World Health Organization. Monograph Series, Number 23, 1966.

Johnson, H. N.: Rabies. *In:* Rivers: Viral and Rickettsial Infections of Man. J. B. Lippincott Company, Philadelphia, 1948.

Kent, J. R., and Finegold, S. M.: Human rabies transmitted by the bite of a bat. With comments on the duck-embryo vaccine. New Eng. J. Med. 263:1058–1065, 1960.

Koch, F. J., Sagartz, J. W., Davison, D. E., and Lawhaswasdi, K.: Diagnosis of human rabies by the cornea test. Am. J. Clin. Path. 63:509–515, 1975.

Koprowski, H.: Mouse inoculation test. *In:* World Health Organization. Monograph Series, Number 23, 1966.

Knutti, R. E.: Acute ascending paralysis and myelitis due to the virus of rabies. J.A.M.A. 93:754–758, 1929.

Leech, R. W.: Electron-microscopic study of the inclusion body in human rabies. Neurology 21:91–94, 1971.

Lennette, E. H., Soave, O. A., Nakamura, K., and Kellogg, G. H., Jr.: A fatal human case of rabies following the bite of a rabid bat (Lasionycteris noctivagans). J. Lab. Clin. Med. 55:89–93, 1960.

Loofbourow, J. C., Cabasso, V. J., Roby, R. E., and Anuskiewicz, W.: Rabies immune globulin (human). Clinical trials and dose determination. J.A.M.A. 217:1825–1831, 1971.

Macrae, A. D.: Rabies in England. Lancet 2:1415–1417, 1969.

Melnick, J. L.: Classification and nomenclature of animal viruses, 1971. Progr. Med. Virol. 13:462–484, 1971.

Meyer, K. F.: Man contracting rabies from man. J.A.M.A. 165:158–159, 1957.

Miller, A., and Nathanson, N.: Rabies: Recent advances in pathogenesis and control. Ann. Neurol. 2:511–519, 1977.

Negri, A.: Beitrag zum studium der aetiologie der tollwuth. Z. Hyg. Infekt.-Kr. 43:507–528, 1903.

Pasteur, L.: Chamberland and Roux. Nouvelle communication sur la rage. Compt. Rend. Acad. Sci. 98:457–463, 1884.

Pasteur, L.: Methode pour prévenir la rage apres morsure. Compt. Rend. Acad. Sci. 101:765–772, 1885.

Pawan, J. L.: Transmission of paralytic rabies in Trinidad by vampire bat (Desmodus rotundus murinus Wagner, 1840). Ann. Trop. Med. 30:101–130, 1936.

Plotkin, S. A., and Wiktor, T.: Vaccination of children with human cell culture rabies vaccine. Pediatrics 63:219–221, 1979.

Porras, C., Barboza, J. J., Fuenzalida, E., Adaros, H. L., de Diaz, A. M. O., and Furst, J.: Recovery from rabies in man. Ann. Intern. Med. 85:44–48, 1976.

Rubin, R. H., Hattwick, M. A. W., Jones, S., Gregg, M. B., and Schwartz, V. D.: Adverse reactions to duck embryo rabies vaccine. Range and incidence. Ann. Intern. Med. 78:643–649, 1973.

Schindler, R.: Studies on the pathogenesis of rabies. Bull. W. H. O. 25:119, 1961.

Shiraki, H., Otani, S., Tamthai, B., Chamuni, A., Chitanondh, H., and Charuchinda, S.: Rabies postvaccinal encephalomyelitis and genuine rabies in human beings. World Neurol. 3:125–146, 1962.

Soave, O. A., Johnson, H. N., and Nakamura, K.: Reactivation of rabies virus infection with adrenocorticotrophic hormones. Science 133:1360–1361, 1961.

Sung, J. H., Hayano, M., Mastri, A. R., and Okajak, T.: A case of human rabies and ultrastructure of the Negri body. J. Neuropath. Exp. Neurol. 35:541–559, 1976.

Tangchai, P., and Vejjajiva, A.: Pathology of the peripheral nervous system in human rabies. A study of nine autopsy cases. Brain 94:299–306, 1971.

Tierkel, E. S.: Diseases Transmitted from Animal to Man. Charles C Thomas, Springfield, Ill., 1963.

Tierkel, E. S.: Rapid microscopic examination for Negri bodies and preparation of specimens for biological test. *In:* World Health Organization. Monograph Series, Number 23, 1966.

Toro, G., Vergara, I., and Roman, G.: Neuroparalytic accidents of antirabies vaccination with suckling mouse brain vaccine. Clinical and pathologic study of 21 cases. Arch. Neurol. 34:694–700, 1977.

Tsiang, H.: Evidence for an intraaxonal transport of fixed and street rabies virus. J. Neuropath. Exp. Neurol. 38:286–296, 1979.

Warrell, D. A., Davidson, N. M., Pope, H. M., Bailie, W. E., Lawrie, J. H., Ormerod, L. D., Kertesz, A., and Lewis, P.: Pathophysiologic studies in human rabies. Am. J. Med. 60:180–190, 1976.

Wiktor, T. J., Plotkin, S. A., and Grella, D. W.: Human cell culture rabies vaccine: Antibody response in man. J.A.M.A. 224:1170–1171, 1973.

Winkler, W. G., Schmidt, R. C., and Sikes, R. K.: Evaluation of human rabies immune globulin and homologous and heterologous antibody. J. Immunol. 102:1314–1321, 1969.

World Health Organization. Monograph Series, Number 23. Laboratory Techniques in Rabies, 1966.

Chapter Seventeen

RUBELLA

In the eighteenth century, German authors wrote of a disease called Rötheln, characterized by mildness of symptoms and a short-lived rash, and one commonly confused with scarlet fever and measles. The illness was generally regarded to be of little consequence to the human race and even its existence as a distinct entity was denied by some. By mid-nineteenth century it had become established as an illness distinct from measles and, in 1866, was first called rubella by an English physician named Henry Veale. Its viral etiology was demonstrated in 1938 by Hiro and Tasaka, who produced the disease in susceptible children by the administration of nasal washings from patients with the illness. It was not until 1962, however, that isolation of the virus in tissue culture was accomplished by Weller and Neva and by Parkman, Buescher, and Artenstein. The ability to isolate and cultivate the virus was soon followed by the development of an effective vaccine and the eventual documentation of new insights into the breadth of the clinical illness.

The long-held concept that rubella was a mild and generally insignificant viral disease was thunderously shaken in 1941 when Norman Gregg of Australia first observed congenital defects in infants born of mothers who had experienced rubella early in pregnancy. This initial association between congenital cataracts and prenatal maternal rubella was soon to be enlarged to include microcephaly, cardiac disease, and deafness in various proportions and was a landmark, not only regarding the significance of acquired rubella, but also in relation to the association between viral disease and congenital defects in general.

Acquired Rubella

Rubella is typically a childhood infection with a peak incidence between ages five and nine years (Horstmann) but, more than with other childhood exanthems, it is not uncommon in older children and even young adults. Antibody studies have shown that 20 to 25 percent of adolescents (Wyll and Grand) and 15 to 18 percent of women of childbearing age remain susceptible to rubella (Sever et al.). Postnatally acquired rubella is rarely observed in infants under one year of age. It is more prevalent in the springtime months, and in the United States has been notable for its periodic occurrence in the form of major epidemics. Large outbreaks in this country occurred in 1935, in 1943, and again in 1964 (Witte et al.).

Acquired rubella is usually a mild illness with transient systemic symptoms. Like many infectious disorders, however, the severity of the illness is a spectrum which ranges from an asymptomatic infection to one with significant and, rarely, even fatal complications. The frequency with which subclinical infection occurs is not known but studies utilizing serologic tests indicate it is not uncommon. Up to 40 percent of cases in certain outbreaks either are asymptomatic or occur without a recognized rash (Brody et al.), emphasizing the difficulty of diagnosis on clinical grounds and the importance of laboratory serologic examinations.

The incubation period of rubella ranges from 14 to 21 days. In the younger child, a rash first appearing on the face is the usual initial manifestation of illness. Prodromal symptoms may precede the rash in patients of any age but are more common in the adolescent age group and in adults. In such patients, malaise, cough, pharyngitis, conjunctivitis, and tender cervical or occipital adenopathy may be present three to five days before the rash supervenes.

Transmission of the illness takes place by the respiratory route. Rubella virus is shed into the nasopharynx of the infected host for a week or more prior to the onset of symptoms and may be conveyed to the susceptible child during this period. Virus reaches the respiratory tract of the susceptible child and is believed to spread by lymphatic channels or viremia to regional lymph nodes where replication occurs (Heggie and Robbins), perhaps accounting for the lymph node enlargement in the suboccipital and cervical regions. By ten days after exposure, the virus can be demonstrated in the blood stream from where it eventually invades the respiratory mucosa, leading to symptoms of coryza and associated with low-grade fever.

The rash is first noted on the face but rapidly descends to involve the trunk, upper limbs, and then the legs. Its duration is quite variable, as is its quality. In the average case, the rash persists for two or three days but in some it is present for not more than several hours. There can also be some degree of variability from hour to hour, and certain events, such as a hot bath, will make it more pronounced. The typical rubella rash is erythematous and macular, but lacking the depth of color seen with the rash with rubeola or the brilliance of the eruption with scarlet fever. The lesions are initially rather discrete but soon coalesce, partially obliterating the separateness of the spots. In addition to the cutaneous eruption, an enanthem referred to as Forchheimer spots has been described in rubella. The lesions involve the soft palate in the form of discrete petechiae but frequently are either absent or not commonly observed.

The pathogenesis of the rubella exanthem remains unclear. Heggie and Robbins pointed out that the onset of the rash coincides with the appearance of circulating antiviral antibody. Rubella virus can be recovered from skin showing the exanthem but also from cutaneous areas unaffected with the rash, indicating that viral replication in the skin is only one factor contributing to the development of the rash (Heggie).

Lymphadenopathy is a constant part of the acquired rubella syndrome and is one of the more important aspects for clinical diagnosis. Suboccipital, postauricular, and posterior cervical nodes are primarily involved and may or may not be associated with tenderness to palpation. In unusual instances in which marked tenderness is present, nuchal rigidity may occur, erroneously suggesting the possibility of bacterial meningitis. Lymphadenopathy precedes the rash in most cases but is frequently not observed until examination is performed because of low-grade fever, mild conjunctivitis, or the appearance of the exanthem.

Rubella is usually a mild illness causing little discomfort and with a total duration of symptoms of only a few days. Older children are frequently more ill than those younger and, occasionally, the illness is complicated by either thrombocytopenia, arthritis, or meningoencephalitis. Thrombocytopenia is well known in newborn infants with congenital rubella but is an infrequent manifestation of the acquired disease (Steen and Torp). It is usually noted within a week after the onset of the rash and rarely persists longer than two weeks. The degree of platelet reduction is variable but may be sufficiently pronounced to cause epistaxis, melena, hematuria, or purpura. Ackroyd described one child with rubella complicated by thrombocytopenic purpura who died from a cerebral hemorrhage. Morse et al. also reported a single fatal case of intracranial bleeding secondary to thrombocytopenia. Thrombocytopenia secondary to acquired rubella has been found to be more common in girls than in boys, and, in contrast to rubella arthritis, is more often observed in children than in adults (Ferguson). Certain authors have suggested that some cases of idiopathic thrombocytopenic purpura in childhood may result from inapparent rubella infection (Ozsoylu et al.). The cause of platelet damage by the rubella virus remains speculative.

Arthralgia or arthritis is the most common complication of rubella in the adult female. It is infrequently seen in children and rarely observed in males. The onset of joint manifestations coincides with the appearance of the rash in some cases or develops within the next five to seven days in others. The metacarpophalangeal and proximal interphalangeal joints are most often affected but knee, ankle, and wrist joints are also commonly involved. There is considerable variation in the severity of joint symptoms, and the duration may be measured in days or up to two weeks. Affected joints sometimes are without objective signs on examination, while in other patients, redness, swelling, and increased heat to palpation is associated with intense pain similar to that of rheumatic fever. Even a migratory component to the inflammatory process has been observed in some persons. Numbness and tingling suggestive of peripheral nerve involvement has been described in conjunction with arthritis (Lee), and a carpal tunnel syndrome has also been mentioned (Fry et al.). Whether the arthritis of rubella is due to viral invasion of the joint or represents an immune response is not known. While it may cause severe discomfort, it is regarded to be a transient and benign complication of the disease.

Diagnosis

Diagnosis of an isolated case of rubella on the basis of clinical findings alone is not reliable because an identical rash can be provoked by other viral agents. Recognition is facilitated when the illness occurs in epidemic fashion, in which case the most useful clinical signs include the presence of enlarged suboccipital and retroauricular lymph nodes plus the distribution of the exanthem. No specific findings in the usual blood studies are to be expected, although leukopenia is frequently present.

Confirmation of the diagnosis of rubella in the usual childhood case would be of little significance except for the knowledge that the child has had the disease, which provides permanent immunity, and because of the importance of exposure to the illness of susceptible pregnant women. The status of immunity of the young adult female and especially the pregnant female has become of greater importance since the recognition of the possible effects of the disease on the fetus and since the development of an effective vaccine.

Four methods are available for the detection of rubella antibody, including the hemagglutination inhibition (HI) antibody test, neutralization antibody test, complement fixation test, and the indirect fluorescent antibody test (Sever et al. 1967). The hemagglutination inhibition test developed by Stewart et al. is the most useful technique both for diagnosis of the disease and for determination of immunity. Rubella HI antibody is detectable in serum within a few days after onset of the rash and reaches peak levels within two weeks (Ziring et al.). The antibody titer then declines gradually over a period of years

but remains at detectable levels for life in most persons. This is not true in children with congenital rubella, in whom the HI antibody titer may disappear at variable times after infancy. By five years of age, approximately 20 percent of children with intrauterine-acquired rubella no longer have detectable antibody (Ziring et al.). Because of the lifelong persistence of rubella HI antibody after postnatally acquired rubella, the test is most valuable for determining the status of immunity in the adult female and has special value in pregnancy. Routine performance of the rubella hemagglutination inhibition test has become a part of the initial prenatal evaluation in obstetrical clinics. The presence of rubella HI antibody indicates previous infection and thus immunity, while its absence indicates susceptibility to the disease.

Within a few days after onset of the rubella rash, neutralizing antibodies can be demonstrated in serum, but rising to lower levels than HI antibodies. Complement-fixing antibodies generally develop several days after antibodies detected by other tests. Peak titers persist for several months but then decline to become undetectable after a few years. Thus, the complement fixation test is less useful for determination of the state of immunity than are the other techniques. The complement fixation test is most useful when the first serum specimen is obtained from the patient more than one or two weeks after subsidence of the rash. While the HI titer may have reached a plateau, a subsequent serum specimen may still reveal a significant titer rise of complement-fixing antibodies, thus confirming the diagnosis of recent infection.

Virus isolation techniques can also be helpful in diagnosis of the acute disease but are not widely used because of the expense involved plus the specificity of the serologic tests. Rubella virus can usually be isolated from the pharynx for a week before onset of the rash and up to two weeks after the rash has resolved. Virus may be isolated from serum a week prior to the rash but usually disappears from blood about the time of onset of the rash. Although virus isolation techniques are infrequently used in acquired rubella, they can be important in establishing the period of infectivity of the infant with congenital rubella. Whenever fluid is obtained from affected joints in patients with rubella, or whenever cerebrospinal fluid is obtained because of an encephalitic complication, attempts at viral isolation should be made.

Rubella Vaccine and Its Complications

The first effective rubella vaccine was developed by Meyer, Parkman and Panos, who attenuated the virus by 77 passages in tissue cultures of green monkey kidney cells. Additional live, attenuated, rubella virus vaccines have subsequently been developed and experience has demonstrated their relative safety and extreme effectiveness (Cherry et al., DuPan et al., Farquhar et al., Lepow et al.). Among 119 children without rubella antibodies given the vaccine, 97 percent experienced infection as demonstrated by an antibody response (Parkman et al.). The importance of the vaccine is ultimately to prevent fetal death or damage from the disease, a goal hopefully achieved by widespread immunization of children, resulting in a decrease in the prevalence of the virus in the population, thereby preventing exposure of pregnant women.

Live rubella virus vaccine in the form of a single injection is now recommended for children between one year of age and puberty. Although virus may be shed from the pharynx for two weeks after vaccination, there has been little evidence of communicability from this source. Fleet et al. studied 67 school teachers susceptible to rubella before an immunization campaign was carried out among their pupils. None of the 67 teachers developed serologic evidence of infection, indicating absence of spread of the vaccine virus. Among another group of women given rubella vaccine in the immediate postpartum period, none of their infants demonstrated serologic evidence of exposure to the rubella virus, even though some of the infants were breast-fed (Farquhar).

Rubella vaccine should not be administered to immunocompromised patients or to women during pregnancy because of the potential hazard to the fetus. Studies in which vaccine has been administered in early pregnancy before legal abortion have shown a significant percentage of placental or fetal invasion by the vaccine virus (Vaheri et al.). Modlin et al. evaluated the risks of rubella vaccination shortly before or after conception. Among 145 women who had inadvertently received rubella vaccine in whom pregnancy was subsequently terminated by therapeutic abortion, rubella vaccine virus was recovered from the products of conception in nine. Of 72 infants carried to term following maternal rubella vaccination around the time of conception, none had clinical or serologic evidence of infection with the virus. Modlin and colleagues estimated from these studies that the maximal risk of fetal infection after maternal rubella immunization is 5 to 10 percent, and, in reality, is probably less. It is now recommended that rubella vaccine be limited to non-pregnant women in whom susceptibility has been proved by HI antibody tests. The recipient must agree to adhere to an acceptable contraceptive program for two months following immunization. Rubella vaccination of the susceptible female in the immediate postpartum period has become popular because of the diminished risk of pregnancy during this period.

Complications of rubella vaccine are not uncommon. They are usually mild and transient when they do occur and not of the magnitude that should inhibit proper use of the vaccine (Chin et al.). A brief, rubella-like illness is infrequently seen in children following administration of the vaccine but occurs more often in the adult female. Weibel et al. gave HPV-77 rubella vaccine to 35 susceptible adult females and observed illness to some extent in 20. Rash, malaise, adenopathy, arthralgia, and arthritis were the usual symptoms but were mild in almost all. Arthralgia or arthritis has been the most notable adverse reaction to the vaccine and, as expected from experience with the acquired disease, has been much more prominent in adult women than in children. For reasons that are not clear, joint involvement has been more common with HPV-77 vaccine prepared in dog kidney cells than with either the Cendehill vaccine or HPV-77 grown in duck-embryo tissue culture (Horstmann). Vaccine-induced arthralgia or arthritis can be severe but has been transient in most cases. Spruance et al., however, have described recurrent joint symptoms in children for as long as eight months after receiving rubella vaccine. Joint pain in these patients usually began soon after rising in the morning, involved mainly the knees, and would result in a limp with the affected leg held in a position of partial flexion. Episodes lasted one to seven days and recurred at intervals of twice per week up to once every three months.

Certain patients with joint complications secondary to rubella vaccine also experience numbness or paresthesias, usually confined to the distal portion of the upper limbs (Chin et al., Spruance et al.). Kilroy and colleagues stated that two syndromes in children could be recognized following rubella vaccination, although the common occurrence of mixed cases suggested they were different expressions of a single pathogenic mechanism. In one group of children, recurrent pain in the wrists and hands lasting up to an hour was described which began from 10 days to several weeks after vaccination. The pain characteristically awakened the child from sleep and often was associated with numbness or paresthesias in the hands and fingers. Younger children were frequently observed rubbing their hands during the episodes of discomfort. In the second group, the interval from vaccination to onset of symptoms varied from 29 to 70 days, with a mean of 45 days. The outstanding complaint was pain in the popliteal fossa, usually bilateral, and more pronounced during the waking hours than at night. These children presented with a crouched posture with partial flexion of the knees and exhibited a tendency to walk on their toes. Signs of joint inflammation were consistently absent and the illness was transient. In both groups, motor nerve conduction velocities in the upper extremities were frequently abnormally slowed, suggesting a polyneuropathy.

Similar complications of rubella vaccine in children were described by Gilmartin et al. under the terms brachial radiculoneuritis and lumbosacral radiculoneuritis. Children with the upper extremity syndrome were usually abruptly awakened from sleep by painful dysesthesias or shooting pains in arms or hands. The symptoms recurred, sometimes several times per night, and lasted up to 30 minutes. Those with the lower extremity syndrome described aching or pain in the legs, usually more intense in the morning hours shortly after arising. Such patients exhibited a crouched gait with flexed knees, similar to that described by Kilroy et al. Symptoms persisted for several weeks in most patients, and, in some, evidence of associated arthritic involvement became apparent. While the mechanism by which rubella vaccine produces symptoms described by these authors is not clear, the evidence available is compatible with some form of peripheral nerve dysfunction from which recovery is expected. Acute myelitis complicating rubella vaccination has also been described but is rare (Hanissian et al., Holt et al.).

Rubella Meningoencephalitis

Encephalitis or meningoencephalitis has been regarded to be a rare complication of acquired rubella, in contrast to its more frequent occurrence with rubeola (measles). Whether the acute central nervous system disorder in reported cases of rubella is an encephalitis with actual viral invasion of brain tissue, an encephalopathy in which there is a cerebral response to the presence of the virus elsewhere, or the result of an inflammatory vasculopathy has not been clarified. Virus has not been isolated from the brain in such cases and what little neuropathology has been described is not conclusive. For simplicity, the illness will here be referred to as rubella encephalitis, recognizing that the pathogenesis of the disorder remains in doubt.

How often rubella is complicated by encephalitic signs is unknown, and some have suggested that certain outbreaks have been more notable for this complication than others. Davison and Friedfeld postulated that the epidemic in 1935 was associated with an increased incidence of neurologic complications as compared with previous outbreaks. From the Detroit rubella epidemic in 1942, Margolis et al. estimated that encephalomyelitis occurred in one of 6,000 cases, while Sherman et al. judged that central nervous system complications occurred in one in 5,000 cases in the 1964 outbreak. Although these two estimates are comparable, their accuracy is open to question. Virtually all cases reported of rubella complicated by encephalitis have been in patients with rash indicative of the disease. Until recent years, the presence of the exanthem was almost a necessity for diagnosis because serologic methods were not available. Since rubella without rash is not unusual, it is possible that some cases diagnosed as acute viral encephalitis of unknown type in children or adults could be due to this virus. It would seem reasonable, therefore, to include a rubella HI antibody test among serologic studies in patients with acute encephalitis in whom the cause is not evident.

Encephalitis complicating acquired rubella is not age-limited but authors have suggested that it seems to occur more frequently in adolescence or adulthood than would be expected on the basis of the usual age distribution of rubella (Davison and Friedfeld). The initial encephalitic manifestations usually begin one to six days after the onset of the rash. Characteristically, the first evidence of cerebral involvement has been three or four days after the rash was initially observed, by which time the eruption has usually faded (Bradford, Davison and Friedfeld, Margolis et al., Mitchell and Pampiglione). Similar to other exanthems, the onset of neurologic signs can even precede the appearance of the rash (Holliday).

The onset of neurologic manifestations with rubella encephalitis is usually abrupt but there is considerable variation in the presenting symptoms. Headache, lethargy, irritability, and vomiting are the most common initial complaints. The child reported by Briggs was seemingly recovering from rubella when he was noted to be dysphasic. Later the same day he developed a right hemiparesis and then experienced recurrent convulsions leading to death one day later. One of the cases described by Connelly et al. had the onset with recurrent generalized convulsions followed by right hemiplegia, which was found to be the result of left internal carotid artery thrombosis. In other patients, the encephalitic symptoms are ushered in by the sudden development of convulsions followed by coma.

The neurologic signs present after the onset of the disease likewise are quite variable, although fever and evidence of meningeal irritation are usual, convulsions are common, and long tract signs are occasionally observed. Confusion, disorientation, and tremulousness may precede a state of unresponsiveness. Marked hyperthermia and an irregular respiratory pattern are poor prognostic signs but are not incompatible with possible complete recovery. Various cranial nerve deficits have been described, including peripheral facial palsy. Profound cerebellar ataxia is the most striking neurologic deficit in some instances (Holliday). In other patients, spinal cord dysfunction may precede or occur coincidentally with encephalitic signs. Pampiglione et al. described a 13-year-old girl who developed paresthesias and weakness of the legs in addition to urinary retention three days after the occurrence of the rash. The illness resulted in a sensory level at the level of the sixth cervical segment and was compounded by bilateral optic neuritis. Encephalitic signs were minimal and recovery of spinal cord function was only partial.

As opposed to the leukopenia that is usual with uncomplicated rubella, the patient with acute rubella encephalitis is likely to reveal a significant leukocytosis with an increase in immature granulocytes. Cerebrospinal fluid findings generally include clear fluid which contains ten to 100 cells per cu. mm., most of which are lymphocytes. Total absence of cells in the cerebrospinal fluid, however, is not incompatible with the diagnosis. The glucose content is normal or elevated and the same is true of the CSF protein content.

Whether the illness is mild or severe, the acute stage of rubella encephalitis is brief and permanent sequelae are infrequent (Margolis et al.). Either complete recovery occurs within a few days after the first signs of neurologic involvement or death ensues rapidly. Among the four fatal cases reported by Margolis and colleagues, death occurred in all within three days after the onset of encephalitic symptoms. Up to 1956, Steen and Torp were able to find 88 published cases of rubella encephalitis or meningoencephalitis, 17 of which had resulted in death. While sequelae have been described, most survivors appear to recover completely and exhibit no lasting deficits (Kenny et al.).

Pathologic studies from patients with rubella encephalitis have been sparse and have not clarified the precise nature of the process. Considerations in regard to pathogenesis have included the possibility of direct viral invasion of the brain by the rubella virus, activation of a latent virus by the basic illness, a demyelinating process similar to that with postvaccinal encephalomyelitis, or "toxic" encephalopathy in which there is an abnormal brain response to unknown factors associated with the systemic viral illness. None of the above has been completely excluded, although significant myelin disruption has not been observed and the relative infrequency of sequelae would seem to remove the disorder from the "allergic" category in which perivenous demyelination is characteristic. Examples of postnatally acquired rubella encephalitis in which the virus is recovered from the CSF support the concept that viral invasion of the brain does occur in some cases (Squadrini et al.). It is probable, also, that in some instances, an inflammatory cerebral vasculitis is a major factor accounting for acute neurologic signs complicating rubella (Connolly et al.).

The available neuropathologic observations have generally described minimal to mild inflammatory cell infiltration of the meninges, and some degree of perivascular infiltration in the brain with lymphocytes and plasma cells (Briggs, Davison and Friedfeld, Margolis et al.). More than slight perivenous demyelination has not been observed (Davison and Friedfeld, Sherman et al.), and neuronal changes have not been specific. Sherman and colleagues attempted unsuccessfully to isolate the virus from brain tissue after death and emphasized the lack of specific histologic changes indicative of viral invasion of the brain, or of demyelination. These authors proposed to call the disorder an encephalopathy rather than encephalitis and agree that the mechanism of origin is unclear.

Treatment of acquired rubella encephalitis is supportive, with important measures including the control of convulsions, prevention of hyperthermia, and maintenance of fluid and electrolyte metabolism. Corticosteroids have been used in some cases but the benefit therefrom remains unclear.

Congenital Rubella

The teratogenic effect of the rubella virus was first recorded by Norman Gregg in 1941, subsequent to his observation of an unusual number of infants with congenital cataracts following a rubella outbreak in Sydney, Australia. In addition to ocular abnormalities, Dr. Gregg made mention of cardiac defects and low birth weight in the original publication in the *Transactions of Ophthalmological Society of Australia*. His observations were soon confirmed by other reports (Swan) and in 1944, Gregg added deafness and developmental retardation to the components of the congenital rubella syndrome.

Soon after the initial reports, the combination of cataracts and other ocular abnormalities, congenital cardiac disease, deafness, microcephaly, and reduced birth weight became well known as the cardinal manifestations of the congenital rubella syndrome. It was evident that not all of these abnormalities occurred in every affected child but that the illness in the newborn represents a spectrum in regard to degree of involvement, with variation in part depending on when in the first trimester fetal infection occurs. The early studies proclaimed what subsequently became evident to be an exaggeration of the degree of risk to the fetus when rubella occurred in the first trimester, largely because the investigations were directed primarily to the identification of abnormalities in the infant. Thus, many mothers who had the illness during pregnancy but gave birth to normal progeny were overlooked and not included in the estimates. In 1943, Swan and colleagues stated that if rubella occurred in the first two months of pregnancy, there was a 100 percent chance of fetal abnormality and that the risk was reduced to 50 percent if the maternal illness occurred in the third month of gestation. Additional reports expressed

marked variations in the degree of fetal risk with first trimester maternal rubella (Ingalls, Jackson and Fisch, Pitt, Swan et al.). It is now generally stated that the risk of congenital malformations when rubella affects the mother in the first trimester of pregnancy is at least 15 to 20 percent (Horstmann, Lundström, Tartakow) and probably higher if follow-up evaluation is extended for several years after birth.

Fetal infection is not limited to those mothers who have had an overt illness but can also occur secondary to subclinical maternal infection (Avery et al. 1965). Although fetal involvement may occur when maternal rubella occurs in the fourth gestational month (Sever et al. 1969), the incidence is lower than when the disease occurs earlier. Hardy et al. demonstrated that fetal infection with subsequent lasting deficits can result from second trimester maternal rubella. Of 24 women with documented rubella between the fourteenth and thirty-first weeks of pregnancy, two suffered fetal death and 15 gave birth to infants believed to show clinical abnormalities. The authors emphasized the more subtle clinical expressions of illness among infants infected during the second trimester of pregnancy and indicated that the manifestations were more those associated with chronic viral infection than with faulty organogenesis, as occurs with first trimester involvement. It is also now recognized that the illness can result in spontaneous abortion or stillbirth, or that the affected live newborn may exhibit signs that range from severe multiple organ system involvement to very mild abnormalities, or may even appear normal at birth. Multiple and severe organ system involvement is greatest when fetal infection occurs in the first eight weeks of pregnancy, while single organ system dysfunction is more likely when fetal infection occurs later.

Despite the presence and persistence of specific antibody, the affected infant will often shed the virus for months after birth, thus creating a hazard to susceptible nurses and other adults. Among 376 children with congenital rubella, pharyngeal viral excretion was found in the first month of life in 84 percent, from one to four months in 62 percent, from five to eight months in 33 percent, and from nine to 12 months in 11 percent. Three percent continued to shed virus between 13 and 20 months after birth (Cooper et al.). That the infant shedding rubella virus is capable of infecting adults was shown by Schiff and Dine and has been documented by many other investigators. These authors studied eight susceptible nurses exposed to affected newborns and noted an attack rate exhibited by titer rise in six of the eight women. How long viral persistence and shedding can continue is speculative, but perhaps they extend even into adulthood. Menser and collaborators reported virus excretion in the urine of a 29-year-old female with congenital rubella, possibly representing chronic infection since intrauterine life.

The rubella epidemic in the United States in 1964 was followed by the birth of many infants with congenital defects of the type previously recognized to be characteristic of the syndrome. Many newborn infants, however, were observed to have additional abnormalities that had not previously been included in the congenital rubella syndrome. Thrombocytopenia, purpura, hepatosplenomegaly, jaundice, pneumonitis, myocardial damage, skeletal lesions, anemia, large or full anterior fontanel, and meningoencephalitis in the neonate led to the designation of the "expanded" rubella syndrome (Dudgeon, Korones et al., Rudolph et al., Sever et al. 1965). As in previous experiences, there was a wide variation in the expression of the disease in this outbreak, but, in general, the earlier in pregnancy fetal infection occurred, the more extensive were the abnormalities in the newborn. The mortality rate was high in infants with the "expanded form" of congenital rubella, and ranged from 20 to 32 percent (Rudolph et al.). Although many of the systemic manifestations in the newborn period observed in the 1964 epidemic were judged to be "new," White et al. reported that similar clinical findings had been observed previously. The lack of previous recognition, they assumed, was in part due to the lesser frequency with which such infants were seen in the non-epidemic years plus the previous lack of awareness that the newborn syndrome represented a chronic and continuing infectious disease. Most authors have favored the concept that a difference in clinical expression of the intrauterine-acquired illness did occur with the 1964 epidemic, but the explanation for the altered manifestations has not been clarified.

Clinical Manifestations

The development of viral isolation techniques and serologic diagnostic methods has resulted in a remarkable broadening of our awareness of the varied modes of appearance of the newborn and young infant with intrauterine-acquired rubella. It is now known that the disease is a chronic infectious process, that virus will persist in many structures for weeks or months after birth, and that evidence of infection or organ damage may be present at birth, first appear days or weeks after birth, or not be identified for years thereafter. Multiple organ system involvement of either major or minor proportions is characteristic of the illness but with variation from case to case (Fig. 17–1). One of the more constant features of the congenital rubella syndrome is intrauterine growth retardation followed by postnatal growth failure. The pathogenesis of growth deficiency is probably multifactorial in infants with brain and heart disease but appears not to be due to endocrine dysfunction (Michaels and Kenny). Disturbances at the cellular level due to inhibitory effects of the intracellular virus may reduce the size but not the number of cells within various tissues.

Cooper et al. (1969) analyzed the major defects in 376 affected children and found hearing loss in 66 percent, cardiac disease in 48 percent, psychomotor retardation in 45 percent, cataracts in 28 percent, and neonatal thrombocytopenia in 22 percent. Deafness occurred as an isolated defect in 18 percent of the cases. Among 109 infants with congenital rubella, Plotkin and associates (1967) observed a birth weight below 2,500 grams in 47 percent, heart disease in 57 percent, ocular defects of one type or another in 53 percent, deafness in 51 percent, and mental retardation in 42 percent. Approximately one-half of those judged to be mentally retarded were microcephalic. The correlation between stage of pregnancy when the rash occurred and resulting defects was not precise among these patients, but the tendency was that ocular and cardiac defects were more often associated with infection in the first gestational month, while deafness and mental retardation were more related to infection during the third month of pregnancy. Others have found that cataract and patent ductus are infrequent when fetal rubella is contracted beyond the second month of gestation (Ueda et al.). In still another series of 41 children with congenital rubella assessed several years after birth (Forrest and Menser, 1970), ocular abnormalities were present in 90 percent, deafness in 76 percent, congenital heart disease in 37 percent, and central nervous system involvement in 32 percent. The birth weight

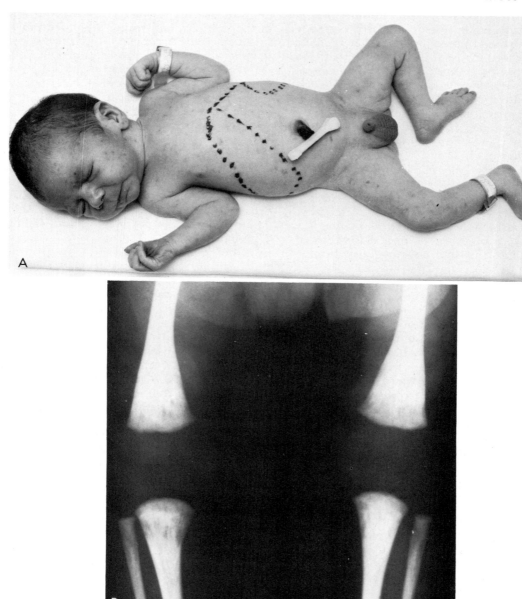

Figure 17–1. Congenital rubella. *A,* Three-day-old infant with a birth weight of 2640 grams. The child's mother was exposed to rubella in the first trimester of pregnancy but had no clinical illness. On the first day of life, the infant was found to have a platelet count of 8,000 per cu. mm., multiple petechial skin lesions, hepatosplenomegaly, a patent ductus arteriosus, and a cataract in the left eye. Rubella encephalitis was manifested by convulsions on the second day of life and a CSF lymphocytic pleocytosis. *B,* Skeletal lesions in the same child. There are multiple linear areas of radiolucency in the metaphyses of the distal femurs and proximal tibiae.

was abnormally low in 41 percent of the patients in this group. From these and other similar studies, it is apparent that different investigators have observed essentially the same organ systems being involved, but at considerable variance in regard to the frequencies. In addition, the follow-up reports provide better data on those defects that are fixed and repeatedly observable and provide less information about the transient neonatal abnormalities, including petechiae, jaundice, pneumonitis, and encephalitis.

Hematologic Defects. Neonatal thrombocytopenia is the most notable hematologic abnormality of the congenital rubella syndrome and has been observed in from 35 percent (Cooper et al.) to 65 percent (Banatvala et al.) of cases since 1964. A petechial or purpuric eruption often accompanies the reduced platelet count but skin lesions have been observed in affected infants with normal platelet counts. The rash is usually generalized but the face and upper thorax are selectively involved in some cases. Thrombocytopenia is frequently identified in the first day of life although it can develop days or even weeks later. A single case described by Reiss and Pryles was unusual in that thrombocytopenia was first observed at nine months of age, remitted but recurred two months later. Severe thrombocytopenia may result in umbilical or gastrointestinal bleeding, in addition to cutaneous lesions, and is a contraindication to circumcision or intramuscular injection of medications. The platelet count usually reverts to normal a few weeks after birth in infants with congenital rubella but in exceptional cases will remain abnormally low for up to six months (Zinkham et al.).

The pathogenesis of neonatal thrombocytopenia in the congenital rubella syndrome is not entirely clear. Bone marrow aspirates reveal a decreased number of megakaryocytes in some cases but are normal in others. Zinkham et al. studied the bone marrow of infants with this illness and found that cellularity was often generally reduced, and in some there was an increase in the number of histiocytes, many of which were actively phagocytic.

A less common abnormality is anemia with reticulocytosis, normoblastemia, and abnormal red cell morphology. The Coombs tests are negative in such infants and the cause of the shortened red cell survival remains obscure. Leukopenia also may be present but is usually transient. Still less common is dermal erythropoiesis (Klein and Markarian), the mechanism of origin of which is also obscure. Finally, chromosomal breaks in cultured leukocytes from children with congenital rubella have been identified by some authors (Kuroki et al., Nusbacher et al.) but not confirmed by others (Wolman et al.).

Cardiac and Cardiovascular Defects. Patent ductus arteriosus has long been assumed to be the most common cardiac defect in children with congenital rubella (Campbell). The addition of angiographic examination to clinical evaluation, however, has provided evidence that constriction or hypoplasia of the pulmonary arteries or their peripheral branches is at least as characteristic of the congenital rubella syndrome. Hastreiter and colleagues studied 37 infants with cardiac anomalies associated with congenital rubella and found all to have some degree of involvement of the pulmonary arteries or their peripheral branches. Patent ductus was present in 76 percent and coarctation of the aortic isthmus in 16 percent. Peripheral pulmonary artery narrowing is bilateral in most patients but one side can be more severely affected than the other. Additional defects of an intracardiac type have been described but are considered to be unusual. Ventricular septal defect, tetralogy of Fallot, and atrioventricular communis have only infrequently been related to this syndrome.

Myocardial damage resulting in abnormal electrocardiographic findings occurs in some infants and may cause or contribute to cardiac failure. Korones et al. illustrated the extensive and severe myocardial necrosis with minimal inflammatory response in two fatal cases and indicated that the process is progressive, leading to death in some infants but reversible in others. Nodular sclerosis of the cardiac valves which contain deposits of mucopolysaccharide has also been described (Singer et al.).

Vascular lesions, including proliferation of the arterial intima, play a significant role in the systemic as well as in the pulmonary circulation in rubella embryopathy (Esterly and Oppenheimer, 1969). Large vessels, including the aorta (Siassi et al.), are more consistently affected but medium-sized arteries can also be involved. Renal artery stenosis can be sufficiently severe to cause renal ischemia and subsequent hypertension (Esterly and Oppenheimer, 1967).

Ocular Defects. Ophthalmologic abnormalities of the congenital rubella syndrome contribute significantly to the disabilities of the affected child but are also important diagnostic signals, enhancing recognition of the disorder in those without other characteristic features in the newborn period. The principal ocular deficits include cataracts, microphthalmia, iris hypoplasia, congenital glaucoma and retinopathy (Roy et al.) (Fig. 17–2). Zimmerman emphasized the presence of an active iridocyclitis as a characteristic feature of the ocular involvement of this disease, a finding little mentioned by other authors.

Rubella cataracts are the end result of viral damage of the developing lens between the fourth and seventh embryonic weeks. The typical cataract is usually present bilaterally

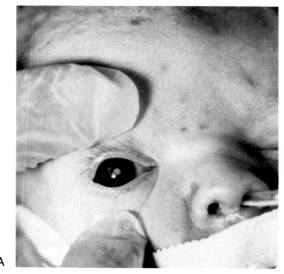

A

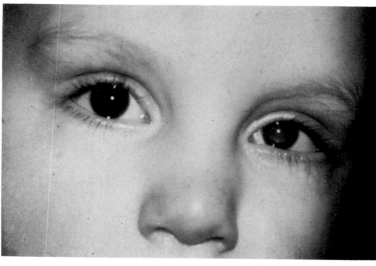

B

Figure 17–2. Cataracts with congenital rubella. *A,* One-day-old infant with bilateral dense cataracts. The child also has hepatosplenómegaly, thrombocytopenia, rash, and cardiomegaly. *B,* Cataract in a 2-year-old child with congenital rubella.

and is apparent either at birth or in the next few weeks. A peculiar sign often observed in infants with bilateral cataracts from rubella and other causes has been called the oculodigital phenomenon of Franceschetti (Roy et al.). This consists of the repetitive habit of applying pressure with the thumbs or index finger on the eyes, perhaps to produce some form of retinal stimulation. Descriptively, the cataract in congenital rubella is a densely white or pearly central lesion with a peripheral zone with a less dense appearance. Continued evolution of the process after birth may result in partial or total resorption of the lens material, forming a membranous cataract. The unique growth pattern and avascular character of the ocular lens appears to favor prolonged survival of the rubella virus.

Menser et al. (1967) were able to isolate the virus from cataractous material removed from a child aged two years and eleven months.

Microphthalmia may coexist with congenital cataracts and is more often observed when lens changes are unilateral. Microphthalmia is said to be present when the diameter of the cornea is 10 millimeters or less (Roy et al.). Iris hypoplasia is commonly found in the microphthalmic eye, in addition to esotropia and nystagmus.

Congenital glaucoma is the least common of the major ocular abnormalities of congenital rubella and is easily overlooked unless proper examination is performed. Haziness of the cornea secondary to edema, and rupture of Descemet's membrane are important signs indicative of rubella glaucoma, while corneal enlargement is often absent. Diagnosis is established by intraocular pressure measurements.

The retinopathy of congenital rubella is more common than is generally appreciated, although its precise incidence is not known. It consists of small, black deposits of variable size, predominantly involving the posterior pole of the retina and especially the macular region (Stark). The pigmentation tends to fade toward the periphery of the retina and is usually absent in the most peripheral regions. The optic discs are not usually abnormal on ophthalmoscopic examination. The retinopathy is probably present at birth in affected children but has rarely been identified earlier than four months of age. It is not believed to be progressive and does not seem to interfere with visual acuity or peripheral vision (Kresky and Nauheim). Other ocular defects of fetal rubella are usually present, and whether retinopathy occurs as an isolated manifestation of the congenital rubella syndrome is not known.

Deafness. Disturbances of hearing have been claimed to be the most common manifestation of the congenital rubella syndrome by certain investigators (Cooper et al., Lundström). Deafness is usually the last defect to be identified in the afflicted child and may require periodic testing for several years after birth before its presence is recognized. Maternal rubella during the latter part of the second and throughout the third months of pregnancy is especially prone to result in deafness in the newborn child. No time early in pregnancy is spared and even second trimester rubella can result in auditory defects (Borton and Stark, Hardy et al.). Damage to the inner ear structures ranges from mild to severe, thus leading to a wide variation in the degree of hearing loss. In addition to its presence in children with multiple defects, deafness secondary to intrauterine rubella may exist as an isolated disturbance, requiring a high index of suspicion for its etiologic identification (Karmody).

Most authors have attributed hearing impairment to sensorineural disturbances but some have postulated additional conduction defects due to middle ear damage (Richards). Borton and Stark studied 80 subjects with hearing deficits from congenital rubella and confirmed the variable degree of severity and also found that sensorineural deafness was the most common type. In addition, they found that a small percentage of patients had audiometric evidence of mixed deficits, suggesting middle ear pathology in combination with inner ear disease.

Pulmonary Complications. Respiratory involvement has become recognized as part of the "expanded" rubella syndrome but is rarely a predominant feature unless due to cardiac failure. In certain children, however, respiratory distress is severe and is a significant factor determining the outcome of the illness in the weeks or months after birth. Among 17 newborns with congenital rubella studied by Korones et al. (1965), six had roentgenographic evidence of pneumonia.

Pulmonary involvement is in the form of a subacute or chronic interstitial pneumonia. Auscultatory findings may be minimal even though bilateral interstitial infiltrates persist or even progress on x-ray examination for several weeks. Histologically, the inflammatory reaction consists of infiltrates of lymphocytes and large mononuclear cells in addition to variable numbers of plasma cells (Singer et al.). Alveolar septal thickening from edema or fibrosis and alveolar exudate are also frequently seen.

The variable clinical course of congenital rubella pneumonia has been stressed by Phelan and Campbell. Cough, tachypnea, and subcostal retractions indicate a pulmonary inflammatory response in the immediate newborn period in some. In others, clinical evidence of pneumonia does not develop until weeks or months after birth and may then progress rapidly, causing death soon thereafter. Respiratory disease in infants with congenital rubella is generally believed to be due to viral invasion of the lungs. Identical clinical and roentgenographic abnormalities in infants with congenital rubella can be produced by pneumonia due to *Pneumocystis carinii* (Phelan and Campbell, Lingeman et al.), an organism which occurs more often in children with immunoglobulin disorders or reticuloendothelial malignancies.

Hepatic Disease. Hepatomegaly, hepatosplenomegaly, and jaundice in the newborn became known to be common features of the congenital rubella syndrome following the 1964 epidemic. Among 22 patients, Korones et al. (1965) found liver enlargement in nine, splenomegaly in five, and jaundice in three. In one child in this group, rubella virus was isolated from the liver two months after birth. Hepatic involvement was present in 20 of 25 affected newborns reported by Rudolph et al.

The presence of rubella hepatitis is reflected by an elevated direct-reacting serum bilirubin, the development of jaundice in the first few days after birth, and elevation of the serum glutamic oxaloacetic transaminase levels and other hepatic enzymes. The hepatic pathology in such cases reveals variable alterations both in degree and in type (Esterly et al. 1967). Focal necrotic lesions with cholestasis have frequently been described, but, more recently, multinucleated giant-cell transformation has been recognized by several investigators (Esterly et al. 1967, Plotkin et al. 1965, Stern and Williams). The giant-cell abnormalities in these cases of neonatal rubella are identical to those with "neonatal hepatitis" of unknown cause. Strauss and Bernstein observed giant-cell hepatitis in infants with congenital rubella in whom some features of extrahepatic biliary obstruction also were present. These observations suggested to the authors the interesting possibility that the rubella virus contracted in utero might lead to biliary atresia as well as causing parenchymal hepatic disease.

Less well known than hepatic involvement with congenital rubella is the occurrence of interstitial pancreatitis (Bunnell and Monif, Donowitz and Gryboski). The long-term importance of this lesion remains unknown. Diabetes mellitus has developed in both children and adults with congenital rubella at a rate greater than expected and may be the end result of the effects on islet-cell function (Forrest et al., Johnson and Tudor).

Skeletal Disease. The discovery of long bone lesions on roentgenographic examination by Rudolph and colleagues in 1965 opened new dimensions to the transplacental rubella syndrome and provided the clinician with a new diagnostic method for recognition of the illness. The skeletal defects have been shown to exist in both upper and lower limbs in the newborn infant but are especially pronounced in the distal femoral and proximal tibial metaphyses. Roentgenographically, they consist of linear areas of radiolucency in the metaphyses with their longitudinal axis running parallel to the long axis of the bone. In comparison, the diaphyses of the long bones remain unaffected. The metaphyseal lucencies are best seen in the newborn period and frequently disappear between one and three months of age. The osseous lesions rarely persist longer than three months but have remained for as long as ten months in one reported case (Reiss and Pryles). The pathogenesis of these so-called "celery-stalk" lesions in congenital rubella has been speculative but there is little supporting evidence

of an active, viral osteomyelitis. Histologic study has shown that osteoporotic zones in the metaphyses correspond to the radiolucencies and that an active inflammatory process is not apparent (Reed).

The association of long bone lesions in infants with congenital rubella with other systemic active inflammatory and hematologic manifestations was made clear by the study of Rudolph et al. Their series of 75 patients was divided into three groups. Group one included those with the "expanded" rubella syndrome; group two, those with the "classic" syndrome with congenital cardiac defects and cataracts; and group three, those infants who were apparently normal but with a history of maternal rubella during pregnancy. Characteristic long bone lesions were found in 84 percent (27 of 32) in group one, in 21 percent (7 of 33) in group two, and in none in group three. The skeletal lesions described above occur in few other conditions and, thus, are highly characteristic of congenital rubella. Virtually identical bone changes, however, have recently been described in a newborn with cytomegalovirus disease (Graham et al.). Congenital syphilis and hypophosphatasia have also been mentioned in differential diagnosis (Rabinowitz et al.).

The newborn skull may also reveal roentgenographic abnormalities in the form of a large anterior fontanel with forward extension of its anterior dimensions into the region of the metopic suture (Singleton et al.). Mineralization within brain parenchyma sufficient to be observed on x-ray has not been considered part of the rubella syndrome and is more typical of either neonatal toxoplasmosis or cytomegalovirus disease. Cerebral mineralization has been shown microscopically (Peters and Davis) and recently has been demonstrated roentgenographically in a newborn infant with congenital rubella (Rowen et al.).

Immunologic Aspects. The paradox of persistent viral excretion in infants with congenital rubella despite large quantities of specific antibody has stimulated interest and study of the immune mechanisms involved. After several years of investigations, the most striking aspect of the available literature regarding the immunologic status of these infants is the variability and inconsistency of the results. Simons has recently reviewed the status of the problem and attempted to explain many of the discrepancies found in the various published studies. He questioned the presence of a consistent immunologic deficit in infants with intrauterine-acquired rubella and suggested that circulating antibody can only eliminate the rubella virus once the virus is released from cells. It is possible, therefore, that eventual termination of infection is primarily determined by the longevity of the infected cell.

Investigations by Singer and co-workers demonstrated that tissues associated with immunologic competence were able to undergo morphologic changes secondary to congenital rubella infection. Their findings included precocious development of germinal centers and plasma cells in lymph nodes and spleen in affected infants, similar to those often observed with other forms of congenital infection. Phytohemagglutinin stimulation and other antigenic studies of lymphocytes for evaluation of cellular immunity have been positive in certain studies (Singer et al., Simons) but abnormal in others (Olson et al., White et al.). Determinations of serum immunoglobulins in rubella infants have shown various abnormalities, the most common being a moderate elevation of IgM. The usual trend is for the serum IgM to remain elevated during the first few months of life but to decline thereafter (Michaels).

Schimke et al. described a child with congenital rubella with an immune defect typical of dysgammaglobulinemia type I. Concentration of IgM was profoundly elevated in this child, while IgG was reduced and IgA was undetectable. Germinal centers were absent in peripheral lymph nodes and no responses were seen with any of the antigens expected to produce wheal and flare cutaneous response. Despite the persistence of the immune abnormality, continued shedding of the virus did not occur. Similar immunoglobulin abnormalities were found in the case reported by Hancock et al. in which maternal rubella did not occur until the seventeenth week of pregnancy and abnormalities in the infant did not appear until three months of age. Treatment with the antiviral agent amantadine was believed to have produced clinical improvement. Claman and colleagues presented a similar child with rubella embryopathy with dysgammaglobulinemia, consisting of elevation of the IgM content but low to absent IgG and IgA levels. The importance of this case was the presence of lymphadenopathy, which revealed a marked histiocytic response on microscopic examination. The authors postulated that the histiocytic proliferative reaction was a tissue response to persistent viral infection in the presence of altered immune mechanisms. Still another infant with congenital rubella described by Plotkin et al. (1966) had hypogammaglobulinemia with decreased IgG and absent IgA and IgM serum levels. Virus was recovered from the blood and CSF at five months of age. Virus excretion was not affected by amantadine therapy in this child. More recently, hypoplasia of the thymus and thymus-dependent lymphoid tissue has been demonstrated in two infants with congenital rubella (Garcia et al.).

Central Nervous System Involvement. Information pertaining to the neurologic aspects of congenital rubella is surprisingly sparse compared to that pertaining to other organ systems. While there is no doubt that the rubella virus contracted in utero can and frequently does adversely affect the central nervous system, the incidence of involvement and the range of various types of structural injury remain in question. A chronic meningoencephalitis with persistence of the virus in brain and CSF is now undisputed as the most common type of brain disease in the newborn and young infant with congenital rubella. Malformations of the brain have often been attributed to this illness but substantiation is difficult to find. Friedman and Cohen (1947) reported a child with agenesis of the corpus callosum possibly due to intrauterine rubella, but the evidence of rubella was marginal. Hydrocephalus has often been mentioned as a sequel of intrauterine rubella but documented examples are uncommon. Sarwar et al. described a three-year-old child with congenital rubella with aqueductal occlusion demonstrated by air and positive contrast ventriculography. Although the lateral ventricles were distended, the head size was not enlarged, raising doubt that total obstruction of the aqueduct had been present in the first year of life. The "external" hydrocephalus referred to by several authors appears to have had reference to excessive quantities of fluid over the cerebral convexities, thus suggestive of cerebral atrophy rather than hydrocephalus. While the relative lack of well-documented cases does not categorically exclude the possibility, the present available evidence suggests that hydrocephalus is not an established component of the congenital rubella syndrome. Other types of cerebral malformations have been attributed to maternal rubella (Gray) but were not well substantiated and have not appeared in recent and detailed pathologic examinations (Rorke and Spiro, Singer et al.).

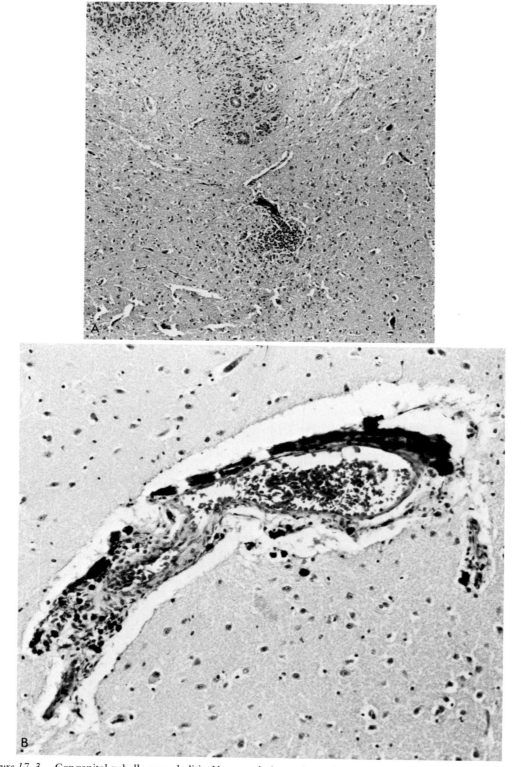

Figure 17–3. Congenital rubella encephalitis. Neuropathology of a 10-week-old infant with birth weight of 2250 grams and multiple organ involvement. *A,* Section through the midbrain demonstrates gliosis of the aqueduct of Sylvius, near the upper central part of the photograph. Just below the center of the photograph is an area of dense perivascular inflammation. *B* and *C,* Dystrophic mineralization of blood vessel walls in the brain with surrounding cerebral ischemic changes.

Illustration continued on opposite page

The intracranial pathology that has been well documented in the congenital rubella syndrome includes a chronic leptomeningitis and degenerative vascular lesions resulting in focal ischemic necrosis of cerebral parenchyma (Desmond et al. 1967, Rorke and Spiro, Singer et al.) (Fig. 17–3). Meningeal infiltration with large mononuclear cells, lymphocytes, and plasma cells may be the only significant histologic abnormality but more often coexists with other types of parenchymal damage. The vulnerability of blood vessels in tissues generally in the rubella syndrome is shared by the cerebral vasculature where variable degrees of destruction of vessel walls lead to disturbance of blood flow and subsequent areas of ischemic necrosis. In the studies by Rorke and Spiro, the vascular changes were most marked in the deep white matter and in the corpus striatum and thalamus. Vascular alterations were associated with areas of softening in the cerebral white matter, which, on histologic examination, varied from regions showing proliferation of astroglia and microglia to areas with frank necrosis. Some myelin depletion with axonal sparing was observed in infants who survived longer than one month after birth. Vascular degenerative alterations in the brain were also observed in the cases of Peters and Davis. Mineralization in vessel walls and perivascular spaces was most striking in the putamen in these patients.

Microcephaly has been repeatedly stressed as the clinical hallmark of neurologic involvement in congenital rubella. The degree of abnormality of the infant's head size, however, becomes less distinct when it is compared to the somatic size rather than when it is compared only to that expected for the chronological age of the child. Somatic growth retardation of major degree is a common feature of the illness (Michaels and Kenny) and renders analysis of the head circumference more difficult. Furthermore, evaluation of intellectual skills is complicated when limitations include visual loss and deafness. Although it is not surprising that brain growth may be compromised by the prenatal cerebral insults described above, the use of the term microcephaly as a summarization of the clinical neurologic deficits is an oversimplification. As pointed out by Macfarlane et al., many children with congenital rubella with head circumferences small for their chronological age are, in fact, small children in whom the small head is proportionate to their small stature.

The most extensive review of the clinical features of the neurologic aspects of congenital rubella is that by Desmond and colleagues (1967). Among 100 patients with congenital

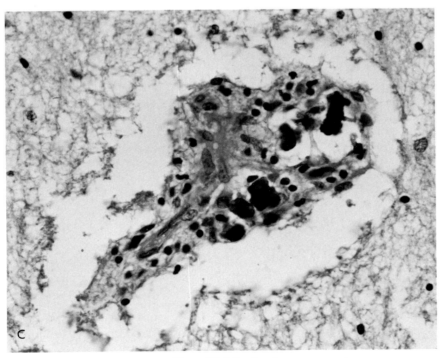

Figure 17–3 Continued

rubella, neurologic abnormalities were found in 81 at some time between birth and age 18 months. The most frequent pattern they observed included hypotonia and lethargy in the newborn period in association with a large and full anterior fontanel. Irritability became more evident weeks or months after birth and was manifested by excessive crying, continuous motor activity, and photophobia. Weight gain was poor and head lag persisted beyond four months of age. A smaller number of infants exhibited similar signs but were hypertonic from early infancy or even maintained a posture of opisthotonus. In some, back arching was notably a posture the baby assumed with tactile stimulation. Still other affected infants had recurrent convulsions superimposed upon tone abnormalities, lethargy, or irritability. Two infants in the series of Desmond et al. (1967) departed from the usual clinical course of congenital rubella by the abrupt appearance of a meningitis-like illness between two and three months of age. Another was said to have developed normally until seven months of age, when the onset of seizures was followed by the loss of motor and social skills. Excessive size and fullness of the anterior fontanel was an important aspect of the physical findings in this group, being present in 45 percent. It was most noticeable during the first three months and was usually no longer present by six months after birth.

Follow-up information in regard to neurologic function of infants with congenital rubella is difficult to assess. Approximately 30 to 50 percent are left with some variety of neurologic handicap, other than visual or auditory (Desmond et al., Forrest and Menser). As expected, impairments extend from mild in degree to those that preclude development of speech, ambulation, or self-care of any type. Children with congenital rubella with normal intellectual skills commonly have many problems with academic achievement and require special attention in the school setting (Desmond et al. 1978). Inattentiveness, short attention span, visual or hearing handicaps, and deficits of tactile perception are all factors in such children which impede the learning process even though intellect may be normal.

The most recent observation in children with congenital rubella has been the occurrence of a progressive rubella panencephalitis similar to subacute sclerosing panencephalitis caused by the measles virus (Townsend et al. 1975, Weil et al.). Cases in children known to have had intrauterine-acquired ru-

bella have had their onset with a progressive deteriorative neurologic illness between eight and 14 years of age. The clinical findings have included gradual intellectual and motor deterioration, ataxia, and seizures. The CSF examinations in these children have revealed a modest lymphocytic pleocytosis, an increased protein content, and elevation of the gamma globulin content. Serum and CSF rubella antibody have been markedly increased. Various electroencephalographic abnormalities have been described but the suppression-burst pattern characteristic of subacute sclerosing panencephalitis has not been found. Rubella virus has not been recovered from the CSF but has been isolated from the brain (Cremer et al., Weil et al.). Neuropathologic examination has revealed diffuse neuronal loss in the cortical areas and perivascular cuffing by lymphocytes and plasma cells in atrophic white matter (Townsend et al. 1976). Inclusion bodies have not been described.

In addition to the occurrence of a late onset type of chronic progressive encephalitis in children with congenital rubella, a similar illness has been described in two cases in which rubella had been acquired in early childhood (Lebon and Lyon, Wolinsky et al.). In these cases also, the serum and CSF rubella antibody titers were elevated, as was the CSF gamma globulin content. These cases indicate, therefore, that the rubella virus, like the measles virus, can persist in latent fashion in the brain for lengthy periods of time, with the eventual production of a chronic, progressive encephalitic disorder.

Cerebrospinal fluid examination in the newborn period of infants with congenital rubella is usually characterized by some degree of elevation of the protein content and a lymphocytic pleocytosis. Such findings are present in most neonates with clinical evidence of rubella meningoencephalitis but are found in some that are spared of signs of cerebral disease. Unlike many types of viral encephalitis in infants or children in which recovery of virus from CSF is unusual, the encephalitis of congenital rubella is notable for the high frequency with which viral isolation is possible (Monif and Sever). Korones et al. (1965) isolated the virus from the CSF in six of 13 infants ranging in age from birth to three and one-half months. In three of the virus-positive CSF specimens, the protein and cell contents were normal. Desmond et al. (1967) obtained positive isolations in 25 of 99 CSF specimens from infants up to three months of age. Virus persisted in the CSF throughout the first year in nine patients and until 18 months after birth in one child.

Diagnosis of Congenital Rubella

Congenital rubella is suspected when there is a history of maternal exposure or infection during pregnancy or physical signs in the newborn or young infant suggestive of the disease. Diagnosis is confirmed by viral isolation studies on nasopharyngeal secretions, stool, or CSF, in addition to serial serologic tests of blood from both the patient and the mother. The child with signs of congenital infection such as jaundice, thrombocytopenia, and cataracts is easily recognized to be a candidate for this diagnosis, but diagnostic studies for the disease should be extended to include other illnesses perhaps less readily suggestive of intrauterine-acquired rubella. For example, the child with obstructive jaundice appearing within weeks after birth whose primary differential diagnosis includes biliary atresia and giant-cell hepatitis should be surveyed for rubella infection. The previously normal infant who develops recurrent convulsions in the early weeks of life or the infant with myoclonic seizures and a hypsarrhythmic electroencephalogram also is a candidate for serologic examinations. The latter disorder is not generally considered one that results from intrauterine rubella but, since the etiology in many cases remains unestablished, congenital infections warrant consideration. The young infant who acquires an interstitial pneumonitis or who develops unexplained myocardial failure also deserves rubella serologic tests.

With the exception of viral isolation procedures, the usual laboratory method of identification of rubella infection in the infant is with the hemagglutination inhibition or neutralization tests. The HI antibody titer is elevated at birth in the infected child, representing the sum of antibody passively transferred from the mother and that actively produced by the fetus. By four to six months after birth, the maternal passively transferred antibody is usually undetectable. Persistence of antibody thereafter and up to two or three years of age can be assumed to be evidence of congenital rubella infection. Unless the virus is isolated from the infant, a single positive titer in the first few months of life cannot be considered diagnostic. For this reason, serial titers are indicated, with a persisting or rising titer after maternal antibody has been expected to disappear being of diagnostic importance.

Unlike postnatally acquired rubella, which usually produces a lasting elevation in HI antibody titer, congenital rubella is frequently followed by a progressively declining titer and occasionally by the eventual absence of detectable antibody. Hardy et al. found that of 20 children with intrauterine-acquired rubella, six had titers as high as 1:512 between six and 12 months of age, but between 20 and 40 months, titers in the range of 1:8 or 1:16 were usual. By just over three years of age, seven children had no demonstrable antibody titer. The low or absent antibody levels therefore render diagnosis difficult if the affected child is three years of age or older when first seen. Furthermore, a low titer after three years of age could possibly be due to previously acquired, natural rubella. Cooper et al. (1971) likewise found that some children with congenital rubella subsequently became antibody-negative by four or five years of age. In addition, they showed that seronegative children with congenital rubella often exhibited no seroconversion when given rubella vaccine (HPV-77). This lack of serologic response to rubella vaccine has been proposed as a diagnostic aid in older children suspected of having congenital rubella but with absent HI antibody titers. Among normal seronegative children, the great majority will show a significant rise in rubella HI antibody within a month after immunization.

An additional method that has been used as a screening test for the presence of intrauterine infection of several types is the determination of IgM content in cord blood or blood obtained in the neonatal period (Alford et al.). Since IgM antibodies do not normally cross the placenta from mother to fetus, the normal newborn infant has low levels of this type of immunoglobulin. High IgM levels at birth indicate an active immune response of the fetus and have been found in infants with toxoplasmosis, cytomegalovirus disease, syphilis, and rubella. Production of rubella IgM antibody continues for one to three months after birth in infants with congenital rubella. Although an elevated IgM level in the newborn infant can be used as evidence of an intrauterine infectious illness, the absence of elevated levels does not exclude the possibility. McCracken et al. accepted values of IgM above 20 mg. per 100 ml. to be abnormal in the neonatal period and found that only 18 percent of infants with congenital rubella had abnormal levels.

Many of those with high levels were severely affected and would have been readily identified by other methods. Thus, the procedure may have some value as a screening test in the newborn period for intrauterine infection but cannot be considered to consistently identify all such infants.

REFERENCES

Ackroyd, J. F.: Three cases of thrombocytopenic purpura occurring after rubella. Quart. J. Med. 42:299, 1949.

Alford, C. A., Schaefer, J., Blankenship, W. J., Straumfjord, J. V., and Cassady, G.: A correlative immunologic, microbiologic and clinical approach to the diagnosis of acute and chronic infections in newborn infants. New Eng. J. Med. 277:437–449, 1967.

Alford, C. A., Jr., Foft, J. W., Blankenship, W. J., Cassady, G., and Benton, J. W., Jr.: Subclinical central nervous system disease of neonates: A prospective study of infants born with increased levels of IgM. J. Pediat. 75:1167–1178, 1969.

Avery, G. B., Monif, G. R. G., Sever, J. L., and Leikin, S. L.: Rubella syndrome after inapparent maternal illness. Am. J. Dis. Child. 110:444–446, 1965.

Banatvala, J. E., Horstmann, D. M., Payne, M. C., and Gluck, L.: Rubella syndrome and thrombocytopenic purpura in newborn infants. New Eng. J. Med. 273:474–478, 1965.

Borton, T. E., and Stark, E. W.: Audiological findings in hearing loss secondary to maternal rubella. Pediatrics 45:225–229, 1970.

Bradford, R. I. C.: Two cases of rubella meningoencephalitis. Brit. Med. J. 1:312–313, 1943.

Briggs, J. F.: Meningoencephalitis following rubella. J. Pediat. 7:609–612, 1935.

Brody, J. A., Sever, J. L., McAlister, R., Schiff, G. M., and Cutting, R.: Rubella epidemic on St. Paul Island in the Pribilofs, 1963. I. Epidemiologic, clinical and serological findings. J.A.M.A. 191:619–623, 1965.

Bunnell, C. E., and Monif, G. R. G.: Interstitial pancreatitis in the congenital rubella syndrome. J. Pediat. 80:465–466, 1972.

Campbell, M.: Place of maternal rubella in the aetiology of congenital heart disease. Brit. Med. J. 1:691–696, 1961.

Cherry, J. D., Bobinski, J. E., and Comerci, G. D.: A clinical trial with live attenuated rubella virus vaccine (Cendehill 51 strain). J. Pediat. 75:79–86, 1969.

Chin, J., Werner, S. B., Kusumoto, H. H., and Lennette, E. H.: Complications of rubella immunization in children. Calif. Med. 114:7–12, 1971.

Claman, H. N., Suvatte, V., Githens, J. H., and Hathaway, W. E.: Histiocytic reaction in dysgammaglobulinemia and congenital rubella. Pediatrics 46:89–95, 1970.

Connolly, J. H., Hutchinson, W. M., Allen, I. V., Lyttle, J. A., Swallow, M. W., Dermott, E., and Thomson, D.: Carotid artery thrombosis, encephalitis, myelitis and optic neuritis associated with rubella virus infections. Brain 98:583–594, 1975.

Cooper, L. Z., Florman, A. L., Ziring, P. R., and Krugman, S.: Loss of rubella hemagglutination inhibition antibody in congenital rubella. Failure of seronegative children with congenital rubella to respond to

HPV-77 rubella vaccine. Am. J. Dis. Child. 122:397–403, 1971.

Cooper, L. Z., Green, R. H., Krugman, S., Giles, J. P., and Mirick, G. S.: Neonatal thrombocytopenic purpura and other manifestations of rubella contracted in utero. Am. J. Dis. Child. 110:416–427, 1965.

Cooper, L. Z., Ziring, P. R., Ockerse, A. B., Fedun, B. A., Kiely, B., and Krugman, S.: Rubella. Clinical manifestations and management. Am. J. Dis. Child. 118:18–29, 1969.

Cremer, N. E., Oshiro, L. S., Weil, M. L., Lennette, E. H., Itabashi, H. H., and Carnay, L.: Isolation of rubella virus from brain in chronic progressive panencephalitis. J. Gen. Virol. 29:143–153, 1975.

Davison, C., and Friedfeld, L.: Acute encephalomyelitis following German measles. Am. J. Dis. Child. 55:496–510, 1938.

Desmond, M. M., Fisher, E. S., Vorderman, A. L., Schaffer, H. G., Andrew, L. P., Zion, T. E., and Catlin, F. I.: The longitudinal course of congenital rubella encephalitis in nonretarded children. J. Pediat. 93:584–591, 1978.

Desmond, M. M., Wilson, G. S., Melnick, J. L., Singer, D. B., Zion, T. E., Rudolph, A. J., Pineda, R. G., Ziai, M. H., and Blattner, R. J.: Congenital rubella encephalitis. Course and early sequelae. J. Pediat. 71:311–331, 1967.

Donowitz, M., and Gryboski, J. D.: Pancreatic insufficiency and the congenital rubella syndrome. J. Pediat. 87:241–243, 1975.

Dudgeon, J. A.: Maternal rubella and its effect on the foetus. Arch. Dis. Childh. 42:110–125, 1967.

Du Pan, R. M., Huygelen, C., Peetermans, J., and Prinzie, A.: Clinical trials with a live attenuated rubella virus vaccine. Cendehill 51 strain. Am. J. Dis. Child. 115:658–662, 1968.

Esterly, J. R., and Oppenheimer, E. H.: Pathological lesions due to congenital rubella. Arch. Path. 87:380–388, 1969.

Esterly, J. R., and Oppenheimer, E. H.: Vascular lesions in infants with congenital rubella. Circulation 36:544–554, 1967.

Esterly, J. R., Slusser, R. J., and Ruebner, B. H.: Hepatic lesions in the congenital rubella syndrome. J. Pediat. 71:676–685, 1967.

Farquhar, J. D.: Follow-up on rubella vaccinations and experience with subclinical reinfection. J. Pediat. 81:460–465, 1972.

Farquhar, J. D., Plotkin, S. A., and Schoengold, R. J.: Cendehill strain of rubella vaccine: Clinical evaluation. J. Pediat. 75:412–417, 1969.

Ferguson, A. W.: Rubella as a cause of thrombocytopenic purpura. Pediatrics 25:400–408, 1960.

Fleet, W. F., Jr., Schaffner, W., Lefkowitz, L. V., Jr., Murphy, C. D., and Karzon, D. T.: Exposure of susceptible teachers to rubella vaccinees. Am. J. Dis. Child. 123:28–30, 1972.

Forrest, J. M., and Menser, M. A.: Congenital rubella in school children and adolescents. Arch. Dis. Childh. 45:63–69, 1970.

Forrest, J. M., Menser, M. A., and Burgess, J. A.: High frequency of diabetes mellitus in young adults with congenital rubella. Lancet 2:332–334, 1971.

Friedman, M., and Cohen, P.: Agenesis of the corpus callosum as a possible sequel to maternal rubella during pregnancy. Am. J. Dis. Child. 73:178–185, 1947.

Fry, J., Dillane, J. B., and Fry, L.: Rubella in 1962. Brit. Med. J. 2:833–834, 1962.

Garcia, A. G. P., Olinto, F., and Fortes, T. G. O.: Thymic

hypoplasia due to congenital rubella. Arch. Dis. Childh. 49:181–185, 1974.

Gilmartin, R. C., Jr., Jabbour, J. T., and Duenas, D. A.: Rubella vaccine myeloradiculoneuritis. J. Pediat. 80:406–412, 1972.

Graham, C. B., Thal, A., and Wassum, C. S.: Rubella-like bone changes in congenital cytomegalic inclusion disease. Radiology 94:39–43, 1970.

Gray, M. J.: Conception during rubella incubation period. Obstet. Gynec. 23:526–527, 1964.

Gregg, N. M.: Congenital cataract following German measles in the mother. Trans. Ophthal. Soc. Aust. 3:35–45, 1941.

Gregg, N. M. A.: Further observations on congenital defects in infants following maternal rubella. Trans. Ophthal. Soc. Aust. 4:119–131, 1944.

Hancock, M. P., Huntley, C. C., and Sever, J. L.: Congenital rubella syndrome with immunoglobulin disorder. J. Pediat. 72:636–645, 1968.

Hanissian, A. S., Martinez, A. J., Jabbour, J. T., and Duenas, D. A.: Vasculitis and myositis secondary to rubella vaccination. Arch. Neurol. 28:202–204, 1973.

Hardy, J. B., McCracken, G. H., Jr., Gilkeson, M. R., and Sever, J. L.: Adverse fetal outcome following maternal rubella after the first trimester of pregnancy. J.A.M.A. 207:2414–2420, 1969.

Hardy, J. B., Sever, J. L., and Gilkeson, M. R.: Declining antibody titers in children with congenital rubella. J. Pediat. 75:213–220, 1969.

Hastreiter, A. R., Joorabchi, B., Pujatti, G., van der Horst, R. L., Patacsil, G., and Sever, J. L.: Cardiovascular lesions associated with congenital rubella. J. Pediat. 71:59–65, 1967.

Heggie, A. D.: Pathogenesis of the rubella exanthem: Distribution of rubella virus in the skin during rubella with and without rash. J. Infect. Dis. 137:74–77, 1978.

Heggie, A. D., and Robbins, F. C.: Natural rubella acquired after birth. Clinical features and complications. Am. J. Dis. Child. 118:12–17, 1969.

Hiro, Y., and Tasaka, S.: Die Röteln sind eine viruskrankheit. Mschr. Kinderheilk. 76:328–332, 1938.

Holliday, P. B., Jr.: Pre-eruptive neurological complications of the common contagious diseases—rubella, rubeola, roseola, and varicella. J. Pediat. 36:185–198, 1950.

Holt, S., Hudgins, D., Krishnan, K. R., and Critchley, E. M. R.: Diffuse myelitis associated with rubella vaccination. Brit. Med. J. 2:1037–1038, 1976.

Horstmann, D. M.: Rubella: The challenge of its control. J. Infect. Dis. 123:640–654, 1971.

Horstmann, D. M.: Rubella and the rubella syndrome. New epidemiologic and virologic observations. Calif. Med. 102:397–403, 1965.

Ingalls, T. H.: German measles and German measles in pregnancy. Am. J. Dis. Child. 93:555–558, 1957.

Jackson, A. D. M., and Fisch, L.: Deafness following maternal rubella: Results of a prospective investigation. Lancet 2:1241–1244, 1958.

Johnson, G. M., and Tudor, R. B.: Diabetes mellitus and congenital rubella infection. Am. J. Dis. Child. 120:453–455, 1970.

Karmody, C. S.: Subclinical maternal rubella and congenital deafness. New Eng. J. Med. 278:809–814, 1968.

Kenny, F. M., Michaels, R. H., and Davis, K. S.: Rubella encephalopathy. Later psychometric, neurologic, and encephalographic evaluation of seven survivors. Am. J. Dis. Child. 110:374–380, 1965.

Kilroy, A. W., Schaffner, W., Fleet, W. F., Jr., Lefkowitz, L. B., Jr., Karzon, D. T., and Fenichel, G. M.: Two syndromes following rubella immunization. Clinical observations and epidemiological studies. J.A.M.A. 214:2287–2292, 1970.

Klein, H. Z., and Markarian, M.: Dermal erythropoiesis in congenital rubella. Clin. Pediat. 8:604–607, 1969.

Korones, S. B., Ainger, L. E., Monif, G. R. G., Roane, J., Sever, J. L., and Fuste, F.: Congenital rubella syndrome: New clinical aspects with recovery of virus from affected infants. J. Pediat. 67:166–191, 1965.

Korones, S. B., Ainger, L. E., Monif, G. R. G., Roane, J., Sever, J. L., and Fuste, F.: Congenital rubella syndrome: Study of 22 infants. Myocardial damage and other new clinical aspects. Am. J. Dis. Child. 110:434–440, 1965.

Kresky, B., and Nauheim, J. S.: Rubella retinitis. Am. J. Dis. Child. 113:305–310, 1967.

Kuroki, Y., Makino, S., Aya, T., and Nayagama, T.: Chromosome abnormalities in cultured leukocytes from rubella patients. Jap. J. Human Genet. 11:17–23, 1966.

Lebon, P., and Lyon, G.: Non-congenital rubella encephalitis. Lancet 2:468, 1974.

Lee, P. R.: Arthritis and rubella. Brit. Med. J. 2:925, 1962.

Lepow, M. L., Veronelli, J. A., Hostetler, D. D., and Robbins, F. C.: A trial with live attenuated rubella vaccine. Am. J. Dis. Child. 115:639–647, 1968.

Lingeman, C. H., Schulz, D. M., and Lukemeyer, J. W.: *Pneumocystis carinii* pneumonia in congenital rubella. Am. J. Dis. Child. 113:585–587, 1967.

Lundström, R.: Rubella during pregnancy: Follow-up study of children born after epidemic of rubella in Sweden, 1951, with additional investigation on prophylaxis and treatment of maternal rubella. Acta Pediat. 51 (Suppl. 133):1–110, 1962.

Macfarlane, D. W., Boyd, R. D., Dodrill, C. B., and Tufts, E.: Intrauterine rubella, head size, and intellect. Pediatrics 55:797–801, 1975.

Margolis, F. J., Wilson, J. L., and Top, F. H.: Postrubella encephalomyelitis. J. Pediat. 23:158–165, 1943.

McCracken, G. H., Jr., Hardy, J. B., Chen, T. C., Hoffman, L. S., Gilkeson, M. R., and Sever, J. L.: Serum immunoglobulin levels in newborn infants. II. Survey of cord and follow-up sera from 123 infants with congenital rubella. J. Pediat. 74:383–392, 1969.

Menser, M. A., Forrest, J. M., Slinn, R. F., Nowak, M. J., and Dorman, D. C.: Rubella viruria in a 29-year-old woman with congenital rubella. Lancet 2:797–798, 1971.

Menser, M. A., Harley, J. D., Hertzberg, R., Dorman, D. C., and Murphy, A. M.: Persistence of virus in lens for three years after prenatal rubella. Lancet 2:387–388, 1967.

Meyer, H. M., Jr., Parkman, P. D., and Panos, T. C.: Attenuated rubella virus: II. Production of an experimental live virus vaccine and clinical trial. New Eng. J. Med. 275:575–580, 1966.

Michaels, R. H.: Immunologic aspects of congenital rubella. Pediatrics 43:339–350, 1969.

Michaels, R. H., and Kenny, F. M.: Postnatal growth retardation in congenital rubella. Pediatrics 43:251–259, 1969.

Mitchell, W., and Pampiglione, G.: Neurological and mental complications of rubella. Lancet 2:1250–1253, 1954.

Modlin, J. F., Herrmann, K., Brandling-Bennett, A. D., Eddins, D. L., and Hayden, G. F.: Risk of congenital abnormality after inadvertent rubella vaccination of pregnant women. New Eng. J. Med. 294:972–974, 1976.

Monif, G. R. G., and Sever, J. L.: Chronic infection of the central nervous system with rubella virus. Neurology 16:111–112, 1966.

Morse, E. E., Zinkham, W. H., and Jackson, D. P.: Thrombocytopenic purpura following rubella infection in children and adults. Arch. Intern. Med. 117:573–579, 1966.

Nusbacher, J., Hirschhorn, K., and Cooper, L. Z.: Chromosomal abnormalities in congenital rubella. New Eng. J. Med. 276:1409–1413, 1967.

Olson, G. B., Dent, P. B., Rawls, W. E., South, M. A., Montgomery, J. R., Melnick, J. L., and Good, R. A.: Abnormalities of in vitro lymphocyte responses during rubella virus infections. J. Exp. Med. 128:47–68, 1968.

Ozsoylu, S., Kanra, G., and Savas, G.: Thrombocytopenic purpura related to rubella infection. Pediatrics 62:567–569, 1978.

Pampiglione, G., Young, S. E. J., and Ramsay, A. M.: Neurological and electroencephalographic problems of the rubella epidemic of 1962. Brit. Med. J. 2:1300–1302, 1963.

Parkman, P. D., Buescher, R. L., and Artenstein, M. S.: Recovery of rubella virus from army recruits. Proc. Soc. Exp. Biol. Med. 111:225–230, 1962.

Parkman, P. D., Hopps, H. E., and Meyer, H. M., Jr.: Rubella virus, isolation, characterization, and laboratory diagnosis. Am. J. Dis. Child. 118:68–77, 1969.

Peters, E. R., and Davis, R. L.: Congenital rubella syndrome: Cerebral mineralizations and subperiosteal new bone formation as expressions of this disorder. Clin. Pediat. 5:743–746, 1966.

Phelan, P., and Campbell, P.: Pulmonary complications of rubella embryopathy. J. Pediat. 75:202–212, 1969.

Pitt, D. B.: Congenital malformations and maternal rubella. Progress report. Med. J. Aust. 1:881–890, 1961.

Plotkin, S. A., Cochran, W., Lindquist, J. M., Cochran, G. G., Schaffer, D. B., Scheie, H. G., and Furukawa, T.: Congenital rubella syndrome in late infancy. J.A.M.A. 200:435–441, 1967.

Plotkin, S. A., Klaus, R. M., and Whitely, J. P.: Hypogammaglobulinemia in an infant with congenital rubella syndrome; failure of 1-adamantanamine to stop virus excretion. J. Pediat. 69:1085–1091, 1966.

Plotkin, S. A., Oski, F. A., Hartnett, E. M., Hervada, A. R., Friedman, S., and Gowing, J.: Some recently recognized manifestations of the rubella syndrome. J. Pediat. 67:182–191, 1965.

Rabinowitz, J. G., Wolf, B. S., Greenberg, E. I., and Rausen, A. R.: Osseous changes in rubella embryopathy. (Congenital rubella syndrome.) Radiology 85:494–500, 1965.

Reed, G. B., Jr.: Rubella bone lesions. J. Pediat. 74:208–213, 1969.

Reiss, J. S., and Pryles, C. B.: Thrombocytopenia in congenital rubella. New Eng. J. Med. 275:264–265, 1966.

Richards, C. S.: Middle ear changes in rubella deafness. Arch. Otolaryng. 80:48–59, 1964.

Rorke, L. B., and Spiro, A. J.: Cerebral lesions in congenital rubella syndrome. J. Pediat. 70:243–255, 1967.

Rowen, M., Singer, M. I., and Moran, E. T.: Intracranial calcification in the congenital rubella syndrome. Am. J. Roentgenol. 115:86–91, 1972.

Roy, F. H., Hiatt, R. L., Korones, S. B., and Roane, J.: Ocular manifestations of congenital rubella syndrome. Recovery of virus from affected infants. Arch. Ophthal. 75:601–607, 1966.

Rudolph, A. J., Singleton, E. B., Rosenberg, H. S., Singer, D. B., and Phillips, C. A.: Osseous manifestations of the congenital rubella syndrome. Am. J. Dis. Child. 110:428–433, 1965.

Rudolph, A. J., Yow, M. D., Phillips, C. A., Desmond, M. M., Blattner, R. J., and Melnick, J. L.: Transplacental infection in newly born infants. J.A.M.A. 191:843–846, 1965.

Sarwar, M., Azar-Kia, B., Schechter, M. M., Valsamis, M., and Batnitzky, S.: Aqueductal occlusion in the congenital rubella syndrome. Neurology 24:198–201, 1974.

Schiff, G. M., and Dine, M. S.: Transmission of rubella from newborns. A controlled study among young adult women and report of an unusual case. Am. J. Dis. Child. 110:447–451, 1965.

Schimke, R. N., Bolano, C., and Kirkpatrick, C. H.: Immunologic deficiency in the congenital rubella syndrome. Am. J. Dis. Child. 118:626–633, 1969.

Sever, J. L., Fuccillo, D. A., Gitnick, G. L., Huebner, R. J., Gilkeson, M. R., Ley, A. C., Tzan, N., and Traub, R. G.: Rubella antibody determinations. Pediatrics 40:789–797, 1967.

Sever, J. L., Hardy, J. B., Nelson, K. B., and Gilkeson, M. R.: Rubella in the collaborative perinatal research study. II. Clinical and laboratory findings in children through 3 years of age. Am. J. Dis. Child. 118:123–132, 1969.

Sever, J. L., Nelson, K. B., and Gilkeson, M. R.: Rubella epidemic, 1964: Effect on 6,000 pregnancies. Am. J. Dis. Child. 110:395–407, 1965.

Sever, J. L., Schiff, G. M., Bell, J. A., Kapikian, A. Z., Huebner, R. J., and Traub, R. G.: Rubella: frequency of antibody among children and adults. Pediatrics 35:996–998, 1965.

Sherman, F. E., Michaels, R. H., and Kenny, F. M.: Acute encephalopathy (encephalitis) complicating rubella. J.A.M.A. 192:675–681, 1965.

Siassi, B., Klyman, G., and Emmanouilides, G. C.: Hypoplasia of the abdominal aorta associated with the rubella syndrome. Am. J. Dis. Child. 120:476–479, 1970.

Simons, M. J.: Congenital rubella: An immunological paradox? Lancet 2:1275–1278, 1968.

Singer, D. B., Rudolph, A. J., Rosenberg, H. S., Rawls, W. E., and Boniuk, M.: Pathology of the congenital rubella syndrome. J. Pediat. 71:665–675, 1967.

Singer, D. B., South, M. A., Montgomery, J. R., and Rawls, W. E.: Congenital rubella syndrome. Lymphoid tissue and immunologic status. Am. J. Dis. Child. 118:54–61, 1969.

Singleton, E. B., Rudolph, A. J., Rosenberg, H. S., and Singer, D. B.: The roentgenographic manifestations of the rubella syndrome in newborn infants. Am. J. Roentgenol. 97:82–91, 1966.

Spruance, S. L., Klock, L. E., Jr., Bailey, A., Ward, J. R., and Smith, C. B.: Recurrent joint symptoms in children vaccinated with HPV-77DK12 rubella vaccine. J. Pediat. 80:413–418, 1972.

Spruance, S. L., and Smith, C. B.: Joint complications associated with derivatives of HPV-77 rubella virus vaccine. Am. J. Dis. Child. 122:105–111, 1971.

Squadrini, F., Taparelli, F., De Rienzo, B., Giovannini, G., and Pagani, C.: Rubella virus isolation from cerebrospinal fluid in postnatal rubella encephalitis. Brit. Med. J. 2:1329–1330, 1977.

Stark, G.: Rubella retinopathy. An account of six cases. Arch. Dis. Childh. 41:420–423, 1966.

Steen, E., and Torp, K. H.: Encephalitis and thrombocytopenic purpura after rubella. Arch. Dis. Childh. 31:470–473, 1956.

Stern, H., and Williams, B. M.: Isolation of rubella virus in a case of neonatal giant-cell hepatitis. Lancet 1:293–295, 1966.

Stewart, G. L., Parkman, P. D., Hopps, H. E., Douglas, R. D., Hamilton, J. P., and Meyer, H. M., Jr.: Rubella-virus hemagglutination-inhibition test. New Eng. J. Med. 276:554–557, 1967.

Strauss, L., and Bernstein, J.: Neonatal hepatitis in congenital rubella. A histopathologic study. Arch. Path. 86:317–327, 1968.

Swan, C.: A study of three infants dying from congenital defects following maternal rubella in the early stages of pregnancy. J. Path. Bact. 56:289–295, 1944.

Swan, C., Tostevin, A. L., and Black, G. H. B.: Final observations on congenital defects in infants following infectious diseases during pregnancy with special reference to rubella. Med. J. Aust. 2:889–908, 1946.

Swan, C., Tostevin, A. L., Mayo, H., and Black, G. H. B.: Congenital defects in infants following infectious diseases during pregnancy. Med. J. Aust. 2:201–210, 1943.

Tartakow, I. J.: The teratogenicity of maternal rubella. J. Pediat. 66:380–391, 1965.

Townsend, J. J., Baringer, J. R., Wolinsky, J. S., Malamud, N., Mednick, J. P., Panitch, H. S., Scott, R. A. T., Oshiro, L. S., and Cremer, N. E.: Progressive rubella panencephalitis. Late onset after congenital rubella. New Eng. J. Med. 292:990–993, 1975.

Townsend, J. J., Wolinsky, J. S., and Baringer, J. R.: The neuropathology of progressive rubella panencephalitis of late onset. Brain 99:81–90, 1976.

Ueda, K., Nashida, Y., Oshima, K., and Shepard, T. H.: Congenital rubella syndrome: Correlation of gestational age at time of maternal rubella with type of defect. J. Pediat. 94:763–766, 1979.

Vaheri, A., Vesikari, T., Oker-Blom, N., Seppala, M., Parkman, P. D., Veronelli, J., and Robbins, F. C.: Isolation of attenuated rubella-vaccine virus from human products of conception and uterine cervix. New Eng. J. Med. 286:1071–1074, 1972.

Veale, H.: History of an epidemic of Rötheln, with observation on its pathology. Edin. Med. J. 12:404–414, 1866.

Weibel, R. E., Stokes, J., Jr., Buynak, E. B., and Hilleman, M. R.: Rubella vaccination in adult females. New Eng. J. Med. 280:682–685, 1969.

Weil, M. L., Itabashi, H. H., Cremer, N. E., Oshiro, L. S., Lennette, E. H., and Carnay, L.: Chronic progressive panencephalitis due to rubella virus simulating subacute sclerosing panencephalitis. New Eng. J. Med. 292:994–998, 1975.

Weller, T. H., and Neva, F. A.: Propagation in tissue culture of cytopathic agents from patients with rubella-like illness. Proc. Soc. Exp. Biol. Med. 111:215–225, 1962.

White, L. R., Leikin, S., Vallavicenco, O., Abernathy, W., Avery, G., and Sever, J. L.: Immune competence in congenital rubella? Lymphocyte transformation, delayed hypersensitivity, and response to vaccination. J. Pediat. 73:229–234, 1968.

White, L. R., Sever, J. L., and Alepa, F. P.: Maternal and congenital rubella before 1964: Frequency, clinical features, and search for isoimmune phenomena. J. Pediat. 74:198–207, 1969.

Witte, J. J., Karchmer, A. W., Case, G., Herrmann, K. L., Abrutyn, E., Kassanoff, R., and Neill, J. S.: Epidemiology of rubella. Am. J. Dis. Child. 118:107–111, 1969.

Wolinsky, J. S., Berg, B. O., and Maitland, C. J.: Progressive rubella panencephalitis. Arch. Neurol. 33:722–723, 1976.

Wolman, S. R., McMorrow, L. E., Ziring, P. R., and Cooper, L. Z.: Lack of chromosomal breakage in congenital rubella. Pediatrics 52:213–220, 1973.

Wyll, S. A., and Grand, M. G.: Rubella in adolescents. Serologic assessment of immunity. J.A.M.A. 220:1573–1575, 1972.

Zimmerman, L. E.: The histopathologic basis for the ocular manifestations of the congenital rubella syndrome. Proceedings of the Institute of Medicine of Chicago, Vol. 26, No. 8, March, 1967.

Zinkham, W. H., Medearis, D. N., Jr., and Osborn, J. E.: Blood and bone-marrow findings in congenital rubella. J. Pediat. 71:512–524, 1967.

Ziring, P. R., Florman, A. L., and Cooper, L. Z.: The diagnosis of rubella. Pediat. Clin. N. Amer. 18:87–97, 1971.

Chapter Eighteen

CHRONIC VIRAL INFECTIONS OF THE CENTRAL NERVOUS SYSTEM

Research in the past two decades has resulted in the recognition that a group of chronic, progressive neurologic diseases of man are caused by viral agents (Gajdusek, Horta-Barbosa et al., Johnson and Gibbs, Weiner et al.). The terms chronic, latent, or slow virus infection have been applied to these conditions with the descriptive terms having reference to the tempo of the clinical illness rather than to the biological characteristics of the infecting organisms. To the present date, there is evidence strongly supporting a viral etiology of five chronic neurologic diseases of man and several that attack various animal species. Those involving man include kuru, Creutzfeldt-Jakob disease, progressive multifocal leukoencephalopathy, subacute sclerosing panencephalitis, and chronic rubella panencephalitis.

The infectious agents that cause these chronic conditions in humans and animals have been categorized as conventional and unconventional agents (Table 18–1). The conventional viruses have structural, chemical, and biological characteristics of classic, well-known viruses and are incriminated in the cause of subacute sclerosing panencephalitis, progressive rubella encephalitis, and progressive multifocal leukoencephalopathy in man, as well as visna and canine distemper in animals. The unconventional agents have not been isolated and are believed to exhibit

biological and physicochemical properties exceptional for any known infectious agent (ter Meulen and Hall). Viruses causing kuru and Creutzfeldt-Jakob disease in humans and scrapie and transmissible mink encephalopathy in animals are classified as unconventional agents. This group of disorders caused by the unconventional agents is collectively referred to as subacute spongiform encephalopathies, a term coined by Nevin et al. in 1960 because of histopathologic abnormalities common to them (Asher et al.).

Kuru is an exotic progressive disease with prominent cerebellar signs that occurs in natives in New Guinea and probably is transmitted by the habit of cannibalism practiced in that region. Its viral etiology has been doc-

Table 18–1. Chronic ("Slow") Virus Disorders of the Central Nervous System of Man and Animals—Infectious Agents

Conventional agents
  Subacute sclerosing panencephalitis
  Progressive rubella panencephalitis
  Progressive multifocal leukoencephalopathy
  Visna
  Canine distemper encephalomyelitis
Unconventional agents
  Kuru
  Creutzfeldt-Jakob disease
  Scrapie
  Transmissible mink encephalopathy

umented by its transmissibility to chimpanzees and to New World monkeys. Creutzfeldt-Jakob disease is also a progressive spongiform encephalopathy which has been transmitted from patient to chimpanzee, hamsters, and mice. It is manifested by progressive dementia, myoclonus, extrapyramidal signs, signs of anterior horn cell degeneration, and eventual death. In neither kuru nor Creutzfeldt-Jakob disease has a virus yet been isolated. Progressive multifocal leukoencephalopathy is a demyelinating condition in which the virus seems to attack oligodendroglia primarily and which occurs most often in adults with leukemia, Hodgkin's disease, or other debilitating illnesses. It begins insidiously and usually advances to death within a few months after onset. Evidence now exists that the disease is caused by members of the papova group of viruses. Subacute sclerosing panencephalitis is a disease primarily of childhood manifested by progressive intellectual deterioration, myoclonic seizures, characteristic electroencephalographic abnormalities, and death months or years after onset. The possible relationship of this disorder to the measles virus was suggested by Bouteille and colleagues in 1965 when they observed tubular structures within intranuclear inclusions, similar in morphology to the nucleocapsids of myxoviruses. Subsequent cultivation of the measles virus from the brain of affected patients confirmed these findings.

Following the discovery of a chronic progressive encephalitic disorder caused by the measles virus in children without clinically apparent immunologic disease, another variant form of measles encephalitis was identified in children with disease associated with immunologic dysfunction (Aicardi et al., Agamanolis et al., Breitfeld et al., Murphy and Yunis, Pullen et al.). This subacute, progressive form of measles encephalitis differs from acute measles encephalitis by the longer time interval of two to six months between the primary measles infection and the onset of neurologic signs, by its occurrence in patients immunosuppressed because of leukemia or renal transplantation, and by features primarily of a progressive, degenerative nature. It is different from the usual pattern observed with SSPE in the shorter period between the primary measles infection and onset of neurologic signs, its more rapid clinical course, the lack of consistent elevation of CSF measles antibody titer, and, again, its occurrence in the immunosuppressed patient. Subacute measles encephalitis in the immunosuppressed patient is characterized by progressive deterioration of mentation and the occurrence of seizures, most often in the form of segmental myoclonus or epilepsia partialis continua. Death occurs within several weeks after onset in most and the neuropathology includes eosinophilic inclusions in neurons and glial cells, giant cells, but not the extensive neuronal damage seen with subacute sclerosing panencephalitis. Ultrastructural studies reveal tubular aggregates consistent with myxovirus infection and confirmed by immunofluorescence (Pollan et al., Wolinsky et al.).

Echo virus has also now been associated with an atypical form of subacute progressive encephalitis in patients with immunodeficiency disease (Bardelas et al., Bodensteiner et al., Wilfert et al.). Patients with this disorder frequently have a dermatomyositis-like syndrome associated with a progressive, deteriorative encephalopathy but with few clinical inflammatory signs. The CSF reveals a lymphocytic pleocytosis and Echo virus can usually be recovered from the CSF. In addition, chronic, progressive central nervous system disease has been described in immunosuppressed children following poliovirus vaccination (Davis et al.).

These atypical, progressive encephalitic disorders in clinically immunosuppressed children have definite similarities to the chronic encephalitic conditions in clinically normal individuals and represent a link with the latter. Their occurrence adds information to the concept that some of the "slow" virus infections of the nervous system are dependent on some alteration of the host's immune mechanism to what in most instances are common viruses and are thereby manifested in atypical fashion.

Although "slow" virus infections of the nervous system are not common, the discovery of a viral cause has stimulated renewed interest in the possibility that other chronic neurologic disorders, such as multiple sclerosis, amyotrophic lateral sclerosis, and paralysis agitans, might also be viral-induced. Multiple sclerosis appears especially likely to be a disease with chronic viral persistence in view of epidemiologic, serologic, and virologic investigations. Epidemiologic studies have shown that persons migrating from high-risk to low-risk areas after adolescence retain a higher risk of developing the disease, while those that move from low-risk to high-risk regions retain a lower risk (Kurtzke et al.). This risk pattern is consistent with exposure to an infectious agent in the childhood years.

Several different viruses have been proposed as the possible offender in multiple sclerosis, with greatest attention being directed toward paramyxoviruses and vaccinia virus because of abnormal antibody responses to these viruses in patients with this disease (Adams and Imagawa, Clarke et al., Miyamoto et al., Sever et al., Thompson et al., Weiner et al.). In addition, paramyxovirus-like nucleocapsids have been observed within brain tissue by electron microscopy (Prineas, Raine et al., Tanaka et al.), and, with cell fusion techniques, a paramyxovirus has been isolated from brain tissue of multiple sclerosis patients (ter Meulen et al.). While the etiology of multiple sclerosis remains unproven, a viral cause now appears to be the most likely possibility. If it is established to be a chronic viral infection, the mechanism by which the virus produces demyelination will still be unexplained.

That viruses might affect the human brain in a fashion leading to chronic and progressive neurologic dysfunction has come as no surprise since chronic, deteriorative neurologic disease caused by viruses in animals had been identified long ago. After several years of experience with chronic viral infections of sheep, Sigurdsson, in 1954, defined slow virus infection as one in which the agent continues to multiply and produces progressive abnormality over a period of months or years, usually with localization of the infection to a single organ system, and in most instances with a very prolonged incubation period. The best known chronic viral neurologic infections of animals include visna, scrapie, and transmissible mink encephalopathy.

Visna is a chronic, afebrile, demyelinating disease of sheep first observed in Iceland in 1935. It is caused by an enveloped RNA virus characterized as a conventional agent and can be transmitted from sheep to sheep by intracerebral inoculation of brain tissue from a diseased animal (Sigurdsson et al.). Following an incubation period of months to years after intracerebral inoculation, the animal develops weakness which progresses to eventual quadriplegia and subsequent death. Unlike most other chronic viral infections, a marked lymphocytic pleocytosis and increase in the protein content of the cerebrospinal fluid occurs long before onset of the neurologic signs (Griffin et al., Nathanson et al.). During this period of incubation, virus can be isolated from brain or cerebrospinal fluid and complement-fixing antibodies can be found in serum and cerebrospinal fluid. This clinically silent meningoencephalitis persists for several weeks or months and is followed by a prolonged latent period during which the virus can be recovered by cocultivation from leukocytes in the peripheral blood (Griffin). The cerebral pathology consists of meningeal and perivascular inflammation, in addition to focal areas of myelin destruction (Sigurdsson et al.). Similar changes are seen in the brain stem and spinal cord.

Scrapie is a slowly progressive neurologic disease of sheep and goats which is one of the four subacute transmissible spongiform encephalopathies caused by unconventional agents. It is manifested by incoordination of gait, scraping and rubbing against fixed objects, hyperexcitability, and tremulousness. The disease was first transmitted to healthy sheep in 1936 by inoculation of brain tissue of affected animals (Cuillé and Chelle) and is characterized by a prolonged incubation period followed by an afebrile symptomatic phase lasting up to a year. The scrapie agent, which is resistant to heat, formalin and irradiation, has not yet been isolated, although particles believed to be related to the virus have been observed in dilated post-synaptic processes of scrapie-infected brain by electron microscopy (Baringer and Prusiner). A most interesting aspect of the natural disease is its apparent hereditary predisposition, despite its transmissibility by intracerebral inoculation (Beck et al. 1964). The pathology of scrapie is remarkable because of the absence of inflammation, a prominent astrocytic gliosis, and the presence of vacuolated nerve cells and astrocytes, resulting in a spongiform appearance, especially in the pons and medulla (Palmer), within which have been seen accumulations of virus-like particles (Bignami and Parry).

Transmissible mink encephalopathy is a progressive, fatal spongiform encephalopathy first identified in mink in Wisconsin and subsequently in Idaho and elsewhere. The disorder has many similarities to scrapie and it is possible that both are caused by the same agent (Kimberlin and Marsh, Marsh and Kimberlin). Inoculation of mink with the scrapie agent results in a disease identical to transmissible mink encephalopathy (Hanson et al.). Transmissible mink encephalopathy is characterized by an incubation period extending up to a year followed by a clinical illness with ataxia, excitability, convulsions, and eventual coma, leading to death within a few months after onset of neurologic signs.

It can be transmitted from mink to mink and also from mink to squirrel monkey by inoculation of brain tissue of the infected animal (Eckroade et al., Grabow et al.). The pathology of the disease is limited to the central nervous system and consists of diffuse vacuolation of the gray matter, widespread neuronal degeneration, and extensive astrocytosis.

Kuru

Kuru is a subacute, progressive neurologic disease of the Fore people of the Eastern Highlands of New Guinea. The term kuru in Fore language means "trembling with fear," a characteristic sign almost always observed during the progression of the illness. The disease was introduced to the medical community in 1957 by Gajdusek and Zigas and subsequently was identified to be the first chronic degenerative disease affecting the human brain with an established viral etiology and transmissibility. Early studies by Gajdusek and Zigas and others (Hornabrock, Neumann et al.) revealed the disease to be most prevalent among adult women and children of either sex. The onset is characteristically insidious and, in most cases, death occurs within a year after the first symptoms appear.

Observers of patients with kuru have described the remarkably constant manner in which symptoms and signs appear and evolve. Gajdusek (1967) eloquently wrote about the manner in which affected natives recognized their own slight tremulousness or shivering and very minimal disturbance of balance before such signs could be detected even by an experienced examiner. A remarkable early sign was mentioned by Hornabrock who noted that the normal even rhythm of the thigh-length beaten bark skirts of the women while walking would reveal very slight disturbances of rhythm, thus betraying the earliest sign of gait incoordination. Trivial symptoms, once developed, often persist for months with little change, but eventually a conspicous disturbance of gait becomes evident. Staggering and lurching, in association with tremulousness of the hands and facial musculature, are accompanied by slurred speech and intermittent headache. Strabismus develops in some children with the disease, but nystagmus is unusual. Mentation and alertness remain unaffected until the late stages when progressive dementia supervenes. By this stage of the illness, the individual has usually completely lost ability to ambulate, is often hypotonic but hyperreflexic, and exhibits a pattern of lethargy or agitation. In general, the symptoms and signs from onset until near the terminal stages of the disease are those of cerebellar dysfunction, with or without brain stem abnormalities.

The pathology of kuru is limited to the central nervous system and consists of diffuse neuronal degeneration, microglial proliferation, hypertrophy of astrocytes throughout the brain, status spongiosus of the cerebral cortex and basal ganglia, and minimal to mild demyelination. With special stains, round, homogeneously stained plaques are usually abundant throughout the brain (Kakulas et al., Neumann et al.).

Although the possibility that kuru might be an infectious illness was entertained from the time of the initial investigations, the absence of cells in the cerebrospinal fluid and the lack of significant perivascular cuffing or other inflammatory changes in the brain seemed to weigh heavily against this type of etiology. The eventual demonstration of transmissibility of the disease to chimpanzees and then to spider monkeys secured the illness among the chronic viral infectious diseases of the nervous system (Beck et al. 1966, 1973, Gajdusek and Gibbs, Lampert et al.). As in the natural disease, the principal lesions in experimental kuru are found in the cerebral cortex, the caudate and putamen, the hypothalamus, and the cerebellum (Beck et al. 1975). A virus has not yet been isolated and serum antibody titer rises have not been demonstrated.

The mechanism of natural spread of the virus among the Fore people is a fascinating chapter of the story of this exotic disease. Various theories that were proposed seemed unlikely to adequately explain the predisposition of young women and children until attention was directed to the ritualistic custom of cannibalism commonly practiced by the natives in the endemic area. This habit of consumption of flesh of their kinsmen after death apparently was primarily a gesture of respect for the departed. When it was recognized that cannibalism was practiced almost entirely by women and children and only rarely by adult males, the probable mode of transmission of the infecting agent became obvious. Clinical disease is now believed to ensue between four and 20 years after ingestion of virus-laden human tissue and is rarely seen in the male because of his distaste for cannibalistic habits (Mathews et al. 1968). With the decline in cannibalism in the early 1950's, kuru subsequently declined in frequency and has continued to do so to the present time. The disease is not currently occurring in children in New Guinea (Gajdusek et al. 1970, King 1975), and perhaps will disappear entirely.

Creutzfeldt-Jakob Disease

In 1920, Creutzfeldt of Berlin described an unusual type of neurologic disorder associated with progressive dementia. The following year his countryman Alfons Jakob published the first of a series of reports of a similar disorder, which thereafter became known as Creutzfeldt-Jakob disease. For several decades, the condition was shelved in the ill-defined category of the presenile dementias, along with Alzheimer's and Pick's disease. The puzzling combination of dementia, long tract signs, and extrapyramidal signs allowed its clinical separation from these latter disorders, as did the pathology, which departed primarily because of the absence of certain characteristic features present with the other, better known forms of presenile dementia. Authors doubted the justification for the existence of Creutzfeldt-Jakob disease as a distinct entity and the result was the development of a variety of subclassifications and many synonyms for the disease, the best known being spastic pseudosclerosis and corticostriatal-spinal degeneration. The so-called Heidenhain variant of Creutzfeldt-Jakob disease is characterized by the early onset of cortical visual loss in association with progressive dementia and eventually with other signs.

The appropriate position of Creutzfeldt-Jakob disease among progressive neurologic diseases remained unsettled until 1968 when Gibbs and coworkers were successful in transmitting the disease to the chimpanzee, thus demonstrating that it is caused by a transmissible, although unconventional, agent. Creutzfeldt-Jakob disease is now categorized among the transmissible subacute spongiform encephalopathies, along with kuru, scrapie, and transmissible mink encephalopathy. Evidence now supports the concept that it is a subacute viral encephalopathy, although little is known about the biological characteristics of the infecting agent. The natural mechanism of spread and the reservoir of the Creutzfeldt-Jakob disease infectious agent remain unknown. Iatrogenic transmission of the disease has been documented in one case via a transplanted, infected cornea (Duffy et al. 1974), and in two others secondary to the use of electrodes contaminated by their implantation in a patient with the disease (Bernoulli et al.).

Creutzfeldt-Jakob disease is an uncommon progressive dementing disease of adults of either sex, predominantly occurring in the fifth and sixth decades of life. The youngest reported cases have been persons in the early twenties (Creutzfeldt, Stender) but onset under age 40 years is considered unusual. The disease has been identified in many parts of the world, and the majority of cases have developed in sporadic fashion although familial cases have on rare occasions been recognized (Jakob et al. 1950, May et al.). The familial occurrence of Creutzfeldt-Jakob disease (Galvez et al.) as well as the familial clustering of cases among Libyan-born Israelis (Neugut et al.) has suggested the possibility of a genetically determined predisposition to develop the disease. There appear to be no predisposing or clinically apparent immunologic compromising factors related to the onset of this disorder. The usual duration of the disease from onset of symptoms to death varies from one to 15 months and occasionally can be somewhat longer. The average length of the illness in the series reviewed by Roos et al. was just over seven months and in that of Galvez was 6.3 months. The annual incidence of Creutzfeldt-Jakob disease on the basis of deaths per million people has been found to be 0.26 per million in the United States (Masters et al. 1978) and 0.31 per million in Chile (Galvez et al.). The average annual incidence in Paris has been calculated to be 1.1 cases per million people (Brown and Cathala). The most striking departure from these approximately similar figures is among Jewish immigrants from Libya, in whom the incidence has been estimated to be 31.3 per million (Kahana et al.).

The onset of symptoms is insidious in the majority of cases and frequently begins with fatigue, feelings of depression, and weight loss, symptoms recognized to be the forerunner of the more specific neurologic abnormalities only in retrospect (Brown et al.). Mental abnormalities are the common first definite signs of the disease and include disturbances of memory, impairment of judgment, behavior and personality alterations, or more specific deficits of higher cortical function. Self-neglect, apathy, and mood swings in the early stages sometimes lead observers to consideration of a primary psychiatric disorder until other neurologic signs become manifest. Disturbances of coordination are common early features of Creutzfeldt-Jakob disease, and, in some patients, progressive cerebellar ataxia is the first observed neurologic deficit (Gomori et al.), even preceding dementia.

Within weeks or a few months after onset, long tract signs, such as hyperreflexia, clonus, and pathologic reflexes, are added to signs of extrapyramidal dysfunction. The degree of basal ganglia involvement varies from patient to patient but may include cog-wheel rigidity, bradykinesia with loss of facial expression, tremor, or other dyskinesias of variable type. Myoclonus, often provoked by sensory stimuli, is a common part of the evolution of the disease while generalized convulsions are observed less frequently. Some patients eventually show evidence of anterior horn cell degeneration, manifested by fasciculations, weakness, and atrophy. Rarely, these findings will be the presenting feature of the illness, thus resembling motor neuron disease until the other characteristic features become apparent (Allen et al.).

Visual disturbances, paresthesias, hallucinations, dysarthria, and various other neurologic signs are noted in some as the illness proceeds to its terminal stage. Total incapacitation from the mental and motor standpoint is eventually reached, by which time disability is profound and death soon follows. Thus, the typical picture of Creutzfeldt-Jakob disease includes the gradual onset of disturbances of mentation in a patient between 40 and 60 years of age, followed by progressive deterioration with the development of signs of spasticity, extrapyramidal signs, and myoclonus. Amyotrophy is occasionally observed as the disease proceeds relentlessly to death six to eight months after onset.

The cerebrospinal fluid in most cases is normal or reveals only a mild elevation in the protein content. The electroencephalogram is consistently abnormal and generally shows progressive worsening coinciding with the clinical course. During the initial clinical stage of the illness, normal rhythms are gradually replaced by diffuse slow theta and delta activity and occasionally with periodic bursts. In the fully developed stage of the disease, periodic discharges consisting of diffuse high voltage biphasic or triphasic bursts with spike and slow activity are commonly present. Chiofalo et al. found periodic bursts in 25 of 27 patients with Creutzfeldt-Jakob disease and noted that the duration of the periodic complexes ranged from 200 to 600 milliseconds, with the duration of the intervals between the bursts always being less than 2.5 seconds. Periodic activity is usually intermittent when first developed but eventually may become continuous, a finding indicating that death will probably soon follow (Burger et al.).

As might be anticipated from the character of the clinical signs, the pathology of Creutzfeldt-Jakob is widespread throughout the central nervous system (Beck et al. 1969, Gonatas et al. Katzman et al., Silberman et al.). The cerebral cortex is usually visibly atrophic and contains loss of nerve cells in all layers with considerable astrocytic proliferation, some of the gemistocytic type. Spongiform changes, especially of the deeper cortical layers, are a conspicuous microscopic finding in most cases, evident in the form of small, round or oval clear vacuoles in the neurophil (Fig. 18–1). Although the pathogenesis of this characteristic alteration remains unclear, the spongiform appearance has been found to be the result of distention within cell processes. Neuronal loss and astrocytic proliferation are also prominent in the caudate, the putamen, and certain thalamic nuclei. Atrophic cerebellar changes consist of loss of granule cells and usually dense fibrous gliosis throughout all layers of the cerebellar cortex. Despite the cortical changes, demyelination within the cerebrum or cerebellum remains slight in most cases. Brain stem and spinal cord abnormalities likewise are common. Masters and Richardson found that among patients with Creutzfeldt-Jakob disease who died less than five months after onset of symptoms, there were quantitatively more spongiform changes within the brain than neuronal loss or gliosis. In those with longer survival, the spongiform changes gradually decreased while neuronal depletion and gliosis became more prominent. Characteristically absent in Creutzfeldt-Jakob disease are senile plaques and neurofibrillary tangles, an important criterion distinguishing this condition from other presenile dementias, such as Alzheimer's disease. Astrocytic nuclear bodies of similar type have been observed in both Creutzfeldt-Jakob disease and in Alzheimer's disease by ultrastructural techniques (Grunnet). Argentophilic plaques are generally not considered typical in Creutzfeldt-Jakob disease but have been described on rare occasion (Hirano et al.).

Membership among the chronic viral infections of the nervous system was achieved by Creutzfeldt-Jakob disease in 1968 when its transmissibility to chimpanzees was demonstrated by Gibbs and colleagues. The experiment has subsequently been reproduced (Gibbs and Gajdusek, Lampert et al.) and more recently the disease has been transmit-

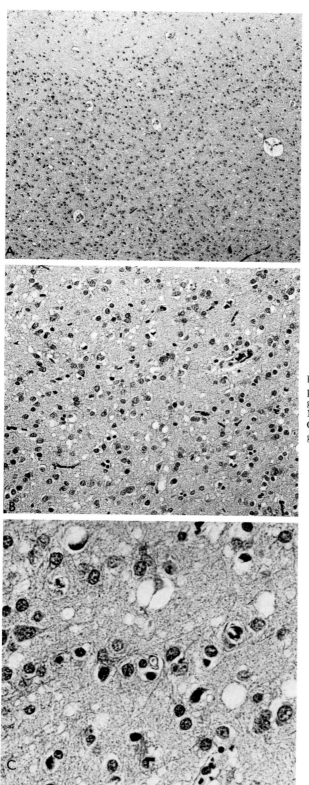

Figure 18–1. Creutzfeldt-Jakob disease. *A,* Cerebral cortex, trichrome, 80×. There is neuronal depletion and marked gliosis with relatively mild spongiform change. *B,* Cerebral cortex, trichrome, 200×. Neuronal loss, gliosis, and moderate vacuolization. *C,* Cerebral cortex, trichrome, 500×. Gliosis with spongiform appearance.

ted to New World monkeys (Zlotnik et al.), to hamsters (Manuelidis et al. 1977), and to mice (Manuelidis et al. 1978), with the result being that the infected animals develop a progressive neurologic disorder after a prolonged incubation period. Transmission of Creutzfeldt-Jakob disease to mice results in a scrapie-like syndrome in the infected rodents with histopathologic findings which resemble those of mice infected with the scrapie agent (Manuelidis et al. 1978). The significance of this observation remains unclear but suggests that the two agents may be identical.

The pathology of the experimentally transmitted disease in monkeys, as in man, is primarily one with spongiform changes of the cortical gray matter and neuronal loss and gliosis mainly of the cerebral cortex and basal ganglia. Masters et al. (1976) observed that microscopic lesions were present in the brain of experimentally infected monkeys soon after inoculation and long before there was evidence of clinically detectable disease. Although virus-like particles have been observed in brain tissue of patients with Creutzfeldt-Jakob disease (Bots et al., Vernon et al.), the virus yet remains to be isolated and identified.

The documentation of iatrogenic transmission of Creutzfeldt-Jakob disease has brought about considerable concern among medical and laboratory workers about the possible hazard that might be associated with patient care, diagnostic tests requiring needle electrodes, surgical procedures, and postmortem examinations. Manuelidis et al. (1978) have demonstrated that there is a viremic stage in experimental Creutzfeldt-Jakob disease, suggesting that it might be possible to transmit the illness by blood transfusion. In addition to the infectiousness of multiple visceral organs and possibly of blood, it is also believed that CSF contains the virus and could be infectious under certain circumstances (Gajdusek et al. 1977). In the cases reported by Bernoulli et al. (1977), the disease was transmitted to two young adults who underwent surgical removal of epileptogenic foci after the intracerebral implantation of silver electrodes which had, more than two years previously, been implanted in a patient subsequently proven to have Creutzfeldt-Jakob disease. The electrodes had been sterilized with 70 percent alcohol and formaldehyde vapor following their use in the original demented patient but this had failed to inactivate the infectious agent. The report by

Duffy et al. demonstrated that the disease could be transmitted person-to-person by transplantation of a cornea from an infected donor, an event documented experimentally in guinea pigs by Manuelidis et al. (1977).

As a result of these observations and because it is known that the infectious agent resists inactivation by boiling in water and by exposure to 10 percent formalin, 70 percent alcohol, and ionizing and ultraviolet radiation, Gajdusek et al. (1977) and Baringer et al. (1980) have proposed guidelines for management of patients with progressive, dementing disease and for the handling of their tissues. Patients with dementing illness should not be used for blood or tissue donors, and instruments or electrodes used on such patients for electroencephalography, electromyography, or during surgical procedures should be autoclaved for one hour at 121°C and 20 psi, which will inactivate the agent. The virus can also be inactivated with 5 percent hypochlorite or 0.03 percent permanganate. The additional precautions that should be taken with patients who have or might have Creutzfeldt-Jakob disease are elaborated in detail in the publication by Gajdusek and colleagues (1977).

Progressive Multifocal Leukoencephalopathy

Progressive multifocal leukoencephalopathy (PML) is a rare subacute demyelinating disease of the brain first described by Aström and colleagues in 1958. The disorder occurs primarily in adults with Hodgkin's disease and chronic lymphocytic leukemia but has also been observed in association with other malignancies, sarcoidosis, tuberculosis, and a variety of other chronic illnesses treated with immunosuppressive agents (Lyon et al., Richardson 1974, Sponzilli et al.). A few cases have been observed in renal transplant recipients (McCormick et al., ZuRhein and Varakis). Although the disease has generally been regarded to be one confined to the adult age group, it has been identified in an 11-year-old boy with severe combined immunodeficiency (ZuRhein et al. 1978). Because of the decided predilection for progressive multifocal leukoencephalopathy to occur in immunosuppressed individuals, it is no surprise that occasional instances are found in which the disease is simultaneously associated with

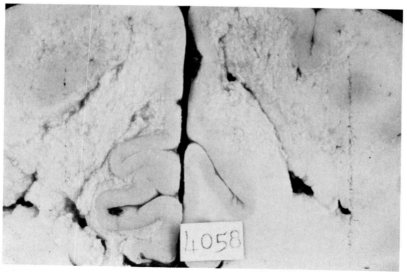

A

Figure 18–2. Progressive multifocal leukoencephalopathy. *A,* Coronal section of the brain showing widespread demyelinating lesions bilaterally, extending to the cortical margin. *B,* Giant bizarre astrocytes, one (large cell at the top) containing type B inclusions.

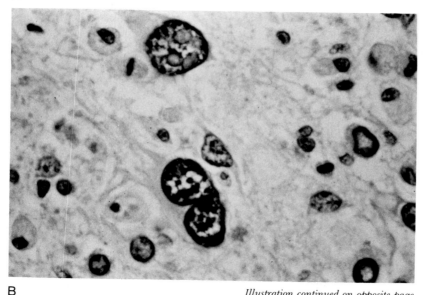

B

Illustration continued on opposite page

infection caused by other opportunistic infectious agents (Malas and Weiss, Mathew et al. 1976, McCormick et al.). Progressive multifocal leukoencephalopathy on rare occasion has occurred in healthy persons (Bolton and Rozdilsky, Faris and Martinez, Fermaglich et al.). The clinical course of the disease is usually fairly rapid, with death occurring one to six months after onset of neurologic symptoms in most cases. Variations can occur, as exemplified by the case described by Hedley-Whyte et al., in which the symptoms of the illness persisted for five years.

The clinical pattern is generally a progressive one after onset of neurologic manifestations, but the course is often punctuated by the abrupt appearance of certain abnormalities. The symptoms and signs reflect the diffuseness of cerebral, cerebellar, and brain stem involvement as well as the multifocal and usually asymmetric character of the pathology (Richardson, Sibley and Weisberger, Woolsey and Nelson). Impairment of memory, confusion, and disorientation are common early signs, which gradually progress to severe dementia. Hemiparesis is another frequent early finding. Long tract signs, initially evident on one side of the body, eventually are present bilaterally. Visual disturbances develop during progression of the disorder in many patients, sometimes leading to complete blindness. Cerebellar deficits, brain stem signs, and seizures are occasionally described, depending on the distribution of the lesions. The spinal cord can be involved pathologically, but clinical signs of spinal cord dysfunction are rare.

The disease causes neurologic dysfunction that is obvious to the examiner, but the multiplicity of signs appearing in progressive fashion is diagnostically confusing. The case described by Mancall was exceptional in this respect in that the patient was essentially asymptomatic from the neurologic standpoint except for a single convulsion a few days prior to death. The cerebrospinal fluid is normal in many patients with progressive multifocal leukoencephalopathy, but a modest lymphocytic pleocytosis can occur and the protein content can be mildly increased. Although the diagnosis is sometimes suspected clinically, it can be confirmed only by pathological examination of brain tissue, obtained either by brain biopsy or at postmortem examination. The combination of the gross and microscopic findings is highly characteristic and not produced by any other disease yet identified.

Cranial computed tomography adds another dimension which can increase the degree of suspicion of the possibility of progressive multifocal leukoencephalopathy, although the abnormalities demonstrated by this technique are not specific for this disorder. Microscopic foci of demyelination would not be demonstrable by computed tomography but large lesions result in low density areas in white matter which do not enhance and do not exhibit a mass effect (Carroll et al.). With progression of the disease, the hypodense areas are expected to become somewhat larger in size and may coincide with some degree of ventricular enlargement. Radionuclide scans are normal in most patients with progressive multifocal leukoencephalopathy although rare exceptions have been described (Mathews et al. 1976, Mosher et al.).

The pathology of progressive multifocal leukoencephalopathy is most striking in the cerebral hemispheres and to a lesser degree in the cerebellum and brain stem. It consists of disseminated foci of demyelination with relative preservation of axis cylinders. Many foci are solitary and of variable size, while others appear to have enlarged and coalesced with adjacent areas of demyelination. Microscopically, oligodendroglia are depleted in the center of the focus of demyelination but those at the periphery show nuclear enlargement, some with eosinophilic intranuclear inclusions. Alterations of astrocytes are less constant but a variety of changes occur. Some become bizarre, gigantic forms with multiple nuclei and even atypical mitotic figures, resembling neoplastic "transformation" (Fig. 18–2). Inclusion bodies can sometimes be observed in astrocytes and less often in neurons.

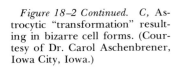

Figure 18–2 Continued. C, Astrocytic "transformation" resulting in bizarre cell forms. (Courtesy of Dr. Carol Aschenbrener, Iowa City, Iowa.)

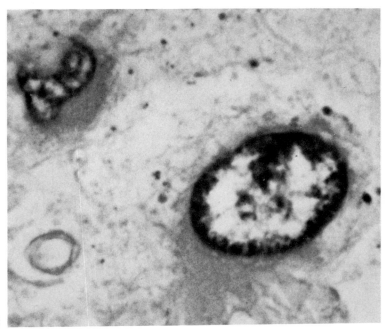

C

Intranuclear inclusions have also been found in renal tubular cells (Martin and Banker). Inflammation is usually minimal or absent in the brain.

It is generally believed that the primary insult in this disease is upon the oligodendroglia, whose destruction is followed by patchy demyelination without axonal dissolution. The bizarre astrocytic alterations are assumed to represent a secondary response, although the character of the astrocytic changes has provoked considerable interest because of the neuro-oncogenicity in animals of certain of the papovaviruses. Intracerebral inoculation of hamsters with the JC virus almost consistently results in malignant brain tumors (Padgett et al. 1977). These observations have raised the question and have provoked investigation of the possible role of the papovaviruses in human brain tumors (Greenlee et al., Meinke et al.).

That progressive multifocal leukoencephalopathy might be a viral-induced disease occurring in persons with relative immunologic unresponsiveness was suggested by Cavanagh and colleagues in 1959 and again by Richardson in 1961. The evidence of immunologic abnormalities in patients with progressive multifocal leukoencephalopathy has largely been on the basis of its occurrence with neoplastic or other disorders known to be associated with immunosuppression. Ellison did demonstrate immunologic hyporeactivity of the delayed type in a patient with progressive multifocal leukoencephalopathy, and, more recently, Knight et al. have described the condition in a 22-year-old man without neoplastic disease but with chronic deficiencies of both humoral and cell-mediated immunity.

The presence of intranuclear inclusions suggested to many workers a possible viral cause, and in 1965 ZuRhein and Chou and, independently, Silverman and Rubinstein were able to demonstrate with ultrastructural techniques the presence of virus-like particles within inclusions in oligodendroglia. These particles were believed to belong to the deoxyribonucleic acid–containing papovaviruses, and because of their morphology, to the polyoma subgroup of papovaviruses called Simian virus 40 (SV40). Up to that time, papovaviruses were not known to be pathogenic for man except for the production of warts by the human papilloma virus, although papovaviruses had been recognized to have oncogenic properties in animals.

In 1971, Padgett et al. successfully isolated an agent from the brain of a patient with progressive multifocal leukoencephalopathy that was felt to be a new papovavirus, one termed the JC virus, so labeled after the initials of the patient from whom it was isolated. The same virus was retrieved by Weiner et al. (1973) and subsequently has been found to be the offender in the great majority of cases of progressive multifocal leukoencephalopathy (Narayan et al.). The JC virus has been found to be prevalent among the population, with a high rate of acquisition in the childhood years. By middle age, 70 to 75 percent of the population possess antibody against this virus (Padgett and Walker 1973). The properties of this and other papovaviruses have been reviewed by Padgett and Walker (1976). An SV40 virus of the polyoma virus subgroup of the papovaviruses also has been cultivated from diseased human brain tissue by Weiner et al. (1972). A third papovavirus, the BK virus, has been isolated from the urine of a renal allograft patient but has not been implicated as a cause of progressive multifocal leukoencephalopathy (Gardner et al.).

Of interest also is the recent finding by Coleman et al. that, of 74 renal allograft recipients, 10 were found to be excreting polyomavirus in the urine. Hogan et al. (1980) studied 61 immunosuppressed renal transplant patients and found 11 to be excreting JC virus and 9 excreting BK virus in the urine. While none of the patients in their series developed progressive multifocal leukoencephalopathy, there was a higher incidence of transplant-related complications associated with polyomavirus replication, suggesting a wider range of pathogenicity of these viruses than is generally recognized.

To the present time, progressive multifocal leukoencephalopathy is the only demyelinating disease of man in which a viral infection primarily affecting oligodendroglia has been documented. It is not yet known whether the causative papovaviruses represent latent particles in the brain that have become activated or are viruses normally nonpathogenic that gain entrance to and produce infection in a compromised host. Marriot et al. reported remission of the illness following treatment with cytosine arabinoside, although other reports describe lack of significant effect of transfer factor, cytosine arabinoside (Van Horn et al.), or adenine arabinoside (Rand et al.).

Subacute Sclerosing Panencephalitis

In 1933 and again in 1934, Dawson described a type of chronic, progressive encephalitis in children in which he observed the presence of intranuclear and, less often, intracytoplasmic inclusion bodies similar to those associated with certain other viral infections. Because of the presence of inclusions, he suggested the possibility of a viral cause for the illness, but efforts to recover an infectious agent were unsuccessful. Thereafter, the disease became known as Dawson's subacute inclusion body encephalitis. Pette and Doring later published similar cases and the term nodular panencephalitis of Pette and Doring became popular for a period of time. In 1945, van Bogaert drew attention to a disorder he considered to be similar but emphasized the predominant involvement of the cerebral white matter in his cases and referred to the condition as subacute sclerosing leukoencephalitis. With continued clinical and pathological observations, it became evident that the different descriptions had reference to a single entity, now known as subacute sclerosing panencephalitis, the name proposed by Greenfield in 1950.

As more reports became available, the scope of the clinical pattern of the disease gradually emerged but its categorization among other progressive brain diseases in children remained unclear. Its true character began to unfold in 1965 when Bouteille and workers with the electron microscope demonstrated nucleocapsids resembling those of the paramyxovirus group in the brain of patients with subacute sclerosing panencephalitis, a discovery soon duplicated by other workers (Freeman et al., Dayan et al., Shaw et al., Tellez-Nagel and Harter). Two years later, Connolly et al. reported the presence of elevated titers of measles (rubeola) antibody in serum and cerebrospinal fluid of children with the disease, a finding subsequently verified many times. Measles antigen was demonstrated in the cerebral cortex by immunofluorescence (Connolly et al., Lennette et al.) and finally, in 1969, several groups of investigators in different laboratories succeeded in cultivating measles virus or a measles-like virus from brain tissue of patients with subacute sclerosing panencephalitis (Chen et al., Horta-Barbosa, Payne et al., ter Meulen et al.). Demonstration of transmissibility of the infection to animals (Katz et al., Lehrich et al.) established a relationship between subacute sclerosing panencephalitis and a virus which is or is very much like the measles virus. The SSPE-infectious agent has now been transmitted from human brain tissue to ferrets (Katz et al.), hamsters (Lehrich et al.), and dogs (Notermans et al.), as well as to calves and lambs (Thein). The experimentally transmitted illness is an encephalitic disorder with a prolonged incubation period, and, interestingly enough, the afflicted animals do not exhibit a rise in measles antibody as occurs in the human with subacute sclerosing panencephalitis.

Despite these remarkable advances in knowledge acquired over a relatively short period of time, complete understanding of all the mechanisms involved in the occurrence of this disease has not been achieved. Discoveries provoked new questions, and certain bits of information regarding pathogenesis have been variously interpreted. Some investigators proposed the theory that the disease results from random reactivation of an incomplete or mutant measles virus that has lain dormant in the brain for several years (Fields, Johnson). Others believed that other factors, perhaps genetic or environmental, may be involved, in part because of the occurrence, albeit infrequent, of familial cases of subacute sclerosing panencephalitis (Clark and Best, Kennedy, Lorand et al.). The most intriguing example of sibling occurrence was described by Ch'ien et al. of two brothers who had contracted classic rubeola at the same time and later developed subacute sclerosing panencephalitis simultaneously. Twin studies have been virtually nonexistent, with the exception of the report by Whitaker et al. in which only one of identical twins developed the illness. In a follow-up report of the same children seven years after the first report, the unaffected twin had remained healthy (Houff et al.).

Other postulates regarding etiology and pathogenesis of the disease arose from results of epidemiologic investigations (Brody and Detels, Detels et al., Jabbour et al. 1972). Such studies have shown that males acquire subacute sclerosing panencephalitis at a rate between three and four times that of females, and that children from rural communities are much more often affected than are those from urban areas. In addition, measles often occurs at an unusually early age in children who later develop subacute sclerosing panencephalitis. Studies of large numbers of patients with subacute sclerosing panencephalitis have demonstrated that, on the average, they are at least three years younger than controls when they experience natural measles. Approximately 45 to 50 percent are under two years of age and 25 percent are under one year when measles occurs, and the mean time period from the occurrence of natural measles until the onset of symptoms of subacute sclerosing panencephalitis is seven years (Modlin et al. 1977). Jabbour et al. (1972) found the average interval between natural measles infection and the onset of subacute sclerosing panencephalitis to be five years. Approximately 15 percent have no history of clinical measles, although household exposure has usually existed (Brody and Detels, Detels et al.).

As an explanation for these findings, Brody and Detels postulated that subacute sclerosing panencephalitis occurs among persons in whom there is an abnormal balance between the measles virus and the immune mechanism of the host, which allows viral persistence within brain cells following the natural infection. This might be initiated by the acquisition of the measles virus early in life, at a time when passive maternal antibody is still present, thus possibly accounting for the high incidence of inapparent infections. Because of the male predominance and the striking association of the disease with children from a rural environment, the authors also suggested that the eventual precipitating event in subacute sclerosing panencephalitis is an infection with an animal virus, perhaps a papova-like agent, which might act as a so-called helper virus. The possibility of a second virus which might activate a measles or measles-like virus or somehow collaborate with it to produce subacute sclerosing panencephalitis has received support by the observation of structures resembling papovaviruses within cytoplasm of brain cell cultures from patients with subacute sclerosing panencephalitis (Barbanti-Brodano et al., Koprowski et al., Müller et al.).

Subacute sclerosing panencephalitis has also been found to occur in patients coincident with an acute Epstein-Barr virus infection (Feorino et al., Hochberg et al.). In these unusual instances, the pathological changes have been characteristic of subacute sclerosing panencephalitis, and raised levels of measles antibody were identified in blood and CSF. The role played by the Epstein-Barr virus in these cases is uncertain but it is postulated that mononucleosis-associated transient immunosuppression may be responsible

for activation of latent measles virus in brain, resulting in the clinical syndrome.

Possible immunologic abnormalities or variations which might predispose one to the development of this condition have been widely discussed but remain unproven (Gerson and Haslam, Jabbour et al. 1969, Kolar, Lennette et al., Saunders et al.). Blocking factors against the cellular immune response have been found in the sera of some patients with subacute sclerosing panencephalitis, although the nature and significance of these factors has not been clarified (Steele et al., Swick et al.). Most children who acquire the disease have been clinically previously normal. Since 1969, the incidence of subacute sclerosing panencephalitis in the United States has substantially declined as a result of a decrease in the occurrence of natural measles secondary to the use of measles vaccine (Modlin et al. 1977). The illness has been found in children who had received measles vaccine and without a history of natural measles, but the risk following vaccine is believed to be much lower than the risk after the natural infection (Baguley and Glasgow, Parker et al., Schneck). Modlin et al. (1977) found the risk of development of subacute sclerosing panencephalitis following measles vaccination to be 0.5 to 1.1 cases per million while the risk following natural measles is 5.2 to 9.7 cases per million cases of measles.

Thus, our present state of knowledge allows us to accept subacute sclerosing panencephalitis as a subacute or chronic viral infection of the brain in which measles (rubeola) or a measles-like virus is implicated in the pathogenesis. Other factors—genetic, immunologic, or environmental—or second viruses probably are prerequisites for the development of the disease but clarification awaits continued research.

Clinical Manifestations

Subacute sclerosing panencephalitis is a world-wide disease which affects children in the majority of instances. In the United States, the greatest concentration of cases has been found in the southeastern and central parts of the country. The age range in most series is between two and 20 years with the mean affected age being nine years. Of the 453 cases reviewed by Modlin et al. (1979) 85 percent of patients had the onset of the illness between five and 14 years of age. Exceptional cases proposed to be subacute sclerosing panencephalitis in infancy include the child reported by Dayan and Cumings with onset of disease at two months and death at five months of age, and the infant described by Bhettay et al. with onset of convulsions at eight months and death at 10 months of age. At the other end of the spectrum is the patient reported by Cape et al. in whom symptoms first appeared at 32 years of age. Most children have had previously uncomplicated measles, only remarkable because of the generally earlier occurrence than is customary.

The common pattern of the illness is a fairly steady progressive one with a duration from onset to death of six to 24 months. Variations are not infrequent, however, and some cases follow a rapid and fulminating course leading to death only weeks after onset. Gilden et al. described two patients with subacute sclerosing panencephalitis in whom the clinical course was unusually short from onset to death. In the first, the patient became comatose nine days after onset of neurologic symptoms and died one month later. The second child went into coma 13 days after onset, with death occurring one month after the first symptoms were observed. Others gradually progress in the usual fashion but then assume a stable pattern or even show spontaneous improvement for a period of

time (Resnick et al.) (Fig. 18–3). Of 118 patients with subacute sclerosing panencephalitis in the Middle East, Risk et al. (1978) described spontaneous long-term improvement in six (5 percent). The extent of recovery of function in these children was substantial in that they went from a bedridden condition to the ability to ambulate and care for their own basic needs. The possibility of a prolonged existence with apparent stability is more often seen in the later stages of the disease, after advanced mental and motor disability has been reached. On rare occasion, the patient may linger for as long as eight years before death intervenes (Landau and Luse).

The clinical course of subacute sclerosing panencephalitis has been divided into three stages by many authors (Freeman) and into four stages by some (Jabbour et al. 1969), although the manifestations should be thought of as a continuum, with variations that are considerable. The first symptoms of the disease in many cases are subtle changes of intellectual function, behavior, or personality. The teacher may notice decline of academic achievement or disinterest in school activities. Forgetfulness, distractibility, temper outbursts, or recurrent night terrors are sometimes initially regarded to be emotional in

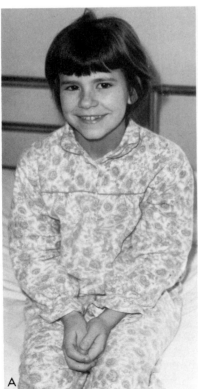
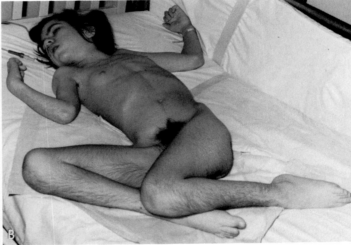

Figure 18–3. Subacute sclerosing panencephalitis. *A,* Eight-year-old girl with a 2-month history of memory loss and gradual decline in school performance. Nightmares, crying spells, and myoclonic seizures began 4 to 6 weeks after onset. Physical examination at this time was unremarkable except for mild mental confusion and other signs of dementia. The diagnosis was established on the basis of blood and CSF measles (rubeola) antibody titers, and characteristic electroencephalographic abnormality. The illness was gradually progressive and within 1 year after onset the child could no longer ambulate or communicate verbally. Her extremities became spastic, and myoclonic seizures occurred frequently in repetitive fashion. *B,* At 11 years of age, she exhibited a spastic quadriparesis with distal muscle atrophy, and was unresponsive to most forms of stimulation. She was last seen at 17 years of age and remains essentially unchanged.

origin until other signs appear. Although most affected children have been assumed to be normal prior to onset, Pettay and colleagues were impressed with the high frequency of long-standing poor school performance before onset of the more definitive abnormalities. They suggested that this might also represent the earliest, almost imperceptible, effect of the virus on the brain.

While gradual onset and progressive deterioration of intellectual function has been widely recognized as the classic mode of onset of the disease, other presenting symptoms have not uncommonly been described. In some cases, the first observed abnormalities have been clumsiness, poor coordination, myoclonus, akinetic attacks, or even grand mal seizures. A rare presenting symptom is the abrupt onset of a unilateral movement disorder in the form of dystonic or hemiballismic activity of one extremity. Several children have been reported in whom visual disturbances or acute onset of blindness secondary to a retinopathy or maculopathy heralded other features of the illness (Andriola and Karlsberg, Bove and Shelburne, Cape et al., Nelson et al., Parker et al.). An unusual but diagnostically confusing presentation is with symptoms of increased intracranial pressure accompanied by papilledema (Glowacki et al.). Progression of the illness is often quite rapid in such cases and can be accelerated by unwarranted air contrast procedures.

Within weeks or a few months after the initial complaints, most patients with this illness begin to exhibit periodic "spasms," referred to as myoclonus. Once developed, seizures of this type often are repetitive, occurring in repeated fashion at intervals between 10 and 60 seconds. A sensory stimulus can sometimes provoke such attacks. A characteristic feature of the myoclonic jerk is the tempo of each, which consists of shock-like onset of flexion of the head, trunk, and extremities, followed by a slower, more gradual relaxation phase (Metz et al.). By this stage of the disease, the electroencephalogram has usually developed a characteristic suppression-burst pattern, thus allowing a clinical diagnosis with a reasonable degree of accuracy. Another type of repetitive seizure that can occur early in the course of the illness is akinetic or "drop" attacks (Risk and Haddad). When this type of seizure occurs in the young child with this illness before there are mental or behavioral changes, one is not likely to consider the diagnosis unless it is suggested by the electroencephalographic abnormality.

As mental capabilities continue to regress, motor disturbances become more obvious in the form of spasticity, tremor, athetoid activity, or ataxia. Basal ganglia dysfunction is usually not prominent clinically but infrequently can be striking. Mossakowski and Mathieson reported one such case in which rhythmic tremor, slowed gait, and rigidity were sufficiently marked that the child at first was considered to have postencephalitic parkinsonism. Ocular abnormalities of various types are commonly observed in children with subacute sclerosing panencephalitis. Papilledema occurs in those with brain swelling with associated increased intracranial pressure, while others develop primary optic atrophy with visual loss. Nystagmus and cortical visual loss also complicate the disorder in some. The best known ocular disturbance is a focal chorioretinitis that often affects the macular area and is present without an associated vitreous reaction (Andriola and Karlsberg, Font et al., Landers and Klintworth, Nelson et al., Robb and Watters). In unusual cases, the macular pigmentary abnormality is associated with peripheral chorioretinal involvement (Morgan et al.). Maculopathy with visual loss is usually identified during the course of the disease but can be the very first complaint.

Within weeks or months after onset, the child becomes mentally bankrupt, minimally responsive, and bedridden with hypertonicity and either a decorticate or decerebrate posture. At this advanced stage of the illness, unexplained episodes of hyperthermia and profuse diaphoresis are seen, while myoclonus may at this point abate or disappear. Many will die soon thereafter but an occasional child will remain in this advanced state of debilitation for months or even years.

Laboratory and Other Diagnostic Studies

The diagnosis of subacute sclerosing panencephalitis can be presumed in a child with acquired and progressive intellectual decline combined with characteristic myoclonic seizures. Confirmation, however, is on the basis of laboratory findings, the typical electroencephalographic abnormality, and the pathologic demonstration of an encephalitis associated with intranuclear and intracytoplasmic eosinophilic inclusion bodies. An almost invariable finding is the presence in serum and cerebrospinal fluid of elevated complement-fixing or hemagglutinating measles (rubeola) antibody titers which usually reach levels as high or even much higher than occur during convalescence from natural measles (Griffin and Katz, Legg, Sever and Zeman). With uncomplicated natural measles, the serum complement fixation titer usually declines from an average of 1:260 at the time of the acute infection to a range from 1:8 or 1:20 by two or more years later (Adels et al., Jabbour et al. 1969). In children with subacute sclerosing panencephalitis, titers in serum range from 1:64 to 1:2,048 and sometimes show gradual rise during the course of the disease. Cerebrospinal fluid measles antibody titers range from 1:8 to 1:64 in most cases. Negative measles antibody titers in children believed to have subacute sclerosing panencephalitis are decidedly unusual but have been reported (Bove and Shelburne).

Cerebrospinal fluid analysis generally reveals clear fluid containing either no cells or a modest lymphocytic pleocytosis. The glucose content is normal and the protein content is normal or mildly increased. Protein levels between 50 and 80 mg. per 100 ml. represent the usual range. The CSF colloidal gold curve, now infrequently done, shows a paretic, or first zone, elevation. With the exception of the elevated measles antibody titer, the most valuable cerebrospinal fluid finding in subacute sclerosing panencephalitis is an elevation of gamma globulin content, which accounts for 20 to 50 percent of the total protein within the CSF. Immunoelectrophoresis has shown that the increased gamma globulin is predominantly IgG (Link et al.) and that the elevated CSF content is the result of local production by cells within the central nervous system (Cutler et al.). The elevated first zone colloidal gold reaction reflects the increased gamma globulin content of cerebrospinal fluid. An additional diagnostic method is the possible detection of measles-virus antigen in cells in CSF by immunofluorescence (Dayan and Stokes).

The electroencephalogram shows typical abnormalities in the early stages of the disease, sometimes even before repetitive myoclonic spasms have entered the picture (Cobb and Hill, Ibrahim and Jeavons, Radermecker). It is possible for the disorder to become far advanced before the characteristic EEG changes occur but this is unusual. The customary and best known abnormality is referred to as the suppression burst pattern, in which background activity becomes slow with low voltage and is interrupted at intervals of three to 30 seconds but most often every five to seven seconds by high-voltage slow complexes, often immediately preceded by sharp, spike, or polyspike discharges (Markand and Panszi) (Fig. 18–4). The periodic discharges

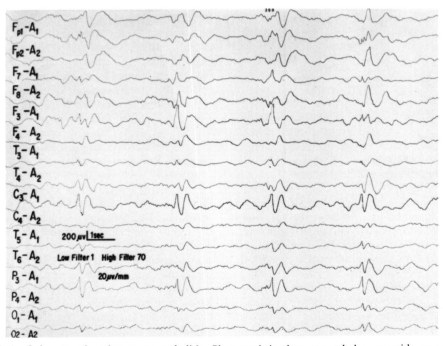

Figure 18–4. Subacute sclerosing panencephalitis. Characteristic electroencephalogram with suppression burst pattern. Low-voltage activity in all leads is interrupted at periodic intervals by brief high-voltage complexes.

last from one to three seconds, are classically bilateral and synchronous, and may be associated with myoclonus observed clinically. In some patients, periodic complexes on the electroencephalogram are activated only during sleep (Westmoreland et al.). In the late stages of the illness, the periodic pattern may disappear, corresponding to disappearance of the myoclonic spasms. When this occurs, the electroencephalogram remains severely abnormal, with diffuse high-voltage slow activity arising from all leads. The typical periodic burst complexes are of particular diagnostic importance in children in whom the mode of presentation of the disease is different from the customary. For example, in the child with recent personality changes associated with increased pressure symptoms, this type of EEG disturbance provides evidence that the process is a diffuse intracranial disturbance and thus virtually eliminates a solitary mass from consideration.

Brain biopsy has been used as a diagnostic method in which the histologic findings of encephalitis plus the presence of Cowdry type A intranuclear inclusions have been accepted as indicative of the disease, assuming that the clinical course is compatible. The high degree of diagnostic reliability of serum and CSF measles antibody titers plus the typical electroencephalographic pattern have reduced the need for tissue confirmation of the disease. In addition, inclusions are not always found in biopsy material in children subsequently proven to have subacute sclerosing panencephalitis.

Pathology

The neuropathology of subacute sclerosing panencephalitis is that of a viral encephalitis in which both gray and white matter are involved to a variable degree. In general, more chronic cases usually reveal more extensive white matter gliosis and demyelination, while intranuclear inclusion bodies are more readily demonstrated in those with a shorter clinical course. Perivascular and leptomeningeal lymphocytic and plasma cell infiltrates, neuronal cell loss, neuronophagia, and scattered microglial nodules are nonspecific reactions, common to viral encephalitis generally.

The most notable feature of the pathology of this disease is the presence of intranuclear and intracytoplasmic eosinophilic inclusions, best seen in oligodendroglia and to a lesser degree in neurons. Inclusions are not invar-

iably found and, especially in brain biopsy material, may be impossible to identify. They vary in size from a diameter of two to 10 microns, with larger inclusions virtually completely occupying the cell nucleoplasm (Herndon and Rubinstein). Among patients with prolonged survival, Alzheimer neurofibrillary changes can sometimes be found in the cerebral cortex and basal ganglia (Mandybur et al.). The pathology of the disorder is widespread in the brain but is virtually confined to the nervous system and retina. Myopathic changes associated with structures resembling inclusions have been observed in the diaphragm and the intercostal muscles (Bove and Shelburne).

Treatment

Treatment of subacute sclerosing panencephalitis includes measures to maintain nutrition to the degree possible, appropriate skin care, and efforts to control seizures. Past experience has indicated that the myoclonic jerks characteristic of this disorder respond poorly to the conventional anticonvulsants in most cases. Phenobarbital or phenytoin is generally prescribed but the results are not usually favorable. Diazepam occasionally offers some benefit, and haloperidol in certain cases can have a significant effect on the reduction of myoclonus (De Giacomo et al.).

Many different therapeutic approaches have been attempted to influence the course of subacute sclerosing panencephalitis, but, to date, none have consistently or effectively altered the eventual outcome. Kolar et al. described improvement in a child with subacute sclerosing panencephalitis after thymectomy but further reports have not appeared. Corticosteroids, 5-iodo-2-deoxyuridine, 5-bromo-2-deoxyuridine, amantadine, and pyran copolymer have received trials but with little success (Freeman, Haslam et al.), and sometimes with adverse effects (Leavitt et al.). Poly I/C administered intracerebrally has been shown to favorably modify SSPE virus encephalitis in hamsters (Kriel and Wulff), but the agent has not been shown to be beneficial in the natural disease in humans. Recent therapeutic trials have largely been with isoprinosine, an antiviral agent with in vitro activity against a wide range of RNA viruses. In some reports, beneficial effects have been attributed to isoprinosine therapy (Huttenlocher and Mattson), while others have not documented improvement or significant alterations on the course of the illness (Haddad and Risk, Silverberg et al.).

Chronic Rubella Panencephalitis

In 1974, Lebon and Lyon in Paris published a brief note in Lancet which described a slowly progressive encephalitic disorder with onset at age eight years in a child who had been previously normal. The illness was characterized clinically by progressive dementia and prominent cerebellar signs, while the CSF revealed a lymphocytic pleocytosis and an elevated protein content, 30 to 50 percent of which was gamma globulin. Rubella antibody titers in serum and CSF were remarkably high, which led the authors to conclude that the chronic, progressive illness was the result of infection with rubella virus.

In 1975, simultaneous publications by Weil et al. and by Townsend et al. described a very similar illness beginning in later childhood in patients with the congenital rubella syndrome. The child reported by Weil et al. had the onset of progressive dementia at eight years of age, followed by the development of ataxia, choreiform activity, myoclonus, and perimacular pigmentary retinopathy at 11 years of age. The CSF contained a slight lymphocytic pleocytosis and a striking increase in gamma globulin content. Rubella antibody titers were markedly elevated in the serum and CSF, and rubella virus was isolated from a brain biopsy specimen (Cremer et al.). The paper of Townsend and colleagues (1975) included three patients, all with a previous history compatible with congenital rubella. The first patient experienced the beginning of intellectual decline at age 12 years, followed by progressive ataxia and spasticity six years later. The other two children had the onset of a gait abnormality at 12 years of age and all three were found to have high serum and CSF rubella antibody titers. Rubella virus could not be isolated from brain tissue or CSF in these cases. The neuropathology, described in a separate paper by Townsend et al. (1976), included a diffuse destructive inflammatory process of white matter but without inclusion bodies, and extensive atrophy of the cerebellum. Both reports by Weil et al. and Townsend et al. (1975) commented on the similarity of this condition caused by the rubella virus to subacute sclerosing panencephalitis which results from the measles virus. It is presumed that rubella virus had remained latent in the brain following

intrauterine infection in these cases, although there is no explanation as to why the virus became activated in later childhood, resulting in a progressive encephalitic disorder. An additional similar example was reported by Jan et al. (1979), which included an unsuccessful trial with isoprinosine therapy.

Another report by Wolinsky et al. described a child with natural, postnatal rubella at seven years of age which was followed 11 years later by the onset of ataxia and subsequent dementia. Laboratory tests were similar to those in the previously reported cases, including elevated rubella antibody titers in blood and CSF. While progressive rubella encephalitis is admittedly rare, the above cases document the existence of the disorder, both in children with congenital rubella and in children with previous postnatally acquired rubella. It resembles subacute sclerosing panencephalitis clinically, although the pathology of the disease is somewhat different and the periodic complexes on the electroencephalogram characteristic of subacute sclerosing panencephalitis are not seen with progressive rubella panencephalitis.

REFERENCES

Adams, J. M., and Imagawa, D. T.: Measles antibodies in multiple sclerosis. Proc. Soc. Exp. Biol. Med. 111:562–566, 1962.

Adels, B. R., Gajdusek, D. C., Gibbs, C. J., Jr., Albrecht, P., and Rogers, N. G.: Attempts to transmit subacute sclerosing panencephalitis and isolate a measles related agent, with a study of the immune response in patients and experimental animals. Neurology 18:30–51, 1968.

Agamanolis, D. P., Tan, J. S., and Parker, D. L.: Immunosuppressive measles encephalitis in a patient with a renal transplant. Arch. Neurol. 36:686–690, 1979.

Aicardi, J., Goutieres, F., Arsenio-Nunes, M-L., and Lebon, P.: Acute measles encephalitis in children with immunosuppression. Pediatrics 59:232–239, 1977.

Allen, I. V., Dermott, E., Connolly, J. H., and Hurwitz, L. J.: A study of a patient with the amyotrophic form of Creutzfeldt-Jakob Disease. Brain 94:715–724, 1971.

Andriola, M., and Karlsberg, R. O.: Maculopathy in subacute sclerosing panencephalitis. Am. J. Dis. Child. 124:187–189, 1972.

Asher, D. M., Gibbs, C. J., Jr., and Gajdusek, D. C.: Pathogenesis of subacute spongiform encephalopathies. Ann. Clin. Lab. Sci. 6:84–103, 1976.

Aström, K-E., Mancall, E. L., and Richardson, E. P., Jr.: Progressive multifocal leuko-encephalopathy. A hitherto unrecognized complication of chronic lymphatic leukemia and Hodgkin's disease. Brain 81:93–111, 1958.

Baguley, D. M., and Glasgow, G. L.: Subacute sclerosing panencephalitis and Salk vaccine. Lancet 2:763–765, 1973.

Barbanti-Brodano, G., Oyanagi, S., Katz, M., and Koprowski, H.: Presence of two different viral agents in brain cells of patients with subacute sclerosing panencephalitis. Proc. Soc. Exp. Biol. Med. 134:230–235, 1970.

Bardelas, J. A., Winkelstein, J. A., Seto, D. S. Y., Tsai, T., and Rogel, A. D.: Fatal ECHO 24 infection in a patient with hypogamma-globulinemia: Relationship to dermatomyositis-like syndrome. J. Pediat. 90:396–399, 1977.

Baringer, J. R., Gajdusek, D. C., Gibbs, C. J., Jr., Masters, C. L., Stern, W. E., and Terry, R. D.: Transmissible dementias: Current problems in tissue handling. Neurology 30:302–303, 1980.

Baringer, J. R., and Prusiner, S. B.: Experimental scrapie in mice: Ultrastructural observations. Ann. Neurol. 4:205–211, 1978.

Beck, E., Bak, I. J., Christ, J. F., Gajdusek, D. C., Gibbs, C. J., Jr., and Hassler, R.: Experimental kuru in the spider monkey. Histopathological and ultrastructural studies of the brain during early stages of incubation. Brain 98:595–612, 1975.

Beck, E., Daniel, P. M., Alpers, M., Gajdusek, D. C., and Gibbs, C. J., Jr.: Experimental "Kuru" in chimpanzees. A pathological report. Lancet 2:1056–1059, 1966.

Beck, E., Daniel, P. M., Asher, D. M., Gajdusek, D. C., and Gibbs, C. J., Jr.: Experimental kuru in the chimpanzee. A neuropathologic study. Brain 96:441–462, 1973.

Beck, E., Daniel, P. M., Matthews, W. B., Stevens, D. L., Alpers, M. P., Asher, D. M., Gajdusek, D. C., and Gibbs, C. J., Jr.: Creutzfeldt-Jakob disease. The neuropathology of a transmission experiment. Brain 92:699–716, 1969.

Beck, E., Daniel, P. M., and Parry, H. B.: Degeneration of the cerebellar and hypothalamo-neurohypophyseal systems in sheep with scrapie; and its relationship to human system degenerations. Brain 87:153–176, 1964.

Bernoulli, C., Siegfried, J., Baumgartner, G., Regli, F., Rabinowicz, T., Gajdusek, D. C., and Gibbs, C. J., Jr.: Danger of accidental person-to-person transmission of Creutzfeldt-Jakob disease by surgery. Lancet 1:478–479, 1977.

Bhettay, E., Kipps, A., and McDonald, R.: Early onset of subacute sclerosing panencephalitis. J. Pediat. 89:271–272, 1976.

Bignami, A., and Forno, L. S.: Status spongiosus in Creutzfeldt-Jakob disease. Electron microscopic study of a cortical biopsy. Brain 93:89–94, 1970.

Bignami, A., and Parry, H. B.: Electron microscopic studies of the brain of sheep with natural scrapie. I. The fine structure of neuronal vacuolation. Brain 95:319–326, 1972.

Bignami, A., and Parry, H. B.: Electron microscopic studies of the brain of sheep with natural scrapie. II. The small nerve processes in neuronal degeneration. Brain 95:487–494, 1972.

Bodensteiner, J. B., Morris, H. H., Howell, J. T., and Schochet, S. S.: Chronic ECHO type 5 virus meningoencephalitis in X-linked hypogammaglobulinemia: Treatment with immune plasma. Neurology 29:815–819, 1979.

Bolton, C. F., and Rozdilsky, B.: Primary progressive multifocal leukoencephalopathy. A case report. Neurology 21:72–77, 1971.

Bots, G. T. A. M., de Man, J. C. H., and Verjaal, A.: Virus-like particles in Creutzfeldt-Jakob disease. Acta Neuropath. 18:267–270, 1971.

Bouteille, M., Fontaine, C., Bedrenne, C., and Delarue, J.: Sur un cas d'encephalite subaigue a inclusions: Etude anatomoclinique et ultrastructurale. Rev. Neurol. 113:454–458, 1965.

Bove, K. E., and Shelburne, S. A., Jr.: Subacute inclusion body encephalitis associated with myopathy. Arch. Neurol. 27:42–44, 1972.

Breitfeld, V., Hashida, Y., Sherman, F. E., Odagiri, K., and Yunis, E. J.: Fatal measles infection in children with leukemia. Lab. Invest. 28:279–291, 1973.

Brody, J. A., and Detels, R.: Subacute sclerosing panencephalitis: A zoonosis following aberrant measles. Lancet 2:500–501, 1970.

Brown, P., and Cathala, F.: Creutzfeldt-Jakob disease in France: I. Retrospective study of the Paris area during the ten-year period 1968–1977. Ann. Neurol. 5:189–192, 1979.

Brown, P., Cathala, F., Sadowsky, D., and Gajdusek, D. C.: Creutzfeldt-Jakob disease in France: II. Clinical characteristics of 124 consecutive verified cases during the decade 1968–1977. Ann. Neurol. 6:430–437, 1979.

Burger, L. J., Rowan, A. J., and Goldensohn, E. S.: Creutzfeldt-Jakob disease. An electroencephalographic study. Arch. Neurol. 26:428–433, 1972.

Cape, C. A., Martinez, A. J., Robertson, J. T., Hamilton, R., and Jabbour, J. T.: Adult onset of subacute sclerosing panencephalitis. Arch. Neurol. 28:124–127, 1973.

Carroll, B. A., Lane, B., Norman, D., and Enzmann, D.: Diagnosis of progressive multifocal leukoencephalopathy by computed tomography. Radiology 122:137–141, 1977.

Cavanagh, J. B., Greenbaum, D., Marshall, A. H. E., and Rubinstein, L. J.: Cerebral demyelination associated with disorders of the reticuloendothelial system. Lancet 2:524–529, 1959.

Chen, T. T., Watanabe, I., Zeman, W., and Mealey, J., Jr.: Subacute sclerosing panencephalitis: Propagation of measles virus from brain biopsy in tissue culture. Science 163:1193–1194, 1969.

Ch'ien, L. T., Wilborn, W. H., Carey, J. H., Ceballos, R., Benton, J. W., and Alford, C. A.: The simultaneous occurrence of subacute sclerosing panencephalitis in two brothers. I. Clinical, virologic, and histopathologic studies. J. Infect. Dis. 125:123–128, 1972.

Chiofalo, N., Fuentes, A., and Galvez, S.: Serial EEG findings in 27 cases of Creutzfeldt-Jakob disease. Arch. Neurol. 37:143–145, 1980.

Clark, N. S., and Best, P. V.: Subacute sclerosing (inclusion body) encephalitis. Arch. Dis. Childh. 39:356–362, 1964.

Clarke, J. K., Dane, D. S., and Dick, G. W. A.: Viral antibody in the cerebrospinal fluid and serum of multiple sclerosis patients. Brain 88:953–962, 1965.

Cobb, W., and Hill, D.: Electroencephalogram in subacute progressive encephalitis. Brain 73:392–404, 1950.

Coleman, D. V., Gardner, S. D., and Field, A. M.: Human polyomavirus infection in renal allograft recipients. Brit. Med. J. 3:371–375, 1973.

Connolly, G. H., Allen, I. V., and Hurwitz, L. J.: Measles virus antibody and antigen in SSPE. Lancet 1:542–544, 1967.

Cremer, N. E., Oshiro, L. S., Weil, M. L., Lennette, E. H., Itabashi, H. H., and Carnay, L.: Isolation of rubella virus from brain in chronic progressive panencephalitis. J. Gen. Virol. 29:143–153, 1975.

Creutzfeldt, H. G.: Über eine eigenartige herdformige Erkrankung des Zentralnervensystems. Z. Ges. Neurol. Psychiat. 57:1–18, 1920.

Cuillé, J., and Chelle, P. L.: Pathologie animale—la maladie dite tremblante du mouton est-elle inoculable? Compt. Rend. Acad. Sci. 203:1552–1554, 1936.

Cutler, R. W. P., Merler, E., and Hammerstad, J. P.: Production of antibody by the central nervous system in subacute sclerosing panencephalitis. Neurology 18:129–132, 1968.

Cutler, R. W. P., Watters, G. V., Hammerstad, J. P., and Merler, E.: Origin of cerebrospinal fluid gamma globulin in subacute sclerosing leukoencephalitis. Arch. Neurol. 17:620–628, 1967.

Davis, L. E., Bodian, D., Price, D., Butler, I. J., and Vickers, J. H.: Chronic progressive poliomyelitis secondary to vaccination of an immunodeficient child. New Eng. J. Med. 297:241–245, 1977.

Dawson, J. R., Jr.: Cellular inclusions in cerebral lesions of lethargic encephalitis. Am. J. Path. 9:7–15, 1933.

Dawson, J. R., Jr.: Cellular inclusions in cerebral lesions of epidemic encephalitis: Second report. Arch. Neurol. Psychiat. 31:685–700, 1934.

Dayan, A. D., and Cumings, J. N.: An infantile case of subacute sclerosing panencephalitis with an abnormal ganglioside pattern in the brain. Arch. Dis. Childh. 44:187–196, 1969.

Dayan, A. D., Gostling, J. V. T., Greaves, J. L., Stevens, D. W., and Woodhouse, M. A.: Evidence of a pseudomyxovirus in the brain in subacute sclerosing leucoencephalitis. Lancet 1:980–981, 1967.

Dayan, A. D., and Stokes, M. I.: Immunofluorescent detection of measles-virus antigens in cerebrospinal-fluid cells in subacute sclerosing panencephalitis. Lancet 1:891–892, 1971.

De Giacomo, P., Cappiello, J., and Perniola, T.: Haloperidol in subacute sclerosing leucoencephalitis. Lancet 2:1095, 1967.

Detels, R., Brody, J. A., McNew, J., and Edgar, A. H.: Further epidemiological studies of subacute sclerosing panencephalitis. Lancet 2:11–14, 1973.

Duffy, P., Wolf, J., Collins, G., De Voe, A. G., Strecter, B., and Cowen, D.: Possible person-to-person transmission of Creutzfeldt-Jakob disease. New Eng. J. Med. 290:692–693, 1974.

Eckroade, R. J., Zu Rhein, G. M., Marsh, R. F., and Hanson, R. P.: Transmissible mink encephalopathy: Experimental transmission to the squirrel monkey. Science 196:1088–1090, 1970.

Ellison, G. W.: Progressive multifocal leukoencephalopathy (PML). I. Investigation of the immunologic status of a patient with lymphosarcoma and PML. J. Neuropath. Exp. Neurol. 28:501–506, 1969.

Faris, A. A., and Martinez, A. J.: Primary progressive multifocal leukoencephalopathy. A central nervous system disease caused by a slow virus. Arch. Neurol. 27:357–360, 1972.

Feorino, P. M., Humphrey, D., Hockberg, F., and Chilicote, R.: Mononucleosis-associated subacute sclerosing panencephalitis. Lancet 2:530–532, 1975.

Fermaglich, J., Hardman, J. M., and Earle, K. M.: Spontaneous progressive multifocal leukoencephalopathy. Neurology 20:479–484, 1970.

Fields, B. N.: Genetic manipulation of reovirus—a model for modification of disease? New Eng. J. Med. 287:1026–1033, 1972.

Font, R. L., Jenis, E. H., and Tuck, K. D.: Measles maculopathy associated with subacute sclerosing panencephalitis. Immunofluorescent and immuno-ultrastructural studies. Arch. Path. 96:168–174, 1973.

Freeman, J. M.: The clinical spectrum and early diagnosis of Dawson's encephalitis. With preliminary notes on treatment. J. Pediat. 75:590–603, 1969.

Freeman, J. M.: Treatment of Dawson's encephalitis with 5-bromo-2-deoxyuridine. Double-blind study. Arch. Neurol. 21:431–434, 1969.

Freeman, J. M.: Treatment of subacute sclerosing panencephalitis with 5-bromo-2-deoxyuridine and pyran copolymer. Neurology 18:176–180, 1968.

Freeman, J. M., Magoffin, R. L., Lennette, E. H., and Herndon, R. M.: Additional evidence of the relation between subacute inclusion-body encephalitis and measles virus. Lancet 2:129–131, 1967.

Gajdusek, D. C.: Slow virus diseases of the central nervous system. Am. J. Clin. Path. 56:320–330, 1971.

Gajdusek, D. C.: Slow-virus infections of the nervous system. New Eng. J. Med. 276:392–400, 1967.

Gajdusek, D. C., and Gibbs, C. J., Jr.: Transmission of two subacute spongiform encephalopathies of man (kuru and Creutzfeldt-Jakob disease) to New World monkeys. Nature 230:588–591, 1971.

Gajdusek, D. C., Gibbs, C. J., Jr., Asher, D. M., Brown, P., Diwan, A., Hoffman, P., Nemo, G., Rohwer, R., and White, L.: Precautions in medical care of, and in handling materials from, patients with transmissible virus dementia (Creutzfeldt-Jakob disease). New Eng. J. Med. 297:1253–1258, 1977.

Gajdusek, D. C., Sorenson, E. R., and Meyer, J.: A comprehensive cinema record of disappearing kuru. Brain 93:65–76, 1970.

Gajdusek, D. C., and Zigas, V.: Degenerative disease of the central nervous system in New Guinea. The endemic occurrence of "kuru" in the native population. New Eng. J. Med. 257:974–978, 1957.

Gajdusek, D. C., and Zigas, V.: Kuru. Clinical, pathological and epidemiological study of an acute progressive degenerative disease of the central nervous system among natives of the Eastern Highlands of New Guinea. Am. J. Med. 26:442–469, 1959.

Galvez, S., Masters, C., and Gajdusek, C.: Descriptive epidemiology of Creutzfeldt-Jakob disease in Chile. Arch. Neurol. 37:11–14, 1980.

Gardner, S. D., Field, A. M., Coleman, D. V., and Hulme, B.: New human papovavirus (BK) isolated from urine after renal transplantation. Lancet 1:1253–1257, 1971.

Gerson, K. L., and Haslam, R. H. A.: Subtle immunologic abnormalities in four boys with subacute sclerosing panencephalitis. New Eng. J. Med. 285:78–82, 1971.

Gibbs, C. J., Jr., and Gajdusek, D. C.: Infection as the etiology of spongiform encephalopathy (Creutzfeldt-Jakob disease). Science 165:1023–1025, 1969.

Gibbs, C. J., Jr., Gajdusek, D. C., Asher, D. M., Alpers, M. P., Beck, E., Daniel, P. M., and Matthews, W. B.: Creutzfeldt-Jakob disease (spongiform encephalopathy): Transmission to the chimpanzee. Science 161:388–389, 1968.

Gilden, D. H., Rorke, L. B., and Tanaka, R.: Acute SSPE. Arch. Neurol. 32:644–646, 1975.

Glowacki, J., Guazzi, G. C., and van Bogaert, L.: Pseudotumoural presentation of certain cases of subacute sclerosing panencephalitis. J. Neurol. Sci. 4:199–215, 1967.

Gomori, A. J., Partnow, M. J., Horoupian, D. S., and Hirano, A.: The ataxic form of Creutzfeldt-Jakob disease. Arch. Neurol. 29:318–323, 1973.

Gonatas, N. K., Terry, R. D., and Weiss, M.: Electron microscopic study in two cases of Jakob-Creutzfeldt disease. J. Neuropath. Exp. Neurol. 24:575–598, 1965.

Grabow, J. D., Zu Rhein, G. M., Eckroade, R. J., Zollman, P. E., and Hanson, R. P.: Transmissible mink encephalopathy agent in squirrel monkeys. Serial electroencephalographic, clinical and pathologic studies. Neurology 23:820–832, 1973.

Greenfield, J. G.: Encephalitis and encephalomyelitis in England and Wales during the last decade. Brain 73:141–166, 1950.

Greenlee, J. E., Becker, L. E., Narayan, O., and Johnson, R. T.: Failure to demonstrate papovavirus tumor antigen in human cerebral neoplasms. Ann. Neurol. 3:479–481, 1978.

Griffin, D. E., Narayan, O., Bukowski, J. F., Adams, R. J., and Cohen, S. R.: The cerebrospinal fluid in visna, a slow viral disease of sheep. Ann. Neurol. 4:212–218, 1978.

Griffith, J. F., and Katz, S. L.: Subacute sclerosing panencephalitis; laboratory findings in 6 cases. Neurology 18:98–100, 1968.

Grunnet, M. L.: Nuclear bodies in Creutzfeldt-Jakob and Alzheimer's diseases. Neurology 25:1091–1093, 1975.

Haddad, F. S., and Risk, W. S.: Isoprinosine treatment in 18 patients with subacute sclerosing panencephalitis: A controlled study. Ann. Neurol. 7:185–188, 1980.

Hanson, R. P., Eckroade, R. J., Marsh, R. F., Zu Rhein, G. M., Kanitz, C. L., and Gustafson, D. P.: Susceptibility of mink to sheep scrapie. Science 712:859–861, 1971.

Haslam, R. H. A., McQuillen, M. P., and Clark, D. B.: Amantadine therapy in subacute sclerosing panencephalitis. A preliminary report. Neurology 19:1080–1086, 1969.

Hedley-Whyte, E. T., Smith, B. P., Tyler, H. R., and Peterson, W. P.: Multifocal leukoencephalopathy with remission and five year survival. J. Neuropath. Exp. Neurol. 25:107–116, 1966.

Herndon, R. M., and Rubinstein, L. J.: Light and electron microscopy observations on the development of viral particles in the inclusions of Dawson's encephalitis (subacute sclerosing panencephalitis). Neurology 18:8–20, 1968.

Hirano, A., Ghatak, N. R., Johnson, A. B., Partnow, M. J., and Gomori, A. J.: Argentophilic plaques in Creutzfeldt-Jakob disease. Arch. Neurol. 26:530–542, 1972.

Hochberg, F. H., Lehrich, J. R., Richardson, E. P., Jr., Feorino, P., and Aström, K. E.: Mononucleosis-associated subacute sclerosing panencephalitis. Acta Neuropath. 34:33–40, 1976.

Hogan, T. F., Borden, E. C., McBain, J. A., Padgett, B. L., and Walker, D. L.: Human polyomavirus infections with JC virus and BK virus in renal transplant patients. Ann. Intern. Med. 92:373–378, 1980.

Hornabrook, R. W.: Kuru–A subacute cerebellar degeneration. The natural history and clinical features. Brain 91:53–74, 1968.

Horta-Barbosa, L., Fucillo, D. A., London, W. T., Jabbour, J. T., Zeman, W., and Sever, J. L.: Isolation of measles virus from brain cell cultures of two patients with subacute sclerosing panencephalitis. Proc. Soc. Exp. Biol. Med. 132:272–277, 1969.

Horta-Barbosa, L., Fucillo, D. A., and Sever, J. L.: Chronic viral infections of the central nervous system. J.A.M.A. 218:1185–1188, 1971.

Horta-Barbosa, L., Fucillo, D. A., Sever, J. L., and Zeman, W.: Subacute sclerosing panencephalitis: isolation of measles virus from a brain biopsy. Nature 221:974, 1969.

Houff, S. A., Madden, D. L., and Sever, J. L.: Subacute sclerosing panencephalitis in only one of identical

twins. A seven-year follow-up. Arch. Neurol. 36:854–856, 1979.

Huttenlocher, P. R., and Mattson, R. H.: Isoprinosine in subacute sclerosing panencephalitis. Neurology 29:763–771, 1979.

Ibrahim, M. M., and Jeavons, P. M.: The value of electroencephalography in the diagnosis of subacute sclerosing panencephalitis. Dev. Med. Child Neurol. 16:295–307, 1974.

Jabbour, J. T., Duenas, D. A., Sever, J. L., Krebs, H. M., and Horta-Barbosa, L.: Epidemiology of subacute sclerosing panencephalitis (SSPE). A report of the SSPE registry. J.A.M.A. 220:959–962, 1972.

Jabbour, J. T., Garcia, J. H., Lemmi, H., Ragland, J., Duenas, D. A., and Sever, J. L.: Subacute sclerosing panencephalitis. A multidisciplinary study of eight cases. J.A.M.A. 207:2248–2254, 1969.

Jabbour, J. T., Roane, J. A., and Sever, J. L.: Studies of delayed dermal hypersensitivity in patients with subacute sclerosing panencephalitis. Neurology 19:929–931, 1969.

Jakob, A.: Über eigenartige Erkrankungen des Zentralnervensystems mit bemerkenswertem anatomischem Befunde (spastische Pseudosklerose-encephalomyelopathie mit disseminierten Degenerationsherden). Deutsch. Z. Nervenheilk. 70:132–146, 1921.

Jakob, H., Pyrkosch, W., and Strube, H.: Die erbliche Form der Creutzveldt-Jakobschen Krankheit. Arch. Psychiat. Nervkrankh. 184:653–674, 1950.

Jan, J. E., Tingle, A. J., Donald, G., Kettyls, M., Buckler, W. S. J., and Dolman, C. L.: Progressive rubella panencephalitis: Clinical course and response to 'isoprinosine.' Dev. Med. Child Neurol. 21:648–652, 1979.

Johnson, R. T.: Subacute sclerosing panencephalitis. J. Infect. Dis. 121:227–230, 1970.

Johnson, R. T., and Gibbs, C. J., Jr.: Koch's postulates and slow infections of the nervous system. Arch. Neurol. 30:36–38, 1974.

Kahana, E., Alter, M., Braham, J., and Sofer, D.: Creutzfeldt-Jakob disease: Focus among Libyan Jews in Israel. Science 183:90–91, 1974.

Kakulas, B. A., Lecours, A.-R., and Gajdusek, D. C.: Further observations on the pathology of kuru. (A study of the two cerebra in serial section.) J. Neuropath. Exp. Neurol. 26:85–97, 1967.

Katz, M., Rorke, L. B., Masland, W. S., Brodano, G. B., and Koprowski, H.: Subacute sclerosing panencephalitis: Isolation of a virus encephalitogenic for ferrets. J. Infect. Dis. 121:188–195, 1970.

Katz, M., Rorke, L. B., Masland, W. S., Koprowski, H., and Tucker, S. H.: Transmission of an encephalitogenic agent from brains of patients with subacute sclerosing panencephalitis to ferrets. New Eng. J. Med. 279:793–798, 1968.

Katzman, R., Kagan, E. H., and Zimmerman, H. M.: A case of Jakob-Creutzfeldt disease. I. Clinicopathological analysis. J. Neuropath. Exp. Neurol. 20:78–94, 1961.

Kennedy C.: A ten-year experience with subacute sclerosing panencephalitis. Neurology 18:58–59, 1968.

Kimberlin, R. H., and Marsh, R. F.: Comparison of scrapie and transmissible mink encephalopathy in hamsters. I. Biochemical studies of brain during development of disease. J. Infect. Dis. 131:97–103, 1975.

King, H. O. M.: Kuru. Epidemiological developments. Lancet 2:761–763, 1975.

Knight, A., O'Brien, P., and Osoba, D.: "Spontaneous"

progressive multifocal leukoencephalopathy. Immunologic aspects. Ann. Intern. Med. 77:229–233, 1972.

Kolar, O.: Immunopathologic observations in subacute sclerosing panencephalitis. Neurology 18:107–111, 1968.

Kolar, O., Obrucnik, M., Behounkova, L., Musil, J., and Penickova, V.: Thymectomy in subacute sclerosing leucoencephalitis. Brit. Med. J. 3:22–24, 1967.

Koprowski, H., Barbanti-Brodano, G., and Katz, M.: Interactions between papova-like virus and paramyxovirus in human brain cells: A hypothesis. Nature 225:1045–1047, 1970.

Kriel, R. L., and Wulff, H.: SSPE virus infections in suckling hamsters. Modification by intracerebral administration of poly IC. Arch. Neurol. 30:238–241, 1974.

Kurtzke, J. F., Kurland, L. T., and Goldberg, I. D.: Mortality and migration in multiple sclerosis. Neurology 21:1186–1197, 1971.

Lampert. P. W., Earle, K. M., Gibbs, C. J., Jr., and Gajdusek, D. C.: Experimental kuru encephalopathy in chimpanzees and spider monkeys. Electron microscopic studies. J. Neuropath. Exp. Neurol. 28:353–370, 1969.

Lampert, P. W., Gajdusek, D. C., and Gibbs, C. J., Jr.: Experimental spongiform encephalopathy (Creutzfeldt-Jakob disease) in chimpanzees. J. Neuropath. Exp. Neurol. 30:20–32, 1971.

Landau, W. M., and Luse, S. A.: Relapsing inclusion body encephalitis (Dawson's type) of eight years' duration. Neurology 8:669–676, 1958.

Landers, M. B., III, and Klintworth, G. K.: Subacute sclerosing panencephalitis (SSPE). A clinicopathologic study of the retinal lesions. Arch. Ophthal. 86:156–163, 1971.

Leavitt, T. J., Merigan, T. C., and Freeman, J. M.: Hemolytic-uremic-like syndrome following polycarboxylate interferon induction. Am. J. Dis. Child. 121:43–47, 1971.

Lebon, P., and Lyon, G.: Non-congenital rubella encephalitis. Lancet 2:468, 1974.

Legg, N. J.: Virus antibodies in subacute sclerosing panencephalitis: a study of 22 patients. Brit. Med. J. 3:350–352, 1967.

Lehrich, J. R., Katz, M., Rorke, L. B., Barbanti-Brodano, G., and Koprowski, H.: Subacute sclerosing panencephalitis. Encephalitis in hamsters produced by viral agents isolated from human brain cells. Arch. Neurol. 23:97–102, 1970.

Lennette, E. H., Magoffin, R. L., and Freeman, J. M.: Immunologic evidence of measles virus as an etiologic agent in subacute sclerosing panencephalitis. Neurology 18:21–29, 1968.

Link, H., Panelius, M., and Salmi, A. A.: Immunoglobulins and measles antibodies in subacute sclerosing panencephalitis. Demonstration of synethesis of oligoclonal IgG with measles antibody activity within the central nervous system. Arch. Neurol. 28:23–30, 1973.

Lorand, B., Nagy, T., and Tariska, S.: Subacute progressive panencephalitis. World Neurol. 3:376–390, 1962.

Lyon, L. W., McCormick, W. F., and Schochet, S. S., Jr.: Progressive multifocal leukoencephalopathy. Arch. Intern. Med. 128:420–426, 1971.

Malas, D., and Weiss, S.: Progressive multifocal leukoencephalopathy and cryptococcal meningitis with systemic lupus erythematosus and thymoma. Ann. Neurol. 1:188–191, 1977.

Mancall, E. L.: Progressive multifocal leukoencephalopathy. Neurology 15:693–699, 1965.

Mandybur, T. I., Nagpaul, A. S., Pappas, Z., and Niklowitz, W. J.: Alzheimer neurofibrillary change in subacute sclerosing panencephalitis. Ann. Neurol. 1:103–107, 1977.

Manuelidis, E. E., Angelo, J. N., Gorgacz, E. J., Kim, J. H., and Manuelidis, L.: Experimental Creutzfeldt-Jakob disease transmitted via the eye with infected cornea. New Eng. J. Med. 296:1334–1336, 1977.

Manuelidis, E. E., Angelo, J. N., Gorgacz, E. J., and Manuelidis, L.: Transmission of Creutzfeldt-Jakob disease to syrian hamster. Lancet 1:479, 1977.

Manuelidis, E. E., Gorgacz, E. J., and Manuelidis, L.: Viremia in experimental Creutzfeldt-Jakob disease. Science 200:1069–1071, 1978.

Manuelidis, E. E., Gorgacz, E. J., and Manuelidis, L.: Transmission of Creutzfeldt-Jakob disease with scrapie-like syndromes to mice. Nature 271:778–779, 1978.

Markand, O. N., and Panszi, J. G.: The electroencephalogram in subacute sclerosing panencephalitis. Arch. Neurol. 32:719–726, 1975.

Marriott, P. J., O'Brien, M. D., Mackenzie, I. C. K., and Janota, I.: Progressive multifocal leukoencephalopathy: remission with cytarabine. J. Neurol. Neurosurg. Psychiat. 38:205–209, 1975.

Marsh, R. F., and Kimberlin, R. H.: Comparison of scrapie and transmissible mink encephalopathy in hamsters. II. Clinical signs, pathology, and pathogenesis. J. Infect. Dis. 131:104–110, 1975.

Martin, J. B., and Banker, B. Q.: Subacute multifocal leukoencephalopathy with widespread intranuclear inclusions. Arch. Neurol. 21:590–602, 1969.

Masters, C. L., Harris, J. O., Gajdusek, C., Gibbs, C. J., Jr., Bernoulli, C., and Asher, D. M.: Creutzfeldt-Jakob disease: Patterns of worldwide occurrence and the significance of familial and sporadic clustering. Ann. Neurol. 5:177–188, 1979.

Masters, C. L., Kakulas, B. A., Alpers, M. P., Gajdusek, D. C., and Gibbs, C. J., Jr.: Preclinical lesions and their progression in the experimental spongiform encephalopathies (Kuru and Creutzfeldt-Jakob disease) in primates. J. Neuropath. Exp. Neurol. 35:593–605, 1976.

Masters, C. L., and Richardson, E. P., Jr.: Subacute spongiform encephalopathy (Creutzfeldt-Jakob disease). The nature and progression of spongiform change. Brain 101:333–334, 1978.

Mathews, J. D., Glasse, R., and Lindenbaum, S.: Kuru and cannibalism. Lancet 2:449–452, 1968.

Mathews, T., Wisotzkey, H., and Moossy, J.: Multiple central nervous system infections in progressive multifocal leukoencephalopathy. Neurology 26:9–14, 1976.

May, W. W., Itabashi, H. H., and DeJong, R. N.: Creutzfeldt-Jakob disease. II. Clinical, pathologic, and genetic study of a family. Arch. Neurol. 19:137–149, 1968.

McCormick, W. F., Schochet, S. S., Jr., Sarles, H. E., and Calverley, J. R.: Progressive multifocal leukoencephalopathy in renal transplant recipients. Arch. Intern. Med. 136:829–834, 1976.

Meinke, W., Goldstein, D. A., and Smith, R. A.: Simian virus 40-related DNA sequences in a human brain tumor. Neurology 29:1590–1594, 1979.

Metz, H., Gregoriou, M., and Sandifer, P.: Subacute sclerosing panencephalitis. A review of 17 cases with special reference to clinical diagnostic criteria. Arch. Dis. Childh. 39:554–557, 1964.

Miyamoto, H., Walker, J. E., Ginsberg, A. H., Burks, J. S., McIntosh, K., and Kempe, C. H.: Antibodies to vaccinia and measles viruses in multiple sclerosis patients. Arch. Neurol. 33:414–417, 1976.

Modlin, J. F., Jabbour, J. T., Witte, J. J., and Halsey, N. A.: Epidemiologic studies of measles, measles vaccine, and subacute sclerosing panencephalitis. Pediatrics 59:505–512, 1977.

Modlin, J. F., Halsey, N. A., Eddins, D. L., Conrad, J. L., Jabbour, J. T., Chien, L., and Robinson, H.: Epidemiology of subacute sclerosing panencephalitis. J. Pediat. 94:231–236, 1979.

Morgan, B., Cohen, D. N., Rothner, A. D., and Williamson, R.: Ocular manifestations of subacute sclerosing panencephalitis. Am. J. Dis. Child. 130:1019–1021, 1976.

Mosher, M. B., Schall, G. L., and Wilson, J.: Progressive multifocal leukoencephalopathy. Positive brain scan. J.A.M.A. 218:226–228, 1971.

Mossakowski, M. J., and Mathieson, G.: A parkinsonian syndrome in the course of subacute encephalitis. Neurology 11:461–469, 1961.

Müller, D., ter Meulen, V., Katz, M., and Koprowski, H.: Cytochemical evidence for the presence of two viral agents in subacute sclerosing panencephalitis. Lab. Invest. 25:337–342, 1971.

Murphy, J. V., and Yunis, E. J.: Encephalopathy following measles infection in children with chronic illness. J. Pediat. 88:937–942, 1976.

Narayan, O., Penney, J. B., Jr., Johnson, R. T., Herndon, R. M., and Weiner, L. P.: Etiology of progressive multifocal leukoencephalopathy. Identification of papovaviruses. New Eng. J. Med. 289:1278–1282, 1973.

Nathanson, N., Petursson, G., Georgsson, G., Palsson, P. A., Martin, J. R., and Miller, A.: Pathogenesis of visna. IV. Spinal fluid studies. J. Neuropath. Exp. Neurol. 38:197–208, 1979.

Nelson, D. A., Wiener, A., Yanoff, M., and dePeralta, J.: Retinal lesions in subacute sclerosing panencephalitis. Arch. Ophthal. 84:613–621, 1970.

Neugut, R. H., Neugut, A. I., Kahana, E., Stein, Z., and Alter, M.: Creutzfeldt-Jakob disease: Familial clustering among Libyan-born Israelis. Neurology 29:225–231, 1979.

Neumann, M. A., Gajdusek, D. C., and Zigas, V.: Neuropathologic findings in exotic neurologic disorders among natives of the highlands of New Guinea. J. Neuropath. Exp. Neurol. 23:486–507, 1964.

Nevin, S., McMenemy, W. H., Behrman, S., and Jones, D. P.: Subacute spongiform encephalopathy—a subacute form of encephalopathy attributable to vascular dysfunction (spongiform cerebral atrophy). Brain 83:519–564, 1960.

Notermans, S. L. H., Tijl, W. F. J., Willems, F. T. C., and Slooff, J. L.: Experimentally induced subacute sclerosing panencephalitis in young dogs. Neurology 23:543–553, 1973.

Padgett, B. L., and Walker, D. L.: New human papovaviruses. Prog. Med. Virol. 22:1–35, 1976.

Padgett, B. L., and Walker, D. L.: Prevalence of antibodies in human sera against JC virus, an isolate from a case of progressive multifocal leukoencephalopathy. J. Infect. Dis. 127:467–470, 1976.

Padgett, B. L., Walker, D. L., Zu Rhein, G. M., Eckroade, R. J., and Dessel, B. H.: Cultivation of papova-like virus from human brain with progressive multifocal leucoencephalopathy. Lancet 1:1257–1260, 1971.

Padgett, B. L., Walker, D. L., Zu Rhein, G. M., and Var-

akis, J. N.: Differential neuroöncogenicity of strains of JC virus, a human polyoma virus, in newborn syrian hamsters. Cancer Res. 37:718–720, 1977.

Palmer, A. C.: Distribution of vacuolated neurons in brains of sheep affected with scrapie. J. Neuropath. Exp. Neurol. 19:102–110, 1960.

Parker, J. C., Jr., Klintworth, G. K., Graham, D. G., and Griffith, J. F.: Uncommon morphologic features in subacute sclerosing panencephalitis (SSPE). Report of two cases with virus recovery from one autopsy brain specimen. Am. J. Path. 61:275–284, 1970.

Payne, F. E., Baublis, J. V., and Itabashi, H. H.: Isolation of measles virus from cell cultures of brain from a patient with subacute sclerosing panencephalitis. New Eng. J. Med. 281:585–589, 1969.

Pettay, O., Donner, M., Halonen, H., Palosuo, T., and Salmi, A.: Subacute sclerosing panencephalitis: Preceding intellectual deterioration and deviant measles serology. J. Infect. Dis. 124:439–444, 1971.

Pette, H., and Doring, G.: Über einheimische panencephalomyelitis vom charakter der encephalitis japonica. Deutsch. Z. Nervenheilk. 149:7–44, 1939.

Prineas, J. W.: Paramyxovirus-like particles associated with acute demyelination in chronic relapsing multiple sclerosis. Science 178:760–762, 1972.

Pullan, C. R., Noble, T. C., Scott, D. J., Wisniewski, K., and Gardner, P. S.: Atypical measles infections in leukaemic children on immunosuppressive treatment. Brit. Med. J. 1:1562–1565, 1976.

Radermecker, J.: Aspects electroencephalographiques dans trois cas d'encephalite subaique. Acta Neurol. Belg. 49:222, 1949.

Raine, C. S., Powers, J. M., and Susuki, K.: Acute multiple sclerosis. Confirmation of "paramyxovirus-like" intranuclear inclusions. Arch. Neurol. 30:39–46, 1974.

Rand, K. H., Johnson, K. P., Rubinstein, L. J., Wolinsky, J. S., Penney, J. B., Walker, D. L., Padgett, B. L., and Merigan, T. C.: Adenine arabinoside in the treatment of progressive multifocal leukoencephalopathy: Use of virus-containing cells in the urine to assess response to therapy. Ann. Neurol. 1:458–462, 1977.

Resnick, J. S., Engel, W. K., and Sever, J. L.: Subacute sclerosing panencephalitis. Spontaneous improvement in a patient with elevated measles antibody in blood and spinal fluid. New Eng. J. Med. 279:126–129, 1968.

Richardson, E. P., Jr.: Our evolving understanding of progressive multifocal leukoencephalopathy. Ann. N.Y. Acad. Sci. 230:358–364, 1974.

Richardson, E. P., Jr.: Progressive multifocal leukoencephalopathy. New Eng. J. Med. 265:815–823, 1961.

Risk, W. S., and Haddad, F. S.: The variable natural history of subacute sclerosing panencephalitis. A study of 118 cases from the Middle East. Arch. Neurol. 36:610–614, 1979.

Risk, W. S., Haddad, F. S., and Chemali, R.: Substantial spontaneous long-term improvement in subacute sclerosing panencephalitis. Six cases from the Middle East and a review of the literature. Arch. Neurol. 35:494–502, 1978.

Robb, R. M., and Watters, G. V.: Ophthalmic manifestations of subacute sclerosing panencephalitis. Arch. Ophthal. 83:426–435, 1970.

Roos, R., Gajdusek, D. C., and Gibbs, C. J., Jr.: The clinical characteristics of transmissible Creutzfeldt-Jakob disease. Brain 96:1–20, 1973.

Saunders, M., Knowles, M., Chambers, M. E., Caspary,

E. A., Gardner-Medwin, D., and Walker, P.: Cellular and humoral responses to measles in subacute sclerosing panencephalitis. Lancet 1:72–74, 1969.

Schneck, S. A.: Vaccination with measles and central nervous system disease. Neurology 18:79–82, 1968.

Sever, J. L., Kurtzke, J. F., Alter, M., Schumacher, G. A., Gilkeson, M. R., Ellenberg, J. H., and Brody, J. A.: Virus antibodies and multiple sclerosis. Arch. Neurol. 24:489–494, 1971.

Sever, J. L., and Zeman, W.: Serological studies of measles and subacute sclerosing panencephalitis. Neurology 18:95–97, 1968.

Shaw, C. M., Buchan, G. C., and Carlson, C. B.: Myxovirus as a possible etiologic agent in subacute inclusion-body encephalitis. New Eng. J. Med. 277:511–515, 1967.

Sibley, W. A., and Weisberger, A. S.: Demyelinating disease of the brain in chronic lymphatic leukemia. Occurrence of a case in the husband of a patient with multiple sclerosis. Arch. Neurol. 5:300–307, 1961.

Sigurdsson, B.: Observations on three slow infections of sheep. I. Maedi, slow progressive pneumonia of sheep: epizoological and pathological study. II. Paratuberculosis (Johne's disease) of sheep in Iceland: immunological studies and observations on its mode of spread. III. Rida, chronic encephalitis of sheep, with general remarks on infections which develop slowly and some of their special characteristics. Brit. Vet. J. 110:7–9, 255–270, 307–322, 341–354, 1954.

Sigurdsson, B., Palsson, P. A., and Grimsson, H.: Visna, a demyelinating transmissible disease of sheep. J. Neuropath. Exp. Neurol. 16:389–403, 1957.

Sigurdsson, B., Palsson, P. A., and van Bogaert, L.: Pathology of Visna. Transmissible demyelinating disease in sheep in Iceland. Acta Neuropath. 1:343–362, 1962.

Silberman, J., Cravioto, H., and Feigin, I.: Cortico-striatal degeneration of the Creutzfeldt-Jakob type. J. Neuropath. Exp. Neurol. 20:105–118, 1961.

Silverman, L., and Rubinstein, L. J.: Electron microscopic observations in a case of progressive multifocal leukoencephalopathy. Acta Neuropath. 5:215–224, 1965.

Silverberg, R., Brenner, T., and Abramsky, O.: Inosiplex in the treatment of subacute sclerosing panencephalitis. Arch. Neurol. 36:374–375, 1979.

Sponzilli, E. E., Smith, J. K., Malamud, N., and McCulloch, J. R.: Progressive multifocal leukoencephalopathy: A complication of immunosuppressive treatment. Neurology 25:664–668, 1975.

Steele, R. W., Fucillo, D. A., Hensen, S. A., Vincent, M. M., and Bellanti, J. A.: Specific inhibitory factors of cellular immunity in children with subacute sclerosing panencephalitis. J. Pediat. 88:56–62, 1976.

Stender, A.: Weitere beiträge zum kapital "spastische pseudosklerose Jakobs." Ztschr. Neurol. Psychiat. 128:528, 1930.

Swick, H. M., Brooks, W. H., Roszman, T. L., and Caldwell, D.: A heat-stable blocking factor in the plasma of patients with subacute sclerosing panencephalitis. Neurology 26:84–88, 1976.

Tanaka, R., Iwasaki, Y., and Koprowski, H.: Paramyxovirus-like structures in brains of multiple sclerosis patients. Arch. Neurol. 32:80–83, 1975.

Tellez-Nagel, I., and Harter, D. H.: Subacute sclerosing leukoencephalitis: Ultrastructure of intranuclear and intracytoplasmic inclusions. Science 154:899–901, 1966.

ter Meulen, V., and Hall, W. W.: Slow virus infections of the nervous system: Virological, immunological and pathogenetic considerations. J. Gen. Virol. 41:1–25, 1978.

ter Meulen, V., Katz, M., Käckell, Y-M., Barbanti-Brodano, G., Koprowski, H., and Lennette, E. H.: Subacute sclerosing panencephalitis: In-vitro characterization of viruses isolated from brain cells in culture. J. Infect. Dis. 126:11–17, 1972.

ter Meulen, V., Koprowski, H., Iwasaki, Y., Käckell, Y. M., and Müller, D.: Fusion of cultured multiple-sclerosis brain cells with indicator cells: Presence of nucleocapsids and virions and isolation of para-influenzae-type virus. Lancet 2:1–5, 1972.

Thein, P., Mayr, A., ter Meulen, V., Koprowski, H., Käckell, M. Y., Müller, D., and Meyermann, R.: Subacute sclerosing panencephalitis. Transmission of the virus to calves and lambs. Arch. Neurol. 27:540–548, 1972.

Thompson, J. A., Glasgow, L. A., and Bray, P. F.: Evaluation of central nervous system vaccinia antibody synthesis in multiple sclerosis patients. Neurology 27:227–229, 1977.

Townsend, J. J., Baringer, J. R., Wolinsky, J. S., Malamud, N., Mednick, J. P., Panitch, H. S., Scott, R. A. T., Oshiro, L. S., and Cremer, N. E.: Progressive rubella panencephalitis. Late onset after congenital rubella. New Eng. J. Med. 292:990–993, 1975.

Townsend, J. J., Wolinsky, J. S., and Baringer, J. R.: The neuropathology of progressive rubella panencephalitis of late onset. Brain 99:81–90, 1976.

van Bogaert, L.: La leukoencephalite sclerosante subaigue. J. Neurol. Neurosurg. Psychiat. 8:101–120, 1945.

Van Horn, G., Bastian, F. O., and Moake, J. L.: Progressive multifocal leukoencephalopathy: Failure of response to transfer factor and cytarabine. Neurology 28:794–797, 1978.

Vernon, M. L., Horta-Barbosa, L., Fucillo, D. A., Sever, J. L., Baringer, J. R., and Birnbaum, G.: Virus-like particles and nucleoprotein-type filaments in brain tissue from two patients with Creutzfeldt-Jakob disease. Lancet 1:964–966, 1970.

Weil, M. L., Itabashi, H. H., Cremer, N. E., Oshiro, L. S., Lennette, E. H., and Carnay, L.: Chronic progressive panencephalitis due to rubella virus simulating subacute sclerosing panencephalitis. New Eng. J. Med. 292:994–998, 1975.

Weiner, H. L., Cherry, J., and McIntosh, K.: Decreased lymphocyte transformation to vaccinia virus in multiple sclerosis. Neurology 28:415–420, 1978.

Weiner, L. P., Herndon, R. M., Narayan, O., Johnson, R. T., Shah, K., Rubinstein, L. J., Preziosi, T. J., and Conley, F. K.: Isolation of virus related to SV40 from patients with progressive multifocal leukoencephalopathy. New Eng. J. Med. 286:385–431, 1972.

Weiner, L. P., Johnson, R. T., and Herndon, R. M.: Viral infections and demyelinating diseases. New Eng. J. Med. 288:1103–1110, 1973.

Weiner, L. P., Narayan, O., Penney, J. B., Jr., Herndon, R. M., Feringa, E. R., Tourtellotte, W. W., and Johnson, R. T.: Papovavirus of JC type in progressive multifocal leukoencephalopathy. Rapid identification and subsequent isolation. Arch. Neurol. 29:1–3, 1973.

Westmoreland, B. F., Gomez, M. R., and Blume, W. T.: Activation of periodic complexes of subacute sclerosing panencephalitis by sleep. Ann. Neurol. 1:185–187, 1977.

Whitater, J. N., Sever, J. L., and Engel, W. K.: Subacute

sclerosing panencephalitis in only one of identical twins. New Eng. J. Med. 287:864–866, 1972.

Wilfert, C. M., Buckley, R. H., Mohanakumar, T., Griffith, J. F., Katz, S. L., Whisnant, J. K., Eggleston, P. A., Moore, M., Treadwell, E., Oxman, M. N., and Rosen, F. S.: Persistent and fatal central-nervous-system Echovirus infections in patients with agammaglobulinemia. New Eng. J. Med. 296:1485–1489, 1977.

Wolinsky, J. S., Berg, B. O., and Maitland, C. J.: Progressive rubella panencephalitis. Arch. Neurol. 33:722–723, 1976.

Wolinsky, J. S., Swoveland, P., Johnson, K. P., and Baringer, J. R.: Subacute measles encephalitis complicating Hodgkin's disease in an adult. Ann. Neurol. 1:452–457, 1977.

Woolsey, R. M., and Nelson, J. S.: Progressive multifocal leukoencephalopathy. Neurology 15:662–666, 1965.

Zlotnik, I., Grant, D. P., Dayan, A. D., and Earl, C. J.: Transmission of Creutzfeldt-Jakob disease from man to squirrel monkey. Lancet 2:435–438, 1974.

Zu Rhein, G. M., and Chou, S. M.: Particles resembling papova viruses in human cerebral demyelinating disease. Science 148:1477–1479, 1965.

Zu Rhein, G. M., Padgett, B. L., Walker, D. L., Chun, R. W. M., Horowitz, S. D., and Hong, R.: Progressive multifocal leukoencephalopathy in a child with severe combined immunodeficiency. New Eng. J. Med. 299:256–257, 1978.

Zu Rhein, G. M., and Varakis, J.: Progressive multifocal leukoencephalopathy in a renal-allograph recipient. New Eng. J. Med. 291:798, 1974.

Miscellaneous Infections of the Nervous System

Chapter Nineteen

FUNGAL INFECTIONS

Introduction

Medical mycology is a difficult category of infectious disease for most clinicians, primarily because of the complex taxonomy and the bewildering array of terms peculiar to the description of the morphologic characteristics and methods of reproduction of the organisms. Emmons et al. estimate that there are approximately 100 species of fungi recognized to be pathogenic to man, almost half of which cause diseases primarily of cutaneous and subcutaneous tissues. Classification of the fungi is not uniform from author to author and has been altered considerably with the passage of time. As the method of reproduction of certain fungi has been clarified, a number of fungi have been removed from one class and placed in another by recent authors (Emmons et al.). Members of the Actinomycetales are discussed among the fungi by tradition, largely because the diseases they produce resemble certain of the mycoses, but are more appropriately classified as bacteria. They form branched filaments like the higher filamentous fungi but their size is nearer that of true bacteria and they fragment readily into bacillary or coccoid elements. In addition, Actinomyces and Nocardia species are sensitive to penicillin and sulfonamides respectively, in contrast to the higher fungi. Among the Eumycotina, or true fungi, several species of the Phycomycetes (Zygomycetes) and Ascomycetes are pathogenic in man. Many human pathogens are also included in the class Deuteromycetes (Fungi Imperfecti) (Table 19–1).

The true fungi are microorganisms that are larger than bacteria and exist in two forms in tissue and culture, referred to as molds and yeasts, terms that are descriptive but have no taxonomic significance. Molds are represented by the filamentous form and are made up of tubular filaments that are sometimes branched and are called hyphae. The mold filaments may be divided into segments by transverse septa and are referred to as septate hyphae, characteristic of Aspergillus species. A notable feature of fungi of the class Phycomycetes is broad hyphae that are nonseptate. With continued growth of mold on artificial media, the hyphae branch, fuse, and result in a dense, dry mat of growth called the mycelium. The portion of the growth that extends above the substrate is referred to as the aerial mycelium. From the

Table 19–1. Fungi and Actinomycetes that Cause Neurologic Disease in Man

Actinomycetes
  Actinomyces
  Nocardia
Phycomycetes (Zygomycetes)
  Mucor
  Rhizopus
  Absidia
Ascomycetes
  Histoplasma
  Candida
  Blastomyces
  Allescheria (Petriellidium)
Basidiomycetes
  Cryptococcus neoformans
Deuteromycetes (Fungi imperfecti)
  Coccidioides
  Aspergillus
  Penicillium
  Cladosporium
  Sporothrix

hyphae of certain fungi specialized branches develop, which produce conidia and other types of spores.

Yeasts and yeast-like fungi are unicellular and mononucleated organisms which form moist or mucoid colonies in culture. They characteristically possess a thick cell wall, and, with Cryptococcus neoformans, the cell wall is surrounded by a well-defined capsule. Some yeasts reproduce asexually by a process by which a new cell is formed that is called a bud (blastospore), which then separates from the mother cell. When the blastospore fails to break free from the parent cell, it elongates and eventually produces another bud which undergoes the same process. This results in elongated budding structures referred to as pseudohyphae and is characteristic of Candida species but can be seen with other organisms as well. Reproduction of Coccidioides immitis in tissue is by a different mechanism in which endospores develop within the parent spherule, which, with maturity, gradually enlarges until rupture of the membrane of the spherule liberates young endospores into the adjacent tissue, each of which subsequently matures to form another endosporulating spherule.

Yeasts of importance causing neurologic disease in man include Cryptococcus neoformans, Histoplasma capsulatum, several Candida species, and, less commonly, Torulopsis glabrata and Blastomyces dermatitidis. A method of laboratory differentiation of yeast pathogens on the basis of the germ tube test, morphologic examination, and sugar assimilation and fermentation has recently been outlined by Dolan. Several fungi pathogenic for man are referred to as dimorphic, or diphasic, in that they are molds when grown on some artificial media at room temperature but yeast-like when seen in tissue. Examples of dimorphic fungi include Histoplasma capsulatum, Blastomyces dermatitidis, Coccidioides immitis, and Sporothrix schenckii. Cryptococcus neoformans is a budding yeast both in vivo and in vitro, while Aspergillus species are usually filamentous in vivo and in vitro.

Clinical Spectrum of Fungal Disease of the Nervous System

Except for cryptococcosis and coccidioidomycosis, fungal disease of the nervous system in past years was rarely observed or identified, and generally was considered in the class of medical curiosities. The growth of Neuropathology as a medical specialty, the prolongation of life in patients with metabolic and neoplastic diseases, the advent of organ transplantation, and the widespread use of corticosteroid, cytotoxic and antimetabolic drugs for such conditions has now radically changed the significance of human fungal infections. Additive factors enhancing secondary invasion in such patients include the administration of antibiotics or corticosteroids, or the presence of marked and persistent leukopenia, due to either the underlying disease or its treatment. Chronic corticosteroid therapy has been stressed by some authors as one of the most important factors predisposing the patient to disseminated fungal infection (Mirsky and Cuttner). Mechanisms of steroid action resulting in diminished resistance to infection include the suppression of reticuloendothelial function decreasing antibody synthesis, reduction in neutrophil migration to areas of inflammation, and the stabilization of lysosomal membranes, thus inhibiting release of catabolic enzymes.

Approximately 50 percent of patients with leukemia or lymphoma in some series have been found to have significant fungal infection of one type or another at autopsy (Gruhn and Sanson, Singer et al.). In a series of 51 autopsies on renal transplant patients, Rifkind et al. found 45 percent to have systemic fungal infections. Of 31 patients with cardiac transplants, 16 percent were identified to have fungal disease of the brain on postmortem examination (Schober and Herman). The terms "predisposed," "compromised," and "immunosuppressed" have now become applicable to individuals harboring a whole host of mycotic organisms and their effect on the brain.

Candida and Aspergillus species have become recognized to be the most common fungi invading the patient with leukemia or lymphoma, or complicating other conditions associated with immunosuppression. Cryptococcus neoformans, Nocardia species, Torulopsis glabrata, Cladosporium trichoides, Sporothrix schenckii, and, rarely, even Histoplasma capsulatum and Allescheria boydii are now exhibiting their opportunistic qualities as secondary invaders of the compromised and debilitated patient. Among cases of Cryptococcus infection of the central nervous system, it is estimated that 30 to 50 percent occur in predisposed hosts, especially those with leukemia, lymphoma, or diabetes mellitus. Members of the class Phycomycetes (Zygomycetes), especially genus Rhizopus and Mucor, are included in this enterprising list of fungi but show a greater tendency to invade the acidotic diabetic than the patient with malignancy. Coccidioidomycosis has traditionally been considered to be an infection in which the race of the infected patient is a more important factor in determining the severity of the illness than are immunologic defects secondary to an underlying disease or its treatment. This infection, also, has recently been shown to occur in the compromised host and is especially likely to result in disseminated disease in such persons (Deresinski and Stevens). With any of the fungi mentioned above, opportunistic infection can be confined to one locale, especially the respiratory tract, or it can be in the form of widespread, disseminated disease, with or without neurologic infiltration.

Deep-seated fungal infections in the otherwise normal individual are most often caused by Cryptococcus neoformans, Coccidioides immitis, Histoplasma capsulatum and Blastomyces dermatitidis, the latter two being rare causes of neurologic disease. In a consecutive autopsy series including all age groups Parker et al. found Candida species to be the single most common fungus identified within the brain. Candida species accounted for 49 percent of all cerebral mycoses, and was more than twice as common as Cryptococcus neoformans, the second most common offender.

The natural habitats, and thus the source, of many of the fungi that cause human disease are now known. Aspergillus species and members of the class Phycomycetes, order Mucorales, are ubiquitous saprophytes that are widespread in soil and decaying vegetable matter. Likewise, Sporothrix, Nocardia, and Allescheria are widespread in nature and readily accessible to humans. Histoplasma capsulatum exists in soil contaminated with bird droppings and Cryptococcus is found where pigeons contaminate the earth's surface. Coccidioides immitis resides in arid, desert regions where rainfall is limited and climatic temperatures are high, conditions especially common to the southwestern part of this country. Candida species are readily accessible, being commonly found inhabiting the human oral cavity, intestinal tract, or skin. Blastomyces dermatitidis has been a notable holdout among pathogenic fungi in regard to revealing its habitat in nature. It generally cannot be isolated from soil, does not normally inhabit the body in non-pathogenic fashion, and is not a common cause of disease in animals. Whether it is rare in nature or, more likely, simply elusive, remains to be seen.

Portal of entry and usual primary site of infection of the fungi described herein vary, but most enter the body by inhalation. Histoplasma capsulatum, Cryptococcus neoformans, Coccidioides immitis, Blastomyces dermatitidis, and Aspergillus species are all respiratory pathogens primarily. Histoplasma capsulatum is commonly disseminated during the initial, acute phase but does so in benign, self-limited fashion in the majority of cases. When spread occurs from the lungs with Cryptococcus or Coccidioides, the brain is the site of predilection. With Blastomyces dermatitidis, dissemination from the lung is most often to the skin or to bone, and only rarely to the central nervous system. When brain or spinal cord involvement does occur, it is either by hematogenous spread or by direct extension into the epidural space from overlying cranial or vertebral blastomycotic osteomyelitis. Mucorales also enters the body by respiratory inhalation but the nasal mucosa and paranasal sinuses represent additional primary sites of entry. Sporothrix is usually a primary pathogen of skin, introduced by direct inoculation in most cases. In the few reports of meningitis caused by this organism, the portal of entry has not been known, since disease elsewhere has not been present. Allescheria boydii is best known as one of many causes of cutaneous mycetoma (maduromycosis); however, when it attacks the compromised host, the initial involvement is usually within the lungs. Of the few reported cases of meningitis or brain abscess caused by Allescheria boydii, some, but not all, have complicated underlying immunocompromising disorders. Most cases of chromoblastomycosis also are primary cutaneous disorders, but in cases of meningitis due to Cladosporium trichoides, the organism's site of primary entry has not been clarified. Candida species can reach the brain from numerous sources since the organisms are readily available from a variety of sites and are especially prone to colonize intravascular catheters or other indwelling foreign bodies.

The tissue response within the brain following invasion by fungi varies somewhat with different organisms but includes a meningeal inflammatory reaction, multiple microabscesses, solitary abscess, granuloma formation, either multiple or solitary, and

Table 19–2. Types of Fungal Infections of the Nervous System

Meningitis (acute, subacute, chronic)
Meningoencephalitis
Abscess (solitary, multiple, microabscesses)
Granuloma (solitary, multiple, microgranuloma)
Arterial thrombosis (ischemic infarction)

infarctional lesions (Table 19–2). Combinations of these pathologic forms may develop secondary to infection with individual fungal agents. The characteristic feature of Mucorales infection is vascular invasion leading to thrombotic occlusion and ischemic infarction. Major vessels, such as the internal carotid artery or cavernous sinus, as well as more peripheral cerebral arterioles can be invaded by members of this Order. Direct cerebral infiltration can also occur with these non-septated organisms, with or without an associated in-

flammatory reaction. Aspergillus species and Penicillium also show a decided predisposition to invade vascular structures.

Meningitis of the subacute or chronic type can occur with many fungi but is the usual response to intracranial involvement with Cryptococcus neoformans, Coccidioides immitis, and Histoplasma capsulatum. Abscess formation—either microabscesses or larger suppurative lesions—is the customary reaction to Candida species, Nocardia, Actinomyces, and Aspergillus. Solitary cerebral or cerebellar granulomas have been described with infection caused by Cryptococcus, Coccidioides, Histoplasma, Nocardia, Actinomyces, and Aspergillus species. These solid lesions can be quite large, and when solitary, may simulate an intracranial neoplasm from the clinical standpoint. The most common type of central nervous system infection with blastomycosis is meningitis, although almost

Table 19–3. Disease and Form of Organism in Tissues

Actinomycosis—suppurative tissue reaction. Sulfur granules may be sparse in tissue. Sulfur granules with hematoxylin and eosin stain in the form of round bodies up to 300 μ in diameter with peripheral radiate structures. Gram-positive on gram stain, branched filaments.

Nocardiosis—narrow hyphae, 1μ or less in diameter, up to 25μ in length. Branched hyphae, often grouped in clusters. Hyphae not easily demonstrable by hematoxylin and eosin stain but are visualized by gram stains and methenamine silver stain.

Phycomycosis—short, broad, nonseptate hyphae that are haphazardly branched. Hyphae are variable in width, sometimes collapsed or partially distorted. Marked tendency for vascular invasion. Hyphae usually very well stained with hematoxylin and eosin stain, less well delineated by special stains.

Aspergillosis—broad, septate hyphae, dichotomous branching in "tree-like" fashion. Hyphae often irregularly stained, smaller in diameter than hyphae of Phycomycetes. The characteristic fruiting body, the conidiophore, not seen in brain tissue but can be observed in pulmonary cavities.

Cryptococcosis—oval, budding yeast of variable size, 2–15μ in diameter, distinctive thick, mucoid capsule, A clear halo sometimes separates the yeast from the cytoplasm of the cell in which it is contained. Hyphae not seen, pseudohyphae can occasionally be observed.

Candidiasis—yeast usually readily identified within cerebral granulomata or microabscesses with he-

matoxylin and eosin stain and with Gridley stain. Round or oval blastospores, 2–4μ in diameter. Pseudohyphae of variable length.

Torulopsiasis—clumped yeast, oval or round cells with pseudohyphae.

Histoplasmosis—oval budding yeast with a rigid cell wall. Yeast measures 2–5μ in diameter and presents a distinct pseudocapsule resulting from retraction of the protoplasm away from the cell wall during fixation. Organisms are especially seen within macrophages or reticuloendothelial cells.

Coccidioidomycosis—large spherical cells (spherules) within granulomas. Mature spherule containing endospores often seen in tissue with methenamine silver or Gridley stains.

Blastomycosis—yeast, 8–15μ in diameter with well-defined cell wall. Protoplasm often retracted away from the wall, leaving a small clear space. Single bud with a broad-based attachment often seen.

Sporotrichosis—difficult to demonstrate in histologic sections. Yeast within microabscesses or granulomas. Asteroid body is the most distinctive feature but is rarely observed. Asteroid consists of a central, oval, yeast-like structure bounded by a substance with a radiate periphery.

Cladosporiosis—round or oval yeast forms approximately 10μ in diameter, some with budding and some with hyphae with distinct cross walls, and infrequent or no branching. A dimorphic fungus.

equally common is the total number of cases of cerebral, cerebellar, or brain stem abscess or granuloma, or cerebral or spinal epidural abscess.

The microscopic form the fungus assumes in brain tissue is important because of its diagnostic implications (Table 19–3). Although absolute diagnosis depends on cultural morphology, direct histologic examination of fungi in tissue or pus can provide a presumptive diagnosis in many instances, especially when the findings are correlated with the clinical information and the presence of mycotic disease elsewhere. Many fungi that infect the nervous system can be easily seen with the conventional hematoxylin and eosin preparations, but some are better demonstrated with Grocott's silver methenamine stain, the Gridley stain, or the periodic acid–Schiff stain. Hyphae of the Phycomycetes are an exception in this regard in that they are well defined with the hematoxylin and eosin stain but poorly demonstrated by the customary special stains. The India ink examination is an important tool for identification of Cryptococcus neoformans in cerebrospinal fluid.

Other diagnostic methods such as skin tests or serologic reactions are generally of limited value in the patient with systemic or neurologic fungal disease. The histoplasmin skin test is useful to survey large numbers of persons for evidence of prior infection but should be avoided as a diagnostic method with acute disease. The blastomycin skin test is negative in most patients with widespread blastomycosis and, therefore, is also of little value. Likewise, the skin test in patients with coccidioidal meningitis is very often non-reactive during the acute stage of the illness.

Serologic diagnostic tests are valuable in histoplasmosis, including the complement fixation reaction to yeast and mycelial phase antigens, and the determination of precipitin bands to histoplasmin antigen. Precipitin and complement-fixing antibodies in serum and cerebrospinal fluid are also of diagnostic importance in patients with coccidioidal meningitis. Countercurrent immunoelectrophoresis is an additional method that shows promise for the diagnosis of a variety of forms of coccidioidomycosis (Aguilar-Torres et al.). Determination of cryptococcal polysaccharide antigen in blood or cerebrospinal fluid by the complement fixation test has reasonable reliability and is now widely utilized. Complement fixation tests have not been rewarding for the diagnosis of infections caused by Blastomyces dermatitidis.

Treatment

The treatment regimen of the patient with a central nervous system fungal infection is usually a long-term affair, using potentially

Table 19–4. Sample Flow Sheet—Treatment with Amphotericin B

NAME OF PATIENT—AGE 15 YEARS
WT. IN KILOGRAMS—70
DATE OF ONSET OF TREATMENT—15 MAY, 1980

	Amph. B (mg./dose IV)	Amph. B (mg. total to date)	Urinalysis	BUN-Cr.	Serum Electrolytes	Hb-Plat. Count	CSF	CSF Cryptococcal Antigen
June 1	35	500	Cells: 0 Protein: 0	20–1.8	Na 138 Cl 102 K 3.8	14–200,000		
June 2	35	535	Cells: 4 Protein: 0	20–1.6			OP 180 Cells 28 Protein 210 Glucose 30 India ink(-)	1/16
June 3	35	570	Cells: 4 Protein: trace	22–2.0	Na 136 Cl 102 K 3.8	14–200,000		
June 4								
June 5								
June 6								

toxic antimicrobial drugs, and is one which requires the skills of persons in a variety of medical disciplines. These aspects, as well as the need for specialized laboratory facilities capable of performing the appropriate serologic tests, sensitivity tests on organisms isolated, and certain neuroradiologic procedures, indicate the desirability for the management of such patients to be in a referral medical center.

The antifungal drugs are generally notable for their potential toxicity on either the hematopoietic system or the kidneys. Periodic laboratory examinations should be performed to anticipate the occurrence of such adverse effects. Because of the long duration of treatment of these infections, the laboratory results as well as the details of the drug regimen should be graphically charted on a flow sheet to enable rapid observation of the status of the treatment program and its complications (Table 19–4). The cerebrospinal fluid should be examined at frequent intervals, as this provides one of the best indices of the progress of the illness. The frequent occurrence of hydrocephalus, especially with cryptococcal and coccidioidal infections, warrants the performance of cranial computed tomography at one- or two-week intervals. Should hydrocephalus occur and become progressive, some type of diversionary procedure is frequently indicated.

The antifungal agents most widely used at present include amphotericin B, 5-fluorocytosine, and miconazole (Table 19–5). Amphotericin B has the broadest spectrum and is generally regarded to be the mainstay of antifungal therapy despite its nephrotoxic qualities. Five-fluorocytosine possesses a more narrow spectrum of activity and is ordinarily used in combination with amphotericin B for cryptococcal and candida neurologic infections. Miconazole is usually reserved for susceptible organisms that have proved to be treatment failures with the other drugs. Sulfonamides, sulfonamides in combination with cycloserine, or trimethoprim-sulfamethoxazole are used for nocardial infections, while penicillin is the drug of choice for infections caused by Actinomyces species. In rare instances, surgical treatment in concert with drug therapy is indicated. Fungal epidural or large cerebral abscesses can be aspirated and solitary granulomatous lesions of large size can occasionally be excised.

The use of transfer factor, a dialyzable extract of immune white blood cells capable of transferring delayed-type hypersensitivity, is

Table 19–5. Drugs Used for Treatment of Central Nervous System Fungal Infections

Amphotericin B
Cryptococcus neoformans
Coccidioides immitis
Candida species
Histoplasma capsulatum
Mucorales (order)
Blastomyces dermatitidis
Sporotrichum schenckii
Aspergillus species (?)
5-Fluorocytosine
Cryptococcus neoformans
Candida species
Cladosporium trichoides
Torulopsis glabrata (?)
Aspergillus species (?)
Miconazole
Cryptococcus neoformans
Coccidioides immitis
Allescheria boydii
Candida species
Sulfonamides
Nocardia asteroides
Penicillin
Actinomyces israelii, bovis

in the investigational stage as a method of treatment of certain intractable fungal infections and has shown promise for coccidioidal, cryptococcal, and candida infections (Feigin et al., Gross et al., Steele et al.).

Amphotericin B. Amphotericin B was discovered in 1956 and since has been the drug of choice for numerous invasive fungal infections. The drug is a polyene antibiotic with a mechanism of action which involves binding to ergosterol of the fungal cell membrane, thus resulting in an increased permeability of the cell membrane leading to leakage of intracellular contents and eventual death of the cell. To enhance the solubility of the compound, the commercial preparation of amphotericin B (Fungisone) contains sodium deoxycholate. The preparation for intravenous use cannot be mixed with saline but is diluted with 5 percent dextrose in water, with the concentration of the drug being not greater than one mg. per 10 ml. of fluid. The solution should be used promptly after preparation, although little decomposition appears to occur during the 4- to 6-hour infusion period. Peak serum levels persist for at least 6 to 8 hours following the intravenous infusion of the drug and then usually decline to approximately one-half the initial level by 24 hours (Drutz et al.). Amphotericin B methyl ester is considerably more water-soluble and less nephrotoxic than amphotericin B; however, its antifungal action is believed to be less than that of the parent compound (Huston and Hoeprich).

Although amphotericin B is the single most widely used and most effective drug available for treatment of most fungal infections of the nervous system, it has major disadvantages in being a highly toxic drug and one in which there is limited penetration into the CSF and brain when given systemically. It is known that amphotericin B has a very slow disappearance rate from serum and urine after a single dose or following termination of therapy. The route of excretion of the drug, how much tissue storage occurs, or whether there is metabolic conversion to other yet undetected compounds remains unclear. A certain amount of the drug has been shown to be excreted in the urine and via the biliary system but the fate of approximately 60 to 70 percent of an administered dose remains undetermined (Atkinson and Bennett, Craven et al.).

For most fungal infections of the central nervous system, amphotericin B is first administered intravenously, at least until it is shown that this route is not adequate or until its use must be curtailed because of toxic effects. With coccidioidal meningitis, however, it is necessary to give the drug both intravenously and intrathecally. Recommendations for intravenous use have varied considerably but, in general, the dose and duration of therapy have been largely determined by the toxicity of the drug, and especially the nephrotoxicity. The most widely used regimen is initiation of therapy with an intravenous dose of 0.1 mg. per kilogram per day for mildly ill patients and 0.25 mg. per kilogram per day for those more severely affected, with each infusion being given over a 4- to 6-hour period. The daily dose is gradually increased to a maximum of 1.0 mg. per kilogram per day by 10 to 14 days. Relatively few adults will tolerate a dose of 1.0 mg. per kilogram per day and, in most, progressive compromise in renal function will require a reduction in the dose or temporary discontinuation of therapy. When therapy is resumed, the dose administered is usually in the range of 0.5 to 0.6 mg. per kilogram per day, which is often the maximum level that can be tolerated. Some seem to do better on doses of 0.6 to 0.8 mg. per kilogram given every second day, and experience improvement clinically and by laboratory testing in regard to the status of the infection.

Drutz et al. designed a therapeutic regimen in which the dose of amphotericin B was based on serum level determinations. The goal of therapy was to give sufficient amphotericin B to achieve a peak serum level that was twice the in vitro sensitivity of the most resistant fungi isolated in their series. The serum level required was 1.56 micrograms per ml. and this was achieved in most by the administration of 20 to 40 mg. of amphotericin B, an amount which presumably would be 0.3 to 0.6 mg. per kilogram per day. The clinical and laboratory response to treatment by this method was favorable and toxicity was minimized, suggesting perhaps that lower doses of the drug might be adequate than are generally assumed. Using this method, the authors arbitrarily chose a total duration of therapy of 10 weeks, rather than determining the duration on the basis of a predetermined total dosage. The alternate approach is to give the drug until a fixed, total quantity has been administered, such as a cumulative dose of 1,500 to 2,000 mg. per 1.7 square meters of body surface.

Except in the special instance of treatment of coccidioidal meningitis, intrathecal amphotericin B is usually reserved for certain patients seriously ill at the onset of therapy, especially those who for other reasons already have compromised renal function, for those patients who show an inadequate response to a reasonable trial with intravenous therapy, and those who continue to relapse after an adequate course of intravenous therapy. The initial intrathecal injection should be a test dose in the adult of 0.1 mg. or less to be certain that the drug is tolerated. Thereafter, the intrathecal dose of amphotericin B in the adult is 0.25 to 0.5 mg. mixed in 5 ml. of distilled water or spinal fluid and administered slowly every other day. Alazraki et al. have advised the intrathecal use of a hyperbaric solution of amphotericin B in 10 percent dextrose in water, with the patient placed in the Trendelenburg position after its injection. The increased density of the solution along with the head-down position was advised to improve transport of the drug through the spinal canal and to the basilar cisterns, the usual site of dense exudate in most fungal infections of the nervous system. To minimize side effects, some authors recommend the addition of 15 mg. of hydrocortisone to the mixture to be injected intrathecally.

Adverse reactions to lumbar intrathecal amphotericin B are common and sometimes sufficiently severe to require discontinuation of this route of administration. Pain in the back or legs, or aseptic meningitis with meningeal signs are the most common complications, while arachnoiditis can be the most devastating. A subcutaneous reservoir for direct intraventricular instillation of the drug has been used but it, too, has been beset with numerous and limiting complications (Diamond and Bennett, Graybill and Ellenbogen). Amphotericin B administered intrathecally is removed from the CSF by bulk flow through the arachnoid villi (Atkinson and Bindschadler). Even in the absence of systemically administered amphotericin B, that injected into the CSF will gain entrance into the circulation and can contribute to systemic toxic effects.

Toxic effects of systemically administered amphotericin B are both numerous and common and often require a compromise in the dosage that can safely be given. Immediate reactions frequently observed include chills, fever, nausea, and vomiting. Febrile reactions to the drug can often be successfully managed by pre-medication with diphenhydramine, and vomiting can be curtailed with the use of chlorpromazine. Hypokalemia is occasionally observed but can be corrected by supplemental oral potassium intake. More troublesome are phlebitis at the site of injection, anemia, and nephrotoxicity (Utz et al.). Phlebitis can be prevented in some instances by the addition of heparin in dose of 5 mg. to the infusion. Reactions that are less common but serious are those considered idiosyncratic such as anaphylactoid shock, acute hepatic failure, convulsions, ventricular fibrillation, and cardiac arrest.

Anemia is a frequent side effect of chronic amphotericin B therapy and is of the normocytic, normochromic type believed by some to be secondary to reversible bone marrow suppression (Butler). More recent studies suggest that amphotericin B produces anemia by inhibiting erythropoietin production rather than by direct suppression on bone marrow activity (MacGregor et al.). Anemia is usually of limited severity and in most cases does not curtail treatment. In certain instances, however, the degree of hemoglobin drop may be sufficient to require blood transfusion (Wilson and Feldman).

Nephrotoxicity secondary to amphotericin B is the greatest deterrent to its effective use (Iovine et al., Cherry et al.). In the series reported by Utz et al., over 80 percent of patients developed abnormalities of renal function and many retained decreased renal function after termination of therapy.

Among 24 children described by Wilson and Feldman, 23 developed azotemia during treatment with amphotericin B, but in none was it necessary to discontinue therapy more than temporarily. Because of the predilection for renal toxicity, urine examination and renal function tests should be done at frequent intervals during the course of treatment. Renal impairment is detected by the appearance of red or white blood cells in the urine, casts in the urine, a rising blood urea nitrogen and creatinine, or a decrease in creatinine clearance. When renal impairment develops, it is usually managed by administration of the drug on alternate days instead of daily or by complete cessation of therapy for a few days until laboratory evidence of improvement is established. The adjustment of dosage in the patient who develops compromised renal function is best determined by the results of blood level determinations.

Five-fluorocytosine. Five-fluorocytosine is a fluorinated pyrimidine first shown to have antifungal activity in mice in 1964 (Grunberg et al.). The drug is well absorbed when given orally and has excellent penetration into the CSF, resulting in CSF levels approximately 50 to 70 percent of the serum level. Approximately 90 percent of the orally administered dose is excreted unchanged in the urine. The mode of its intracellular action is not fully understood, although within cells of sensitive fungi the compound is converted to 5-fluorouracil. Recent studies have indicated that conversion of 5-fluorocytosine to 5-fluorouracil also occurs within human cells and may account for its toxic manifestations in certain patients (Diasio et al.).

The role of 5-fluorocytosine in the treatment of invasive fungal infections remains controversial. Its spectrum of activity is narrow, primarily including activity against Cryptococcus neoformans, Candida species, and Torulopsis glabrata (Fass and Perkins, Vandevelde et al.). Because of the frequent occurrence of pretreatment resistance of Candida species to 5-fluorocytosine in addition to the common development of resistance of Cryptococcus neoformans during treatment, the drug is seldom used alone but generally is combined with amphotericin B. The combination has successfully eradicated candida meningitis in newborn and young infants (Chesney et al., Lilien et al.). Montgomerie and colleagues demonstrated synergism of amphotericin B and 5-fluorocytosine, even among Candida strains that were highly resistant to 5-fluorocytosine. The combination of the two drugs is also recommended for moderately or seriously ill patients with cryptococcal meningitis (Bennett et al., Harder and Hermans, Utz et al.). The theoretical advantage of the combination is the synergism that has been partly attributed to the ability of amphotericin B to increase the permeability of yeast cell membranes to 5-fluorocytosine, allowing a reduction of the dose of amphotericin B and thereby reducing its nephrotoxicity.

Because 5-fluorocytosine is almost entirely excreted by the kidneys, compromise of renal function will result in high serum levels unless the dose is appropriately adjusted (Dawborn et al.). While blood level determinations are important in all patients so that the oral dose can be altered to result in serum levels of 60 to 80 micrograms per ml., they are imperative when 5-fluorocytosine is used in combination with amphotericin B. This is because of the common occurrence of nephrotoxicity associated with amphotericin B therapy, which will require reduction of the dose of 5-fluorocytosine so that levels will be retained within the desired range. When renal function is intact, the usual oral dose of 5-fluorocytosine is 100 to 150 mg. per kilogram per day in four divided doses with adjustments being made to keep the serum level in the therapeutic range.

Adverse effects of 5-fluorocytosine are less frequent than with amphotericin B, although fatal aplastic anemia has been described (Bryan and McFarland, Meyer and Axelrod). The mechanism of bone marrow suppression is unclear but is believed to be related to the blood level and is seen with levels exceeding 125 micrograms per ml. (Kauffman and Frame). In most instances, evidence of marrow suppression is reversible following reduction of the dose or discontinuation of the drug. Other side effects include diarrhea, hallucinations, and hepatic dysfunction reflected by laboratory studies.

Miconazole. Miconazole is an imidazole derivative which is sparingly soluble in water, highly protein-bound, and has broad-spectrum, membrane-active antifungal activity. First described in 1972 (Brugmans et al., Van Cutsem and Thienpont), the drug represents the most recent important addition to the available antimicrobials for treatment of certain central nervous system fungal infections. The mechanism of action of miconazole is the inhibition of purine transport and cell-wall synthesis. The drug has been used mainly for patients with sensitive invasive fungal infections that have not responded to adequate trials with amphotericin B or in patients who cannot tolerate amphotericin B. Miconazole is effective against Coccidioides immitis, Cryptococcus neoformans, Histoplasma capsulatum, and Candida species (Deresinski et al., Stevens et al., Sung et al.). It is, perhaps, the drug of choice for serious infections caused by Allescheria (Petriellidium) boydii.

Because of the poor CSF penetration of miconazole when given systemically, treatment of most fungal infections of the nervous system requires intrathecal administration. The most commonly recommended intravenous dose is 30 mg. per kilogram per day given in divided doses every eight hours over approximately 30 minutes. In the first day of treatment, the dose should be reduced to approximately 20 percent of the recommended dose to be certain it is tolerated. The intrathecal dose for the adult is 20 mg. Side effects are generally mild and include nausea, anemia, increase or decrease of the platelet count, pruritic skin eruptions, phlebitis, and hyperlipidemia (Bagnarello et al., Drutz and Catanzaro). In an evaluation of 183 patients treated with miconazole, nausea or vomiting or both occurred in 25 percent, and central nervous system toxicity including tremors, confusion, dizziness, or seizures were described in 16 percent (Jordon et al.).

CRYPTOCOCCAL MENINGOENCEPHALITIS

Cryptococcosis is a cosmopolitan infectious disorder with a decided predisposition for central nervous system involvement in the form of a subacute or chronic meningoencephalitis. The causative organism is Cryptococcus neoformans (Torula histolytica), which is a budding, encapsulated yeast that exists as a saprophyte in nature and is capable of producing disease in a variety of animals as well as in man. The presence of the capsule is important for the morphologic diagnosis of this organism in tissue and fluid specimens, and may also play a role in its virulence by bringing about inhibition of phagocytosis of the yeast cell by leukocytes (Bulmer and Sans). Cryptococcus neoformans is widely identified in soil and has been found abundantly in pigeon and other avian excreta, a probable source of some human infections.

The respiratory tract is believed to be the portal of entry of most cases. When hematogenous dissemination occurs therefrom, it is usually to the nervous system although, less commonly, other viscera may also be affected. Skeletal involvement is infrequent but can occur with disseminated cryptococcosis, and can rarely be the only site of extrapulmonary infection (Poliner et al.). An unusual example of the possible widespread dissemination of this disease is the two-year-old child described by Siewers and Cramblett in whom lymph nodes, lungs, liver, spleen, and bone marrow were affected. An additional rare expression of the disease is multiple lymph node involvement, referred to as lymphonodular cryptococcosis, in the absence of pulmonary or central nervous system infection (Fusner and McClain).

Among patients with cryptococcal meningoencephalitis, pulmonary involvement may have been present earlier but healed, may be asymptomatic but evident roentgenographically, or, less often, can be both symptomatic and apparent on x-ray. Roentgenographically, invasive pulmonary cryptococcosis is characterized by a predilection for involvement of the lower lobes of the lung, only infrequent cavitation, little tendency for calcification, and inconspicuous hilar lymphadenopathy. Recent clinical observations suggest that Cryptococcus neoformans is possibly a common saprophyte of the tracheobronchial tree and that many persons harbor the organism in a completely benign fashion (Tynes et al., Warr et al.). In addition, certain pulmonary diseases may predispose to the development of this fungus in the tracheobronchial tree, such as chronic bronchitis, tuberculosis, and pulmonary alveolar proteinosis (Sunderland et al.). In patients with symptomatic pulmonary cryptococcosis without clinical evidence of other organ system disease, studies should include culture on appropriate media of blood, urine, and cerebrospinal fluid. Isolation of Cryptococcus neoformans from these specimens is considered evidence of serious disease even in the absence of symptoms (Tynes et al.).

Cryptococcal meningoencephalitis spares no age group but is uncommon in the first decade of life. Eighty to 85 percent of cases are between 20 and 60 years of age and approximately 70 percent of reported cases have been males (Butler et al., Edwards et al.). In children, especially, past reports of cryptococcosis of the central nervous system have largely been in those without predisposing disease. When all age groups are considered, estimates have varied widely but it is generally believed that an immunosuppressive or debilitating condition is present in 30 to 50 percent of cases in this country (Butler et al., Diamond and Bennett, Sarosi et al., Tay et al.). Hodgkin's disease and leukemia are the most common malignant diseases in which there is an enhanced susceptibility, while diabetes mellitus and collagen-vascular disease are the most common non-neoplastic disorders with an increased risk to this infection. Immunosuppression following renal transplantation is an additional predisposing cause of cryptococcal meningoencephalitis (Schröter et al.). Chronic corticosteroid therapy for any purpose, but especially in patients with debilitating disease, increases the danger of invasive cryptococcal infection. In addition, cryptococcosis can occur in a patient with another fungal disease, such as disseminated histoplasmosis (Morris et al.) or candidiasis (Spicer et al.).

Clinical Manifestations

Neurologic infection with Cryptococcus neoformans in most instances is a subacute or chronic meningoencephalitis, similar to that caused by the tubercle bacillus but generally with a more protracted clinical course. It is usually a gradually progressive disease although some cases may show remissions and exacerbations, even without therapy. A much less common form is characterized by signs of a focal expanding mass, possibly simulating either cerebral abscess or neoplasm (Hassin). Although most reported cases have been in the adult age group, cryptococcosis of the nervous system should be considered to be unusual but not rare in children (Emanuel et al., McDonald et al., Siewers and Cramblett). In all age groups, the illness has been recognized with increasing frequency in recent years and is judged to be the most common type of mycotic meningitis in otherwise normal, or non-immunosuppressed, individuals (Littman and Walker, Rose et al.).

The patient with cryptococcal meningoencephalitis has symptoms of insidious onset followed by gradual worsening. Most are symptomatic for several weeks or a few months before diagnosis is made. Exceptional cases are well known in which the disease has persisted for one or more years, repeatedly defying or escaping diagnostic efforts. The most remarkable example of the possible chronicity of neurologic cryptococcosis is the case described by Beeson, which extended over a 16-year period in the pre-amphotericin B era.

Headache is the most common initial complaint. It gradually becomes more persistent and severe, and is associated with nausea, vomiting, lethargy, and weight loss. As the illness worsens, mental symptoms including memory loss and disorientation are added to the earlier complaints. Ocular abnormalities of one type or another frequently develop during evolution of the disease and were present in 40 percent in the series of 40 cases described by Butler et al. Some patients experience blurred vision, diplopia, or photophobia. Either optic atrophy or papilledema may be found, or more localizing deficits such as internuclear ophthalmoplegia (Gonyea and Heilman), indicative of brain stem involvement. Low-grade fever is intermittently present but is not a prominent feature of the illness. Children often respond with greater temperature elevations than adults but the illness can run its course with only modest temperature elevations. Likewise, clear-cut signs of meningeal irritation are present in fewer than half of all patients with cryptococcal meningoencephalitis (Edwards et al.). As symptoms progress, a variety of neurologic signs often appear, including hemiparesis or hyperreflexia, facial paralysis, or recurrent convulsions. Unless the diagnosis is established and treatment begun, leth-

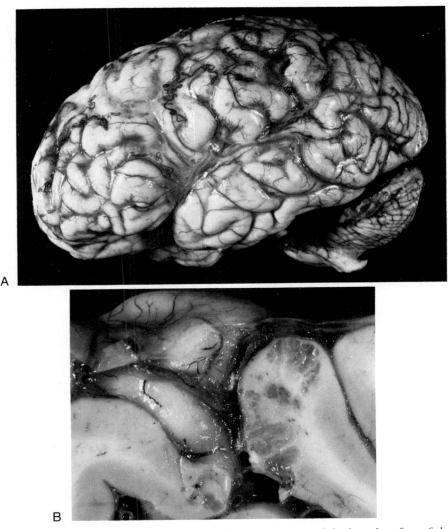

Figure 19–1. Cryptococcal meningoencephalitis. *A,* Gross appearance of the lateral surface of the left cerebral hemisphere. Gelatinous, glistening leptomeningeal thickening with exudate is present, best seen in the region of the Sylvian fissure. *B,* Expansile lesions in the cerebral cortex replacing normal tissue. These areas are heavily yeast-laden on microscopic examination. Note the thickened leptomeninges containing exudate.

argy proceeds to coma, and death eventually ensues. Although headache, lethargy, papilledema and other pressure signs can be accounted for on the basis of brain swelling and the meningeal inflammatory response, certain patients with this disease develop communicating hydrocephalus, which compounds the problem and is not likely to be recognized unless specifically searched for (Edwards et al., Tay et al.). Hydrocephalus is presumed to be secondary to the gelatinous basilar exudate characteristic of this disease and can be a significant factor leading to clinical deterioration and eventual death.

Much less often, cryptococcal infection of the nervous system presents with symptoms of an expanding mass due to a localized cryptococcal granuloma or abscess. Lesions of this

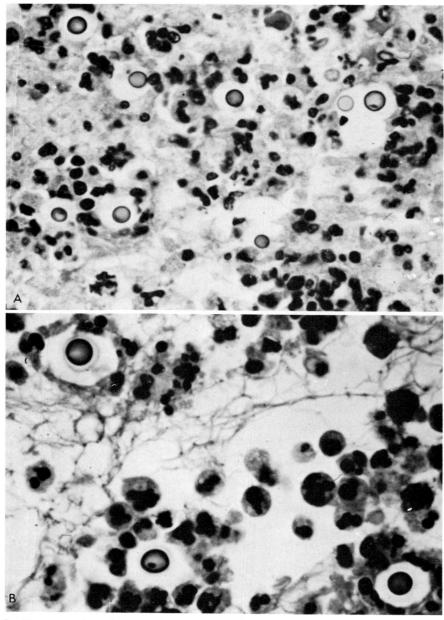

Figure 19–2. Cryptococcal meningoencephalitis. *A* and *B*, Cryptococcus neoformans is a circular encapsulated yeast surrounded by a broad, clear halo. Many darkly stained inflammatory cells are present.

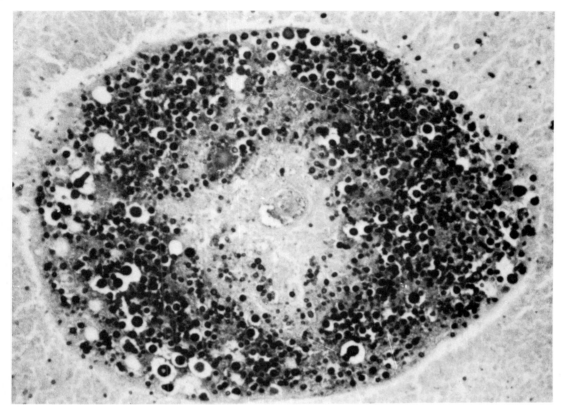

Figure 19–3. Cryptococcal meningoencephalitis. Clusters of cryptococci of variable size are located in perivascular space within brain tissue. Note the clear halo encircling many of the yeast cells and the relative absence of an inflammatory reaction surrounding the collection of organisms.

type can be either single or multiple and may or may not be associated with evidence of meningeal involvement (Roberts et al., Selby and Lopes, Vijayan et al.). In addition to gradually increasing intracranial pressure, the manifestations of intracranial cryptococcal granulomas are those of progressive focal deficits and recurrent seizures, depending on the location of the lesion. Such patients can be assumed to have a cerebral neoplasm or pyogenic abscess, with the correct diagnosis being established only after craniotomy and biopsy or removal of the lesion. Focal cryptococcal granuloma has also been described within the spinal cord and cauda equina (Skultety).

The neuropathology of cryptococcal meningoencephalitis in fatal cases is variable, but in some cases gross observation of the brain reveals few abnormalities. In others, diffuse or localized meningeal opacification is present in addition to small tubercle-like nodules on the cortical surface, and ventricular distention of mild or moderate degree (Fig.

19–1). Histologically, one finds meningeal infiltration with cryptococci which are oval or circular encapsulated yeast-like organisms five to 15 microns in diameter, usually well demonstrated by the periodic acid–Schiff stain or the Gomori methenamine silver stain (Fig. 19–2). The mucicarmine stain is particularly useful to demonstrate the capsular material of the organism, which stains bright red on this preparation. Clusters of cryptococci are seen lodged in bubble-like cavities within the brain, which in many instances represent distended perivascular spaces (Fig. 19–3). These cystic spaces may be sufficiently large to be identified on gross observation or so small that they can be recognized only microscopically. A characteristic feature in tissue is the presence of a clear halo surrounding the organism, sometimes as broad as the diameter of the fungus itself. Cellular reaction to the infection is minimal in some cases, either in the meninges or the brain, and when present, consists of perivascular infiltration with lymphocytes, macrophages, and plasma cells. Masses of cryptococci are frequently seen in distended Virchow-Robin spaces adjacent to the cortical surface.

Differential Diagnosis

Cryptococcal meningoencephalitis resembles a number of disorders associated with a progressive course and a lymphocytic pleocytosis in the cerebrospinal fluid. When it develops in a patient with an underlying predisposing disease such as malignancy or diabetes mellitus, the infectious process can be obscured by or confused with the manifestations of the primary or predisposing illness. The greatest diagnostic difficulty is the differentiation of cryptococcal disease of the nervous system from tuberculous meningitis. Symptoms and signs are similar in the two disorders, although the rate of progression is usually somewhat more rapid in patients with tuberculous meningitis. The greater tendency for pulmonary tuberculosis to involve the upper lobes and cryptococcosis to affect the lower lobes of the lungs is of less diagnostic value in the child than in the adult. With either disease, the chest x-ray can be entirely normal or cryptococcal meningitis can occur in one with pulmonary tuberculosis (Emanuel et al.). Furthermore, the cerebrospinal fluid alterations are virtually the same in the two illnesses, and, in both, identification or isolation of the causative organism can be difficult or require several weeks.

Medulloblastoma or ependymoma of the fourth ventricle in the child on rare occasion is associated with a cellular pleocytosis, neck stiffness, and a gradually deteriorating course due to increased intracranial pressure, which can be confused with a subacute infectious process. It is even possible for the cerebrospinal fluid glucose content to be reduced in such cases, although this is the unusual exception. Other neoplastic diseases which enter the differential diagnosis of cryptococcal meningitis include diffuse meningeal invasion with metastatic carcinoma or melanoma. The less common form of cryptococcal neurologic disease in which focal signs result from a localized cryptococcal granuloma resembles either a cerebral or cerebellar glioma or pyogenic abscess and often can be differentiated only by tissue examination.

Cryptococcal meningitis and sarcoidosis of the nervous system have many clinical features in common but, in children, neurologic involvement with sarcoidosis is unusual. An

other disorder that can resemble a subacute granulomatous meningitis is granulomatous angiitis of the brain. This rare illness is believed to be an autoimmune condition which primarily affects adults (Sandhu et al.). It is an inflammatory process of blood vessels of the brain and results in progressive neurologic deterioration with signs of diffuse cerebral dysfunction along with a CSF lymphocytic pleocytosis and increased protein content in most cases (Kolodny et al.). Diagnosis depends on microscopic examination of brain tissue. The clinical course can be similar to that of cryptococcal meningoencephalitis, which is excluded on the basis of negative stains and cultures of the CSF and the absence of CSF polysaccharide antigen. Partially treated pyogenic meningitis is an additional condition that might cause diagnostic confusion but can usually be differentiated on the basis of the history of the illness and response to intravenous antibiotic therapy.

Laboratory Diagnosis

Cryptococcal disease of the central nervous system is suspected in the patient with a subacute and progressive illness in whom the signs point to a diffuse cerebral process in association with signs of increased intracranial pressure. History of exposure to pigeons, the existence of an underlying predisposing disease, and the presence of an inflammatory pulmonary illness are further points suggestive of cryptococcal meningoencephalitis. The white blood cell count can be either normal or elevated, as can the erythrocyte sedimentation rate.

Cerebrospinal fluid examination is one of the most valuable diagnostic procedures, but findings are subject to variation from patient to patient, or even in the same patient on serial examinations. In rare instances the cerebrospinal fluid is normal or shows only a few cells but with a modest increase in the protein content. In most, however, the opening pressure is elevated, the fluid is clear or turbid on gross observation and contains 40 to 1,000 cells, with an average of 150 to 300 cells per cu. mm. The cellular response is mainly lymphocytic but early in the course of the disease neutrophils may temporarily predominate. Elevation of the protein content is one of the more constant findings, with ranges between 60 and 400 mg. per 100 ml. in most cases. Cerebrospinal fluid glucose values are reduced to 10 to 40 mg. per 100 ml. in the majority, but normal glucose levels are not inconsistent with the diagnosis. Although there is limited information yet available about CSF lactic acid levels in cryptococcal meningitis, the few reports that do exist indicate that the CSF lactic acid content is increased in this disease (Brook et al., Komorowski et al.). The diagnostic value of this determination in fungal disease of the nervous system is not clear, but it may prove to be useful as a guide to the degree of response to treatment, in conjunction with other CSF studies. Demonstration of alcohol in the cerebrospinal fluid has been recommended as a diagnostic method for cryptococcal meningoencephalitis (Dawson and Taghavy); however, other yeasts produce alcohol, and strains of Cryptococcus neoformans vary markedly in alcohol production (Louria). For these reasons the test is no longer considered diagnostically useful.

The most rapid diagnostic method is the demonstration of the fungus in cerebrospinal fluid by the India ink preparation. Since Cryptococcus neoformans is the only oval, encapsulated yeast-like organism to invade the brain, its identification by the India ink method virtually confirms the diagnosis. Failure to identify cryptococci with India ink preparations, even on several CSF specimens, does not exclude the possibility of the disease. Of 35 patients with cryptococcal meningitis reported by Butler et al., the organism was found on direct smear of the CSF in only 57 percent. Large volume CSF specimens, as much as 30 ml., are more likely to yield positive results on smear and culture than small volume specimens, and in some instances, cisternal or ventricular fluid samples will be positive when lumbar fluid is negative (Gonyea). In cases in which cryptococcal meningitis is strongly suspected from the clinical standpoint but the diagnosis cannot be proved by examination of lumbar CSF, a cisternal tap should be considered, but only performed after computed tomography has been done to be certain that advanced hydrocephalus is not present. If hydrocephalus is definitely present, a shunt is probably indicated and ventricular fluid specimens can be obtained when the procedure is done.

The India ink examination is performed by placing one 3-millimeter loopful of India ink on a clean glass slide, mixed with one loopful of sterile distilled water. The CSF specimen is centrifuged for 15 minutes and a drop of the sediment is mixed on the slide with the diluted India ink. The preparation is covered with a clean coverslip, taking care to eliminate air bubbles, which may be confused with yeast cells. On microscopic examination, Cryptococcus neoformans is identified as a round or oval structure about the size of or slightly larger than the erythrocyte. The capsule will repel the ink particles and is surrounded by a smooth, broad halo.

Additional diagnostic methods on CSF include culture on Sabouraud's media and mouse inoculation. These examinations also are not entirely reliable and, furthermore, several weeks may be required for confirmation of the diagnosis by cultural methods. On Sabouraud's media, colonies of cryptococci are mucoid, glistening, and brown in color. Microscopic examination of the growth reveals thick-walled, budding encapsulated yeasts without mycelia or endospores. In addition to cerebrospinal fluid, blood and urine should also be submitted for fungus cultures in the patient suspected of having cryptococcosis. The urine is one of the most frequently overlooked sites for attempted isolation of Cryptococcus neoformans, and is second only to CSF as a source for positive cultures in patients with cryptococcal meningitis (Butler et al.).

Skull x-rays and electroencephalogram are primarily of value to exclude other possible diagnostic considerations. In certain patients with cryptococcal meningitis, progressive decline in responsiveness, worsening ataxia, or increasing papilledema suggests the possibility of communicating hydrocephalus secondary to the inflammatory process. This complication has now been shown to be a very important feature of this disease, which often requires shunt therapy (Richardson et al., Wilhelm et al.), and should be searched for at periodic intervals during the treatment regimen. While clinical signs in some cases will provide evidence suggesting the possible development of hydrocephalus, in others who are obtunded or unresponsive it can only be recognized by the performance of serial radiologic studies. Cranial computed tomography now provides a means of early identification of ventricular enlargement, as well as the possible existence of abscess or granulomatous mass lesions of significant size. Periodic scans at intervals of one to two weeks during the course of treatment will enhance diagnosis of these complications and facilitate the needed therapeutic measures (Fig. 19–4).

Because of the significant numbers of negative India ink tests and negative cerebrospinal fluid cultures in patients with cryptococcal

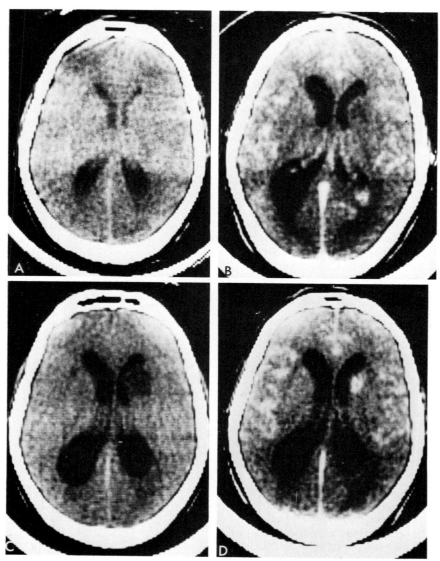

Figure 19–4. Cryptococcal meningoencephalitis complicated by progressive communicating hydrocephalus. *A,* Computed tomogram with contrast infusion 2 weeks after onset of symptoms of meningeal infection. The left lateral ventricle is somewhat larger than the right and the occipital horns are mildly distended bilaterally. *B,* Computed tomogram with contrast enhancement 8 weeks after onset of illness. The ventricles have become larger and there is an irregular area of decreased density in the region of the right caudate nucleus immediately adjacent to the right frontal horn. *C,* Computed tomogram without contrast infusion 10 weeks after onset of symptoms. The anterior horns of the lateral ventricles have continued to enlarge and the hypodense area in the right caudate region has expanded and now compresses the right lateral ventricle. *D,* Computed tomogram with contrast infusion 10 weeks after onset of illness. There is marked enhancement of the lesion in the right caudate area and also a "cortical" pattern of enhancement bilaterally suggestive of altered vascular permeability secondary to inflammation in the cortical areas. Although the CSF had shown improvement with antifungal treatment during this time, the patient had become more listless and drowsy from 6 to 10 weeks after onset of his illness. At 10 weeks, he was treated with a ventriculoperitoneal shunt and improved soon thereafter. Biopsy of the right caudate lesion that is demonstrated on the scans revealed it to be a cryptococcal granuloma.

meningoencephalitis, serologic methods of diagnosis of the disease have been of increasing importance. Detection of anticryptococcal antibody by the indirect fluorescence test is occasionally positive but generally has been disappointing because of its inconsistency. Cryptococcal polysaccharide antigen in blood or cerebrospinal fluid is detected by latex agglutination or complement fixation tests since the original report by Bloomfield et al. and these tests are of reasonable diagnostic reliability, although false negatives can occur (Goodman et al., Bindschadler and Bennett). False positive reactions can also occur (Mackinnon et al.) and are usually related to the presence of rheumatoid factor (Dolan). The latex agglutination method is generally considered to be more sensitive than the complement fixation technique, and some feel that diagnostic accuracy of the serologic methods can be improved by performance of both tests (Snow and Dismukes). A latex agglutination titer on CSF of 1 to 8 or greater is considered significant and provides strong evidence for the diagnosis of cryptococcal meningitis. The antigen titer, if elevated before therapy, is expected to decline during effective treatment and disappear within a few months thereafter. Thus, detection of cryptococcal antigen in cerebrospinal fluid not only is of diagnostic value before treatment but is also useful in follow-up fashion as a gauge of persistence of the infection, and of relapses or remission.

In summary, it can be stated that the clinical picture and cerebrospinal fluid findings are usually sufficiently characteristic to suggest the diagnosis of cryptococcal meningitis, but laboratory confirmation of the disease can be difficult, even on repeated attempts. Because of the importance of early initiation of treatment, certain authors have recommended cisternal tap or burr holes and ventricular tap, since fluid samples from these areas may be positive on India ink preparation and culture when CSF obtained by lumbar puncture has been repeatedly negative (Edwards et al., Gonyea). This approach would seem useful in particularly difficult cases not otherwise solvable. In cases in which there is a high probability of cryptococcal meningitis but in which the diagnostic methods have repeatedly failed, meningeal and brain biopsy is an additional consideration. Even this is not entirely dependable because the meningeal infection is not always uniform.

Treatment

Before the availability of current therapeutic methods, cryptococcal meningoencephalitis was nearly uniformly fatal, with 90 percent of patients dying within one year after onset of symptoms (Butler). With modern treatment, 70 to 80 percent are expected to recover (Butler et al., Edwards et al.), some with variable degrees of residual deficits. Predictors of a less favorable prognosis include occurrence of the disease in a patient with lymphoreticular malignancy or on corticosteroid therapy, the isolation of cryptococci from extraneural sites, and high cryptococcal antigen titers in the CSF and serum at the time of diagnosis (Diamond and Bennett).

Treatment of cryptococcal meningitis is a long and arduous task which requires diligent attention to many details, including the proper administration of antimicrobial therapy and monitoring the possible occurrence of side effects from the drug therapy, as well as a continual search for complications of the disease process itself. The response, or lack of response, to treatment should be followed by periodic CSF examinations, with results of these and appropriate blood studies graphically charted on a flow-sheet. The possibility of the development of progressive communicating hydrocephalus is sufficiently great that cranial computed tomograms should be obtained at periodic intervals. Its occurrence will require placement of an intraventricular reservoir or a ventriculoperitoneal shunt in some cases, with clinical improvement often occurring thereafter (Edwards et al., Tay et al., Wilhelm et al.).

Amphotericin B is the primary drug for treatment of cryptococcal disease of the nervous system and is used either alone or in combination with 5-fluorocytosine. Past experience has demonstrated that amphotericin B has markedly altered the prognosis of the illness, although the drug has the drawbacks of poor penetration into the CSF and a high frequency of toxic side effects, especially on renal function. It is given intravenously in mildly ill patients in an initial dose of 0.1 mg per kilogram per day and in moderately or severely ill patients in a dose of 0.25 mg. per kilogram per day. Each daily dose is mixed in a quantity of 5 percent dextrose in water and the infusion is given over a four- to six-hour period. If this dose is tolerated, the daily dosage is gradually increased to 1.0 mg. per kilogram per day after several days. While children may tolerate daily injections of 1.0 mg. per kilogram per day (Wilson and Feldman), most older persons will soon develop nephrotoxicity on this dosage, requiring its temporary discontinuation with eventual resumption of therapy with a dosage of 0.5 to 0.6 mg. per kilogram per day, or in some cases, even every second day. The total amount of amphotericin B that is administered must be altered from patient to patient, depending on side-effects and response of the infection, but is usually in the range of 1,500 to 2,000 mg. per 1.7 square meters of body surface.

During the course of treatment, laboratory tests to be done at two- to three-day intervals include hemoglobin, white blood cell count, platelet count, urinalysis, serum electrolytes, blood urea nitrogen and creatinine, and creatinine clearance. Despite the fact that penetration of the drug into the cerebrospinal fluid is poor, the intravenous route has been shown to be effective in many patients, assuming the drug is tolerated. Of 36 patients in the series reported by Butler et al., 31 improved with amphotericin B treatment. Five died, all of whom had some form of coexisting disease. Seventeen of the 31 improved patients remained well but 11 subsequently experienced one or more relapses with meningeal infection.

Intrathecal amphotericin B combined with intravenous administration is reserved for patients seriously ill at the onset of therapy or for those who continue to deteriorate in the face of continuing intravenous therapy. Intrathecal therapy is also often used in those who experience a relapse. In patients who develop nephrotoxicity following intravenous therapy, it is sometimes possible to continue treatment with intrathecal administration of the drug alone until there is laboratory evidence of improvement of renal function. The intrathecal dose of amphotericin B in the adult is 0.25 to 0.5 mg. mixed in 5 ml. of distilled water or spinal fluid and administered slowly every other day. The initial intrathecal injection should be a test dose of 0.1 mg. or less to be certain that the drug is tolerated by this route. To minimize side effects, some authors recommend the addition of 15 mg. of hydrocortisone to the mixture to be injected intrathecally. Adverse reactions to lumbar intrathecal amphotericin B are common and sometimes sufficiently severe to require discontinuation of this route of administration. Pain in the back or legs and aseptic meningitis with meningeal signs are the most common complications, while arachnoiditis can be the most devastating. A subcutaneous reservoir for direct intraventricular instillation of the drug has been used, but it, too, has been beset with numerous and limiting complications (Diamond and Bennett).

Five-fluorocytosine has been shown to add a significant contribution to the treatment of cryptococcal meningitis and is now recommended in combination with amphotericin B for patients moderately or seriously ill with the disease (Harder and Hermans, Hermans, Steer et al., Utz et al.). The combined use of the two drugs allows a modest reduction in the daily dosage of amphotericin B, thus decreasing the probability of nephrotoxicity. In addition, because 5-fluorocytosine is well absorbed and blood and CSF levels are rapidly obtained, its use establishes effective therapy quickly in the early time period before the dose of amphotericin B has been elevated to maintenance levels. Should nephrotoxicity to amphotericin B require its temporary discontinuation, 5-fluorocytosine provides continued antimicrobial therapy during the interval. The disadvantage of 5-fluorocytosine is the frequent occurrence or eventual emergence of resistant organisms to it, but its use may bring about considerable improvement in the critical early stage of treatment before resistance occurs (Bennett). Bennett and colleagues compared one group of patients with cryptococcal meningitis treated with amphotericin B for 10 weeks with a second group treated with a combination of amphotericin B and 5-fluorocytosine administered for six weeks. Combined therapy resulted in more rapid sterilization of the CSF, was associated with fewer relapses and with less nephrotoxicity, and brought about a higher percentage of patients improved or cured.

The drug has far fewer side effects than amphotericin B but is not entirely free of adverse reactions. Bone marrow depression, rash, diarrhea, and alteration of liver function tests can occur and warrant appropriate laboratory examinations at periodic intervals. Because the drug is largely excreted by the kidneys, impairment of renal function requires a reduction in the oral dosage (Dawborn et al.). Precise dosage is best determined by blood level assay (Diasio et al., Kauffman et al.), with optimal therapeutic levels being between 60 and 80 micrograms per ml. Bone marrow toxicity appears to be blood level–related and has been found to occur with levels over 125 micrograms per ml. (Kauffman and Frame). Initial dose is usually

50 mg. per kilogram per day given orally every six hours, and, if tolerated, is rapidly increased to 100 to 150 mg. per kilogram per day.

Miconazole is an additional drug that has been used in the treatment of cryptococcal meningitis and can be considered to be an alternative for patients who have shown an inadequate response to the more commonly used antifungal agents. Experience with the drug for this disease is limited to this date, with available reports indicating both favorable responses (Deresinski et al., Sung et al.) and failure of response (Fisher et al.). Miconazole is well tolerated by most patients and has been found to have relatively few side effects. It penetrates into the CSF poorly, a characteristic which usually requires both systemic and intrathecal administration for patients more than mildly ill. The most commonly recommended intravenous dose is 30 mg. per kilogram per day given in divided doses every eight hours over 30 minutes. In the first day of treatment, the dose should be reduced to approximately 20 percent of the above recommended daily dosage to be certain that the drug is adequately tolerated. The intrathecal dose for the adult is 20 mg.

Following recovery and cessation of therapy, the patient with cryptococcal meningitis should be followed intermittently at least for two years (Sarosi et al.) with periodic lumbar punctures to exclude the possibility of relapse and with serial evaluations of blood count and renal function. Certain abnormalities of cerebrospinal fluid may persist for years after completion of treatment, even in the absence of clinical signs of illness (Butler). In some patients who are seriously ill at the time of hospital admission, initiation of treatment is advisable before one can entirely differentiate cryptococcal from tuberculous meningeal disease. Treatment for both diseases must be given until one diagnosis or the other is established.

COCCIDIOIDOMYCOSIS

Coccidioidomycosis is a disease with varied clinical manifestations which is caused by the biphasic fungus, Coccidioides immitis. The requirements for growth of this organism limit its natural distribution to regions characterized by arid climates. Long, hot summers with limited rainfall and relatively warm winters are required, in addition to wind and dust, which aid exposure of the mold to humans. Endemic regions in the United States include parts of California, especially the San Joaquin Valley where the infection rate is distinctly high, southern Nevada and the southwestern corner of Utah, central and western portions of Arizona, the most southern parts of New Mexico, and through western and southwestern Texas. A high rate of infection occurs across the northern part of Mexico and in Venezuela, and the disease is also seen in Paraguay and Argentina. Although most infections with Coccidioides immitis occur in populations indigenous to the endemic areas, even limited exposure to spore-containing dust by travel through or brief stays in the area can be sufficient to contract the illness. Because of the current mobility of the population and the availability of rapid transportation, coccidioidomycosis cannot be thought of as a totally regional disease but may be encountered anywhere in this country in persons who have toured or transiently visited endemic areas. Cases encountered in regions remote from the endemic parts of the country are likely to result in diagnostic confusion or error since the disease will be less well known elsewhere or, perhaps, not considered in the differential diagnosis at all.

The vegetative or saprophytic phase of Coccidioides immitis is characterized by chlamydospores and arthrospores. Arthrospores are readily separated from hyphae by only slight mechanical disturbance and, in nature, become air-borne. When inhaled into the lungs of the susceptible host, the highly infectious spores rapidly convert to the parasitic phase, consisting of endosporulating spherules, which are thick-walled, round or oval-shaped organisms 10 to 60 microns in diameter. Unlike the arthrospore phase, the spherules and endospores are not transmissible and thus man-to-man transmission is not expected. When taken from tissue, pus, sputum, or other specimens and placed in appropriate culture media, the spherules form mycelia, which are again converted into myriads of spores, or the saprophytic phase.

Inhalation of spores into the respiratory tract is the portal of entry in the vast majority of human cases. Direct man-to-man transmission probably does not occur and placental transmission from mother to fetus has not been documented. Studies utilizing skin tests in endemic areas have shown that infection with Coccidioides immitis increases directly with the length of time spent in the region. Approximately 10 to 15 percent of newly arrived residents contract the infection within the first year and almost 90 percent do so within 10 years (Smith et al.). In approximately 40 percent, the acquisition of the disease is associated with symptoms, while 60 percent remain subclinical, being identified by the emergence of skin hypersensitivity to coccidioidin (Smith et al., Smith). The majority of symptomatic cases are manifested by a transient respiratory illness associated with influenza-like symptoms. Generalized dissemination of the disease occurs in approximately one in 400, or 0.25 percent, of both asymptomatically and symptomatically infected white males and one in 2,000 infected white females (Littman et al.). Dark-skinned races seem to be much more susceptible to serious and widespread disease than is the case with the white race. It is estimated that dissemination of the infection occurs at a rate 10 times higher in the black than in the white male and 150 to 200 times higher in the Filipino compared to the white. Pregnancy is an additional factor that is believed to increase the risk of dissemination of coccidioidal disease.

Coccidioidomycosis usually occurs in sporadic fashion but localized outbreaks are well known. Teel et al. reported two families comprising 10 people who spent a day together in Texas. Nine of the 10 persons developed the illness soon thereafter. An epidemic on a larger scale occurred when 61 of 103 archeology students developed the illness after excavating in northern California (Werner et al.). One remarkable aspect of this particular outbreak was that 77 percent of acquired infections were symptomatic. Infection caused by Coccidioides immitis is largely determined by lack of immunity and significant exposure to the organism. Unlike Cryptococcus neoformans, Candida, or Aspergillus species, Coccidioides immitis is not a prominent cause of disease in the immunologically compromised host (Hart et al.), although reactivation of coccidioidomycosis can occur with the use of immunosuppressive agents or high-dose corticosteroid therapy (Deresinski and Stevens). In such patients, the skin tests are likely to be of limited value.

Clinical Manifestations

As mentioned above, more than half the cases of infection with this organism are believed to remain asymptomatic and are identified only by skin test reactivity. Symptomatic infections fall within one of three types, with the majority being in the form of an acute respiratory illness of variable severity. The second type is a localized, cutaneous coccidioidal granuloma, which usually results from direct inoculation secondary to trauma. The third and most severe form of the disease is disseminated coccidioidomycosis. This is a chronic granulomatous process which sometimes involves multiple organs but in other cases is characterized by spread to one vital area, such as the meninges and the brain. Coccidioidomycosis spares no age group and has been described in infants as young as three weeks of age (Christian et al., Hyatt, Townsend and McKey). The disease appears to be poorly tolerated in infants in whom dissemination is manifested by miliary pulmonary involvement, congestive heart failure, hepatomegaly, and neurologic signs. The disease is seen throughout the year, but the highest seasonal incidence of acute coccidioidomycosis is during the summer and early fall.

Following entry of the organism into the respiratory tract, the incubation period varies from seven to 28 days, with an average of 10 to 14 days. The acute, respiratory form of the illness associated with erythema nodosum or erythema multiforme has long been known by clinicians in the San Joaquin Valley as "valley fever" or "desert fever." The onset is usually abrupt with fever, cough, and chest pain, in addition to generalized symptoms such as anorexia, malaise, and muscle aches (Dennis and Hansen). Rash is present in some cases, but the time of onset and type of eruption appears to have some regional variations. In the localized outbreak of 61 cases in northern California, Werner et al. observed a generalized maculopapular eruption soon after onset of the illness in almost one-half the patients. Erythema multiforme was noted in approximately 50 percent within days after onset of symptoms in children from the Tucson, Arizona area (Richardson et al.). In cases from the San Joaquin Valley, Faber et al. stressed the occurrence of erythema nodosum, which appeared one to three weeks after onset of the acute illness, was most prominent on the anterior tibial surfaces, and was sometimes associated with arthritic signs involving the knees and ankles.

The acute pulmonary illness is self-limited in the majority of cases, with recovery occurring after a symptomatic period of a few days up to two or three weeks. Roentgenograms of the chest during the acute phase reveal infiltrates, hilar adenopathy, a pleural reaction, or pleural effusion. In certain cases, pulmonary coccidioidomycosis becomes chronic, resulting in a clinical course and roentgenographic findings similar to those of tuberculosis (Sarosi et al.). The primary pulmonary infection with Coccidioides immitis is frequently associated with an eosinophilic response in the peripheral blood. In most, eosinophils account for 5 to 10 percent of the total white blood cell count, and the peak elevation is usually found between the second and third weeks after onset.

Disseminated coccidioidomycosis is an infrequent but serious complication of the acute form of the disease and carries a significant mortality rate. Almost any part of the body may be affected, but there is a predilection for dissemination to involve the lungs, bone, skin, and meninges. Lymph nodes, myocardium, and liver can also be implicated. Spread throughout the lungs occurs in miliary fashion similar to that of tuberculosis. Coccidioidal osteomyelitis favors the radius, ulna, tibia, and sometimes the skull. In the extremities, skeletal lesions are especially common at sites of ligamentous insertion. Coccidioidal infection of the vertebrae can include involvement of the body and laminar arches but usually with sparing of the disc space, and is often associated with paraspinous abscess formation. Widespread, rapidly developing osteolytic skeletal lesions have been described on rare occasion and can create diagnostic confusion in some instances (Bayer et al.). Dissemination to the nervous system most often gives rise to a chronic granulomatous meningitis but localized granulomas can behave like a mass lesion within the brain or cause a spinal cord compression syndrome (Ingham, Jackson et al., Rand).

Extrapulmonary dissemination is believed to occur primarily in the early stages of the disease. If dissemination is going to occur, it usually does so within eight weeks after infection is acquired. "Late" dissemination is not entirely denied but is considered to be unusual if it occurs at all, except in the immunosuppressed patient. Colwell and Tillman observed that the occurrence of disseminated disease during the acute stage can be suspected if weight loss accompanies the illness or if marked leukocytosis and anemia are present. Prolonged symptoms and paratracheal adenopathy are additional findings suggestive of extrapulmonary spread of the infection. In patients with coccidioidal meningitis, however, historical evidence of the preceding acute pulmonary illness is often completely lacking. Because the early manifestations of intracranial involvement with Coccidioides immitis are non-specific, any patient suspected to have dissemination of any type should have a cerebrospinal fluid examination.

Coccidioidal Meningitis

In most instances, Coccidioides immitis reaches the nervous system by hematogenous spread from the lungs. Less often, intracranial or intraspinal involvement is secondary to direct extension from adjacent skull or vertebral osteomyelitis. Most intracranial infections are manifested by a subacute or chronic meningitis (Jenkins and Postlewaite, Norman and Miller, Reeves and Baisinger), but, on rare occasion, a focal coccidioidal granuloma of the cerebrum or cerebellum will give rise to progressive symptoms indicative of a focal mass lesion (Storts).

Symptoms of coccidioidal meningitis in some cases will evolve almost in direct relationship with those of the primary pulmonary infection. After two to four weeks of fever, cough, chest pain, and weight loss, the patient develops headache and is found to be listless or perhaps intermittently confused. Neurologic symptoms and signs are thereafter likely to be progressive until diagnosis is established by examination of the cerebrospinal fluid. In others, the illness assumes the form of a chronic, smoldering meningeal inflammatory process that begins gradually, without an obvious preceding illness. Intractable headaches, personality change, and ease of fatigue may last for weeks or many months with little else to suggest the potential seriousness of the infection (Caudill et al.). Signs of meningeal irritation are often conspicuously absent even though headaches are severe and disturbances in mentation are advanced. Convulsions are added to the picture in some, in addition to a variety of neurologic signs such as cranial nerve deficits or coordination abnormalities. Focal neurologic signs in some instances can be attributed to cerebrovascular occlusion secondary to coccidioidal vasculitis (Kobayashi et al.).

In cases of chronic meningitis, hydrocephalus eventually develops secondary to the thick basilar exudate, which leads to obstruction at the level of the incisura or of the outlet foramina of the fourth ventricle. Symptoms and signs of meningitis, which may have been long-standing and only slowly progressive, are frequently accelerated when ventricular expansion occurs (Ramseyer et al.). Headaches are more intense, visual loss and dementia become more severe, and papilledema may now be added to other neurologic signs already present. Deterioration in all aspects is likely to proceed to death if treatment is not begun. Without treatment, coccidioidal meningitis is a fatal illness, although the length of survival is exceedingly variable. Several weeks to a few months is the usual duration of the untreated disease but exceptional cases will go on for years before death intervenes (Norman and Miller).

The cerebrospinal fluid is consistently abnormal in patients with coccidioidal meningitis, although proof of the disease by isolation of the organism therefrom is often

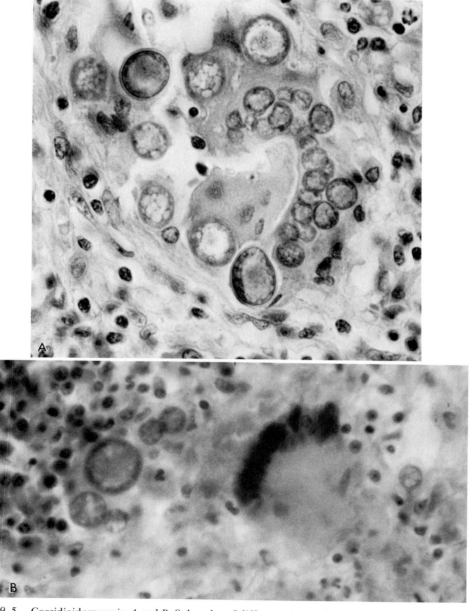

Figure 19–5. Coccidioidomycosis. *A* and *B*, Spherules of different sizes and in variable stages of endosporulation. In *A*, the circular, bubble-like structures within certain spherules are endospores. *B* shows spherules associated with inflammatory cells and a multinucleated giant cell.

Illustration continued on opposite page

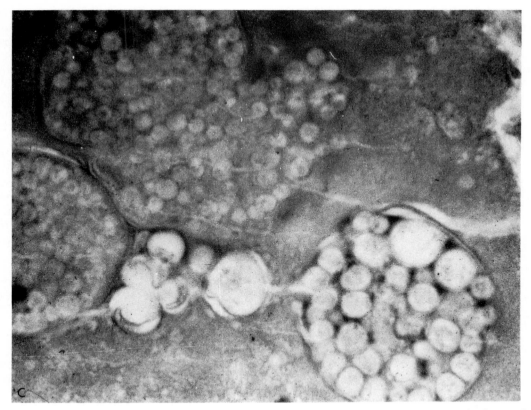

Figure 19–5 Continued. C, Mature spherules (sporangium) packed with endospores. Two at the bottom have ruptured, liberating endospores which subsequently will mature to spherules, thus repeating the cycle.

difficult. The cellular response in most cases before treatment is between 50 and 500 cells per cu. mm. with 50 to 90 percent being lymphocytes. CSF eosinophilia is found in some cases and is an important clue to the diagnosis when subacute meningitis occurs in a patient from an endemic zone. Protein elevation is reasonably constant and most values are in the range of 100 to 500 mg. per 100 ml. The glucose content of the CSF is reduced to 10 to 35 mg. per 100 ml. in most cases, but occasionally normal levels are found. While the presence of a granulomatous meningeal process is consistently evident in fluid obtained by lumbar puncture, the ventricular fluid is subject to greater variation and generally is of less diagnostic value (Goldstein et al.).

The pathology of coccidioidal meningitis is that of a granulomatous meningeal process which is most extensive at the base of the brain. Diffuse leptomeningeal thickening is present in addition to multiple, small granulomata in the meninges and on the cortical surface. Ventricular enlargement is usually evident on gross inspection of the sectioned brain, and, in some, granulomatous lesions within the parenchyma of the cerebrum or cerebellum can be as large as several centimeters in diameter. Chronic ependymitis produces a shaggy, roughened appearance to the ependymal surfaces. Microscopically, the granulomatous reaction consists of an abundant cellular infiltrate composed of neutrophils, lymphocytes, plasma cells, multinucleated giant cells, and organisms of variable size. Vascular changes are pronounced in the exudate and consist of extensive endothelial proliferation and perivascular cellular infiltration, often with organisms seen within the vessel wall. Spherules in different stages of endosporulation and ruptured spherules liberating endospores into tissue can be observed within the inflammatory reaction (Fig. 19–5).

Diagnosis

Coccidioidal meningitis should be suspected in a patient from an endemic area or in a patient who has been in an endemic area and subsequently develops persistent headaches and other signs of meningeal inflammation. A preceding acute pulmonary illness enhances the possibility, as does the occurrence of erythema nodosum during the respiratory stage, but their absence does not exclude the diagnosis. Cerebrospinal fluid examination nearly always shows significant abnormalities, but if Coccidioides immitis is not isolated, the findings can be viewed only as compatible with but not diagnostic of coccidioidomycosis. From a summary of prior experience, it is estimated that Coccidioides immitis can be recovered in 20 to 40 percent of cases of coccidioidal meningitis (Drutz and Catanzaro). The subacute or chronic history, plus the cerebrospinal fluid abnormalities, stimulates a differential diagnosis which includes tuberculous meningitis, cryptococcal meningoencephalitis as well as other fungal infections, partially treated bacterial meningitis, parameningeal suppurative infections, sarcoidosis, and carcinomatous or melanoma infiltration of the meninges. Rarely, a primary posterior fossa tumor in a child is associated with meningeal signs, cells in the cerebrospinal fluid, and a reduced glucose content, thus resembling a chronic granulomatous process.

Skin hypersensitivity to Coccidioides immitis is ascertained by the intracutaneous injection of 0.1 ml. of 1:100 dilution of coccidioidin, a polysaccharide substance prepared from the culture filtrates of the arthrospore phase of Coccidioides immitis grown in synthetic media. When tests with this strength are negative but the disease remains a possibility, 1:10 dilution is then used, although with this concentrated form there may be cross-reactivity in persons who have had histoplasmosis. The reaction is interpreted at 24 and 48 hours, with induration of 5 millimeters or more being a positive response. Skin sensitivity may be established by one week after onset of symptoms and is almost always positive by three weeks, unless anergy occurs in association with overwhelming infection. The coccidioidin skin test does not alter the results of serologic tests used to establish the diagnosis of active infection. Caution is advised with the use of coccidioidin in patients with erythema nodosum, in whom the skin test may exacerbate the cutaneous lesions or provoke local necrotizing changes (Drutz and Catanzaro). The skin test is a valuable method for surveying the incidence of previous infection but is frequently negative with disseminated coccidioidomycosis, and especially with coccidioidal meningitis (Caudill et al.).

The more recently developed skin test material called spherulin is a soluble material that is liberated from Coccidioides immitis spherules produced in vitro (Levine et al.). Spherulin has been found to detect prior infection with this fungus substantially more often than does coccidioidin, but, like the latter, carries the same risks in patients with erythema nodosum and does not appear to significantly affect serologic test results. The value of the spherulin skin test in the recognition of the disseminated form of the disease remains unclear, although it has been suggested that positive reactions are more frequent with this substance than occur with coccidioidin (Drutz and Catanzaro).

Serologic methods of diagnosis include determination of precipitin and complement-fixing antibodies in serum and in cerebrospinal fluid in suspected meningitis cases. Precipitin antibodies in serum rise early in the infection and usually disappear within five months, regardless of the course of the disease. Complement-fixing antibodies appear in the circulation more slowly than precipitin antibodies, and, in patients with asymptomatic infection, an antibody response by this method may not occur at all. Positive or rising titers can be demonstrated by four to eight weeks after onset of symptoms. Unless dissemination of the disease occurs, the complement fixation antibody titer gradually decreases and disappears by six to eight months. Persistence of complement-fixing antibodies or a titer of 1:32 or greater is indicative of disseminated disease. Complement-fixing antibodies cannot always be found in the cerebrospinal fluid in patients with coccidioidal meningitis (Caudill et al.) and thus a negative test does not exclude the possibility. A positive complement fixation test on CSF is diagnostic of coccidioidal meningitis, and serial tests of both serum and CSF can be helpful as an indicator of the response to treatment. Countercurrent immunoelectrophoresis has also been performed on serum and CSF to identify this disease. Preliminary results have been promising, although false negative tests can occur in patients with coccidioidal meningitis (Aguilar-Torres et al.).

Absolute confirmation of the diagnosis of coccidioidomycosis is by isolation of the organism or its identification in tissue by microscopic examination. Endosporulating spherules are best demonstrated by the Grocott methenamine silver stain. Fluorescent antibody techniques have also been developed for identification of the fungus in tissue specimens (Kaplan and Kraft). Clinical specimens are cultured on Sabouraud's agar, on which the colony develops rapidly with aerial mycelia with a cottony, white appearance. Cultures of Coccidioides immitis should be handled with extreme caution by laboratory personnel because of the infectious nature of the material. Precautions that have been recommended to protect laboratory workers are that petri dishes should not be used for inoculation of fungi that might be Coccidioides immitis; suspected cultures should be transferred with utmost care in an adequately ventilated hood, and the filamentous mat should be moistened before removing cultures from the hood (Omieczynski). Microscopic examination of the growth reveals arthrospores along the course of the hyphae. The resulting growth is further identified by intraperitoneal injection in mice in whom typical spherules will develop.

Treatment

Primary pulmonary coccidioidomycosis is usually a benign, self-limited illness which is managed without antifungal therapy except in certain instances in patients with conditions which predispose to dissemination. Extrapulmonary spread represents a serious complication of the disease, with life-threatening possibilities, and is a definite indication for antifungal therapy. Amphotericin B is the drug of choice and, in patients with coccidioidal meningitis, is administered both intravenously and intrathecally. The initial intrathecal dose should be very low, perhaps 0.1 mg. for the first two or three injections, and then gradually increased to doses of 0.25 to 0.5 mg. given three or four times per week. Treatment of coccidioidal meningitis must be prolonged because of the nature of the disease and the susceptibility to relapse. Some authors recommend weekly intrathecal injections of amphotericin B for indefinite periods of time even after recovery. After a few weeks of therapy, when clinical and CSF improvement have occurred, it is usually possible to decrease the daily intravenous dose of amphotericin B and eventually to change to an every-other-day or twice-per-week regimen. During the course of the illness, the appropriate clinical observations and periodic computed cranial tomography should be performed to identify the development of hydrocephalus. Hydrocephalus that is progressive and more than mild in degree may require shunting therapy, although such procedures carry the hazard of further extracranial spread of the infection (Ramseyer et al.). When hydrocephalus occurs, an intraventricular reservoir is sometimes used for direct intraventricular instillation of amphotericin B.

Miconazole is an imidazole derivative that shows promise as an alternative drug for treatment of coccidioidal meningitis in patients unable to tolerate or who do not respond adequately to amphotericin B (Stevens et al., Sung et al.). It appears to have fewer side effects than amphotericin B but, like the latter, is highly protein-bound and penetrates into the CSF poorly. Preliminary experience has indicated that treatment of coccidioidal meningitis with miconazole requires both systemic and intrathecal administration. Because of the obvious limitations and potential adverse effects of the available antifungal drugs for treatment of coccidioidal meningitis, other modes of treatment of the disease have been considered. The use of transfer factor appears to have beneficial effects but will require additional investigation before its role is clarified (Graybill, Steele et al.).

CANDIDA MENINGOENCEPHALITIS

Candida species are common inhabitants of the oral cavity, intestinal tract, and vagina and can be cultured from these sites in 35 to 40 percent of normal persons (Conant). Candida is a common cause of dermatitis or oral lesions in the newborn infant (Fig. 19–6) and of vulvovaginitis in the adult, but in the great majority of cases these are benign lesions that respond promptly to local treatment. A rare disorder involving cellular immunodeficiency is referred to as chronic mucocutaneous candidiasis, in which approximately one-half of the cases are associated with endocrinopathies such as hypoparathyroidism, hypoadrenalism, pernicious anemia, and diabetes mellitus (Blizzard and Gibbs, Landau). Familial chronic mucocutaneous candidiasis is inherited as an autosomal recessive trait and on only rare occasion is associated with endocrine dysfunction (Kroll et al., Wuepper and Fudenberg). Recurrent mucocutaneous

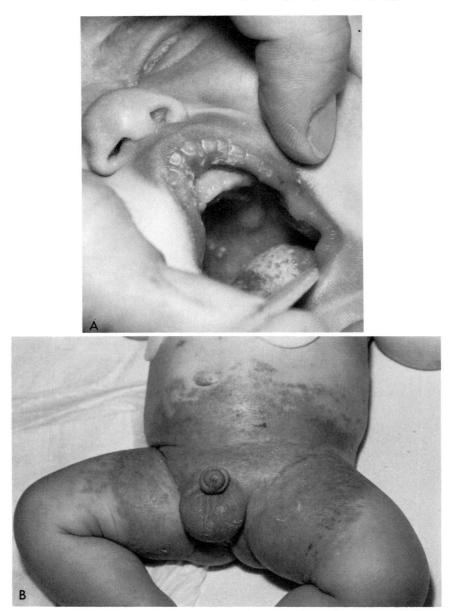

Figure 19–6. Candida surface lesions in normal infants. *A,* Candida infection of the tongue ("thrush") in a normal 14-day-old infant. The white nodules on the hard palate are submucosal epithelial retention cysts called Epstein's pearls and not foci of infection. *B,* Candida dermatitis in an otherwise normal 5-month-old infant. It is a diffuse, scaling, erythematous eruption with satellite lesions, characteristic of monilial infection.

candidiasis is also seen with the DiGeorge syndrome, a disorder characterized by absence or hypoplasia of the thymus and parathyroid glands (Cleveland et al., Gatti et al.).

Under certain circumstances, Candida species can produce serious systemic disease in the human, either with sepsis and disseminated involvement of multiple organs, or with tissue invasion that is relatively isolated to either the brain, lungs, or kidneys. Disseminated infections due to this fungus have increased remarkably in the past 15 to 20 years, and at present, Candida species are the most common cause of fungal infection in the compromised host (Bodey, Hart et al., Rifkind et al.). Of the 72 immunologically compromised patients with fungal infections reported by Hart and colleagues, Candida species were the offending organisms in 42. Candida species have also been found to be the most common fungus found in the brain in a consecutive autopsy series which included all age groups (Parker et al.). In this study, Candida species accounted for 49 percent of all fungal infections of the central nervous system and were more than twice as common as Cryptococcus neoformans, the second most common offender.

Conditions and circumstances associated with disseminated candidiasis include leukemia and other hematologic malignancies (Gruhn and Sanson, Henig et al.), renal transplantation (Rifkind et al.), immunosuppressive treatment with antimetabolic or cytotoxic agents for any purpose, prolonged antibiotic therapy, and prolonged administration of corticosteroids (Fig. 19–7). Candida meningitis has been described in a child as a complication of multiple antibiotic therapy for acute bacterial meningitis (Shurtleff et al.). Serious and debilitating diseases such as burns, hepatic cirrhosis, and systemic lupus erythematosus can also be associated with generalized candida infections. An important factor associated with the recent increase in systemic candida infection in infants is the widespread use of indwelling catheters in the umbilical vessels (Adler et al.) and of prolonged central venous catheterization for parenteral alimentation (Ashcraft and Leape, Boeckman and Krill, Curry and Quie, Isac-

son et al.). Candida is the most common fungus isolated from patients with indwelling catheters for central feeding (Heird et al.) but, in addition to the intravascular foreign body itself, other factors are usually present with such infants that predispose to fungal infection. Many children who require parenteral feeding have received multiple antibiotics and many have had some form of gastrointestinal disorder requiring surgery, thereby providing a potential source of hematogenous invasion by Candida species. On rare occasion, Candida species will colonize a ventricular shunt, resulting in meningitis or ventriculitis (Bayer et al., Rodgers et al.). An additional rare event is fetal infection with Candida species following premature rupture of membranes (Levin et al.). Transplacental transmission of Candida species is not believed to occur.

Reasons for the enhanced susceptibility of systemic fungal, including candida, infections in patients with the various factors outlined above are only partially known. With leukemia and certain other malignancies, both the basic disease and the drugs used for treatment of the disease disturb the immune defense mechanisms, thus favoring infections ordinarily checked naturally by the normal person. Multiple and prolonged antibiotics alter the normal bacterial flora, especially of the gastrointestinal tract, thereby allowing candida to flourish locally. Systemic invasion

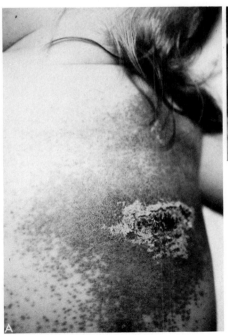
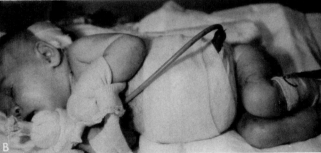

Figure 19–7. Candida sepsis in predisposed infants. *A,* Candida dermatitis in a 2-year-old child with Down's syndrome with leukemia. Blood cultures were positive for Candida species. *B,* Candida sepsis and meningitis in a 7-week-old infant with gastroschisis managed surgically a few hours after birth. Because of recurrent intestinal obstruction, the child had several additional operative procedures, a central feeding catheter, numerous peripheral venous catheters, and multiple antibiotics.

therefrom is particularly likely when operative intervention on the bowel is required or when there is intestinal mucosal injury secondary to the effects of chemotherapeutic agents. Having gained entrance into the blood stream, fungal organisms are most likely to result in serious generalized disease if intravenous or intracardiac foreign bodies are present on which colonization occurs and from which perpetual seeding is possible. The mechanism by which corticosteroids increase the predisposition to candida infections is speculative but may in part be related to stabilization of lysosomal membranes induced by these drugs. The inhibition of release of lysosomal enzymes secondary to membrane stabilization diminishes digestion of phagocytized organisms, permitting the infecting agent to multiply and eventually destroy the cell (Epstein et al.).

Regardless of the pathogenesis, the great majority of systemic or cerebral infections due to Candida species occur in persons with an underlying condition which enhances the patient's susceptibility to opportunistic infection. Its occurrence in a previously normal person is infrequent, and even then some form of acutely acquired immune disturbance is often suspected (Kohlschütter and Pelet). Lehrer and Cline studied an otherwise healthy adult with disseminated candida infection and discovered that neutrophils of the patient lacked detectable levels of the lysosomal enzyme myeloperoxidase, an enzyme believed necessary for the killing of candida organisms by white blood cells after phagocytosis. Although Candida albicans remains the most commonly identified species in patients with serious candida infections, other species can also be pathogenic, including Candida tropicalis, krusei, parakrusei, and guilliermondii (Bodey, Hurley, Louria et al., Richart and Dammin). In the study by Bodey of fungal infections in acute leukemia, of 54 Candida species identified, 52 were either Candida albicans or Candida tropicalis.

Clinical Manifestations and Pathology

Systemic candida infection in certain patients remains limited to the blood stream without clinical or laboratory evidence of other organ system involvement. In some, a single organ is almost selectively affected while, in others, the infectious process becomes widespread with invasion of multiple structures. The kidneys are the most consis-

tently involved organs in disseminated candidiasis, followed by the heart, lungs, intestinal tract, brain, and liver (Louria et al.). In leukemic patients with systemic candida infection, the gastrointestinal tract is almost consistently involved at autopsy, and macroscopic lesions in the liver and spleen are frequently surprisingly large in size (Myerowitz et al.) (Fig. 19–8).

There is no characteristic constellation of clinical findings indicative of systemic candida infection and, thus, the disease is often identified fortuitously, for example, on blood cultures done periodically because of the presence of a central feeding catheter. In leukemic patients or those following organ transplantation, cerebral involvement with Candida is occasionally found unexpectedly at necropsy.

Fever is the most consistent finding in children with candida sepsis or disseminated infection, often accompanied by irritability, lethargy, vomiting, and weight loss, especially in infants. The infant who develops systemic candidiasis may also exhibit hepatosplenomegaly and soft tissue edema, with or without other evidence of congestive heart failure. Petechiae are observed in some and can be associated with intestinal bleeding or, rarely, even consumption coagulopathy (Philippidis et al.). Tachypnea and tachycardia are seen in those with cardiorespiratory involvement, and a variety of neurologic signs appear when the brain is invaded.

Endophthalmitis secondary to candidemia has been observed with increasing frequency in recent years (Haning et al., Meyers et al.), both clinically and at necropsy. In addition, candida endophthalmitis has been found to occur in infants receiving intravenous hyperalimentation without signs of systemic candida infection, and in some cases, in the absence of positive blood cultures for Candida species (Montgomerie and Edwards). Intraocular candida infection usually causes blurred vision and frequently is associated with conjunctival erythema. The hallmark of candida endophthalmitis is a focal, glistening-white, retinal lesion, which can be either solitary or multiple, and which is often associated with vitreous inflammation (Edwards et al., Fishman et al.). In illicit drug users, candida endophthalmitis can be manifested by severe vitreous involvement and anterior uveitis without the typical retinal lesion, and in the absence of evidence of systemic candidiasis (Aquilar et al.).

Another complication of candida sepsis

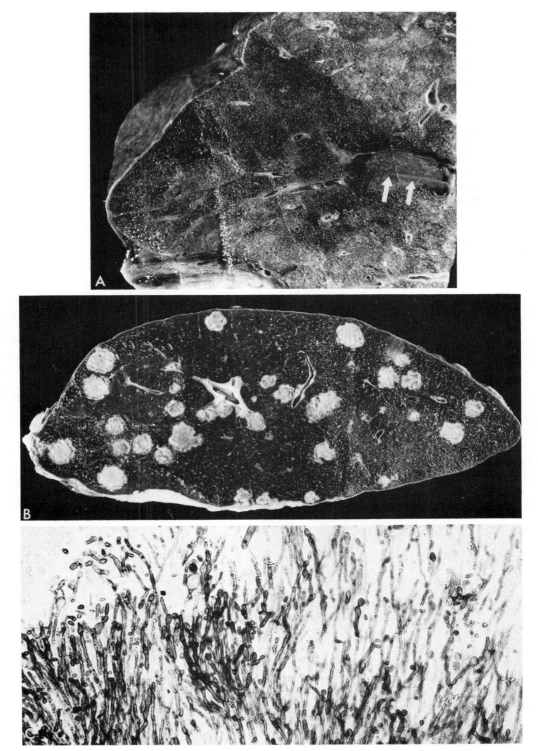

Figure 19–8. Disseminated candidiasis in a child with leukemia. *A,* Cut section of the lung shows a hemorrhagic infarct distal to a thrombosed vessel (white arrows), occluded by Candida albicans invasion of the vascular wall. *B,* Multiple, cannonball-like Candida albicans granulomata in the spleen of the same patient. *C,* Pseudohyphae and mycelial forms of Candida albicans from the spleen (PASH stain, 500×).

now recognized, especially in infants, is acute arthritis (Adler et al., Klein et al., Pruitt et al.). Monarticular involvement is possible but, in addition, the process can involve multiple joints in symmetrical fashion manifested by joint pain, tenderness, and swelling. Erythema or warmth are not usually found with candida arthritis. Roentgenographically, there is joint effusion and either metaphyseal irregularity or a frank destructive metaphysitis resembling that of congenital syphilis (Fig. 19–9). Articular involvement can occur in the acute stage of disseminated candida infection or can be delayed for several weeks after the subsidence of the generalized illness (Murray et al.).

Candida infection of the central nervous system can often be diagnosed in life but is not rare as an unexpected autopsy finding in immunocompromised patients or in those with chronic debilitating illnesses requiring long-term intravascular catheterization. A literature review by Black revealed 42 published cases of cerebral candidiasis published up to 1970. Thirty-five of the 42 had some type of underlying condition which increased susceptibility to fungal infection, while in seven patients no demonstrable predisposing factor could be found. In 27 patients the intracranial infection was predominantly meningitic, and in 15 candida produced either cerebral abscess, multiple microabscesses, or granulomatous lesions. Twelve of the 42 cases involved infants less than one month of age. Males are affected with candida meningoencephalitis more than females (Black, DeVita et al.), although the reason for this is unexplained. In almost one-half of the reported cases of candida meningoencephalitis, oral thrush or localized candidiasis elsewhere was found.

Symptoms and signs of candida meningoencephalitis depend to some degree on whether the infection is primarily meningeal, both meningeal and parenchymal, or consists of a cerebral abscess or multiple microabscesses. Fever, vomiting, convulsions, and lethargy or coma are the commonly described manifestations, in association with neck stiffness, papilledema, and various focal neurologic deficits. When the process is in the form of a solitary large cerebral abscess, the re-

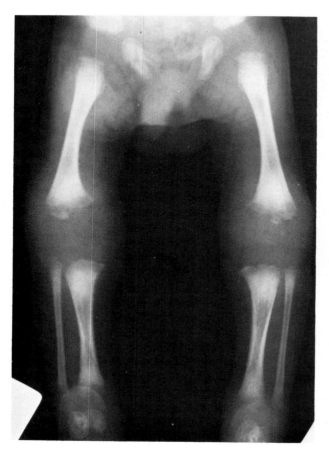

Figure 19–9. Candida metaphysitis. Widespread, bilateral destructive metaphyseal lesions in a 1-month-old infant with disseminated candidiasis. The infant had intestinal obstruction treated surgically on the first day of life and subsequently received parenteral alimentation and antibiotics. Skeletal lesions healed with antifungal therapy.

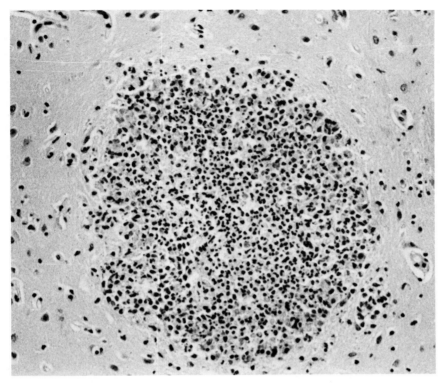

Figure 19–10. Candida encephalitis. Microabscess within the brain. The lesion is composed of densely packed inflammatory cells and macrophages.

sulting focal signs, progressive course, and positive brain scan can closely resemble either a neoplasm or suppurative abscess of bacterial origin (Black). Cerebrospinal fluid findings vary, also depending considerably on whether the brunt of the infection is meningeal or parenchymal. When the meninges are infected, the cerebrospinal fluid usually shows a cellular response, which more often is neutrophilic than lymphocytic. The protein content is significantly elevated and the glucose value is either reduced or is normal. Candida sometimes can be seen on gram stain as a gram-positive organism and is obtained on culture of the CSF in most cases. In contrast, abscess, microabscesses, or granulomatous lesions within the brain with little meningeal involvement produce few distinctive cerebrospinal fluid changes and the organism cannot usually be recovered therefrom. Cells may be few or absent and the protein value is normal or perhaps only slightly increased.

The neuropathology of candida infections of the central nervous system includes meningeal opacification and venous congestion, along with a variable degree of cerebral swelling. Cerebral lesions, when present, consist of multiple abscesses of different sizes, some

being several centimeters in diameter while others are sufficiently small that they can be recognized only by microscopic examination (Roessman and Friede) (Fig. 19–10). Microabscesses are found widely disseminated in the brain and consist of necrotic foci surrounded by polymorphonuclear leukocytes and macrophages. Solitary, massive abscess formation in one cerebral hemisphere is a less common manifestation of cerebral candidiasis (Black), and, as in large abscesses in general, is associated with surrounding edema and the possibility of internal herniations. Other lesions, particularly small ones, are granulomatous in appearance, being composed of inflammatory cells, histiocytes, and multinucleated giant cells, some of which contain organisms (Fig. 19–11). Yeast-like organisms with pseudohyphae are readily demonstrable in parenchymal lesions and in the meningeal exudate by use of Grocott's methenamine silver or periodic acid–Schiff stains. Both meningeal and cerebral vessels are frequently involved in the inflammatory process, some of which become thrombosed, leading to infarction of surrounding tissue. Arteritis is generally less striking with candida meningitis than occurs with tissue inva-

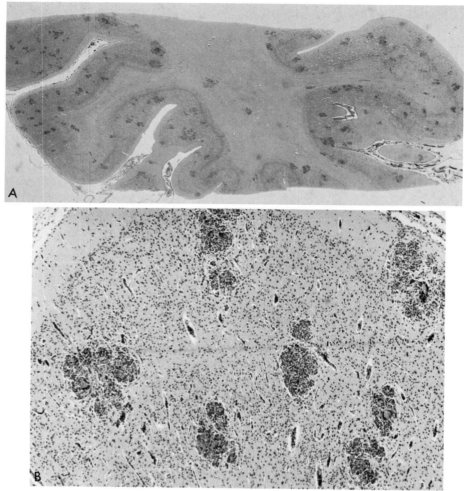

Figure 19–11. Disseminated candidiasis with Candida encephalitis in an infant. *A,* Large number of fungal granulomatous lesions widespread through the cerebral cortex and much more sparse in the white matter. *B,* Close-up view of the cortical granulomata.

Illustration continued on opposite page

sion with Aspergillus species or the Phycomycetes, but in some instances extensive candida granulomatous angiitis of major intracranial vessels with intimal thickening and fibrinoid necrosis of the media will be found (Edelson et al.). Intracranial mycotic aneurysm secondary to vascular invasion by Candida albicans has been described but is rare (Goldman et al.).

Diagnosis

The occurrence of unexplained fever, neurologic signs, or pulmonary infiltrates in the immunologically compromised host, especially when leukopenic, in the patient on prolonged corticosteroid or antibiotic therapy, or the patient with intravascular catheters should suggest the possibility of opportunistic infection, such as candidiasis. Confirmation of the diagnosis is established by isolation of the yeast from blood, joint effusion, or spinal fluid cultures. It is possible, however, to have widespread visceral involvement with candida, and yet not be able to isolate the fungus on repeated blood cultures. As with other types of fungal meningitis, isolation of Candida species from the CSF is more likely to be successful when a relatively large CSF sample can be submitted to the laboratory (Edelson et al.). When captured, Candida species grow well on the media used routinely for blood cultures but grow most readily on Sabouraud's agar. On this medium, Candida albicans results in soft, cream-colored colonies with a distinctive yeast-like odor. Candida isolated from properly collected urine may be indicative of systemic infection, and especially so if the same organism is obtained from both blood and urine. Children with urinary catheters, however, are frequently found to have candida in the urine, which promptly disappears after the catheter is removed. Likewise, in some blood culture–positive children with intravascular catheters, the organisms vanish without additional treatment once the catheter is eliminated.

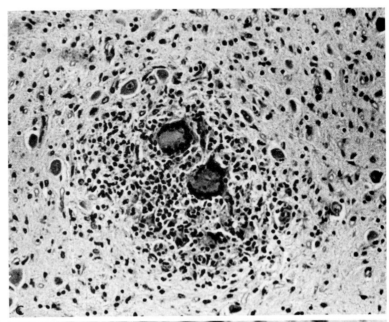

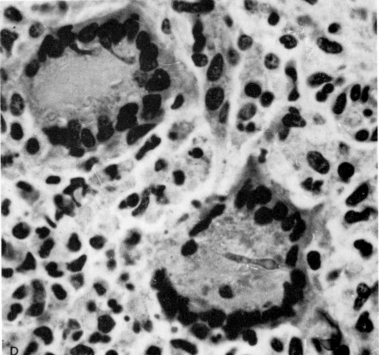

Figure 19–11 Continued. C, Multinucleated giant cells within a granulomatous lesion. *D,* Higher power reveals pseudohyphae of Candida species within the giant cell.

The significance of a yeast in tissue is best determined by examination of tissue stained with Grocott's methenamine silver technique. Candida is identified as an oval, budding yeast with pseudomycelia. Yeasts from tissue, blood, cerebrospinal fluid, or other specimens can be identified as Candida albicans by inoculation on chlamydospore or corn meal agar. Within 24 hours, this organism will reveal thick-walled spores referred to as chlamydospores. If the organism is found to be one of Candida species but not Candida albicans, specific species identification is accomplished by fermentation studies (Martin et al.).

Serologic methods of diagnosis of candidiasis are not widely available but can be of value in certain instances. A four-fold or greater rise of precipitating or agglutinating antibodies in serum during the course of a febrile illness is strongly suggestive of systemic candidiasis (Preisler et al., Rosner et al.). The agglutinating antibody titer is believed to be the more reliable of the two methods and is probably not rendered positive by the presence of candida on skin or mucous membranes (Preisler et al.). In a study of 115 high-risk patients of whom 69 were identified to have systemic candidiasis, Kozinn et al. found true positive precipitin reactions in 65 of the 69 and false negative responses in four. False positive reactions occurred in seven instances. It has been recommended that patients at risk to the development of systemic candida infections have serologic tests at periodic intervals as an aid to early diagnosis. In addition, children with indwelling central feeding catheters should have routine blood cultures for bacteria and fungi once or twice per week.

Treatment

Disseminated candida infection, especially when accompanied by meningoencephalitis, must always be regarded as a serious and life-threatening illness, but a successful therapeutic outcome has been recorded on numerous occasions (Fass and Perkins, Haning et al., Isacson et al., Klein et al., Roe and Haynes, Steer et al., Vandevelde et al.). With treatment, the prognosis of cerebral candidiasis is considerably better if the symptoms and signs are those primarily of meningeal involvement and much worse in those with encephalitic involvement. In patients with indwelling vascular catheters who develop positive blood cultures for candida, immediate removal of the catheter is indicated and sometimes this alone results in subsidence of the infection. Catheters removed because of symptoms or signs indicative of infection should always be cultured for bacterial and fungal pathogens, as this may provide evidence of the offending organism.

Amphotericin B has been the most widely used drug for treatment of systemic candida infections, including meningitis, and remains the mainstay of therapy. There has been increasing popularity in recent years of the combined use of amphotericin B and 5-fluorocytosine. Advantages of the combination are that the dose of amphotericin can be reduced somewhat because of the presumed synergistic effect of the two drugs, and the excellent penetration of 5-fluorocytosine into the CSF compared to the rather poor entry of amphotericin B. Five-fluorocytosine is not recommended alone because of the pretreatment resistance of 10 to 20 percent of Candida strains, and due to the rapid emergence of resistant organisms among those previously sensitive during therapy (Hill et al.). Studies of Montgomerie et al., however, have shown that synergism occurs with combined therapy, even though many of the Candida isolates were very resistant to 5-fluorocytosine. These authors suggested that at achievable serum levels of amphotericin B and 5-fluorocytosine, the synergistic effect is often cidal for Candida species, whereas the effect of either drug given alone would only be inhibitory. Combined therapy with amphotericin B and 5-fluorocytosine has successfully eradicated candida meningitis in a premature newborn infant (Lilien et al.) as well as in older children (Chesney et al.) and is recommended as the regimen of choice by a number of authors. Duration of therapy is determined by clinical and laboratory response and is often influenced by toxic effects of the drugs. In most instances of candida meningitis, therapy is continued for six to 12 weeks. The use of prophylactic antifungal therapy in high-risk patients has not been extensively investigated. Limited studies have suggested that concomitant use of oral amphotericin B with antibacterial antibiotics may decrease the occurrence of gastrointestinal invasion and dissemination of Candida species in patients with hematologic malignancies (Ezdinli et al.).

Miconazole is an additional drug which has received preliminary trials for parenteral use for candida infections (Balk et al., Fischer et al.). There is little known to date regarding its value in treatment of candida meningitis, although the drug penetrates into the CSF rather poorly following intravenous administration.

ASPERGILLOSIS

Aspergillosis is an infrequently encountered fungal disease clinically but one now seen with increasing frequency pathologically. It is stated that aspergillosis now is second only to candidiasis among the mycoses in cancer patients (Young et al.). It is an illness with a clinical spectrum which varies in severity from an almost incidental, saprophytic relationship of organism and host to a fulminating and lethal infection. Infection with this organism spares no age group but adults make up the majority of reported cases. Members of the genus Aspergillus are ubiquitous, filamentous, saprophytic fungi that are commonly found in soil and decaying vegetable matter but can sometimes be found even in a hospital environment (Aisner et al.). The genus includes numerous species, of which Aspergillus fumigatus and Aspergillus flavus have been most often incriminated as causes of human infection. Much less often, Aspergillus niger, Aspergillus oryzae, and many other species have produced disease in the human. Aspergillus species are recognized microscopically as broad, branching, septate hyphae that are 3 to 4 microns in width, often irregularly stained.

In past years, pulmonary aspergillosis was considered to be a rare occupational hazard of bird handlers, hair sorters, millers, or other workers dealing with grain dust. With continued observations, the spectrum of infection with Aspergillus species has been expanded to include primary and secondary forms (Finegold et al.), with gradually increasing awareness of the importance of leukemia and other debilitating diseases as contributing factors to the disseminated type of disease (Table 19–6). As applied to disease caused by Aspergillus species, the term primary refers to infestation with the fungus in the absence of underlying anatomic, immunologic, or other predisposing conditions. Secondary aspergillosis may be either localized or disseminated, but occurs in the individual with some underlying condition which enhances susceptibility to invasive fungal infection.

Table 19–6. Classification of Aspergillosis*

I. Primary aspergillosis—in the absence of underlying disease or other predisposing factors

  A. Localized
    1. Abscesses or granulomas (including mycetoma)
    2. Allergic—bronchitis with asthma and/or eosinophilia

  B. Invasive
    1. Acute—usually bronchopneumonic
    2. Chronic granulomatous disease—usually pulmonary

  C. Disseminated—widespread abscesses or granulomas

II. Secondary aspergillosis—associated with local process, debilitating illness, impaired host defenses, or complicating antibacterial and/or corticosteroid hormone therapy

  A. Localized—usually pulmonary
    1. Saprophytic relationship
      a. Abscess (or mycetoma)
      b. Focal infiltration
    2. Chronic, low-grade infection or granuloma

  B. Invasive—usually bronchopneumonic

  C. Disseminated
    1. Endocarditis
    2. Multiple abscesses or granulomas

*From Finegold et al.

Primary aspergillosis affects the lungs in one form or another in the majority of cases and only rarely spreads to other organs. Disseminated and fatal disease has occurred in early infancy without a predisposing cause (Allan and Anderson), and hematogenous cerebral involvement from pulmonary lesions has been described in the primary form (Linares et al.). Primary pulmonary aspergillosis results in granulomatous lesions or abscesses in many cases but, rarely, the process can be invasive, leading to bilateral pneumonitis, with or without associated abscesses and with a rapidly fatal course (Hertzog et al.). Strelling and colleagues described fulminating primary pulmonary aspergillosis in two siblings and assumed that both children had inhaled the fungus from cattle-cake with which they had played.

An additional unusual form of pulmonary involvement with this fungus is referred to as allergic bronchopulmonary aspergillosis (Hinson et al., Simon et al.). The majority of cases have been observed in patients known to be asthmatic and, to a lesser degree, the disorder represents a complication of cystic fibrosis. The lesions in this condition are not invasive but are confined to the bronchial tree. The manifestations are believed to result from hypersensitivity of the tissues of the host to the fungus. Exudation within the bronchial lumen leads to bronchial obstruction, which gives rise to atelectasis or localized emphysema. Without treatment, the recurrent pulmonary inflammatory reaction associated with this disorder results in progressive pulmonary damage, eventually leading to bronchiectasis and pulmonary fibrosis. Clinically, there are recurrent episodes of acute asthmatic-like respiratory distress, fever, cough, and peripheral eosinophilia. Elevation of the serum immunoglobulin E is an important diagnostic feature of the disorder, and has also been shown to be an indicator of disease activity once treatment has been begun (Hart et al., Rosenberg et al.). Treatment includes the use of corticosteroids, which presumably are effective because of their suppressive effect on the antigen-antibody reactions which give rise to this illness.

Secondary forms of aspergillosis have come to be of much greater medical importance and have been recognized with increasing frequency in recent years (Carbone et al., Kammer and Utz, Meyer et al.), especially in association with leukemia. A finding repeatedly noted in the patient with hematologic malignancy who acquires invasive disease with this fungus is leukopenia, although other factors most likely are also contributory. Aspergillosis in the immunocompromised host may be either pulmonary or disseminated in type and is not often suspected or recognized during the life of the patient.

One form of secondary localized pulmonary aspergillosis is referred to as an aspergilloma or mycetoma, which is a non-invasive, saprophytic fungal mass that develops in bronchiectatic bronchi or within pre-existent cavitary lung lesions. Focal aspergilloma is an important complication of pulmonary sarcoidosis, forming within the cystic cavities and possibly giving rise to fever, cough, and recurrent hemoptysis (Israel and Ostrow). The lesion can be suspected by the characteristic roentgenographic appearance of a round density within a cavitary lesion, with a clear crescent topping the fungal mass. Such lesions are often better demonstrated by tomography than by conventional films. Aspergillomas can also occur in cavitary lung lesions secondary to tuberculosis, pneumoconiosis, or emphysema.

Another predisposing condition associated with an increased incidence of aspergillus infection in recent years is cardiac valvular disease. Aspergillus endocarditis represents a complication of cardiac surgery in most reported cases (Doughten and Pearson, Kammer and Utz), although it can occur as part of disseminated disease without previous valvular damage (Luke et al., Zimmerman). Noteworthy characteristics of aspergillus endocarditis have been the striking infrequency with which the organism has been isolated in blood culture and the tendency for the infection to result in infected embolization to the brain, kidneys, or extremities (Kammer and Utz).

The most common condition associated with secondary, and especially disseminated, aspergillosis is leukemia and, to a lesser degree, other hematologic or solid malignancies (Gruhn and Sanson). Young and colleagues reported 98 patients with aspergillosis, of whom 71 had leukemia of one type or another. Of 22 cases of secondary aspergillosis reviewed by Carbone et al., 20 occurred in patients with neoplastic disease, of whom 16 had acute leukemia. Among 92 cases of aspergillosis complicating neoplastic disease reported by Meyer et al., 50 were in association with leukemia, most often of the acute variety. In addition to hematologic malignant conditions, virtually any disorder treated with immunosuppressive drugs, corticosteroids, or antibiotics for a prolonged period increases the risk of infection caused by Aspergillus species. Aspergillosis has been observed following renal transplantation (Burton et al.), cardiac transplantation (Schober and Herman), secondary to aplastic anemia (Gerstl et al.), and complicating a variety of other chronic debilitating diseases (Young et al.).

Secondary aspergillosis in the compromised or chronically ill host is often confined to the lungs, but therein produces severe and invasive disease. When hematogenous dissemination occurs, virtually any organ can be implicated, but the brain, intestinal tract, liver, kidneys, and heart are preferred sites (Williams) (Fig. 19–12). Among the 98 immunocompromised patients with aspergillosis reported by Young et al., 92 had pulmonary involvement, 21 experienced infection of the gastrointestinal tract, 13 had brain involvement, and in 12 the liver was invaded. Symptoms and signs are variable, depending on which structures are affected, but are often non-specific and intermixed with those of associated bacterial infection or

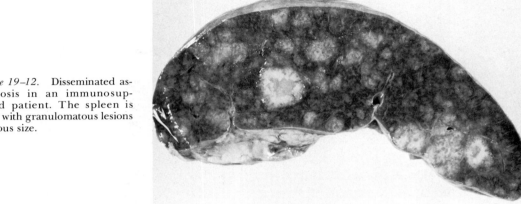

Figure 19–12. Disseminated aspergillosis in an immunosuppressed patient. The spleen is packed with granulomatous lesions of various size.

those resulting from the underlying or predisposing illness. Unremitting fever and the development of pulmonary infiltrates which show no response to antibiotic therapy is the commonest clinical pattern of secondary aspergillosis. Endophthalmitis and intraorbital granulomas have also been described with disseminated aspergillus infections (McCormick et al., Naidoff and Green). Predisposition of the fungus for arterial invasion, repeated failure to isolate the organism on blood culture, and difficulty establishing an antemortem diagnosis are all characteristic features of secondary aspergillosis. The infection represents a serious complication in the debilitated patient and, when identified at autopsy, its occurrence is usually believed to have contributed significantly to death of the patient (Meyer et al.).

Aspergillosis of the Central Nervous System

Aspergillosis of the brain usually occurs in concert with pulmonary involvement and infection of other organs in an immunosuppressed patient. In a few reports, neurologic symptoms and signs have predominated, with little evidence of disease elsewhere (Burston and Blackwood, Jackson et al., Mukoyama et al.) or in patients without a predisposing illness (Linares et al.). The disease is rarely suspected in life but more often is found at autopsy, especially in association with acute leukemia or secondary to immunosuppressive or corticosteroid therapy. The influence of corticosteroids in enhancing dissemination of the infection to the brain has been demonstrated experimentally by intranasal inoculation of control and cortisone-treated mice (Epstein et al.). Drug abuse is an additional debilitating condition which has been complicated by central nervous system aspergillus infections (Gordon et al., Kaufman et al.).

Hematogenous spread of Aspergillus species to the brain results in either a solitary granuloma (Linares et al.) or abscess (Amromin and Gildenhorn, Mukoyama et al.) or, more often, multiple such lesions (Hughes, Meyer et al.) (Fig. 19–13). Meningeal infiltration and inflammation is also present in some cases, but the major impact of the infection is within the parenchyma of the brain. Rarely, aspergillus infection will appear to be limited to the meninges, resulting in a subacute or chronic granulomatous meningitis (Gordon et al.). The cerebral reaction observed microscopically depends on the acuteness of the illness and also varies in different parts of the brain. In the acute stage, the fungi provoke an inflammatory response that is often associated with tissue infarction secondary to vascular occlusion resulting from blood vessel invasion by the organism. Even major arterial structures, such as the internal carotid artery, can be affected in this fashion (McCormick et al.). Arterial invasion by Aspergillus species can also damage the vessel wall, leading to aneurysm formation, which may give rise to spontaneous subarachnoid or cerebral hemorrhage (Horten et al.).

More chronic lesions are granulomatous in character and are composed of fibrous tissue, inflammatory cells, plasma cells, organisms, and an occasional giant cell. Other lesions consist of large areas of frank necrosis with variable amounts of hemorrhage. The clinical manifestations of aspergillosis of the brain are not distinctive, but with diffuse involve-

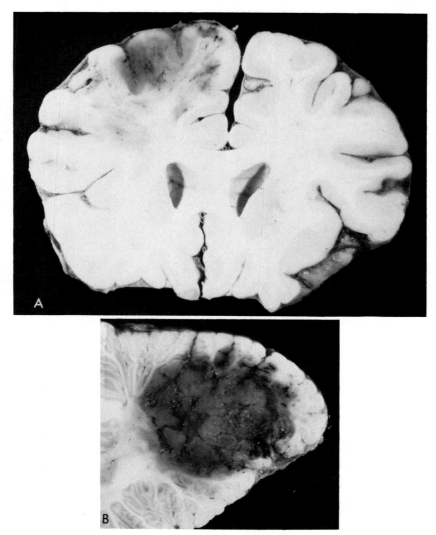

Figure 19–13. Aspergillus encephalitis in an immunosuppressed child. *A,* Coronal section through the frontal lobes demonstrates a hemorrhagic infarct secondary to Aspergillus species vascular invasion resulting in vascular occlusion. *B,* Large cerebellar hemisphere Aspergillus granuloma with hemorrhage.

Illustration continued on opposite page.

ment include such signs as headache, lethargy, confusion, convulsions, and variable focal signs. The unusual occurrence of a large solitary lesion gives rise to a progressive syndrome characterized by increased intracranial pressure and focal neurologic deficits, the type depending on the localization of the lesion. Still another type of neurologic syndrome can complicate aspergillus endocarditis or aspergillus infection of a cardiac valve prosthesis (Dayal et al.). Fungal embolic episodes from the intracardiac site are common in such cases, with a preference for cerebral involvement (Kammer and Utz). Embolic oc-

clusion of a major cerebral vessel precipitates a stroke-like picture but is associated with fever, chills, and other signs of infection.

Cerebrospinal fluid findings with cerebral aspergillosis are of little diagnostic help and are quite variable. The cerebrospinal fluid may be entirely normal or reveal a cellular response, which can be either predominantly polymorphonuclear or mononuclear in type. The glucose content is normal while the protein value is often moderately increased. Isolation of the fungus from the cerebrospinal fluid cannot usually be accomplished, although positive cultures have been reported on rare occasion (Gordon et al., Horten et al.).

Diagnosis

The infrequency of clinical diagnosis of aspergillosis is largely explained by the limited ability in life to isolate the organism in culture. With disseminated disease, the fungus can rarely be obtained from blood or cerebrospinal fluid. Even cultures of sputum or tracheal secretions are often unrewarding, despite the presence of pulmonary infection. Furthermore, in patients with cerebral aspergillosis, the cerebrospinal fluid commonly reveals only a few cells and little else except an elevated protein content which might otherwise be explained by the predisposing illness. Because of the unreliability of cultural meth-

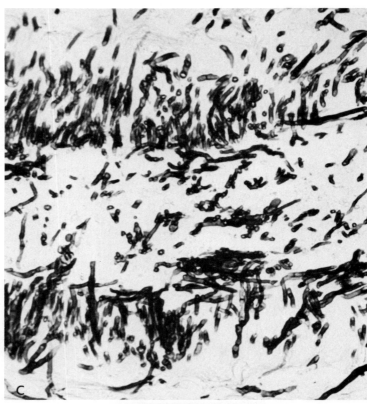

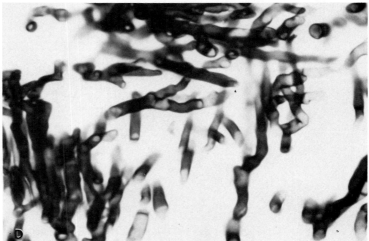

Figure 19–13 Continued. C, Aspergillus species abundantly invading the walls of a cerebral blood vessel. *D,* High-power view shows the acute branching, septations, and variable staining qualities characteristic of Aspergillus species.

ods as a means to establish a premortem diagnosis, some authors recommend percutaneous needle biopsy of the lung or open thoracotomy as a diagnostic method in the immunosuppressed patient who develops an unexplained pulmonary infiltrate with fever that does not respond to antibiotics (Burton et al.). Serodiagnosis of aspergillosis by determination of serum precipitins by an immunodiffusion test (Coleman et al.) has been claimed useful by some (Hefferman and Asper) but is felt to be of limited value by others. Meyer et al. found that a positive serum precipitin reaction to aspergillus antigen indicated invasive aspergillosis, but a negative test could not be accepted as evidence excluding the disease.

Aspergillosis is, therefore, often unexpectedly identified at autopsy on the basis of the morphologic characteristics of the fungus in tissue and the associated tissue reaction. The hyphae are broad, accept methenamine silver stain in a less than uniform fashion, and are notably branched, usually in a "tree-like" fashion (Fig. 19–14). The presence of the characteristic conidiophores virtually confirms a tissue diagnosis, but they are seen only infrequently in tissue. The hyphae of Aspergillus species can usually be differentiated from those of the Phycomycetes, since the latter are non-septated and somewhat more irregular in width. Both fungi exhibit a decided predilection for blood vessel invasion.

Candida species are recognized as round or oval yeast forms with pseudohyphae with much less lateral branching and generally with more uniform staining than aspergillus. In the absence of conidiophores, aspergillus cannot usually be distinguished morphologically from Penicillium species but the latter is a much less common cause of human infection. Nocardia asteroides is easily distinguished because of the multiplicity of forms and the much smaller size of the filamentous elements as compared to aspergillus. While morphologic identification of Aspergillus species in tissue is reasonably reliable, final identification is on the basis of culture on appropriate media.

Treatment

Pulmonary aspergillosis has been successfully treated with amphotericin B in some cases (Aisner et al., Burton et al.), but disseminated disease generally responds poorly to drug therapy. Amphotericin B has been regarded to be the drug of choice, and, for cerebral aspergillosis, probably should be given by both systemic and intrathecal administration. Five-fluorocytosine administered orally has recently been found to be effective against Aspergillus species (Steer et al.) but to a lesser degree than with Candida species or Cryptococcus neoformans. Infection lim-

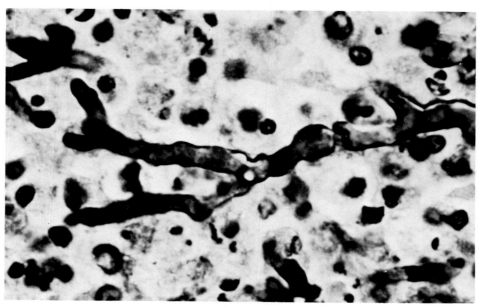

Figure 19–14. Aspergillus species in tissue. Broad, septate, branched hyphae are somewhat irregularly stained (Grocott's methenamine silver stain).

ited to the lung responds more favorably but meningeal infection also has been successfully eliminated with this drug (Atkinson and Israel, Gordon et al.). The combined use of amphotericin B and 5-fluorocytosine has been recommended for invasive aspergillus infections (Codish et al., Kammer and Utz) and would seem desirable because of the limited success with previous therapeutic experience with this infection. Studies by Kitahara et al. have demonstrated that the combination of amphotericin B and 5-fluorocytosine or amphotericin B and rifampin is synergistic against certain aspergillus isolates.

HISTOPLASMOSIS

Histoplasmosis is primarily a pulmonary infection but is an illness with a wide spectrum of possible manifestations, with involvement of a single organ system asymptomatically or seriously, or multiple organs in disseminated fashion. The disease has been identified in many parts of the world, and in the United States occurs endemically in the northeast and along the Ohio, Mississippi, and lower Missouri valleys. The high incidence of infection in these regions is reflected by a rate of skin test reactivity among adults as high as 80 percent (Edwards and Palmer). The disease is caused by Histoplasma capsulatum, a commonly found inhabitant of soil, which, in tissue, is a round or oval intracellular yeast measuring 2 to 5 microns and with a distinct pseudocapsule. The pseudocapsular appearance is explained by the retraction of the protoplasm away from the rigid cell wall that occurs with fixation. This results in the formation of a clear space that simulates a capsule but represents an artifact of laboratory preparation.

The organism was discovered in 1905 by Samuel Darling, a pathologist working in Panama, who chose the name, Histoplasma capsulatum because of its predisposition to invade the histiocyte and because of its morphologic similarity to plasmodium-like organisms. Initially considered to be a protozoan by Darling, the organism is now known to be a dimorphic fungus, which, when cultured on Sabouraud's agar, is notably slow-growing and results in septate hyphae bearing round chlamydospores on short pedicles. Subculturing to blood agar slant converts the filamentous culture to a yeast-like phase, analogous to that which occurs in tissue. The designation chosen by Darling, Histoplasma capsu-

latum, has remained in use despite the fact that the organism is not related to plasmodia and is not encapsulated.

Histoplasmosis is acquired by respiratory inhalation of air-borne spores in the vast majority of cases, although entry of spores via the gastrointestinal tract from contaminated drinking water has been proposed (Ritter). Man-to-man transmission is not known to occur. In many instances a specific source of the fungus is not apparent, but in others the infected individual has been in close contact with chicken coops or excreta of pigeons, other birds, or bats. Histoplasmosis is more common in adult males than females, perhaps because of occupational exposure to sources of the organism. In children there is no apparent sex predisposition. The primary disease in the majority of cases is asymptomatic or sufficiently mild that it is etiologically unrecognized. Evidence of prior infection in such patients is either by skin test reactivity or on the basis of the characteristic, multiple calcified pulmonary lesions seen on chest x-ray.

Most acute cases with respiratory symptoms occur sporadically, but several large outbreaks have been described. In 1970, 384 students and faculty in Ohio developed clinical illness after cleaning a school courtyard which had been a roost for starlings and blackbirds (Brodsky et al.). Eighty-seven adults developed acute pulmonary histoplasmosis in Mason City, Iowa, in 1964 following the removal of trees and brush which had served as a starling roost (Medeiros et al.). Another outbreak affected 23 of 29 persons who explored a bat-infested limestone cave in Florida (Morbidity and Mortality Reports, Vol. 22, 1973), and an additional one involved 42 persons who helped to cut and remove a fallen oak tree in Nashville, Tennessee (Ward et al.).

Acute pulmonary histoplasmosis usually occurs in otherwise normal persons and does not show a predisposition to develop in association with malignancies or immunosuppression. The simultaneous occurrence of pulmonary histoplasmosis and tuberculosis in adults is higher than expected by coincidence (Vanek and Schwarz, Ahn et al.). Progressive, disseminated forms of the disease, estimated to occur in less than one per thousand patients with histoplasmosis, are most commonly seen in the very young, the elderly, or those with some type of immunosuppressing illness (Reddy et al., Furcolow). Disseminated histoplasmosis has been described with leu-

Table 19–7. Classification of Symptomatic
Histoplasmosis

A. Pulmonary histoplasmosis
    Acute pulmonary
    Focal lesion (histoplasmoma)
    Chronic pulmonary
B. Disseminated histoplasmosis
C. Other forms (cutaneous, pericardial, laryngeal,
    hepatic)

---

kemia (Cox and Hughes, Bodey, Smith and
Utz), with reticuloendothelial malignancies
(Ende et al., Furcolow, Murray and Sladden),
and in patients immunosuppressed with non-
neoplastic disorders (Couch et al., Rifkind et
al., Watson et al.) or on chronic corticosteroid
therapy (Reddy et al.).

Clinical Manifestations

Symptomatic primary pulmonary histoplasmosis is characterized by its abrupt onset
with respiratory and influenza-like symptoms
and tends to follow unusually heavy exposure
to the infectious agent. Most common symptoms include fever, chills, headache, myalgia,
fatigue, chest pain, and cough. Erythema
multiforme and erythema nodosum have
been notable in certain outbreaks (Meideiros
et al., Sellers et al.), but are not considered to
be common manifestations of the disease.
The pulmonary infiltrates seen on chest x-ray
in the acute phase are usually bilateral and
often manifested in a nodular fashion (Fig.
19–15). The nodules are larger than those in
miliary tuberculosis and appear soft, with
poorly defined margins (Christoforidis).

The primary illness is benign and self-limited in the majority of instances but can be
complicated by pericarditis (Friedman et al.,
Vanek and Schwarz) or by regional lymph
node enlargement, which sometimes results
in compression of adjacent bronchi or vascular structures. With healing, pulmonary
and lymph node lesions show a marked predisposition to undergo calcium deposition, a
process that can occur within a few months
after the primary infection or require several
years to develop. Despite the benign and
transient nature of primary pulmonary histoplasmosis in most cases, hematogenous but
self-limited spread of the organism at the
time of the initial infection is a common event
(Friedman et al., Vanek and Schwarz). In unusual cases, pulmonary histoplasmosis assumes a progressive course, resulting in

chronic, cavitary pulmonary disease, similar
to that of tuberculosis (Ahn et al., Parker et
al.). Chronic, progressive pulmonary histoplasmosis is currently assumed to represent
an opportunistic infection usually occurring
in persons with pre-existent chronic obstructive pulmonary disease. An additional rare
expression of the primary disease is an acute
granulomatous hepatitis (Lanza et al.).

Progressive, disseminated histoplasmosis is
an infrequent but serious disease which is
seen either in infancy (Holland and Holland)
or in persons with some predisposing or debilitating condition. Common manifestations
in the infant include fever, anemia, thrombocytopenia, and leukopenia (Fig. 19–16).
Hepatosplenomegaly, pulmonary infiltrates,
and destructive adrenal involvement are associated with rapid clinical deterioration and
eventual death unless treatment is begun
early in the illness. Neurologic involvement
can accompany the disseminated form of the
disease, but, as mentioned subsequently, occurs in only a small percentage of such cases.

Histoplasmosis of the Central Nervous System

Clinical manifestations of histoplasmosis of
the central nervous system are rarely seen,
although cerebral invasion by the organism
following dissemination from the lungs is
probably more common than is generally recognized. Schulz reviewed autopsies of 120
cases of histoplasmosis and found lesions or
organisms in the brain or meninges in 12.
Three of the patients were children two years
of age or less and nine were adults. Although
the total number of cases of histoplasmosis of
the central nervous system reported to this
date is relatively small, until recently the majority occurred in non-immunosuppressed
patients. The more current literature indicates a change in this regard in that most
cases with neurologic involvement described
recently are in patients with underlying diseases, such as Hodgkin's disease, leukemia,
post-renal transplantation, or hypogammaglobulinemia (Couch et al., Karalakulasingam
et al., Kauffman et al.). Even in immunosuppressed individuals with disseminated disease
with Histoplasma capsulatum, only the minority appear to develop neurologic involvement. Of the 54 such cases reviewed by
Kauffman et al., only five were found to have
central nervous system histoplasmosis.

Neurologic histoplasmosis can occur in a

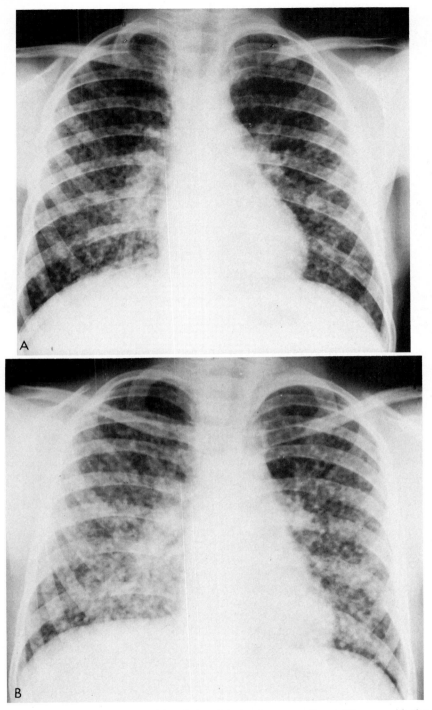

Figure 19–15. A and B, Acute pulmonary histoplasmosis in brothers, ages 8 and 10 years, with simultaneous and nearly identical acute respiratory illnesses. Symptoms of 2 weeks' duration included malaise, headache, cough, spiking fever, and exertional dyspnea. Histoplasma capsulatum was isolated on culture from the bone marrow of both patients. Spontaneous recovery occurred within 8 weeks after onset. Chest roentgenograms show bilateral, extensive, coarse nodular infiltrates and hilar adenopathy.

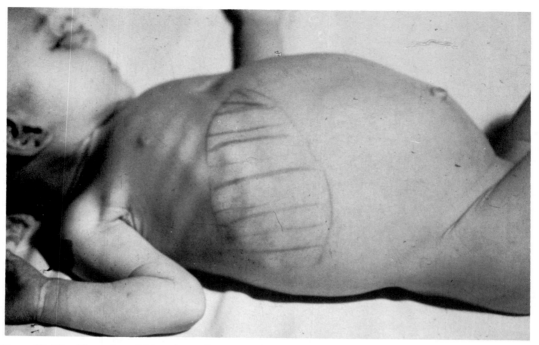

Figure 19–16.   Disseminated histoplasmosis. Four-month-old infant with a history of abdominal distention for 2 months, pallor for 1 month, and poor weight gain. Physical findings included tachypnea and tachycardia, marked hepatosplenomegaly, soft tissue edema, and decreased muscle tone. Hemoglobin 4.3 gm. per 100 ml., white blood count 3,800 per cu. mm., platelet count 14,000. Total serum protein 2.3 gm. per 100 ml. Provisional diagnosis at the time of hospital admission was acute leukemia, but bone marrow examination revealed histiocytes heavily parasitized with Histoplasma capsulatum. Death occurred at age 5 months.

variety of forms, including leptomeningitis, multiple miliary granulomas of the meninges or brain, and a solitary focal granulomatous lesion of the parenchyma of the brain (Fig. 19–17). In the great majority of cases in which the central nervous system is involved, the primary infection is believed to be in the lungs, and in many instances other organ systems are also involved. Reports which describe histoplasmosis of the central nervous system alone are exceedingly limited (Gilden et al., Juba). Histoplasma meningitis develops in acute, rapidly progressive fashion in some cases (Nelson et al.) and as a subacute or chronic granulomatous process in others (Gerber et al., Snyder and White, Sprofkin et al., Tynes et al.). Focal, granulomatous lesions may occur within the cerebrum, cerebellum, or brain stem and give rise to a progressive syndrome with localized neurologic deficits and increased intracranial pressure, thus simulating an intracranial neoplasm or abscess (Greer et al., White and Fritzlen). In other cases, both meningeal and parenchymal invasion with histoplasma results in signs of meningeal irritation in addition to a variety of signs of neurologic dysfunction. Without

treatment, neurologic histoplasmosis is associated with a high mortality rate, although the duration of the illness is subject to remarkable variation.

The cerebrospinal fluid in patients with histoplasmosis of the nervous system is usually abnormal, although exceptions do exist (Cooper and Goldstein). The cellular response is often predominantly neutrophilic, but in some cases both neutrophils and lymphocytes are present. Elevation of the cerebrospinal fluid protein content is perhaps the most consistent abnormality, while the glucose value may be normal but more often is reduced. Isolation of histoplasma from the cerebrospinal fluid is generally difficult and may be impossible, even on multiple attempts. It is recommended that the fluid specimen be centrifuged for 30 minutes before inoculation of the sediment into the appropriate culture medium.

Histoplasmosis of the leptomeninges produces a thick, yellowish exudate, most striking at the base of the brain. Discrete, gray opacities that resemble tubercles are often seen adjacent to vessels over the cerebral convexities. Miliary, granulomatous lesions are

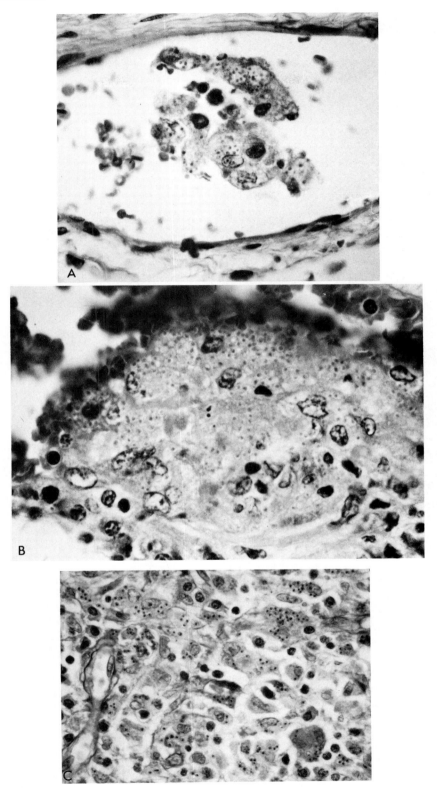

Figure 19–17. Cerebral histoplasmosis. *A,* Numerous yeast-like organisms in macrophages within a cerebral blood vessel. *B,* Histoplasma capsulatum in a small mural thrombus in a cerebral vessel. *C,* Histoplasma capsulatum in macrophages within brain tissue.

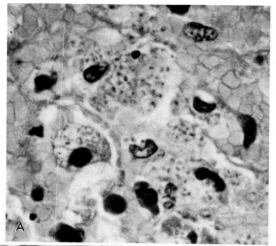

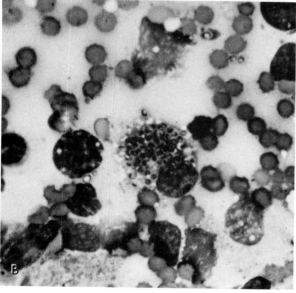

Figure 19–18. Histoplasmosis. *A,* Histoplasma capsulatum in the spleen in an infant with disseminated histoplasmosis. Organisms are small intracytoplasmic bodies within macrophages (H & E). *B,* Yeast within a histiocyte in bone marrow (Giemsa stain).

sometimes scattered throughout the brain. Histologically, the meningeal exudate is composed of macrophages, neutrophils, and lymphocytes and is associated with a pronounced perivascular inflammatory reaction. The fungus stained with methenamine silver is a round or ovoid body, 2 to 5 microns in diameter, often in clusters within the cytoplasm of macrophages. Within liver and spleen, the yeast parasitize reticuloendothelial cells, and in bone marrow they are observed clustered in histiocytes (Fig. 19–18).

Diagnosis

Hematogenous dissemination of histoplasma to the nervous system is suggested by the development of meningeal or neurologic signs along with cerebrospinal fluid abnormalities in the patient known to have extraneural histoplasmosis. Proof of the illness is on the basis of isolation of the organism from the cerebrospinal fluid, although this is frequently unsuccessful. When the organism cannot be cultured from cerebrospinal fluid in the patient with evidence of granulomatous meningeal inflammation, meningeal biopsy can be diagnostic in some cases and warrants consideration. Isolation of the yeast from blood or bone marrow, histologic identification of the organism in bone marrow, or microscopic identification and isolation in culture of the yeast from excised lymph node tissue are more dependable diagnostic methods. Davies et al. have stressed the importance of trephine bone marrow biopsy, which yields tissue for identification of fungi on stained preparations and in culture, as well as adequate tissue for microscopic examination for granulomas or proliferation of macrophages, findings suggestive of disseminated histoplasmosis. Histoplasma capsulatum can be cultured on the commonly used laboratory media. On Sabouraud's agar, the colony is initially cottony white in appearance and becomes brown with age.

The histoplasmin skin test is of value for population surveys to identify frequency of past infection but is of limited usefulness to identify active, disseminated disease. The skin test is frequently negative in the presence of disseminated histoplasmosis (Cooper and Goldstein, Reddy et al.). Since the skin test antigen can stimulate mycelial phase antibodies (Campbell and Hill) and thus disturb interpretation of diagnostic serologic tests, it should not be used when one is considering the possibility of active disease, whether pulmonary or disseminated. Tests on serum indicative of active infection with Histoplasma capsulatum include the presence of precipitin bands to histoplasmin antigen (Heiner) and complement fixation to yeast and mycelial phase antigens. Complement-fixing antibodies to the yeast phase antigen rise three to four weeks after the primary infection is acquired and decline several weeks later unless disseminated disease follows. While serologic tests are of great value in the diagnosis of histoplasmosis in the patient with normal immune mechanisms, they are often not helpful in the immunocompromised host (Kauffman et al.).

Treatment

Primary pulmonary histoplasmosis is managed conservatively, even in cases in which the organism is isolated from blood or bone marrow. Recovery is expected in the majority of such cases within one to several weeks. The progressive, disseminated form of the disease is treated with amphotericin B. In patients with histoplasma meningitis, amphotericin B is administered intravenously in the initial course, but if relapse occurs or if the infection is intractable, intrathecal therapy should be considered. Adrenal insufficiency complicates some cases with widespread disease and requires replacement therapy when identified. Disseminated histoplasmosis without therapy carries a high mortality rate, but many examples of successful treatment with amphotericin B have been recorded (Cox and Hughes, Nelson et al., Reddy et al., Snyder and White, Tynes et al.).

BLASTOMYCOSIS

Blastomycosis, also known as Gilchrist's disease or North American blastomycosis, is an infectious disease with a clinical spectrum that remains incompletely defined and which is caused by a yeast whose source in nature has been elusive to investigators for years. Blastomyces dermatitidis is a dimorphic fungus which is a spherical, thick-walled, budding yeast in exudate or tissue. The first description is credited to Gilchrist, who, in 1894, identified large, oval organisms obtained from a lesion on the hand of a patient. The nature of the infection was not entirely clear at that time, but four years later the infecting organism was recognized as a fungus and named Blastomyces dermatitidis by Gilchrist and Stokes. The history of identification of the organism and the early concepts of the pathologic conditions produced by Blastomyces dermatitidis were eloquently reviewed in 1939 by Martin and Smith of the Duke University School of Medicine. Their extensive summarization of the literature compiled to that date and addition of 13 cases represented a major contribution to the understanding and awareness of this mycotic disease.

Previously believed to be confined to the United States and Canada, infection caused by Blastomyces dermatitidis has been described in Mexico and South America, and more recently in many other countries (Emmons et al.). In the United States, most cases are found in the Ohio and Mississippi River valleys, and in southern and southeastern states (Harrell and Curtis). Blastomycosis is a disease mainly of adults and affects males considerably more often than females, especially men with outdoor occupations. In most instances, the illness occurs in sporadic fashion but a few outbreaks involving several persons have been described (Smith et al. 1955, Tosh et al.). The illness does not have a predisposition for the immunologically compromised patient.

Blastomycosis originally was believed to be primarily a cutaneous disease which resulted from direct inoculation of the fungus into the skin. Extracutaneous manifestations were subsequently observed, but, in many cases, visceral or skeletal infection was assumed to be the result of spread from the initial cutaneous site of infection. In 1951, Schwarz and Baum presented evidence that the portal of entry in most cases is by inhalation and that respiratory infection is the customary initial form of disease. Lymphatic and hematogenous dissemination therefrom can result in other organ involvement, such as the skin, oral or nasal mucosa, genitourinary tract, bone, or, rarely, the central nervous system. This concept of primary respiratory involvement in blastomycosis is now generally accepted. The majority of cutaneous infections are secondary from spread from other organs and only rarely is the skin primarily affected by direct inoculation from the external environment (Witorsch and Utz).

Subsequent to these observations, blastomycosis became known as a chronic pulmonary disease with symptoms almost identical to those of pulmonary tuberculosis except for the much greater susceptibility of Blastomyces dermititidis to spread to the skin. The decided predisposition for dissemination became obvious and, although the illness followed a chronic course, it was assumed that it was a prognostically serious condition in the majority of cases. More recent studies have suggested, however, that blastomycosis affects man in a much broader clinical spectrum than had previously been recognized, and that it has many features in common with histoplasmosis and coccidioidomycosis. One unexplained difference is the relative lack of blastomycotic infection in the very young, as occurs occasionally with histoplasmosis and to a lesser extent with coccidioidomycosis. With the latter disorder, meningeal involvement is much more common, and, unlike histoplasmosis, healed pulmonary blastomycosis is not associated with radiologically evident calcified lesions. The ability to identify the mild, transient, or asymptomatic form of respiratory blastomycosis has been hampered by the limited value and unpredictability of the skin test and the complement fixation reaction.

It is now known that blastomycosis has a clinical spectrum that extends from asymptomatic pulmonary infection to severe, life-threatening disseminated disease (Sarosi et al.). Between the extremes are cases with acute, self-limited symptomatic infection in which the process is confined to the respiratory tract and from which complete recovery occurs. In addition, an acute, severe, rapidly progressive form of pulmonary blastomycosis can also occur but has only rarely been described (Palmer and McFadden). What remains to be determined is the relative frequency of occurrence of asymptomatic or mild infections caused by this fungus in comparison to the more readily identifiable chronic pulmonary and disseminated forms of the disease.

Although it is now accepted that man acquires Blastomyces dermatitidis by inhalation, the source of the organism remains obscure. Neither man-to-man nor animal-to-man transmission has been identified. Attempts to isolate the organism from nature have largely been unsuccessful (Furcolow and Smith), and only rarely has Blastomyces dermatitidis been recovered from soil at a case site (Denten et al.). Nonetheless, it is still assumed that, in the majority of instances, man acquires the fungus from contaminated soil (Sarosi and Davies).

Clinical Manifestations

As mentioned above, blastomycosis is believed to be acquired by inhalation of the fungus, which leads to pulmonary infection of variable severity and duration. The incubation period has not been established. Disseminated infection is not uncommon with this illness, sometimes provoking symptoms or signs of disease of other organs with minimal or only roentgenographic evidence of pulmonary involvement. Secondary sites of predilection include the skin and skeletal structures. Among a series of 40 cases of blastomycosis published by Witorsch and Utz, approximately two-thirds had infection involving two or more organ systems. Of 63 cases of blastomycosis reported by Duttera and Osterhout, cutaneous lesions were found in 57 percent, pulmonary infection was identified in 52 percent, bone involvement in 19 percent, and central nervous system involvement in 6 percent. Most cases of this disease are sporadic but a few small-scale epidemics have been described (Smith et al., Sarosi et al.).

The initial pulmonary infection in some individuals is a benign, transient, influenza-like illness with chills and fever, headache, myalgia, and a hacking cough with the production of mucopurulent sputum. The illness is complicated by pleural effusion in some cases (Powell and Schuit). In other cases, pulmonary infection becomes chronic, bearing similarity to pulmonary tuberculosis, and complicated by eventual manifestations of dissemination to other sites. In some patients, manifestations of the pulmonary infection have subsided weeks or months before secondary lesions appear elsewhere. The skin is the most frequently involved secondary site, where solitary or multiple lesions may develop (Turner and Wadlington). The cutaneous lesion begins as a small papule which, over a period of weeks to months, enlarges to an elevated, indurated, crusted lesion with a violaceous color and irregular borders. Removal of the crust reveals granulomatous tissue intermixed with multiple small abscesses. Satellite lymphadenopathy is associated with surface lesions, similar to that with sporotrichosis.

Skeletal lesions of disseminated blastomycosis are osteolytic in type with irregular margins and sometimes associated with contiguous soft tissue abscesses (Fig. 19–19). When the osteomyelitic process affects the skull or vertebrae, an adjacent abscess extending to the epidural space results in cerebral or spinal cord compression. In addition to metastatic spread to the skin or bony structures, the infection may involve the genitourinary tract, lymph nodes, liver, and less often, various other structures. Widespread, disseminated blastomycosis is characterized by its chronicity, tendency for abscess formation, and poor eventual outcome. The sedimentation rate is usually elevated and blood leukocytosis is often present.

Blastomycosis of the Nervous System

Central nervous system infection is a serious but unusual complication of blastomycosis which, as with other forms of the disease, has occurred predominantly in adults. Most cases are the result of hematogenous spread from the lungs, and the majority are associated with clear-cut evidence of extraneural blastomycotic infection. Blastomyces dermatitidis has a propensity to spread to the posterior elements of the vertebrae and, for this reason, spinal epidural abscess or granuloma with cord compression is relatively frequent among cases with central nervous system involvement (Gonyea, Greenwood and Voris). Intracranial epidural abscess can likewise complicate cranial osteomyelitic lesions. Within the parenchyma of the cerebrum or cerebellum, blastomycotic abscess or granuloma produces focal neurologic signs, in ad-

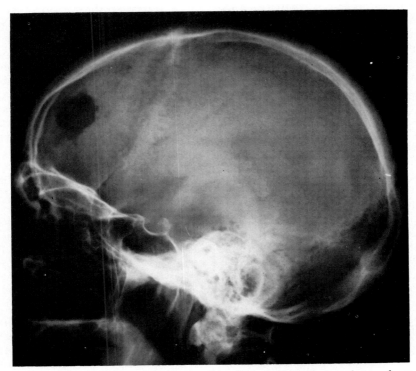

Figure 19–19.   Blastomycosis. Blastomycotic osteomyelitis of the skull. Skull x-ray shows a large osteolytic lesion in the frontal area with irregular margins, secondary to dissemination from the lungs.

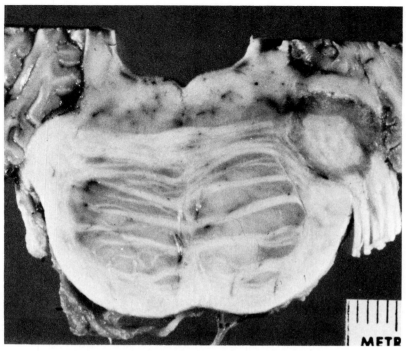

Figure 19–20.   Blastomycosis. Solid granuloma within the pons at the level of the trigeminal nerve.

dition to signs of increased intracranial pressure, thus simulating an intracranial neoplasm (Leers et al., Waisbren and Ullrich). Such focal lesions may occur anywhere in the brain, brainstem, or spinal cord and can either be single or multiple (Fig. 19–20). Meningitis is the most common type of central nervous system blastomycosis, manifested by headache, vomiting, confusion, and neck rigidity (Carmody and Tappen, Friedman and Signorelli, Loudon and Lawson). The clinical pattern of blastomycotic meningitis can be either acute or chronic, with considerable variation in the severity or rate of progression of symptoms. Almost all reported cases have been in persons with prior evidence of blastomycotic disease elsewhere, although Gonyea has described cases with meningeal involvement in the absence of evidence of other organ system disease. As in other forms of granulomatous meningitis, relapse can occur following apparently successful therapy.

The cerebrospinal fluid in patients with blastomycotic meningitis is usually under increased pressure and shows a cellular pleocytosis, usually lymphocytic in type, a mild to moderate increase in protein content, and frequently, a modest reduction in the glucose value. Yeast forms may be seen on stained smear of a centrifuged specimen, although

proof of the diagnosis on smear or culture of cerebrospinal fluid is often difficult. Gonyea has emphasized the greater likelihood of isolation of organisms from cisternal or ventricular fluid specimens as compared to lumbar spinal fluid for blastomycotic as well as other granulomatous meningeal infections. Meningeal biopsy for microscopic examination and for culture is an additional important measure for consideration when fungal infection of the meninges is suspected but cannot be proved by the customary methods. The tissue response to this infection is either a granulomatous or suppurative reaction in meninges or brain, or a combination of both. In the blastomycotic granuloma, the presence of inflammatory cells, epithelioid cells, and multinucleated giant cells resembles that in tuberculous lesions. Without treatment, meningitis or brain abscess caused by Blastomyces dermatitidis is assumed to be uniformly fatal.

Diagnosis

Diagnosis of blastomycosis can be established only by cultural identification of Blastomyces dermatitidis from tissue, secretions, or exudate. Sputum, pus, cerebrospinal fluid, or excised tissue should be cultured on brain-heart infusion glucose agar or Sabouraud's glucose agar, on which identifiable colonies will develop within a week. On Sabouraud's agar, growth is initially smooth and yeast-like but rapidly develops aerial projections. Eventually, the majority of the growth becomes filamentous with the mold being white in color. Microscopic examination of the growth shows many spherical spores, 4 to 8 microns in diameter, attached directly to the hyphae (Conant). On glucose blood agar, the fungus retains its yeast form, as in tissue. In tissue sections or direct examination of exudates, Blastomyces dermatitidis is readily seen with the hematoxylin and eosin stain as well as the methenamine silver stain. The yeast can be found either in free form or within multinucleated giant cells or monocytes, as with Histoplasma capsulatum. It is a round or oval thick-walled organism, 6 to 15 microns in diameter, often with a single bud with a broad-based attachment (Fig. 19–21). The broad attachment of the single bud to the parent cell is distinctive of Blastomyces dermatitidis, although budding cells are sometimes difficult to find in infected tissues. Rapid examination of pus or sputum can also be accomplished by mixing the specimen on a glass slide with a drop of 10 percent potassium hydroxide. The refractile wall of the yeast can be observed by this method. Intraperitoneal inoculation of mice or the guinea pig is an additional laboratory diagnostic method. The pathologic response in the animal is the formation of peritoneal abscesses or granulomatous adenopathy, which can be demonstrated approximately four weeks after inoculation.

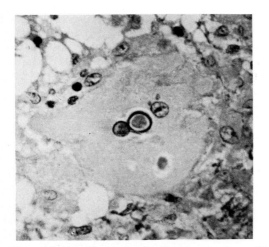

Figure 19–21. Blastomycosis. Blastomyces dermatitidis in tissue is a round or oval, thick-walled yeast with a single bud. Note the broad-based attachment of the bud to the parent cell (H & E).

The blastomycin skin test is subject to variable results and generally has not been found to be a useful diagnostic tool. The test is performed by the intradermal injection of 0.1 ml. of blastomycin and interpreted 24 and 48 hours thereafter. An indurated area greater than 5 millimeters is a positive response. Cross reactions with histoplasmin appear to be common (Furcolow et al.), while the test is frequently negative in patients known to have clinical disease (Witorsch and Utz). Likewise, the complement fixation test is not consistently reliable and remains negative in certain patients proved to have blastomycosis. When antibody titers do rise, they rarely exceed 1:128, and more often titers of 1:32 or less are found (Harrell and Curtis). Titer elevations that do occur are transient.

Treatment

Treatment of disseminated blastomycosis requires long-term chemotherapy in addition to the judicious application of surgical removal of solid granulomatous lesions or drainage of abscesses when tissue compression occurs therefrom. Drugs effective for this illness include 2-hydroxystilbamidine and amphotericin B, with the latter generally preferred in recent years.

Blastomycosis of the central nervous system is always a serious condition but is not invariably fatal if early and appropriate treatment is rendered (Gonyea, Rainey and Harris). Solitary granulomas have been successfully removed from the brain in conjunction with amphotericin B treatment (Waisbren and Ullrich). Osteomyelitis of the skull (Turner and Wadlington) and blastomycotic meningitis (Carmody and Tappen) have also been successfully treated with amphotericin B, but meningitis carries a particularly poor prognosis.

PHYCOMYCOSIS (MUCORMYCOSIS)

Phycomycosis (mucormycosis, zygomycosis) refers to one of several forms of fungal disease which have variable clinical expressions but with a predisposition for central nervous system involvement and for vascular invasion, producing thrombosis by the causative organism. Among fungal infections, mucormycosis varies from most in that it is often a rapidly progressive illness with death occurring one to three weeks after onset. Like several other mycotic disorders, it shows a definite predisposition to attack the compromised host. No other fungal disease, however, exhibits the predilection for the diabetic patient that mucormycosis shows. Infections in this category are caused by fungi in the class Phycomycetes (Zygomycetes), and the vast majority are in the order Mucorales, family Mucoraceae, genus Rhizopus, Mucor, or Absidia (Table 19–8). The commonly used term, mucormycosis, is correctly applicable to mycotic infection caused by members of the order Mucorales. It does not necessarily imply, however, that the offending organism is of the genus Mucor, since Rhizopus is a more common cause of the condition than are species of the genus Mucor. Although mucormycosis is a designation universally and largely appropriately used, some have preferred the broader term, phycomycosis, since rare reports exist of human disease due to Basidiobolus, which is a member of the order Entomophthorale (Joe et al.). The non-septate hyphae of all the species in these groups are nearly identical and cannot usually be differentiated by microscopic examination of the organism in tissue.

Fungi of the order Mucorales are ubiquitous saprophytes often found in decaying vegetable matter or soil and on rare occasion can be recovered from nasal or throat cultures of normal individuals. In addition, they are common laboratory contaminants. They have limited capability to produce disease in the normal person and only rarely has visceral involvement been described in an otherwise healthy individual (DeWeese et al.). With certain predisposing conditions, however, these fungi become invasive pathogens, often giving rise to rapidly progressive and life-threatening disease. In infancy, disseminated mucormycosis can complicate severe debilitating illnesses associated with dehydra-

tion, acidosis, or uremia (Borland, Hale, Martin et al.). In older children and adults, diabetes mellitus, and especially acute diabetic acidosis, is the major precipitating factor and accounts for over 50 percent of all cases reported to date in patients beyond the infant age group (Abramson et al., DeWeese et al., Landau and Newcomer, Long and Weiss, McCall and Strobos, Merriam and Tedeschi, Prockop and Silva-Hutner, Sandler et al., Smith et al.). Leukemia, lymphoma, other forms of cancer, and the immunosuppressive drug therapy used for these conditions also enhance the risk of invasive disease caused by this group of fungi (Carpenter et al., Hart et al., Hutter). Mucormycosis has occurred in patients with severe burns (Baker), in narcotic addicts (Hameroff et al.), complicating septic abortion (McBride et al.), cardiac and renal transplantation (Hammer et al., Schober and Herman), and a variety of other serious debilitating and nutritional disorders, especially when treatment has included corticosteroids or antibiotic agents (Agger and Maki).

Mucormycosis is not a common illness but, like other diseases caused by opportunistic invaders, it has been recognized with increasing frequency in the past two decades. The disease spares no age group and has been described in early infancy as well as in the elderly. Mucormycosis, rarely, can be a localized, cutaneous infection involving the external ear canals, the skin adjacent to the fingernails, or skin elsewhere. Cutaneous mucormycosis has also occurred as a nosocomial infection in which skin inoculation has been attributed to contaminated bandages (Gartenberg et al., Sheldon and Johnson). Skeletal involvement with Phycomycetes is often present as an infection contiguous to sinus or orbital invasion with the fungus, but osteomyelitis as an independent infection has only

Table 19–8.   Classification of Fungi Causing Phycomycosis (Mucormycosis)

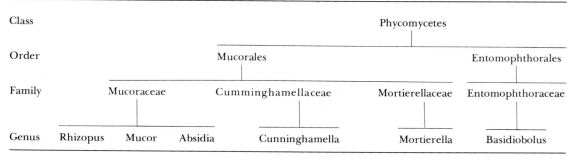

Class				Phycomycetes			
Order		Mucorales				Entomophthorales	
Family	Mucoraceae		Cumminghamellaceae		Mortierellaceae	Entomophthoraceae	
Genus	Rhizopus	Mucor	Absidia	Cunninghamella	Mortierella	Basidiobolus	

Table 19–9.   Classification of Phycomycosis

Cutaneous
Pulmonary
Gastrointestinal
Rhinocerebral
Cerebral
Disseminated

rarely been described (Echols et al.). The more common and more widely recognized infections with these fungi are those with visceral involvement, in which the portal of entry is either respiratory, gastrointestinal, or within the nasal cavity or paranasal sinuses.

Pulmonary mucormycosis is most frequently identified at autopsy in persons with leukemia, lymphoma, or other malignancies, but can occur, rarely, as an occupational disease in handlers of flour and grain (Murphy and Bornstein). Inhaled spores penetrate the bronchial wall and invade the lung parenchyma and pulmonary blood vessels, giving rise to pneumonitis and vascular thromboses with secondary tissue infarction. Pulmonary mucormycosis can occur without other organ involvement, but identical pulmonary pathology can result from hematogenous spread from other structures or from aspiration of infected secretions from the paranasal sinuses. The gastrointestinal tract is much less commonly affected than the lungs as the primary target organ but can become secondarily infected in other forms of the disease. Fungi can reach the gastrointestinal tract by hematogenous spread in disseminated mucormycosis, by direct invasion from infected mediastinal structures, from swallowed material from lesions in the nasal cavity or paranasal sinuses, or, rarely, by direct oral ingestion of spores from the external environment. Within the stomach or intestine, the lesions produced are either ulcerative or infarcts that are secondary to mucorthrombosis.

The most widely recognized form of mucormycosis is that in which the primary impact of the infection is upon facial and intracranial structures, a disorder referred to as rhinocerebral or orbitocerebral mucormycosis. This condition has been described in an otherwise normal child (DeWeese et al.) and secondary to leukemia, but it has its strongest association with diabetes mellitus and especially with poorly controlled diabetes with ketoacidosis. The portal of entry of the fungus is either via the nasal mucosa or the paranasal

sinuses, from which it rapidly spreads to the homolateral orbital structures, adjacent vascular channels, and into the brain. It is this form in which the brain is most commonly involved, although cerebral invasion can also be part of the disseminated disease in which multiple organs are implicated in the immunologically compromised or debilitated patient.

Rhinocerebral (Orbitocerebral) Mucormycosis

Phycomycotic infection originating within the nasal cavity or paranasal sinus and spreading to the orbit and subsequently to the brain is the most common and most distinctive form of disease produced by this group of fungi. Most cases have developed in uncontrolled diabetics but the disorder can also occur in other conditions with acidosis and dehydration, as well as in a variety of neoplastic disorders. The disease has also been described as a complication of severe craniocerebral trauma for which treatment included corticosteroids and antibiotics (Dean et al.). Most cases follow a remarkably consistent pattern, with the patient's hospital admission being for an acute complication of his basic, predisposing disease. The first manifestations of fungal invasion are usually local symptoms such as unilateral face pain or pain in the region of the orbit in association with erythema and proptosis. Facial or periorbital swelling on the affected side rapidly progresses to discoloration and firm induration (Fig. 19–22). Rapidly progressive proptosis with conjunctival edema and erythema is followed by drooping of the eyelid, dilatation of the pupil, and external ophthalmoplegia. Precipitous loss of vision may accompany the other ocular findings. Funduscopic examination at this stage may reveal normal findings, evidence of retinal ischemia, or distended retinal veins. Within days after onset, persistent orbitofacial pain is accompanied by facial paralysis and disturbances of superficial sensation on the same side of the face. In some cases, an initial bloody nasal discharge progresses to the formation of black necrotic turbinates and nasal mucosa, leading to partial nasal obstruction.

Evidence of intracranial involvement can appear simultaneously with the development of the facial and orbital abnormalities, but, more often, neurologic signs follow the man-

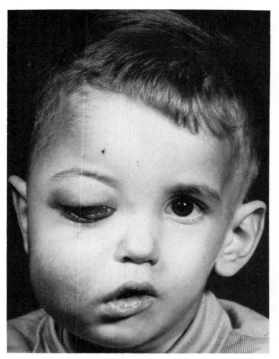

Figure 19–22. Mucormycosis in a 3-year-old boy without preceding illness or a predisposing cause. The initial symptoms were malaise and anorexia, followed by right facial swelling, proptosis, external ophthalmoplegia, and visual loss on the right. Mucorales was isolated from tissue obtained by biopsy of the right maxillary sinus. The child subsequently experienced right carotid artery thrombosis, intracranial extension of infection, and death.

ifestations described above by several days. The brain is implicated by direct extension of infection through the orbital walls or the cribriform plate, and secondarily by fungal invasion of the internal carotid artery or other vascular structures. Vascular invasion causing thrombotic occlusion is an outstanding characteristic of the Mucorales, with the end result being massive cerebral infarction in some cases. The clinical correlates of the cerebral pathology include headache, progressive lethargy, disorientation, convulsions, and hemiparesis. Mild neck stiffness is observed in some but rarely is marked. Cerebral swelling secondary to ischemic infarction can give rise to progressive obtundation and papilledema. Unless complicated by a secondary bacterial infection, temperature elevation is mild or absent, although exceptions do occur. The course of the illness is usually one with gradual deterioration and it has a high mortality rate unless response occurs to early initiation of therapy. Death can occur within a

week after onset or be delayed for several weeks, largely depending on the severity of the cerebral involvement.

The peripheral white blood cell count is generally elevated in the rhinocerebral form of mucormycosis, sometimes reaching levels as high as 40,000 per cu. mm. Sinus x-rays demonstrate clouding or opacification of the maxillary and ethmoid sinuses on the affected side, without a fluid level but with bony destructive changes of the sinuses and the walls of the orbit. Carotid angiography is useful in certain patients, providing evidence of carotid artery narrowing or even total occlusion secondary to vascular mycotic invasion (Courey et al.). Cerebrospinal fluid examination reveals variable findings and may be entirely normal despite considerable cerebral pathologic involvement. The opening pressure is usually elevated and the fluid is either clear or xanthochromic, depending on whether bleeding has occurred in infarcted brain tissue. Cells are frequently absent but may number up to 1,000 per cu. mm. and be predominantly polymorphonuclear leukocytes. The glucose content is normal or increased in the patient with diabetes with hyperglycemia and ketoacidosis. The protein value in most cases is significantly elevated. Phycomycetes cannot be isolated from the cerebrospinal fluid. Computed cranial tomography is a valuable technique to demonstrate the size and distribution of infarctional lesions in the brain and to reveal the degree of ventricular shift, if present.

The brain in fatal cases of rhinocerebral mucormycosis shows softened and sometimes hemorrhagic lesions, usually confined to one hemisphere, that are secondary to internal carotid and other vessel thrombosis. In some cases, nearly all major vessels at the base of the brain are occluded, producing extensive, bilateral infarctional necrosis of the cerebral hemispheres (Borland). An inflammatory infiltrate surrounds some infected, thrombosed vessels. Occasionally, the arterial wall is weakened to the point of mycotic aneurysm formation, with possible bleeding into the brain or the subarachnoid space. Broad, branching, non-septate hyphae can be seen within thrombosed arterial lumens and sometimes free in adjacent brain tissue (Fig. 19–23). In some areas, Mucorales hyphae are observed within tissue but with an absence of an inflammatory response, while in other areas a moderate inflammatory cell infiltration is present, composed primarily of polymorphonuclear cells. Massive granuloma formation

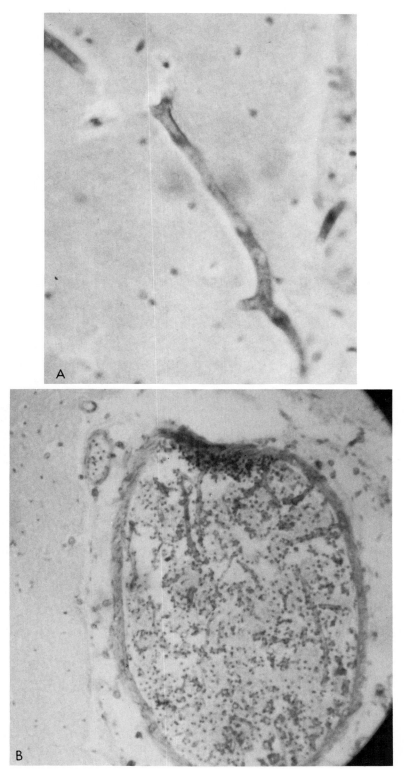

Figure 19–23. Mucormycosis. *A,* Nonseptate hyphae of Mucor species lying free within brain tissue with minimal surrounding inflammatory response. *B,* Many nonseptate, branched hyphae within the lumen of a thrombosed cerebral blood vessel.

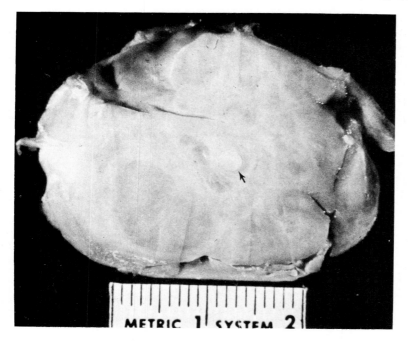

Figure 19–24. Mucormycosis due to Mucor species. Large granuloma encasing and compressing the optic nerve (arrow).

containing hyphae, fibrous tissue, and inflammatory cells may occupy the cavernous sinus or orbit, surround the optic nerve (Fig. 19–24), or be found within the cerebral parenchyma. Meningeal inflammation and infiltration with hyphae varies from slight to moderate in degree.

Diagnosis

The rhinocerebral or orbitocerebral forms of phycomycosis can be suspected clinically in the diabetic or otherwise predisposed patient by the rapid evolution of unilateral facial swelling proceeding to panophthalmitis with proptosis and followed by neurologic signs. Suppurative orbital cellulitis or cavernous sinus thrombosis manifest similar findings but are usually associated with a higher degree of fever, and the latter more often exhibits bilateral ocular signs. Roentgenographic findings, including the absence of a fluid level in the infected maxillary sinus and the bony destruction of the sinus and orbital walls, are more indicative of mucormycosis than a bacterial process. Cerebral mucormycosis without ocular infection, occurring as part of widespread disseminated disease, cannot usually be diagnosed clinically unless the organism is identified in other sites. In such cases, the opportunistic fungal infestation is found at autopsy, having been previously un-suspected. Even in cases with hematogenous spread to the brain, Mucorales exhibits a conspicuous predisposition to invade and occlude vascular channels. The basilar artery as well as the carotid or its branches can be affected in such patients (Carpenter et al.).

Because of the usual rapid clinical course characteristic of this fungal infection and owing to the usual inability to recover the organism from blood or cerebrospinal fluid, clinical diagnosis in life depends upon identification of Mucorales from infected tissue. Useful skin tests and serologic tests are not available. In the rhinocerebral form, biopsy tissue specimens from the nasal mucosa, palate, paranasal sinuses, or orbit are examined for the non-septated, branching hyphae 15 to 25 microns in width that are characteristic of the order Mucorales. They are readily seen with the usual hematoxylin and eosin stain but often are less well demonstrated with the Gridley stain, periodic acid–Schiff method, and silver methenamine stain. In culture, members of the Phycomycetes grow on a variety of commonly used media under aerobic conditions. On Sabouraud's glucose agar, there is rapid growth resulting in an abundant, fluffy white colony which darkens a few days later.

The genus of the Mucorales observed in tissue cannot usually be determined by microscopic examination. Certain differences are seen when the organisms are grown on artificial media, which do allow the genus identification by an expert observer. Members of the genus Rhizopus produce long aerial hyphae, called stolons, which curve down to come in contact with the surface of the medium and along which are small nodes giving rise to non-branching sporangiophores. Opposite to the node are rhizoids, or finger-like filaments that attach the stolon to the media. The genus Mucor also has sporangiophores arising from stolons; however, they branch profusely and rhizoids are absent. Fungi of the genus Absidia have stolons with rhizoids, but their relation to the sporangiophore is different from that which occurs with Rhizopus.

Treatment

Cerebral phycomycosis is a serious and life-threatening condition which, without therapy, is virtually uniformly fatal. Carpenter et al. found 63 reported cases with cerebral involvement up to 1968. Only eight survived and death occurred in 55. Up to 1971, Hale was able to identify 36 reported cases in infants and young children, 34 of which proved fatal.

The possibility of survival from this illness is enhanced by prompt diagnosis, correction to the degree possible of the underlying predisposing factors, and early initiation of amphotericin B therapy. The potential value of intensive amphotericin B treatment has been documented by reported cures (Landau and Newcomer, McCall and Strobos, Meyers et al., Prockop and Silva-Hutner, Sandler et al.). Dexamethasone or other corticosteroids should not be used as antiedema agents in patients with cerebral swelling associated with this illness. Among those who recover, residual deficits such as visual loss or hemiparesis are not uncommon.

RARE FUNGAL DISEASES INVOLVING THE NERVOUS SYSTEM

Sporotrichosis

Sporotrichosis is an uncommon infection caused by the diphasic aerobic fungus, Sporothrix schenckii (Syn. Sporotrichum schenckii), first identified by Schenck in 1898. In tissue, the fungus provokes a combination of suppurative and granulomatous reactions similar to several other mycotic infections. The fungus cells are difficult to identify in tissue, and, when observed, are in a variety of forms. The most typical microscopic structure associated with Sporothrix infection is the asteroid body; however, it is often not demonstrable. The asteroid body is characterized by a radiate periphery with a round or oval body located centrally which assumes a yeast-like appearance, sometimes with budding, with special fungus stains. In vitro, the yeast phase is sustained at incubation temperature, but at room temperature the fungus forms a mycelial colony which becomes dark brown in color. Hyphae are branched, narrow in diameter, and with conidiophore formation arising at right angles or obliquely from the hyphae.

The great majority of human cases of sporotrichosis follow direct inoculation of the organism into the skin or subcutaneous tissues and are manifested by a chronic ulcerative lesion at the site of inoculation associated with subcutaneous nodules along the course of the draining lymphatics (Orr and Riley, Chandler et al.). Sporothrix schenckii has a wide saprophytic existence and can be implanted into the skin by a scratch from a variety of foreign objects, prick of a rosebush, contact with contaminated sphagnum moss, or contamination of a break in the skin surface with infected soil. Extracutaneous sporotrichosis is far less frequent than the cutaneous form but has been described with involvement of the lungs, bones, urinary tract, and eye (Wilson et al.). Intraocular involvement with Sporothrix schenckii in the form of a necrotizing, granulomatous retinochoroiditis can result from direct extension from inoculation sporotrichosis of the eyelids or conjunctivae, or as part of widespread hematogenous dissemination of the fungus. Unifocal infection of the intraocular structures has also been described on rare occasion in the absence of an obvious primary source of the illness (Cassady and Foerster, Font and Jakobiec). Systemic sporotrichosis with cutaneous, pulmonary, and articular invasion has also been recognized in adults with debilitating and immunocompromised conditions, indicating the opportunistic capability of this fungus (Lynch et al.). The portal of entry in such cases is unproved but is assumed to be via the lungs.

Central nervous system sporotrichosis is extremely rare, with only a few cases described to date, and these have been in adults (Collins, Klein et al., Shoemaker et al.). The portal of entry of the organism has been unknown in these cases, although in the adult with meningitis described in Ewing et al., the primary infection appeared to be within the lungs, with hematogenous dissemination to the meninges. The central nervous system pathologic condition has been either a chronic granulomatous meningoencephalitis or multiple cerebral microabscesses or granulomata. The few cases reported have generally had a fatal outcome except for the case described by Klein et al. and that of Freeman and Ziegler. Cerebrospinal fluid findings have included a modest reduction of glucose, an elevation in protein content, and a lymphocytic pleocytosis. Isolation of the organism from cerebrospinal fluid has been successful in some cases but has required repeated cultures obtained over the course of several weeks. In the patient described by Freeman and Ziegler, culture of repeated specimens of lumbar cerebrospinal fluid remained negative but the fungus was finally isolated by culture of fluid obtained by cisternal tap.

Diagnosis of sporotrichosis of any site depends on isolation of the organism in culture on Sabouraud's glucose agar, since it can rarely be identified by direct examination of pus or stained infected tissue. Diagnosis can be made in some cases by fluorescent antibody staining of the fungus in smears prepared from exudates of lesions (Kaplan and Ivens). Serologic diagnostic tests have been developed but are subject to variable results (Wilson et al.). Amphotericin B is the drug of choice for disseminated, pulmonary, or neurologic sporotrichosis. The adult with Sporothrix meningitis successfully treated by Freeman and Ziegler received intravenous as well as intraventricular amphotericin B, the latter by way of an indwelling ventricular reservoir.

Torulopsosis

Torulopsis glabrata is a yeast of the family Cryptococcaceae which occasionally inhabits the oral cavity, urinary tract, or lower intestinal tract in non-pathogenic fashion. In recent years, it has become recognized that Torulopsis glabrata can be an opportunistic pathogen in patients with diabetes mellitus or those with underlying disease treated with antibiotics, corticosteroids, or immunosuppressive drugs (Marks et al.). Fungemia with fever and hypotension resembling bacterial sepsis has been the most notable syndrome attributed to the organism when it attacks the compromised host but widespread tissue invasion can occur. Isolation of the fungus from the tracheobronchial tree or lungs is common in such patients, and, in some, rapidly progressive or fatal pneumonia will occur (Aisner et al.). Another form of infection with this organism is pyelonephritis without other organ system involvement, especially in the diabetic patient (Kauffman and Tan). Torulopsis glabrata fungemia has also been related to intravenous hyperalimentation in adults (Valdivieso et al.).

Cerebral involvement has not generally been observed in cases with systemic infection but most likely can be expected in the future by detailed neuropathologic examination. Minkowitz reported a 15-year-old girl treated with multiple antibiotics who at autopsy had multiple glial nodules in the cerebrum, brain stem, and spinal cord, with Torulopsis glabrata within vessels in the abnormal foci. In tissue, the organism is a round or oval budding yeast, 2 to 4 microns in diameter, without mycelia or a capsule. It remains yeast-like on Sabouraud's media, resulting in smooth, shiny colonies that are light in coloration. There is little information to date regarding treatment of infection due to this organism but sensitivity to 5-fluorocytosine has been suggested (Marks et al., Vandevelde et al.).

Allescheria (Petriellidium) boydii Infections

Allescheria boydii is a filamentous fungus of the class Ascomycetes. It is best known as one of the causes of mycetoma (maduromycosis, "Madura foot"), a chronic mycotic infection of warm climates characterized by swelling and protracted draining sinuses, which usually occur at the site of soft tissue injury. The fungus is a soil saprophyte with a world-wide distribution (Ajello), and has generally been regarded to be of low pathogenicity from the standpoint of visceral disease. Allescheria boydii was first identified in its imperfect (asexual) form by Tarozzi in 1909 and was named Monosporium apiospermum by Saccardo in 1911. In 1921, Boyd and Crutchfield isolated a "new" fungus of the ascomycete family, and one year later the organism was named Allescheria boydii by Shear. Emmons, in 1944, demonstrated that subcultures of a strain of Monosporium apiospermum previously isolated from a patient with maduromycosis produced perithecia like those of Allescheria boydii, thus establishing that the two fungi represent different forms of the same organism. It is now accepted that Monosporium apiospermum is the imperfect (asexual) stage and Allescheria boydii is the perfect (sexual, ascocarpic) stage of the fungus. In 1970, Malloch proposed that the genus of this organism be termed Petriellidium.

Allescheria boydii in tissue stained with methenamine silver is in the form of broad, septate hyphae. The tissue form bears close morphologic similarity to Aspergillus, with which it is easily confused unless cultures are examined. Culture on Sabouraud's medium produces rapid growth with colonies that are initially white but soon become smoky-gray with a dark reverse side.

Reports of systemic infection caused by Allescheria boydii have been relatively few, and describe adults rather than children. In some of the reported cases, the infection occurred as a primary one and the portal of entry of the organism was not identified. In others, the invasive fungal infection occurred in immunocompromised patients who had been treated with antibiotic or corticosteroid therapy (Lutwick et al.), or as a complication of a chronic illness, such as diabetes mellitus or collagen vascular disease. The lungs have been the most common extracutaneous site of infection produced by Allescheria boydii (Alture-Werber et al., Louria et al., Lutwick et al., Scharyj et al., Tong et al.). Keratitis (Ernest and Rippon, Levitt and Goldstein), endophthalmitis (Glassman et al.), and chronic otomycosis (Blank and Stuart) are additional, although rare, manifestations of infection with this organism. Gluckman et al. reported a case of Allescheria boydii sinusitis in a 58-year-old diabetic man on chronic hemodialysis. The illness in this individual closely resembled the more common rhinocerebral form of phycomycosis.

The first report of neurologic disease due to Allescheria boydii was that of Wolf et al. in 1948. The patient was an adult female from Trinidad who developed meningitis four weeks following spinal anesthesia. The organism was isolated from cerebrospinal fluid on several occasions in this case, and death occurred approximately nine months after onset of illness. A chronic granulomatous leptomeningeal exudate was found at autopsy. The same case was published again in more detail by Benham and Georg, and the neuropathology was extensively described by Aronson et al. Rosen and colleagues reported a 19-year-old woman with subacute glomerulonephritis treated with corticosteroids and azathioprine who was found at autopsy to have two cerebral abscesses and a thyroid abscess caused by Allescheria boydii. A similar case with mycotic cerebral and thyroid infection in a patient with lupus erythematosus was subsequently reported by Forno and Billingham. Other reports of neurologic disease secondary to Allescheria boydii included a previously healthy adult female who developed paraplegia resulting from a thoracic epidural granuloma (Selby) and a few immunosuppressed adults with brain abscesses (Lutwick et al., Walker et al., Winston et al.).

The severity of central nervous system infection caused by this organism is apparent from the fact that all the above cases expired except that reported by Selby, in which the infection involved the spinal cord. The authors have seen a three-year-old leukemic child with a frontal lobe abscess caused by Allescheria boydii who survived without neurologic deficits following surgical drainage and amphotericin B therapy (Bell and Myers). The isolate from this lesion was resistant in vitro to amphotericin B even though recovery occurred concomitant with its use. The available data regarding in vitro sensitivity of Allescheria boydii isolates to amphotericin B are fragmentary but in most instances the organism has been found to be resistant (Mohr and Muchmore, Nielsen). Preliminary studies suggest that miconazole may be a useful drug for treatment of infection caused by Allescheria boydii but further studies are needed (Lutwick et al.).

Penicilliosis

Penicillium is another fungus that rarely causes human disease, but in the patient with leukemia or lymphoma or one treated with steroids or antimetabolic drugs, it can become an opportunistic pathogen. As a ubiquitous organism and a common contaminant, the isolation of Penicillium from certain specimens, such as sputum, does not necessarily mean that disease is caused by the isolate (Emmons et al.). Penicillium is in the same class of fungi as Aspergillus and Allescheria boydii and bears considerable morphologic similarity to them. The organism is readily seen in hematoxylin and eosin stained sections or with the methenamine silver stain. In tissue, Penicillium species have broad, branched hyphae with occasional septa but with less frequent septations than occur with Aspergillus. On Sabouraud's agar, Penicillium is characterized by an aerial mycelium with spore-bearing hyphae with brush-like, fruiting heads.

The most commonly affected organ by this fungus in the predisposed patient is the respiratory tract. Central nervous system infection with Penicillium is rare, although some cases attributed to Aspergillus species may have been due to this organism. Huang and Harris described a leukemic adult treated with corticosteroids and antibiotics whose clinical course included mental confusion and convulsions. Disseminated infection with Penicillium was found at autopsy. The brain revealed a well-defined cortical hemorrhagic infarct which contained the fungus. Another patient with cerebral involvement due to Penicillium was reported by Morriss and Spock. The patient, an 11-year-old child, had no preceding illness but developed maxillary sinusitis after a dental extraction. Following a protracted course during which he received antibiotics and corticosteroids, the child experienced a subarachnoid hemorrhage and eventually died. Necrotizing, granulomatous lesions harboring Penicillium were found in the maxillary and ethmoid sinuses and at the base of the brain. Vessels of the circle of Willis were thrombosed by fungal invasion, and a ruptured mycotic aneurysm of the left internal carotid artery was identified. The clinical findings and vascular invasion by Penicillium in this case bear striking similarity to the rhinocerebral form of mucormycosis. Experience regarding treatment of infections caused by Penicillium is limited but amphotericin B has been recommended as the drug of choice.

Chromoblastomycosis

Chromoblastomycosis is a localized mycotic infection of the skin and subcutaneous tissue caused by the dematiaceous fungi, a group of fungi with dark-colored hyphae. The illness most commonly occurs in tropical and subtropical areas and can result from one of several fungi, including Phialophora verrucosa, Phialophora compacta, Phialophora dermatitidis, and Cladosporium carrionii (Emmons et al., 1977). Most cases have been in adults, although the disease has been described in a child in the United States (Hughes). The surface lesions of chromoblastomycosis are usually located on one lower extremity and are ulcerative or granulomatous in appearance with secondary spread along regional lymphatics. Hematogenous dissemination from the local infection is possible but is extraordinarily rare.

Neurologic infection resulting from the naturally pigmented fungi has only rarely been reported and has been designated by a confusing and only partially correct variety of terms, including cerebral chromoblastomycosis, cerebral dematiomycosis, and cladosporiosis. Among published cases of central nervous system infection caused by the dematiaceous fungi, most that have been identified etiologically have been due to Cladosporium trichoides (Duque, Musella and Collins, Riley and Mann, Symmers) but a few have been caused by Phialophora pedrosoi (Lucasse et al.) and Phialophora dermatitidis (Tsai et al.). Cladosporium trichoides is not believed to be a cause of the cutaneous form of the disease referred to as chromoblastomycosis, and thus the designation of cerebral chromoblastomycosis when caused by this organism is less than entirely accurate. The term cladosporiosis is applicable to those cases in which cerebral involvement with Cladosporium trichoides is proved by cultural methods but not the lesser number in which the offender is Phialophora species. Likewise, many of the previously reported cases in which the organism was classified among the pigmented fungi only on the basis of the morphology of the fungus in tissue cannot be labeled cladosporiosis since Cladosporium trichoides cannot be differentiated from other members without culture verification. These semantic complexities relative to neurologic infections with this group of fungi have been discussed by Bennett et al.

Up to 1973, Bennett and colleagues identified 34 previously published cases from countries throughout the world and added one additional example of neurologic infection caused by dematiaceous fungi. As noted earlier, Cladosporium trichoides has been the causative agent in most of the etiologically proven cases, and the majority have been in the form of encapsulated cerebral abscesses. The portal of entry of the fungus is not usually apparent since extracranial involvement is generally absent, although initial infection by respiratory inhalation has been suspected in some instances. Most affected patients have been previously normal with nothing to suggest the possibility of predisposing immunologic abnormalities. The location of the abscess or abscesses dictates the character of the clinical signs, which usually include a variety of focal neurologic deficits, seizures, and signs of increased intracranial pressure. The illness is usually progressive in rapid or subacute fashion, and most patients die within one year or less of the onset of symptoms (Middleton et al.). Diagnosis of Cladosporium trichoides brain abscess has been established during life in some cases by isolation of the fungus from pus aspirated surgically and in others at the time of autopsy.

Subacute or chronic meningitis is a much less common manifestation of infection with this group of fungi but is no less serious from the prognostic standpoint (Duque, Bennett et al.). The 17-year-old boy with chronic Cladosporium meningitis described by Bennett et al. had symptoms of 11 months' duration at the time of his death. On post-mortem examination, the abnormalities were confined to the central nervous system where a gray purulent exudate was found at the base of the brain, along with diffuse ependymitis. Multinucleated giant cells and pigmented, septate hyphae were found within the leptomeningeal exudate. The cerebrospinal fluid in such cases contains a polymorphonuclear leukocytosis, a moderate to marked degree of protein elevation, and, in some instances, a modest reduction of cerebrospinal fluid glucose content.

With hematoxylin-eosin and with methenamine silver staining, Cladosporium trichoides in tissue is in the form of pigmented, smooth-walled hyphae, 2 to 4 microns in diameter, with occasional branching and irregularly placed septations. It is distinguished from other dematiacious fungi by growth on Sabouraud's agar on which colonies are smooth and olive gray-black in color.

Treatment of central nervous system infection caused by Cladosporium trichoides or other pigmented fungi has generally been unsatisfactory, with eventual death being the usual outcome of the illness. A localized cerebral abscess is surgically aspirated or excised, followed by long-term drug therapy. There is in vitro evidence of possible effectiveness of 5-fluorocytosine (Block et al.) and also clinical evidence of benefit of the drug in treatment of cutaneous chromoblastomycosis (Nsanzumuhire et al.). Its use for intracranial infection with this group of fungi has

been limited, but thus far results have not been encouraging (Middleton et al.).

Actinomycosis

Actinomycosis is a chronic suppurative disorder in which there is a marked predisposition for the formation of abscesses and sinus tracts, often leading to multiple cutaneous fistulas. Most human infections are caused by Actinomyces israelii, an anaerobic, gram-positive, non–acid fast bacterium, which, along with Nocardia asteroides, is a member of the family Actinomycetaceae. Actinomyces israelii can be part of the normal flora of the oral cavity, especially in persons with poor oral hygiene and dental caries, and of the gastrointestinal tract. A notable feature of the organism in tissue or pus is the formation of yellowish granules which can achieve a diameter of 2 or more millimeters and which are referred to as "sulfur granules." These colonies are best stained with hematoxylin and eosin or methenamine silver and consist of a central basophilic area surrounded at the perimeter by radially placed filaments which assume a club- or bullet-shaped appearance (Fig. 19–25). Granules are often sparse in exudate or tissue specimens and, for this reason, establishment of the diagnosis of actinomycosis is frequently delayed (Brown). When cultured anaerobically, the colony is pale or white in color and with a lobulated surface. Other bacteria, such as *Actinobacillus actinomycetemcomitans, Staphylococcus* species, or *Streptococcus* species, are commonly found in actinomycotic infected lesions, and can play a role in the chronicity of the process (Weese and Smith).

Human actinomycosis was recognized in the latter part of the nineteenth century, although, until recent years, Actinomyces species were often not differentiated from the aerobic actinomycete, Nocardia asteroides. Actinomycosis is a world-wide disease, which has only infrequently been described in children. The disorder has been divided into three types, including the cervicofacial type, the thoracic type, and the abdominal type (Cope). Cervicofacial actinomycosis is the most common and also the most favorable in regard to prognosis.

Central nervous system actinomycosis is considered rare and is almost always secondary to actinomycotic disease elsewhere. It can result from direct spread from cervicofacial

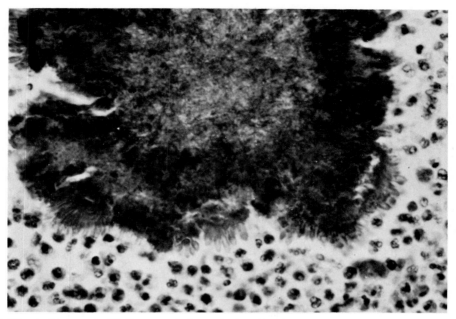

Figure 19–25.   Actinomycosis. "Sulfur granule," or colonies of Actinomyces species, composed of a dense mat of filaments centrally, surrounded by club-shaped filamentous structures in a radial distribution.

involvement, or by hematogenous dissemination from other locations, especially from the lungs. Cerebral abscess is the most common form of neurologic infection with this organism (Eckhoff, Jacobson and Cloward, Lewin and Morgan, Maltby, McDowell et al., Stevens), although a diffuse meningoencephalitis can also occur (Cann and Holles, Edwards et al.). Intracranial lesions, referred to as actinomycomas, have also been described, consisting of a solitary gelatinous mass giving rise to either intraventricular obstruction or a mass effect when in the cerebral parenchyma (Cope).

Mediastinal infection is sometimes complicated by osteomyelitic involvement of the vertebral spine, in which direct extension intraspinally gives rise to spinal epidural abscess (Krumdieck and Stevenson, Lane et al.). Vertebral actinomycosis is usually a chronic disorder with recurrent fever, malaise, and back pain, and associated with the formation of subcutaneous abscesses or draining sinuses. Epidural extension gives rise to signs of spinal cord compression of variable severity. Intracranial epidural abscess can likewise result from actinomycotic invasion of the skull by contiguous spread of adjacent soft tissue infection. Exudate from actinomycotic abscess in brain or epidural space has been described in most cases to be thick, and with a gray-green color.

Central nervous system actinomycosis must be considered a prognostically serious disease, although recovery has been described with a combination of surgical and antibiotic therapy (Schneider and Rand). The possible value of penicillin for treatment of actinomycosis was mentioned as early as 1941 (Abraham et al.), and its clinical importance was documented by 1948 (Nichols and Herrell). Penicillin is now the drug of choice for actinomycotic infections; however, long-term administration of the antibiotic is required.

Nocardiosis

Nocardiosis is an uncommon disease, especially in children, with a clinical spectrum that includes acute or chronic pulmonary disease, a chronic granulomatous or suppurative disorder of the skin or bones, a disease predominated by central nervous system signs, and a widely disseminated illness with multiple organ system involvement. Nocardia is pathogenic for the presumably normal host, and in most of the early reports the disease occurred in previously uncompromised persons. In the past two decades, there has been an increased awareness of the association of nocardial infections with immunosuppression or secondary to other types of chronic debilitating disease (Rosett and Hodges).

Among 13 adult patients with infections caused by Nocardia asteroides reported by Palmer et al. (1974), seven had an underlying illness associated with an immunocompromised state. Nocardiosis has been described in children with chronic granulomatous disease (Bujak et al.); in adults with systemic lupus erythematosus (Hathaway and Mason), sarcoidosis (Raich et al.), pulmonary alveolar proteinosis (Supena et al.), and renal transplantation (Cohen et al.); and in both children and adults with underlying neoplastic disease treated with chemotherapy or radiation (Cox and Hughes, Young et al., Hart et al.). Thus, Nocardia has been established as a significant opportunistic pathogen but not with the prevalence seen with Candida species, Aspergillus, or certain viral agents.

Nocardia was first isolated from infected cattle by Nocard in 1888. Two years later, Eppinger reported the first isolate of this organism from a human with widespread disease, including a brain abscess, which he referred to as "pseudotuberculosis." The pathogenic species are now classified among the bacteria in the family Actinomycetaceae. Criteria for their classification as bacteria include their size of one micron or less in diameter, their gram-positive and occasional acid-fast staining reactions, and the tendency for their vegetative mycelium to fragment into bacillary and coccoid elements (Conant). Nocardia are ubiquitous in nature, being commonly found in soil in almost all parts of the world. They are filamentous forms in tissue, with fine branching hyphae that measure one centimeter or less in diameter, are up to 20 microns in length (Fig. 19–26), and are easily cultivated on Sabouraud's or beef infusion glucose agar. A period of one to four weeks may be required for the organisms to form their characteristic cultural morphology.

The majority of human infections are caused by Nocardia asteroides but Nocardia brasiliensis is also a known pathogen, especially in Central and South America where it is best known as one of the causes of mycetoma. In this country, Nocardia brasiliensis has been a rarely identified cause of a variety of infections, including mycetoma, cutaneous abscesses, lymphocutaneous infection resembling sporotrichosis, and disseminated infection with pulmonary and brain abscesses (Berd). Still less common is infection resulting from Nocardia caviae. In the few case reports that have been published, this species has caused disseminated infection in immunosuppressed adults (Arroyo et al., Causey et al.). The human is colonized with Nocardia species by respiratory inhalation in the majority of cases.

Nocardiosis is most commonly a pulmonary infection, either acute or chronic, and with symptoms which include fever, cough, night sweats, and weight loss. It thus resembles tuberculosis and often has been confused diagnostically with this disease. Anemia and

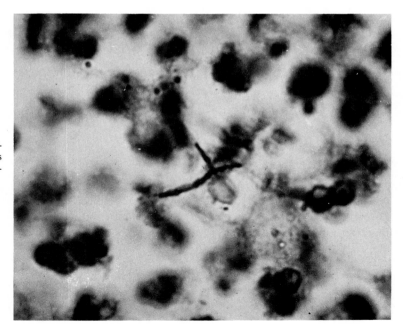

Figure 19–26. Nocardia asteroides. Small, filamentous forms with fine, branching hyphae (Grocott's silver methenamine stain).

leukocytosis are common laboratory findings with this illness, which, when associated with pleural effusion, can lead to an erroneous diagnosis of staphylococcal pneumonia. Within the lungs, Nocardia gives rise to a suppurative process with the formation of multiple abscesses of different sizes. Adults have represented the majority of reported cases of pulmonary nocardiosis but the disease has been described in children as well (Stites and Glezen). The infection can remain confined to the lungs, although metastatic spread occurs with considerable frequency. Hematogenous dissemination in some cases is widespread (Ballenger and Goldring), but in other instances affects only a single secondary organ system, such as the brain. Although disseminated infection with Nocardia most commonly arises from pulmonary involvement, spread to other organs can also result from primary soft tissue or bone lesions (Frazier et al.).

In regard to predisposed sites, the brain is exceeded only by the lung with infection caused by Nocardia. The majority of intracranial infections identified thus far have been caused by Nocardia asteroides, although on rare occasion other Nocardia species have been isolated from brain abscesses (Arroyo et al., Berd). Most cerebral or cerebellar lesions are multiloculated solitary or multiple abscesses that are poorly or partially encapsulated and contain thick yellow or green purulent exudate (Idriss et al., Shuster et al., Rankin and Javid) (Fig. 19–27). Adjacent to the abscess, one sees chronic granulomatous changes in which inflammatory cells and an occasional giant cell can be observed. Nocardia in tissue is not demonstrated by the hematoxylin and eosin stain but can be identified by the methenamine silver method. Meningitis infrequently will coexist with parenchymal abscess or, more rarely, can occur alone.

Clinical features in the patient with a Nocardia brain abscess include a brief and rapidly progressive course, focal neurologic deficits that are dictated by the location of the lesion or lesions, and signs of increased intracranial pressure. The cerebrospinal fluid reveals few abnormalities, except for possible pressure elevation, unless meningitis coexists. In this case, polymorphonuclear cells are present, the protein is elevated, and the fungus may be recovered in culture. Intraspinal Nocardia granuloma or abscess causing spinal cord compression has been reported

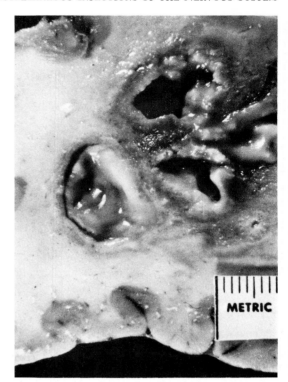

Figure 19–27. Nocardial brain abscess. Multiloculated, poorly encapsulated abscess surrounded by a heavy granulomatous reaction.

but is far less common than intracranial involvement (Welsh et al.). Diagnosis of central nervous system Nocardia infection is dependent on recovery of the organism from the abscess contents, an accomplishment achieved only at autopsy in a number of previously reported cases. The probability that a focal cerebral suppurative lesion is caused by Nocardia is obviously enhanced in the predisposed patient with a pulmonary lesion which is proved to be nocardial in origin. Isolation of this organism from sputum is unusual, however, so that diagnosis in life is usually dependent on specimens obtained by pulmonary brush biopsy, percutaneous needle biopsy, or open lung biopsy. Isolation of the fungus on blood culture has been reported in patients with disseminated infection (Roberts et al.).

Supena and colleagues were able to identify approximately 150 reported cases of nocardiosis up to 1974, of which 30 percent had central nervous system involvement. Of the 49 reported cases in which the brain was affected, only nine patients had survived. Treatment of Nocardia brain abscess includes surgical drainage and long-term chemotherapy, usually in the range of six to 12 months. More abbreviated antimicrobial treatment can be followed by recurrence of intracranial infection as late as one year later (Byrne et al.). In cases with multiple brain abscesses, surgical drainage of each lesion is not feasible and treatment depends on antimicrobial therapy (Kirmani et al.).

Sulfonamides have been the mainstay of therapy for nocardial infections for a number of years and are given in dosage sufficient to maintain a serum level of 12 to 15 mg. per 100 ml. A combination of sulfonamide and cycloserine has also been successfully used in treatment of infections caused by this fungus (Hoeprich et al., Palmer et al.). Cycloserine is said to diffuse well into most tissues, including the brain, and can be used as an alternate drug in patients allergic to sulfa preparations. Possible neurotoxic effects of the drug include mental confusion, hallucinations, and convulsions. Trimethoprim-sulfamethoxazole is an additional drug regimen that has been reported with success for the treatment of Nocardia species brain abscess (Baikie et al., Maderazo and Quintiliani). Other drugs that have been recommended for nocardial infections include minocycline, and ampicillin plus erythromycin (Bach et al.). Further experience is needed to determine which of the above represents optimal treatment for Nocardia infection of the nervous system but combined drug therapy would seem logical. Nocardia species have been shown to be sensitive to amikacin in vitro (Dalovisio and Panky, Wallace et al.) but its value in human infections remains to be seen. The poor penetration of the aminoglycosides into cerebrospinal fluid and brain would limit their use in patients with intracranial nocardial infection.

REFERENCES

Abraham, E. P., Chain, E., Fletcher, C. M., Gardner, A. D., Heatley, N. G., Jennings, M. A., and Florey, H. W.: Further observations on penicillin. Lancet 2:177–189, 1941.

Abramson, E., Wilson, D., and Arky, R. A.: Rhinocerebral phycomycosis in association with diabetic ketoacidosis. Report of two cases and a review of clinical and experimental experience with amphotericin B therapy. Ann. Intern. Med. 66:735–742, 1967.

Adler, S., Randall, J., and Plotkin, S. A.: Candidal osteomyelitis and arthritis in a neonate. Am. J. Dis. Child. 123:595–596, 1972.

Agger, W. A., and Maki, D. G.: Mucormycosis. A complication of critical care. Arch. Intern. Med. 138:925–927, 1978.

Aguilar, G. L., Blumenkrantz, M. S., Egbert, P. R., and McCulley, J. P.: Candida endophthalmitis after intravenous drug abuse. Arch. Ophthalmol. 97:96–100, 1979.

Aguilar-Torres, F. G., Jackson, L. J., Ferstenfeld, J. E., Pappagianis, D., and Rytel, M. W.: Counterimmunoelectrophoresis in the detection of antibodies against Coccidioides immitis. Ann. Intern. Med. 85:740–744, 1976.

Ahn, C., Kilman, J. W., Vasko, J. S., and Andrews, N. C.: The therapy of cavitary pulmonary histoplasmosis. J. Thorac. Cardiovasc. Surg. 57:42–51, 1969.

Aisner, J., Schimpff, S. C., Bennett, J. E., Young, V. M., and Wiernik, P. H.: Aspergillus infections in cancer patients. Association with fireproofing materials in a new hospital. J.A.M.A. 235:411–412, 1976.

Aisner, J., Schimpff, S. C., Sutherland, J. C., Young, V. M., and Wiernik, P. H.: Torulopsis glabrata infections in patients with cancer. Increasing incidence and relationship to colonization. Am. J. Med. 61:23–28, 1976.

Aisner, J., Schimpff, S. C., and Wiernik, P. H.: Treatment of invasive aspergillosis: Relation of early diagnosis and treatment to response. Ann. Intern. Med. 86:539–543, 1977.

Ajello, L.: The isolation of Allescheria boydii Shear, an etiologic agent of mycetomas, from soil. Am. J. Trop. Med. Hyg. 1:227–238, 1952.

Alazraki, N. P., Fierer, J., Halpern, S. E., and Becker, R. W.: Use of a hyperbaric solution for administration of intrathecal amphotericin B. New Eng. J. Med. 290:641–646, 1974.

Allan, G. W., and Andersen, D. H.: Generalized aspergillosis in an infant 18 days of age. Pediatrics 26:432–440, 1960.

Alture-Werber, E., Edberg, S. C., and Singer, J. M.: Pulmonary infection with Allescheria boydii. Am. J. Clin. Path. 66:1019–1024, 1976.

Amromin, G. D., and Gildenhorn, V. B.: Massive cerebral aspergillus abscess in a leukemic child. Case report. J. Neurosurg. 35:491–494, 1971.

Aronson, S. M., Benham, R., and Wolf, A.: Maduromycosis of the central nervous system. J. Neuropath. Exp. Neurol. 12:158–168, 1953.

Arroyo, J. C., Nichols, S., and Carroll, G. F.: Disseminated Nocardia caviae infection. Am. J. Med. 62:409–412, 1977.

Ashcraft, K. W., and Leape, L. L.: Candida sepsis complicating parenteral feeding. J.A.M.A. 212:454–456, 1970.

Atkinson, A. J., Jr., and Bennett, J. E.: Amphotericin B pharmacokinetics in humans. Antimicrob. Agents Chemother. 13:271–276, 1978.

Atkinson, A. J., Jr., and Bindschadler, D. D.: Pharmacokinetics of intrathecally administered amphotericin B. Am. Rev. Respir. Dis. 99:917–924, 1969.

Atkinson, G. W., and Israel, H. L.: 5-fluorocytosine treatment of meningeal and pulmonary aspergillosis. Am. J. Med. 55:496–504, 1973.

Bach, M. C., Gold, O., and Finland, M.: Activity of minocycline against Nocardia asteroides: Comparison with tetracycline in agar-dilution and standard disc-diffusion tests and with sulfadiazine in an experimental infection of mice. J. Lab. Clin. Med. 81:787–793, 1973.

Bach, M. C., Monaco, A. P., and Finland, M.: Pulmonary

nocardiosis: Therapy with minocycline and with erythromycin plus ampicillin. J.A.M.A. 224:1378–1381, 1973.

Bagnarello, A. G., Lewis, L. A., McHenry, M. C., Weinstein, A. J., Naito, H. K., McCullough, A. J., Lederman, R. J., and Gavan, T. L.: Unusual serum lipoprotein abnormality induced by the vehicle of miconazole. New Eng. J. Med. 296:497–499, 1977.

Baikie, A. G., MacDonald, C. B., and Mundy, G. R.: Systemic nocardiosis treated with trimethoprim and sulphamethoxazole. Lancet 2:261, 1970.

Baker, R. D.: Pulmonary mucormycosis. Am. J. Path. 32:287–313, 1956.

Balk, M. W., Crumrine, M. H., and Fischer, G. W.: Evaluation of miconazole therapy in experimental disseminated candidiasis in laboratory rats. Antimicrob. Agents Chemother. 13:321–325, 1978.

Ballenger, C. N., Jr., and Goldring, D.: Nocardiosis in childhood. J. Pediat. 50:145–169, 1957.

Bayer, A. S., Edwards, J. E., Jr., Seidel, J. S., and Guze, L. B.: Candida meningitis. Report of seven cases and review of the English literature. Medicine 55:477–486, 1976.

Bayer, A. S., Yoshikawa, T. T., Galpin, J. E., and Guze, L. B.: Unusual syndromes of coccidioidomycosis: Diagnostic and therapeutic considerations. Medicine 55:131–152, 1976.

Beeson, P. B.: Cryptococcic meningitis of nearly sixteen years' duration. Arch. Intern. Med. 89:797–801, 1952.

Bell, W. E., and Myers, M. G.: *Allescheria (Petriellidium) boydii* brain abscess in a child with leukemia. Arch. Neurol. 35:386–388, 1978.

Benham, R. W., and Georg, L. K.: Allescheria boydii, causative agent in a case of meningitis. J. Invest. Derm. 10:99–110, 1948.

Bennett, J. E.: Chemotherapy of systemic mycoses. New Eng. J. Med. 290:30–31, 320–323, 1974.

Bennett, J. E., Bonner, H., Jennings, A. E., and Lopez, R. I.: Chronic meningitis caused by *Cladosporium trichoides*. Am. J. Clin. Path. 59:398–407, 1973.

Bennett, J. E., Dismukes, W. E., Duma, R. J., Medoff, G., Sande, M. A., Gallis, H., Leonard, J., Fields, B. T., Bradshaw, M., Haywood, H., McGee, Z. A., Cate, T. R., Cobbs, C. G., Warner, J. F., and Alling, D. W.: A comparison of amphotericin B alone and combined with flucytosine in the treatment of cryptococcal meningitis. New Eng. J. Med. 301:126–131, 1979.

Berd, D.: Nocardia brasiliensis infection in the United States: A report of nine cases and a review of the literature. Am. J. Clin. Path. 60:254–258, 1973.

Bindschadler, D. D., and Bennett, J. E.: Serology of human cryptococcosis. Ann. Intern. Med. 69:45–62, 1969.

Black, J. T.: Cerebral candidiasis: case report of brain abscess secondary to Candida albicans, and review of the literature. J. Neurol. Neurosurg. Psychiat. 33:864–870, 1970.

Blank, F., and Stuart, E. A.: Monosporium apiospermum Sacc., 1911, associated with otomycosis. Canad. Med. Assoc. J. 72:601, 1955.

Blizzard, R. M., and Gibbs, J. H.: Candidiasis: Studies pertaining to its association with endocrinopathies and pernicious anemia. Pediatrics 42:231–237, 1968.

Block, E. R., Jennings, A. E., and Bennett, J. E.: Experimental therapy of cladosporiosis and sporotrichosis with 5-fluorocytosine. Antimicrob. Agents Chemother. 3:95–98, 1973.

Bloomfield, N., Gordon, M. A., and Elmendorf, D. F.,

Jr.: Detection of Cryptococcus neoformans antigen in body fluids by latex particle agglutination. Proc. Soc. Exp. Biol. Med. 114:64–67, 1963.

Bodey, G. P.: Fungal infections complicating acute leukemia. J. Chronic Dis. 19:667–687, 1966.

Boeckman, C. R., and Krill, C. E., Jr.: Bacterial and fungal infections complicating parenteral alimentation in infants and children. J. Pediat. Surg. 5:117–126, 1970.

Borland, D. S.: Mucormycosis of the central nervous system. Am. J. Dis. Child. 97:852–856, 1959.

Boyd, M. F., and Crutchfield, E. D.: A contribution to the study of mycetoma in North America. Am. J. Trop. Med. 1:215–289, 1921.

Brodsky, A. L., Gregg, M. B., Loewenstein, M. S., Kaufman, L., and Mallison, G. F.: Outbreak of histoplasmosis associated with the 1970 Earth Day activities. Am. J. Med. 54:333–342, 1973.

Brook, I., Bricknell, K. S., Overturf, G. D., and Finegold, S. M.: Measurement of lactic acid in cerebrospinal fluid of patients with infections of the central nervous system. J. Infect. Dis. 137:384–390, 1978.

Brown, J. R.: Human actinomycosis. A study of 181 subjects. Hum. Path. 4:319–330, 1973.

Brugmans, J., Van Cutsem, J., Keykants, J., Schuermans, V., and Thienpont, D.: Systemic antifungal potential, safety, biotransport and transformation of miconazole nitrate. Eur. J. Clin. Pharmacol. 5:93–99, 1972.

Bryan, C. S., and McFarland, J. A.: Cryptococcal meningitis. Fatal marrow aplasia from combined therapy. J.A.M.A. 239:1068–1069, 1978.

Bujak, J. S., Ottesen, E. A., Dinarello, C. A., and Brenner, V. J.: Nocardiosis in a child with chronic granulomatous disease. J. Pediat. 83:98–100, 1973.

Bulmer, G. S., and Sans, M. D.: Cryptococcus neoformans. III. Inhibition of phagocytosis. J. Bact. 95:5–8, 1968.

Burston, J., and Blackwood, W.: A case of aspergillus infection of the brain. J. Path. Bact. 86:225–228, 1963.

Burton, J. R., Zachery, J. B., Bessin, R., Rathbun, H. K., Greenough, W. B., III, Sterioff, S., Wright, J. R., Slavin, R. E., and Williams, G. M.: Aspergillosis in four renal transplant recipients. Diagnosis and effective treatment with amphotericin B. Ann. Intern. Med. 77:383–388, 1972.

Butler, W. T.: Pharmacology, toxicity, and therapeutic usefulness of amphotericin B. J.A.M.A. 195:371–375, 1966.

Butler, W. T., Alling, D. W., Spickard, A., and Utz, J. P.: Diagnostic and prognostic value of clinical and laboratory findings in cryptococcal meningitis. A follow-up study of forty patients. New Eng. J. Med. 270:59–67, 1964.

Byrne, E., Brophy, B. P., and Perrett, L. V.: Nocardia cerebral abscess: New concepts in diagnosis, management, and prognosis. J. Neurol. Neurosurg. Psychiat. 42:1038–1045, 1979.

Campbell, C. C., and Hill, G. B.: Further studies on development of complement-fixing antibodies and precipitins in healthy histoplasmin-sensitive persons following single histoplasmin skin test. Am. Rev. Resp. Dis. 90:927–934, 1964.

Cann, L. W., and Hollis, G. J.: A case of actinomycotic cerebrospinal meningitis associated with aural actinomycosis. Lancet 1:130–131, 1931.

Carbone, P. P., Sabesin, S. M., Sidransky, H., and Frei, E., III: Secondary aspergillosis. Ann. Intern. Med. 60:556–567, 1964.

Carmody, E. J., and Tappen, W.: Blastomycosis meningitis: Report of a case successfully treated with amphotericin B. Ann. Intern. Med. 51:780–791, 1959.

Carpenter, D. F., Brubaker, L. H., Powell, R. D., Jr., and Valsamis, M. P.: Phycomycotic thrombosis of the basilar artery. Neurology 18:807–812, 1968.

Cassady, J. R., and Foerster, H. C.: *Sporotrichum schenckii* endophthalmitis. Arch. Ophthal. 85:71–74, 1971.

Caudill, R. G., Smith, C. E., and Reinarz, J. A.: Coccidioidal meningitis. A diagnostic challenge. Am. J. Med. 49:360–365, 1970.

Causey, W. A., Arnell, P., and Brinker, J.: Systemic Nocardia caviae infection. Chest 65:360–362, 1974.

Chandler, J. W., Jr., Kriel, R. L., and Tosh, F. E.: Childhood sporotrichosis. Am. J. Dis. Child. 115:368–372, 1968.

Cherry, J. D., Lloyd, C. A., Quilty, J. F., and Laskowski, L. F.: Amphotericin B therapy in children. A review of the literature and a case report. J. Pediat. 75:1063–1069, 1969.

Chesney, P. J., Teets, K. C., Mulvihill, J. J., Salit, I. E., and Marks, M. I.: Successful treatment of candida meningitis with amphotericin B and 5-fluorocytosine in combination. J. Pediat. 89:1017–1019, 1976.

Christian, J. R., Sarre, S. G., Peers, J. H., Salazar, E., and de Rosario, J.: Pulmonary coccidioidomycosis in a twenty-one-day-old infant. Report of a case and review of the literature. Am. J. Dis. Child. 92:66–74, 1956.

Christoforidis, A. J.: Radiologic manifestations of histoplasmosis. Am. J. Roentgenol. 109:478–490, 1970.

Cleveland, W. W., Fogel, B. J., Brown, W. T., and Kay, H. E. M.: Foetal thymic transplant in a case of DiGeorge's syndrome. Lancet 2:1211–1214, 1968.

Codish, S. D., Tobias, J. S., and Hannigan, M.: Combined amphotericin B-flucytosine therapy in aspergillus pneumonia. J.A.M.A. 241:2418–2419, 1979.

Cohen, M. L., Weiss, E. B., and Monaco, A. P.: Successful treatment of Pneumocystis carinii and Nocardia asteroides in a renal transplant patient. Am. J. Med. 50:269–276, 1971.

Coleman, R., Marie, R., and Kaufman, L.: The use of the immunodiffusion test in the serodiagnosis of aspergillosis. Appl. Microbiol. 23:301–308, 1972.

Collins, W. T.: Disseminated ulcerating sporotrichosis with widespread visceral involvement: report of a case. Arch. Derm. Syph. 56:523–528, 1947.

Colwell, J. A., and Tillman, S. P.: Early recognition and therapy of disseminated coccidioidomycosis. Am. J. Med. 31:676–691, 1961.

Conant, N. F.: Medical mycology. *In:* Dubos and Hirsch: Bacterial and Mycotic Infections of Man. J. B. Lippincott, Philadelphia, 1965.

Cooper, R. A., Jr., and Goldstein, E.: Histoplasmosis of the central nervous system. Report of two cases and review of the literature. Am. J. Med. 35:45–57, 1963.

Cope, V. Z.: Actinomycosis. Oxford University Press, London, 1938.

Couch, J. R., Abdou, N. I., and Sagawa, A.: Histoplasma meningitis with hyperactive suppressor T cells in cerebrospinal fluid. Neurology 28:119–123, 1978.

Courey, W. R., New, P. F. J., and Price, D. L.: Angiographic manifestations of craniofacial phycomycosis. Report of 3 cases. Radiology 103:329–334, 1972.

Cox, F., and Hughes, W. T.: Disseminated histoplasmosis and childhood leukemia. Cancer 33:1127–1133, 1974.

Cox, F., and Hughes, W. T.: Contagious and other aspects of nocardiosis in the compromised host. Pediatrics 55:135–138, 1975.

Craven, P. C., Ludden, T. M., Drutz, D. J., Rogers, W.,

Haegele, K. A., and Skrdlant, H. B.: Excretion pathways of amphotericin B. J. Infect. Dis. 140:329–341, 1979.

Curry, C. R., and Quie, P. G.: Fungal septicemia in patients receiving parenteral hyperalimentation. New Eng. J. Med. 285:1221–1225, 1971.

Dalovisio, J. R., and Panky, G. A.: In vitro susceptibility of *Nocardia asteroides* to amikacin. Antimicrob. Agents Chemother. 13:128–129, 1978.

Darling, S. T.: Protozoan general infection producing pseudotubercles in lungs and focal necrosis in liver, spleen, and lymph nodes. J.A.M.A. 46:1283–1285, 1906.

Davies, S. F., McKenna, R. W., and Sarosi, G. A.: Trephine biopsy of the bone marrow in disseminated histoplasmosis. Am. J. Med. 67:617–622, 1979.

Dawborn, J. K., Page, M. D., and Schiavone, D. J.: Use of 5-fluorocytosine in patients with impaired renal function. Brit. Med. J. 4:382–384, 1973.

Dawson, D. M., and Taghavy, A. A.: A test for spinal-fluid alcohol in torula meningitis. New Eng. J. Med. 269:1424, 1963.

Dayal, Y., Weindling, H. K., and Price, D. L.: Cerebral infarction due to fungal embolus. A complication of aspergillus infection on an aortic valve prosthesis. Neurology 24:76–79, 1974.

Dean, D. F., Ajello, L., Irwin, R. S., Woelk, W. K., and Skarulis, G. J.: Cranial zygomycosis caused by *Saksenaea vasiformis.* J. Neurosurg. 46:97–103, 1977.

Dennis, J. L., and Hansen, A. E.: Coccidioidomycosis in children. Pediatrics 14:481–484, 1954.

Denton, J. F., McConough, E. S., Ajello, L., and Auscherman, R. J.: Isolation of Blastomyces dermatitidis from soil. Science 133:1126–1127, 1961.

Deresinski, S. C., Lilly, R. B., Levine, H. B., Galgiani, J. N., and Stevens, D. A.: Treatment of fungal meningitis with miconazole. Arch. Intern. Med. 137:1180–1185, 1977.

Deresinski, S. C., and Stevens, D. A.: Coccidioidomycosis in compromised hosts. Experience at Stanford University Hospital. Medicine 54:377–395, 1974.

DeVita, V. T., Utz, J. P., Williams, T., and Carlone, P. P.: Candida meningitis. Arch. Intern. Med. 117:527–535, 1966.

DeWeese, D. D., Schleuning, A. J., II, and Robinson, L. B.: Mucormycosis of the nose and paranasal sinuses. Laryngoscope 75:1398–1407, 1965.

Diamond, R. D., and Bennett, J. E.: A subcutaneous reservoir for intrathecal therapy of fungal meningitis. New Eng. J. Med. 288:186–188, 1973.

Diamond, R. D., and Bennett, J. E.: Prognostic factors in cryptococcal meningitis. A study of 111 cases. Ann. Intern. Med. 80:176–181, 1974.

Diasio, R. B., Lakings, D. E., and Bennett, J. E.: Evidence for conversion of 5-fluorocytosine to 5-fluorouracil in humans: Possible factor in 5-fluorocytosine clinical toxicity. Antimicrob. Agents Chemother. 14:903–908, 1978.

Diasio, R. B., Wilburn, M. E., Shadomy, S., and Espinel-Ingroff, A.: Rapid determination of serum 5-fluorocytosine levels by high-performance liquid chromatography. Antimicrob. Agents Chemother. 13:500–504, 1978.

Dolan, C. T.: A practical approach to identification of yeast-like organisms. Am. J. Clin. Path. 55:580–590, 1971.

Dolan, C. T.: Specificity of the latex-cryptococcal antigen test. Am. J. Clin. Path. 58:358–364, 1972.

Doughten, R. M., and Pearson, H. A.: Disseminated intravascular coagulation associated with aspergillus endocarditis. J. Pediat. 73:576–582, 1968.

Drutz, D. J., and Catanzaro, A.: Coccidioidomycosis. Part I. Am. Rev. Resp. Dis. 117:559–585, 1978.

Drutz, D. J., and Catanzaro, A.: Coccidioidomycosis. Part II. Am. Rev. Resp. Dis. 117:727–771, 1978.

Drutz, D. J., Spickard, A., Rogers, D. E., and Koenig, M. G.: Treatment of disseminated mycotic infections. A new approach to amphotericin B therapy. Am. J. Med. 45:405–418, 1968.

Duque, O.: Meningo-encephalitis and brain abscess caused by Cladosporium and Fonsecaea. Review of the literature, report of two cases, and experimental studies. Am. J. Clin. Path. 36:505–517, 1961.

Duttera, M. J., Jr., and Osterhout, S.: North American blastomycosis. A survey of 63 cases. Southern Med. J. 62:295–301, 1969.

Echols, R. M., Selinger, D. S., Hallowell, C., Goodwin, J. S., Duncan, M. H., and Cushing, A. H.: Rhizopus osteomyelitis. A case report and review. Am. J. Med. 66:141–145, 1979.

Eckhoff, N. L.: Actinomycosis of the central nervous system: Report of two cases. Lancet 1:7–8, 1941.

Edelson, R. N., McNatt, E. N., and Porro, R. S.: Candida meningitis with cerebral arteritis. N. Y. J. Med. 75:900–904, 1975.

Edwards, C., Elliott, W. A., and Randall, K. J.: Spinal meningitis due to Actinomyces bovis treated with penicillin and streptomycin. J. Neurol. Neurosurg. Psychiat. 14:134–136, 1951.

Edwards, J. E., Montgomerie, J. Z., Foos, R. Y., Shaw, V. K., and Guze, L. B.: Experimental hematogenous endophthalmitis caused by candida albicans. J. Infect. Dis. 131:649–657, 1975.

Edwards, P. Q., and Palmer, C. W.: Nationwide histoplasmin sensitivity and histoplasma infection. Pub. Health Rep. 78:241, 1963.

Edwards, V. E., Sutherland, J. M., and Tyrer, J. H.: Cryptococcosis of the central nervous system. Epidemiological, clinical and therapeutic features. J. Neurol. Neurosurg. Psychiat. 33:415–425, 1970.

Emanuel, B., Ching, E., Lieberman, A. D., and Goldin, M.: Cryptococcus meningitis in a child successfully treated with amphotericin B, with a review of the pediatric literature. J. Pediat. 59:577–591, 1961.

Emmons, C. W.: *Allescheria boydii* and *Monosporium apiospermum*. Mycologia 36:188–193, 1944.

Emmons, C. W., Binford, C. H., Utz, J. P., and Kwon-Chung, K. J.: Medical Mycology. Lea and Febiger, Philadelphia, 1977.

Ende, N., Pizzolato, P., and Ziskind, J.: Hodgkin's disease associated with histoplasmosis. Cancer 5:763–769, 1952.

Eppinger, H.: Ueber eine neue pathogene cladothrix und eine durch sie heruorgerufene pseudotuberculosis. Wien. Klin. Wschr. 3:321–323, 1890.

Epstein, S. M., Miale, T. D., Moossy, J., Verney, E., and Sidransky, H.: Experimental intracranial aspergillosis. J. Neuropath. Exp. Neurol. 27:473–482, 1968.

Epstein, S. M., Verney, E., Miale, T. D., and Sidransky, H.: Studies on the pathogenesis of experimental pulmonary aspergillosis. Am. J. Path. 51:769–788, 1967.

Ernest, J. T., and Rippon, J. W.: Keratitis due to Allescheria boydii (monosporium apiospermum). Am. J. Ophthal. 62:1202–1204, 1966.

Ewing, G. E., Bosl, G. J., and Peterson, P. K.: Sporothrix schenckii meningitis in a farmer with Hodgkin's disease. Am. J. Med. 68:455–457, 1980.

Ezdinli, E. Z., O'Sullivan, D. D., Wasser, L. P., Kim, U., and Stutzman, L.: Oral amphotericin for candidiasis in patients with hematologic neoplasms. An autopsy study. J.A.M.A. 242:258–260, 1979.

Faber, H. K., Smith, C. E., and Dickson, E. C.: Acute coccidioidomycosis with erythema nodosum in children. J. Pediat. 15:163–171, 1939.

Fass, R. J., and Perkins, R. L.: 5-fluorocytosine in the treatment of cryptococcal and candida mycoses. Ann. Intern. Med. 74:535–539, 1971.

Feigin, R. D., Shackelford, P. G., Eisen, S., Spitler, L. E., Pickering, L. K., and Anderson, D. C.: Treatment of mucocutaneous candidiasis with transfer factor. Pediatrics 53:63–70, 1974.

Finegold, S. M., Will, D., and Murray, J. F.: Aspergillosis. A review and report of twelve cases. Am. J. Med. 27:463–482, 1959.

Fisher, J. F., Duma, R. J., Markowitz, S. M., Shadomy, S., Espinel-Ingroff, A., and Chew, W. H.: Therapeutic failures with miconazole. Antimicrob. Agents Chemother. 13:965–968, 1978.

Fischer, T. J., Klein, R. B., Kershnar, H. E., Borut, T. C., and Stiehm, E. R.: Miconazole in the treatment of chronic mucocutaneous candidiasis: A preliminary report. J. Pediat. 91:815–819, 1977.

Fishman, L. S., Griffin, J. R., Sapico, F. L., and Hecht, R.: Hematogenous candida endophthalmitis—A complication of candidemia. New Eng. J. Med. 286:675–681, 1972.

Font, R. L., and Jakobiec, F. A.: Granulomatous necrotizing retinochoroiditis caused by *Sporotrichum schenkii*. Report of a case including immunofluorescence and electron microscopical studies. Arch. Ophthal. 94:1513–1519, 1976.

Forno, L. S., and Billingham, M. E.: *Allescheria boydii* infection of the brain. J. Pathol. 106:195–198, 1972.

Frazier, A. R., Rosenow, E. C., and Roberts, G. D.: Nocardiosis. A review of 25 cases occurring during 24 months. Mayo Clin. Proc. 50:657–663, 1975.

Freeman, J. W., and Ziegler, D. K.: Chronic meningitis caused by Sporotrichum schenckii. Neurology 27:989–992, 1977.

Friedman, J. L., Baum, G. L., and Schwarz, J.: Primary pulmonary histoplasmosis. Associated pericardial and mediastinal manifestations. Am. J. Dis. Child. 109:298–303, 1965.

Friedman, L. L., and Signorelli, J. J.: Blastomycosis: A brief review of the literature and a report of a case involving the meninges. Ann. Intern. Med. 24:385–400, 1946.

Furcolow, M. L.: Opportunism in histoplasmosis. Lab. Invest. 11:1134–1139, 1962.

Furcolow, M. L., Schwarz, J., Hewell, B. A., and Grayston, J. T.: Incidence of tuberculin, histoplasmin, and blastomycin reactors among a group of school children. Am. J. Pub. Health 43:1523–1531, 1953.

Furcolow, M. L., and Smith, C. D.: A new hypothesis on the epidemiology of blastomycosis and the ecology of Blastomyces dermatitidis. Trans. N. Y. Acad. Sci. 35:421–430, 1973.

Fusner, J. E., and McClain, K. L.: Disseminated lymphonodular cryptococcosis treated with 5–fluorocytosine. J. Pediat. 94:599–601, 1979.

Gartenberg, G., Bottone, E. J., Keusch, G. T., and Weitzman, I.: Hospital-acquired mucormycosis (Rhizopus rhizopodiformis) of skin and subcutaneous tissue. Epidemiology, mycology and treatment. New Eng. J. Med. 299:1115–1118, 1978.

Gatti, R. A., Gershanik, J. J., Levkoff, A. H., Wertelecki, W., and Good, R. A.: DiGeorge syndrome associated with combined immunodeficiency. J. Pediat. 81:920–926, 1972.

Gerber, H. J., Schoonmaker, F. W., and Vazquez, M. D.: Chronic meningitis associated with histoplasma endocarditis. New Eng. J. Med. 275:74–76, 1966.

Gerstl, B., Weidman, W. H., and Newmann, A. V.: Pulmonary aspergillosis: report of two cases. Ann. Intern. Med. 28:662–671, 1948.

Gilchrist, T. C.: Protozoan dermatitis. J. Cutan. Genitourin. Dis. 12:496, 1894.

Gilchrist, T. C., and Stokes, W. R.: A case of pseudolupus vulgaris caused by blastomyces. J. Exp. Med. 3:53–78, 1898.

Gilden, D. H., Miller, E. M., and Johnson, W. G.: Central nervous system histoplasmosis after rhinoplasty. Neurology 24:874–877, 1974.

Glassman, M. I., Henkind, P., and Alture-Werber, E.: Monosporium apiospermum endophthalmitis. Am. J. Ophthal. 76:821–824, 1973.

Gluckman, S. J., Ries, K., and Abrutyn, E.: *Allescheria (Petriellidium) boydii* sinusitis in a compromised host. J. Clin. Microbiol. 5:481–484, 1977.

Goldman, J. A., Fleischer, A. S., Leifer, W., Parent, A., Schwarzman, S. W., and Raggio, J.: *Candida albicans* mycotic aneurysm associated with systemic lupus erythematosus. Neurosurgery 4:325–328, 1979.

Goldstein, E., Winship, M. J., and Pappagianis, D.: Ventricular fluid and the management of coccidioidal meningitis. Ann. Intern. Med. 77:243–246, 1972.

Gonyea, E. F.: Cisternal puncture and cryptococcal meningitis. Arch. Neurol. 28:200–201, 1973.

Gonyea, E. F.: The spectrum of primary blastomycotic meningitis: A review of central nervous system blastomycosis. Ann. Neurol. 3:26–39, 1978.

Gonyea, E. F., and Heilman, K. M.: Neuro-ophthalmic aspects of central nervous system cryptococcosis. Internuclear and supranuclear ophthalmoplegia. Arch. Ophthal. 87:164–168, 1972.

Goodman, J. S., Kaufman, L., and Koenig, M. G.: Diagnosis of cryptococcal meningitis. Value of immunologic detection of cryptococcal antigen. New Eng. J. Med. 285:434–436, 1971.

Gordon, M. A., Holzman, R. S., Senter, H., Lapa, E. W., and Kupersmith, M. J.: Aspergillus oryzae meningitis. J.A.M.A. 235:2122–2123, 1976.

Graybill, J. R.: Transfer factor in coccidioidomycosis. Clin. Res. 23:304A, 1975.

Graybill, J. R., and Ellenbogen, C.: Complications with the Ommaya reservoir in patients with granulomatous meningitis. J. Neurosurg. 38:477–480, 1973.

Greenwood, R. C., and Voris, H. C.: Systemic blastomycosis with spinal cord involvement. Case report. J. Neurosurg. 7:450–454, 1950.

Greer, H. D., III, Geraci, J. E., Corbin, K. B., Miller, R. H., and Weed, L. A.: Disseminated histoplasmosis presenting as a brain tumor and treated with amphotericin B: Report of case. Mayo Clin. Proc. 39:490–494, 1964.

Gross, P. A., Patel, C., and Spitler, L. E.: Disseminated cryptococcus treated with transfer factor. J.A.M.A. 240:2460–2462, 1978.

Gruhn, J. G., and Sanson, J.: Mycotic infections in leukemic patients at autopsy. Cancer 16:61–73, 1963.

Grunberg, E., Titsworth, E., and Bennet, M.: Chemotherapeutic activity of 5-fluorocytosine. Antimicrob. Agents Chemother. 1963:566–568, 1964.

Hale, L. M.: Orbital-cerebral phycomycosis. Report of a case and a review of the disease in infants. Arch. Ophthal. 86:39–43, 1971.

Hameroff, S. B., Eckholdt, J. W., and Lindenberg, R.: Cerebral phycomycosis in a heroin addict. Neurology 20:261–265, 1970.

Hammer, G. S., Bottone, E. J., and Hirschman, S. Z.: Mucormycosis in a transplant recipient. Am. J. Clin. Path. 64:389–398, 1975.

Haning, H. A. L., Johnston, R., Touloukian, R., and Margolis, C. Z.: Successfully treated candida endophthalmitis in a child. Pediatrics 51:1027–1031, 1973.

Harder, E. J., and Hermans, P. E.: Treatment of fungal infections with flucytosine. Arch. Intern. Med. 135:231–237, 1975.

Harrell, E. R., and Curtis, A. C.: North American blastomycosis. Am. J. Med. 27:750–766, 1959.

Hart, P. D., Russell, E., Jr., and Remington, J. S.: The compromised host and infection. II. Deep fungal infection. J. Infect. Dis. 120:169–191, 1969.

Hart, R. J., Patterson, R., and Sommers, H.: Hyperimmunoglobulinemia E in a child with allergic bronchopulmonary aspergillosis and bronchiectasis. J. Pediat. 89:38–41, 1976.

Hassin, G. B.: Torulosis of the central nervous system. J. Neuropath. Exp. Neurol. 6:44–60, 1947.

Hathaway, B. M., and Mason, K. N.: Nocardiosis. Study of fourteen cases. Am. J. Med. 32:903–909, 1962.

Hefferman, A. G. A., and Asper, S. P., Jr.: Insidious fungal disease. Bull. Johns Hopkins Hosp. 118:10–26, 1966.

Heiner, D. C.: Diagnosis of histoplasmosis using precipitin reactions in agar gel. Pediatrics 22:616–627, 1958.

Heird, W. C., Driscoll, J. M., Jr., Schullinger, J. N., Grebin, B., and Winters, R. W.: Intravenous alimentation in pediatric patients. J. Pediat. 80:351–372, 1972.

Henig, E., Djaldetti, M., Pinkhas, J., and DeVries, A.: Candida tropicalis meningitis in Hodgkin's disease. J.A.M.A. 199:182–215, 1967.

Hermans, P. E.: Antifungal agents used for deep-seated mycotic infections. Mayo Clin. Proc. 52:687–693, 1977.

Hertzog, A. J., Smith, T. S., and Goblin, M.: Acute pulmonary aspergillosis. Pediatrics 4:331–335, 1949.

Hill, H. R., Mitchell, T. G., Matsen, J. M., and Quie, P. G.: Recovery from disseminated candidiasis in a premature neonate. Pediatrics 53:748–752, 1974.

Hinson, K. F. W., Moon, A. J., and Plummer, N. S.: Bronchopulmonary aspergillosis. A review and a report of eight new cases. Thorax 7:317–333, 1952.

Hoeprich, P. D., Brandt, D., and Parker, R. H.: Nocardial brain abscess cured with cycloserine and sulfonamides. Am. J. Med. Sci. 255:208–216, 1968.

Holland, P., and Holland, N. H.: Histoplasmosis in early infancy. Hematologic, histochemical, and immunological observations. Am. J. Dis. Child. 112:412–421, 1966.

Horten, B. C., Abbott, G. F., and Porro, R. S.: Fungal aneurysms of intracranial vessels. Arch. Neurol. 33:577–579, 1976.

Huang, S. N., and Harris, L. S.: Acute disseminated penicilliosis. Report of a case and review of pertinent literature. Am. J. Clin. Path. 39:167–174, 1963.

Hughes, W. T.: Chromoblastomycosis: Successful treatment with topical amphotericin B. J. Pediat. 71:351–356, 1967.

Hughes, W. T.: Generalized aspergillosis. A case involving the central nervous system. Am. J. Dis. Child. 112:262–265, 1966.

Hurley, R.: Acute disseminated (septicaemic) moniliasis in adults and children. Postgrad. Med. 40:644–653, 1964.

Huston, A. C., and Hoeprich, P. D.: Comparative susceptibility of four kinds of pathogenic fungi to amphotericin B and amphotericin B methyl ester. Antimicrob. Agents Chemother. 13:905–909, 1978.

Hutter, R. V. P.: Phycomycetous infection (mucormycosis) in cancer patients: a complication of therapy. Cancer 12:330–350, 1959.

Hyatt, H. W., Sr.: Coccidioidomycosis in a 3-week-old infant. Am. J. Dis. Child. 105:93–98, 1963.

Idriss, Z. H., Cunningham, R. J., and Wilfert, C. M.: Nocardiosis in children: Report of three cases and review of the literature. Pediatrics 55:479–484, 1975.

Ingham, S. D.: Coccidioidal granuloma of the spine with compression of the spinal cord. Bull. Los Angeles Neurol. Soc. 1:41–45, 1936.

Iovine, G., Berman, L. B., Halikis, D. N., Mowrey, F. H., Chappelle, E. H., and Gierson, H. W.: Nephrotoxicity of amphotericin B. A clinical-pathologic study. Arch. Intern. Med. 112:853–862, 1963.

Isacson, M., Noah, Z., Faber, J., Herishano, Y., and Gottfried, L.: Use of 5-fluorocytosine in systemic candidiasis in infancy. Arch. Dis. Childh. 47:954–959, 1972.

Israel, H. L., and Ostrow, A.: Sarcoidosis and aspergilloma. Am. J. Med. 47:243–250, 1969.

Jackson, F. E., Kent, D., and Clare, F.: Quadriplegia caused by involvement of cervical spine with Coccidioides immitis. J. Neurosurg. 21:512–515, 1964.

Jackson, I. J., Earle, K. M., and Kuri, J.: Solitary aspergillus granuloma of the brain. Report of 2 cases. J. Neurosurg. 12:53–61, 1955.

Jacobson, J. R., and Cloward, R. B.: Actinomycosis of the central nervous system. J.A.M.A. 137:769–771, 1948.

Jenkins, V. E., and Postlewaite, J. C.: Coccidioidal meningitis: report of four cases with necropsy findings in three cases. Ann. Intern. Med. 35:1068–1084, 1951.

Joe, L. K., Eng, N. I. T., Pohan, A., Van der Meulen, H., and Emmons, C. W.: Basidiobolus ranarum as a cause of subcutaneous mycosis in Indonesia. Arch. Derm. 74:378–383, 1956.

Jordon, W. M., Bodey, G. P., Rodriquez, V., Ketchell, S. J., and Henney, J.: Miconazole therapy for treatment of fungal infections in cancer patients. Antimicrob. Agents Chemother. 16:792–797, 1979.

Juba, A.: Uber eine seltene mykose (durch Histoplasma capsulatum verursachte meningoencephalitis) des zentralnervensystems. Psychiat. Neurol. 135:260–268, 1958.

Kammer, R. B., and Utz, J. P.: Aspergillus species endocarditis. The new face of a not so rare disease. Am. J. Med. 56:506–521, 1974.

Kaplan, W., and Ivens, M. S.: Fluorescent antibody staining of Sporotrichum schenckii in cultures and clinical materials. J. Invest. Dermatol. 35:151–159, 1960.

Kaplan, W., and Kraft, D. E.: Demonstration of pathogenic fungi in formalin-fixed tissues by immunofluorescence. Am. J. Clin. Path. 52:420–432, 1969.

Karalakulasingam, R., Arora, K. K., Adams, G., Serratoni, F., and Martin, D. G.: Meningoencephalitis caused by Histoplasma capsulatum. Occurrence in a renal transplant recipient and a review of the literature. Arch. Intern. Med. 136:217–220, 1976.

Kauffman, C. A., Carleton, J. A., and Frame, P. T.: Simple assay for 5-fluorocytosine in the presence of amphotericin B. Antimicrob. Agents Chemother. 9:381–383, 1976.

Kauffman, C. A., and Frame, P. T.: Bone marrow toxicity associated with 5-fluorocytosine therapy. Antimicrob. Agents Chemother. 11:244–247, 1977.

Kauffman, C. A., Israel, K. S., Smith, J. W., White, A. C., Schwarz, J., and Brooks, G. F.: Histoplasmosis in immunosuppressed patients. Am. J. Med. 64:923–932, 1978.

Kauffman, C. A., and Tan, J. S.: Torulopsis glabrata renal infection. Am. J. Med. 57:217–223, 1974.

Kaufman, D. M., Thal, L. J., and Farmer, P. M.: Central nervous system aspergillosis in two young adults. Neurology 26:484–488, 1976.

Kirmani, N., Tuazon, C. U., Ocuin, J. A., Thompson, A. M., Kramer, N. C., and Geelhoed, G. W.: Extensive cerebral nocardiosis cured with antibiotic therapy alone. Case report. J. Neurosurg. 49:924–929, 1978.

Kitahara, M., Seth, V. K., Medoff, G., and Kobayashi, G. S.: Activity of amphotericin B, 5-fluorocytosine, and rifampin against six clinical isolates of aspergillus. Antimicrob. Agents Chemother. 9:915–919, 1976.

Klein, J. D., Yamauchi, T., and Horlick, S. P.: Neonatal candidiasis, meningitis, and arthritis: Observations and a review of the literature. J. Pediat. 81:31–34, 1972.

Klein, R. C., Ivens, M. S., Seabury, J. H., and Dascomb, H. E.: Meningitis due to Sporotrichum schenckii. Arch. Intern. Med. 118:145–149, 1966.

Kobayashi, R. M., Coel, M., Niwayama, G., and Trauner, D.: Cerebral vasculitis in coccidioidal meningitis. Ann. Neurol. 1:281–284, 1977.

Kohlschutter, A., and Pelet, B.: Pulmonary candidiasis treated with 5-fluorocytosine. Arch. Dis. Childh. 49:154–156, 1974.

Kolodny, E. H., Rebeiz, J. J., Caviness, V. S., Jr., and Richardson, E. P., Jr.: Granulomatous angiitis of the central nervous system. Arch. Neurol. 19:510–524, 1968.

Komorowski, R. A., Farmer, S. G., Hanson, G. A., and Hause, L. L.: Cerebrospinal fluid lactic acid in diagnosis of meningitis. J. Clin. Microbiol. 8:89–92, 1978.

Kozinn, P. J., Galen, R. S., Taschdjian, C. L., Goldberg, P. L., Protzman, W., and Kozinn, M. A.: The precipitin test in systemic candidiasis. J.A.M.A. 235:628–629, 1976.

Kroll, J. J., Einbinder, J. M., and Merz, W. G.: Mucocutaneous candidiasis in a mother and son. Arch. Dermatol. 108:259–262, 1973.

Krumdieck, N., and Stevenson, L.: Spinal epidural abscess associated with actinomycosis. Arch. Path. 30:1223–1226, 1940.

Landau, J. W.: Chronic mucocutaneous candidiasis—associated immunologic abnormalities. Pediatrics 42:227–230, 1968.

Landau, J. W., and Newcomer, V. D.: Acute cerebral phycomycosis (mucormycosis). Report of a pediatric patient successfully treated with amphotericin B and cycloheximide and review of the pertinent literature. J. Pediat 61:363–385, 1962.

Lane, T., Goings, S., Fraser, D. W., Ries, K., Pettrozzi, J., and Abrutyn, E.: Disseminated actinomycosis with spinal cord compression: Report of two cases. Neurology 29:890–893, 1979.

Lanza, F. L., Nelson, R. S., and Somayaji, B. N.: Acute granulomatous hepatitis due to histoplasmosis. Gastroenterology 58:392–396, 1970.

Leers, W–D., Russell, N. A., and Laroye, G.: Cerebellar abscess due to Blastomyces dermatitidis. Canad. Med. Assoc. J. 107:657–660, 1972.

Lehrer, R. I., and Cline, M. J.: Leukocyte myeloperoxidase deficiency and disseminated candidiasis: the role of myeloperoxidase in resistance to Candida infection. J. Clin. Invest. 48:1478–1488, 1969.

Levin, S., Zaidel, L., and Bernstein, D.: Intrauterine infection of fetal brain by candida. Am. J. Obstet. Gynecol. 130:597–599, 1978.

Levine, H. B., Gonzales-Ochoa, A., and Ten Eyck, D. R.: Dermal sensitivity to Coccidioides immitis. A comparison of responses elicited in man by spherulin and coccidioidin. Am. Res. Resp. Dis. 107:379–386, 1973.

Levitt, J. M., and Goldstein, J.: Keratomycosis due to Allescheria boydii. Am. J. Ophthal. 71:1190–1191, 1971.

Lewin, W., and Morgan, A. D.: Actinomycosis of the brain. J. Neurol. Neurosurg. Psychiat. 10:163–170, 1947.

Lilien, L. D., Ramamurthy, R. S., and Pildes, R. S.: Candida albicans meningitis in a premature neonate successfully treated with 5-fluorocytosine and amphotericin B: A case report and review of the literature. Pediatrics 61:57–61, 1978.

Linares, G., McGarry, P. A., and Baker, R. D.: Solid solitary aspergillotic granuloma of the brain. Report of a case due to Aspergillus candidus and review of the literature. Neurology 21:177–184, 1971.

Littman, M. L., Horowitz, P. L., and Swadey, J. G.: Coccidioidomycosis and its treatment with amphotericin B. Am. J. Med. 24:568–592, 1958.

Littman, M. L., and Walter, J. E.: Cryptococcosis: Current status. Am. J. Med. 45:922–932, 1968.

Long, E. L., and Weiss, D. L.: Cerebral mucormycosis. Am. J. Med. 26:625–635, 1959.

Loudon, R. G., and Lawson, R. A., Jr.: Systemic blastomycosis. Recurrent neurological relapse in a case treated with amphotericin B. Ann. Intern. Med. 55:139–147, 1961.

Louria, D. B.: Deep-seated mycotic infections, allergy to fungi and mycotoxins. New Eng. J. Med. 277:1065–1071, 1967.

Louria, D. B., Lieberman, P. H., Collins, H. S., and Blevins, A.: Pulmonary mycetoma due to Allescheria boydii. Arch. Intern. Med. 117:748–751, 1966.

Louria, D. B., Stiff, D. P., and Bennett, B.: Disseminated moniliasis in the adult. Medicine 41:307–337, 1962.

Lucasse, C., Chardome, J., and Magis, P.: Mycose cérébrale par Cladosporium trichoides chez un indigène du Congo Belge. Ann. Soc. Belg. Med. Trop. 34:475–484, 1954.

Luke, J. L., Bolande, R. P., and Gross, S.: Generalized aspergillosis and aspergillus endocarditis in infancy. Report of a case. Pediatrics 31:115–122, 1963.

Lutwick, L. I., Galgiani, J. N., Johnson, R. H., and Stevens, D. A.: Visceral fungal infections due to Petriellidium boydii (Allescheria boydii). Am. J. Med. 61:632–640, 1976.

Lynch, P. J., Voorhees, J. J., and Harrell, E. R.: Systemic sporotrichosis. Ann. Intern. Med. 73:23–30, 1970.

MacGregor, R. R., Bennett, J. E., and Erslev, A. J.: Erythropoietin concentration in amphotericin B-induced anemia. Antimicrob. Agents Chemother. 14:270–273, 1978.

MacKinnon, S., Kane, J. G., and Parker, R. H.: False-positive cryptococcal antigen test and cervical prevertebral abscess. J.A.M.A. 240:1982–1983, 1978.

Maderazo, E. G., and Quintiliani, R.: Treatment of nocardial infection with trimethoprim and sulfamethoxazole. Am. J. Med. 57:671–675, 1974.

Malloch, D.: New concepts in the microascaceae illustrated by two new species. Mycologia 62:727–740, 1970.

Maltby, G. L.: Intracranial actinomycosis: Report of an unusual case. J. Neurosurg. 8:674–678, 1951.

Marks, M. I., Langston, C., and Eickhoff, T. C.: Torulopsis glabrata—An opportunistic pathogen in man. New Eng. J. Med. 283:1131–1135, 1970.

Martin, D. S., Jones, C. P., Yao, K. F., and Lee, L. E., Jr.: A practical classification of the monilias. J. Bact. 34:99–129, 1937.

Martin, D. S., and Smith, D. T.: Blastomycosis. I. A re-view of the literature. Am. Rev. Tuberc. 39:275–304, 1939.

Martin, D. S., and Smith, D. T.: Blastomycosis. II. A report of thirteen new cases. Am. Rev. Tuberc. 39:488–515, 1939.

Martin, F. P., Lukeman, J. M., Ranson, F. R., and Geppert, L. J.: Mucormycosis of the central nervous system associated with thrombosis of the internal carotid artery. J. Pediat. 44:437–442, 1954.

McBride, R. A., Corson, J. M., and Dammin, G. J.: Mucormycosis. Two cases of disseminated disease with cultural identification of Rhizopus; review of the literature. Am. J. Med. 28:832–846, 1960.

McCall, W., and Strobos, R. R. J.: Survival of a patient with central nervous system mucormycosis. Neurology 7:290–292, 1957.

McCormick, W. F., Schochet, S. S., Jr., Weaver, P. R., and McCrary, J. A.: Disseminated aspergillosis. Aspergillus endophthalmitis, optic nerve infarctions and carotid artery thrombosis. Arch. Pathol. 99:353–359, 1975.

McDonald, R., Greenberg, E. N., and Kramer, R.: Cryptococcal meningitis. Arch. Dis. Childh. 45:417–420, 1970.

McDowell, D. E., Ulmer, J. L., Velo, A. G., Ekren, W. S., and Kriz, J. P.: Cerebral abscess due to Actinomyces israeli. Southern Med. J. 58:227–230, 1965.

Medeiros, A. A., Marty, S. D., Tosh, F. E., and Chin, T. D. Y.: Erythema nodosum and erythema multiforme as clinical manifestations of histoplasmosis in a community outbreak. New Eng. J. Med. 274:415–420, 1966.

Merriam, J. C., Jr., and Tedeschi, C. G.: Cerebral mucormycosis. A fatal fungus infection complicating other disease. Neurology 7:510–515, 1957.

Meyer, R., and Axelrod, J. L.: Fatal aplastic anemia resulting from flucytosine. J.A.M.A. 228:1573, 1974.

Meyer, R. D., Young, L. S., Armstrong, D., and Yu, B.: Aspergillosis complicating neoplastic disease. Am. J. Med. 54:6–15, 1973.

Meyers, B. R., Lieberman, T. W., and Ferry, A. P.: Candida endophthalmitis complicating candidemia. Ann. Intern. Med. 79:647–653, 1973.

Meyers, B. R., Wormser, G., Hirschman, S. Z., and Blitzer, A.: Rhinocerebral mucormycosis. Premortem diagnosis and therapy. Arch. Intern. Med. 139:557–560, 1979.

Middleton, F. G., Jurgenson, P. F., Utz, J. P., Shadomy, S., and Shadomy, H. J.: Brain abscess caused by Cladosporium trichoides. Arch. Intern. Med. 136:444–448, 1976.

Minkowitz, S., Koffler, D., and Zak, F. G.: Torulopsis glabrata septicemia. Am. J. Med. 34:252–255, 1963.

Mirsky, H. S., and Cuttner, J.: Fungal infection in acute leukemia. Cancer 30:348–352, 1972.

Mohr, J. A., and Muchmore, H. G.: Susceptibility of Allescheria boydii to Amphotericin B. Antimicrob. Agents Chemother. 1969: 429–430, 1968.

Montgomerie, J. Z., and Edwards, J. E., Jr.: Association of infection due to Candida albicans with intravenous hyperalimentation. J. Infect. Dis. 137:197–201, 1978.

Montgomerie, J. Z., Edwards, J. E., Jr., and Guze, L. B.: Synergism of amphotericin B and 5-fluorocytosine for candida species. J. Infect. Dis. 132:82–86, 1975.

Morbidity and Mortality Weekly Reports. Vol. 22, No. 15, 14 April 1973.

Morris, J. H., MacAulay, M., and Poser, C. M.: Systemic cryptococcosis and histoplasmosis in the same patient. A case report. Neurology 14:147–153, 1964.

Morriss, F. H., Jr., and Spock, A.: Intracranial aneurysm

secondary to mycotic orbital and sinus infection. Report of a case implicating Penicillium as an opportunistic fungus. Am. J. Dis. Child. 119:357–362, 1970.

Mukoyama, M., Gimple, K., and Poser, C. M.: Aspergillosis of the central nervous system. Report of a brain abscess due to A. fumigatus and review of the literature. Neurology 19:967–974, 1969.

Murphy, J. D., and Bornstein, S.: Mucormycosis of the lung. Ann. Intern. Med. 33:442–453, 1950.

Murray, H. W., Fialk, M. A., and Roberts, R. B.: Candida arthritis. A manifestation of disseminated candidiasis. Am. J. Med. 60:587–595, 1976.

Murray, P. J. S., and Sladden, R. A.: Disseminated histoplasmosis following long-term steroid therapy for reticulosarcoma. Brit. Med. J. 2:631–632, 1965.

Musella, R. A., and Collins, G. H.: Cerebral chromoblastomycosis. Case report. J. Neurosurg. 35:219–222, 1971.

Myerowitz, R. L., Pazin, G. P., and Allen, C. M.: Disseminated candidiasis. Changes in incidence, underlying diseases, and pathology. Am. J. Clin. Path. 68:29–38, 1977.

Naidoff, M. A., and Green, W. R.: Endogenous aspergillus endophthalmitis occurring after kidney transplant. Am. J. Ophthalmol. 79:502–509, 1975.

Nelson, J. D., Bates, R., and Pitchford, A.: Histoplasma meningitis. Recovery following amphotericin B therapy. Am. J. Dis. Child. 102:218–223, 1961.

Nichols, D. R., and Herrell, W. E.: Penicillin in the treatment of actinomycosis. J. Lab. Clin. Med. 33:521–525, 1948.

Nielsen, H. S.: Effects of Amphotericin B in vitro on perfect and imperfect strains of Allescheria boydii. Appl. Microbiol. 15:86–91, 1967.

Nocard, E.: Note sur la maladie des boeufs de la Guadelope connue sous le nom de farcin. Ann. Inst. Pasteur. 2:293–302, 1888.

Norman, D. D., and Miller, Z. R.: Coccidioidomycosis of the central nervous system: a case of ten years duration. Neurology 4:713–717, 1954.

Nsanzumuhire, H., Vollum, D., and Poltera, A. A.: Chromomycosis due to Cladosporium trichoides treated with 5-fluorocytosine. Case report. Am. J. Clin. Path. 61:257–263, 1974.

Omieczynski, D. T.: Safe isolation of Coccidioides immitis from clinical specimens. Health Lab. Sci. 7:227–232, 1970.

Orr, E. R., and Riley, H. D., Jr.: Sporotrichosis in childhood: Report of ten cases. J. Pediat. 78:951–957, 1971.

Palmer, D. L., Harvey, R. L., and Wheeler, J. K.: Diagnostic and therapeutic considerations in Nocardia asteroides infection. Medicine 53:391–401, 1974.

Palmer, P. E., and McFadden, S. W.: Blastomycosis. Report of an unusual case. New Eng. J. Med. 279:979–983, 1968.

Parker, J. C., Jr., McCloskey, J. J., and Lee, R. S.: The emergence of candidosis. The dominant postmortem cerebral mycosis. Am. J. Clin. Path. 70:31–36, 1978.

Parker, J. D., Sarosi, G. A., Doto, I. L., Bailey, R. E., and Tosh, F. E.: Treatment of chronic pulmonary histoplasmosis. A national communicable disease center cooperative mycoses study. New Eng. J. Med. 283:225–229, 1970.

Philippidis, P., Naiman, J. L., Sibinga, M. S., and Valdes-Dapena, M. A.: Disseminated intravascular coagulation in Candida albicans septicemia. J. Pediat. 78:683–686, 1971.

Poliner, J. R., Wilkins, E. B., and Fernald, G. W.: Localized osseous cryptococcosis. J. Pediat. 94:597–599, 1979.

Powell, D. A., and Shuit, K. E.: Acute pulmonary blastomycosis in children: Clinical course and follow-up. Pediatrics 63:736–740, 1979.

Preisler, H. D., Hasenclever, H. F., Levitan, A. A., and Henderson, E. S.: Serologic diagnosis of disseminated candidiasis in patients with acute leukemia. Ann. Intern. Med. 70:19–30, 1969.

Prockop, L. D., and Silva-Hutner, M.: Cephalic mucormycosis (phycomycosis). A case with survival. Arch. Neurol. 17:379–386, 1967.

Pruitt, A. W., Achord, J. L., Fales, F. W., and Patterson, J. H.: Glucose-galactose malabsorption complicated by monilial arthritis. Pediatrics 43:106–110, 1969.

Raich, R. A., Casey, F., and Hall, W. H.: Pulmonary and cutaneous nocardiosis. Am. Rev. Resp. Dis. 83:505, 1961.

Rainey, R. L., and Harris, T. R.: Disseminated blastomycosis with meningeal involvement. Report of a patient cured by amphotericin B without resort to intrathecal administration. Arch. Intern. Med. 117:744–747, 1966.

Ramseyer, J. C., Baker, R. N., and Tomiyasu, U.: Ventriculovenous shunt in treatment of obstructive hydrocephalus due to coccidioidomycotic meningitis. Neurology 16:701–708, 1966.

Rand, C. W.: Coccidioidal granuloma: two cases simulating tumor of spinal cord. Arch. Neurol. Psychiat. 23:502–511, 1930.

Rankin, J., and Javid, M.: Nocardiosis of the central nervous system. Neurology 5:815–820, 1955.

Reddy, P., Gorelick, D. F., Brasher, C. A., and Larsh, H.: Progressive disseminated histoplasmosis as seen in adults. Am. J. Med. 48:629–636, 1970.

Reeves, D. L., and Baisinger, C. F.: Primary chronic coccidioidal meningitis: a diagnostic neurosurgical problem. J. Neurosurg. 2:269–280, 1945.

Richardson, H. B., Jr., Anderson, J. A., and McKay, B. M.: Acute pulmonary coccidioidomycosis in children. J. Pediat. 70:376–382, 1967.

Richardson, P. M., Mohandas, A., and Arumugasamy, N.: Cerebral cryptococcosis in Malaysia. J. Neurol. Neurosurg. Psychiat. 39:330–337, 1976.

Richart, R., and Dammin, G. J.: Candida tropicalis as a pathogen for man. New Eng. J. Med. 263:474–477, 1960.

Rifkind, D., Marchiaro, T. L., Schneck, S. A., and Hill, R. B.: Systemic fungal infections complicating renal transplantation and immunosuppressive therapy. Am. J. Med. 43:28–38, 1967.

Riley, O., Jr., and Mann, S. H.: Brain abscess caused by Cladosporium trichoides. Review of 3 cases and report of fourth case. Am. J. Clin. Path. 33:525–531, 1960.

Ritter, C.: Studies of the viability of Histoplasma capsulatum in tap water. Am. J. Pub. Health 44:1299, 1959.

Roberts, G. D., Brewer, N. S., and Hermans, P. E.: Diagnosis of nocardiosis by blood culture. Mayo Clin. Proc. 49:293–296, 1974.

Roberts, M., Rinaudo, P. A., Tilton, R. C., and Valinskas, J.: Treatment of multiple intracerebral cryptococcal granulomas with 5-fluorocytosine. Case report. J. Neurosurg. 37:229–232, 1972.

Rodgers, B. M., Vries, J. K., and Talbert, J. L.: Laparoscopy in the diagnosis and treatment of malfunctioning ventriculoperitoneal shunts in children. J. Pediat. Surg. 13:247–253, 1978.

Roe, D. C., and Haynes, R. E.: Candida albicans meningitis successfully treated with amphotericin B. Am. J. Dis. Child. 124:926–929, 1972.

Roessmann, U., and Friede, R. L.: Candidal infection of the brain. Arch. Path. 84:495–498, 1967.

Rose, F. C., Grant, H. C., and Jeanes, A. L.: Torulosis of the central nervous system in Britain. Brain 81:542–555, 1958.

Rosen, F., Deck, J. H. N., and Rewcastle, N. B.: Allescheria boydii—unique systemic dissemination to thyroid and brain. Canad. Med. Assoc. J. 93:1125–1127, 1965.

Rosenberg, M., Patterson, R., and Roberts, M.: Immunologic responses to therapy in allergic bronchopulmonary aspergillosis: Serum IgE value as an indicator and predictor of disease activity. J. Pediat. 91:914–917, 1977.

Rosett, W., and Hodges, G. R.: Recent experiences with nocardial infections. Am. J. Med. Sci. 276:279–285, 1978.

Rosner, F., Gabriel, F. C., Taschdjian, C. L., Cuesta, M. B., and Kozinn, P. J.: Serologic diagnosis of systemic candidiasis in patients with acute leukemia. Am. J. Med. 51:54–62, 1971.

Saccardo, P. A.: Omnium hucusque cognitorum. Sylloge Fungorum. 22:1287, 1911.

Sandhu, R., Alexander, S., Hornabrook, R. W., and Stehbens, W. E.: Granulomatous angiitis of the CNS. Arch. Neurol. 36:433–435, 1979.

Sandler, R., Tallman, C. B., Keamy, D. G., and Irving, W. R.: Successfully treated rhinocerebral phycomycosis in well controlled diabetes. New Eng. J. Med. 285:1180–1182, 1971.

Sarosi, G. A., and Davies, S. F.: Blastomycosis. Am. Rev. Resp. Dis. 120:911–938, 1979.

Sarosi, G. A., Hammerman, K. J., Tosh, F. E., and Kronenberg, R. S.: Clinical features of acute pulmonary blastomycosis. New Eng. J. Med. 290:540–543, 1974.

Sarosi, G. A., Parker, J. D., Doto, I. L., and Tosh, F. E.: Amphotericin B in cryptococcal meningitis. Long-term results of treatment. Ann. Intern. Med. 71:1079–1087, 1969.

Sarosi, G. A., Parker, J. D., Doto, I. L., and Tosh, F. E.: Chronic pulmonary coccidioidomycosis. A national communicable disease center cooperative mycoses study. New Eng. J. Med. 283:325–329, 1970.

Scharyj, M., Levene, N., and Gordon, H.: Primary pulmonary infection with Monosporium apiospermum. Report of a case with clinical, pathologic and mycologic data. J. Infect. Dis. 106:141–148, 1960.

Schenck, B. R.: On refractory subcutaneous abscesses caused by a fungus possibly related to the Sporotricha. Bull. Johns Hopkins Hosp. 2:286–290, 1898.

Schneider, R. C., and Rand, R. W.: Actinomycotic brain abscess. Complete excision with recovery. J. Neurosurg. 6:255–259, 1949.

Schober, R., and Herman, M. M.: Neuropathology of cardiac transplantation. Survey of 31 cases. Lancet 1:962–967, 1973.

Schroter, G. P. J., Temple, D. R., Husberg, B. S., Weil, R., III, and Starzl, T. S.: Cryptococcosis after renal transplantation: Report of ten cases. Surgery 79:268–277, 1976.

Schulz, D. M.: Histoplasmosis of the central nervous system. J.A.M.A. 151:549–551, 1953.

Schwarz, J., and Baum, G. L.: Blastomycosis. Am. J. Clin. Path. 21:999–1029, 1951.

Selby, R.: Pachymeningitis secondary to Allescheria boydii. Case report. J. Neurosurg. 36:225–227, 1972.

Selby, R. C., and Lopes, N. M.: Torulomas (cryptococcal granulomata) of the central nervous system. J. Neurosurg. 38:40–46, 1973.

Sellers, T. E., Jr., Price, W. N., Jr., and Newberry, W. M., Jr.: Epidemic of erythema multiforme and erythema nodosum caused by histoplasmosis. Ann. Intern. Med. 62:1244–1262, 1965.

Shear, C. L.: Life history of an undescribed ascomycete from a granular mycetoma of man. Mycologia 14:239–243, 1922.

Sheldon, D. L., and Johnson, W. C.: Cutaneous mucormycosis. Two documented cases of suspected nosocomial cause. J.A.M.A. 241:1032–1034, 1979.

Shoemaker, E. H., Bennett, H. D., Fields, W. S., Whitcomb, F. C., and Halpert, B.: Leptomeningitis due to Sporotrichum schenckii. Arch. Path. 64:222–227, 1957.

Shurtleff, D. B., Peterson, W., and Sherris, J. C.: Systemic Candida tropicalis infection treated with amphotericin. New Eng. J. Med. 269:1112–1115, 1963.

Shuster, M., Klein, M. M., Pribor, H. C., and Kozub, W.: Brain abscess due to Nocardia. Report of a case. Arch. Intern. Med. 120:610–614, 1967.

Siewers, C. M. F., and Cramblett, H. G.: Cryptococcosis (torulosis) in children. A report of four cases. Pediatrics 34:393–400, 1964.

Simon, H. B., Guerry, D., Breslow, A., and Kirkpatrick, C. H.: Opportunistic pathogens in the immunologically hyperresponsive host. Pneumocystis carinii infection in a patient with allergic bronchopulmonary aspergillosis. Am. J. Med. 55:856–864, 1973.

Singer, C., Kaplan, M. H., and Armstrong, D.: Bacteremia and fungemia complicating neoplastic disease. A study of 364 cases. Am. J. Med. 62:731–742, 1977.

Skultety, F. M.: Cryptococcic granuloma of the dorsal spinal cord. A case report. Neurology 11:1066–1070, 1961.

Smith, C. E.: Diagnosis of pulmonary coccidioidal infections. Calif. Med. 75:385–391, 1951.

Smith, C. E., Beard, R. R., Whiting, E. G., and Rosenberger, H. G.: Varieties of coccidioidal infection in relation to the epidemiology and control of the diseases. Am. J. Public Health 36:1394–1402, 1946.

Smith, C. E., Whiting, E. G., Baker, E. E., Rosenberger, H. G., Beard, R. R., and Saito, M. T.: The use of coccidioidin. Am. Rev. Tuberc. 57:330, 1948.

Smith, J. G., Jr., Harris, J. S., Conant, N. F., and Smith, D. T.: An epidemic of North American blastomycosis. J.A.M.A. 158:641–646, 1955.

Smith, J. W., and Utz, J. P.: Progressive disseminated histoplasmosis—a prospective study of 26 patients. Ann. Intern. Med. 76:557–565, 1972.

Smith, M. E., Brunham, D. K., and Black, M. B.: Cerebral mucormycosis. Report of a case. Arch. Path. 66:468–473, 1958.

Snow, R. M., and Dismukes, W. E.: Cryptococcal meningitis. Diagnostic value of cryptococcal antigen in cerebrospinal fluid. Arch. Intern. Med. 135:1155–1157, 1975.

Snyder, C. H., and White, R. S.: Successful treatment of histoplasma meningitis with amphotericin B. A case report. J. Pediat. 58:554–558, 1961.

Spicer, C., Hiatt, W. O., and Kessel, J. F.: Candida albicans and Cryptococcus neoformans occurring as infective agents in an eight-year-old boy. J. Pediat. 33:761–769, 1948.

Sprofkin, B. E., Shapiro, J. L., and Lux, J. J.: Histoplasmosis of the central nervous system. A case report of histoplasma meningitis. J. Neuropath. Exp. Neurol. 14:288–296, 1955.

Steele, R. W., Sieger, B. E., McNitt, T. R., Gentry, L. O.,

and Moore, W. L., Jr.: Therapy for disseminated coccidioidomycosis with transfer factor from a related donor. Am. J. Med. 61:283–286, 1976.

Steer, P. L., Marks, M. I., Klite, P. D., and Eickhoff, T. C.: 5-fluorocytosine: An oral antifungal compound. Ann. Intern. Med. 76:15–22, 1972.

Stevens, D. A., Levine, H. B., and Deresinski, S. C.: Miconazole in coccidioidomycosis. II. Therapeutic and pharmacologic studies in man. Am. J. Med. 60:191–202, 1976.

Stevens, H.: Actinomycosis of nervous system. Neurology 3:761–772, 1953.

Stites, D. P., and Glezen, W. P.: Pulmonary nocardiosis in childhood. A case report. Am. J. Dis. Child. 114:101–105, 1967.

Storts, B. P.: Coccidioidal granuloma simulating brain tumor in child of four years. J.A.M.A. 112:1334–1335, 1935.

Strelling, M. K., Rhaney, K., Simmons, D. A. R., and Thomson, J.: Fatal acute pulmonary aspergillosis in two children of one family. Arch. Dis. Childh. 41:34–43, 1966.

Sunderland, W. A., Campbell, R. A., and Edwards, M. J.: Pulmonary alveolar proteinosis and pulmonary cryptococcosis in an adolescent boy. J. Pediat. 80:450–456, 1972.

Sung, J. P., Campbell, G. D., and Grendahl, J. G.: Miconazole therapy for fungal meningitis. Arch. Neurol. 35:443–447, 1978.

Supena, R., Karlin, D., Strate, R., and Cramer, P. G.: Pulmonary alveolar proteinosis and Nocardia brain abscess. Report of a case. Arch. Neurol. 30:266–268, 1974.

Symmers, W. S. C.: A case of cerebral chromoblastomycosis (cladosporiosis) occurring in Britain as a complication of polyarteritis treated with cortisone. Brain 83:37–51, 1960.

Tarozzi, G.: Ricerche anatome-patologiche, bacteriologiche, e sperimentali spora un caso di actinomicosi del piede. Arch. Sci. Med. 33:553–632, 1909.

Tay, C. H., Chew, W. L. S., and Lim, L. C. Y.: Cryptococcal meningitis: Its apparent increased incidence in the Far East. Brain 95:825–832, 1972.

Teel, K. W., Yow, M. D., and Williams, T. W., Jr.: A localized outbreak of coccidioidomycosis in southern Texas. J. Pediat. 77:65–73, 1970.

Tong, J. L., Valentine, E. H., Durrance, J. R., Wilson, G. M., and Fischer, D. A.: Pulmonary infection with Allescheria boydii. Report of a fatal case. Am. Rev. Tuberc. 78:604–609, 1958.

Tosh, F. E., Hammerman, K. J., Weeks, R. J., and Sarosi, G. A.: A common source epidemic of North American blastomycosis. Am. Rev. Resp. Dis. 109:525–529, 1974.

Townsend, T. E., and McKey, R. W.: Coccidioidomycosis in infants. Am. J. Dis. Child. 86:51–53, 1953.

Tsai, C. Y., Lü, Y. C., Wang, L–T., Hsu, T. L., and Sung, J–L.: Systemic chromoblastomycosis due to Hormodendrum dermatitidis (Kano) Conant. Report of the first case in Taiwan. Am. J. Clin. Path. 46:103–114, 1966.

Turner, D. J., and Wadlington, W. B.: Blastomycosis in childhood: Treatment with amphotericin B and a review of the literature. J. Pediat. 75:708–717, 1969.

Tynes, B., Mason, K. N., Jennings, A. E., and Bennett, J. E.: Variant forms of pulmonary cryptococcosis. Ann. Intern. Med. 69:1117–1125, 1968.

Tynes, B. S., Crutcher, J. C., and Utz, J. P.: Histoplasma meningitis. Ann. Intern. Med. 59:615–621, 1963.

Utz, J. P., Bennett, J. E., Brandriss, M. W., Butler, W. T., and Hill, G. J.: Amphotericin B toxicity. Ann. Intern. Med. 61:334–354, 1964.

Utz, J. P., Garriques, I. L., Sande, M. A., Warner, J. F., Mandell, G. L., McGehee, R. F., Duma, R. J., and Shadomy, S.: Therapy of cryptococcosis with a combination of flucytosine and amphotericin B. J. Infect. Dis. 132:368–373, 1975.

Valdivieso, M., Luna, M., Body, G. P., Rodriquez, V., and Gröschel, D.: Fungemia due to Torulopsis glabrata in the compromised host. Cancer 38:1750–1756, 1976.

Van Cutsem, J. M., and Thienpont, D.: Miconazole, a broad-spectrum antimycotic agent and antibacterial activity. Chemotherapy 17:392–404, 1972.

Vandevelde, A. G., Mauceri, A. A., and Johnson, J. E., III: 5-fluorocytosine in the treatment of mycotic infections. Ann. Intern. Med. 77:43–51, 1972.

Vanek, J., and Schwarz, J.: The gamut of histoplasmosis. Am. J. Med. 50:89–104, 1971.

Vijayan, N., Bhatt, G. P., and Dreyfus, P. M.: Intraventricular cryptococcal granuloma. A case report with review of the literature. Neurology 21:728–734, 1971.

Waisbren, B. A., and Ullrich, D.: An isolated blastomycetoma of the posterior cranial fossa treated successfully with surgery and amphotericin B. Am. J. Med. 32:621–624, 1962.

Walker, D. H., Adamec, T., and Krigman, M.: Disseminated petriellidosis (allescheriosis). Arch. Path. Lab. Med. 102:158–160, 1978.

Wallace, R. J., Jr., Septimus, E. J., Musher, D. M., and Martin, R. R.: Disk diffusion susceptibility testing of *Nocardia* species. J. Infect. Dis. 135:568–576, 1977.

Ward, J. I., Weeks, M., Allen, D., Hutcheson, R. H., Jr., Anderson, R., Fraser, D. W., Kaufman, L., Ajello, L., and Spickard, A.: Acute histoplasmosis: Clinical, epidemiologic and serologic findings of an outbreak associated with exposure to a fallen tree. Am. J. Med. 66:587–595, 1979.

Warr, W., Bates, J. H., and Stone, A.: The spectrum of pulmonary cryptococcosis. Ann. Intern. Med. 69:1109–1116, 1968.

Watson, J. I., Mandl, M. A. J., and Rose, B.: Disseminated histoplasmosis occurring in association with systemic lupus erythematosus. Canad. Med. Assoc. J. 99:958–962, 1968.

Weese, W. C., and Smith, I. M.: A study of 57 cases of actinomycosis over a 36-year-period. A diagnostic 'failure' with good prognosis after treatment. Arch. Intern. Med. 135:1562–1568, 1975.

Welsh, J. D., Rhoades, E. R., and Jaques, W.: Disseminated nocardiosis involving the spinal cord. Arch. Intern. Med. 108:73–79, 1961.

Werner, S. B., Pappagianis, D., Heindl, I., and Mickel, A.: An epidemic of coccidioidomycosis among archeology students in northern California. New Eng. J. Med. 286:507–512, 1972.

White, H. H., and Fritzlen, T. J.: Cerebral granuloma caused by Histoplasma capsulatum. J. Neurosurg. 19:260–263, 1962.

Wilhelm, J. P., Siegel, B. A., and James, A. E., Jr.: Brain scanning and cisternography in cryptococcosis. Radiology 109:121–124, 1973.

Williams, A. H.: Aspergillus myocarditis. Am. J. Clin. Path. 61:247–256, 1974.

Wilson, D. E., Mann, J. J., Bennett, J. E., and Utz, J. P.: Clinical features of extracutaneous sporotrichosis. Medicine 46:265–279, 1967.

Wilson, R., and Feldman, S.: Toxicity of amphotericin B in children with cancer. Am. J. Dis. Child. 133:731–734, 1979.

Winston, D. J., Jordan, M. C., and Rhodes, J.: Allescheria boydii infections in the immunosuppressed host. Am. J. Med. 63:830–835, 1977.

Witorsch, P., and Utz, J. P.: North American blastomycosis: A study of 40 patients. Medicine 47:169–200, 1968.

Wolf, A., Benham, R., and Mount, L.: Maduromycotic meningitis. J. Neuropath. Exp. Neurol. 7:112–113, 1948.

Wuepper, K. D., and Fudenberg, H. H.: Moniliasis, 'autoimmune' polyendocrinopathy, and immunologic family study. Clin. Exp. Immunol. 2:71–82, 1967.

Young, L. S., Armstrong, D., Blevins, A., and Liberman, P.: Nocardia asteroides infection complicating neoplastic disease. Am. J. Med. 50:356–367, 1971.

Young, R. C., Bennett, J. E., Vogel, C. L., Carbone, P. P., and De Vita, V. T.: Aspergillosis. The spectrum of the disease in 98 patients. Medicine 49:147–173, 1970.

Zimmerman, L. E.: Candida and aspergillus endocarditis. Arch. Path. 50:591, 1950.

Chapter Twenty

PARASITIC INFECTIONS

Neurologic disease caused by parasites is relatively uncommon in this country compared to certain other parts of the world, but international air travel has enhanced the possibility of encountering anywhere diseases ordinarily geographically restricted. These disorders, in general, go hand in hand with poverty and poor living conditions, and, as a result, public health measures and public education in more highly developed countries keep most parasitic disorders at a minimum. Toxoplasmosis is the most significant parasitic illness causing brain disease in the United States. It is a cause of a severe, destructive encephalitis leading to mental retardation when acquired in utero. It has also become an important secondary invader in persons immunosuppressed after renal transplantation or in patients on chemotherapy or corticosteroid treatment for a variety of neoplastic diseases. Another protozoal infection that only rarely affects the brain is Entamoeba histolytica. Multiple brain abscesses can complicate abdominal visceral disease with this parasite (Hughes et al., Lombardo et al.). Of greater interest and importance is the recognition in recent years of primary amebic meningoencephalitis caused by members of the genus Naegleria or Acanthamoeba. Most reported cases thus far have affected children or young adults, have occurred after the patient was swimming, and probably are explained by entry of the organism into the brain via the olfactory bulbs. It is one of the few causes of nonbacterial meningoencephalitis in which the cerebrospinal fluid is purulent. The disease has been fatal in almost all recorded cases to date.

Roundworm (nematode) infestations giving rise to neurologic disease are uncommon but do occur with toxocariasis, trichinosis, Angiostrongylus cantonensis, and Strongyloides stercoralis, the latter in the presence of defects in cell-mediated immunity. Toxocara encephalitis occurs mainly in small children who acquire the infective ova from dogs that harbor the adult worm in the intestinal tract. The parasite is better known as a cause of visceral larva migrans, in which liver and lung disease predominate in association with hypereosinophilia.

An acute or subacute meningitic disorder characterized by an eosinophilic response in the CSF and referred to as "eosinophilic meningitis" is recognized in Hawaii, other Pacific islands, and parts of Southeast Asia (Char and Rosen, Rosen et al.). The illness occurs in both adults and children and most cases are caused by the nematode lungworm of rats, Angiostrongylus cantonensis. Humans are believed to acquire the infection by the consumption of raw or poorly cooked crustaceans, terrestrial snails, or slugs, which serve as the intermediate host (Kuberski and Wallace). The acute illness varies in severity, with most recovering without sequelae. Less often, the illness is more intense and can lead to death (Rosen et al.). A marked eosinophilic response in CSF is usually found, and, in some cases, Angiostrongylus cantonensis can be recovered from the CSF (Yii et al.).

Punyagupta and colleagues studied 484

cases of "eosinophilic meningitis" in Thailand and recognized two separate syndromes, each believed to be caused by a different parasite. One type was referred to as typical eosinophilic meningitis, manifested by headache, vomiting, meningeal signs, and seizures on occasion. The onset was usually acute and the majority recovered completely after a brief illness. Angiostrongylus cantonensis was believed to be the causative agent of this form of illness. The second variety was called eosinophilic myeloencephalitis and was associated with severe nerve root pain followed by paralysis of extremities and often with a sudden change in sensorium. Hemorrhagic or xanthochromic CSF characterized these cases, which the authors felt were caused by Gnathostoma spinigerum, a nematode, the adult worm being found in the stomach wall of dogs and cats in many Asian countries. Man is infected by eating raw or poorly cooked frogs or fish. The brain and spinal cord in such cases reveal multiple areas of hemorrhage and necrotic tracts resulting from the migration of the parasite through central nervous system tissue (Bunnag et al.).

Infection with the nematode Strongyloides stercoralis is usually benign and limited to the intestinal tract. Dissemination is possible in rare instances, especially in patients with impaired cell-mediated immunity. Hematogenous spread to the brain has been described in immunosuppressed adults, resulting in widespread microinfarcts and petechial hemorrhages, sometimes in concert with gram-negative bacterial meningitis (Meltzer et al.,

Table 20–1. Parasites that Cause Neurologic Disease in Man

1 Helminths
  A Nemathelminthes (roundworms)
    Toxocara canis, cati
    Trichinella spiralis
    Onchocerca volvulus
    Angiostrongylus cantonensis
    Strongyloides stercoralis
  B Platyhelminthes (tapeworms and flukes)
    Taenia solium (cysts)
    Taenia multiceps
    Echinococcus granulosus (hydatid cyst)
    Schistosoma
    Paragonimus westermani
2 Protozoa
    Toxoplasma gondii
    Naegleria (ameba)
    Acanthamoeba (ameba)
    Entamoeba histolytica
    Plasmodium falciparum, vivax
    Trypanosoma gambiense
    Trypanosoma rhodesiense

Neefe et al.). Thiabendazole is recommended for infection caused by this parasite, although the mortality rate in disseminated strongyloidiasis is high.

Neurologic disease in the form of intracranial cystic lesions can occur from the larval stage of three tapeworms. These include the hydatid cyst of Echinococcus granulosus, the cysticercus of Taenia solium, and the coenurus of Multiceps multiceps. Echinococcosis is contracted by ingestion of ova excreted by the infected dog. The embryo penetrates the intestinal wall and is transmitted by the blood stream to tissues where the echinococcus cyst eventually develops. The liver and the lungs are the most common infested site and the brain is only rarely implicated. Children are infected more often than adults, and in the brain, echinococcus cysts are usually large single lesions but may have secondary or daughter cysts (Griponissiotis). Hydatid cysts are usually parietal or occipital in location and give rise to a progressive syndrome resembling a cerebral neoplasm in the same region. The brain is at greater risk with cysticercosis, in which either single or multiple cystic lesions can occur in the cerebrum, cerebellum, or within the ventricular system. The most characteristic manifestation of intracranial cysticercosis is the formation of a racemose cysticercus within the fourth ventricle, giving rise to obstructive hydrocephalus and signs of cerebellar dysfunction. Coenurosis of the brain is the least common of the group and has only rarely been reported in humans. The intracranial cyst in this disease is usually solitary and shows a predilection for the CSF pathways and especially the posterior fossa. The most striking histologic difference between the coenurus and the cysticercus is the presence of multiple scolices in the former and a single scolex in the latter.

Parasitic diseases in other parts of the world that can be associated with neurologic complications include paragonimiasis, malaria, schistosomiasis, and trypanosomiasis. Paragonimiasis is a common pulmonary disease in the Far East but dissemination to the cerebrum is not infrequent. The cystic lesions produce seizures and other signs of focal, cerebral dysfunction and are eventually identifiable by roentgenographic examination because of their tendency to calcify. With malaria and schistosomiasis, the development of neurologic involvement is more common in persons previously unimmune to the disease. Thus, in addition to children, persons most susceptible are those foreign to the endemic area but becoming exposed during temporary residence there.

HELMINTH INFECTIONS

Toxocariasis (Visceral Larva Migrans)

Toxocariasis is a worldwide parasitic infection caused by the larval stage of the common dog roundworm, Toxocara canis, and to a much less extent, by the larval form of Toxocara cati, the cat ascarid. The adult nematode is 7 to 12 centimeters in length and is harbored in the intestine of dogs and cats where eggs are produced and excreted in stools. After a brief period of embryonation, the ovum contains an infective larva. When the eggs are subsequently ingested by other dogs or cats, they hatch in the intestine of the animal and larvae burrow into the intestinal wall, reaching portal venous blood and migrating to the liver and the lung. Further migration up the bronchial tree to the trachea is followed by re-entry into the intestinal tract. A common method of infection in dogs is prenatal transmission to the fetus, resulting in a much higher percentage of intestinal infection in puppies than in older dogs. For this reason, puppies create a greater potential source of infection to children than do older canines.

When Toxocara canis ova are swallowed by man, the larvae emerge from the eggs within the intestine, penetrate the bowel wall, and pass via portal blood to the liver and lungs and sometimes to other organs. The parasites are poorly adapted to the human host, however, and within man they do not complete their life cycle beyond the second larval stage. In the larval stage, they can survive for many months within tissue, causing granulomatous lesions in one or many organs. Because of the anomalous life cycle within man, adult worms do not occur within the human intestine and thus ova are not excreted in the stool.

Toxocara canis larvae were first identified in tissues of a child with visceral larva migrans by Beaver et al. in 1952. The disease has become recognized as one affecting children most commonly between one and six years of age. It is more common in boys than girls, and, in most reported cases, either intimate contact with dogs or a history of pica has been described. Children who acquire toxocara ova by eating dirt or other foreign materials are also susceptible to a variety of additional problems, such as other parasitic disorders or lead poisoning (Moore).

Symptoms and signs in the child with toxocariasis largely result from involvement of the liver and lungs, which are the most commonly affected organs (Snyder). Less often, the organism extends to the eye, giving rise to unilateral ocular disease of one type or another. Invasion of the brain with nematodes of this type has been described on only a few occasions. Cutaneous and skeletal lesions (Snyder), granulomatous disease of the urinary bladder (Perlmutter et al.), and myocardial infestation (Woodruff) are additional rare manifestations. Of unknown frequency is the occurrence of toxocara infection in children manifested only by a persistent eosinophilia (Zinkham).

Common symptoms and signs of the disease include lassitude, anorexia, poor weight gain, and intermittent fever. Cough or wheezing is frequent, and in exceptional cases the pulmonary inflammatory response is severe, producing respiratory distress of life-threatening proportion (Beshear and Hendley). Hepatomegaly is the most common physical sign and is associated with splenic enlargement in some patients.

A significant degree of anemia is usual in children with toxocara infection, as is peripheral leukocytosis. Eosinophilia is the most constant laboratory finding, although it is likely to be absent in children with toxocara ocular disease without significant liver involvement. Eosinophils account for at least 30 percent of the white blood cells in children with visceral larva migrans, and in some cases will reach 90 percent. Hyperglobulinemia is present in more severe cases, mainly owing to increase in the gamma globulin content. Pulmonary infiltrations identified on chest x-ray may be sparse or extensive and usually correlate with the severity of the respiratory symptoms. The diffuse, bilateral mottling of both lungs in severe cases is roentgenographically similar to that of miliary tuberculosis.

Visceral larva migrans is usually a transient and benign disease from which most children recover within a few weeks after onset. Blood eosinophilia will persist in some cases for weeks or even months after other abnormalities have resolved. Death is very infrequent and lasting sequelae are usually seen only in children with ocular involvement. The possibility that epilepsy may result from dissemination to the brain in the acute stage has been mentioned but remains speculative (Huntley et al., Woodruff).

During migration of toxocara larvae through liver, lung, and other tissues, the tracts of their passage are marked by inflammatory lesions. When migration terminates and the nematode dies, the tissue involved responds by the formation of focal granulomas within which the organism is encased. Surrounding the parasites, the cellular infiltrate includes lymphocytes and eosinophils as well as a variable number of foreign body giant cells (Fig. 20–1).

Ocular and Neurologic Involvement

Intraocular nematode infestation gained attention in 1950 when Wilder found larvae in sections of eyes removed from children with retinal masses believed preoperatively to be retinoblastomas. Many childhood cases of ocular involvement with Toxocara canis have subsequently been described and the eye is now recognized to be the most frequently affected site, other than the liver and lungs. In the majority of published cases, invasion of the eye with toxocara has occurred without the typical findings of visceral larva migrans or the characteristic blood changes (Brown). In addition, children with ocular disease due to this parasite are usually somewhat older than those with symptoms and signs of abdominal visceral involvement (Zinkham). Only one eye is affected in most cases, and the usual initial symptoms are failing vision and strabismus.

The inflammatory process with intraocular toxocara includes a diffuse endophthalmitis

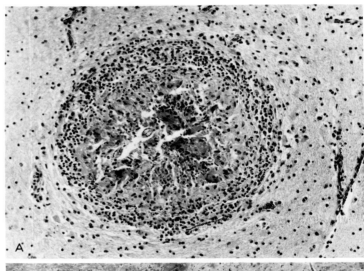

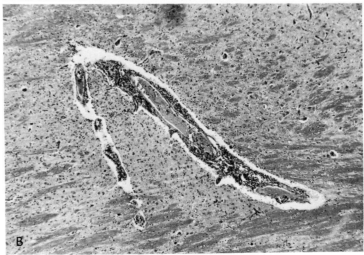

Figure 20–1. Toxocariasis. *A,* Granuloma in the cerebral white matter. *Toxocara canis* larvae are present in the center of the lesion. *B,* Perivascular inflammatory reaction in a child with toxocara encephalitis. (Courtesy of Dr. Sidney Schochet, Oklahoma City, Oklahoma; Neurology, 17: 227–229, 1967.)

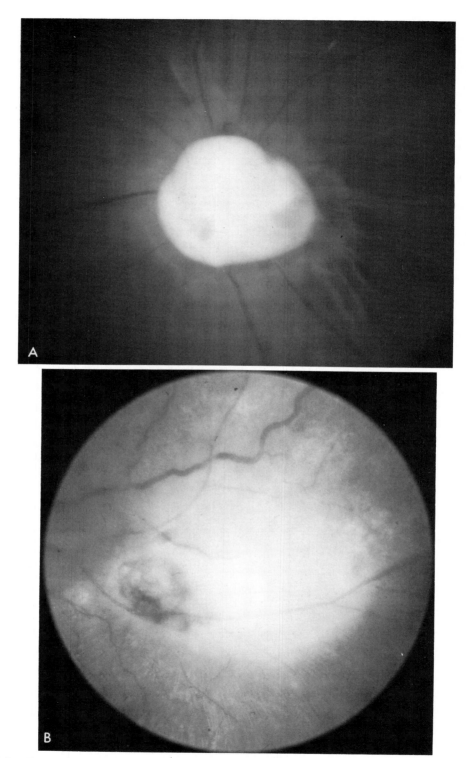

Figure 20-2.   Toxocariasis, ocular. *A*, Granulomatous mass with a white, elevated appearance which obscures the optic disc. The inflammatory lesion contains the nematode, *Toxocara canis. B*, Chronic granuloma in the macular region.

or focal lesions in the form of peridiscal or macular granulomas (Wilkinson and Welch) (Fig. 20–2). More peripheral retinal inflammatory masses are occasionally seen, and optic neuritis less often is present (Bird et al.). Children with diffuse nematode endophthalmitis have extensive unilateral intraocular inflammation with profound visual loss, vitreous inflammation, and retinal detachment. Visual disturbance also accompanies posterior pole granulomas, which usually present as a pale, elevated mass that is one or two disc diameters in size.

Symptomatic neurologic disease caused by toxocara is rare and only a few cases have been reported in which parasites have been found in the brain (Beautyman and Woolf, Moore, Schochet). Neurologic disturbances such as convulsions, lethargy, or neck stiffness have been encountered in other children with severe abdominal visceral involvement, but the pathogenesis in cases with survival is obscure (Huntley et al.). Anderson et al. reported an 18-month-old child with serologic evidence of acute toxocara infection in whom there was a rapidly progressive spastic hemiparesis. Laboratory findings included a blood eosinophilia as well as an eosinophilic pleocytosis in the CSF. Of the few cases in which toxocara have been observed in brain tissue, the cause of death was usually attributable to another disease (Moore, Beautyman and Woolf). For this reason, the significance of toxocara larvae within the brain is difficult to assess. In the case described by Schochet, the affected child rapidly became comatose and had recurrent convulsions. The cerebrospinal fluid revealed a modest lymphocytic pleocytosis, and at necropsy multiple cerebral granulomas were seen, one of which contained toxocara larvae. No other cause for the neurologic manifestations was found and toxocara encephalitis was assumed to be the primary factor causing death.

Diagnosis and Treatment

Diagnosis of visceral larva migrans due to Toxocara canis or cati should be clinically suspected in the young child with hepatomegaly associated with hypereosinophilia and hyperglobulinemia. Elevated serum titers of anti-A and anti-B isohemagglutinins add further supporting evidence of a parasitic infection. Liver biopsy by the open technique can either support or confirm the diagnosis, although identification of nematode larvae has been found to be very difficult on biopsy material.

Sections will reveal the inflammatory, granulomatous lesions left following the migration of the parasite through tissue, but a large sample and a diligent search may be required to find the larval organism itself.

The intradermal skin test using toxocara antigen is helpful (Woodruff et al. 1964), although false positive reactions can occur in persons with other helminthic infections (Woodruff 1970). Serologic techniques for the diagnosis of visceral larva migrans caused by toxocara include the indirect hemagglutination test, bentonite flocculation test, enzyme-linked immunosorbent assay, and double diffusion in agar (Glickman et al., Heiner and Kevy). Of the various methods, the enzyme-linked immunosorbent assay using a larval antigen has been judged to be the most sensitive test and is the one of choice (Glickman et al.).

The above laboratory abnormalities and diagnostic methods are applicable to the child with abdominal visceral disease due to toxocara but are not reliable for most cases with intraocular toxocariasis. These patients do not usually have evidence of widespread tissue involvement and the laboratory findings are not helpful. Diagnosis rests on age of the patient, history of exposure to puppies or dogs, and the ophthalmologic findings of endophthalmitis or a posterior pole granuloma. Unless the eye is surgically removed, diagnosis usually remains presumptive.

Treatment of visceral larva migrans in the past was with diethylcarbamazine and corticosteroids. Improvement with such medications was noted by some authors (Snyder), although the degree of effectiveness has been controversial. Thiabendazole has been recommended more recently but it, too, remains to be proved in the treatment of toxocariasis (Nelson et al., Aur et al.). The use of the drug in conjunction with corticosteroids is recommended for moderate or severe illness due to toxocara, especially with respiratory or myocardial involvement. Both drugs have been recommended for ocular toxocara infection, but when severe ocular damage has occurred, enucleation may be necessary. The recommended dose of thiabendazole is 50 mg. per kilogram per day given orally in three divided doses.

Preventive measures to curtail infections in children depend upon the termination of pica and proper care of household pets to eliminate intestinal parasitic infestation. Advice about these measures should be provided to the family whenever one child with toxocara infection is identified so that other siblings will not likewise become infected.

Trichinosis

Trichinoisis is the most prevalent helminthic infestation of man, but the overwhelming majority of infected persons are asymptomatically parasitized. In the United States, there has been a gradual decline in reported cases since 1947, a tendency paralleled by the decrease in swine trichinosis during the same period. The decline in trichinosis is attributed to laws enacted in 1952 prohibiting the feeding of raw garbage to hogs, as well as increased public awareness of the hazard of eating uncooked or poorly cooked pork (Fig. 20–3). Federal inspection of pork to be used for domestic consumption does not include examination for Trichinella spiralis larvae. Of 6200 human cases reported from 1947 to 1972, the mortality rate was 2 percent (Annual Summary, 1972). It is important to note that those reported represent symptomatic cases, thus allowing their identification. Countless more individuals acquire the parasite with minimal or no symptoms. Fatality in this large group would be expected to be nonexistent. In view of the importance of cellular immunity in the host defense against nematode infections, it is presumed that trichinosis might be unusually severe in the immunosuppressed patient (Jacobson and Jacobson).

The causative organism is Trichinella spiralis, which differs from other roundworms in that its life cycle is devoid of a free-living existence at any stage. An animal, or man, acts as both the intermediate and final host, harboring the adult nematode temporarily and the larvae for much longer periods. To complete the life cycle, flesh infected with the encysted larvae must be eaten by another host. The pig is the best-known host, in addition to being the commonest source of infection for man, but other carnivorous animals also may be infected. Pigs become infected by consumption of uncooked flesh in garbage or by feeding on meat scraps from slaughterhouses or other sources.

Man acquires the parasite by eating uncooked or poorly cooked pork or other larvae-containing flesh. For this reason, infants and young children are infrequently infected as compared to older children and adults. The encysted larvae that are ingested pass into the small intestine where, within a few

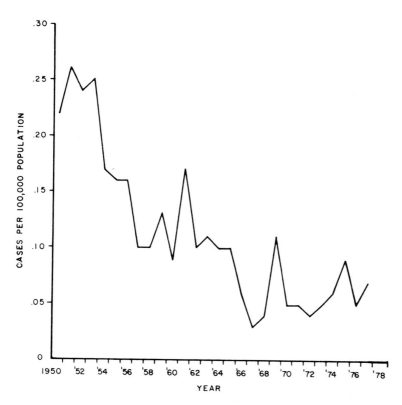

Figure 20–3. Trichinosis. Reported cases per 100,000 population by year in United States, 1950–1977. (From: Morbidity and Mortality Weekly Report, Annual Summary, 1977, Volume 26, No. 53, Sept. 1978.)

hours, the capsule is dissolved, leaving them free to invade the intestinal mucosa. Sexual maturation occurs rapidly, mating follows, and the male eventually dies and is eliminated. The female survives and remains burrowed in the intestinal wall where, five to seven days later, she begins to deposit larvae into the mucosa. Larval production continues for up to six weeks, at which time the adult female nematode also dies and is eliminated from the intestinal tract. The larvae penetrate the intestinal lymphatics and lymph nodes, are transmitted to the thoracic duct, and enter the blood stream, where they become widely disseminated throughout the body but with an obvious preference for striated muscle tissue. Myocardial infiltration can occur, but the heart somehow seems to provide a poor shelter for larvae and encystment rarely occurs. The brain also can be affected but symptomatic involvement is rarely seen. Heaviest muscle infiltration occurs in the diaphragm and intercostal muscles, in addition to the masseter, extraocular, biceps, and gastrocnemius muscles. Encapsulation of the larvae within muscle begins within two to three weeks and is completed by three months. Mineralization of the encysted larvae begins several months later. The time sequences of the changes in muscle allow certain estimates as to age of the infestation, especially with biopsy material. If encapsulation has not occurred, parasitization in muscle can be dated to less than four or five weeks. If encapsulated larvae are non-calcified, infection has occurred within the previous four to six months.

Clinical Manifestations

The clinical manifestations of trichinosis in man have been divided into three phases corresponding to (1) intestinal invasion by the adult parasite, (2) larval migration and tissue invasion, and (3) larval encystment in tissues, particularly muscle. The incubation period between consumption of the infected meat and onset of gastroenteritis is between one and two weeks in most cases. Symptoms in the initial stage of intestinal invasion by the nematode can be totally absent or manifested by abdominal pain, vomiting, or diarrhea, which lasts from one to four days. The classic symptoms and signs of trichinosis occur during the second stage of larval migration, which begins soon after the manifestations of gastrointestinal irritation. The severity of the disease varies considerably, depending in part on the magnitude of the infecting dose. In the majority of cases, the infection is light and gives rise to no symptoms or only very mild complaints. Rarely, the illness is overwhelming and leads to a fatal outcome. Symptoms during the stage of larval migration persist from one to four weeks and are characterized by fever, periorbital and facial edema, headache, muscle tenderness, pain, and weakness. In unusually heavy infestations, the myopathic process can be severe, with exquisite tenderness and profound, generalized weakness (Davis et al.). Local pain on extraocular movement is particularly troublesome to some patients. Conjunctivitis, cutaneous eruptions, and subungual splinter hemorrhages are additional possible findings.

Many of the symptoms and signs observed during the second phase of the disease are explained on the basis of the host's allergic tissue reaction to the migrating larvae. Disturbance of myocardial function is not uncommon at this time and is manifested by electrocardiographic changes. The most frequently encountered abnormalities are T-wave changes or low voltage QRS complexes. It has been estimated that electrocardiographic abnormalities have occurred in approximately 20 percent of published cases of trichinosis (Metzler et al.); however, such changes are temporary and normal patterns are expected within a few weeks. Reports of hepatic involvement in trichinosis are rare (Kennedy and Rege). Cases that have been described exhibited hepatomegaly and liver function derangements but eventual healing occurred in most.

Within two to four weeks after the beginning of systemic signs, there is a gradual diminution of soft tissue swelling and muscle pain. Neurologic signs can persist or appear for the first time at this stage, but in most patients gradual recovery ensues.

Eosinophilia ranging from 10 to 40 percent is present in most patients, but the degree does not correlate well with the severity of the infection. The total white blood cell count is variable, being normal in some and modestly elevated in other cases. The erythrocyte sedimentation rate is normal or even low in many cases, a point of diagnostic value in differentiation of trichinosis from dermatomyositis or periarteritis nodosa. In severe cases, hypoalbuminemia is found, although the mechanism causing it is unclear (Rachon et al.). Reduction in serum albumin may contribute to peripheral edema but does not account for the periorbital and facial swelling, which is more likely a hypersensitivity vascular response to the migrating and infiltrating larvae. Serum creatine phosphokinase is usually elevated in patients with symptoms of muscle involvement (Bouree et al., Doege et al.).

Central Nervous System Manifestations

Central nervous system involvement has been well documented in certain cases of trichinosis (Dalessio and Wolff, Gray et al., Kennedy and Rege, Kramer and Aita, Perot et al.), although the incidence and the pathogenesis of this complication have not been clarified. Headache and neck pain are frequent symptoms in the first week of the illness, but distinct and significant signs of cerebral disease are infrequent. Neurologic manifestations during the first week of the symptomatic phase are those of a meningoencephalitis, with headache, lethargy, confusion, or other behavioral abnormalities. When focal neurologic signs occur, they usually make their appearance between two and four weeks after the onset of the systemic illness. Virtually any area of the brain can be implicated, giving rise to many possible types of deficits, either singly or in combination. Localized convulsions, hemiparesis, dysphasia, or cerebellar disturbances indicate focal involvement and are usually accompanied by other clinical or electroencephalographic evidence of more diffuse cerebral dysfunction. The cerebrospinal fluid in patients with trichinosis encephalitis can be entirely normal, or can reveal a modest lymphocytic pleocytosis, increased protein content, or elevated pressure. In some cases, larvae have been identified in the cerebrospinal fluid (Evers).

Whether the inflammatory response to disseminated larvae or an associated allergic reaction to the parasite accounts for neurologic signs is still unestablished. The allergic concept has received support from reported cases showing beneficial response to corticosteroid therapy. It is likely, however, that both factors are important in regard to pathogenesis. The neuropathology includes scattered punctate hemorrhages, cerebral edema, and granulomatous nodules, some of which contain larvae. Perivascular lymphocytic infiltration can be found in meninges as well as within the brain.

Diagnosis and Treatment

Clinical diagnosis of trichinosis should be suspected in a patient with an acute myositis with eosinophilia, especially when more than one member of a family or group is affected and when there is a history of consumption of raw or poorly cooked pork. The intradermal skin test using antigen prepared from trichinella larvae is of some diagnostic value, although both false negative and false positive results have been described. A positive test is characterized by a wheal greater than 5 millimeters in diameter surrounded by a zone of erythema. The skin test does not become positive until two to four weeks after onset of systemic symptoms and then remains positive for several years. Other available diagnostic procedures include the complement fixation test, the precipitin test, and the bentonite flocculation test, none of which become positive until the third or fourth week of the illness. These tests are not entirely reliable since false positives may occur. Search for ova and parasites in the stool is unrewarding in this disease, but in cases with central nervous system involvement, the cerebrospinal fluid should be examined for larvae.

Muscle biopsy is a valuable diagnostic method, which is most helpful if done after the third week of the illness and if the biopsy is obtained from the most painful accessible muscle. Identification of noncalcified encapsulated larvae surrounded by inflammatory cells provides evidence of recent infection. In some cases, larvae cannot be found but one sees areas of mononuclear cell infiltration associated with vasculitis. The latter can be viewed as consistent with the diagnosis of trichinosis but not confirmatory, and confirmation would depend on other tests.

Treatment of mildly affected patients with trichinosis is probably not necessary except for symptomatic measures such as antipyretics and analgesics. For more severe infections, thiabendazole is recommended in an oral dosage of 50 mg. per kilogram per day (Stone et al.). Experience has suggested beneficial effects from this drug. Because of the possibility of toxic effects, its use should be restricted to patients with significant signs of disease. Evidence of cerebral involvement is an indication for corticosteroid therapy, initially in high dosage. Numerous authors have commented on improvement from corticosteroid therapy, at times of dramatic proportions (Davis et al., Dalessio and Wolff, Perot et al.). Treatment of severe infestations of Trichinella spiralis with thiabendazole can result in acute, massive dissolution of larvae, producing a Herxheimer reaction (Campbell and Blair). This may be prevented by the concomitant use of corticosteroids.

Cysticercosis

Cysticercosis is caused by Cysticercus cellulosae, the larval form of the pork tapeworm, Taenia solium. Man is the only definitive host, harboring the adult tapeworm in the upper part of the small intestine. Proglottids laden with eggs are periodically eliminated in feces and subsequently consumed by the intermediate host, the hog. Within the gut of the hog, ova become larval forms which penetrate the intestinal wall, gaining entrance to lymphatics and veins, thus leading to dissemination to muscles and other organs. The human becomes infected by ingestion of uncooked, infected pork flesh. The consumed cysticercus with its evaginated scolex attaches to the jejunal mucosa and develops into the adult worm in the intestine of man, thus completing the life cycle.

The above cycle accounts for human intestinal infestation with the adult tapeworm, but acquisition of the larval form which produces cysticercosis is by a different method. This type of infection is acquired by ingestion of Taenia solium eggs in food or water contaminated by human feces. The ova can also be acquired by oral transmission by the unclean hands of a carrier of the adult tapeworm. Finally, internal autoinfection is possible by regurgitation of eggs from the jejunum into the stomach by reverse peristalsis. The ingested ova hatch into larval forms called oncospheres, which penetrate the intestinal wall, gain entrance to lymphatics and blood vessels, and become disseminated to muscle and possibly other tissues. Here, they become the mature cysticercus, an oval translucent cyst with a single scolex bearing four suckers. Complete maturation into the cysticercus occurs in 10 to 12 weeks, the size and structure of the cystic structure being determined somewhat by the type of tissue it has invaded. In man, cysticerci show a preference for striated muscle but can also develop in brain, ocular structures, liver, lung, heart, and subcutaneous tissues.

Taenia solium infection, and thus cysticercosis, is relatively rare in the United States, largely because hogs have limited access to human excreta. Infection with this parasite is common, however, in Mexico, South America, India, and certain European countries such as Poland. It has been stated that cerebral cysticercosis has been found in 2.6 to 3.6 percent of all autopsies in Mexico (Lombardo and Mateos). Cysticercosis is occasionally encountered in certain border states, such as Texas and California, and can be seen elsewhere because of the ease of world-wide travel.

Clinical Manifestations

During the stage of dissemination and invasion, there are usually no symptoms or only mild muscle pain. Striated muscle is the most commonly affected site where hundreds of cysticerci may develop. As cysts enlarge in muscle and subcutaneous tissue, their presence in some cases is reflected by multiple non-tender nodules of variable size. An unusual response to the presence of cysts in muscle is a pseudohypertrophic myopathy manifested by progressive muscle weakness and generalized muscular enlargement (Jacob and Mathew, Sawhney et al.). Subcutaneous and muscular cystic lesions may eventually calcify and be visualized roentgenographically.

The brain is the next most predisposed site and can harbor one or many parasitic cysts. Symptoms or signs of cerebral involvement do not usually occur until the death of the parasite evokes an inflammatory response. For this reason, clinical neurologic signs are usually delayed for five to 20 years after the infection is acquired. Ocular involvement with cysticercosis can result from cyst formation within extraocular muscles or within the orbit itself (Reddy and Satyendran). Orbital lesions have been found in the retina or vitreous, and less often in the anterior ocular segment.

Intracranial infestation is the most serious component of the disease, although it is possible for cysts to be present in the brain without associated symptoms. In the cerebral hemispheres, the cysticercus shows preference for gray matter localization (Fig. 20–4). Cysts may also be located in the brain stem, cerebellum or meninges, and, much less often, within the intraspinal canal. In addition, they can establish themselves within the ventricular system or in the cerebellopontine

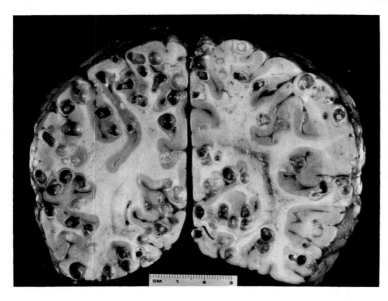

Figure 20–4. Cerebral cysticercosis. Very extensive widespread cystic involvement. Note the predilection for the disease to be localized to the cortex. This case is atypical because of the severity of the process.

angle. The size and histologic structure of the cysticercus depends to considerable degree on its intracranial location (Trelles). Within the brain parenchyma, the cysticercus stimulates an inflammatory response, which leads to the formation of a connective tissue membrane that encapsulates and limits the size of the lesion. Adjacent blood vessels are affected by the inflammatory reaction, with endothelial proliferation causing narrowing or frank occlusion of the involved vessels.

As opposed to cystic lesions in the brain parenchyma, the cysticercus within the ventricular system is able to enlarge and proliferate, giving rise to a racemose cyst, one with projections and loculations. Bickerstaff et al. have suggested that the unchecked growth of the intraventricular cyst is explained by the relative absence of an inflammatory response, which elsewhere is the stimulus for encapsulation. The racemose cysticercus is a large, thin-walled, translucent, and multilocular structure whose shape is adapted to the area of the ventricular system it occupies. Secondary reactions to the presence of intracranial cysticerci are ependymitis and chronic leptomeningitis of variable degree (Kuper et al.) (Fig. 20–5).

Symptoms and signs produced by intracranial cysticercosis are dependent on the size, number, and location of the lesions. The single most common clinical expression of cerebral cysticercosis is recurrent seizures, often focal in type, and sometimes followed by transient postictal paralysis. The clinical manifestations in certain instances can be-

come quite complex because obstruction from posterior fossa lesions may occur in concert with supratentorial signs owing to multiple cysts in the cerebral hemispheres (Bickerstaff et al., Kuper et al., Lombardo and Mateos). In addition, brain stem dysfunction can coexist with signs of ventricular obstruction or with signs of recurrent and chronic meningitis (Tomiyasu et al.). Common features of cysticerci within the cerebrum include recurrent convulsions, progressive dementia in some patients, visual disturbances, and variable other localizing signs, depending on the site of the lesions. If basilar arachnoiditis develops, increased pressure signs will be engrafted upon the above-mentioned focal disturbances. The picture may become even more complex by the development of a cauda equina syndrome, manifested by pain, sensory loss, and lower motor neuron weakness in the lower extremities. Intraspinal cysticercosis with spinal cord involvement has only rarely been described. Most have been extramedullary lesions (Firemark) although intramedullary cord lesions have also been identified (Cabieses et al., Queiroz et al.).

In some patients, the outstanding features are those of a posterior fossa syndrome caused by a racemose cysticercus within the fourth ventricle. Headache, vomiting, papilledema, and ataxia are the cardinal features, but many patients have had a prior history of seizures or other cerebral signs before the posterior fossa localization becomes evident. In a number of cases with cysts of the fourth ventricle, intermittent attacks of obstructive hydrocephalus, sometimes with vertigo, are precipitated by abrupt movements of the head. Such attacks are known as Bruns syndrome since the description by Bruns in 1906.

The cerebrospinal fluid is abnormal in most patients with intracranial cysticercosis. Lymphocytic pleocytosis is the most constant abnormality and, in some patients, both lymphocytes and eosinophils are present. Cysticercosis is one of several parasitic diseases that can be associated with a striking CSF eosinophilic pleocytosis (Tasker and Plotkin). The protein content is raised to 50 to 100 mg. per 100 ml. and the glucose content is occasionally normal but more often is reduced to 20 to 40 mg. per 100 ml. Elevation of the blood eosinophil count is frequent but is not always found. Roentgenograms of the skull are normal in many cases but in others show evidence of increased intracranial pressure or irregular areas of calcification, which are believed to represent calcium deposition within the capsule and the scolex.

Diagnosis and Treatment

Clinical diagnosis of intracranial cysticercosis can frequently be made in parts of the world where the disease is prevalent. Elsewhere, the disease may not be suspected until the cysticercus is identified after surgery or at autopsy. When subcutaneous nodules are present, they provide an available source of the parasite for histologic examination. Also, multiple calcified soft tissue lesions seen on x-ray in a patient with a characteristic clinical syndrome provides support for the probable diagnosis. Clinical diagnosis should be suspected when the patient resides or has lived in an area known for the occurrence of the illness, has multifocal signs of intracranial disease, and with cerebrospinal fluid which shows a chronic lymphocytic pleocytosis with modest reduction in the glucose content. Serologic diagnosis is on the basis of a serum indirect hemagglutination test, which is available at the Center for Disease Control and a few other reference laboratories in this country. A cerebrospinal fluid complement fixation test has been developed. The reliability of this test has been supported by some workers (Nieto) but questioned by others because of overlapping reactivity with other cestode infestations, including coenurosis and echinococcus cysts of the brain (Hermos et al.). Cranial computed tomography is a valuable method of demonstration of the intracranial pathology in cysticercosis and for the illustration of the number and size of the cystic lesions (Latovitzki et al., Schultz and Ascherl). Cysts within the substance of the cerebrum are usually clearly demarcated from the adjacent brain and have a CSF density. They are not large in most instances and vary in number. A modest degree of contrast enhancement may be seen around the perimeter of the cystic lesion. Small intraventricular cysts can be missed by standard computed tomography and sometimes require metrizamide computed tomography for their demonstration.

The natural history of cysticercosis of the nervous system is quite variable and depends to some degree on the location and number of the cystic lesions. The disease may be characterized by exacerbations and remissions but can be terminated by sudden death. In patients with posterior fossa obstructive lesions, the course is one of progressive worsening unless altered by a surgical procedure. Treatment is generally unsatisfactory in that antihelminthic agents are of little value. Posterior fossa cysts can be attacked surgically but total removal is difficult. Contamination of the ventricular system with the contents of the cysticercus can produce an acute inflammatory response possibly leading to death. In some, increased pressure symptoms are controlled by shunt procedures but this also is of temporizing value only. Single cerebral parenchymal cysts can sometimes be successfully excised; however, multiple lesions dispersed throughout the brain cannot be dealt with surgically.

Echinococcosis (Hydatid Cyst)

Echinococcosis occurs throughout the world, with most cases reported from Australia, New Zealand, Argentina, Uruguay, Turkey, and Spain, all sheep-raising countries. The disease is not common in the United States, but is not to be disregarded since it can be seen in immigrants and among the American Indians in the Southwest. The disorder is also a problem of considerable magnitude among the aboriginal population of Alaska who have frequent and close contact with dogs (Wilson et al.), the most common definitive host. Echinococcus granulosus is a tape worm which, as an adult in the intestinal tract of the dog, measures less than one centimeter in length. The scolices of the

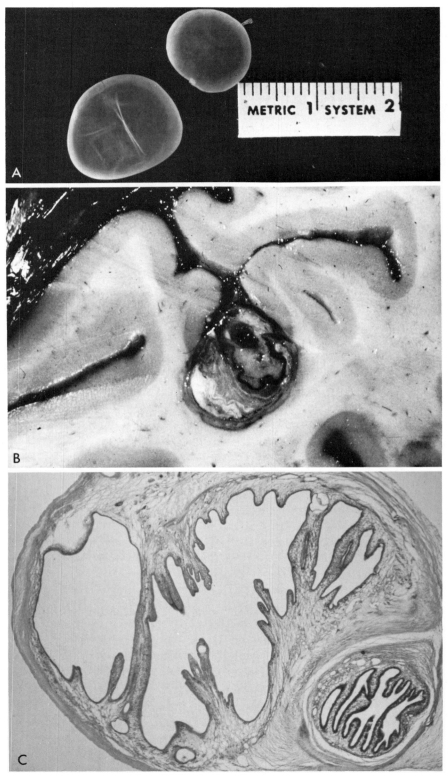

Figure 20–5. See legend on opposite page

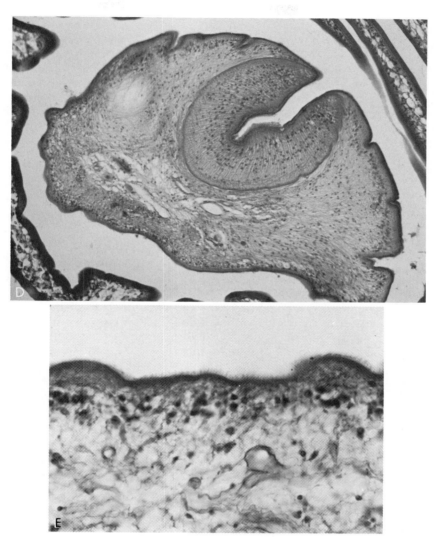

Figure 20–5. Cerebral cysticercosis. *A,* Two relatively small cysticerci removed from the lateral ventricle of a patient with the ventricular form of racemose cysticercosis. *B,* Coronal section of the brain with the parenchymatous form of cysticercosis. An inflammatory reaction surrounds the dead cysticercus. Such a reaction does not occur while the parasites are still viable. *C,* Cross-section through a viable cysticercus removed surgically from the ventricle of a child with hydrocephalus. There is no inflammation associated with this living organism (H&E, 70×). *D,* Section demonstrates the scolex of a viable cysticercus. The rostellum with its hooklets is not visible in this section (trichrome, 100×). *E,* Section illustrates the wall of a viable cysticercus demonstrating the typical 3 layers, with cilia over the dense cuticular layer. The middle nuclear layer and the inner parenchymatous layer are also clearly seen. The cilia are considered vital to the nutritional maintenance of the cysticercus and possibly for motility as well (H&E, 200×).

adult parasite attach to the dog's intestinal mucosa by hooks and suckers. Egg-laden segments are excreted in the feces, which are infective for man, sheep, cattle, and many other animals. Human infection occurs by direct contact with excreta of dogs or by consumption of uncooked foods contaminated with egg-bearing feces of dogs. Eggs hatch in the human duodenum, resulting in larvae which penetrate the intestinal wall. They then pass by a hematogenous route to the liver and lungs where most are filtered, accounting for the common occurrence of hydatid cyst formation in these two organs. Some successfully escape the filtering effect of the liver or lungs and are transmitted to other structures, including the brain, spleen, or other viscera.

Involvement of the brain has been estimated to occur in only 1 to 2 percent of all cases of echinococcosis, although 50 to 75 percent of all cases with cerebral hydatid cysts occur in children (Pearl et al.). The majority of intracranial hydatid cysts are large, single, subcortical lesions located in the parieto-occipital region and are oval or spherical in shape. Multiple cerebral cystic lesions are far less frequent and are more likely to occur by dissemination of scolices by ventricular cannulation of the cyst during ventriculography or by rupture of the cyst at the time of surgical removal. Spontaneous rupture of an intracardiac cyst can also result in multiple intracerebral lesions by direct embolization. The brain tends to accommodate the slowly enlarging mass quite well for a long period of time. Gradual displacement of brain tissue without invasion and with little inflammatory response allows the lesion to become remarkably large in most cases (Arana-Iniguez and Julian, Kaya et al.).

Clinical signs in children with cerebral hydatid cysts are usually chronic in duration, slowly progressive, and characterized by manifestations of increased intracranial pressure and a variety of signs of focal cerebral dysfunction, thus resembling slow-growing neoplastic lesions. Headache, vomiting, papilledema, and suture separation or asymmetrical head enlargement in young children represent evidence of long-standing intracranial hypertension secondary to the mass effect of the lesion. Hemiparesis, hemisensory defects, and focal seizures are localizing signs, and their presence depends on the site of the mass. Intraspinal cysts resulting in spinal cord compression are far less common than those within the head but have been described, extending from their primary site in the posterior mediastinum (Carrea et al., Rakower and Milwidsky).

Diagnosis

Cerebral echinococcus cyst is suspected in a child from an endemic region who is found to have a single, large intracerebral cystic lesion without a solid component. The presence of a peripheral blood eosinophilia is suggestive of a parasitic disorder but is often not present in patients with echinococcosis (Kaya et al.). The Carsoni intradermal test and the Weinberg complement fixation test have been used since 1909 but are generally regarded to be unreliable. An immunofluorescent technique on sera using scolices obtained from hydatid fluid of infected sheep has been proposed as a reliable diagnostic method for preoperative identification of this disease (Florez et al.).

Localization of the intracranial cystic mass is best accomplished by computed cranial tomography, sometimes in conjunction with carotid angiography. Computed tomography would be expected to outline the size, shape, and position of the lesion precisely, with the spherical mass containing fluid of CSF density and without a solid component on enhancement. The cerebral hydatid cyst is larger and more spherical than the lesions of cysticercosis and is much less often associated with calcium deposition. Angiography demonstrates the mass in the form of an avascular lesion with stretching and distortion of the adjacent vessels (Arana-Iniguez and Julian). Ventriculography is claimed to be contraindicated owing to the danger of inadvertent puncture of the cyst with resultant widespread contamination by scolices of the adjacent brain and subarachnoid space, leading to multiple cyst formation. Absolute diagnosis is on the basis of pathologic demonstration of parts of the parasite and the characteristic membranes of the cyst following its surgical removal.

Treatment

Treatment of cerebral hydatid cysts is surgical removal through a craniotomy flap, which is made slightly larger than the size of the cyst (Carrea et al.). Authors have repeatedly stressed the importance of delivery of the cystic mass intact without perforation or puncture (Griponissiotis, Kaya et al.). Spillage of the hydatid cyst fluid in the subarachnoid space can result in the eventual formation of multiple new implants but can also precipitate an acute reaction with profound hyperthermia, meningeal signs, or anaphylactic shock (Kaya et al.). Methods to assist removal of the lesion include lowering of the head of the operating table once the cyst is exposed through a transcortical incision, gentle irrigation with fluid through the cleavage plane between the cyst and the surrounding brain, and cautious injection of air into the opposite lateral ventricle which forces the mass to the surface. In addition to surgical methods, mebendazole is a potent antihelminthic which has been stated to be effective in the treatment of this disease (Chevis).

Coenurosis

Coenurosis in the human is a disease caused by the larval phase of the tapeworm Multiceps (Taenia) multiceps. It is well known as a cause of intracerebral cysts in sheep and other animals in certain foreign countries such as South Africa but rarely produces neurologic disease in man. Hermos et al. were able to find published reports of 53 human cases in the world literature up to 1970. The adult tapeworm measures up to 60 centimeters in length and inhabits the intestinal tract of dogs, foxes, or coyotes, from which eggs are intermittently shed in the stools. These animals become infected by consumption of sheep's brains which are provided to them after the carcasses have been otherwise disposed of (Becker and Jacobson). Man is an intermediate host and becomes infected with the larval stage following oral ingestion of the ova from the feces of dogs. Oncospheres hatch in the intestine, penetrate the intestinal wall to reach the circulation, and are then distributed to the brain, spinal cord, or other tissues where the larva becomes a coenurus. Except for enlodgement in the brain, direct visceral involvement is infrequent. Other sites of infestation may be within the abdominal cavity, the pleura, or intramuscular connective tissue. Unlike the cysticercus, which has a single scolex, the coenurus has multiple scolices invaginated in its wall. In addition, the coenurus becomes considerably larger, measuring up to 4 or 5 centimeters in diameter.

Clinical Manifestations

Coenurosis of the nervous system of man is a very rare disease and only a limited number of human infestations have been reported. Most identified cases have been in adult males but Hermos et al. described a two-year-old child in this country with a multiloculated coenurus in the posterior fossa, which proved to be a fatal lesion.

In most reported cases, the cyst has occurred in the region of the fourth ventricle or basilar cisterns, giving rise to an illness of weeks or months in duration and manifested by signs of increased intracranial pressure due to obstructive hydrocephalus in combination with disturbances of cerebellar function. Whether the lesions are located above or below the tentorium, there is a decided predilection for their occurrence within the CSF pathways, either within the ventricular system or in the major CSF pathways external to the brain. There is a single report in which paraplegia secondary to an intramedullary coenurus in the thoracic cord occurred in a 14-year-old child (Landells). The cerebral hemispheres also can be the site of cyst formation but only a few examples have been described. Intraocular cysts are likewise extremely rare (Epstein et al.). Regardless of the location of the lesion in the central nervous system, the cerebrospinal fluid usually reveals a mononuclear cell reaction and moderate to marked elevation in the protein content.

The coenurus within the cerebral hemisphere is unilocular and oval or circular in shape, while that in the fourth ventricle may become irregular and racemose, thus resembling the cysticercus. When the cyst is multilocular, only one of the racemose projections will contain scolices while the rest are sterile (Robinson). Dozens of scolices visible as small white spots on the delicate, transparent bladder characterize the coenurus, differentiating the coenurus from the cysticercus, which has only a single scolex.

Clinical diagnosis prior to surgery or autopsy is not usually possible and most reported patients have died without surgical intervention. With surgically removed tissue, when one or more scolices cannot be found, a specific diagnosis cannot be established except for its identification as a parasitic cyst. Hydatid cysts are generally larger in size and, with their smaller hooks and characteristically laminated membrane, can usually be distinguished from either a coenurus or a cysticercus. Treatment is unsatisfactory in most cases of intracranial coenurosis. Cases with obstructive hydrocephalus due to posterior fossa lesions are candidates for craniectomy and attempted removal of the lesion. Racemose cysts extending through the foramen magnum or located in the basilar cisterns cannot usually be completely excised.

Schistosomiasis

Human schistosomiasis is caused by three species of blood flukes: Schistosoma haematobium, which is found primarily in Africa and the Middle East; Schistosoma mansoni, which occurs in Africa, South America and the West Indies, and Schistosoma japonicum which occurs mainly in Southeast Asia. The life cycle of the schistosome is complex. Man serves as the primary host and the water snail is the secondary host. Schistosoma haematobium resides within pelvic veins in the human, and Schistosoma mansoni and japonicum are found within mesenteric veins. Eggs are passed to venules where a larval form, the miracidium, develops within the egg, which then ruptures through the wall of the venule gaining entrance to the lumen of the urinary bladder or the intestine and is subsequently excreted in the urine or feces. On entry into water, the miracidia hatch from the eggs and penetrate a snail, from which the next stage, the forked-tailed cercariae, eventually emerge. The free-swimming cercariae either die or come in contact with man, entering by burrowing through the skin. The cercariae eventually come to reside in the portal venous system. After a few weeks, the adult worms migrate to the mesenteric and pelvic venules, where they shed their eggs.

Transient pruritis and rash may occur when the skin is penetrated by cercariae. With liver invasion, clinical features include recurrent urticaria, edema, respiratory distress, and eosinophilia in the peripheral blood. Hepatomegaly and liver tenderness develop in two to three weeks, associated with fever, abdominal pain, and diarrhea.

Since Schistosoma haematobium is found mainly in pelvic veins, its deposited eggs produce inflammatory lesions in the bladder and genitalia, and, to a lesser degree, in the distal intestine. Increased frequency, pain on micturition, and hematuria are the customary symptoms. Changes in the bladder mucosa or urethra complicated by secondary bacterial infection can lead to upper urinary tract disease with hydronephrosis. Chronic local irritation from schistosoma eggs appears to predispose to bladder wall malignancy.

Schistosoma japonicum and mansoni are harbored in mesenteric veins and their eggs invade the intestinal wall. Eggs are commonly carried back through the portal system into the liver and the lungs. The resulting inflammatory process leads to hepatosplenomegaly, eventual hepatic cirrhosis, and portal hypertension with hypersplenism. Inflammatory disease of the intestinal tract is evoked by the eggs discharged through its wall, leading to mucosal ulcers, polyps, and strictures. Schistosoma japonicum provokes the most severe inflammatory reactions, probably because it produces many times more eggs than Schistosoma mansoni.

Clinical diagnosis of schistosomiasis is suspected in endemic areas or patients from endemic areas by the presence of allergic eruptions, hepatic signs, and gastrointestinal disturbances. After the initial stages of the illness, characteristic schistosome eggs can be found in the feces or urine, although large quantities and, often, repeated specimens must be examined. Other diagnostic methods include rectal or bladder mucosal biopsy and serum complement fixation tests.

Neurologic Manifestations

Symptomatic neurologic complications of schistosomiasis are exceedingly rare compared to the estimated number of persons who harbor these parasites. Up to 1963, Marcial-Rojas and Fiol found reports of 97 patients with neurologic involvement. Schistosoma japonicum was the cause in 60 cases, 58 of which involved the brain and only two the spinal cord. Schistosoma haematobium was the causative organism in 11 cases, and in eight of the 11 the spinal cord was affected. Schistosoma mansoni accounted for 26 cases with neurologic involvement, and in 17 of the 26 the spinal cord was the site of disease. The factors related to the occurrence of variations from the customary pattern of schistosomal disease are unclear but probably include the degree of pre-existent immunity of the individual and the magnitude of the initial schistosomal invasion (Bird). In an endemic region with a population whose acquired immunity is high, it is possible that even wide dissemination of ova may produce no symptoms. If natural immunity plays such a protective role, it is possible that dissemination of ova to the nervous system resulting in symptomatic neurologic disease might occur more often in persons foreign to endemic areas but residing there temporarily.

The mechanism by which schistosomiasis causes brain or spinal cord disease is not yet settled. Some authors have suggested that the adult female worm migrates to cerebral or intraspinal venous channels, causing mechanical venous obstruction, and at the same time deposits eggs, which provoke an inflammatory response. A more widely held concept is that ova are transmitted from mesenteric or pelvic veins to nervous tissue, either via the vertebral venous plexus of Batson or through more systemic channels. Ova have been observed within damaged brain or spinal cord tissue in a number of reports. In addition to possible brain or spinal cord involvement in schistosomiasis, a myopathic process has been described (Mansour and Reese). Features include generalized muscle wasting and weakness, most severe in the lower extremities, while histologic examinations have revealed variation in muscle fiber size, increase in sarcolemmic nuclei, and some degree of infiltration with macrophages and lymphocytes. The pathogenesis of the myopathy remains unclear.

Cerebral schistosomiasis is much more common than spinal cord involvement and the majority of cases are caused by Schistosoma japonicum. The onset of cerebral disease can be early, within two or three months after exposure, in which case the manifestations usually appear abruptly and resemble an encephalitic process (Blankfein and Chirico). Fever, headache, lethargy, pain on neck flexion, and long tract signs are common, while coma, seizures, and specific focal deficits are less frequent. Peripheral blood leukocytosis with a definite eosinophilia is found in most of this group. In others, the onset of cerebral signs does not occur until more than six months after the initial signs of systemic disease. Late onset of this type is more likely to be associated with focal neurologic signs resembling those of a space-occupying lesion. Unilateral motor or sensory deficits, focal seizures, and papilledema are more common in this group, while leukocytosis and eosinophilia are less marked than in those with earlier onset. Death from cerebral schistosomiasis is unusual, but lasting neurologic deficits are not uncommon.

The typical lesion in the brain is one or more focal granulomas which grossly resemble a tuberculoma. Microscopically, the lesions consist of schistosoma ova in brain surrounded by gliosis, inflammatory cells, macrophages, and multinucleated giant cells. Granulomas are of variable size, number, and location, and with different degrees of tissue injury.

Spinal cord disease caused by schistosoma ova may be in the form of a focal intramedullary granuloma that can usually be localized with myelography, or a more diffuse inflammatory myelopathy. In most reported cases, the low thoracic or lumbar spinal cord has been the affected site (Bird, Marcial-Romas and Fiol, Pepler and Lombaard, Wakefield et al.). Clinically, the onset is with low back discomfort and cramp-like pain in the legs followed by the rapid development of paraplegia, with sensory loss below the level of the lesion. Sphincter disturbances are added to the above signs as the disease progresses. The maximal degree of neurologic deficit is usually reached within several days to a few weeks after onset but, in exceptional cases, the course is much more slowly evolving. Damage to the spinal cord is severe in most cases, and, while improvement is expected, complete recovery of function does not usually occur. On rare occasion, the spinal cord can be extensively damaged, leading to widespread necrosis of the cord and ending fatally (Queiroz et al.).

The cerebrospinal fluid in schistosomiasis of the nervous system is usually abnormal, with a lymphocytic pleocytosis and elevation of the protein content. In cases with a spinal cord lesion producing a complete block, the protein content will become markedly increased. Eosinophils have been observed in the spinal fluid in neurologic schistosomal disease, but this is the rare exception (Wakefield et al.). Niridazole is currently the drug of choice for treatment of schistosomiasis (Mahmoud) and some have also recommended corticosteroids for patients with neurologic complications of the disease (Lechtenberg and Vaida).

Paragonimiasis

Paragonimiasis is primarily a pulmonary disease endemic in the Far East and caused by the lung fluke, Paragonimus westermani. Man is the definitive host, operculated snails the first intermediate host, and fresh-water crabs the second intermediate host. Man becomes infected by eating uncooked crabs or crayfish. An additional source of infection of children in Korea is the administration of crushed crayfish juice as a mode of therapy for measles. The parasite resides in the lungs where ova are excreted from the host into the sputum and the feces. The ovum develops into the free-swimming meracidium, which survives if it penetrates a suitable snail, in which it becomes a sporocyst. After several weeks, this matures into the cercaria, which emerges from the snail to penetrate a fresh-water crab or crayfish, in which the larval metacercaria becomes encysted. Following ingestion of the uncooked crustacean by man, the capsules of the metacercariae are dissolved within the stomach and the parasite penetrates the intestinal wall to gain entrance into the peritoneal cavity. The adolescent worms then burrow through the diaphragm and pleura to reach the lungs where, in cystic abscess-like cavities, they become adult worms in approximately six weeks. During the migration from the abdominal cavity, extrapulmonary localization sometimes occurs, with the brain being the most common site. Except for the effect on the brain or spinal cord, extrapulmonary lesions generally are of minimal clinical importance.

Symptoms resulting from pulmonary involvement have an insidious onset and in the majority of instances the respiratory disease is a chronic one but remains benign. Males are affected considerably more often than females. Older children and young adults are involved in the majority of cases, and, in general, the disease occurs more frequently in persons of poorer socioeconomic groups. A dry cough eventually becomes productive of blood-tinged, rusty-brown sputum. Fever, chest pain, and pleural effusion occur in some infested patients.

Diagnosis of paragonimiasis is suspected by the presence of chronic cough with hemoptysis in a patient with low-grade eosinophilia and a history of eating raw crabs or crayfish. Chest x-ray abnormalities are usual but must be differentiated from those of tuberculosis. The most valuable diagnostic method is the identification of eggs in sputum, stool, or, less often, from aspirated fluid from the pleural cavity. The intradermal skin test is useful as a screening technique but does have cross reactivity with the antigen of Clonorchis sinensis. Cross sensitivity with other parasites is also a problem with the complement fixation test, but it is of value when combined with sputum and stool examination for ova. The complement fixation test is usually positive in the spinal fluid in patients with cerebral paragonimiasis.

Neurologic Manifestations

The most common and most serious extrapulmonary site of involvement in paragonimiasis is the brain. The route by which the parasite reaches the brain has been in dispute. Some authors have favored hematogenous spread, but the most commonly accepted concept is that larvae enter the brain through connective tissue surrounding the jugular vein (Yokogawa and Suemori). After reaching the cerebrum, the larvae mature into adult worms and deposit their ova locally. As in the pulmonary form of the disease, cerebral paragonimiasis occurs predominantly in people less than 30 years of age. Most have had pulmonary symptoms preceding neurologic signs, sometimes of several years' duration.

Recurrent seizures are the most common initial neurologic disturbance, although an occasional patient has had one or more meningitic episodes before convulsions have made their appearance (Higashi et al., Kim, Oh). In some patients, chronic meningitis with headache, vomiting, weight loss, neck stiffness, and fever proceed gradually to a disorder with signs of a localized cerebral mass accompanied by papilledema. In others, recurrent seizures, commonly Jacksonian in type, are followed by abrupt and persistent hemiplegia, leading to the identification of a focal granulomatous cerebral lesion. The type of seizures as well as the signs found on neurologic examination depends largely on the localization and size of the cerebral lesion. Progressive dementia is observed in some adult cases, while the incidence of mental retardation is much higher in children with cerebral paragonimiasis than in the average population (Kim). Primary optic atrophy often associated with decreased visual acuity is an additional finding observed in some patients.

For reasons unexplained, paragonimiasis shows a predilection for the posterior part of the cerebral hemispheres. The posterior temporal and parieto-occipital regions are the customary sites of one of two types of cerebral lesions. The first is a solid granulomatous mass whose center consists of necrotic debris in which are found parasitic ova, inflammatory cells, and giant cells. The shape is roughly round or oval and the lesion is frequently surrounded by an area of gliosis as well as plasma cells, lymphocytes, and eosinophils. In chronic lesions, punctate or perivascular calcific deposits are seen. The second

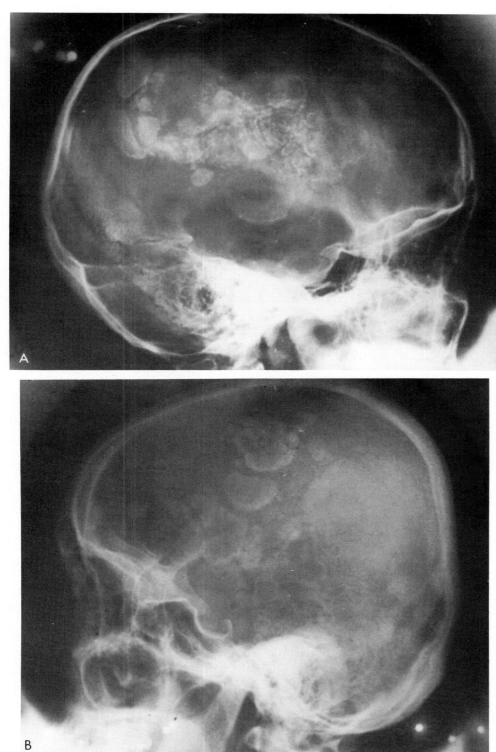

Figure 20–6. Cerebral paragonimiasis. Characteristic roentgenographic appearance with multiple round or oval lesions with increased density at their peripheral margins. (Courtesy of Dr. Shin Joong Oh, Birmingham, Alabama; Radiology, 90:292–299, 1968.)

type of cerebral lesion is a poorly encapsulated abscess which harbors thick, yellowish purulent material. Paragonimus ova can be readily identified in most instances on the inner surface of the thin capsule. Despite the ease of demonstration of paragonimus ova in lesions in the brain, the adult fluke is only rarely identified, probably because of its rapid disintegration.

In addition to the diagnostic tests indicative of pulmonary infestation with this parasite, certain examinations are useful in persons with neurologic paragonimiasis. The cerebrospinal fluid is not invariably abnormal but may reveal a lymphocytic pleocytosis and, less frequently, a certain number of eosinophils (Oh). When the clinical picture is that of a localized mass lesion, the opening pressure is often elevated and the protein content increased. Intracranial calcification has been described in greater than 50 percent of cases and is more consistently present in those with neurologic complaints of long standing. The characteristic roentgenographic pattern in cerebral paragonimiasis is one resembling a "soap bubble" configuration with a round or oval shape highlighted by an increased peripheral density (Fig. 20–6).

Cases in which the granuloma or abscess assumes the form of a localized mass are managed by surgical excision or drainage. Bithionol has recently been shown to be effective in the treatment of pulmonary paragonimiasis and may be useful in the early stages of cerebral infestation (Oh).

PROTOZOAL INFECTIONS

Toxoplasmosis

The spectrum of human toxoplasmosis has gradually unfolded since the reports of Wolf, Cowan, and Paige in 1939. It became widely known as a devastating congenital infection leading to hydrocephalus, cerebral calcification, and chorioretinitis, and only recently has it been recognized that this represents one of the least common forms of infection with this parasite. Congenital infection with isolated ocular involvement (Fair), asymptomatic acquired infection, and acquired infection in the immunosuppressed host (Vietzke et al.) are now recognized to be the more common manifestations of toxoplasmosis. With prolonged survival of patients with hematologic malignancies and the wide-scale use of immunosuppressive drugs for a variety of disorders, Toxoplasma gondii has become an important opportunistic invader with a definite propensity for cerebral involvement.

Toxoplasma gondii is an obligatory intracellular parasite first identified by Nicolle and Manceaux in 1908 in a North African rodent, the gondi. The organism was subsequently found to exist in a wide range of birds and mammals, including man, in which virtually any cell except the non-nucleated erythrocyte can be infected. Free trophozoites are usually concentric or oval in shape in tissue and measure 4 to 7 microns in length. With Giemsa or Wright stains, the nucleus assumes a pink to red appearance and the cytoplasm is pale blue. In tissue, toxoplasmas are characteristically seen in clusters surrounded by a limiting membrane, the so-called encysted form. These structures were earlier called pseudocysts because it was believed that the outer wall was derived from the host rather than from the parasite. It is now believed that the parasite contributes significantly to the formation of the wall and for this reason they are considered to be "true" cysts (Frenkel, Garnham et al.). Within tissue, encysted toxoplasmas can remain viable for many years. Liberation of the organisms from the confines of the cyst by one means or another has been considered to be the explanation for recurrences of activity of the disease in certain situations.

The methods by which human infection with toxoplasmosis is contracted have gradually become clarified even though certain details remain unestablished. Man-to-man transmission probably does not occur, with the notable exception of transplacental infection from the mother to her fetus. This results from maternal blood stream infection resulting in placental lesions from which parasites gain entrance to the fetal circulation. While this mode of transmission is beyond doubt, the time-relationships during pregnancy when it can occur are still in dispute. Experimental and clinical observations have suggested that consumption of uncooked or poorly cooked infected meat accounts for some acquired human infections with Toxoplasma gondii. The most convincing demonstration of this was by Desmonts et al. who found a high rate of seroconversion in hospitalized children fed poorly cooked mutton. More recently, the cat has been incriminated as a source of human toxoplasmosis (Frenkel et al., Teutsch et al.). Initial studies suggested that toxoplasmas could be transmitted within Toxocara cati ova in the feline feces, but more recent observations indicate that fecal transmission can occur without toxocara ova. The role of the cat as a source of this parasite has prompted some to outline specific recommendations regarding exposure and care of cats by the pregnant woman and immunodeficient patients (Krogsted et al., Swartzberg and Remington). Additional methods by which the human can acquire the disease include transmission by leukocyte transfusions (Siegel et al.) and by contamination in the laboratory in which live toxoplasmas are used for diagnostic tests (Sexton et al., Ström).

Acquired Toxoplasmosis

Epidemiologic studies summarized by Feldman indicate that toxoplasmosis is a world-wide disease but with considerable variation in its incidence among different population groups. It is believed that, in this country, one-third to one-fourth of adults have positive dye-test antibody titers, indicating previous infection with Toxoplasma gondii. Other estimates are that approximately 50 percent of the population in the United States is infected with Toxoplasma gondii in asymptomatic form and that there are approximately 3000 congenitally infected infants born per year in this country (Krick and Remington). In England, approximately 50 percent of blood donors have been found to have positive dye-test titers (Robertson). The majority of acquired infections with this organism are either asymptomatic or so mild that studies are not accomplished and the illness is not identified. Even in mild or asymptomatic cases, the parasites are widely distributed throughout the body during the acute stage. They become encased within cysts which persist in tissue with minimal surrounding cellular reaction and may remain for the lifetime of the individual. It is postulated that encystment occurs in response to the development of antibodies by the host. Once encysted, the parasite becomes only weakly antigenic so that antibody titers eventually decline to low levels despite the persistence of viable toxoplasmas within the cystic structures (Remington and Cavanaugh).

Acquired toxoplasmosis in previously normal persons most often results in subclinical illness. Symptomatic acquired toxoplasmosis can present in one of many forms but is usually a benign and transient illness. In some patients the illness is characterized by a diffuse maculopapular rash associated with malaise and muscle pain. Rarely, the rash is petechial in quality, resembling that of rickettsial disease (Pinkerton and Henderson). In others, the illness is manifested by lymphadenopathy with or without fever and with a negative heterophil reaction, representing one type of heterophil-negative mononucleosis. Myocarditis can complicate the disorder but is unusual (Ström). Still another infrequent type of acquired toxoplasma infection is acute hepatitis, which clinically resembles viral hepatitis (Vischer et al.), or granulomatous hepatitis in conjunction with acute lymphadenopathic involvement (Weitberg et al.). Meningoencephalitis is a rare expression of acquired toxoplasmosis in otherwise normal persons but has been observed in previously normal children (Neumann et al., Sabin) and in adults (Koeze and Klingen). The neurologic findings may coexist with either rash or generalized adenopathy and can follow a self-limited course or prove fatal. A relationship between acute infection with Toxoplasma gondii and polymyositis/dermatomyositis has been debated for several years. Recent reports have indicated that such disorders can be associated with infection with this parasite on rare occasion (Greenlee et al., Hendrickx et al.).

The role of Toxoplasma gondii as a cause of postnatally acquired ocular disease has been a disputed topic and one still unsettled. Bilateral chorioretinitis is one of the hallmarks of congenital toxoplasmosis and in some instances will represent the only clinical abnormality of this form of the disease. Since encysted parasites are able to remain viable within the retina for many years, recurrent activity of the inflammatory process can become manifest by rupture of the cysts and liberation of the organisms. Some have felt that active ocular inflammation first identified in the older child or adult is always on this basis and does not represent a postnatally acquired infection. However, there are now well-documented cases of acquired toxoplasmosis in older persons in which acute chorioretinitis has occurred (Masur et al., Nicholson and Wolchok). The current general consensus of opinion is that chorioretinitis can complicate acquired toxoplasmosis in the adult but that it should be considered to be an unusual event (Hogan). An older child seen for the first time and found to have visual loss and bilateral macular chorioretinitis can be assumed to have had the onset of the process before four years of age, and thus probably prenatally, if ocular examination reveals definite pendular nystagmus.

Toxoplasmosis and the Immunocompromised Host

Certain gram-negative and gram-positive bacteria, viruses of the herpes group, fungi including Candida and Aspergillus species, and Toxoplasma gondii have emerged as important opportunistic pathogens in patients with impaired immunologic mechanisms. Pneumocystis carinii can be added to this list of common secondary invaders, but unlike the organisms above, is not known to cause neurologic disease in the immunologically compromised host.

Toxoplasmosis has been described in patients with a variety of malignant disorders but is a special hazard in patients with hematologic malignancies receiving immunosuppressive or corticosteroid therapy. It is seen in children with acute leukemia and neuroblastoma, in patients with Hodgkin's disease and other lymphomas, in multiple myeloma and a variety of solid tumors, and in patients with collagen-vascular disorders (Abell and Holland, Carey et al., Gleason and Hamlin, Ruskin and Remington, Theologides et al., Vietzke et al.). It is likewise a hazard in compromised patients following renal transplantation (Reynolds et al., Ghatak et al.) and cardiac transplantation (Remington, 1970). A remarkable feature of severe and often fatal infection with Toxoplasma gondii in immunosuppressed patients is the coexistence of cytomegalovirus or herpesvirus infections with surprising frequency (Luna and Lichtiger, Vietzke et al.). The explanation for the susceptibility of patients with neoplastic disease to toxoplasmosis is not entirely clear but it appears that circulating antibodies alone do not provide protection against serious infection with this parasite. It has been suggested that the vulnerability of the brain is partly due to the lack of ability of antibody to gain entrance to the central nervous system because of the blood-brain barrier. At least one factor of importance in such suppressed patients is a defect in delayed hypersensitivity, although disturbances in other immune mechanisms are probably also operative. Toxoplasmosis in the immunosuppressed patient can be the result of either reactivation of latent infection or dissemination of a primarily acquired infection.

Toxoplasmosis associated with malignancy or in other immunologically compromised patients may affect a variety of organ systems but the disease displays a decided predilection for central nervous system involvement in the form of a diffuse meningoencephalitis, a progressive cerebral mass lesion or a combination of the two. Rarely, a toxoplasmic cerebral lesion presents as an abscess with ring enhancement on computed tomography and purulent material obtained on needle aspiration (McLeod et al.). In some cases, the infection is essentially limited to the brain (Ghatak).

Clinical findings in such patients are quite variable, but in many cases the patient's gradual decline and eventual demise is attributed to the underlying malignant disease, and toxoplasmosis is unexpectedly found at necropsy (Gleason and Hamlin). Persistent or recurrent fever is often the first sign of the illness, eventually complicated by symptoms and signs of either diffuse or focal cerebral disease. Headache, drowsiness, and disorientation are associated with a variety of signs indicative of diffuse cerebral and brain stem involvement. An occasional patient will exhibit signs of increased intracranial pressure along with progressive focal deficits, indicative of a mass lesion and resembling a cerebral neoplasm. In such patients, computed tomography or angiography may demonstrate a focal cerebral lesion, again simulating a cerebral neoplasm. With severe neurologic involvement with toxoplasmosis, the course is usually one of progressive deterioration terminating in coma and subsequently in death within weeks or a few months after onset. Cerebrospinal fluid findings include an elevated pressure in some patients and an increased protein content in most. The glucose value is usually within normal limits. The cell count may be normal but more often is modestly elevated and is composed predominantly of mononuclear cells.

The cerebral pathology is that of a necrotizing toxoplasmic encephalomyelitis but usually with only minimal meningeal changes. In certain cases, gross inspection of the sectioned brain reveals a large, localized necrotic lesion in which abundant toxoplasmas can be seen microscopically, both free and in cyst form (Fig. 20–7). In others, the process is multifocal, with multiple areas of discoloration which on gross inspection resemble metastatic neoplastic lesions (Fig. 20–8). Still others show minimal gross changes but patchy areas of tissue necrosis on microscopic examination, in addition to perivascular round

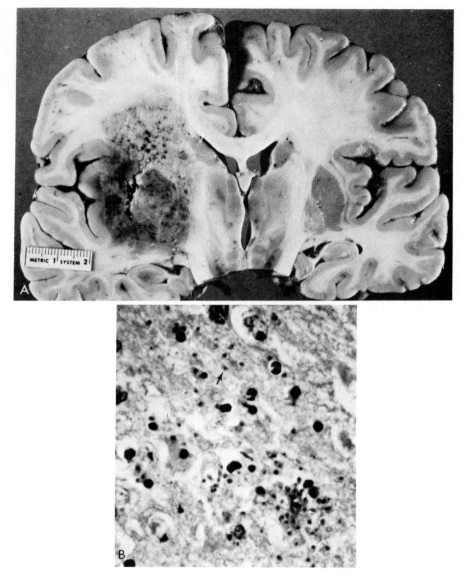

Figure 20–7. Cerebral toxoplasmosis in a leukemic child treated with corticosteroids and antimetabolic drugs. *A,* Coronal section of the brain with an extensive, necrotic lesion in the white matter of one cerebral hemisphere. *B,* Microscopic examination demonstrates toxoplasmas singly and in clusters, some within cytoplasm of macrophages. The parasites are small, rounded or oval bodies with dark-stained nuclei and indistinct cytoplasm (arrow). Some assume a fusiform or lunate shape. Larger, dark circular structures are glial nuclei.

cell infiltration and toxoplasmas in various forms disseminated in brain tissue. Encysted parasites are sometimes found in the brain without an associated inflammatory reaction (Fig. 20–9). Morphologic identification of the toxoplasma cyst is not difficult since the organisms it resembles do not usually show a predisposition to affect the brain of the immunosuppressed host (Ghatak et al.). When microscopic diagnosis is in question, electron microscopic examination can be useful since

the fine structure of toxoplasma is now well recognized (Garnham et al.).

Toxoplasma encephalitis in the compromised host represents a life-threatening complication which is important to identify because response to therapy is possible. Survival is not likely once definite and advanced neurologic signs have developed but can occur with treatment begun in the early stages of the condition. Of 20 patients with immunosuppressive disorders complicated by toxo-

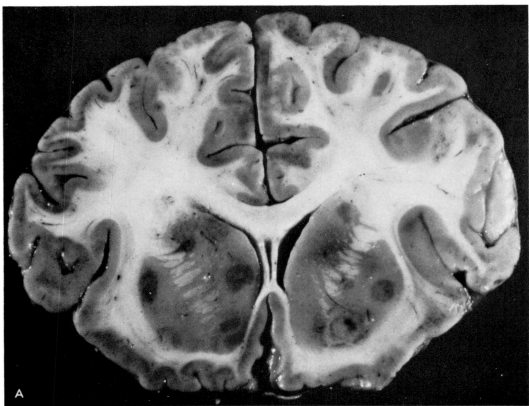

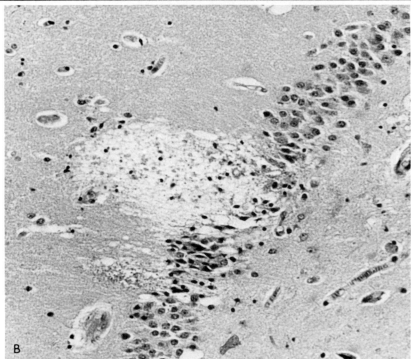

Figure 20–8. Cerebral toxoplasmosis in a child on immunosuppressive therapy for reticuloendothelial malignancy. *A,* Coronal section of the brain through the frontal lobes, which contain multiple, discrete foci of discoloration and softening caused by toxoplasma encephalitis. The lesions are most conspicuous in the striata. *B,* Photomicrograph of the hippocampus demonstrating a discrete area of tissue rarefaction impinging upon the dentate fascia.

Illustration continued on opposite page

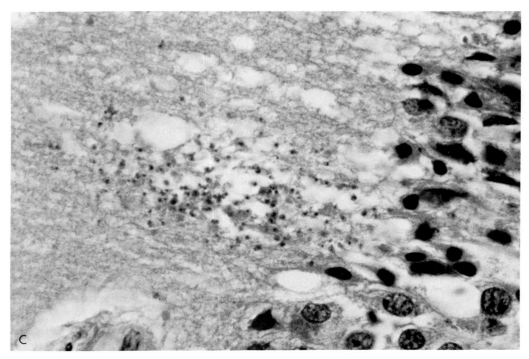

Figure 20–8 Continued. C, Higher magnification of the necrotic focus seen in B. Many free toxoplasma organisms with darkly stained nuclei are present within the damaged area.

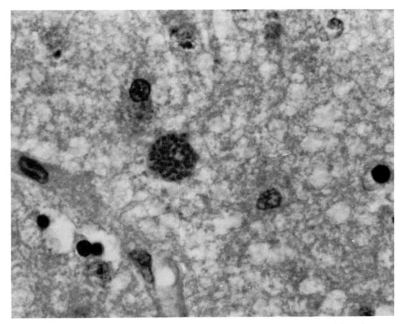

Figure 20–9. Toxoplasma encephalitis. Encysted parasites within the brain of a child on immunosuppressive drug therapy. Note the absence of an inflammatory response to the encysted organisms.

plasmosis, treatment with sulfadiazine and pyrimethamine resulted in marked improvement or complete remission in 80 percent (Ruskin and Remington). The importance of rapid diagnosis has been stressed by Ruskin and Remington. These authors recommend early consideration of brain biopsy in the immunocompromised patient with persistent fever and otherwise unexplained progressive neurologic dysfunction. Demonstration of toxoplasmas in the trophozoite stage in biopsy specimens is confirmatory of the diagnosis. Despite the immunologic effects of both the underlying neoplastic disease and the therapy used for the basic disease, antibody response providing serologic evidence of the infection occurs in most patients. Because serologic diagnosis is complicated by the high incidence of toxoplasma antibodies in the adult population, Feldman has advised that toxoplasma serologic tests be performed on all patients who are to be placed on immunosuppressing drug therapy so that subsequent test results at the time of occurrence of febrile illnesses can be more logically analyzed.

Congenital Toxoplasmosis

Transplacental transmission of Toxoplasma gondii from the mother to the fetus can result in abortion, stillbirth, an asymptomatic but infected neonate, or a newborn infant with signs of disease expressed in variable fashion and severity. Because the most easily recognized form of the disease in the infant is the least common and since the maternal infection is asymptomatic in the majority of cases, the incidence of congenital toxoplasmosis is uncertain. The prevalence of clinically recognizable cases in this country has been estimated to be at least one in 3000 to 4000 births (Miller et al.), and in France it is judged to be approximately one per 1,000 births (Couvreur and Desmonts). Other studies have suggested that the incidence of toxoplasma infections in pregnant women may be as high as four to six per 1,000 but that fetal infection occurs in less than half and many of these are inapparent infections (Stern et al.). Desmonts and Couvreur (1974) recently reported 378 pregnant women with either high initial toxoplasma antibody titers (195 cases) or seroconversion (183 cases) during pregnancy. Of the 183 women who acquired the infection during pregnancy, toxoplasma was isolated from the placenta in 25 percent.

Of the 378 pregnancies, 11 ended in abortion and seven infants were either stillborn or died shortly after birth. Most, but not all, of these latter 18 cases were infected. Of the 183 women who acquired toxoplasmosis during pregnancy, congenital toxoplasmosis occurred in only approximately one-third. Among 59 infected infants, tissue injury was severe in nine and the manifestations were mild in 11. The congenital infection remained subclinical in 39. Couvreur and colleagues have shown that when twins are affected with congenital toxoplasmosis, the clinical pattern is usually similar in each of monozygotic twins but displays considerable variability in dizygotic twins. This suggests that a different degree of placental involvement in the dizygotic pairs is important in determining the extent of parasitization and thus the severity of tissue injury in the fetus.

The time during pregnancy when acquired maternal toxoplasmosis creates the greatest risk to the fetus has been another disputed point. It is probable that transmission of the organisms to the fetus can occur anytime during pregnancy. Couvreur and Desmonts found that the most serious fetal infections resulted from acquired maternal toxoplasmosis between the second and sixth months of pregnancy. In their more recent review in 1974, Desmonts and Couvreur confirmed their earlier finding that fetal death or severe disease occurred only as a result of infection with toxoplasma acquired from the second to the sixth fetal months. No cases of congenital toxoplasmosis were observed when maternal infection was acquired before or approximately at the time of conception, while those acquired in the last trimester resulted in no disease or subclinical disease in the newborn infant. It is agreed by most authors that only toxoplasma infection acquired during pregnancy endangers the fetus. Previously acquired infections are believed to be insignificant in regard to the effects on the fetus, and, likewise, when fetal infection has occurred during a pregnancy, subsequent pregnancies should not be at risk. There are rare exceptions, however, and a few examples of repeated congenital infections with toxoplasma have been described (Garcia, Langer). Repeated infections with subsequent pregnancies are best explained on the basis of encysted parasites established in the uterine wall during the primary infection. Because of the prolonged survival of organisms in the cyst form, it is possible for placental and fetal infection to occur long after the primary systemic infection. Stern and Romano described two siblings, one eight years older than the other, each with chorioretinitis believed to be secondary to congenital toxoplasmosis.

Clinical Manifestations

The classic triad of hydrocephalus, intracranial calcification, and bilateral chorioretinitis in the newborn infant is now recognized to be only part of the clinical spectrum of intrauterine-acquired toxoplasmosis. Furthermore, the same combination of findings can result from cytomegalovirus, and probably other viral infections acquired by transplacental infection. In general, the earlier the onset of clinical signs after birth, the more severe is the infection and the greater is the likelihood of neurologic involvement. In some cases, the infant appears normal at birth and develops signs of ocular, neurologic, or hepatic disease weeks or months thereafter (Glasser and Delta). The child may seemingly be normal for a period of time after birth until convulsions and increasing head size dictate the need for medical diag-nostic evaluation. Chorioretinitis is the only manifestation of the disease in certain cases (Fair, Hogan) and may not be identified until later in childhood. (Fig. 20–10).

In the study by Couvreur and Desmonts of 300 symptomatic patients of various ages with congenital toxoplasmosis, 76 percent had chorioretinitis, 51 percent had neurologic dysfunction of some type, and 26 percent had an abnormality of intracranial volume, either hydrocephalus or microcephaly. Thirty-two percent of the patients were found to have intracranial calcification on x-ray. Among the patients less than five months of age with congenital toxoplasmosis, 27 percent had been jaundiced and almost 19 percent had enlargement of the liver or spleen.

With the severe form of congenital toxoplasmosis, the infant is obviously ill at birth and exhibits signs of multiple organ system disease which can be rapidly fatal or lead to permanent and severe neurologic and ocular sequelae. As in other intrauterine-acquired infections, the frequency of prematurity is considerably higher than in the average population. Hepatomegaly, jaundice, and diffuse soft tissue edema can simulate erythroblas-

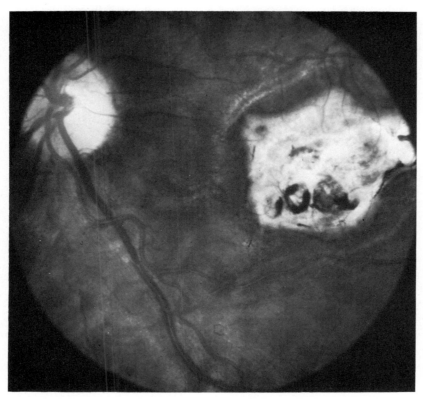

Figure 20–10.   Macular chorioretinitis in a child with congenital toxoplasmosis. The optic disc is atrophic and the child had severe visual loss.

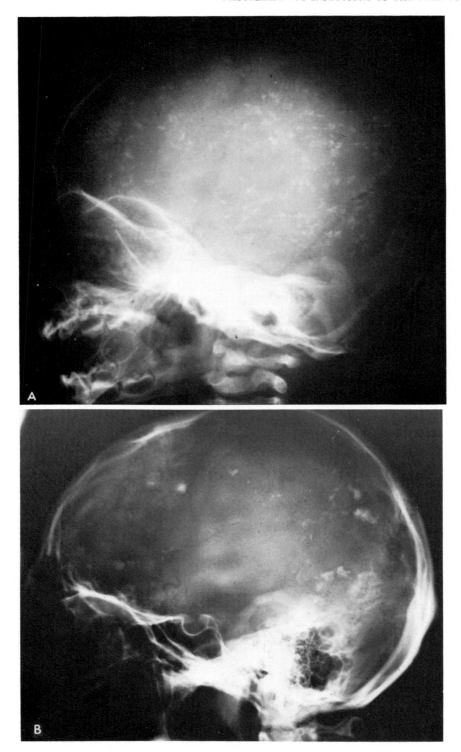

Figure 20–11. Congenital toxoplasmosis with intracranial calcification. *A,* Lateral skull x-ray of an infant with hydrocephalus, chorioretinitis, and multiple, punctate calcifications scattered diffusely in the brain. (Courtesy of Dr. Robert Groover, Rochester, Minnesota.) *B* and *C,* Skull x-rays of a 15-year-old boy with mild microcephaly, chorioretinitis, and a history of generalized convulsions. Irregular, dense, calcific lesions are diffusely present.

Illustration continued on opposite page

tosis until the diagnosis is clarified by laboratory studies (Bain et al.). The full spectrum of the neonatal disease in its classic form includes severe neurologic involvement associated with hydrocephalus, or even hydranencephaly (Altshuler), and diffuse cerebral calcifications observed on x-ray. The cerebral calcifications are generally multiple and are scattered indiscriminately in the brain (Fig. 20–11). Less often, only one or two small calcific lesions are seen on x-ray. This diffuse pattern of calcification is in contrast to that associated with congenital cytomegalovirus encephalitis in which calcification is more often periventricular in location. Microcephaly is less common than hydrocephalus, but regardless of whether the head size is abnormally large or small, abnormality of head size indicates a diffuse and usually necrotizing encephalitis, which will be followed by developmental and mental retardation. Other common findings in the newborn with generalized infection include petechiae or purpura, jaundice, and hepatic enlargement. Immune complex nephrosis with generalized edema and ascites is a rare complication of congenital toxoplasmosis (Shahin et al.). Bilateral chorioretinitis may be present in early infancy or develop subsequently. Microphthalmia is less frequent but can be observed in severely affected patients (Manschot and Daamen). Placental involvement with encysted parasites seen microscopically or with placental hydrops observed on gross inspection can be of diagnostic value in the congenital form of the disease (Altshuler).

Laboratory findings in the neonate with widely disseminated toxoplasmosis vary, but common abnormalities include thrombocytopenia and elevations of both the direct and indirect serum bilirubin levels. Increased serum IgM levels are present in some cases, as with other types of congenital infections. Infants with toxoplasmic encephalitis with hydrocephalus often have xanthochromic ventricular or lumbar cerebrospinal fluid, which contains a protein content of several hundred milligrams percent. Cells in the cerebrospinal fluid vary from a few up to 300 per cu. mm. and can be either neutrophils or mononuclear in type. By examination of Wright-stained preparations of cerebrospinal fluid sediment, toxoplasma can occasionally be identified (dos Santos, Feldman).

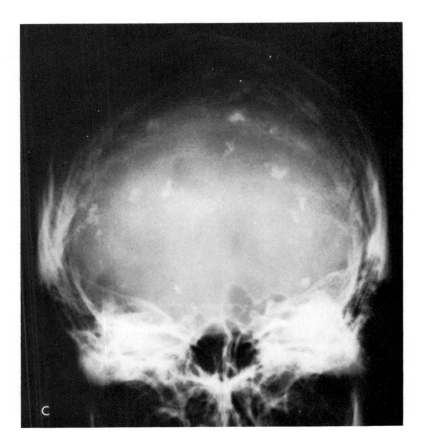

Figure 20–11 Continued

The neuropathology of this disorder is a diffuse or multifocal necrotizing encephalitis, with or without ventricular enlargement. A frequent observation on gross inspection of the infected brain is the presence of diffuse leptomeningeal cloudiness and multiple yellowish opacities on the cortical surface or in the leptomeninges (Wolf and Cowen). Coronal sections of the cerebrum show loss of the normal architectural markings and areas of degeneration and discoloration that are often sharply demarcated. Microscopically, the leptomeningeal exudate is composed of lymphocytes and plasma cells with a lesser number of neutrophils. Areas of cerebral discoloration represent variable degrees of coagulation necrosis and inflammation, with foci of calcification in the most damaged regions. Parasite-laden cysts and free toxoplasmas can usually be found in less damaged areas of brain tissue as well as in the meningeal exudate. Encysted parasites are commonly seen in brain tissue with virtual absence of an inflammatory response in their vicinity. Ventricular distention, when present, can be partially explained on the basis of the encephaloclastic inflammatory process but is primarily the result of ependymal granulations within the aqueduct, and periaqueductal granulomas which lead to aqueductal occlusion.

Diagnosis

Diagnosis of toxoplasmosis is suspected clinically in the newborn infant by the signs of disseminated infection described above, or in the older child by the presence of chorioretinitis, with or without intracranial calcifications. In the older child or adult with immunosuppression, it is the occurrence of persistent, unexplained fever or the development of a progressive neurologic disorder with diffuse inflammatory features that raises the possibility of toxoplasmosis. Serologic studies aid in the confirmation of the diagnosis, as does the demonstration of toxoplasmas in tissue or cerebrospinal fluid. Because encysted toxoplasmas can remain viable in tissue for years without producing an inflammatory response, their identification does not necessarily mean that symptoms or signs are the result of their presence. Remington and Cavanaugh were able to demonstrate the parasite in brain or skeletal muscle at autopsy in 10 percent of patients known to be serologically positive, none of whom had clinical evidence of infection.

Several methods of measuring toxoplasma antibodies are now available. The dye test developed by Sabin and Feldman in 1948 has been the one most widely employed and remains one of the most sensitive. The dye test is performed by mixing live toxoplasmas with serial dilutions of the test serum. Following incubation, alkaline methylene blue is added to each mixture and the number of stained and unstained organisms is determined by microscopic examination. Unaffected parasites accept the blue stain while those exposed to antibody plus a human serum component referred to as "activator" remain unstained. The titer of the serum is that dilution in which 50 percent of the parasites are unstained. For serologic diagnosis of recent infection, two serum specimens obtained at least two weeks apart are desirable. A rising titer indicates a recently acquired infection while a stable titer on serial specimens indicates infection sometime in the past. With active toxoplasmosis, titers often rise to over 1:1024. Antibodies may be detected with the dye test within two to three weeks after the onset of clinical symptoms and persist in gradually diminishing titer for many years. Dye-test antibodies that are passively transferred from mother to fetus decrease significantly by four months after birth and disappear by six months. Although the Sabin-Feldman dye test is sensitive and specific, it is technically demanding and hazardous to laboratory workers because it requires the use of live parasites. In addition, it requires a human accessory factor which is sometimes difficult to obtain. For these reasons, its availability is limited to relatively few diagnostic laboratories.

The complement fixation test has the advantage that live organisms are not required. Complement-fixing antibodies develop more slowly than those to the dye test and either decrease markedly or disappear in approximately two years. The value and reliability of the complement fixation test has been disputed, although Kean and Kimball found it to be a useful method to detect recently acquired toxoplasma infection. In their series, the authors found it to be positive in all children with congenital toxoplasmosis tested under two years of age, although it was acknowledged that in some cases, the complement fixation titer can drop into the undetectable range by three to four months in the congenitally infected infant. The hemagglutination test is now used routinely as a screening procedure in some diagnostic laboratories. It is a relatively easy procedure to perform and has the advantage of using a nonviable antigen. It correlates well with the methylene blue dye test in regard to sensitivity.

The most significant developments for serologic diagnosis of toxoplasmosis are the indirect fluorescent antibody method detecting IgG antibodies, and the IgM fluorescent antibody technique for congenital form of the disease (Remington, Remington and Desmonts, Remington et al.). While reactive serologic tests of the conventional type do not differentiate active infection from passive antibody transfer from mother to fetus, the demonstration of specific IgM antibodies in the neonate is diagnostic of congenital toxoplasmosis. With acquired infections, IgM antibodies develop in the first week of infection and peak within a month. Greater than 1:80 is considered to be a high titer and it will generally drop to negative levels within a few months (Krick and Remington).

In addition to the serologic tests described above, Toxoplasma gondii can sometimes be isolated from blood in tissue culture (Chang et al.). With acute acquired toxoplasmosis, lymph node biopsy has been resorted to for diagnostic purposes (Dorfman and Remington). Morphologic changes compatible with toxoplasmosis include reactive follicular hyperplasia associated with irregular clusters of epithelioid histiocytes, located especially in the cortical and paracortical zones.

Treatment

Eyles and Coleman in 1955 demonstrated that sulfadiazine and pyrimethamine (Daraprim) act synergistically to protect mice against experimental toxoplasmosis. The effect of the drugs in human disease remains controversial, although there is some support for benefit in acute, acquired toxoplasmosis. The advisability of treatment with these drugs depends on a variety of circumstances. Treatment of the acquired infection during pregnancy would seem desirable because of the possibility of transplacental infection but is balanced by the possible teratogenic effects of pyrimethamine (Thiersch). Recognition of acquired toxoplasmosis after the fifth or sixth month of pregnancy would warrant a trial with drug therapy. Desmonts and Couvreur,

in France, treated women who exhibited seroconversion during pregnancy with spiramycin, an antibiotic derived from Streptomyces ambofaciens. The authors found fewer infections among offspring of mothers treated with the drug compared to those not treated. They pointed out that the antibiotic probably does not cross the placental barrier and thus is not likely to cure an already infected fetus.

The infected newborn infant with signs of tissue damage is a poor candidate for therapy. In addition, there is concern over the use of sulfadiazine in the newborn infant because of the danger of kernicterus at relatively low bilirubin levels. More important to identify is the asymptomatic or minimally involved child with congenital infection who is susceptible to the development of further tissue damage in the first year of life. Early treatment of this group might significantly reduce morbidity and mortality; however, it is this category of infected infant that is most difficult to identify.

Sulfadiazine and pyrimethamine therapy is indicated in the older individual with acquired toxoplasmosis complicating disorders associated with immunosuppression. Recommended doses include sulfadiazine, 100 mg. per kilogram per day, and pyrimethamine, 1 mg. per kilogram per day but not over 25 mg. per day. Both drugs are believed to adequately penetrate the CSF and brain. Because pyrimethamine is an antifolic acid agent, platelet and white blood cell counts should be performed twice per week during treatment. Except for hematologic suppression, side effects are unusual if the proper dosage schedule is adhered to (TenPas and Abraham). Convulsions have been described as a manifestation of central nervous system toxicity (Grisham).

Primary Amebic Meningoencephalitis

It had been known for many years that Entamoeba histolytica could invade the brain by hematogenous spread from other sites (Lombardo et al.) but free-living soil and water amebae were believed to harmless saprophytes for both animals and man. In 1959, Culbertson and colleagues demonstrated experimentally that amebae belonging to the genus Hartmannella or that of Acanthamoeba were capable of producing an acute, severe meningoencephalitis in mice. This was accomplished by intranasal inoculation of organisms which were shown to invade the brain via the olfactory nerves, resulting in purulent meningitis which was rapidly fatal.

The theoretical possibility of a primary neurologic infection in the human due to the ubiquitous free-living amebae was proved to be a reality in 1964 when the pathological findings of two cases were presented to the Scientific Session of the American Society of Clinical Pathologists (Butt). The following year, Fowler and Carter provided the first published report which included four fatal cases in South Australia of acute pyogenic amebic meningoencephalitis in children. The illnesses in all four were primary in that other viscera were unaffected, and the disease progressed rapidly to death within a few days after onset, and was postulated to result from transmission of the organisms to the brain through the cribriform plate via the olfactory nerves. Free-living amebae of the Hartmannella or Acanthamoeba group were believed to be at fault.

With the appearance of additional publications, a remarkable degree of consistency from case to case became evident. In most instances, the affected patients were previously normal children or young adults; nearly all had fulminating illnesses rapidly leading to death, and in the vast majority, the patient had been swimming or otherwise exposed to stagnant water in some fashion. In unusual cases, exposure to stagnant water was not a factor, but the illness occurred in adults with pre-existent illnesses, including diabetes mellitus (Duma et al. 1978) and chronic alcoholism (Hoffmann et al.). Nearly all authors commented on the probability of transmission of the infection through the nasal mucosa via the olfactory nerves into the brain. In most reports, the cerebrospinal fluid was purulent but without bacterial pathogens, and usually with higher protein and glucose content than is generally found with pyogenic meningitis. In the years since the disease was first recognized, numerous cases have subsequently been identified from widespread parts of the world, including South Australia (Fowler and Carter, Carter), Czechoslovakia (Cerva et al.), Great Britain (Apley et al.), Africa (Bhagwandeen et al.), South America (Martinez et al.), and the United States. In this country, the illness has been identified in Florida (Butt), Texas (Patras and Andujar), Virginia (Duma et al. 1969, Callicott), Pennsylvania (Robert and Rorke), and Louisiana (Hoffmann et al.).

Although the organisms responsible for this disease are clearly free-living amebae that are widely distributed in moist soil and fresh water, the precise classification of the infecting amebae has been confusing. Hartmannella, Acanthamoeba, and Naegleria have all been implicated but the current belief is that the majority of cases of primary amebic meningoencephalitis are caused by members of the genus Naegleria. The case described by Robert and Rorke and those of Martinez et al. are unusual in that the causative organism was demonstrated to be Acanthamoeba species. It is of interest that the clinical course of these patients was more prolonged and was characterized by more focal neurologic abnormalities than in other patients with primary amebic meningoencephalitis. It has been postulated that entrance into the brain of Acanthamoeba species is secondary to metastatic spread from a primary focus in the skin, respiratory tract, or genitourinary system, rather than across the nasal mucosa, as occurs with Naegleria species (Martinez et al.). Also unlike Naegleria infections, those resulting from Acanthamoeba species have notably been in persons with chronic debilitating illnesses or disorders with immunosuppression. In addition, a single case of meningoencephalitis caused by Hartmannella species in an adult has recently been described (Bhagwandeen et al.).

In large part, the controversy over the classification stems from the morphologic similarity of the three organisms. The distinction between them is difficult and especially so in histologic preparations of infected tissues. In tissue, the trophozoites of Naegleria measure approximately 10 to 18 microns, whereas those of Acanthamoeba are somewhat larger. Cysts with a wrinkled double wall in tissue are found only with Acanthamoeba. A distinctive feature of Naegleria is its ability to convert into a flagellate form which can be induced by dilution of the culture with water. In cerebrospinal fluid, the amebae are easily confused with leukocytes but can be identified by an unstained warmed wet preparation. By this method, the trophozoite can be seen to contain a single central or eccentric nucleus with a conspicuous karyosome and characteristic pseudopodia. The wet preparation should be warmed since cooling reduces motility of the organism. By observing a single organism for a minute or so, motility can be detected as the cell undergoes alterations in shape and configuration. Weng et al. advised the addition of a drop of 1 percent cresyl fast violet stain to a drop of cerebrospinal fluid, which aids in visualization of the nucleus by producing a distinct, purple nuclear membrane.

Clinical Manifestations

Primary amebic meningoencephalitis caused by Naegleria species is generally an acute, rapidly progressive disease of children and young adults who had been previously well. Swimming in fresh water one to two weeks before onset of symptoms has been recorded in many cases, and in some instances numerous cases resulted from a common swimming area (Cerva and Novak). The children described by Apley et al. splashed about in a warm mud puddle before onset of the illness and the man reported by Robert and Rorke had worked in his basement two weeks before symptoms began, removing large amounts of water that had collected. The onset of symptoms is usually abrupt and consists of headache, fever, and pharyngitis or symptoms of nasal obstruction or discharge. An occasional complaint in the first day or so is distortion of taste or smell sensation. Headache, vomiting, and fever persist but within two to four days after onset drowsiness, confusion, and neck stiffness develop. Convulsions may occur but have not been pronounced in most cases. Progressive deterioration follows, leading to deep coma but with minimal if any focal neurologic signs. The vast majority of cases have ended fatally one to two weeks after the first symptoms of the disease. Two of the three patients described by Apley and colleagues are exceptional in this regard in that symptoms and signs were milder than expected and recovery occurred.

The peripheral white blood cell count is almost constantly elevated, with a marked increase in polymorphonuclear leukocytes. Some variability in the cerebrospinal fluid findings has occurred, but in most reports the fluid was purulent with a predominance of neutrophils and thus was initially assumed to indicate a bacterial infection. In a few instances, the initial tap early in the illness revealed clear fluid containing a number of erythrocytes along with a modest leukocytic response, findings that might be confused with those of Herpesvirus hominis encephalitis. The protein content is elevated in almost all patients with primary amebic meningoencephalitis, with a range between 100 mg. per 100 ml. and 1000 mg. per 100 ml. The glucose value has been mildly reduced in some cases and normal in others. With wet preparations described above, mobile amebae can be visualized in the cerebrospinal fluid.

Pathology

The significant pathology in almost all reported examples of primary amebic meningoencephalitis has been confined to the nervous system. In the exceptional case of Duma et al. (1969), amebae were cultured from liver, spleen, and lung as well as the brain, and, histologically, acute myocarditis was present although organisms were not found in the heart. On gross observation, the brain shows mild to moderate swelling but usually without internal herniations. A meningeal exudate is generally obvious in the basilar cisterns but is indistinct over the cerebral convexities and is sometimes associated with focal hemorrhages on the surface of the brain. The olfactory bulbs tend to be inflamed, softened, and often adherent to the adjacent cerebral cortex. Microscopically, the purulent meningeal exudate is composed of polymorphonuclear and mononuclear leukocytes with a variable number of amebae. The inflammatory reaction extends to the superficial cortical gray matter, which shows variable degrees of inflammation, neuronal necrosis, hemorrhages, and invasion with amebae, which can be seen with the hematoxylin and eosin stain. The brain stem is also affected by the encephalitic process but shows less inflammatory change than do the cerebral hemispheres. Necrotizing vasculitis is a common feature of amebic meningoencephalitis, and in part accounts for the violent nature of this illness. The pathology in the case described by Jager and Stamm is unusual in that multiple small hemorrhagic abscesses were found in the cerebral hemispheres and cerebellum. The patient was a young adult with Hodgkin's disease treated for several years with immunosuppresive drugs. The causative ameba was not absolutely identified but Hartmannella was suspected because of its size. The adult diabetic reported by Duma et al. (1978) was also unusual in that the brain at autopsy revealed a large frontal lobe abscess and a smaller cerebellar abscess, in addition to diffuse meningitis.

Treatment

Except for the customary supportive measures, such as control of temperature and fluid and electrolyte management, specific therapy in most cases appears to have little influence on the natural course of this illness. Amphotericin B is the drug of choice for Naegleria infections but would be of value only if given early in the course of the illness (Carter). A single case with survival from Naegleria meningoencephalitis has been described from California (Morbidity and Mortality Weekly Reports, Sept. 15, 1978). The patient was a nine-year-old girl treated with intravenous and intrathecal amphotericin B and miconazole, in addition to rifampin. Her recovery was with sequelae. Both amphotericin B and miconazole have been shown to be effective in vitro against Naegleria species, while antimicrobials appear to be less active against Acanthamoeba (Duma and Finley, Lee et al.).

Cerebral Malaria

Malaria is claimed to be the most important parasitic disease of man. It is estimated that 100 million persons are infected with the disease and that one million die from the illness each year (Brown). It is widely distributed in the tropics and subtropics but can now be seen virtually anywhere because of international travel. Man is the only important reservoir of human malaria and acquires the disease by the bite of an infected Anopheles mosquito. The sporozoite inoculated into the human victim enters the liver and becomes the cryptozoite and subsequently the merozoite which ruptures from the liver cell. Invasion of the erythrocyte by the liberated merozoite results in the formation of a ringform, the trophozoite, which evolves into the schizont. With maturation, this form splits into merozoites that are liberated with red cell rupture only to re-enter other erythrocytes to repeat the schizogonic cycle.

Plasmodium falciparum infection is the most common form of malaria and has an incubation period of eight to 20 days. The interval between the infecting mosquito bite and onset of symptoms with vivax infection may be several months, and even longer with ovale and malariae infestations. The initial symptoms are listlessness and headache followed within 12 hours by fever. Rapid elevations of temperature in the young child are sometimes associated with convulsions, even in the absence of specific cerebral involvement by the malarial parasite (Ransome-Kuti). In the first few days of the illness, bouts of fever may be sufficiently prolonged that peaks of temperature elevation almost merge and the characteristic periodicity will not be evident. Eventually, recurrent temperature spikes at 24- to 48-hour intervals become established with falciparum infection. Enlargement of the liver and spleen is not initially present but develops with more prolonged parasitemia. The acute phase of the illness is usually more severe with falciparum malaria and less intense with vivax and quartan infections. The latter illnesses in children assume a more chronic course, with growth failure, lesser grades of fever, anemia, and hepatosplenomegaly. Death in the acute stage, cerebral involvement, and "blackwater fever" are related primarily to infection with Plasmodium falciparum. In addition to infection acquired in the usual fashion, malaria can be a congenital infection manifested by anemia, jaundice, and hepatosplenomegaly, thus being similar to other better known transplacentally transmitted infections (Thompson et al.).

Cerebral malaria is one of the most serious complications of the disease and is claimed to have a mortality rate of approximately 33 percent (Marsden and Bruce-Chwatt). It occurs in higher frequency in persons unimmune to this parasitic condition and, for this reason, is more common in children between six months and four years of age or in adults ordinarily foreign to endemic areas who have their first exposure during temporary residence in a malarial zone. Conversely, protection against cerebral malaria is afforded by possession of the gene for sickle cell trait or disease (Colbourn and Edington), although the precise mechanism accounting for this is unclear. The frequency of cerebral involvement in cases with falciparum malaria is difficult to judge but military statistics suggest it is in the range of 1 to 2 percent (Daroff et al.).

Cerebral malaria in children usually has an abrupt and dramatic onset which occurs in the first few days of the acute illness. After one to several days of headache and fever, the child either exhibits a disturbance in state of responsiveness or suddenly develops prolonged and repeated generalized convulsions. When neurologic abnormalities precede convulsions, they usually consist of disorientation, confusion, obtundation, tremulousness, or other types of movement disorders. Meningeal signs are not expected and strictly focal neurologic deficits are not common but may occur. Death follows episodes of status epilepticus with hyperthermia. With treatment, complete recovery is possible, even in children in deep coma at the peak of the illness. One of the remarkable features of cerebral malaria is that survivors are free of residual disability in most cases, although exceptions do occur (Daroff et al., Simpson and Sagebiel). The cerebrospinal fluid is usually normal except for the possibility of an increased pressure. A mild lymphocytic response is observed in the minority of cases.

The neuropathology of cerebral malaria consists of generalized mild cerebral edema in addition to petechial hemorrhages, especially in the white matter of the cerebrum and cerebellum (Rigdon and Fletcher). Venous congestion is usual with endothelial proliferation and occlusion of some small vessels with parasitized erythrocytes. Endothelial injury of small vessels, especially capillaries, is followed by perivascular necrosis and extensive glial proliferation in the affected region (Schmid). Cerebral dysfunction is attributed to vascular compromise, in addition to associated factors such as anemia and hyperthermia. Toro and Roman have suggested that the cerebral vasculopathy seen only with Plasmodium falciparum is most likely provoked by the formation of circulating antigen-antibody complexes, analogous to the glomerular basement membrane lesion in cases of malarial nephrotic syndrome.

Treatment of cerebral malaria is considered to be a medical emergency (Jelliffe) and includes supportive measures such as correcting anemia, reducing fever, and controlling convulsions. Dexamethasone has been advised by Toro and Roman because of the possible immune aspects of the vascular injury. Antimalarial therapy that is recommended for this crisis includes chloroquine and quinine administered as soon as possible after the presumptive diagnosis is made. Chloroquine is given by slow intravenous injection in a dose of 0.5 mg. per kilogram. Thereafter, it is given in a daily dose of 5 mg. per kilogram by intramuscular injection. The low initial intravenous dose is because of the danger of shock or convulsions that can be precipitated with chloroquine administered via this route. Once improvement is evident, parenteral therapy is stopped and chloroquine is continued by nasogastric tube or oral administration. Some authors advise the combination of chloroquine and quinine for cerebral malaria but the danger of massive hemolysis with hemoglobinuria is enhanced if quinine is added. Quinine can be given orally or through a nasogastric tube in a dose of 20 mg. per kilogram per day.

REFERENCES

Abell, C., and Holland, P.: Acute toxoplasmosis complicating leukemia. Diagnosis by bone marrow aspiration. Am. J. Dis. Child. 118:782–787, 1969.

Altshuler, G.: Toxoplasmosis as a cause of hydranencephaly. Am. J. Dis. Child. 125:251–252, 1973.

Anderson, D. C., Greenwood, R., Fishman, M., and Kagan, I. G.: Acute infantile hemiplegia with cerebrospinal fluid eosinophilic pleocytosis: An unusual case of visceral larva migrans. J. Pediat. 86:247–249, 1975.

Annual Summary—1972. Trichinosis surveillance. Center for Disease Control. Aug. 1973. Public Health Service.

Apley, J., Clarke, S. K. R., Roome, A. P. C. H., Sandry, S. A., Saygi, G., Silk, B., and Warhurst, D. C.: Primary amoebic meningoencephalitis in Britain. Brit. Med. J. 1:596–599, 1970.

Arana-Iniguez, R., and Julian, J. S.: Hydatid cysts of the brain. J. Neurosurg. 12:323–335, 1955.

Aur, R. J. A., Pratt, C. B., and Johnson, W. W.: Thiabendazole in visceral larva migrans. Am. J. Dis. Child. 121:226–229, 1971.

Bain, A. D., Bowie, J. H., Flint, W. F., Beverley, J. K. A., and Beattie, C. P.: Congenital toxoplasmosis simulating haemolytic disease of the newborn. J. Obstet. Gynaec. Brit. Emp. 63:826–832, 1956.

Beautyman, W., and Woolf, A. L.: An ascaris larva in the brain in association with acute anterior poliomyelitis. J. Path. Bact. 63:635–647, 1951.

Beaver, P. C., Snyder, C. H., Carrera, G. M., Dent, J. N., and Lafferty, J. W.: Chronic eosinophilia due to visceral larva migrans. Pediatrics 9:7–19, 1952.

Becker, B. J. P., and Jacobson, S.: Infestation of the human brain with coenurus cerebralis. Lancet 2:198–202, 1951.

Bertoni, J. M., von Loh, S., and Allen, R. J.: The Aicardi syndrome. Report of 4 cases and review of the literature. Ann. Neurol. 5:475–482, 1979.

Beshear, J. R., and Hendley, J. O.: Severe pulmonary involvement in visceral larva migrans. Am. J. Dis. Child. 125:599–600, 1973.

Bhagwandeen, S. B., Carter, R. F., Naik, K. G., and Levitt, D.: A case of Hartmannellid amebic meningoencephalitis in Zambia. Am. J. Clin. Path. 63:483–492, 1975.

Bickerstaff, E. R., Small, J. M., and Woolf, A. L.: Cysticercosis of the posterior fossa. Brain 79:622–634, 1956.

Bird, A. C., Smith, J. L., and Curtin, V. T.: Nematode optic neuritis. Am. J. Ophthal. 69:74–77, 1970.

Bird, A. V.: Acute spinal schistosomiasis. Neurology 14:647–656, 1964.

Blankfein, R. J., and Chirico, A. M.: Cerebral schistosomiasis. Neurology 15:957–967, 1965.

Bouree, P., Bouvier, J. B., Passeron, J., Galanaud, P., and Dormont, J.: Outbreak of trichinosis near Paris. Brit. Med. J. 1:1047–1049, 1979.

Brown, D. H.: Ocular Toxocara canis. Part II. Clinical review. J. Pediat. Ophthal. 7:182–191, 1970.

Brown, H. W.: Basic Clinical Parasitology, 3rd Edition. Appleton-Century-Crofts, New York, 1969.

Bunnag, T., Comer, D. S., and Punyagupta, S.: Eosinophilic myeloencephalitis caused by Gnathostoma spinigerum. Neuropathology of nine cases. J. Neurol. Sci. 10:419–434, 1970.

Butt, C. G.: Primary amoebic meningoencephalitis. Presented at joint annual meeting of American Society of Clinical Pathologists and College of American Pathologists. Bal Harbour, Florida. Oct. 16–24, 1964.

Butt, C. G.: Primary amebic meningoencephalitis. New Eng. J. Med. 274:1473–1476, 1966.

Cabieses, F., Vallenas, M., and Landa, R.: Cysticercosis of the spinal cord. J. Neurosurg. 16:337–341, 1957.

Callicott, J. H., Jr.: Amebic meningoencephalitis due to free-living amebas of the Hartmannella (Acanthamoeba)-Naegleria group. Am. J. Clin. Path. 49:84–91, 1968.

Campbell, W., and Blair, L.: Chemotherapy of Trichinella spiralis infections (a review). Exp. Parasitol. 35:304–334, 1974.

Carey, R. M., Kimball, A. C., Armstrong, D., and Lieberman, P. H.: Toxoplasmosis. Clinical experiences in a cancer hospital. Am. J. Med. 54:30–38, 1973.

Carrea, R., Dowling, E., Jr., and Guevara, J. A.: Surgical treatment of hydatid cysts of the central nervous system in the pediatric age (Dowling's technique). Child's Brain 1:4–21, 1975.

Carter, R. F.: Primary amoebic meningo-encephalitis: Clinical, pathological and epidemiological features of six fatal cases. J. Path. Bact. 96:1–25, 1968.

Carter, R. F.: Sensitivity to amphotericin B of a Naegleria sp. isolated from a case of primary amoebic meningoencephalitis. J. Clin. Path. 22:470–474, 1969.

Cerva, L., and Novak, K.: Amoebic meningoencephalitis: sixteen fatalities. Science 160:92, 1968.

Cerva, L., Zimak, V., and Novak, K.: Amoebic meningoencephalitis. A new amoeba isolate. Science 163:575–576, 1969.

Chang, C., Stulberg, C., Bollinger, R. O., Walker, R., and Brough, A. J.: Isolation of Toxoplasma gondii in tissue culture. J. Pediat. 81:790–791, 1972.

Char, D. F. B., and Rosen, L.: Eosinophilic meningitis among children in Hawaii. J. Pediat. 70:28–35, 1967.

Chevis, R. A. F.: Mebendazole in surgical and non-operative management of hydatid disease. Med. J. Aust. 2:580, 1976.

Colbourn, M. J., and Edington, G. M.: Sickling and malaria in the Gold Coast. Brit. Med. J. 1:784, 1956.

Couvreur, J., and Desmonts, G.: Congenital and maternal toxoplasmosis. A review of 300 congenital cases. Dev. Med. Child Neurol. 4:519–530, 1962.

Couvreur, J., Desmonts, G., and Girre, J. Y.: Congenital toxoplasmosis in twins. A series of 14 pairs of twins: Absence of infection in one twin in two pairs. J. Pediat. 89:235–240, 1976.

Culbertson, C. G., Smith, J. W., Cohen, H. K., and Minner, J. R.: Experimental infection of mice and monkeys by Acanthamoeba. Am. J. Path. 35:185–197, 1959.

Dalessio, D. J., and Wolff, H. G.: Trichinella spiralis infection of the central nervous system. Report of a case and review of the literature. Arch. Neurol. 4:407–417, 1961.

Daroff, R. B., Deller, J. J., Jr., Kastl, A. J., Jr., and Blocker, W. W., Jr.: Cerebral malaria. J.A.M.A. 202:679–682, 1967.

Davis, M. J., Cilo, M., Plaitakis, A., and Yahr, M. D.: Trichinosis: Severe myopathic involvement with recovery. Neurology 26:37–40, 1976.

Desmonts, G., and Couvreur, J.: Congenital toxoplas-

mosis. A prospective study of 378 pregnancies. New Eng. J. Med. 290:1110–1116, 1974.

Desmonts, G., Couvreur, J., Alison, F., Baudelot, J., Gerbeaux, J., and Lelong, M.: Etude epidemiologique sur la toxoplasmose: de l'influence de la cuisson des viandes de boucherie sur la frequence de l'infection humaine. Rev. Franc. Etudes Clin. Biol. 10:952–958, 1965.

Doege, T. C., Thienprasit, P., Headington, J. T., Pongprot, B., and Tarawanich, S.: Trichinosis and raw bear meat in Thailand. Lancet 1:459–461, 1969.

Dorfman, R. F., and Remington, J. S.: Value of lymphnode biopsy in the diagnosis of acute acquired toxoplasmosis. New Eng. J. Med. 289:878–881, 1973.

dos Santos, J. G.: Toxoplasmosis. A historical review, direct diagnostic microscopy, and report of a case. Am. J. Clin. Path. 63:909–915, 1975.

Duma, R. J., Ferrell, H. W., Nelson, E. C., and Jones, M. M.: Primary amebic meningoencephalitis. New Eng. J. Med. 281:1315–1323, 1969.

Duma, R. J., and Finley, R.: In vitro susceptibility of pathogenic Naegleria and Acanthamoeba species to a variety of therapeutic agents. Antimicrob. Agents Chemother. 10:370–376, 1976.

Duma, R. J., Helwig, W. B., and Martinez, A. J.: Meningoencephalitis and brain abscess due to free-living amoeba. Ann. Intern. Med. 88:468–473, 1978.

Epstein, E., Proctor, N. S. F., and Heinz, H. J.: Intraocular coenurus infestation. S. Afr. Med. J. 33:602–604, 1959.

Evers, L. B.: Manifestations of trichinosis in central nervous system: report of a case with larvae in spinal fluid. Arch. Intern. Med. 63:949, 1939.

Eyles, D. E., and Coleman, N.: Evaluation of curative effects of pyrimethamine and sulfadiazine, alone and in combination, on experimental mouse toxoplasmosis. Antibiot. Chemother. 5:529–539, 1955.

Fair, J. R.: Congenital toxoplasmosis—diagnostic importance of chorioretinitis. J.A.M.A. 168:250–253, 1958.

Fair, J. R.: Congenital toxoplasmosis. Chorioretinitis as the only manifestation of the disease. Am. J. Ophthal. 46:135–154, 1958.

Fair, J. R.: Congenital toxoplasmosis. III. Ocular signs of the disease in state schools for the blind. Am. J. Ophthal. 48:165–172, 1959.

Fair, J. R.: Congenital toxoplasmosis. IV. Case finding using the skin test and ophthalmoscope in state schools for mentally retarded children. Am. J. Ophthal. 48:813–819, 1959.

Feldman, H. A.: Toxoplasmosis. New Eng. J. Med. 279:1370–1375, 1431–1437, 1968.

Firemark, H. M.: Spinal cysticercosis. Arch. Neurol. 35:250–251, 1978.

Florez, G., Sanchez, C., and Albala, F.: Immunological diagnosis of echinococcosis. Child's Brain. 4:189–194, 1978.

Fowler, M., and Carter, R. F.: Acute pyogenic meningitis probably due to Acanthamoeba sp.: a preliminary report. Brit. Med. J. 2:740–742, 1965.

Frenkel, J. K.: Pathogenesis, diagnosis and treatment of human toxoplasmosis. J.A.M.A. 140:369–377, 1949.

Frenkel, J. K., Dubey, J. P., and Miller, N. L.: Toxoplasma gondii in cats: Fecal stages identified as coccidian oocysts. Science 167:893–896, 1970.

Garcia, A. G. P.: Congenital toxoplasmosis in two successive sibs. Arch. Dis. Childh. 43:705–710, 1968.

Garnham, P. C. C., Baker, J. R., and Bird, R. G.: Fine structure of cystic form of Toxoplasma gondii. Brit. Med. J. 1:83–84, 1962.

Ghatak, N. R., Poon, T. P., and Zimmerman, H. M.: Toxoplasmosis of the nervous system in the adult. Arch Path. 89:337–348, 1970.

Glasser, L., and Delta, B. G.: Congenital toxoplasmosis with placental infection in monozygotic twins. Pediatrics 35:276–283, 1965.

Gleason, T. H., and Hamlin, W. B.: Disseminated toxoplasmosis in the compromised host. A report of five cases. Arch. Intern. Med. 134:1059–1062, 1974.

Glickman, L., Schantz, P., Dombroske, R., and Cypress, R.: Evaluation of serodiagnostic tests for visceral larva migrans. Am. J. Trop. Med. Hyg. 27:492–498, 1978.

Gray, D. F., Morse, B. S., and Phillips, W. F.: Trichinosis with neurologic and cardiac involvement. Review of the literature and report of three cases. Ann. Intern. Med. 57:230–244, 1962.

Greenlee, J. E., Johnson, W. D., Jr., Campa, J. F., Adelman, L. S., and Sante, M. A.: Adult toxoplasmosis presenting as polymyositis and cerebellar ataxia. Ann. Intern. Med. 82:367–371, 1975.

Griponissiotis, B.: Hydatid cyst of the brain and its treatment. Neurology 7:789–792, 1957.

Grisham, R. S. C.: Central nervous system toxicity of pyrimethamine (Daraprim) in man. Am. J. Ophthal. 54:1119–1121, 1962.

Heiner, D. C., and Kevy, S. V.: Visceral larva migrans; report of the syndrome in 3 siblings. New Eng. J. Med. 254:629, 1956.

Hendrickx, G. F. M., Verhage, J., Jennekens, F. G. I., and van Knapen, F.: Dermatomyositis and toxoplasmosis. Ann. Neurol. 5:393–395, 1979.

Hermos, J. A., Healy, G. R., Schultz, M. G., Barlow, J., and Church, W. G.: Fatal human cerebral coenurosis. J.A.M.A. 213:1461–1464, 1970.

Higashi, K., Aoki, H., Tatebayashi, K., Morioka, H., and Sakata, Y.: Cerebral paragonimiasis. J. Neurosurg. 34:515–528, 1971.

Hoffmann, E. O., Garcia, C., Lundseth, J., McGarry, P., and Coover, J.: A case of primary amebic meningoencephalitis. Light and electron microscopy, and immunohistologic studies. Am. J. Trop. Med. Hyg. 27:29–38, 1978.

Hogan, M. J.: Ocular toxoplasmosis. Trans. Am. Acad. Ophthal. Otolaryn. Jan.–Feb., 7–37, 1958.

Hughes, F. B., Faehnle, S. T., and Simon, J. L.: Multiple cerebral abscesses complicating hepatopulmonary amebiasis. J. Pediat. 86:95–96, 1975.

Huntley, C. C., Costas, M. C., and Lyerly, A.: Visceral larva migrans syndrome. Clinical characteristics and immunologic studies in 51 patients. Pediatrics 36:523–536, 1965.

Jacob, J. C., and Mathew, N. T.: Pseudohypertrophic myopathy in cysticercosis. Neurology 18:767–771, 1968.

Jacobson, E. S., and Jacobson, H. G.: Trichinosis in an immunosuppressed human host. Am. J. Clin. Path. 68:791–794, 1977.

Jager, B. V., and Stamm, W. P.: Brain abscesses caused by free-living amoeba probably of the genus Hartmannella in a patient with Hodgkin's disease. Lancet 2:1343–1345, 1972.

Jelliffe, D. B.: The therapy of cerebral malaria in children. Editorial comment. J. Pediat. 69:483–484, 1966.

Kaya, V., Ozden, B., Turker, K., and Tarcan, B.: Intracranial hydatid cysts. J. Neurosurg. 42:580–584, 1975.

Kean, B. H., and Kimball, A. C.: The complement-fix-

ation test in the diagnosis of congenital toxoplasmosis. Am. J. Dis. Child. 131:21–28, 1977.

Kennedy, F. B., and Rege, V. B.: Trichinosis. Hemiplegia and liver involvement. Arch. Intern. Med. 117:108–112, 1966.

Kim, S. K.: Cerebral paragonimiasis. A report of forty-seven cases. Arch. Neurol. 1:30–38, 1959.

Koeze, T. H., and Klingon, G. H.: Acquired toxoplasmosis. Case with focal neurologic manifestations. Arch. Neurol. 11:191–197, 1964.

Kramer, M. D., and Aita, J. F.: Trichinosis with central nervous system involvement. A case report and review of the literature. Neurology 22:485–491, 1972.

Krick, J. A., and Remington, J. S.: Current concepts in parasitology. Toxoplasmosis in the adult—an overview. New Eng. J. Med. 298:550–553, 1978.

Krogstad, D. J., Juranek, D. D., and Walls, K. W.: Toxoplasmosis. With comments on risk of infection from cats. Ann. Intern. Med. 77:773–778, 1972.

Kuberski, T., and Wallace, G. D.: Clinical manifestations of eosinophilic meningitis due to *Angiostrongylus cantonensis*. Neurology 29:1566–1570, 1979.

Kuper, S., Mendelow, H., and Proctor, N. S. F.: Internal hydrocephalus caused by parasitic cysts. Brain 81:235–242, 1958.

Landells, J. W.: Intramedullary cyst of the spinal cord due to the cestode Multiceps multiceps in coenurus stage, report of a case. J. Clin. Path. 2:61–63, 1949.

Langer, H.: Repeated congenital infection with Toxoplasma gondii. Obstet. Gynec. 21:318–329, 1963.

Latovitzki, N., Abrams, G., Clark, C., Mayeux, R., Ascherl, G., Jr., and Sciarra, D.: Cerebral cysticercosis. Neurology 28:838–842, 1978.

Lee, K. K., Karr, S. L., Jr., Wong, M. M., and Hoeprich, P. D.: In vitro susceptibilities of *Naegleria fowleri* strain HB-1 to selected antimicrobial agents, singly and in combination. Antimicrob. Agents Chemother. 16:217–220, 1979.

Lichtenberg, R., and Vaida, G. A.: Schistosomiasis of the spinal cord. Neurology 27:55–59, 1977.

Lombardo, L., Alonso, P., Arroyo, L. S., Brandt, H., and Mateos, J. H.: Cerebral amebiasis. Report of 17 cases. J. Neurosurg. 21:704–709, 1964.

Lombardo, L., and Mateos, J. H.: Cerebral cysticercosis in Mexico. Neurology 11:824–828, 1961.

Luna, M. A., and Lichtiger, B.: Disseminated toxoplasmosis and cytomegalovirus infection complicating Hodgkin's disease. Am. J. Clin. Path. 55:499–505, 1971.

Mahmoud, A. A.: Schistosomiasis. New Eng. J. Med. 297:1239–1331, 1977.

Manschot, W. A., and Daamen, C. B. F.: Connatal ocular toxoplasmosis. Arch Ophthal. 74:48–54, 1965.

Mansour, S. E. D., and Reese, H. H.: A previously unreported myopathy in patients with schistosomiasis. Neurology 14:355–361, 1964.

Marcial-Rojas, R. A., and Fiol, R. E.: Neurologic complications of schistosomiasis. Review of the literature and report of two cases of transverse myelitis due to S. mansoni. Ann. Intern. Med. 59:215–230, 1963.

Marsden, P. D., and Bruce-Chwatt, L. J.: Cerebral malaria. *In:* Hornabrook, R. W.: Topics on Tropical Neurology. Vol. 12. Contemporary Neurology Series. F. A. Davis Co., Philadelphia, 1975. Pp. 29–74.

Martinez, A. J., Sotelo-Avila, C., Garcia-Tamayo, J., Moron, J. T., Willaert, E., and Stamm, W. P.: Meningoencephalitis due to Acanthamoeba Sp. Pathogenesis and clinico-pathological study. Acta Neuropath. 37:183–191, 1977.

Masur, H., Jones, T. C., Lempert, J. A., and Cherubini, T. D.: Outbreak of toxoplasmosis in a family and documentation of acquired retinochoroiditis. Am. J. Med. 64:396–402, 1978.

McLeod, R., Berry, P. F., Marshall, W. H., Jr., Hunt, S. A., Ryning, F. W., and Remington, J. S.: Toxoplasmosis presenting as brain abscesses. Diagnosis by computerized tomography and cytology of aspirated purulent material. Am. J. Med. 67:711–714, 1979.

Meltzer, R. S., Singer, C., Armstrong, D., Mayer, K., and Knapper, W. J.: Antemortem diagnosis of central nervous system strongyloidiasis. Am. J. Med. Sci. 277:91–98, 1979.

Metzler, M. H., Sahgal, K. K., and Wolff, G. S.: Second degree atrioventricular block in acute trichinosis. Am. J. Dis. Child. 124:598–601, 1972.

Miller, M. J., Seaman, E., and Remington, J. S.: The clinical spectrum of congenital toxoplasmosis: Problems in recognition. J. Pediat. 70:714–723, 1967.

Moore, M. T.: Human Toxocara canis encephalitis with lead encephalopathy. J. Neuropath. Exp. Neurol. 21:201–217, 1962.

Morbidity and Mortality Weekly Reports. Vol. 27, Sept. 15, 1978.

Neefe, L. I., Pinilla, O., Garagusi, V. G., and Bauer, H.: Disseminated strongyloidiasis with cerebral involvement. A complication of corticosteroid therapy. Am. J. Med. 55:832–838, 1973.

Nelson, J. D., McConnell, T. H., and Moore, D. V.: Thiabendazole therapy of visceral larva migrans. A case report. Am. J. Trop. Med. 15:930–933, 1966.

Neumann, C. G., Hilton, C., and Barreda, A.: Acquired toxoplasmosis in a child. Am. J. Dis. Child. 100:117–120, 1960.

Nicholson, D. H., and Wolchok, E. B.: Ocular toxoplasmosis in an adult receiving long-term corticosteroid therapy. Arch. Ophthal. 94:248–254, 1976.

Nicolle, C., and Manceaux, L.: Sur une infection a corps du gondi. C. R. Acad. Sci. (Paris) 147:763–766, 1908.

Nieto, D.: Cysticercosis of the nervous system. Diagnosis by means of the spinal fluid complement fixation test. Neurology 6:725–738, 1956.

Oh, S. J.: Bithionol treatment in cerebral paragonimiasis. Am. J. Trop. Med. 16:585–590, 1967.

Oh, S. J.: Cerebral paragonimiasis. J. Neurol. Sci. 8:27–48, 1968.

Patras, D., and Andujar, J. J.: Meningoencephalitis due to Hartmannella (Acanthamoeba). Am. J. Clin. Path. 46:226–233, 1966.

Pearl, M., Kotsilimbos, D. G., Lehrer, H. Z., Rao, A. H., Fink, H., and Zaiman, H.: Cerebral echinococcosis, a pediatric disease: Report of two cases with one successful five-year follow-up. Pediatrics 61:915–920, 1978.

Pepler, W. J., and Lombaard, C. M.: Spinal cord granuloma due to Schistosoma haematobium. Report of one case. J. Neuropath. Exp. Neurol. 17:656–659, 1958.

Perlmutter, A. D., Edlow, J. B., and Kevy, S. V.: Toxocara antibodies in eosinophilic cystitis. J. Pediat. 73:340–344, 1968.

Perot, P., Lloyd-Smith, D., Libman, I., and Gloor, P.: Trichinosis encephalitis: A study of electroencephalographic and neuropsychiatric abnormalities. Neurology 13:477–485, 1963.

Pinkerton, H., and Henderson, R. G.: Adult toxoplasmosis: A previously unrecognized disease entity simulating the typhus-spotted fever group. J.A.M.A. 116:807–814, 1941.

Punyagupta, S., Juttijudata, P., and Bunnag, T.: Eosin-

ophilic meningitis in Thailand. Clinical studies of 484 typical cases probably caused by Angiostrongylus cantonensis. Am. J. Trop. Med. 24:921–931, 1975.

Queiroz, L. D., Filho, A. P., Callegaro, D., and De Faria, L. L.: Intramedullary cysticercosis. Case report, literature review and comments on pathogenesis. J. Neurol. Sci. 26:61–70, 1975.

Queiroz, L. de S., Nucci, A., Facure, N. O., and Facure, J. J.: Massive spinal cord necrosis in schistosomiasis. Arch. Neurol. 36:517–519, 1979.

Rachon, K., Januszkiewicz, J., and Wehr, H.: Serum proteins in human trichinosis. Am. J. Med. 44:934–938, 1968.

Rakower, J., and Milwidsky, H.: Primary mediastinal echinococcosis. Am. J. Med. 29:73–83, 1960.

Ransome-Kuti, O.: Malaria in childhood. Adv. Pediat. 19:319–340, 1972.

Reddy, P. S., and Satyendran, O. M.: Ocular cysticercosis. Am. J. Ophthal. 57:664–666, 1964.

Remington, J. S.: The present status of the IgM fluorescent antibody technique in the diagnosis of congenital toxoplasmosis. J. Pediat. 75:1116–1124, 1969.

Remington, J. S.: Toxoplasmosis: Recent developments. Ann. Rev. Med. 21:201–218, 1970.

Remington, J. S., and Cavanaugh, E. N.: Isolation of the encysted form of Toxoplasma gondii from human skeletal muscle and brain. New Eng. J. Med. 273:1308–1310, 1965.

Remington, J. S., and Desmonts, G.: Congenital toxoplasmosis. Variability in the IgM-fluorescent antibody response and some pitfalls in diagnosis. J. Pediat. 83:27–30, 1973.

Remington, J. S., Miller, M. J., and Brownlee, I.: IgM antibodies in acute toxoplasmosis: I. Diagnostic significance in congenital cases and a method for their rapid demonstration. Pediatrics 41:1082–1091, 1968.

Reynolds, E. S., Walls, K. W., and Pfeiffer, R. I.: Generalized toxoplasmosis following renal transplantation. Report of a case. Arch. Intern. Med. 118:401–405, 1966.

Rigdon, R. H., and Fletcher, D. E.: Lesions in the brain associated with malaria. Pathologic study on man and on experimental animals. Arch. Neurol. Psychiat. 53:191–198, 1945.

Robert, V. B., and Rorke, L. B.: Primary amebic encephalitis, probably from Acanthamoeba. Ann. Intern. Med. 79:174–179, 1973.

Robertson, J. S.: Toxoplasmosis. Dev. Med. Child Neurol. 4:507–518, 1962.

Robinson, R. G.: Coenurosis of the central nervous system. World Neurol. 3:35–42, 1962.

Rosen, L., Chappell, R., Laqueur, G. L., Wallace, G. D., and Weinstein, P. P.: Eosinophilic meningoencephalitis caused by a metastrongylid lung-worm of rats. J.A.M.A. 179:620–624, 1962.

Ruskin, J., and Remington, J. S.: Toxoplasmosis in the compromised host. Ann. Intern. Med. 84:193–199, 1976.

Sabin, A. B.: Toxoplasmic encephalitis in children. J.A.M.A. 116:801–807, 1941.

Sabin, A. B., and Feldman, H. A.: Dyes as microchemical indicators of a new immunity phenomenon affecting a protozoan parasite (Toxoplasma). Science 108:660–663, 1948.

Sawhney, B. B., Chopra, J. S., Banerji, A. K., and Wahi, P. L.: Pseudohypertrophic myopathy in cysticercosis. Neurology 26:270–272, 1976.

Schmid, A. H.: Cerebral malaria. On the nature and significance of vascular changes. Europ. Neurol. 12:197–208, 1974.

Schochet, S. S.: Human Toxocara canis encephalopathy in a case of visceral larva migrans. Neurology 17:227–229, 1967.

Schultz, T. S., and Ascherl, G. F., Jr.: Cerebral cysticercosis: Occurrence in the immigrant population. Neurosurgery 3:164–169, 1978.

Sexton, R. C., Jr., Eyles, D. E., and Dillman, R. E.: Adult toxoplasmosis. Am. J. Med. 14:366–377, 1953.

Shahin, B., Papadopoulou, Z. L., and Jenis, E. H.: Congenital nephrotic syndrome associated with congenital toxoplasmosis. J. Pediat. 85:366–370, 1974.

Siegel, S. E., Lunde, M. N., Gelderman, A. H., Halterman, R. H., Brown, J. A., Levine, A. S., and Graw, R. G., Jr.: Transmission of toxoplasmosis by leukocyte transfusion. Blood 37:388, 1971.

Simpson, W. M., and Sagebiel, J. L.: Cerebral malaria: A report of 12 cases encountered at U.S. Naval Base Hospital. U.S. Naval Med. Bull. 41:1596–1602, 1943.

Snyder, C. H.: Visceral larva migrans. Ten years' experience. Pediatrics 28:85–91, 1961.

Stern, G. A., and Romano, P. E.: Congenital ocular toxoplasmosis. Possible occurrence in siblings. Arch Ophthal. 96:615–617, 1978.

Stern, H., Elek, S. D., Booth, J. C., and Fleck, D. G.: Microbial causes of mental retardation. The role of prenatal infections with cytomegalovirus, rubella virus, and toxoplasmosis. Lancet 2:443–448, 1969.

Stone, O. J., Stone, C. T., Jr., and Mullens, J. F.: Thiabendazole—probable cure for trichinosis. Report of first case. J.A.M.A. 187:536–538, 1964.

Ström, J.: Toxoplasmosis due to laboratory infection in 2 adults. Acta Med. Scand. 139:244–252, 1951.

Swartzberg, J. E., and Remington, J. S.: Transmission of toxoplasma. Am. J. Dis. Child. 129:777–779, 1975.

Tasker, W. G., and Plotkin, S. A.: Cerebral cysticercosis. Pediatrics 63:761–763, 1979.

TenPas, A., and Abraham, J. P.: Hematological side-effects of pyrimethamine in the treatment of ocular toxoplasmosis. Am. J. Med. Sci. 249:448–453, 1965.

Teutsch, S. M., Juranek, D. D., Sulzer, A., Dubey, J. P., and Sikes, R. K.: Epidemic toxoplasmosis associated with infected cats. New Eng. J. Med. 300:695–699, 1979.

Theologides, A., Osterberg, K., and Kennedy, B. J.: Cerebral toxoplasmosis in multiple myeloma. Ann. Intern. Med. 64:1071–1074, 1966.

Thiersch, J. B.: Effect of certain 2,4-diaminopyridine antagonists of folic acid on pregnancy and rat fetus. Proc. Soc. Exp. Biol. Med. 87:571–577, 1954.

Thompson, D., Pegelow, C., Underman, A., and Powars, D.: Congenital malaria: A rare cause of splenomegaly and anemia in an American infant. Pediatrics 60:209–212, 1977.

Tomiyasu, U., Ramseyer, J. C., and Baker, R. N.: Wernicke-like syndrome with chronic meningitis: A clinical neuropathological study of a patient with cysticercosis. Bull. Los Angeles Neurol. Soc. 31:72–83, 1966.

Toro, G., and Roman, G.: Cerebral malaria. A dissemi-

nated vasculomyelinopathy, Arch. Neurol. 35:271–275, 1978.

Trelles, J. O.: Cerebral cysticercosis. World Neurol. 2:488–494, 1961.

Vietzke, W. M., Gelderman, A. H., Grimley, P. M., and Valsamis, M. P.: Toxoplasmosis complicating malignancy. Experience at the National Cancer Institute. Cancer 21:816–827, 1968.

Vischer, T. L., Bernheim, C., and Engelbrecht, E.: Two cases of hepatitis due to Toxoplasma gondii. Lancet 2:919–921, 1967.

Wakefield, G. S., Carroll, J. D., and Speed, D. E.: Schistosomiasis of the spinal cord. Brain 85:535–552, 1962.

Weitberg, A. B., Alper, J. C., Diamond, I., and Fligiel, Z.: Acute granulomatous hepatitis in the course of acquired toxoplasmosis. New Eng. J. Med. 300:1093–1096, 1979.

Weleber, R. G., Lovrien, E. W., and Isom, J. B.: Aicardi's syndrome. Case report, clinical features, and electrophysiologic studies. Arch Ophthal. 96:285–290, 1978.

Weng, N. K., Wagner, W., and Parker, J. C., Jr.: Primary amebic meningoencephalitis. A potential problem in the Southeastern United States. Southern Med. J. 64:691–694, 1971.

Wilder, H. C.: Nematode endophthalmitis. Trans. Am. Acad. Ophthal. Otolaryng. 55:99, 1950.

Wilkinson, C. P., and Welch, R. B.: Intraocular toxocara. Am. J. Ophthal. 71:921–930, 1971.

Wilson, J. F., Diddams, A. C., and Rausch, R. L.: Cystic hydatid disease in Alaska. A review of 101 autochthonous cases of Echinococcus granulosus infections. Am. Rev. Resp. Dis. 98:1–15, 1968.

Wolf, A., and Cowen, D.: Perinatal infections of the central nervous system. J. Neuropath. Exp. Neurol. 18:191–242, 1959.

Wolf, A., Cowen, D., and Paige, B. H.: Human toxoplasmosis: occurrence in infants as encephalomyelitis: verification by transmission to animals. Science 89:226–227, 1939.

Wolf, A., Cowen, D., and Paige, B. H.: Human toxoplasmic encephalomyelitis: III. A new cause of granulomatous encephalomyelitis due to a protozoan. Am. J. Path. 15:657–694, 1939.

Woodruff, A. W.: Toxocariasis. Brit. Med. J. 3:663–669, 1960.

Woodruff, A. W., Thacker, C. K., and Shah, A. I.: Infection with animal helminths. Brit. Med. J. 1:1001, 1964.

Yii, C-Y., Chen, C-C., Chen, E-R., Hsieh, H-C., Shih, C-C., Cross, J. H., and Rosen, L.: Epidemiologic studies of eosinophilic meningitis in southern Taiwan. Am. J. Trop. Med. 24:447–454, 1975.

Yokogawa, S., and Suemori, S.: An experimental study of the intracranial parasitism of the human lung fluke, Paragonimus westermani. Am. J. Hyg. 1:63–78, 1921.

Zinkham, W. H.: Visceral larva migrans. A review and reassessment indicating two forms of clinical expression: Visceral and ocular. Am. J. Dis. Child. 132:627–633, 1978.

Chapter Twenty-One

SPIROCHETAL INFECTIONS

SYPHILIS

The long and glorious medical history of syphilis contributed much in a descriptive way to our knowledge, but the greatest contributions to our understanding of the disease have evolved since the turn of the present century. The place of origin of the disease has been a topic of debate and dispute since its first recognition. The many theories that were developed by writers of the sixteenth century have been eloquently reviewed by Miller in the Annals of Medical History in 1930. There is general agreement that the illness first appeared in epidemic proportions in Europe in 1495 following the siege of Naples. From Italy, it soon spread throughout Europe and to the British Isles. How it arrived in Naples was the point of greatest controversy but the voyage of Columbus in 1492 has been repeatedly implicated by medical historians. Strong claims and much evidence suggests that sailors aboard the three ships contracted the illness in the West Indies and returned it to Barcelona in 1493 when Columbus presented the discoveries of his trip to the King and Queen of Spain. Among the armies later assembled at Naples, many Spaniards were included in the ranks composed of soldiers of fortune from a number of countries.

The "new disease" became known under many names, one of which was the New Disease. Within five years after its appearance, it is said that the disease had acquired better than 400 designations (Bloch). In France, it was called the Great Pox and Neapolitan Disease, the latter because their countryman had first acquired it in Italy. The Portuguese referred to it as the Spanish Disease and in Russia it was coined the Polish Disease. In England and Scotland, Grandgore was the common designation for over 200 years, and in Germany, the term Bosen Blatten (evil pocks) became popular. In all countries, the traditional name of the maladie in medical circles was Morbus Gallicus. The name syphilis is believed to have been first introduced as a designation for this illness in the title of a poem written in 1521 by Girolamo Fracastoro and published in Venice in 1530. Fracastoro was a physician who achieved international fame as a result of this writing, even though he attributed the origin of the disease "to a malevolent conjunction of the planets" (Montgomery). His poem describes a shepherd named Syphilus who became afflicted by the illness when he rendered sacrificial honors to the King instead of to the Sun, thus provoking the indignation of the Sun God.

The many facets of the disease, which eventually came to be referred to as "the great imitator," gradually unfolded over the following centuries. Syphilis in the newborn infant had been described previously, but it was not until the publication of the essay by Diday in 1858 entitled "On Syphilis in Newborn Children and in Infants at the Breast" that the infantile form of the illness became widely recognized. In 1903, Metchnikoff and Roux were first successful in transmitting syphilis to monkeys, and in 1905, Schaudinn and Hoffmann working in Berlin identified the causative organism to be a spirochete, which they named *Spirochaeta pallida*. One year later, Landsteiner described the dark-field test for detection of the organism, and soon thereafter von Wassermann developed a serologic method for diagnosis of the infection in humans. Documentation that general paresis was a late manifestation of syphilis came in 1913 when Noguchi succeeded in transmitting syphilis to rabbits by inoculation of brain tissue from paretic patients.

In 1910, Dr. Paul Ehrlich introduced arsphenamine (Salvarsan) which replaced the mercurial preparations used since the fifteenth century and subsequently became widely accepted as the drug of choice for treatment of syphilis until penicillin became available more than 30 years later. Arsphenamine was found to be effective in the early stages of syphilis but of limited value in the tertiary stage. Fever therapy by malarial inoculation was introduced by Julius von Wagner-Jauregg in Vienna in 1917 and eventu-

ally achieved wide acclaim around the world leading to the Nobel prize for the discoverer 10 years later. This therapeutic method, also, was subsequently shown to have definite limitations in regard to its effect on the late stages of syphilitic infection. The modern era of treatment of syphilis began in 1943 when Mahoney et al. demonstrated the treponemicidal effect of the little available and then expensive drug, penicillin.

Control of syphilis seemed inevitable following the advent of penicillin therapy, and in the early 1950's a remarkable decline in the incidence of the disease occurred (Fig. 21–1). The infection lost prominence in medical education with deletion of lectures and academic courses concomitant with the decrease in the number of hospitalized syphilitic patients. Syphilis in the newborn infant became so rare that trainees would complete medical school and pediatric residency without having seen a case of congenital syphilis,

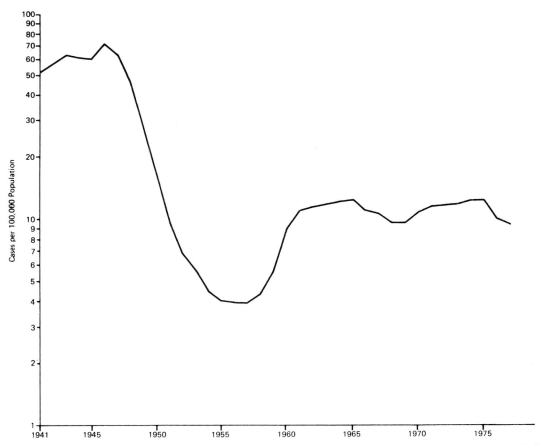

Figure 21–1. Syphilis, primary and secondary. Reported civilian cases per 100,000 population by year in United States, 1941–1977. (From: Morbidity and Mortality Weekly Report, Annual Summary, 1977, Volume 26, No. 53, Sept. 1978.)

and serologic tests often no longer were included in the diagnostic evaluation of a sick neonate. The disease gradually diminished in frequency to reach a low ebb in 1957 but then unexpectedly reappeared and by 1963 the reported cases per year had tripled as compared with six years previously. Although the progressive increase has subsequently been curbed, syphilis has once again become a disease to be taken seriously and pediatricians need to be aware of its potential presence in the neonate.

Natural History of Syphilis

The organism causing syphilis is *Treponema pallidum* which is a member of the order *Spirochaetales* and the family *Treponemataceae*. It is a thin, spiral organism with a length between 5 and 15 microns and can be visualized in the living state by the use of darkfield microscopy. *Treponema pallidum* can pass through mucous membranes or compromised skin and is transmitted in humans by veneral contact in the great majority of cases. The notable exception is transplacental transmission resulting in fetal infection leading to abortion, stillbirth, or congenital syphilis. The untreated disease acquired by veneral contact is remarkably variable from person to person in regard to its natural history. In many, the illness is self-limited after the early stages, but in others it proceeds over the course of many years to lead to devastating consequences in the late or tertiary stage of the disease. Among persons with untreated syphilis, approximately 60 to 70 percent will go through life with little or no physical disability from the disease. Approximately 30 to 35 percent develop significant late lesions, including 17 percent with late benign lesions, 10 percent with cardiovascular syphilitic disease, and 8 to 9 percent with symptomatic neurosyphilis (Termini and Music, Public Health Service Publication No. 1660).

The natural course of the disease is influenced markedly by antibiotic therapy. If adequate treatment is provided after the infection is contracted but before the primary lesion develops, a chancre will probably not appear and the serologic tests will usually remain negative. Treatment during the secondary stage will shorten the duration of the cutaneous lesions and approximately 90 percent will become serologically nonreactive to nontreponemal antigen tests within one to two years. Late disease is usually preventable by treatment in the primary or secondary stages. In congenital syphilis, in which the cutaneous manifestations of the infant represent the secondary stage of the disease, hypersensitivity conditions such as interstitial keratitis and Clutton's joints may still occur subsequently, despite adequate therapy in the neonatal period. Penicillin treatment in the tertiary stage of syphilis is variable in regard to its effects and depends on the degree of tissue damage already sustained. In general, the later in the disease when therapy is administered, the less is the anticipated response. Patients infected for two or three years before receiving treatment may remain seropositive for life.

Primary and Secondary Stages

The primary syphilitic lesion is the chancre, which usually occurs two to four weeks after the infection is acquired and develops at the site of penetration of the spirochetal organisms. In most cases, the chancre is a solitary lesion that varies from one-half to two centimeters in diameter (Fig. 21–2). Its margins are often indurated with a slightly elevated contour and the lesion is usually pain-

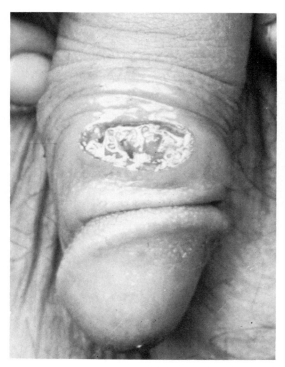

Figure 21–2. Chancre. Primary syphilitic lesion. (Courtesy of Dr. Richard Caplan, Iowa City, Iowa.)

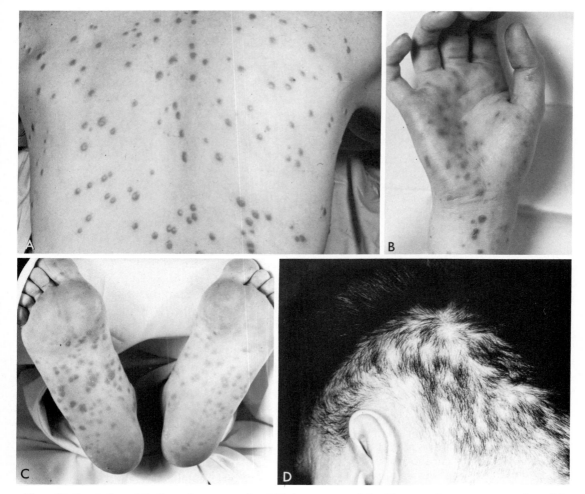

Figure 21–3. *A, B,* and *C,* Secondary stage of syphilis in a young adult with a papulosquamous eruption of the thorax, hands, and feet. Rash on the palms and soles is characteristic of secondary syphilis. *D,* Patchy alopecia in secondary syphilis. (Courtesy of Dr. Richard Caplan, Iowa City, Iowa.)

less. After several weeks, spontaneous healing of the primary lesion without scarring is expected. Within two or three weeks after the appearance of the chancre, serologic tests become positive, indicative of the presence of reagin in serum.

The secondary stage of syphilis makes its appearance within a few weeks up to several months after the primary stage. Cutaneous and mucous membrane lesions of variable type are the hallmark of the secondary stage. Macular and papulosquamous eruptions are most common in adults (Fig. 21–3), but in the newborn, vesicular and bullous lesions more commonly represent the secondary stage. Involvement of the palms and soles is frequently observed, as is patchy alopecia or loss of hair from the eyebrows. Glomerulonephritis has been described on rare occasion in adults with secondary syphilis, with glomerular injury being due to the deposition of treponemal antigen-antibody complexes (Gamble and Reardon). After four to six weeks, the cutaneous manifestations of the secondary stage gradually resolve and eventually disappear. Darkfield examination usually reveals *Treponema pallidum* from specimens from the chancre or from secondary cutaneous lesions. Nontreponemal serologic tests are invariably positive during the secondary stage of the infection, although rarely, when there is excessive production of antibody, undiluted specimens give a negative reaction but testing at higher dilutions give positive test results. This is called the prozone phenomenon and can cause diagnostic error if only undiluted specimens are tested.

Latent Stage

Latent syphilis is a stage of the disease in which the serologic tests are reactive but in the absence of clinical manifestations and with no cerebrospinal fluid abnormalities. In many patients, the disease enters a latent stage following the early symptomatic stages and remains quiescent for the remainder of the individual's life. Latent syphilis has been subdivided into early latent, with a duration up to four years after the secondary stage, and late latent, with a duration of greater than four years. In view of the absence of symptoms and signs, asymptomatic latent syphilis can be diagnosed only by serologic tests and confirmed by treponemal antigen tests.

Late (Tertiary) Neurosyphilis

As mentioned earlier, approximately 8 to 9 percent of patients with untreated syphilis will develop late symptomatic neurosyphilis. The different forms of this tertiary stage include asymptomatic neurosyphilis, meningovascular neurosyphilis, general paresis, and tabes dorsalis. Overlapping of categories can occur in a single patient; for example, clinical signs of both tabes dorsalis and general paresis is referred to as tabo-paresis. Virtually all types of neurosyphilis are preceded by a stage of asymptomatic neurosyphilis, which is usually quite prolonged. During this asymptomatic phase, the patient exhibits no abnormal neurologic signs but the cerebrospinal fluid reveals an increase in mononuclear cells, an increase in protein content, and reactive serologic tests.

An additional late syphilitic lesion is the gumma, which is believed to be the result of "hypersensitivity" to treponemal infection and which can occur in the liver, spleen, bone, intracranial space, and elsewhere. Gummas are generally considered to be relatively benign, although those located intracranially can result in increased intracranial pressure or other signs of a mass lesion. Intracranial gummas may be single or multiple, and most are located over the convexity of the cerebrum or cerebellum with an attachment to the dura. Less often, gummas have been found in the corpus callosum, basal ganglia, brain stem, or in the pituitary gland. They are of tough, rubbery consistency, and can be associated with edema of the adjacent or infiltrated brain tissue. The gumma has considerable collagen within its substance, often with plasma cell and mononuclear cell infiltration, especially at the periphery.

Meningovascular Neurosyphilis. This type of neurosyphilis may assume many forms, resulting in a wide spectrum of clinical neurologic manifestations. Symptomatic meningeal or vascular disease can occur within a year or less after the primary infection or may not develop until many years thereafter. Acute syphilitic meningitis is associated with headache, neck stiffness, and lethargy but with only minimal, if any, febrile response. The cerebrospinal fluid contains a marked increase in mononuclear cells, an increase in protein content, a reduction in the glucose content in some cases, and a positive serologic test for syphilis. It has been described more often in young adults but has also been seen in infants and young children with congenital syphilis (Amesse and Barber). Syphilitic meningitis of a chronic type has also been observed, in which optic atrophy or other cranial nerve deficits become associated with hydrocephalus due to obstruction of cerebrospinal fluid flow at the base of the brain. In the acquired form in the adult, this process is characterized by headache and other increased intracranial pressure signs, but in the infant with congenital syphilis, meningeal proliferative change results in progressive head enlargement.

Chronic syphilitic meningeal inflammation combined with syphilitic vasculitis has occurred mainly in middle-aged and elderly adults and gives rise to a multiplicity of clinical signs, depending on the location and extent of infarcted lesions (Fig. 21–4). Progressive arachnoiditis may produce multiple cranial nerve palsies or a spinal cord syndrome, while occlusive vascular disease can implicate virtually any area of the brain, brain stem, or cerebellum in either acute apoplectic fashion or with chronic, progressive manifestations. Vatz et al. have suggested that syphilitic cerebral angiopathy, as well as certain other non-atherosclerotic vascular lesions, should be suspected in the adult with cerebrovascular disease with angiographic evidence of segmental constriction of the supraclinoid portion of the carotid artery without stenosis of the common carotid or the intracavernous portion of the carotid artery. Syphilitic meningeal involvement can also be associated with an inflammatory myelitis, with clinical signs which include a progressive spastic paraparesis, sensory disturbances, and

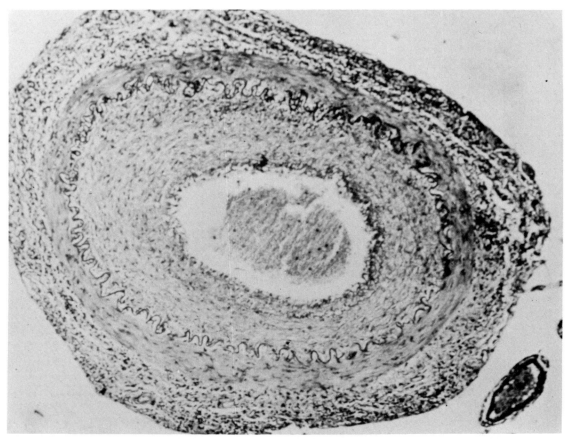

Figure 21–4. Meningovascular neurosyphilis. Syphilitic arteritis with intimal proliferation and inflammatory infiltrate in the adventitia.

neurogenic bladder dysfunction (Fisher and Poser).

Tabes Dorsalis. Tabes dorsalis is a tertiary form of neurosyphilis in which there is atrophy of the dorsal roots and degeneration with demyelination of the posterior columns of the spinal cord. The usual elapse of time between the primary infection and first manifestations of tabes is five to 20 years, although both shorter or longer incubation periods have been described. The pathogenesis of this condition remains unestablished but most investigators have favored the postulate that the primary insult is an inflammatory process within the dorsal rootlets and that dorsal column involvement represents secondary degeneration.

Ataxia is the most characteristic feature of the disease but is not invariably present and causes only mild disability in some. Tabetic ataxia is largely the result of proprioceptive loss and is most profound in the lower extremities. Such patients often have a stagger-

ing wide-based gait in the daytime but are notably more incapacitated in the dark when visual clues compensate less well for proprioceptive dysfunction. Once developed, ataxia can either retain a stable course or relentlessly progress to the point that ambulation becomes impossible. Diminished to absent deep reflexes are customary in the extremities and associated with a decrease in muscle tone, sometimes of profound degree. Loss of the quadriceps stretch reflex in the tabetic patient is referred to as Westphal's sign.

The most notable sensory deficits are those of position and vibration in the distal lower extremities, correlating with the sensory ataxia that is classically part of the disease. Patchy areas of decreased pain and touch sensation, referred to as Hitzig's zones, are also commonly found. Absence of pain on forceful squeezing of the Achilles tendon in the tabetic is known as Abadie's sign. When sensory denervation is severe, articular surfaces of weight-bearing joints become insen-

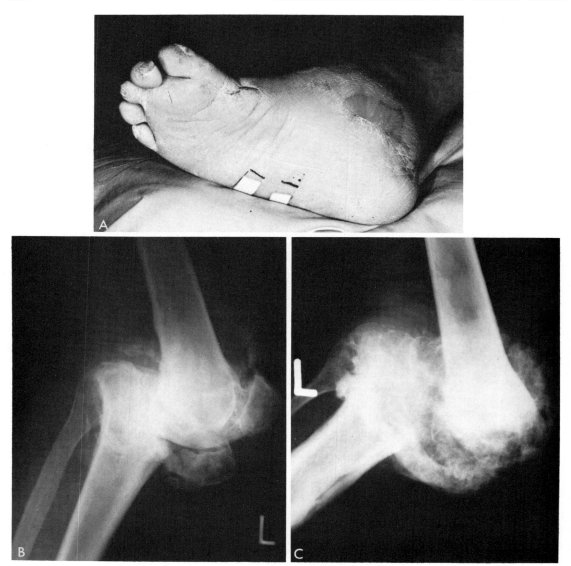

Figure 21–5.   Neuropathic arthropathy. *A,* Charcot joint in a tabetic adult. Deformity of the ankle is associated with dystrophic skin and toenail changes. *B,* Charcot arthropathy of moderate severity affecting the left knee. *C,* The same joint at a later stage showing pronounced joint deformity with destruction of the distal femur and proximal tibia, and marked soft tissue swelling.

sitive and repeated, unrecognized trauma gives rise to neuropathic arthropathy referred to as Charcot joints (Beetham et al.) (Fig. 21–5). The knees and ankles are most often affected but the spine or large joints of the upper limbs can also be involved. In the early stages, the Charcot joint is sometimes warm to palpation and distended by synovial effusion. In the advanced stage, profound joint deformity becomes evident on gross observation and is best demonstrated by roentgenographic examination. Charcot joints have been best known in relation to tabes dor-

salis but, in children, have also been observed with syringomyelia, leprosy, congenital sensory neuropathies, and congenital indifference to pain. Analogous trophic changes of the skin in tabes likewise result from repeated traumatic insults to denervated areas. The end result is a non-healing, perforating ulcer referred to as mal perforans, which is a painless lesion usually located on the weight-bearing surface of one foot.

Tabetic pains are often an early manifestation of tabes dorsalis and, in some cases, precede other signs more diagnostic of the disorder. Pains are usually intermittent, lancinating or lightning-like, and may be located in the limbs or on the trunk. The severity is variable but in an occasional patient the frequency and intensity of tabetic pain are of such magnitude that it becomes disabling. Attacks of visceral pain in the tabetic patient are called tabetic crises and have been described in only about 10 percent of patients with this type of neurosyphilis. The best known are the gastric crises consisting of abrupt onset of severe epigastric pain with recurrent vomiting. Laryngeal crises are less common and are manifested by paroxysms of laryngeal pain and explosive coughing.

Ocular signs are common in tabes dorsalis but can also be seen in any form of late neurosyphilis. Extraocular muscle palsies, ptosis, primary optic atrophy, or visual field defects secondary to vascular occlusive disease may occur in neurosyphilis of any type. Syphilitic optic atropy associated with progressive loss of vision is a common presenting manifestation of neurosyphilis and, in many cases, is the only clinical feature of the disease. The best known and most common type of ocular dysfunction in tabes is the Argyll Robertson pupil described by Douglas Argyll Robertson in 1869. Argyll Robertson pupils are small, irregular pupils that react poorly if at all to light but with preservation of the miotic response to near stimulus. The site of involvement giving rise to Argyll Robertson pupils has been debated for years, with some authors favoring a tectal or pretectal localization and others preferring to place the lesion in the ciliary reflex fibers of the iris itself. Argyll Robertson pupils have their closest association with tabes dorsalis but may be seen with other types of neurosyphilis or even as the only neurologic manifestation of late syphilitic disease. Similar pupillary abnormalities have been described with tectal neoplasms, following encephalitis, or in chronic alcoholics.

Juvenile tabes dorsalis, or tabes complicating congenital syphilis, has been considered one of the rarest forms of late neurosyphilis (Rosenbaum). In past years when congenital syphilis was more common, it was estimated that there were approximately ten cases of juvenile paresis for each case of juvenile tabes dorsalis (Parker). In addition, it was observed that a number of patients who developed tabes dorsalis in the adolescent years subsequently developed progressive dementia leading to the diagnosis of tabo-paresis. Authors also noted that patients with juvenile tabes appeared to have fewer ataxic disturbances than their adult counterpart and that the usual early signs included lightning pains, urinary incontinence, and progressive optic atrophy.

General Paresis. This late form of neurosyphilis develops 15 to 20 years after the primary infection is acquired, is more common in males than females, and is usually gradually progressive ending in death in two to 10 years after onset unless the course is interrupted by penicillin therapy. The disease represents a chronic syphilitic meningoencephalitis in which a variable number of spirochetes can be demonstrated in scattered fashion within the cortical gray matter. The pathology of the disease on gross inspection includes thickening and opacification of meninges, cerebral cortical atrophy, and granular ependymitis. Microscopically, one sees cortical perivascular infiltration with lymphocytes and plasma cells, in addition to degenerative neuronal changes. One of the most characteristic histopathologic alterations is that involving the microglia which become large and elongated and are referred to as rod-cells. Iron deposits in the brain have also been said to be characteristic of this type of neurosyphilis, although the source of iron granules is unclear.

Clinically, general paresis presents in the form of a progressive dementia, often associated with one of a variety of psychiatric syndromes. In addition to memory disturbances and decline in judgment, some paretic patients exhibit euphoria, depression, delusions, or hallucinations. A variety of neurologic signs may accompany the defects of higher intellectual function, such as pupillary abnormalities, dysarthria, movement disorders, and enhanced deep reflexes. A variation of the syndrome in which convulsions and focal neurologic signs are engrafted upon the progressive dementing features is referred to as "Lissauer's general paralysis."

The natural history of the untreated patient with general paresis is usually one of slow, progressive decline of many functional areas, eventually leading to diffuse spasticity and profound retardation. Treatment with penicillin in the early stages may reverse the process entirely, although some patients will continue to worsen despite adequate therapy (Hooshmand et al.).

Juvenile syphilitic encephalitis as a late complication of congenital syphilis was never considered common and has been recognized only with extreme rarity in recent years (Fig.

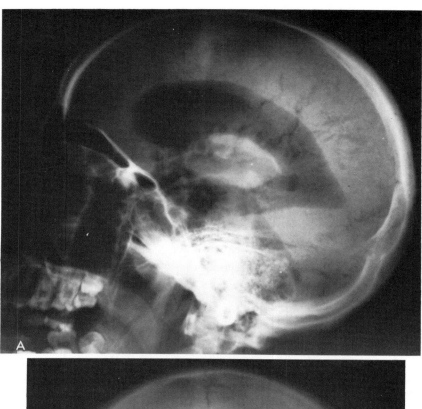

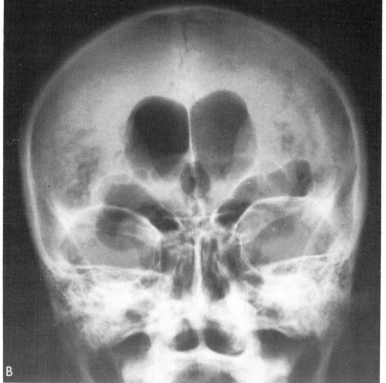

Figure 21–6.   Juvenile syphilitic encephalitis. *A* and *B,* Pneumoencephalogram of a 16-year-old boy with intellectual deterioration beginning at approximately 4 years of age. The illness was characterized by dementia, impulsive and agitated behavior, generalized convulsions, ataxia, and bruxism. Air study demonstrates a moderate degree of generalized cerebrocortical atrophy.

21–6). Cases identified in the past usually became evident in the second decade of life, but, in some, progressive dementia was observed as early as four or five years of age. As with juvenile tabes, patients with juvenile paresis commonly have stigmata of congenital syphilis.

The cerebrospinal fluid in the patient with general paresis is usually abnormal, with an increase in mononuclear cells, an increased protein content, and alteration in gamma globulin content reflected by a first-zone rise in the colloidal gold curve. Cerebrospinal fluid nontreponemal serologic tests are usually, but not always, positive in such cases while the fluorescent treponemal antibody absorption (FTA-ABS) test is virtually always positive.

Laboratory Diagnosis of Syphilis

The darkfield examination is a method of demonstration of spirochetes obtained from surface lesions in the early stages of a syphilitic infection. The test may not be reliable with mouth lesions, however, because other treponemes which are morphologically similar to *Treponema pallidum* can be part of the normal mouth flora. Darkfield examination is performed by obtaining a specimen from an infected lesion, which is then placed on a glass slide, covered with a cover slip, and examined under a darkfield microscope. The latter employs a darkfield condenser which obstructs central light rays but directs light from the periphery upon the object under examination. The result is that the object under study is projected brightly against a dark background. With this method, *Treponema pallidum* is recognized both by its structure and its characteristic motility, consisting of a rotatory action along its long axis in addition to gentle undulations from side to side.

Serologic Tests for Syphilis

Nontreponemal Antigen Tests. Human infection with *Treponema pallidum* results in the eventual production of antibodies of two fundamental types. The first are nonspecific antibodies, or reagins, which usually appear in serum four to six weeks after the infection is acquired. Laboratory tests for reagin are performed with extracts of normal tissue and thus are not specific for syphilitic infection. Such nontreponemal antigen tests are none-

theless valuable because of their wide availability and relative accuracy. The original Wassermann test was a complement fixation reaction in which extract of syphilitic liver tissue was used as the antigen, although normal liver served equally well. As such, the Wassermann test is no longer performed.

The most commonly used nontreponemal antigen tests currently are the Venereal Disease Research Laboratory test (VDRL) and the Kolmer complement fixation test (Sparling). In general, laboratories report the test as the highest dilution of the patient's serum that still gives a positive reaction. Approximately 75 to 80 percent of patients will develop reactive VDRL tests within one to three weeks after the development of a chancre and almost all patients are serologically reactive during the secondary stage. Excessive production of antibody during this stage may give rise to the prozone phenomenon in which a negative reaction occurs with undiluted serum but the reaction becomes positive with further serum dilutions. It is estimated that this response is encountered in 1 to 2 percent of patients with secondary syphilis (Spangler et al.). With adequate treatment of seropositive syphilis in the primary or secondary stage, the VDRL will subsequently decline in titer and will eventually become negative. False positive serum VDRL reactions are sufficiently frequent that the test should never be the only confirmatory method which establishes the diagnosis.

The nontreponemal antigen tests on serum have greater limitations in the diagnosis of tertiary neurosyphilis in which they are often

Table 21–1. Laboratory Tests for Syphilis

A. Nontreponemal antigen tests
  Flocculation (VDRL, Kahn, Kline)
  Complement fixation (Kolmer)

B. Treponemal antigen tests
  Complement fixation
    Reiter protein complement fixation
    Treponema pallidum complement fixation
  Agglutination
    Microhemagglutination (MHA-TP)
  Immobilization
    Treponema pallidum immobilization (TPI)
  Immunofluorescence
    Fluorescent treponemal antibody
      absorption (FTA-ABS)
    IgM-Fluorescent treponema antibody
      absorption (IgM-FTA-ABS)

nonreactive (Hooshmand et al., Smith et al.). The possibility of neurosyphilis on the basis of clinical signs in the face of negative non-treponemal tests, in addition to the biological false-positive serologic reaction, have become two of the main indications for use of the more specific treponemal antigen tests.

Treponemal Antigen Tests. The second type of antibodies that develop in human syphilitic infection are specific antitrepone-mal antibodies which provide the basis for the more recently developed treponemal antigen tests. These tests use as an antigen one of a variety of preparations of the treponeme it-self. The treponemal antigen tests are highly specific of past or present syphilitic infection and false positives are most unusual.

The first treponemal test was developed in 1949 by Nelson and Mayer and is called the *Treponema pallidum* immobilization (TPI) test. The test is expensive and technically difficult and also is invalidated by the presence of an-tibiotics in the serum which inactivate trepo-nemes. The Reiter-protein complement fix-ation (RPCF) test was subsequently devised but was found to be of limited value because it was often nonreactive in patients with late syphilitic disease. The antigen used in this test is a nonpathogenic Reiter strain of trepo-neme.

The most valuable recent developments re-garding specific treponemal tests utilize im-munofluorescent methods. After several modifications, the fluorescent treponemal an-tibody absorption test (FTA-ABS) was re-fined and now is the most widely used trepo-nemal antigen test. The advantages of the test are that it is reactive in most cases of syphilis, even in the primary and tertiary stages, false positive reactions are infrequent, and it has become widely available in most state health department laboratories. Studies have shown that the serum FTA-ABS test is positive in 85 percent of patients with primary syphilis and in 95 to 99 percent of those with all other forms (Deacon et al.) (Table 21–2). Among 163 patients who had been treated more than 10 years earlier with penicillin for latent syphilis or neurosyphilis, Förström and Las-sus found that 92 percent of those with latent syphilis and 96 percent of neurosyphilitic pa-tients were still FTA-ABS reactive while the VDRL was positive in only approximately 60 percent. Investigations have indicated that the FTA-ABS test becomes positive in the early stages of syphilis and remains reactive for many years, even in those who receive treatment. Thus, a positive FTA-ABS test in-dicates that the patient has had syphilis at some time but does not necessarily mean that the disease is active or that treatment is nec-essary. The microhemagglutination test (MHA-TP) is technically simpler than the FTA-ABS test and is as sensitive as the latter for all stages of the disease except the pri-mary stage (Bracero et al.). It has a slightly higher rate of false positive reactions than the FTA-ABS, and has not been applied to CSF examination sufficiently to allow logical inter-pretation.

When an asymptomatic patient is discov-ered to have a reactive serum FTA-ABS test, it is commonplace to examine the cerebro-spinal fluid prior to the initiation of antibiotic therapy. This is done for the purpose of ex-cluding the presence of asymptomatic neu-

Table 21–2.   Comparative Sensitivity of Nontreponemal and Treponemal Tests in Untreated Syphilis*

	APPROXIMATE PERCENT OF SERUMS EXPECTED TO GIVE REACTIVE TEST RESULTS				
	Nontreponemal Tests		*Treponemal Tests*		
STAGE	*VDRL Slide*	*Kolmer*	*FTA-200*	*TPI*	*FTA-ABS*
Primary	76	65	40	53	86
Secondary	100	100	95	98	100
Early Latent	95	95	90	94	99
Late Latent	72	65	68	89	96
Late (Tertiary)	70	60	77	93	97

*From: Public Health Service Publication No. 1660, 1968.

rosyphilis or to indicate the need for periodic CSF examinations following treatment in those with abnormal CSF findings. While the ritual of CSF examination in the asymptomatic individual remains desirable before treatment is begun, the yield of CSF abnormalities in regard to the cell count, protein content, and serologic tests in such persons is quite low (Traviesa et al.). Serologic testing of cerebrospinal fluid has been relied upon for a number of years to provide evidence of the presence or absence of neurosyphilis in asymptomatic patients, and to establish or exclude the diagnosis in the patient with abnormal neurologic signs. Nontreponemal antibody tests on CSF have been considered to be reasonably specific for this purpose with few false positive results but with less than total accuracy in the identification of all cases with neurosyphilis (Burke, Hooshmand et al.). A false positive VDRL on CSF can occur if the specimen is contaminated with seropositive blood from either natural causes or from a traumatic tap. The treponemal antibody tests on CSF (FTA-ABS) have been assumed to be more accurate and have been found by some investigators to be invariably positive in patients with neurosyphilis (Hooshmand et al.). False positive reactions are very infrequent, having occurred in 0.56 percent of specimens in one series (Jaffe et al.). A positive CSF treponemal antibody test in an asymptomatic patient with otherwise normal CSF has been assumed to indicate the presence of asymptomatic neurosyphilis; however, the validity of the concept and the prognostic significance of a positive CSF test in the asymptomatic individual has been questioned by Jaffe and colleagues. These investigators found that the serum titers in such patients with positive CSF tests were usually higher than serum titers in those with negative CSF antibody tests, suggesting the possibility of passive transfer of an immunoglobulin from serum into CSF, which results in a positive test in some cases, perhaps in the absence of neurosyphilitic involvement.

A modification of the FTA-ABS test employs fluorescein-labeled antihuman IgM to detect specific antitreponemal IgM antibodies. This test has been proposed to be useful in the newborn infant as a method to distinguish active infection in an infant from antibody passively transferred from the mother. The value of the procedure has been found to be limited by occasional false positives and a significantly higher rate of occurrence of false negative reactions (Kaufman et al.). The latter are most likely when the fetus has become infected in the later stages of pregnancy.

Congenital Syphilis

Transplacental transmission of syphilis from the mother to the fetus can result in abortion, stillbirth, or active infection in the live neonate, referred to as congenital syphilis. Although congenital syphilis cannot now be considered to be a common disorder, the illness still occurs with sufficient frequency that its possibility should not be disregarded. In some foreign countries, such as South Africa, there persists a high incidence of congenital syphilis among the black population (Rosen and Richardson). In 1960, there were 132 reported infant cases of congenital syphilis in the United States and in 1969 there were 287 cases reported, an increase of better than 100 percent.

Pregnancy beyond the fourth month with the mother in the primary or secondary stage of the disease is more likely to produce fetal death or stillbirth while untreated maternal syphilitic infection subsequent to the secondary stage is more often associated with luetic infection in the newborn infant, which can become symptomatic in one of many forms at variable times after birth. The traditional concept of transplacental transmission of *Treponema pallidum* to the fetus has been that the Langhans cell layer of the placenta provides a temporary barrier protecting the fetus during the first four months of pregnancy. With dissolution of this cell layer at about the sixteenth to eighteenth week of gestation, it has been presumed that the fetus becomes susceptible and remains so for the remainder of the pregnancy. The possibility that this long-held postulate may not be correct is supported by the identification by Harter and Benirschke of spirochetes in tissues of two aborted fetuses of nine and ten weeks' gestational age. The Langhans layer was typically present in both, and in neither was there an inflammatory reaction to the infection. Adequate penicillin treatment of the syphilitic mother in the first four months of pregnancy will prevent fetal infection and, in most cases, treatment of the mother later in pregnancy will bring about cure of the infected fetus. The later in pregnancy one starts treatment, however, the greater are the chances that the infant will subsequently demonstrate certain stigmata of intrauterine-acquired syphilis, even though the active infection is curbed (Fiumara and Lessell).

Clinical Manifestations

Early Stage of Congenital Syphilis. Since *Treponema pallidum* is introduced directly into the fetal circulation by transplacental transmission, there is no primary stage and the lesions present in the infected infant are analogous to those of the secondary stage of syphilis. Most infants with congenital syphilis are normal at birth, although the incidence of prematurity is higher than in the average population. Infants with obvious signs of disease at birth have a poor prognosis for survival, even with antibiotic therapy (Tan). Clinical illness usually appears in the first few weeks or months after birth and may involve one or many different organ systems (Wilkinson and Heller, Woody et al.). In most, the first clinical signs of the disease become apparent between two and eight weeks of age. In others, symptoms are either not recognized or are absent and the disease becomes manifest in the form of late stigmata of congenital syphilis several years later. Some infected infants are first evaluated because of rash or persistent nasal discharge, while others present with anemia, growth failure, or pneumonia. Another common ini-

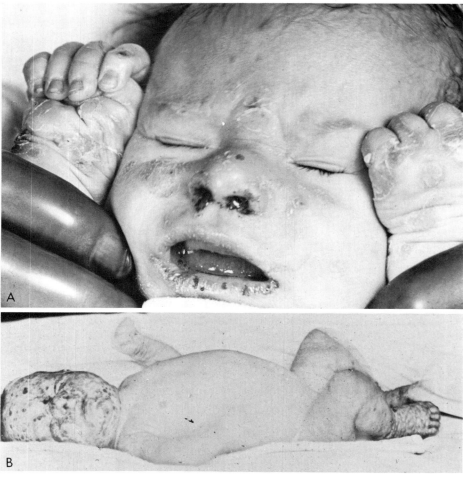

Figure 21–7. Congenital syphilis, cutaneous eruption. *A,* Three-week-old infant with hemorrhagic-mucoid nasal discharge ("snuffles") and extensive eruption involving the skin and oral mucosa. *B,* Photograph taken in 1930 of an infant with congenital syphilis with vesicular and squamous skin lesions affecting mainly the face and distal lower extremities. The cutaneous lesions of congenital syphilis represent the secondary stage of the disease, since spirochetes are introduced directly into the fetal circulation by transplacental transmission.

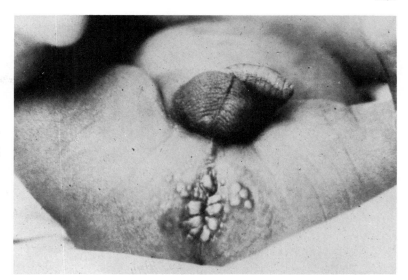

Figure 21–8. Congenital syphilis. Condylomata lata in an infant. Perianal lesions are white, moist, raised plaques teeming with spirochetes.

tial complaint is irritability combined with pain on movement of the limbs, or lack of normal movement of the extremities.

One of the most common manifestations of congenital syphilis is a cutaneous eruption which can assume many different forms (Fig. 21–7). Vesicular or vesiculo-bullous lesions are characteristic of the disease in the infant but papulosquamous lesions may also occur. Cutaneous lesions can be located anywhere on the body, including the palms and soles, but have a predilection for the anogenital region and the face. Extensive cutaneous involvement with denuded areas and bullae in the newborn or young infant resemble pemphigus and should always be an indication for serologic tests for syphilis (Tan). Typical condylomata lata are seen in exceptional cases (Fig. 21–8). A persistent nasal discharge that is initially mucoid but becomes mucopurulent or hemorrhagic is another sign considered to be characteristic of congenital syphilis. This has been referred to as "snuffles" and, like the cutaneous lesions, the nasal discharge is teeming with organisms which render it highly infectious.

Additional common signs in the infant with congenital syphilis include hepatosplenomegaly and lymphadenopathy. Lymph node enlargement is diagnostically non-specific; however, bilateral epitrochlear adenopathy has been considered to be strongly suggestive of congenital syphilis. The majority of infected infants have roentgenographic evidence of skeletal involvement, although only 10 to 20 percent show symptoms therefrom, such as pain on joint motion or soft tissue swelling.

Neurologic signs in the early symptomatic stages are not common even though a significant percentage have a cellular response in the cerebrospinal fluid. In a large series of infants with congenital syphilis studied by Platou et al., of 106 who had cerebrospinal fluid changes attributed to the infection, only six had clinically recognizable neurologic involvement. Acute or subacute syphilitic meningitis can develop after several months in untreated infants. This is accompanied by meningeal signs and bulging of the anterior fontanel, in addition to irritability, convulsions, and 50 to 500 lymphocytes per cu. mm. in the cerebrospinal fluid. Hydrocephalus may complicate this process, but, in past years, hydrocephalus developing several months after birth was recognized as the only clinical sign in some cases of congenital syphilis.

SKELETAL LESIONS. Roentgenographic evidence of skeletal disease is one of the most constant manifestations of congenital syphilis. More than 75 percent of infected newborns are stated to have some type of bony involvement, and in the series of 102 cases described by McLean in 1931, virtually all had such lesions. Multiple bone involvement is characteristic in congenital syphilis, and in severe cases all of the long bone metaphyses can be affected. The most common skeletal process is a destructive metaphysitis or osteochondritis. This is associated with pain on movement in some cases and is the cause of the condition referred to as Parrot's pseudoparalysis. Periostitis is the second and less common type of long bone lesion, and diaphysitis is still more infrequent. Skeletal lesions are sometimes present at birth in infants with congenital syphilis but more often are identified in the second or third postnatal month and can be expected to resolve by one year of age, with or without treatment. One of the most remarkable features of the metaphyseal lesions of congenital syphilis is their ability to heal completely without residual joint deformity or x-ray abnormality.

Syphilitic osteochondritis is seen roentgenographically as lucent or destructive metaphyseal changes, which may be limited to small areas of rarefaction between the end of the shaft and the epiphyseal plate, or involve the entire width of the shaft (Fig. 21–9). When the metaphyseal lesions affect the proximal ends of the tibias, they are usually on the medial aspects, resulting in destructive changes referred to as Wimberger's sign. Periostitis is manifested by periosteal thickening and elevation. It also heals with time but can lead to deformities, such as "sabre shins." Diaphysitis likewise may involve any of the long bones, including the metacarpals or metatarsals. Multiple destructive lesions along the bony shaft produce areas of patchy, moth-eaten rarefaction, sometimes associated with subperiosteal cortical thickening.

The skull is affected in some cases of congenital syphilis with either proliferative changes or destructive lesions that cannot be differentiated from pyogenic osteomyelitis by x-ray examination. The frontal and parietal regions are most often involved, possibly leading to a persistent cranial deformity such as frontal bossing.

HEMATOLOGIC ABNORMALITIES. A certain degree of anemia is common in infants with congenital syphilis, and in some it will be of severe degree. The anemia resembles that of erythroblastosis due to blood group incompatibility but the Coombs test is negative (Whitaker et al.). Hemolysis appears to be the most important causative factor, and, if severe, can even result in fetal hydrops with severe, diffuse edema and pallor (Bulova et al., Tan). Thrombocytopenia has been de-

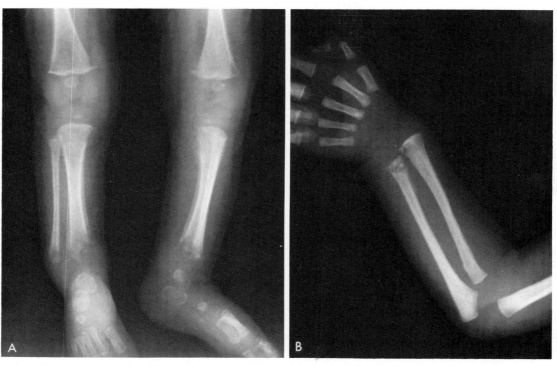

Figure 21–9.   Congenital syphilis, skeletal lesions. *A,* Infant with severe destructive metaphysitis (osteochondritis), especially of the distal tibiae. Metaphyseal changes of the medial aspects of the proximal tibiae are referred to as Wimberger's sign. Skeletal lesions of this type are associated with pain on movement and result in irritability and restricted motion that may suggest paralysis of one or more of the limbs. Periostitis is evident by the periosteal thickening and elevation ("cloaking"). *B,* Typical syphilitic metaphyseal lesions of the distal radius and ulna. (Courtesy of Dr. George Barnes, Jr., Tacoma, Washington.)

scribed in infants with congenital syphilis, although it is not common and the mechanism producing it is not clear (Freiman and Super). When jaundice occurs, the hyperbilirubinemia usually includes elevations of both the conjugated and unconjugated fractions, indicating that hemolysis as well as hepatocellular damage play a role. Splenomegaly is sometimes observed, raising the possibility that certain hematologic abnormalities may be partially attributed to hypersplenism.

RENAL ABNORMALITIES. A rare complication of neonatal syphilis is the nephrotic syndrome (McDonald et al.). It occurs in infants with other manifestations of congenital syphilis and is manifested by the presence of edema and proteinuria. Recent investigations have shown immune complex deposition along the glomerular basement membrane in such cases (Hill et al., Wiggelinkhuizen et al.). These findings, in addition to reduced serum complement, suggest that the pathogenesis of the nephrotic syndrome in congenital syphilis is on an immune basis. In this regard, Suskind and colleagues have reported a child with neonatal syphilis who developed a transient nephrotic state subsequent to adequate penicillin therapy.

Late Stigmata of Congenital Syphilis. Scars or deformities secondary to the early infectious lesions of prenatal syphilis represent stigmata of the active phase of the disease (Fiumara and Lessell, Robinson). Destructive lesions about the lips may leave circumoral radiating scars called rhagades. Retinal scarring in the form of pigmentary retinopathy or chorioretinitis is an occasional residual effect of congenital syphilis and may be associated with optic atrophy and significant visual loss. Bony damage associated with rhinitis in the acute stage is the forerunner of perforations of the nasal septum and the saddle nose deformity. Palatal perforation (Fig. 21–10), maxillary deformities, and cranial bossing are additional skeletal defects resulting from infantile infection.

Dental abnormalities are one of the most distinctive imprints of congenital syphilis, the best known being Hutchinson's teeth and Moon (mulberry) molars. Hutchinson's teeth refers to widely spaced and peg-shaped deformity of the upper central incisors of the permanent dentition and thus are not observed until at least six years of age (Fig. 21–11). The anlage of the permanent upper central incisors is developed between the 15th to 20th fetal weeks as three groups of dental centers. For reasons unknown, only the mid-

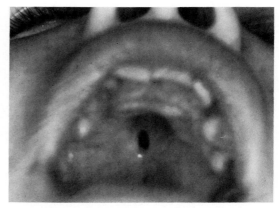

Figure 21–10. Palatal perforation as a late stigmata of congenital syphilis.

dle group is affected by *Treponema pallidum,* resulting in the characteristic notched appearance of the upper central incisors. The Moon, or mulberry, molar is a malformation of the lower first molar in which the tooth has many small cusps instead of the usual four. The enamel is usually poorly developed and, as a result, such teeth are frequently extracted before adolescence. The combination of Hutchinson's teeth, interstitial keratitis, and neural deafness is known as "Hutchinson's triad."

Late "Hypersensitivity" Lesions. Interstitial keratitis, Clutton's joints, and neural deafness are late manifestations of congenital syphilis which are different from the stigmata described above in that they are not believed to be due to inflammation from direct spirochetal invasion but more likely represent tissue hypersensitivity reactions. Penicillin appears to have little influence on these lesions,

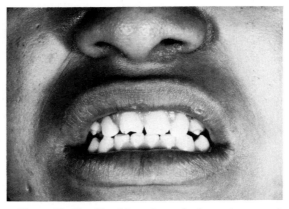

Figure 21–11. Hutchinson's teeth, late stigmata of congenital syphilis. Peg-shaped deformity of the upper central incisors of the permanent dentition.

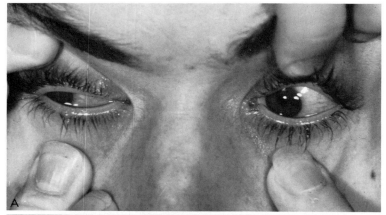

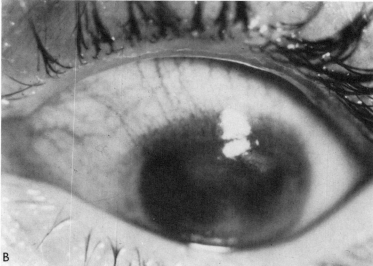

Figure 21–12. Interstitial keratitis, late "hypersensitivity" manifestation of congenital syphilis. *A,* Sixteen-year-old girl with local ocular pain, photophobia, increased lacrimation, and conjunctival infection. *B,* Late stage with marked neovascularity and edema of the cornea, resulting in its ground-glass appearance.

although improvement may occur with corticosteroid therapy, at least with interstitial keratitis and Clutton's joints.

Interstitial keratitis is seen in patients between five and 20 years of age and is more common in females than males (Fig. 21–12). It has been said to occur in 30 to 50 percent of patients with congenital syphilis (Curtis and Philpott). The initial symptoms are ocular pain, photophobia, and lacrimation. At approximately 10 days after onset, increased vascularity extends into the cornea from its margins. Neovascularity and edema produce a reddish, hazy, or ground-glass appearance of the cornea. After weeks or several months, gradual recovery begins, with resolution of the corneal opacities from the periphery extending toward the center. During this period, subjective symptoms diminish and visual acuity improves. If recognized early and

treated with corticosteroids topically, prognosis for recovery of vision is good.

Clutton's joints refers to a painless, symmetrical hydrarthrosis which is more common in females than males and which usually develops between eight and 20 years of age (Clutton). Among 363 patients with congenital syphilis reported by Klauder and Robertson in 1934, 63 developed Clutton's joints, an incidence of 18 percent. The knee joints are the site of involvement in the vast majority of patients. Bony changes do not occur and, after a variable period of time, the serous effusion gradually resolves without residual joint deformity or disability. Authors in the past stressed the similarity between Clutton's joints and interstitial keratitis in regard to the age of onset, female predilection, usual eventual spontaneous resolution, and apparent lack of effect of penicillin therapy. In addition, these two manifestations of congenital syphilis were observed to occur together more often than was expected by chance. Similarly to interstitial keratitis, the treatment of Clutton's joints is with corticosteroids.

Neural deafness also was noted to occur in association with interstitial keratitis in bygone years but was much less common than either interstitial keratitis or Clutton's joints. Hearing loss is usually insidious in onset, almost always bilateral, and frequently with gradual progression leading to significant disability.

Laboratory Diagnosis of Congenital Syphilis

Serologic tests for syphilis are no longer routinely done on newborn or sick infants admitted to hospital in this country (Hoffman and Herweg). Such tests are clearly indicated if the mother gives a history of having had syphilis or treatment for syphilis, or if the infant has clinical manifestations suggestive of the possibility of this infection. Consideration of the need for serologic tests should be raised if prenatal care has been marginal, especially if the child is illegitimate or premature, or if such a child has clinical illness not easily explained on another basis. Persistent nasal discharge or cutaneous rash not otherwise explained should always be warning signals deserving laboratory investigation for prenatally-acquired syphilis. Specimens from surface or mucosal lesions can be diagnostic by darkfield examination if on a syphilitic basis. Any child suspected of harboring a syphilitic infection on clinical grounds or from serologic studies should have long bone and skull x-rays as well as cerebrospinal fluid examination.

A useful but frequently overlooked diagnostic method is the gross and microscopic examination of the placenta. This procedure can be of particular importance if the mother gives a history suggestive of primary syphilis late in pregnancy or if she is admitted in labor having had no prenatal care. The lesions of the syphilitic placenta are quite characteristic (McCord, Russell and Altshuler), and, when present, can be assumed to be associated with fetal infection, regardless of the presence or absence of clinical signs of illness in the infant. The infected placenta is usually abnormally large by weight and to gross observation. Microscopic abnormalities include focal villitis with infiltration of lymphocytes and plasma cells, in addition to perivascular and

endovascular proliferation leading to vascular occlusion (Russell and Altshuler). With special stains, spirochetes can sometimes be identified within the placenta but their absence does not exclude the diagnosis.

Serologic diagnosis of syphilis in the neonate at best is difficult and is complicated by the fact that both reagin and treponemal antibodies cross the placenta. If the mother's serum is reactive, the infant's also will be, with or without neonatal infection. The titer of VDRL antibody that is passively transferred is usually not greater than that of the mother and can be expected to disappear by four months after birth. Thus, with a clinically normal newborn with a reactive serology, one would either have to wait and disprove infection by the gradual disappearance of antibody, or treat without confirmation of the presence of active syphilitic disease. Were the latter approach chosen, many uninfected infants would receive unnecessary penicillin therapy. Diagnostic problems are further compounded by the observation that if the mother acquires syphilis late in pregnancy, both she and the newborn infant may have negative serologic tests.

Passively transferred maternal antibodies resulting in reactive serology in the neonate are contained mainly in the IgG fraction. After it was recognized that the infected fetus in utero can respond by producing specific IgM antibodies, a modification of the FTA-ABS test called the IgM-FTA-ABS test was developed (Scotti et al.). This procedure employs fluorescein-labeled anti-human IgM to detect specific antitreponemal IgM antibodies, and, if reactive in the neonate, should indicate active neonatal infection, since IgM antibodies are not transplacentally transmitted. Studies thus far available indicate that reactive IgM-FTA-ABS tests in the infant are not on the basis of passive antibody transfer (Alford et al., Mamunes et al.). Some investigators believe the test is highly sensitive as an indicator of neonatal syphilitic infection, even in the presymptomatic stage, assuming that the methodology is suitably standardized (Rosen and Richardson), while others believe it is not acceptable for routine use because of the frequency of false negative and false positive results (Taber and Feigin).

Treatment of Congenital Syphilis

The most important aspect of management of maternal and fetal syphilitic infection is preventive, including adequate prenatal care and serologic testing during each pregnancy at the time of the first prenatal visit. If the pregnant female is not seen medically until labor or delivery occurs, the serologic test should be done on cord blood. Adequate penicillin treatment of the infected mother in the first four months of pregnancy will prevent fetal infection, and treatment thereafter during pregnancy will usually cure it. It is still possible for certain late "hypersensitivity" manifestations, such as interstitial keratitis, to occur years later, despite adequate prenatal penicillin treatment.

Treatment of the neonate or infant with congenital syphilis is most effective if given in the presymptomatic phase of the illness. It is very important to examine the cerebrospinal fluid in detail before initiation of antibiotic therapy. In infants with abnormal cerebrospinal fluid indicative of neurologic infection, treatment consists of aqueous penicillin G in a dose of 50,000 units per kilogram per day given intramuscularly or intravenously in two divided doses for a minimum of 10 days. If the cerebrospinal fluid is normal, some recommend the use of benzathine penicillin G in a single intramuscular dose of 50,000 units per kilogram. Benzathine penicillin G, however, gains entrance into the cerebrospinal fluid poorly, if at all (Kaplan and McCracken, Speer et al.) and thus should not be used if there is any question about the possibility of neurosyphilis. For practical reasons, this means that the former regimen with aqueous penicillin G is the preferred one for virtually all cases of congenital syphilis. Even with penicillin doses considered adequate, Ryan et al. demonstrated the persistence after treatment of virulent *Treponema pallidum* in ocular tissues in an infant with congenital syphilis.

Like the adult, the infant with syphilis may experience a Jarisch-Herxheimer reaction following the initiation of penicillin therapy. It is usually observed after the first injection of a treponemicidal agent and is believed to be due to precipitous lysis of spirochetes with liberation of antigenic substances into the blood stream. Transient worsening of cutaneous lesions in addition to fever and irritability occur with this reaction, which is usually benign and transient. The Herxheimer reaction is not an indication for discontinuation of penicillin therapy. Following completion of therapy, the infant should be examined periodically at least for 12 months with ophthalmologic evaluations, serologic tests,

and cerebrospinal fluid examinations at appropriate intervals. The nontreponemal antigen tests usually become nonreactive between four and 12 months after treatment.

LEPTOSPIROSIS

The leptospiroses are a group of diseases characterized by multiorgan involvement with extensive vasculitis and caused by a variety of leptospiral serotypes. Leptospira are aerobic spiral organisms with a length between 4 and 20 microns and a width of approximately 0.2 micron. The various species of the pathogenic leptospira are indistinguishable morphologically but have little in common, either biologically or antigenically, with either the Treponema or the Borrelia group of spirochetes. Human disease caused by leptospira is world-wide and results from transmission of the organism from animal to man by one of several methods. Rats and mice are the most prevalent carriers and shedders of leptospira but cattle, swine, dogs, and other animals may also be infected. Within asymptomatic but infected animals, leptospires become localized in the kidneys leading to urine shedding for long periods of time. Infections in the human result either from direct contact with urine of an affected animal or indirectly through contact with water or soil contaminated by infected animals. Survival of leptospires in water is longer when the water is neutral or slightly alkaline and of shorter duration when it is acidic.

Leptospirosis in children is not common but can occur from *Leptospira canicola* excreted by the dog, or from other species acquired while swimming or wading in contaminated water. Otherwise, risk of contracting the disease is occupationally related and thus affects young males more than any other age group. Persons most vulnerable to infection are agricultural workers, veterinarians, miners, sewer workers, laborers in poultry and fish industries, and swine herdsmen. Military personnel serving in foreign lands may be at risk, in which case the offending serotypes are often different from those present in this country (Berman et al.). In Europe, Asia, and Australia, leptospirosis is most common among persons who work barefoot in rice and cane fields where surface water contains leptospira from urine of rodents. The disease is well known in the Netherlands where most cases are caused by *Leptospira canicola* acquired from contaminated waterways by swimming, accidental immersion, or during occupational activities. In this country, the disease has been observed in all seasons but almost 70 percent occur between the months of July and October (Morbidity and Mortality Report, Vol. 23, 1973).

The long-standing but erroneous concept that "Weil's disease" is synonymous with all types of human leptospirosis had its basis in the historical developments of leptospiral infections. Adolf Weil recognized "spirochaetal jaundice" in 1886 and Stimson, in 1905, was the first to observe leptospires in tissue from a patient who supposedly had died of yellow fever. In 1915, Inada et al. in Japan and Uhlenhuth and Fromme in Germany independently isolated pathogenic organisms from patients with leptospirosis. The first proven case in United States was reported by Wadsworth et al. in 1922. For the next 30 years, the vast majority of cases identified and reported in this country were patients with severe illness associated with jaundice and with a mortality rate of 25 percent (Molner et al.). Thus, for years, the cases that were identified resembled the illness described by Weil in 1886, but it was not yet recognized that this, the severe form, numerically represented a relatively insignificant variant of leptospirosis. Milder and anicteric forms have subsequently become recognized as the common type of leptospirosis (Berman et al.) with only superficial resemblance to the illness depicted by Weil. The mortality rate with leptospirosis is now estimated to be approximately 5 to 10 percent, with almost all fatal cases occurring in persons with severe hepatic or renal involvement (Turner).

Several different species of leptospira cause disease in this country, the most important being *Leptospira icterohemorrhagiae, Leptospira canicola,* and *Leptospira pomona.* Other less important agents include *Leptospira autumnalis, Leptospira bataviae,* and *Leptospira grippotyphosa.* Each serotype is thought to have a primary animal host but almost all serotypes can be harbored and excreted by a variety of animal species. For example, the primary carriers of *Leptospira icterohemorrhagiae* are rats and mice, but swine, dogs, cats, and horses may also be infected. Dogs are the principal carrier of *Leptospira canicola;* however, it has also been isolated from cattle and swine. Swine are the important primary host for *Leptospira pomona.*

Originally it was believed that certain leptospiral species caused different forms of disease in man. "Weil's disease" referred to a severe illness with jaundice due to *Leptospira icterohemorrhagiae;* "canicola fever" was supposedly produced by *Leptospira canicola;* "swine-herd's disease" was felt synonymous with *Leptospira pomona* infection, and "swamp fever" was the term indicating illness secondary to *Leptospira grippotyphosa.* It is now clear that subdividing leptospiral infections into separate categories is unwarranted because the majority of serotypes produce essentially the same type of illness but with some expected variation in severity and sequence of events. Thus, the best designation for this disease is leptospirosis, with an added note of the serotype that is the etiologic cause.

There are two exceptions to this nearly uniform similarity of illness produced by leptospires and in these situations descriptive terms remain useful. "Pretibial fever" or "Fort Bragg fever" is sufficiently different from the usual form of leptospirosis that subdivision seems appropriate. This illness was first observed in troops in North Carolina in 1942 in the form of a benign febrile illness associated with splenomegaly (Daniels and Grennan). Its most characteristic feature is the appearance on about the fourth day of the illness of an erythematous rash usually limited to the pretibial areas bilaterally. The illness was first suspected to have a viral etiology but Gochenour and workers subsequently found it to be caused by a member of the *Leptospira autumnalis* group. The term "Weil's disease" also is descriptively informative but it should be recognized that the syndrome can be caused by a variety of Leptospiral serotypes, including *Leptospira icterohemorrhagiae.* "Weil's disease" refers to a severe leptospiral infection characterized by fever, jaundice, and azotemia, with greater morbidity and higher mortality than the usual leptospiral infections. It should be regarded as an unusual expression of leptospiral infection, perhaps accounting for 5 to 10 percent of cases (Edwards and Domm).

Leptospirosis is not a common disease in any age group in the United States but is especially infrequent in younger children. Older children and young adults are most frequently affected. In 1969, there was 104 cases in all ages reported in this country, and in 1970, there were 52 reported cases. Of 68 human cases reported in 1971, three proved fatal; 76 percent occurred in males, and 36 percent were caused by *Leptospira canicola. Leptospira icterohemorrhagiae* accounted for 16 percent and *Leptospira pomona* for 13 percent of the cases (Morbidity and Mortality Weekly Report, Vol. 20: 1971; Vol. 23: 1973). In 1975, there were 119 cases of human leptospirosis reported in the United States, most not occupationally related. Seventy-one percent occurred in males, 64 percent were identified in the months of July through October, and the case-fatality ratio was 3 percent (Morbidity and Mortality Weekly Report, Vol. 26, 1977).

Clinical Manifestations

As mentioned above, leptospirosis is most prevalent in this country between July and October, corresponding to the peak exposure of people to ponds and lakes, and agricultural workers to surface water in fields and animal pens. Leptospires in the animal host's urine gain entrance into the human by penetration through abraded skin surfaces or via the conjunctivae or mucosal surfaces of the mouth or the nose. The usual range of incubation period is seven to 14 days, with an average of 10 days. Longer incubation periods have been described but are not common.

Symptoms and signs of leptospirosis vary in severity, ranging from a very mild illness manifested only by fever, malaise, and myalgia, to a profound or fatal disease manifested by marked hyperthermia, jaundice, azotemia, coma, and hypotension. The mild form or moderate forms are more common than the very severe type, and most cases fall somewhere between these two variations. Wong and colleagues have pointed out the many similarities between leptospirosis and the mucocutaneous lymph node syndrome and suggested that some reported cases of the latter syndrome may have been unrecognized leptospirosis.

Leptospirosis has been characterized as a biphasic illness with the first or septicemic stage lasting several days up to a week and the second stage largely representing the body's immune response to the infection (Edwards and Domm). The initial phase is that of an acute septic infection during which leptospires are present in blood and usually in cerebrospinal fluid, but without other spinal fluid findings. Antibodies begin to appear in blood about seven or eight days after onset of the illness, and, thereafter, leptospiremia terminates; leptospiruria occurs and may persist for weeks or months, and neurologic or cerebrospinal fluid abnormalities occur in a high percentage of cases.

The first or septic phase of the illness is characterized by an abrupt onset with fever, chills, headache, myalgia, and malaise. Fever assumes a spiking quality and persists for seven to 10 days, when it gradually resolves. Cutaneous rash has been observed in approximately 20 percent of cases by some (Edwards and Domm), and in a higher percentage of cases in other series (Wong et al.). Rash can be maculopapular, petechial, or purpuric in type and can appear at various times during the acute stage of the illness. In cases with extensive and severe vasculitis, especially if associated with systemic hypotension, gangrenous changes can occur in the soft tissues of the distal parts of the extremities (Wong et al.). Headache is customary from soon after the onset of the illness and is both persistent and intense in most patients. Headache in the first stage of the disease cannot be explained on the basis of aseptic meningitis since neck stiffness is absent and the cerebrospinal fluid examination is generally normal at this stage despite the fact that leptospires may be present. Conjunctivitis is one of the most common physical findings in the early part of the illness and usually subsides in the second week after onset. Bradycardia, hypotension or even shock are sometimes observed, and jaundice occurs in 10 percent or less. Evidence of nephritis with oliguria or azotemia is even less frequent but renal involvement manifested by hematuria or proteinuria is seen in a significant percentage of patients. In some cases, gastrointestinal complaints will predominate in the initial stages of the disease (Anderson et al.). Acute, acalculous cholecystitis is one possible cause of abdominal symptoms and can be complicated by severe distention of the gallbladder requiring surgical drainage (Barton et al., Bell et al.). Other complaints are variable but include photophobia, arthralgia, and mental confusion. During the initial, or septic, phase of the illness, blood leukocytosis is common but not invariable, with counts often in the range of 10,000 to 25,000 per cu. mm., and the erythrocyte sedimentation rate is significantly elevated. Serum bilirubin and liver enzymes are invariably elevated in jaundiced patients with hepatitis, but even in the more common anicteric cases, the serum glutamic oxaloacetic transaminase is frequently increased (Berman et al.).

After seven to 10 days, the septic manifestations listed above usually diminish and, in some patients, the illness gradually resolves. In a minority, jaundice and hepatomegaly have complicated the process by this time and the illness assumes a longer and more severe course.

In many patients, a second phase of the disease becomes manifest during the second or third week after onset, with recurrence of fever and the appearance of neurologic manifestations. This is either in the form of cerebrospinal fluid pleocytosis without abnormal physical signs, or aseptic meningitis with signs of meningeal irritation plus cells in the cerebrospinal fluid and increase in the protein content.

Neurologic Aspects

In the first few days of the disease, headache is the most common neurologic manifestation, although drowsiness, confusion, or delirium is observed occasionally. During this stage, the cerebrospinal fluid may contain leptospires but otherwise is normal. Evidence of aseptic meningitis often appears between the fifth and tenth day after onset. Edwards and Domm stated that meningitis will be found in 80 to 90 percent of all cases of leptospirosis if cerebrospinal fluid examination is performed during the second week of the illness. Symptoms and signs vary in intensity, but when present include headache, vomiting, neck stiffness, and visual complaints (Beeson and Hankey, Buzzard and Wylie, Turrell and Hamburger). Rarely, aseptic meningitis represents the only clinical manifestation of leptospirosis, except for preceding fever. Cells are usually present in the spinal fluid in the second week of the illness, regardless of the presence or absence of clinical neurologic involvement (Cargill and Beeson). The cellular response frequently is polymorphonuclear at first followed by a predominance of lymphocytes. The protein and glucose contents may be either normal or mildly elevated. During this period, organisms cannot usually be isolated from the cerebrospinal fluid, adding evidence to the concept that leptospiral meningitis is an expression of an antigen-antibody reaction rather than the result of an inflammatory process directly related to the presence of leptospires.

Encephalitis is much less common than aseptic meningitis and may be followed by permanent sequelae (Gsell and Prader). Ascending myelitis has been recorded in a few cases, either in the acute stage of the disease or several weeks later (Mortensen, Russell). Recovery usually follows in such cases, even when weakness is severe. Peripheral nerve lesions have been described, either early or late, in the form of brachial plexus neuropathy (Middleton, Russell), or involvement of one of a variety of cranial nerves (Edwards and Domm). Regardless of the type of nervous system dysfunction that complicates acute leptospiral infection, a remarkable feature is the degree of neurologic damage that is compatible with eventual complete recovery. Histologic descriptions of neurologic lesions have been sparse but include congestion of meninges, cerebral edema, and perivascular lymphocytic infiltration of the white matter (Arean). Petechial hemorrhages in muscle without significant degenerative changes are seen at autopsy in most cases of leptospirosis.

Laboratory Diagnosis

Diagnosis of leptospirosis depends upon isolation of the organism or on serologic examinations. During the first week of the illness, leptospires may be cultured from blood or cerebrospinal fluid, and thereafter they may be recovered from the urine. Leptospiruria persists for variable periods of time in human infection but can occur as long as 12 to 18 weeks after onset of the illness (Morbidity and Mortality Weekly Report, Vol. 21, 1972). Leptospiral isolates from blood or urine are identified by the addition of specific antiserum. A fluorescent antibody technique can be used for the demonstration of leptospires in urine.

Rise in antibody titer in leptospirosis occurs seven to 10 days after onset of the disease and reaches maximum titers by the third to fourth week. A specific four-fold or greater titer rise demonstrated by the leptospira microscopic agglutination test is considered diagnostic of the disease. In this country, antigens used for routine testing are prepared from *Leptospira icterohemorrhagiae, canicola, pomona,* and *autumnalis.* Cross-reactions are very common, especially between *Leptospira icterohemorrhagiae* and *Leptospira canicola.* With serial titers, the serotype giving the highest titer is usually considered to be the infecting organism.

Prevention and Treatment

Preventive measures are generally limited to obvious factors, such as rodent control and recommendation that susceptible workers wear proper protective clothing to prevent contamination of exposed skin surfaces. Ponds or swimming areas found to harbor pathogenic leptospires which have caused human disease should be closed until the problem subsides.

Supportive measures for the ill patient, such as proper administration of fluids and electrolytes, analgesics for pain, and temperature control are symptomatically helpful. Hepatic and renal function should be carefully watched and appropriately managed should derangements occur. Penicillin in large doses is indicated in the early stages of the disease (Turner), although unequivocal proof of its benefit is lacking. Opinion generally is that penicillin therapy given before the fifth or sixth day of the illness will probably favorably influence its course. Treatment in the second week is not likely to be beneficial since manifestations at this time are more those of an immune response than a septic process. Large doses of penicillin administered early in the disease can precipitate a Herxheimer reaction, another suggestive bit of evidence of the possible effectiveness of antibiotic treatment.

REFERENCES

Alford, C. A., Jr., Polt, S. S., Cassady, G. E., Straumfjord, J. V., and Remington, J. S.: γM-fluorescent treponemal antibody in the diagnosis of congenital syphilis. New Eng. J. Med. 280:1086–1091, 1969.

Amesse, J. W., and Barber, W. W.: Syphilitic meningitis in infants and young children. Am. J. Syph. 11:544, 1927.

Anderson, D. C., Folland, D. S., Fox, M. D., Patton, C. M., and Kaufmann, A. F.: Leptospirosis: A common-source outbreak due to leptospires of the grippotyphosa serogroup. Am. J. Epidem. 107:538–544, 1978.

Arean, V. M.: The pathologic anatomy and pathogenesis of fatal human leptospirosis (Weil's disease). Am. J. Path. 40:393–414, 1962.

Barton, L. L., Escobedo, M. B., Keating, J. P., and Ternberg, J. L.: Leptospirosis with acalculous cholecystitis. Am. J. Dis. Child. 126:350–351, 1973.

Beeson, P. B., and Hankey, D. D.: Leptospiral meningitis. Arch. Intern. Med. 89:575–583, 1952.

Beetham, W. P., Jr., Kaye, R. L., and Polley, H. F.: Charcot's joints. A case of extensive polyarticular involvement, and discussion of certain clinical and pathologic features. Ann. Intern. Med. 58:1002–1012, 1963.

Bell, M. J., Ternberg, J. L., and Feigin, R. D.: Surgical

complications of leptospirosis in children. J. Pediat. Surg. 13:325–330, 1978.

Berman, S. J., Tsai, C., Holmes, K., Fresh, J. W., and Watten, R. H.: Sporadic anicteric leptospirosis in South Vietnam. A study of 150 patients. Ann. Intern. Med. 79:167–173, 1973.

Bloch, M. I.: Der Ursprung der Syphilis. Fischer, Berlin, 1901.

Bracero, L., Wormser, G. P., and Bottone, E. J.: Serologic tests for syphilis: A guide to interpretation in various stages of disease. Mt. Sinai J. Med. 46:289–292, 1979.

Bulova, S. I., Schwartz, E., and Harrer, W. V.: Hydrops fetalis and congenital syphilis. Pediatrics 49:285–287, 1972.

Burke, A. W.: Syphilis in a Jamaican psychiatric hospital: A review of 52 cases including 17 of neurosyphilis. Brit. J. Vener. Dis. 48:249–253, 1972.

Buzzard, E. M., and Wylie, J. A. H.: Meningitis leptospirosa. Lancet 2:417–420, 1947.

Cargill, W. H., Jr., and Beeson, P. B.: The value of spinal fluid examination as a diagnostic procedure in Weil's disease. Ann. Intern. Med. 27:396–400, 1947.

Clutton, H. H.: Symmetrical synovitis of the knee in hereditary syphilis. Lancet 1:391, 1886.

Curtis, A. C., and Philpott, O. S., Jr.: Prenatal syphilis. Med. Clin. N. Amer. 48:707–719, 1964.

Daniels, W. B., and Grennan, H. A.: Pretibial fever. J.A.M.A. 122:361–365, 1943.

Deacon, W. E., Lucas, J. B., and Price, E. V.: Fluorescent treponemal antibody absorption (FTA-ABS) test for syphilis. J.A.M.A. 198:624–628, 1966.

Diday, P.: Syphilis in New-Born Children and Infants at Breast. The New Sydenham Society. London, 1858.

Edwards, G. A., and Domm, B. M.: Human leptospirosis. Medicine 39:117–156, 1960.

Fisher, M., and Poser, C. M.: Syphilitic meningomyelitis. A case report. Arch. Neurol. 34:785, 1977.

Fiumara, N. J., and Lessell, S.: Manifestations of late congenital syphilis. An analysis of 271 patients. Arch. Derm. 102:78–83, 1970.

Förström, L., and Lassus, A.: The fluorescent treponemal antibody absorption test (FTA-ABS) in treated latent and late syphilis. Acta Dermatovener. 49:326–331, 1969.

Freiman, I., and Super, M.: Thrombocytopenia and congenital syphilis in South African Bantu infants. Arch. Dis. Childh. 41:87–90, 1966.

Gamble, C. N., and Reardon, J. B.: Immunopathogenesis of syphilitic glomerulonephritis. Elution of antitreponemal antibody from glomerular immune-complex deposits. New Eng. J. Med. 292:449–454, 1975.

Gochenour, W. S., Jr., Smadel, J. E., Jackson, E. B., Evans, L. B., and Yager, R. H.: Leptospiral etiology of Fort Bragg fever. Public Health Rep. 67:811–813, 1952.

Gsell, O., and Prader, A.: Akute encephalitis durch Leptospira hyos infolge traumatischer infection. Helv. Pediat. Acta 8:318, 1954.

Harter, C. A., and Benirschke, K.: Fetal syphilis in the first trimester. Am. J. Obstet. Gynecol. 124:705–711, 1976.

Hill, L. L., Singer, D. B., Falletta, J., and Stasney, R.: The nephrotic syndrome in congenital syphilis: An immunopathy. Pediatrics 49:260–266, 1972.

Hoffmann, F. D., and Herweg, J. C.: Status of serological testing for congenital syphilis. J. Pediat. 71:686–690, 1967.

Hooshmand, H., Escobar, M. R., and Kopf, S. W.: Neurosyphilis. A study of 241 patients. J.A.M.A. 219:726–729, 1972.

Inada, R., Ido, Y., Hoki, R., Kaneko, R., and Ito, H.: The etiology, mode of infection and specific therapy in Weil's disease (spirochaetosis icterohaemorrhagica). J. Exp. Med. 23:377–402, 1916.

Jaffe, H. W., Larsen, S. A., Peters, M., Jove, D. F., Lopez, B., and Schroeter, A. L.: Tests for treponemal antibody in CSF. Arch. Intern. Med. 138:252–255, 1978.

Kaplan, J. M., and McCracken, G. H., Jr.: Clinical pharmacology of benzathine penicillin G in neonates with regard to its recommended use in congenital syphilis. J. Pediat. 82:1069–1072, 1973.

Kaufman, R. E., Olansky, D. O., and Wiesner, P. J.: The FTA-ABS (IgM) test for neonatal congenital syphilis: A critical review. J. Am. Vener. Dis. Assoc. 1:79–84, 1974.

Klauder, J. V., and Robertson, H. F.: Symmetrical serous synovitis (Clutton's joints). Congenital syphilis and interstitial keratitis. J.A.M.A. 103:236–240, 1934.

Mahoney, J. F., Arnold, R. C., and Harris, A. D.: Penicillin treatment of early syphilis. A preliminary report. Am. J. Pub. Health 33:1387–1391, 1943.

Mamunes, P., Cave, V. G., Budell, J. W., Andersen, J. A., and Steward, R. E.: Early diagnosis of neonatal syphilis. Evaluation of a gamma M-fluorescent treponemal antibody test. Am. J. Dis. Child. 120:17–21, 1970.

McCord, J. R.: Syphilis of the placenta. Am. J. Obstet. Gynecol. 28:743–750, 1934.

McDonald, R., Wiggelinkhuizen, J., and Kaschula, R. O. C.: The nephrotic syndrome in very young infants. Am. J. Dis. Child. 122:507–512, 1971.

McLean, S.: Congenital osseous syphilis. Am. J. Dis. Child. 41:130–152, 363–395, 607–675, 887–992, 1128–1172, 1411–1419, 1931.

Middleton, J. E.: Canicola fever with neurological complications. Brit. Med. J. 2:25–26, 1955.

Miller, J. L.: History of syphilis. Ann. Med. Hist. 2:394–405, 1930.

Molner, J. G., Meyer, K. F., and Raskin, H. A.: Leptospiral infections. A survey. J.A.M.A. 136:814, 1948.

Montgomery, D. W.: Hieronymus Fracastorium. The author of the poem called syphilis. Ann. Med. Hist. 2:406–413, 1930.

Morbidity and Mortality Weekly Report. 20: 25 Dec., 1971.

Morbidity and Mortality Weekly Report. 21: 25 Nov., 1972.

Morbidity and Mortality Weekly Report. 23: 3 Feb., 1973.

Morbidity and Mortality Weekly Report. 26: 28 Jan., 1977.

Mortensen, V.: Nervous complications of Weil's disease. Lancet 1:117–119, 1940.

Nelson, R. A., Jr., and Mayer, M. M.: Immobilization of *Treponema pallidum* in vitro by antibody produced by syphilitic infection. J. Exp. Med. 89:369–393, 1949.

Parker, H. L.: Juvenile tabes. Review of the literature and summary of seven cases. Arch. Neurol. Psychiat. 5:121–130, 1921.

Platou, R. V., Hill, A. J., Jr., Ingraham, N. R., Goodwin, M. S., Wilkinson, E. E., Hansen, A. E., and Heyman, A.: Early congenital syphilis. Treatment of two hundred and fifty-two patients with penicillin. J.A.M.A. 133:10–16, 1947.

Public Health Service Publication No. 1660. Jan., 1968. U. S. Government Printing Office, Washington, D.C.

Robertson, D. A.: Four cases of spinal myosis; with remarks on the action of light on the pupil. Edinburgh Med. J. 15:487–493, 1869.

Robinson, R. C. V.: Congenital syphilis. Arch. Derm. 99:599–610, 1969.

Rosen, E. V., and Richardson, N. J.: A reappraisal of the value of the IgM fluorescent treponemal antibody absorption test in the diagnosis of congenital syphilis. J. Pediat. 87:38–42, 1975.

Rosenbaum, H. A.: Juvenile tabes dorsalis. Report of three cases. Am. J. Dis. Child. 35:866–871, 1928.

Russell, P., and Altshuler, G.: Placental abnormalities of congenital syphilis. A neglected aid to diagnosis. Am. J. Dis. Child. 128:160–163, 1974.

Russell, R. W. R.: Neurological aspects of leptospirosis. J. Neurol. Neurosurg. Psychiat. 22:143–148, 1959.

Ryan, S. J., Hardy, P. H., Hardy, J. M., and Oppenheimer, E. H.: Persistence of virulent Treponema pallidum despite penicillin therapy in congenital syphilis. Am. J. Ophthal. 73:258–261, 1972.

Scotti, A., Logan, L., and Caldwell, J. G.: Fluorescent antibody test for neonatal congenital syphilis: A progress report. J. Pediat. 75:1129–1134, 1969.

Smith, J. L., Singer, J. A., Moore, M. B., Jr., and Yobs, A. R.: Seronegative ocular and neurosyphilis. Am. J. Ophthal. 59:753–763, 1965.

Spangler, A. S., Jackson, J. H., Fiumara, N. J., and Warthin, T. A.: Syphilis with a negative blood test reaction. J.A.M.A. 189:87–90, 1964.

Sparling, P. F.: Diagnosis and treatment of syphilis. New Eng. J. Med. 284:642–653, 1971.

Speer, M. E., Taber, L. H., Clark, D. B., and Rudolph, A. J.: Cerebrospinal fluid levels of benzathine penicillin G in the neonate. J. Pediat. 91:996–997, 1977.

Stimson, A. M.: A note on an organism found in yellow fever tissues. Pub. Health Rep. 22:541, 1907.

Suskind, R., Winkelstein, J. A., and Spear, G. A.: Nephrotic syndrome in congenital syphilis. Arch. Dis. Childh. 48:237–239, 1973.

Taber, L. H., and Feigin, R. D.: Spirochetal infections. Pediat. Clin. N. Amer. 26:377–413, 1979.

Tan, K. L.: The re-emergence of early congenital syphilis. Acta Paediat. Scand. 62:601–607, 1973.

Termini, B. A., and Music, S. I.: The natural history of syphilis: A review. South Med. J. 65:241–245, 1972.

Traviesa, D. C., Prystowsky, S., Nelson, B. J., Johnson, K. P., and Clavan, B. S.: Cerebrospinal fluid findings in asymptomatic patients with reactive serum fluorescent treponemal antibody absorption tests. Ann. Neurol. 4:524–530, 1978.

Turner, L. H.: Leptospirosis. Brit. Med. J. 1:231–235, 1969.

Turner, T. B.: The spirochetes. *In:* Dubos, R. J., and Hirsch, J. D.: Bacterial and Mycotic Infections of Man. J. B. Lippincott, Philadelphia, 1965.

Turrell, R. C., and Hamburger, M.: Canicola fever with meningitis. Am. J. Med. 10:249–253, 1951.

Uhlenhuth, P., and Fromme, W.: Zur aetiologie der sog. Weil'schen krankheit (austeckende gelbsucht). Berl. Klin. Wchnschr. 53:269–273, 1916.

Vatz, K. A., Scheibel, R. L., Keiffer, S. A., and Ansari, K. A.: Neurosyphilis and diffuse cerebral angiopathy: A case report. Neurology 24:472–476, 1974.

Wadsworth, A., Langworthy, H. V., Stewart, F. C., Moore, A. C., and Coleman, M. B.: Infectious jaundice occurring in New York State. Preliminary report of an investigation, with report of a case of accidental infection of the human subject with *Leptospira icterohemorrhagiae* from the rat. J.A.M.A. 78:1120, 1922.

Weil, A.: Über eine eigenthumliche, mit milztumor, icterus and nephritis einhergehende acute infektionskrankheit. Deutsches Arch. Klin. Med. 39:209–232, 1886.

Whitaker, J. A., Sartain, P., and Shaheedy, M.: Hematological aspects of congenital syphilis. J. Pediat. 66:629–636, 1965.

Wiggelinkhuizen, J., Kaschula, R. O. C., Uys, C. J., Kiujten, R. H., and Dale, J.: Congenital syphilis and glomerulonephritis with evidence for immune pathogenesis. Arch. Dis. Childh. 48:375–381, 1973.

Wilkinson, R. H., and Heller, R. M.: Congenital syphilis: Resurgence of an old problem. Pediatrics 47:27–30, 1971.

Wong, M. L., Kaplan, S., Dunkle, L. M., Stechenberg, B. W., and Feigin, R. D.: Leptospirosis: A childhood disease. J. Pediat. 90:532–537, 1977.

Woody, N. C., Sistrunk, W. F., and Platou, R. V.: Congenital syphilis: A laid ghost walks. J. Pediat. 64:63–67, 1964.

Chapter Twenty-Two

RICKETTSIAL DISEASE

ROCKY MOUNTAIN SPOTTED FEVER

Rocky Mountain spotted fever is a tick-borne disease caused by Rickettsia ricketsii and is the most important rickettsial disease in the United States. Approximately 250 to 300 cases per year were reported in this country between 1958 and 1968, but in 1969 the number increased to 498 reported cases, 91 of which occurred in the state of Virginia (Peters). In 1970, 380 cases of Rocky Mountain spotted fever were reported (Morbidity and Mortality Weekly Report, Vol. 19, No. 53 Summary, 1970) and from 1970 thru 1977

the yearly incidence of the disease gradually increased (Fig. 22–1). In 1977, there were 1,115 cases identified in this country, the largest number since reporting began in 1920 (Hattwick et al. 1978). The misleading name of the disease derived from the early belief that it occurred primarily in the Rocky Mountain region subsequent to its discovery in Idaho and Montana in the latter part of the nineteenth century. The illness has now been recognized in almost all states of this country and is more common along the eastern shore than in the Rockies. Delaware, Virginia, North Carolina, the Cape Cod area of Massachusetts, and the eastern section of Long

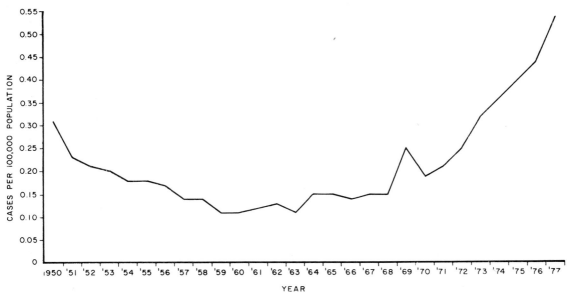

Figure 22–1. Rocky Mountain spotted fever. Reported cases per 100,000 population by year, United States, 1950–1977. (From: Morbidity and Mortality Weekly Report, Annual Summary, 1977, Volume 26, No. 53, Sept. 1978.)

Island have remained strongholds of the disease for several decades (Vianna and Hinman, Hazard et al., Peters). Since 1966, the Rocky Mountain states have accounted for less than 5 percent of the reported cases (Hattwick et al. 1976). Because of its widespread distribution, authors have suggested the illness more appropriately be called tick typhus or spotted fever; however, it remains best known as Rocky Mountain spotted fever.

The tick is the usual vector, transmitting the disease to the human by its bite which conveys the rickettsiae into the recipient's blood stream. Transmission is unlikely unless the tick remains attached for several hours at a minimum. In the western part of the country, *Dermacentor andersoni* (the wood tick) is the common offender, while east of the Rocky Mountains, *Dermacentor variabilis* (the dog tick) is the more frequent agent for transmission of the disease to man. Because of its dependence on the presence of active ticks, Rocky Mountain spotted fever is a seasonal disease which is largely restricted to the spring and summer months. The majority of cases occur between April and September,

with June being the month of greatest prevalence. At least partly because of the geographic differences in the tick vectors, the age groups primarily affected differ in various parts of the country. In the Rocky Mountain region where the wood tick is abundant, spotted fever is more commonly an occupational hazard. Timbermen, forest rangers, trappers, and other adults who work in wooded areas are more frequently affected. Any member of a vacationing family camping in a region harboring infected ticks can likewise contract the disease. In areas where the dog tick is the vector, children are predisposed to the illness, probably because of their greater intimacy of contact with the family pet. It has been estimated that about two-thirds of all cases of Rocky Mountain spotted fever occur in children (Harrell, Hattwick et al. 1976). In addition, cases of laboratory-acquired Rocky Mountain spotted fever have been described in personnel handling the organism (Oster et al.).

The symptoms and signs observed in a child with Rocky Mountain spotted fever result from the generalized proliferative

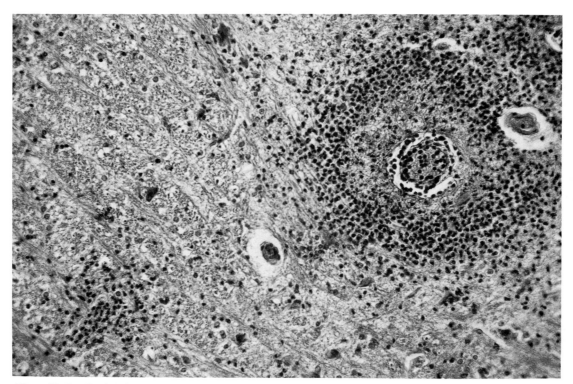

Figure 22–2. Section from the periventricular region of the pons in a fatal case of Rocky Mountain spotted fever. There is severe vasculitis with vessel occlusion, perivascular inflammation, and a separate microglial nodule adjacent to the inflamed vessel. (Courtesy of Dr. James Q. Miller, Charlottesville, Virginia; Neurology, 22:561–566, 1972.)

thrombovasculitis which is similar to that which occurs in typhus fever. Rickettsial invasion of arterioles and capillaries leads to endothelial proliferation, perivascular inflammation, and potential thrombotic occlusion, resulting in tissue ischemia (Hand et al.) (Fig. 22–2). It is a multiple organ system disease which includes vascular involvement of the skin and brain (Harrell, Hassin, Scheinker), accounting for certain clinical features commonly present in children with this disease. In addition to the small vessel and perivascular lesions in the brain, clusters of microglia may be found in scattered fashion, as well as mononuclear cell infiltration of the meninges. Neurologic manifestations of variable degree are present in a high percentage of patients (Bell and Lascari, Miller and Price) and may either provide one with a high degree of suspicion of the correct diagnosis or sufficiently resemble bacterial meningitis or viral encephalitis to mislead one totally, resulting in erroneous and ineffective therapy.

Clinical Manifestations

Rocky Mountain spotted fever may occur in any age group in childhood. The youngest affected in most series is two years with ages four to eight years being the most frequently involved period. The six-month-old infant reported by Jacobs and Chusid is apparently the youngest described case of Rocky Mountain spotted fever. The incubation period, which extends from the tick bite until the onset of symptoms, ranges from two to 12 days, with a mean of seven days. History of recent exposure to ticks or actually finding a tick on the child's body is common, but its absence does not exclude the diagnosis. The onset of symptoms generally is rather abrupt, with fever, vomiting, headache and myalgia being the most common early complaints. Fever rapidly becomes marked, acquiring a spiking quality often reaching levels of 105°F. In some, the morning temperature will drop almost to normal, followed by striking elevations by mid-afternoon. Abdominal pain, vomiting, irritability, and listlessness are added to the symptoms already present, with the degree of illness gradually worsening over the next two to three days. Headache is almost a constant feature of this disease in children who are old enough to describe its presence. Headache is usually diffuse but with bifrontal accentuation and is prone to be

more severe at times that correspond to the highest temperature elevations.

In most cases, the rash appears between the second and fourth day after onset of symptoms and is the single most important sign leading to the correct clinical diagnosis (Fig. 22–3). The development of the rash can be delayed into the second week of the illness and is especially difficult to identify in black patients (Hattwick et al. 1978, Sexton et al.). The eruption is a remarkably constant feature of this disease, present in the majority of patients except perhaps those partially protected by previously administered vaccine (Johnson and Kadull). Among 138 children with this illness described by Bradford and Hawkins, rash was present in 133 while five were not observed to have cutaneous involvement. The rash can be confused with a drug eruption when the child has received antibiotics for fever in the first day or so of the illness. This, also, is a diagnostic pitfall which delays recognition of the illness and increases the possibility of eventual complications or even death. The initial lesions are usually erythematous macules first observed on the wrists and ankles, which then rapidly spread to involve the palms and soles. Within hours to a day or so, the exanthem becomes generalized and often will gradually assume a petechial quality. When extensive, large ecchymotic lesions may develop over certain parts of the body. At the peak of the disease, the rash covers the entire body in variable degree but is almost always more dense over the arms and legs compared to the face and trunk. Its presence on the palms and soles is characteristic of Rocky Mountain spotted fever and is of help differentiating this disease from measles and certain other exanthems. As recovery from the illness occurs, petechiae remain as pigmented spots which only gradually resolve.

As the rash evolves and febrile spikes persist, edema of soft tissues becomes evident, especially of the face and on the dorsal surfaces of the hands and feet (Fig. 22–4). The edema is usually non-pitting and results primarily from the increased permeability of the damaged capillaries and arterioles. Myalgia is severe and is apparent from the irritability and crying which results when muscles are palpated or squeezed. Lymphadenopathy is minimal or absent but splenomegaly is found in about 50 percent of children with this illness (Haynes et al.). A lesser number will have significant enlargement of both the liver and spleen. Some degree of hepatic involve-

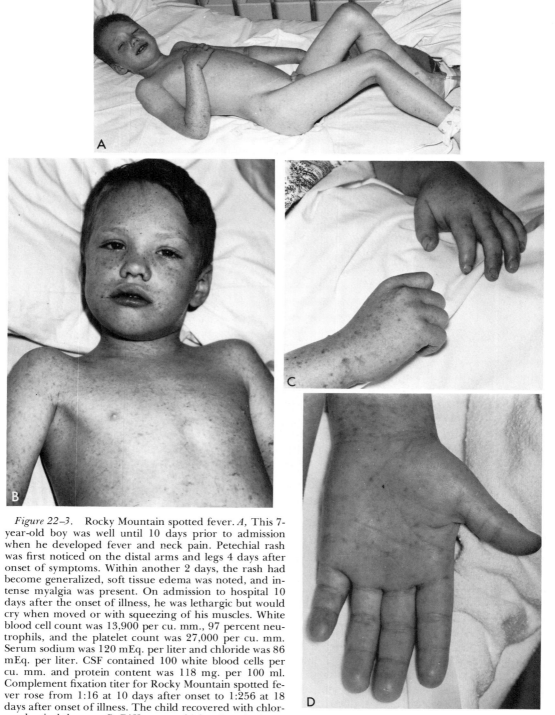

Figure 22–3. Rocky Mountain spotted fever. *A,* This 7-year-old boy was well until 10 days prior to admission when he developed fever and neck pain. Petechial rash was first noticed on the distal arms and legs 4 days after onset of symptoms. Within another 2 days, the rash had become generalized, soft tissue edema was noted, and intense myalgia was present. On admission to hospital 10 days after the onset of illness, he was lethargic but would cry when moved or with squeezing of his muscles. White blood cell count was 13,900 per cu. mm., 97 percent neutrophils, and the platelet count was 27,000 per cu. mm. Serum sodium was 120 mEq. per liter and chloride was 86 mEq. per liter. CSF contained 100 white blood cells per cu. mm. and protein content was 118 mg. per 100 ml. Complement fixation titer for Rocky Mountain spotted fever rose from 1:16 at 10 days after onset to 1:256 at 18 days after onset of illness. The child recovered with chloramphenicol therapy. *B,* Diffuse petechial rash and edema of the lips and eyelids. *C,* Rash and edema of dorsal surface of the hands and fingers. *D,* Rash on the palmar surface of the hands, characteristic of Rocky Mountain spotted fever.

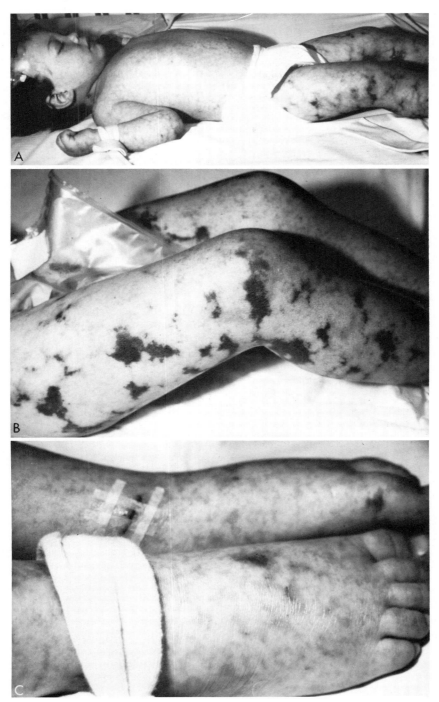

Figure 22–4.   Rocky Mountain spotted fever. *A,* Two-year-old child, 9 days after onset of illness. Several ticks had been removed from his scalp 2 weeks before the onset of symptoms. The illness began with spiking fever and irritability, followed 3 days later by rash, first noticed on the legs and ankles. By 7 days after onset, he was lethargic and irritable, and exhibited severe discomfort when the limbs were moved or the muscles palpated. On admission to the hospital 9 days after onset, the rash was extensive but most intense on the extremities. There was marked edema of the soft tissues of the face, hands, and lower extremities up to the knees. Serum sodium was 118 and chloride 92 mEq. per liter. Platelet count was 38,000 per cu. mm. CSF examination was normal except for 10 cells per cu. mm., all lymphocytes. The child recovered with chloramphenicol therapy. *B,* Petechial and ecchymotic lesions on the legs. *C,* Pedal edema.

ment is common in Rocky Mountain spotted fever, although it is the exceptional case in which hepatic derangement is severe enough to result in jaundice (Ramphal et al.). Compromise of renal function in the early stages of the illness is most often secondary to hypovolemia, although in severe cases renal vasculitis with interstitial nephritis can lead to acute renal failure (Green et al., Walker and Mattern). Myocarditis occurs in certain patients but only rarely does significant cardiomegaly or cardiac failure complicate the illness. An interstitial pneumonitis is occasionally seen on chest x-ray but also is not usually clinically significant. In some instances, pleural effusions complicate the course of the illness and can result in respiratory distress until appropriately managed.

Neurologic manifestations of one type or another are very common and might even be described as uniformly present if headache and myalgia are included in this category. When treatment is initiated within three to four days after onset of fever, further neurologic signs often do not occur. If therapy is not begun, while some children may remain alert and mentally clear, many will develop listlessness, mental confusion, disorientation, or delirium. Gradual decline in awareness is frequently associated with neck stiffness and other signs of neurologic involvement. Hearing loss has been observed during the acute stage of the illness and rarely may persist after recovery. Convulsions are not frequent in children with Rocky Mountain spotted fever but can occur in various patterns. Either generalized clonic seizures or focal motor convulsions may be followed by postictal hemiparesis, coma, or even respiratory arrest. Additional neurologic signs that have been recognized include ataxia, focal motor deficits of various types, tremulousness, and hyperreflexia. Most neurologic signs indicate involvement of the central nervous system although cranial or peripheral nerve dysfunction is not unknown. The sequence of development of neurologic signs in Rocky Mountain spotted fever is variable and is usually modified considerably by the early initiation of specific therapy. In general, headache, lethargy, and mental confusion are seen in the early stages, within two to four days after the appearance of the rash. More severe neurologic manifestations more often evolve four to eight days after development of the eruption.

Ocular abnormalities are notable in some children with Rocky Mountain spotted fever and include conjunctivitis, retinal venous engorgement, and retinal edema or exudates (Raab et al.). Papilledema has been observed, and, at least in some cases, is present despite normal cerebrospinal fluid pressure measured by lumbar puncture (Presley). Such fundus abnormalities most likely result from either increased capillary permeability of retinal vessels or from ischemic changes secondary to endothelial proliferation leading to vascular occlusion.

The clinical course, sequelae, and mortality of Rocky Mountain spotted fever are so clearly determined by the rapidity with which diagnosis is made and specific therapy started that statistics regarding mortality or sequelae have limited meaning. In untreated patients that survive, fever and other symptoms persist for two to four weeks before gradual improvement unfolds. Seriously ill patients have been described who remained comatose for several weeks (Thomas and Berlin). Early and appropriate therapy, conversely, may markedly attenuate the course of the illness, leading to complete recovery within a few days. In the years prior to antibiotics, the mortality rate was said to be 20 to 30 percent compared to approximately 5 to 10 percent currently (Hattwick et al. 1978, Peters). Mortality is higher in persons with delayed appearance of the rash and in black patients, in both instances probably reflecting the importance of the rash in clinical diagnosis and early initiation of therapy (Hattwick et al. 1978). Most deaths that do occur are during the second or third week of the illness and result from shock, hemorrhagic complications, or pulmonary involvement. It is generally agreed that death from spotted fever is most unusual if proper treatment is initiated in the early symptomatic stages. Studies of neurologic sequelae largely date to the pre-antibiotic period (Rosenblum et al., Thomas and Berlin). Although deficits can remain permanently in children seriously ill with the disease, in general, most survivors recover completely or with only minor persisting signs.

Laboratory Findings

During the first few days after onset of symptoms, the white blood cell count is usually normal or slightly reduced, but leukocytosis with an increase of immature forms is expected toward the end of the first week. A minority of children are found to have mild anemia during the second week of the illness, sometimes explained on the basis of gastrointestinal bleeding. Proteinuria associated with oligura and azotemia, in addition to hypoproteinemia, may accompany other metabolic deviations as the illness progresses. In rare cases, frank renal failure will ensue. As is the case with a number of serious childhood infections, serum hyponatremia and hypochloremia can result from recurrent vomiting, from excessive salt loss in the urine, or secondary to inappropriate secretion of antidiuretic hormone. Correction of serum hypoosmolarity is usually prompt following initiation of therapy but may enhance the tendency for convulsions to occur as long as it persists. Pancreatic involvement in some cases can lead to a transient diabetic state with insulin failure resulting in marked hyperglycemia and glucosuria.

Thrombocytopenia has now been widely recognized to be a common finding in Rocky Mountain spotted fever. While not invariable, significant reduction in the platelet count has been observed with surprising frequency when it has been searched for (Hazard et al., Rubio et al.). The petechial character of the rash is not dependent on the presence of thrombocytopenia but cutaneous ecchymoses or intestinal bleeding may result therefrom. Rubio et al. attributed subarachnoid hemorrhage to reduced platelets in a child with Rocky Mountain spotted fever. The cause of thrombocytopenia is not entirely clear but is probably secondary to the underlying vasculitis which provokes platelet clumping as well as intravascular clotting in certain patients. Bone marrow examination exhibits normal megakaryocyte production and thus does not account for decreased platelets in the peripheral blood. In addition to thrombocytopenia, hypofibrinogenemia and other clotting factor abnormalities have been identified (Atkin et al., Trigg), suggesting the existence of intravascular coagulation.

The cerebrospinal fluid examination in the child with Rocky Mountain spotted fever is likely to be helpful mainly in a negative fashion. Among 47 children studied by Haynes and colleagues, the spinal fluid was normal in 27. A lymphocytic pleocytosis is occasionally present but the total number of cells is usually less than 50 per cu. mm. A certain number of red blood cells may be found in the CSF but their number is not sufficient to result in xanthochromia, assuming that the tap was not traumatic. The glucose content remains normal and the protein value is either normal or modestly elevated. Organisms are not seen on gram stain of the fluid specimen.

Additional laboratory abnormalities identified in some include roentgen evidence of an interstitial pneumonia and electrocardiographic findings consistent with myocarditis. Patients with severe myonecrosis and hepatic involvement will have elevations of the serum glutamic oxaloacetic transaminase, creatine phosphokinase, and lactic acid dehydrogenase levels (Green et al., Sexton et al.).

Diagnosis

Diagnosis of Rocky Mountain spotted fever can be divided into two broad categories. The first is the recognition of the probable existence of the disease on the basis of the clinical manifestations, while the second is its confirmation by specific laboratory techniques.

Suspicion of the probability should be aroused in the case of a child with a febrile illness in the spring or summer in whom the characteristic rash develops two to four days after onset. History of exposure to ticks or discovery of a tick attached to the child's body are further points strongly indicative of the possibility of Rocky Mountain spotted fever. The scalp is a favorite site for ticks to take residence, and, especially in girls with abundant hair, they can easily be missed unless an extensive search is made. The evolution of neurologic signs with relatively insignificant CSF changes, along with thrombocytopenia and serum hyponatremia, are further important features that should raise the clinical index of suspicion. Establishment of a presumptive diagnosis on clinical grounds is mandatory because treatment should be started before more definitive studies can confirm the diagnosis. The symptoms and signs, the laboratory findings, and the history of exposure to ticks is usually sufficiently characteristic of the disease that a presumptive clinical diagnosis can be established.

In atypical cases, skin and muscle biopsy is an additional procedure which can be useful in the early stages of the illness. The biopsy should be obtained at the site of a cutaneous lesion and should be processed in emergency fashion. A portion of the tissue is gram-stained and cultured for bacteria while another segment is prepared for microscopic examination. Expected findings in Rocky Mountain spotted fever include lymphocytic cuffing of blood vessels in the dermis and thrombotic occlusion of some vessels in the same region. Giemsa stain discloses the presence of coccobacilli in the endothelium and muscle cells of vascular structures, which is strongly suggestive of the diagnosis. Immunofluorescent study of biopsy material for demonstration of rickettsial organisms is an additional useful diagnostic method if the technique is available (Green et al., Walker and Cain).

Absolute confirmation of the diagnosis of Rocky Mountain spotted fever is on the basis of serologic tests, which do not usually become positive until ten to 14 days or even longer after the onset of symptoms. In some cases, rickettsiae can be isolated during the first several days of the illness by intraperitoneal injection of blood into guinea pigs, or injection into the yolk sac of embryonated eggs.

The Weil-Felix agglutination reaction depends on the presence of an antigen common to rickettsiae and the *Proteus* bacillus and is performed by mixing serum of the patient with OX-19 strain of *Proteus vulgaris*. Although not entirely specific for Rocky Mountain spotted fever, a titer of 1:160 or higher is strong supportive evidence of the disease. A four-fold or greater titer rise during convalescence is of greater diagnostic value than the initial titer alone. The complement fixation test is now a better diagnostic method in that it is specific for Rocky Mountain spotted fever. The test usually becomes positive in the second week of the illness and a four-fold or greater titer rise is virtually diagnostic. Peak titers are usually achieved between two and four weeks after onset of symptoms and slowly decline thereafter.

Differential diagnostic considerations include those febrile disorders associated with a combination of a rash and neurologic manifestations. Meningococcal meningitis or meningococcemia share many common features with Rocky Mountain spotted fever. Likewise, in those with minimal or no rash but with hepatic and renal involvement as well as meningeal signs and a lymphocytic CSF pleocytosis, the disease closely resembles leptospirosis (Ramphal et al.). In the Rocky Mountain region of the United States, Colorado tick fever is frequently confused with Rocky Mountain spotted fever, especially in the initial stages of the illness (Spruance and Bailey). Both diseases are transmitted by the wood tick, occur in the spring or summer months, and begin with fever, malaise, and headache. Rash is much less common with Colorado tick fever and, when it does occur, is more often predominantly located on the trunk. Neurologic manifestations are far less frequent, and marked leukopenia is characteristic of this viral disease. Other types of bacterial meningitis, viral aseptic meningitis or encephalitis, ECHO virus infection, infectious mononucleosis, and rubeola are additional conditions frequently confused with spotted fever. Rat-bite fever caused by *Streptobacillus moniliformis* is a rare disorder in children but is one in which the early clinical features are similar to those of rickettsial disease (Raffin and Freemark). The illness begins with spiking fever and chills, followed by the development of a maculopapular or petechial rash that often involves the palms and soles. Diagnosis is suspected by the history of a rat bite and is proved by the development of a serum titer rise of streptobacillus agglutinins. Bearing close resemblance to Rocky Mountain spotted fever have been the infrequent cases of atypical measles in children exposed to natural rubeola after previous immunization with killed measles vaccine (Nader et al.). This rare illness has been characterized by rash first appearing on the legs, fever, myalgia, and soft-tissue edema, thus similar to the findings with rickettsial disease. Thrombotic thrombocytopenic purpura also may be suspected initially, because of the combination of fever, petechiae, thrombocytopenia, and neurologic abnormalities.

Treatment

As mentioned before, specific therapy is most effective when begun during the first week of the illness, before the diagnosis can be confirmed by serologic tests. Therefore, it is most important that the disease be recognized clinically allowing the initiation of treatment before serious complications are allowed to develop. Either chloramphenicol or tetracycline is effective and the choice must be made on the basis of the personal preference of the physician. Many feel that chloramphenicol has fewer disadvantages in children and prefer its use in a dosage of 100 mg. per kilogram per day administered intravenously. Caution must be exercised, however, with the use of chloramphenicol in this dose in the unusual patient with jaundice and significant compromise of hepatic function. The duration of therapy depends on the course of the illness but most require a minimum of ten days of antibiotic treatment. When therapy is begun in the early stages of the illness, decrease in fever and improvement in general will usually follow within two to four days. If begun in the second week, by which time the child has become "toxic" and with definite neurologic signs, a lag of several days may occur before a favorable response is observed. Sulfonamides are contraindicated, with claims by many authors that they may worsen the disease or even increase the mortality rate.

Additional therapeutic measures are determined by the presence of complications secondary to the generalized vascular inflammatory process. Anemia or hypovolemia leading to shock requires appropriate measures, including fresh whole blood or plasma expanders. In most, however, the presence of soft tissue edema and hypoosmolarity warrants the use of modest fluid restriction until the laboratory findings show improvement (Liu et al.). In the moderately ill or seriously ill patient with this disease, judgments regarding fluid volume requirements are best made on the basis of measurements of central venous pressure determined via a central venous catheter. Documented laboratory evidence of consumption coagulopathy warrants consideration of heparin therapy, although this is most unusual in this disorder. Vitamin K is administered if vitamin K-dependent clotting factors are diminished but should not be given by intramuscular injection when there is significant thrombocytopenia. Corticosteroids have been recommended by certain authors but their value has not been clearly established. In view of the tendency for intestinal bleeding to occur in certain children with Rocky Mountain spotted fever, corticosteroids should probably not be used unless a specific indication arises.

A commercial vaccine is available which is effective in producing considerable modification of the disease, should it occur, but which does not completely prevent it. The vaccine has been used primarily in protecting persons at relatively high risk for the disease, such as laboratory workers who handle the organism and persons in occupations which expose them to potentially infected ticks.

Having identified Rocky Mountain spotted fever in a child, the physician should assume responsibility for notification of the local public health authorities who, in turn, should inform other members of the health profession of the presence of the disease within the community. Subsequent cases are more likely to be recognized early if practitioners have been alerted of the possibility. In addition, when a childhood case is diagnosed, the parents should be advised to make periodic examinations of their other children as well as household pets for the presence of ticks and properly remove them, if found. Vector eradication in communities with identified cases is another component of management which falls under the domain of public health agencies.

REFERENCES

Ailawa, J. K.: Rocky Mountain Spotted Fever. Charles C Thomas, Springfield, Ill., 1966.

Atkin, M. D., Strauss, H. S., and Fisher, G. U.: A case report of "Cape Cod" Rocky Mountain spotted fever with multiple coagulation disturbances. Pediatrics 36:627–632, 1965.

Bell, W. E., and Lascari, A. D.: Rocky Mountain spotted fever. Neurological symptoms in the acute phase. Neurology 20:841–847, 1970.

Bradford, W. D., and Hawkins, H. K.: Rocky Mountain spotted fever in childhood. Am. J. Dis. Child. 131:1228–1232, 1977.

Green, W. R., Walker, D. H., and Cain, B. G.: Fatal viscerotropic Rocky Mountain spotted fever. Am. J. Med. 64:523–528, 1978.

Hand, W. L., Miller, J. B., Reinarz, J. A., and Sanford, J. P.: Rocky Mountain spotted fever. A vascular disease. Arch. Intern. Med. 125:879–882, 1970.

Harrell, G. T.: Rickettsial involvement of the nervous system. Med. Clin. N. Amer. 37:395–422, 1953.

Harrell, G. T.: Rocky Mountain spotted fever. Medicine 28:33–370, 1949.

Hassin, G. B.: Cerebral changes in Rocky Mountain spotted fever. Arch. Neurol. Psychiat. 44:1290–1295, 1940.

Hattwick, M. A. W., O'Brien, R. J., and Hanson, B. F.: Rocky Mountain spotted fever: Epidemiology of an increasing problem. Ann. Intern. Med. 84:732–739, 1976.

Hattwick, M. A. W., Retailliau, H., O'Brien, J., Slutzker, M., Fontaine, R. E., and Hanson, B.: Fatal Rocky Mountain spotted fever. J.A.M.A. 240:1499–1503, 1978.

Haynes, R. E., Sanders, D. Y., and Cramblett, H. G.: Rocky Mountain spotted fever in children. J. Pediat. 76:685–693, 1970.

Hazard, G. W., Ganz, R. N., Nevin, R. W., Nauss, A. H., Curtis, E., Bell, W. J., and Murray, E. W.: Rocky Mountain spotted fever in the eastern United States. Thirteen cases from the Cape Cod area of Massachusetts. New Eng. J. Med. 280:57–62, 1969.

Jacobs, W. M., and Chusid, M. J.: Rocky Mountain spotted fever in an infant: Diagnosis in siblings. Am. J. Dis. Child. 132:928–929, 1978.

Johnson, J. E., III, and Kadull, P. J.: Rocky Mountain spotted fever acquired in a laboratory. New Eng. J. Med. 277:842–847, 1967.

Liu, C. T., Hilmas, D. E., Griffin, M. J., Petersen, C. E., Hadick, C. L., Jr., and Beisel, W. R.: Alterations of body fluid compartments and distribution of tissue water and electrolytes in Rhesus monkeys with Rocky Mountain spotted fever. J. Infect. Dis. 138:42–48, 1978.

McMurry, J. F., Jr.: Review of Rocky Mountain spotted fever. J. Oklahoma Med. Assoc. 59:165–171, 1966.

Miller, J. Q., and Price, T. R.: The nervous system in Rocky Mountain spotted fever. Neurology 22:561–566, 1972.

Morbidity and Mortality Weekly Report, Vol. 19, No. 53, Summary, 1970.

Nader, P. R., Horwitz, M. S., and Rousseau, J.: Atypical exanthem following exposure to natural measles. Eleven cases in children previously inoculated with killed vaccine. J. Pediat. 72:22–28, 1968.

Oster, C. N., Burke, D. S., Kenyon, R. H., Ascher, M. S., Harber, P., and Pedersen, C. E., Jr.: Laboratory-acquired Rocky Mountain spotted fever. The hazard of aerosol transmission. New Eng. J. Med. 297:859–863, 1977.

Peters, A. H.: Tick-borne typhus (Rocky Mountain spotted fever). Epidemiologic trends, with particular reference to Virginia. J.A.M.A. 216:1003–1007, 1971.

Presley, G. D.: Fundus changes in Rocky Mountain spotted fever. Am. J. Ophthal. 67:263–267, 1969.

Raab, E. L., Leopold, I. H., and Hodes, H. L.: Retinopathy in Rocky Mountain spotted fever. Am. J. Ophthal. 68:42–46, 1969.

Raffin, B. J., and Freemark, M.: Streptobacillary rat-bite fever: A pediatric problem. Pediatrics 64:214–217, 1979.

Ramphal, R., Kluge, R., Cohen, V., and Feldman, R.: Rocky Mountain spotted fever and jaundice. Two consecutive cases acquired in Florida and a review of the literature on this complication. Arch. Intern. Med. 138:260–263, 1978.

Rosenblum, M. J., Masland, R. L., and Harrell, G. T.: Residual effects of rickettsial disease on the central nervous system. Results of neurologic examinations and electroencephalograms following Rocky Mountain spotted fever. Arch. Intern. Med. 90:444–455, 1952.

Rubio, T., Riley, H. D., Jr., Nida, J. R., Brooksaler, F., and Nelson, J. D.: Thrombocytopenia in Rocky Mountain spotted fever. Am. J. Dis. Child. 116:88–96, 1968.

Scheinker, I. M.: Histologic observations on the changes in the brain in Rocky Mountain spotted fever. Arch. Path. 35:583–589, 1943.

Sexton, D. J., Banks, P. M., Weig, S., and Roe, C. R.: Late appearance of skin rash and abnormal serum enzymes in Rocky Mountain spotted fever. A case report. J. Pediat. 87:580–582, 1975.

Spruance, S. L., and Bailey, A.: Colorado tick fever. Arch. Intern. Med. 131:288–293, 1973.

Thomas, M. H., and Berlin, L.: Neurologic sequelae of Rocky Mountain spotted fever. Arch. Neurol. Psychiat. 60:574–583, 1948.

Trigg, J. W., Jr.: Hypofibrinogenemia in Rocky Mountain spotted fever. Report of a case. New Eng. J. Med. 270:1042–1044, 1964.

Vianna, N. J., and Hinman, A. R.: Rocky Mountain spotted fever on Long Island. Am. J. Med. 51:725–730, 1971.

Walker, D. H., and Cain, B. G.: A method for specific diagnosis of Rocky Mountain spotted fever on fixed, paraffin-embedded tissue by immunofluorescence. J. Infect. Dis. 137:206–209, 1978.

Walker, D. H., and Mattern, W. D.: Acute renal failure in Rocky Mountain spotted fever. Arch. Intern. Med. 139:443–448, 1979.

Neurologic Conditions Related to Inflammatory or Infectious Disorders

Chapter Twenty-Three

SHUNT INFECTIONS

Diversionary procedures, or shunts, from the ventricular system or lumbar subarachnoid space continue to be the common method of treatment of hydrocephalus in infants and children. Bacterial colonization of a shunt followed by sepsis, ventriculitis, or meningitis is one of the most common and potentially serious complications of this form of treatment. In addition to the effects of the infection itself, bacterial contamination of a shunt or valve mechanism can disrupt its function, exacerbating the hydrocephalic process. Thrombus formation within the cardiac end of the shunt secondary to infection also increases the predisposition to multiple and recurrent pulmonary embolization, possibly leading to eventual pulmonary hypertension and cor pulmonale.

The incidence of shunt infection has been variously estimated but it is generally believed that approximately 15 to 20 percent of patients with vascular shunts will develop this complication at some time or other (Noonan and Ehmke, Luthardt, Morrice and Young). Among 289 children surgically treated for hydrocephalus, Schoenbaum et al. observed that shunt infection occurred in 27 percent. In this series, there was no significant difference between ventriculoatrial and ventriculoperitoneal shunts regarding the incidence of infection, although most previous authors have claimed that peritoneal shunts were less frequently affected than vascular shunts.

Infection of a shunt can occur anytime after its placement but the period of greatest risk is the first four to eight weeks after the operation. *Staphylococcus epidermidis (albus)* is the leading offender, followed by *Staphylococcus aureus* (Bruce et al., Perrin and McLaurin), and, less frequently, other organisms such as *Escherichia coli, Hemophilus influenzae, Pseudomonas, Serratia marcescens,* and *Bacillus cerus* (Leffert et al., Bruce et al., Sells et al.). Visintine et al. described a single case of a ventriculoatrial shunt infection with *Listeria monocytogenes,* and rare cases of ventricular shunt colonization with Candida species have also been reported (Bayer et al., Rodgers et al.). In the series of 77 patients with shunt infections reported by Schoenbaum et al., one-half were caused by *Staphylococcus epidermidis* and one-fourth by *Staphylococcus aureus.* Gram-negative organisms assume greater importance with subarachnoid-ureteral shunts but this type of drainage is now infrequently done.

The high incidence of staphylococcal infection plus the temporal relationship between shunt placement and infection indicates that contamination with organisms from the skin is an important factor regarding pathogenesis. Persistence and difficulty of eradication of staphylococcal colonization of a shunt may be related to the excessive mucoid substance produced by the subtype (S. II) of *Staphylococcus epidermidis* commonly isolated from these patients (Holt, Bayston and Penny). Bacteremia either soon after shunt placement or any time subsequently can also result in colonization of a vascular shunt, with eventual cerebrospinal fluid or systemic infection. An infrequent cause of shunt infection is direct contamination from the surface when the shunt becomes exposed secondary to pressure necrosis of the overlying skin.

Clinical Signs

The clinical manifestations of shunt infection vary considerably, in part depending on the degree of virulence of the infecting or-

647

ganism and whether or not the illness is a septic one, involves only ventricular fluid, or represents a combination of sepsis and meningitis. As a generalization, shunt infection with *Staphylococcus epidermidis* tends to be a more indolent and smoldering process, while that caused by *Staphylococcus aureus* is more likely to be an acute, fulminating one with obvious septic signs. In many instances, fever is the only significant abnormality, while in others fever, lethargy, and vomiting are eventually accompanied by splenomegaly and progressive anemia. Headache and meningeal signs are usually present in those with associated meningeal infection. Cutaneous lesions are not common in children with staphylococcal infected shunts although subungual splinter hemorrhages, petechiae, or even purpura fulminans can occur (Shennan).

Consideration of shunt infection is advised in any child who has a shunt and develops a febrile illness. A significant blood leukocytosis is frequently present but its absence does not exclude the possibility of bacterial sepsis. In the series of infected shunts evaluated by Schoenbaum et al., 25 percent of the patients had white blood cell counts of less than 10,000 per cu. mm. despite active infection. Cutaneous erythema immediately over the shunt tubing is almost certain evidence of infection; however, this is not a common finding. Several blood cultures may be needed in order to isolate the organism, and these are preferably obtained during a febrile spike, or after the valve has been manually compressed several times. Bacteremia is expected and blood cultures are usually positive in patients with infected ventriculoatrial shunts but not in those with colonized ventriculoperitoneal shunts.

Cerebrospinal fluid should be gram-stained and cultured in both aerobic and anaerobic fashion when a shunt infection is suspected; however, ventricular tap is often undesirable because of the possible hazards. Ventricular fluid can be readily obtained if the shunt includes a reservoir (Fig. 23–1) that allows percutaneous tapping and if the proximal (ventricular) end of the tube is patent and terminates within the ventricle. Ventricular fluid can also be obtained by direct aspiration of the shunt tube if the system is patent (Myers and Schoenbaum).

Studies to evaluate methods of prevention

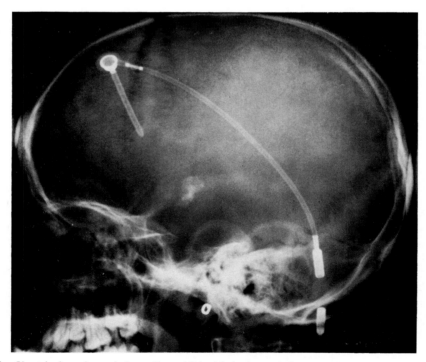

Figure 23–1. Ventriculoperitoneal shunt in a child with hydrocephalus secondary to a calcified hypothalamic mass. The ventricular end of the catheter leads to a reservoir embedded within a frontal burr hole. The presence of the reservoir permits easy assessment of the patency of the proximal end of the tube. It also allows sampling of the ventricular fluid if ventricular infection is considered and provides an accessible route for administration of intraventricular antibiotics should this be necessary.

of shunt infection have yielded conflicting results, although recent investigations provide support for the use of prophylactic antibiotics at the time the shunt procedure is performed (Salmon, McLaurin). Venes noted a significant reduction in shunt infections in children given intravenous oxacillin during induction of anesthesia and repeated six and 12 hours later, but also emphasized the importance of other aspects of the surgical technique. Although sufficient controlled studies have not yet been accomplished, the fact that most early shunt infections stem from the perioperative period and involve a common organism usually sensitive to semisynthetic penicillin would warrant serious consideration of the use of antibiotics at the time the shunt is installed.

Shunt Nephritis

In 1965, Black and colleagues in England identified the association of nephritis in children with infected vascular shunts, a complication now recognized to be an immune-mediated disorder somewhat similar to that of lupus nephritis. Several reports appeared thereafter, although it is generally agreed that shunt nephritis is an unusual complication of ventriculoatrial shunts (Stauffer, Moncrieff et al., McKenzie and Hayden). In most reported cases, shunt colonization and sepsis have been caused by a coagulase-negative staphylococcus, a bacterial agent previously considered not to be pathogenic in man. A few have been secondary to other organisms, such as *Staphylococcus aureus* and *Corynebacterium bovis* (Bolton et al.). The majority of reported cases of shunt nephritis have been in infants or young children, although older persons have been affected as well (Kaufman and McIntosh, Bolton et al.).

Renal manifestations can occur within a month or up to several years after placement of the shunt and often are found in association with signs of septicemia. Spiking fever, night sweats, hepatosplenomegaly, and anemia are followed by positive blood and, sometimes, positive spinal or ventricular fluid cultures. Hematuria is frequently the first renal manifestation of the disorder, which later is associated with proteinuria, systemic hypertension, and azotemia. Several reported cases have presented with features of the nephrotic syndrome, including massive proteinuria, hypoproteinemia, hypercholesterolemia, and edema.

Glomerulonephritis secondary to an infected vascular shunt is now believed to be an immunologic reaction, with the offending antigen being derived from the infecting organism (Stickler et al., Rames et al.). Persistent antigenemia results in nephritogenic immune complex formation with deposition in glomerular capillary walls. Findings indicative of this process include serum complement depletion, cryoglobulinemia, and ultrastructural renal charges (Strife et al., Dobrin et al., Kaufman and McIntosh). Renal pathology consists of diffuse proliferation and swelling of endothelial and mesangial cells with thickened basement membranes (Stickler et al., Bolton et al.). Electron microscopy has revealed granular deposits upon the glomerular basement membrane while immunofluorescent studies have shown the presence of complement and immunoglobulins along the basement membrane (Rames et al., Stickler et al., Kaufman and McIntosh). Cultures of renal tissue obtained at biopsy have been consistently negative.

Treatment

Treatment of shunt infection remains a controversial subject for which there is no established standardized approach. One of the early reviews of the subject suggested that removal of the shunt was required before the infection could be obliterated (Bruce et al.), a concept adhered to by many subsequent authors (Nicholas et al., Schoenbaum et al., Morrice and Young). Experience of McLaurin has questioned this as a universal approach and has indicated that certain select cases can be cured with an intensive course of intravenous and intraventricular antibiotics without removal of the shunt.

Different methods of treatment that have been proposed include systemic antibiotic therapy, systemic and intraventricular antibiotic therapy, antibiotic treatment with shunt removal and immediate replacement in either the same or a different site, and antibiotic therapy with shunt removal with delayed shunt replacement in the same or a different site (Shurtleff et al.). The ideal therapeutic regimen for every case cannot be outlined although it is clear that many, if not most, will require removal of the shunt once it is colonized.

If the infected shunt is a ventriculoatrial one, its removal can be followed by ventricular drainage via a reservoir for a few days and then replaced by a ventriculoperitoneal shunt. In a few instances the removed colonized shunt is found to have been non-functional and the child remains stable without further shunting. When staphylococcal meningitis is also present, as reflected by abnormal cerebrospinal fluid findings including the presence of bacteria, intraventricular methicillin may enhance eradication of the infection. Intraventricular therapy is also important when shunt meningitis is caused by bacteria that are sensitive only to antibiotics that diffuse poorly into the cerebrospinal fluid. For staphylococci resistant to penicillinase-resistant penicillins or for gentamicin-sensitive gram-negative organisms, intraventricular gentamicin in dosage of 1 to 2 mg. per day is recommended (Pickering et al.). Rifampin administered orally, in combination with gentamicin or vancomycin, has also been found to be useful in the treatment of methicillin-resistant staphylococcal shunt infections (Archer et al., Ring et al.). Intravenous therapy is continued for a minimum of three to four weeks and is followed by additional blood and cerebrospinal fluid cultures to be certain the illness is overcome.

The antibiotic of choice depends on the in vitro sensitivity tests but is usually either penicillin or a penicillinase-resistant penicillin derivative. Of the penicillinase-resistant penicillins, methicillin and nafcillin have been the most popular, with little proof of the superiority of one over the other. Methicillin is excreted by the kidneys while nafcillin is excreted primarily by the biliary system. For this reason, nafcillin would be preferable in patients with staphylococcal meningitis complicated by renal failure or shunt nephritis. Methicillin has not been shown to penetrate well into the CSF from serum but nafcillin has been found to achieve CSF concentrations well above minimum inhibitory concentrations for sensitive *Staphylococcus* species (Kane et al., Ruiz and Warner). For this reason, some workers favor nafcillin for treatment of penicillinase-producing staphylococcal meningitis.

REFERENCES

Archer, G. L., Tenenbaum, M. J., and Haywood, H. B.: Rifampin therapy of *Staphylococcus epidermidis*. Use in infections from indwelling artificial devices. J.A.M.A. 240:751–753, 1978.

Bayer, A. S., Edwards, J. E., Jr., Seidel, J. S., and Guze, L. B.: Candida meningitis. Report of seven cases and review of the English literature. Medicine 55:477–486, 1976.

Bayston, R., and Penny, S. R.: Excessive production of mucoid substance in Staphylococcus S.I.I.A.: A possible factor in colonization of Holter shunts. Dev. Med. Child. Neurol. 14(Suppl. 27):25–28, 1972.

Black, J. A., Challacombe, D. N., and Ockenden, B. G.: Nephrotic syndrome associated with bacteraemia after shunt operations for hydrocephalus. Lancet 2:921–924, 1965.

Bolton, W. K., Sande, M. A., Normansell, D. E., Sturgill, B. C., and Westervelt, F. B., Jr.: Ventriculojugular shunt nephritis with Corynebacterium bovis. Am. J. Med. 59:417–423, 1973.

Bruce, A. M., Lorber, J., Shedden, W. I. H., and Zachary, R. B.: Persistent bacteraemia following ventriculo-caval shunt operations for hydrocephalus in infants. Dev. Med. Child. Neurol. 5:461–470, 1963.

Dobrin, R. S., Day, N. K., Quie, P. G., Moore, H. L., Vernier, R. L., Michael, A. F., and Fish, A. J.: The role of complement, immunoglobulin, and bacterial antigen in coagulase-negative staphylococcal shunt nephritis. Am. J. Med. 59:660–673, 1975.

Holt, R.: The classification of staphylococci from colonized ventriculoatrial shunts. J. Clin. Path. 22:475–482, 1969.

Kane, J. G., Parker, R. H., Jordan, G. W., and Hoeprich, P. D.: Nafcillin concentration in cerebrospinal fluid during treatment of staphylococcal infections. Ann. Intern. Med. 87:309–311, 1977.

Kaufman, D. B., and McIntosh, R.: The pathogenesis of the renal lesion in a patient with streptococcal disease infected ventriculoatrial shunt, cryoglobulinemia and nephritis. Am. J. Med. 50:262–268, 1971.

Leffert, H. L., Baptist, J. N., and Gidez, L. I.: Meningitis and bacteremia after ventriculoatrial shunt-revision: Isolation of a lethinase-producing *Bacillus cereus*. J. Infect. Dis. 122:547–552, 1970.

Luthardt, T.: Bacterial infections in ventriculo-auricular shunt systems. Dev. Med. Child. Neurol. 12(Suppl. 22):105–109, 1970.

McKenzie, S. A., and Hayden, K.: Two cases of "shunt nephritis." Pediatrics 54:806–808, 1974.

McLaurin, R. L.: Treatment of infected ventricular shunts. Child's Brain. 1:306–310, 1975.

Moncrieff, M. W., Glasgow, E. F., Arthur, L. J. H., and Hargreaves, H. M.: Glomerulonephritis associated with Staphylococcus albus in a Spitz-Holter valve. Arch. Dis. Childh. 48:69–72, 1973.

Morrice, J. J., and Young, D. G.: Bacterial colonization of Holter valves: A ten-year survey. Dev. Med. Child. Neurol. 16(Suppl. 32):85–90, 1974.

Myers, M. G., and Schoenbaum, S. C.: Shunt fluid aspiration. An adjunct in the diagnosis of cerebrospinal fluid shunt infection. Am. J. Dis. Child. 129:220–222, 1975.

Nicholas, J. L., Kamal, I. M., and Eckstein, H. B.: Immediate shunt replacement in the treatment of bacterial colonization of Holter valves. Dev. Med. Child. Neurol. 12(Suppl. 22):110–113, 1970.

Noonan, J. A., and Ehmke, D. A.: Complications of ventriculovenous shunts for control of hydrocephalus. New Eng. J. Med. 269:70–74, 1963.

Perrin, J. C. S., and McLaurin, R. L.: Infected ventriculoatrial shunts. J. Neurosurg. 27:21–26, 1967.

Pickering, L. K., Ericsson, C. D., Ruiz-Palacios, G., Blevins, J., and Miner, M. E.: Intraventricular and parenteral gentamicin therapy for ventriculitis in children. Am. J. Dis. Child. 132:480–483, 1978.

Rames, L., Wise, B., Goodman, J. R., and Piel, C. F.:

Renal disease with *Staphylococcus albus* bacteremia. J.A.M.A. 212:1671–1677, 1970.

Ring, J. C., Cates, K. L., Belani, K. K., Gaston, T. L., Sveum, R. J., and Marker, S. C.: Rifampin for CSF shunt infections caused by coagulase-negative staphylococci. J. Pediat. 95:317–319, 1979.

Rodgers, B. M., Vries, J. K., and Talbert, J. L.: Laparoscopy in the diagnosis and treatment of malfunctioning ventriculo-peritoneal shunts in children. J. Pediat. Surg. 13:247–253, 1978.

Ruiz, D. E., and Warner, J. F.: Nafcillin treatment of *Staphylococcus aureus* meningitis. Antimicrob. Agents Chemother. 9:554–555, 1976.

Salmon, J. H.: Adult hydrocephalus: Evaluation of shunt therapy in 80 patients. J. Neurosurg. 37:423–428, 1972.

Schoenbaum, S. C., Gardner, P., and Shillito, J.: Infections of cerebrospinal fluid shunts: Epidemiology, clinical manifestations, and therapy. J. Infect. Dis. 131:543–552, 1975.

Sells, C. J., Shurtleff, D. B., and Loeser, J. D.: Gram-negative cerebrospinal fluid shunt-associated infections. Pediatrics 59:614–618, 1977.

Shennan, A. T.: Purpura necrotica as a complication of ventriculoatrial shunts in hydrocephalus. Arch. Dis. Childh. 47:821–823, 1972.

Shurtleff, D. B., Foltz, E. L., Weeks, R. D., and Loeser, J.: Therapy of staphylococcus epidermidis: Infections associated with cerebrospinal fluid shunts. Pediatrics 53:55–62, 1974.

Stauffer, U. G.: Shunt nephritis. Diffuse glomerulonephritis complicating ventriculo-atrial shunts. Dev. Med. Child. Neurol. 12(Suppl. 22):161–164, 1970.

Stickler, G. B., Shin, M. H., Burke, E. C., Hollery, K. E., Miller, R. H., and Seger, W. E.: Diffuse glomerulonephritis associated with infected ventriculoatrial shunt. New Eng. J. Med. 279:1077–1082, 1968.

Strife, C. F., McDonald, B. M., Ruley, E. J., McAdams, A. J., and West, C. D.: Shunt nephritis: The nature of the serum cryoglobulins and their relation to the complement profile. J. Pediat. 88:403–413, 1976.

Venes, J. L.: Control of shunt infections. Report of 150 consecutive cases. J. Neurosurg. 45:311–314, 1976.

Visintine, A. M., Oleske, J. M., and Nahmias, A. J.: *Listeria monocytogenes* infection in infants and children. Am. J. Dis. Child. 131:393–397, 1977.

Chapter Twenty-Four

REYE'S SYNDROME (ACUTE ENCEPHALOPATHY AND FATTY DEGENERATION OF THE VISCERA)

Reye's syndrome is a disorder of acute onset, usually one to several days after a viral upper respiratory infection or varicella, and characterized by manifestations of a diffuse, severe non-inflammatory encephalopathy in addition to derangement of hepatic function. In its severe form, the illness rapidly leads to coma and decerebrate or decorticate rigidity, and often proceeds to cardiorespiratory arrest and death within 48 to 72 hours after onset. Common but not invariable laboratory findings include hypoglycemia and decreased cerebrospinal fluid glucose, marked elevation in serum glutamic oxaloacetic transaminase and ammonia levels, a prolonged prothrombin time, and absence of a cerebrospinal fluid pleocytosis. The pathologic findings are generalized brain swelling without cellular infiltration or other evidence of encephalitis, in addition to fatty degeneration of the liver and sometimes of the kidneys.

Although the etiology and pathogenesis remain speculative, most investigators now feel that Reye's syndrome is best placed in the "post-viral" category and that the encephalopathy is partly but not entirely explained on the basis of hepatic dysfunction which results in hypoglycemia and increased blood and brain levels of toxic substances, including ammonia and lactic acid (Shannon et al.). The pathogenesis of the encephalopathy, however, remains speculative to this date, as is the role of increased intracranial pressure as a factor accounting for certain of the clinical features. Cases have now been observed with deep coma in the absence of intracranial hypertension, and signs of encephalopathy have been observed in children which preceded evidence of hepatic dysfunction (Appelbaum and Thaler).

The disease was recognized as an entity in 1963 by Reye, Morgan and Baral, although it had been described by authors as early as 1929 (Brain et al.). A detailed report by Lyon et al. in 1961 of similar cases emphasized the cerebral manifestations and the dramatic rapidity of the natural course of the illness in most cases. Greater awareness of the syndrome has made it apparent that the disorder is not rare and that variations of its severity occur. The disease has now been recognized in many parts of the world, affects either sex, and has been identified in children from early infancy to 16 years of age with only rare cases in older persons (Varma et al.). Younger children, especially those in the second half of the first decade, are more often affected than older ones, and in those under one year of age the disease has had a particularly high fatality rate. In the original series described by Reye and colleagues, 14 of 21 patients were less than two years of age. Most affected children have been previously normal and the vast majority of reported cases have occurred in isolated fashion within a family. The disease has been described on rare occasion in siblings (Becroft, Glick et al., Hilty et al., Randolph et al.), and also in twins (Thaler et al.).

In this country, Reye's syndrome occurs either sporadically or in clusters, with several cases developing in a community over a limited period of time. The sporadic cases have followed varicella, a nonspecific upper respiratory infection, or one in which a variety of viral agents have been isolated. Cases occurring in small outbreaks have more often been associated with antecedent influenza B infections. Reye's syndrome, or one remarkably similar to it, occurs in endemic fashion in northeastern Thailand, where it is estimated to affect hundreds of children annually and in one large hospital is said to be the leading cause of death in children between one and six years of age (Olson et al.). The strikingly high incidence of the illness in Thailand has been attributed to intoxication with aflatoxin, a substance found in certain foods and believed to be produced by the fungus *Aspergillus flavus*.

Clinical Manifestations

The history, physical findings, and natural course of this disease are fairly uniform from patient to patient, although mild forms of the illness can occur and are identified only by laboratory analysis. In such cases, the preceding viral illness is followed by vomiting and perhaps transient headache or slight depression of awareness, which progresses no further and is followed by uneventful recovery. The most common pattern of this illness with severe clinical manifestations is sufficiently characteristic that clinical diagnosis can usually be made within a few hours after hospital admission. Various forms of clinical staging have been proposed in an attempt to classify the degree of severity of the process at a given moment (Bobo et al., Lovejoy et al., Schubert et al.). The four-stage staging system of DeVivo et al. includes Stage I manifested by vomiting, confusion, and lethargy. Stage II comprises symptoms of agitation, delirium, decorticate posturing, and sometimes hyperventilation. In Stage III, there is

coma with decerebrate posturing, and Stage IV includes flaccidity, apnea, and dilated fixed pupils.

The five-stage system of Bobo et al. and Lovejoy et al. includes Stage I with vomiting, lethargy, and laboratory evidence of liver dysfunction; Stage II with disorientation, combativeness, hyperventilation, hyperreflexia, and presence of responsiveness to noxious stimulation; Stage III with coma, hyperventilation, decorticate rigidity, and preservation of pupillary light and oculovestibular reflexes; Stage IV with deepening coma, decerebrate rigidity, loss of oculocephalic reflexes, and dilated fixed pupils; and Stage V characterized by flaccidity, absence of deep tendon reflexes, and respiratory arrest.

Reye's syndrome is much less common in infancy than in older children, but when it does occur in this age group the clinical manifestations often depart somewhat from the stepwise progression through the different stages described above. Fever, acute onset of respiratory distress with tachypnea, and the rapid emergence of apneic episodes, seizures, and coma are the common presenting manifestations in the infant (Huttenlocher and Trauner). Severe hypoglycemia will be found in most, and vomiting is less striking in the initial stages than is the case in the older child. The mortality rate has been found to be higher when the illness occurs in children less than two years of age, and among survivors there is a higher incidence of residual neurologic damage.

Reye's syndrome in its common form is a biphasic disorder consisting of an initial mild viral illness, usually either as an upper respiratory infection or classic varicella. Following a latent period of one to several days, the second phase develops, most commonly in catastrophic fashion, followed by subsequent deterioration of remarkable rapidity in many instances. When varicella is the preceding illness, the onset of the encephalopathy is usually three to six days after the appearance of the rash. Headache, profuse recurrent vomiting, lethargy and convulsions are the initial manifestations of the encephalopathy which, within hours or a day or so, proceeds to deep coma, sometimes associated with decerebrate or decorticate rigidity (Fig. 24–1). Irritability, delirium, and hyperexcitability are transiently present in some before deep coma supervenes. Recurrent vomiting at frequent intervals is such a notable feature during the early stages of the illness that its absence

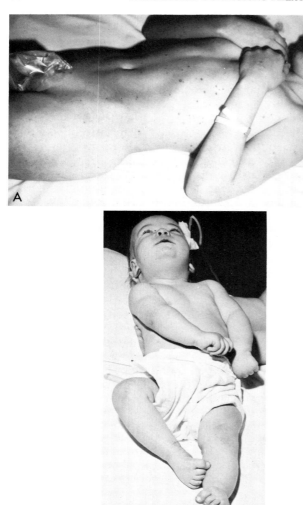

Figure 24–1. Reye's syndrome. *A,* Ten-year-old boy with onset of varicella 4 days before admission. Recurrent vomiting occurred 2 days prior to hospital admission, and the following day the child became lethargic and experienced several convulsions. Physical signs included deep coma, dilated pupils without reaction to light, diffuse hyperreflexia, and labored hyperventilation. Hepatomegaly was present and varicella lesions are evident. Limb posture is that of decorticate rigidity. Serum ammonia and SGOT levels were markedly elevated. The child died after two days of hospitalization. *B,* A febrile respiratory illness developed in this 9-month-old infant 1 week before hospital admission. Four days after onset, vomiting occurred on several occasions. Examinations at the time of admission to hospital revealed an afebrile child with hepatomegaly, hyperventilation, deep coma, and hyperreflexia. Limb posture with the arms rigidly extended is that of decerebrate rigidity. Laboratory studies revealed hypoglycemia and elevation of serum ammonia and SGOT. Death occurred 2 days after admission.

should raise doubt regarding the accuracy of the diagnosis, except in the infant age group. Once the child has become deeply lethargic or unresponsive, the respiratory pattern may be regular and slow or, more commonly, is characterized by rapid and labored breathing, similar to that seen in diabetic acidosis or salicylate intoxication. Muscle tone often fluctuates between hypertonicity and hypotonicity during the progress of the condition. Neck rigidity or other signs of meningeal irritation are not expected unless part of the general posture of increased extensor rigidity. Fever may or may not be present, and in some the illness is complicated by gastrointestinal bleeding.

Owing to the rapid progression of the illness, papilledema frequently is not evident even though increased intracranial pressure secondary to diffuse cerebral edema is present. Hepatomegaly is not always found on the initial physical examination but will develop in more than 50 percent of cases during the clinical course. Acute pancreatitis has been found to complicate the illness in some instances, identified by elevation of the serum amylase level or the occurrence of hypovolemic shock, hypocalcemia, and an increase in the amylase content (Ellis et al.). In some cases, pancreatitis is manifested only by biochemical abnormalities, while in others it contributes to death of the patient. Acute renal failure not explained on the basis of dehydration has also been observed in certain children with Reye's syndrome (Baliga et al.).

Unless the process can be interrupted by prompt and judicious therapy, the majority of cases will progress to a fatal outcome with death from respiratory or cardiorespiratory failure within a few days after onset and sometimes as rapidly as 24 hours after the first appearance of neurologic signs. Among the series of 21 cases described by Norman, over 50 percent were dead within 24 hours after admission to the hospital. Randolph and Gelfman were able to collect reports of 84 cases up to 1968, of which 60 proved fatal. In a more recent series, Lovejoy and colleagues described 17 deaths among 40 patients, a more favorable outcome than most of the previous reports. With recently proposed methods of therapy, the prognosis in Reye's syndrome has become less dismal than earlier statistics suggest. Huttenlocher achieved recovery in eight of 11 patients with a regimen that included exchange transfusions with fresh heparinized blood. Survivors often recover completely but can be left with neurologic sequelae of variable degree, especially when the illness occurs in infants or very young children. In most instances, the illness is a one-time affair, although recurrences have been described (Pichichero and McCabe, van Caillie et al.).

Pathology

The pathology of Reye's syndrome is primarily found in the brain and the liver, although other organs can also be affected (Bourgeois et al., Brown and Madge, Evans et al., Partin et al.). By gross inspection, the leptomeninges appear normal. Diffuse cerebral edema results in flattening of cerebral gyri, reduction of ventricular size, and, often, internal herniations. The most important microscopic finding is the absence of inflammatory cells or other evidence of encephalitic involvement. Anoxic neuronal changes are frequent although nonspecific, possibly reflecting respiratory insufficiency in the terminal stages of the illness, or hypoglycemia commonly present in the initial stages. Intracytoplasmic inclusion bodies in cerebellar Purkinje cells have been identified in one case of Reye's syndrome, although the significance of this finding remains unclear (Turel et al.). Ultrastructural lesions in the brain include neuronal mitochondrial injury which is potentially reversible, astrocytic swelling, and myelin bleb formation (Partin et al. 1975, 1978).

The liver appears swollen and tense and the external surface is characterized by a pale-yellow discoloration. Microscopically, the shape of the hepatocytes is not disturbed but the cells are distended by small-droplet fatty accumulations which surround but do not usually displace the nucleus. Fatty infiltration within the liver is diffuse but is usually most marked in the portal areas. Biochemical analysis of the lipid content in the liver in Reye's syndrome has demonstrated a marked elevation of the triglyceride concentration, a lesser degree of increase in the free fatty acid concentration, and a reduced level of phospholipids compared to control specimens (Chaves-Carballo et al.). Glycogen depletion is frequently striking and correlates well with glucagon-unresponsive hypoglycemia found in some cases. Small, focal areas of necrosis may be present and, rarely, severe generalized hepatocellular necrosis is observed. Ultrastructural examination of the liver in Reye's syndrome by Tang et al. and Partin et al. have revealed mitochondrial pleomorphism and swelling, in addition to proliferation of endoplasmic reticulum. Similar mitochondrial changes have been observed in skeletal muscle (Hanson and Urizar). Fatty infiltration may also be found in the renal tubules and, to a lesser degree, in the heart. Acute renal tubular necrosis with renal failure has also been described (Nicholls et al.). Hemorrhagic pancreatitis has been observed in an occasional case (Glick et al., Stover et al.). Electron microscopic examination of pancreatic acinar cells has revealed intranuclear inclusions that are believed to be a reaction to toxic injury (Collins).

Laboratory Findings

The white blood count is often elevated in children with Reye's syndrome, commonly over 20,000 per cu. mm. Acetone is present in the urine and dehydration may be reflected by elevation of blood urea nitrogen and increased serum osmolarity. Hypoglycemia is present in some children with Reye's syndrome and is much more common when the illness occurs in infants as compared with older children. Blood sugar may be as low as 5 to 10 mg. per 100 ml. and is associated with a reduction in the cerebrospinal fluid glucose content. Hypoglycemia in this illness responds poorly to glucagon and has been shown to occur with low serum insulin levels (Glasgow et al.), indicating that its origin is secondary to disturbed hepatic glucose production.

Biochemical evidence of hepatic dysfunction is now recognized to be a diagnostic hallmark of Reye's syndrome. Serum glutamic oxaloacetic transaminase levels vary from mildly to profoundly elevated, at times to levels of over 2000 mg. per 100 ml., and commonly rises progressively in the early days of the illness. Despite this, serum bilirubin determinations remain normal or show only slight increases and jaundice is not commonly observed clinically. While the elevated serum transaminase levels are assumed to result primarily from hepatic cell injury, in some cases serum creatine phosphokinase of muscle origin is also significantly increased (Roe et al.). Among patients who survive, the serum transaminase levels return to normal within one to three weeks after onset of the illness and this correlates well with rapid dissolution of fatty change within the liver (Powell et al.). Uncomplicated varicella is often associated with significant elevations in the serum glutamic oxaloacetic transaminase levels; however, the serum ammonia and glucose values remain normal in such patients (Pitel et al.). Serum free fatty acids have also been elevated in cases with Reye's syndrome in which they have been measured (Powell et al.), and there is some evidence to suggest that clinical improvement in some way correlates with the rate of clearance of short-chain fatty acids from the serum (Trauner et al.).

Serum ammonia elevation is another manifestation of hepatic injury which is found in Reye's syndrome (Glasgow et al., Huttenlocher et al.) and is believed by some to be one of the main factors provoking cerebral dysfunction. The degree of elevation of the blood ammonia is quite variable, although Glasgow et al. found that patients with the highest blood ammonia levels were the most deeply comatose and that those who survive usually have lower initial serum ammonia levels. Serum ammonia levels greater than 300 μg per 100 ml. have been correlated with an increased case fatality rate (Corey et al. 1977). In addition, the increase of the ammonia content may be very transient and can be missed if the determination is not done early in the course of the disease. Additional evidence of hepatic involvement in some patients includes abnormalities of clotting factors that are liver-dependent (Schwartz). A prolonged prothrombin time is usual with this illness and provides a rapid method of diagnostic testing, as compared to the serum transaminase determination, which requires more time for laboratory analysis. Coagulation abnormalities can be severe in Reye's syndrome, and can include disseminated intravascular

coagulopathy in some instances (Pegelow et al.). Increase in the serum level of certain aminoacids has been found in children with Reye's syndrome and has been proposed as one method of differentiating this disease from acute salicylate intoxication, in which aminoacids remain normal. Hilty et al. identified consistent increases in serum concentrations of glutamine, alanine, alpha-aminobutyrate, and lysine.

Cerebrospinal fluid examination is required in some cases to exclude the possibility of encephalitis or bacterial meningitis. Lumbar puncture is associated with considerable risk, however, when brain swelling is advanced and intracranial pressure is markedly elevated. When the clinical pattern is strongly suggestive of Reye's syndrome, and the biochemical abnormalities support the diagnosis, lumbar puncture is best avoided because of the possibility of provoking internal herniation. The cerebrospinal fluid in Reye's syndrome contains few or no cells, a normal protein content, and a depressed glucose value in those who are hypoglycemic. In exceptional cases, a modest number of cells will be present and cannot be assumed to be incompatible with the diagnosis (Glasgow et al.). The opening pressure can be normal or elevated, depending on the degree of cerebral swelling.

The electroencephalogram reveals bilateral and diffuse slow abnormalities and may be of some predictive or prognostic value when studied in serial fashion (Aoki and Lombroso). Yamada et al. found an unusual association of positive spike bursts superimposed on a background of diffuse delta activity in the early stages of Reye's syndrome. The frequency of the positive spikes varied from seven to 13 cycles per second and were sometimes provoked by noise or other stimuli. Because positive spikes are rare in other forms of coma, the authors proposed that their presence in the comatose child might be of diagnostic value indicative of Reye's syndrome. Trauner et al. have found the degree of electroencephalographic abnormality to correlate with clinical signs and elevations of short-chain fatty acids, but not with serum ammonia levels.

The importance or need for liver biopsy as a diagnostic method for Reye's syndrome is debatable and remains unsettled. Diagnosis on clinical and laboratory grounds has been assumed to be sufficient by some authors (Glasgow et al., Samaha et al.). Others have stressed the clinical similarity of a wide variety of other conditions to Reye's syndrome which do not have the universal small-droplet fatty infiltration of the non-inflamed liver characteristic of Reye's syndrome (Orlowski et al., Schubert). At present, it would seem that the child with the classic features of Reye's syndrome occurring after varicella or within a setting of an influenza outbreak would not require liver biopsy for confirmation of the diagnosis. The procedure would be useful when the illness or the laboratory data are atypical or when clinical differentiation from drug intoxication is not possible.

Differential Diagnosis

Acute viral encephalitis is perhaps the most common initial diagnosis in children with Reye's syndrome, and especially so when the process occurs during the course of a typical varicella infection. Common findings with encephalitis, including meningeal signs and cells in the cerebrospinal fluid, are usually absent in Reye's syndrome, while the presence of hepatomegaly and the above-described metabolic derangements should alert one to the correct diagnosis. Fever is usually present in children with viral encephalitis but also occurs in some cases of Reye's syndrome, and therefore cannot be used as a reliable differential sign. Infectious mononucleosis with encephalitis can simulate Reye's syndrome in that elevation of liver enzymes without jaundice is present in association with signs of diffuse cerebral dysfunction. The peak age of occurrence of the two disorders is somewhat different, as is the chronological pattern of the symptoms leading to coma. Infectious hepatitis with fulminating hepatic coma may be a diagnostic consideration; however, such patients rapidly become icteric, a finding not expected with Reye's syndrome. Atypical cases of acute liver disease with coma have been described which are distinguishable from Reye's syndrome only on the basis of microscopic examination of liver tissue obtained by biopsy (Gall et al.). Acute idiopathic pancreatitis in children has been reported in association with an encephalopathy resembling Reye's syndrome (Morens et al.). Whether the pancreatic insult represents the initial process in these cases or whether they represent examples of Reye's syndrome with unusually severe pancreatic involvement remains unclear. Acute pancreatitis has been recognized in Reye's syndrome (DeVivo and Keating) and can be a significant factor regarding mortality in some instances.

Drug intoxication is an additional consideration sharing features in common with this disorder. This is especially true when the history includes salicylate administration and the physical findings in the comatose child reveal deep, rapid, and labored respirations. Cases that create the greatest degree of confusion are those with a clinical pattern and laboratory findings identical to those of Reye's syndrome, in addition to blood salicylate levels which are in the toxic range (Rosenfeld and Liebhaber). It remains unclear in such cases whether two illnesses are present simultaneously, whether salicylates can potentiate the process of Reye's syndrome once it has been provoked by other factors, or whether in some children, subacute salicylate intoxication can itself give rise to the illness defined as Reye's syndrome. The practical importance of this association is that the intravenous fluid therapy currently recommended for Reye's syndrome with severe cerebral edema is quite different from that instituted for the patient with salicylate intoxication.

Acetaminophen intoxication shares certain common features with Reye's syndrome, although in most instances laboratory evidence of hepatic toxicity precedes signs of encephalopathy by several days, if the latter occurs at all (Rumack and Peterson). With acute, severe acetaminophen intoxication, however, there can be rapid development of coma associated with brain swelling, elevation of serum ammonia and hepatic enzymes, and hypoglycemia (Arena et al., Nogen and Bremner). History of drug ingestion and demonstration of toxic blood levels of acetaminophen must be relied upon to separate the two conditions in such instances. Acute intoxications with pyrrolizidine, an alkaloid found in a number of common plant species (Fox et al.), and with methyl bromide, present in certain insecticides (Shield et al.), have also been reported in children with clinical states resembling Reye's syndrome.

The disorder known as Jamaican vomiting sickness bears many features in common with Reye's syndrome. Both occur predominantly in children, are illnesses of acute onset with rapidly progressive deterioration, are characterized by fatty infiltration of the liver, and are often manifested by vomiting and hypoglycemia. Unlike Reye's syndrome, Jamaican vomiting sickness is not preceded by prodromal symptoms and not uncommonly affects siblings simultaneously. This disorder is believed to be provoked by the ingestion of hypoglycin contained in the unripe akee, a fruit grown in Jamaica. Tanaka et al. have recently demonstrated the presence of methylenecyclopropylacetic acid, a toxic metabolite of hypoglycin A, in the urine of two siblings with Jamaican vomiting sickness, thus differentiating it from Reye's syndrome.

Acute diabetic ketoacidosis may also resemble this disease, with findings often seen in both including coma, hyperpnea, and metabolic acidosis. This diagnostic error is especially possible if the child with Reye's syndrome who is initially hypoglycemic is seen by one physician who administers large quantities of intravenous glucose and subsequently transfers the patient to the care of another.

There are certain rare metabolic disorders characterized by recurrent attacks of hepatic dysfunction which can enter into the differential diagnosis of Reye's syndrome. Systemic carnitine deficiency is manifested by the development of a progressive lipid-storage myopathy in late childhood, but this is sometimes preceded by acute episodes of vomiting, lethargy, hypoglycemia, and hyperammonemia (Karpati et al., Ware et al.). The myopathic features of the disorder usually predominate, thus suggesting the proper diagnosis. Inherited enzyme deficiencies of ornithine transcarbamylase, carbamyl phosphate synthetase, and argininosuccinic synthetase lead to recurrent attacks with hyperammonemia and encephalopathic signs (LaBrecque et al.). The usual early age of onset and the chronological pattern of the illnesses in most cases are quite different from those in Reye's syndrome although exceptions do exist.

Intracranial mass lesions, such as acute subdural or epidural hematoma or cerebral tumor, do not usually create differential diagnostic problems with Reye's syndrome. In exceptional cases, such possibilities may be entertained, particularly when seizures are focal and evidence of liver dysfunction is less marked. The rapid emergence of coma and the signs indicative of diffuse cerebral involvement are usually sufficient to exclude the possibility of a mass lesion. Additional support for a diffuse encephalopathy is usually provided by the electroencephalogram.

Etiology and Pathogenesis

Although the cause of Reye's syndrome remains in the speculative stage, continued epidemiologic, virologic, and biochemical investigations have begun to unravel at least some of the mysteries of the disorder. Exogenous toxins, viral agents, and genetic predisposition have each received etiologic consideration. The intoxication theory has received support from the experience in Thailand where investigators postulate the disease is caused by aflatoxin, a substance present in certain foods (Olson et al.). Other observations suggesting a toxic origin have been the high frequency with which children with this illness have received salicylates, the discovery of isopropyl alcohol in tissues from a child with the disease (Randolph et al.), and the possibility of exposure of another to paint thinner soon before onset of the syndrome (Glasgow and Ferris).

In this country, a presumed etiologic association with viral illness has repeatedly been made and a number of different viral agents have been recovered. Geographically restricted outbreaks of influenza B virus infection have been associated with clusters of cases of Reye's syndrome (Reynolds et al., Riley). Varicella has been recognized by many observers to precede the disorder (Glick et al., Jenkins et al.) and has occurred in 7 to 10 percent of cases of Reye's syndrome (Corey et al., Linnemann et al., 1975). An epidemiologic study by Corey et al. (1976) revealed that when large numbers are analyzed, cases of Reye's syndrome tend to fall into two distinct groups. The first are cases which cluster both temporally and geographically in which children are usually older, with a median age of 11 years, have a preceding upper respiratory infection, and are epidemiologically associated with influenza B infections. The second group includes cases that occur sporadically throughout the year, affect younger children, and are associated with a number of different viral illnesses, varicella being the most common. Other viruses which have been recovered from various tissues or demonstrated otherwise in patients with Reye's syndrome include Coxsackie B (Cullity and Kakulas), Echo (Golden and Duffell), parainfluenza (Powell et al.), Herpes simplex (Becroft), type-1 vaccine-like poliovirus (Brunberg and Bell), adenovirus (Linnemann et al., 1974) and respiratory syncytial virus (Griffin et al.). In only a few cases have viruses been isolated from brain tissue in patients with Reye's syndrome (Becroft, Brunberg and Bell, Cullity and Kakulas, Norman et al.). Virus particles resembling Herpesvirus and myxovirus or paramyxovirus have been described in hepatocytes by electron microscopy by Tang et al., while Partin et al. (1976) were able to isolate influenza virus from liver and muscle biopsy specimens from a child with Reye's syndrome. The Epstein-Barr virus has also been incriminated on the basis of serologic studies but without virus isolation (Dorman et al., Rahal and Henle). In addition, Reye's syndrome has followed simultaneous smallpox and typhoid immunizations (Glick et al.) and has been observed by the authors (unpublished cases) in two siblings shortly after each received smallpox vaccine.

Yet to be answered is how the commonly observed preceding viral infection precipitates the organ system damage which occurs in Reye's syndrome. A popular concept adhered to by some is that the primary brunt of the process is upon the liver, with encephalopathy being mainly secondary to hypoglycemia, hyperammonemia, certain short-chain fatty acids (Trauner et al. 1975), or other yet to be identified toxic substances resulting from hepatic insufficiency. It is generally agreed that this explanation is probably an oversimplification and that Reye's syndrome may represent a response of liver and brain to a variety of different etiologic insults. In one patient with Reye's syndrome, Thaler et al. discovered a partial deficiency of ornithine-transcarbamylase in tissue obtained by liver biopsy. The authors proposed that the enzymatic defect in ammonia metabolism located in mitochondria might be genetically transmitted or induced and that larger than usual amounts of ornithine may be required in such persons for maintenance of conversion of ammonia to urea (Thaler). Illnesses associated with restricted food intake, vomiting, and dehydration could thereby limit the capacity of the urea cycle for removal of ammonia. Thaler and colleagues suggested consideration of treatment with ornithine or arginine to overcome the metabolic block, enhancing elimination of neurotoxic metabolites. Subsequent investigations have demonstrated the frequent occurrence of reductions in hepatic ornithine transcarbamylase and carbamyl phosphate synthetase in the early stages of the illness, which apparently are acquired and are only transiently present (Brown et al., Snodgrass and DeLong). An additional observation of speculative importance in the pathogenesis of this disease is the finding of high levels of endotoxic-like activity in serum and cerebrospinal fluid (Cooperstock et al.). Endotoxin was demonstrated by the Limulus assay in this study and was believed to be derived from the intestinal

tract. The authors postulated that high circulating levels of endotoxin could result from loss of ability to detoxify the substance secondary to hepatic insufficiency.

Decrease in serum hemolytic complement component activities found by Pickering et al. in patients with Reye's syndrome is possibly indicative of a host immune response to the preceding infection. DeVivo has advanced the concept proposed earlier by Partin et al. (1971) that Reye's syndrome is a disorder with primary mitochondrial injury in all tissues, the origin of the insult being obscure. Injury of hepatic mitochondrial enzymes, including ornithine transcarbamylase and carbamyl phosphate synthetase, results in hyperammonemia, while extrahepatic mitochondrial dysfunction disturbs cellular oxidation of fatty acids and pyruvate with accelerated glycolysis leading to excessive production of pyruvate and lactic acid. The postulate by DeVivo also suggests that mitochondrial injury within the brain and walls of cerebral vessels can lead to cerebral swelling and, at the same time, impairment of glucose transport into brain tissue. Thus, the neurologic abnormalities characteristic of Reye's syndrome can be explained on the basis of primary cerebral dysfunction, compounded by inadequate glucose supply to the brain along with the toxic effects on brain tissue of abnormal metabolites resulting from extraneural tissue mitochondrial injury.

Treatment

The method and aggressiveness of treatment of Reye's syndrome are determined to some degree by the severity of the process when the patient is first seen and by the presence or absence, or rate of progression, of the clinical signs. Seizures are controlled with the use of intravenous phenobarbital or diazepam but with constant attention to maintenance of an adequate airway and the prevention of hypoxia and hypercapnea. Hypoglycemia requires immediate correction by glucose infusions and its recurrence can usually be prevented by continued use of glucose-containing solution. DeVivo has pointed out the importance of providing adequate glucose supplies to the brain in this disorder and recommends the intravenous use of 25 percent glucose or otherwise the amount required to maintain blood glucose levels in the range of 300 mg. per 100 ml.

Hemorrhagic complications generally indicate coagulation defects secondary to liver-dependent clotting factors and are combated with vitamin K or with intravenous administration of fresh plasma when severe. Measures should be taken to prevent hyperthermia in this condition because of the increased cerebral metabolic requirements with temperature elevation. Salicylates and other antipyretics should not be used in view of the uncertainty of their possible role in the pathogenesis of this disease. Cessation of oral intake and the oral administration of neomycin in dosage of 250 to 500 mg. every six to eight hours is recommended in view of the uncertain but possible contribution of hepatic dysfunction in regard to neurologic signs.

The mildly affected child with Reye's syndrome manifested only by vomiting and lethargy should be managed with the above-described considerations but closely watched at frequent intervals for progression of the illness. Some degree of fluid restriction would be appropriate, even at this stage, in the hope of forestalling the occurrence of or progression of cerebral edema.

The more seriously ill child with deep lethargy or coma, decorticate or decerebrate posturing, hyperventilation, or pupillary abnormalities can be expected to deteriorate rapidly unless managed intensively. In the past, therapy for this condition was designed with the concept that the encephalopathy was primarily the result of hepatic failure and thus included methods to eliminate toxic materials from the vascular compartment. Peritoneal dialysis was favored by some (Pross et al.) with variable results but with evidence of improvement of the mortality rate in certain reports (Samaha et al.). Others have resorted to exchange transfusions with fresh heparinized blood, also with improved outcomes in some series (Bobo et al., Huttenlocher). The mode of action by which exchange transfusion possibly brings about improvement in this disorder remains unclear. One effect of exchange transfusion is the lowering of the level of intracranial hypertension (Berman et al., Pizzi et al.) and it is possible that improvement is partially explained on this basis. The mechanism by which exchange transfusion reduces intracranial pressure, however, remains unclear.

It is now generally believed by most investigators that the principal cause of death in many cases of Reye's syndrome is not hepatic failure but is the result of massive and rapidly progressive brain swelling with subsequent compromise of cerebral arterial perfusion or internal herniation and brain stem compression. The recognition of the importance of brain swelling and increased intracranial pressure in this disorder has led to the use of intensive regimens to control intracranial pressure, with significant improvement in mortality resulting (Lovejoy et al., Trauner et al. 1978, Venes et al.). For such measures to be effective, it is necessary that treatment be initiated before the child reaches an advanced stage of the disease in which the pupils are dilated and fixed and the limbs have become flaccid and without reflexes.

Vigorous antiedema therapy should be instituted when it is clear that the illness is progressing and has advanced beyond Stage I. Restriction of intravenous fluid administration will enhance the effects of agents used to reduce cerebral edema. Unless clinical signs of dehydration are severe, fluids can be restricted to approximately 50 percent of maintenance requirements. Mannitol in intermittent doses of 0.5 to 1.0 gm. per kilogram given intravenously over a period of 20 to 30 minutes is the most widely used preparation to control cerebral swelling in this condition. How frequently to repeat mannitol infusions and how long and to what degree to continue fluid restriction is difficult to judge clinically but is a critical factor in regard to the hour by hour management. Decisions are best made on the basis of the level of intracranial pressure but this is not always clearly reflected from the clinical signs. The use of one of the recently developed methods of continuous intracranial pressure monitoring provides an accurate estimate of intracranial pressure at frequent intervals and can be maintained for four to six days if necessary (Kindt et al., Pizzi et al.). With the subdural or epidural screw in place, acute rises in pressure can be combated with hyperventilation, followed by periodic infusions of mannitol at intervals of four to six hours. With dehydrating and antiedema therapy, it is important to check periodically the urine output, blood urea nitrogen and creatinine, serum glucose and electrolytes, and the serum osmolarity. An indwelling catheter is required to prevent overdistention of the bladder, and a central venous line or Swan-Ganz catheter is used to monitor central venous pressure or pulmonary wedge pressure, which is maintained at approximately 5 cm. of water. When intracranial pressure monitoring reveals that intracranial hypertension has subsided, intravenous fluid administration is increased in volume and further mannitol infusions are withheld.

Each center has now developed its own aggressive treatment method for severe and progressive Reye's syndrome. While most centers are now realizing a reduction in the case fatality rate by a well-designed therapeutic approach, there is insufficient information yet to determine which particular approach is most effective. The approach to treatment now used by the authors is a complex multidisciplinary one which we feel has significantly improved the chances of survival of the child with this illness, although we do not propose that it is ideal or is necessarily the best form of therapy in the hands of others. Once a child is judged to be a candidate for aggressive therapy, he is moved to the intensive care area where intubation is performed and controlled ventilation is initiated under pancuronium-induced paralysis so that the $PaCO_2$ can be maintained at approximately 25 torr. An arterial line is placed for measurement of arterial blood pressure and to collect arterial blood specimens, and a Swan-Ganz catheter is inserted to provide a measurement of pulmonary artery wedge pressure. The wedge pressure gives an accurate estimate of left atrial filling pressure, which reflects blood volume. An intracranial pressure monitor is instilled via a twist drill burr hole in the right frontal region for continuous intracranial subarachnoid pressure measurement. This allows administration of only that amount of therapy, such as mannitol and fluid restriction, which is necessary to control intracranial hypertension. Lumbar puncture is ordinarily deferred until the intracranial pressure monitor is functional, and can then be done, if necessary, once the intracranial pressure is less than 20 torr.

Intravenous fluids are restricted to approximately 1.5 ml. per kilogram per hour, depending on the pulmonary artery wedge pressure. The wedge pressure is maintained between 3 and 5 torr, and if it falls below this level the intravenous fluid volume is increased. If it rises significantly above this level, diuresis is induced with furosemide. With fluid restriction, the serum osmolarity is maintained between 300 and 320 milliosmoles per liter. Efforts are made to keep the intracranial pressure below 20 torr and to maintain the cerebral perfusion pressure greater than 50. The cerebral perfusion pressure is calculated by subtracting the intracranial pressure from the mean arterial blood pressure. It is generally agreed that as the cerebral perfusion pressure falls progressively below 50, the cerebral microperfusion is progressively compromised and cerebral ischemia results. Controlled ventilation with hypocapnia and fluid restriction alone may control the intracranial pressure but, if not, boluses of mannitol are given intravenously in dosage of 0.5 to 1.0 gm. per kilogram. When intracranial hypertension remains refractory to the above, pentobarbital is added with a loading intravenous dose of 5 mg. per kilogram followed by doses of 2 mg. per kilogram per hour to maintain the barbiturate blood level between 25 and 35 micrograms per ml., which may result in a suppression-burst pattern in the electroencephalogram. The danger of excessively high barbiturate levels is a reduction of cardiac output leading to diminution of tissue perfusion. This can be prevented by altering the dose according to the blood level and by use of a thermodilution method to monitor cardiac output (Freed and Keane). When the above methods fail to control intracranial hypertension, systemic hypothermia is then resorted to.

The clinical course and possible complications of therapy must be analyzed by continuous observations of vital signs, by periodic determinations of serum electrolytes, osmolarity, and glucose, and by accurate measurement of urine output. Serum ammonia, hepatic enzymes, and amylase are repeated at daily intervals, as is the electroencephalogram. Discontinuation of controlled ventilation is on the basis of improvement in hepatic function, improvement in the electroencephalographic findings, and ability to control intracranial pressure. With the patient who has been managed by controlled ventilation for several days, the hours following extubation are a critical time period during which continuous observation is necessary. Upper airway obstruction caused by laryngeal or subglottic edema or web formation is common under these circumstances and can result in sudden CO_2 retention, spikes in intracranial pressure, and hypoxia leading to cardiorespiratory arrest.

REFERENCES

Aoki, Y., and Lombroso, C. T.: Prognostic value of electroencephalography in Reye's syndrome. Neurology 23:333–343, 1973.

Applebaum, M. M., and Thaler, M. M.: Reye syndrome

without initial hepatic involvement. Am. J. Dis. Child. 131:295–296, 1977.

Arena, J. M., Rourk, M. H., Jr., and Sibrack, C. D.: Acetaminophen: Report of an unusual poisoning. Pediatrics 61:68–72, 1978.

Baliga, B., Fleischmann, L. E., Chang, C-H., Sarnaik, A. P., Bidani, A. K., and Arcinue, E. L.: Acute renal failure in Reye's syndrome. Am. J. Dis. Child. 133:1009–1013, 1979.

Becroft, D. M. O.: Syndrome of encephalopathy and fatty degeneration of viscera in New Zealand children. Brit. Med. J. 3:135–140, 1966.

Berman, W., Pizzi, F., Schut, L., Raphaely, R., and Holtzapple, P.: The effects of exchange transfusion on intracranial pressure in patients with Reye syndrome. J. Pediat. 87:887–891, 1975.

Bobo, R. C., Schubert, W. K., Partin, J. C., and Partin, J. S.: Reye syndrome: Treatment by exchange transfusion with special reference to the 1974 epidemic in Cincinnati, Ohio. J. Pediat. 87:881–886, 1975.

Bourgeois, C., Olson, L., Comer, D., Evans, H., Keschamras, N., Cotton, R. Grossman, R., and Smith, R.: Encephalopathy and fatty degeneration of the viscera. A clinicopathologic analysis of 40 cases. Am. J. Clin. Path. 56:558–571, 1971.

Brain, W. R., Hunter, D., and Turnbull, H. M.: Acute meningo-encephalomyelitis of childhood. Report of six cases. Lancet 1:221–227, 1929.

Brown, R. E., and Madge, G. E.: Hepatic degeneration and dysfunction in Reye's syndrome. Am. J. Dig. Dis. 16:1116–1122, 1971.

Brown, T., Hug, G., Lansky, L., Bove, K., Scheve, A., Ryan, M., Brown, H., Schubert, W. K., Partin, J. C., and Lloyd-Still, J.: Transiently reduced activity of carbamyl phosphate synthetase and ornithine transcarbamylase in liver of children with Reye's syndrome. New Eng. J. Med. 294:861–867, 1976.

Brunberg, J. A., and Bell, W. E.: Reye's syndrome. An association with type-1 vaccine-like poliovirus. Arch. Neurol. 30:304–306, 1974.

Chaves-Carballo, E., Ellefson, R. D., and Gomez, M. R.: Hepatic lipids in Reye-Johnson syndrome and in acute encephalopathy without fatty liver. Mayo Clin. Proc. 51:770–776, 1976.

Collins, D. N.: Ultrastructural study of intranuclear inclusions in the exocrine pancreas in Reye's syndrome. Lab. Invest. 30:333–340, 1974.

Cooperstock, M. S., Tucker, R. P., and Baublis, J. V.: Possible pathogenic role of endotoxin in Reye's syndrome. Lancet 1:1272–1274, 1975.

Corey, L., Rubin, R. J., Bregman, D., and Gregg, M. B.: Diagnostic criteria for influenza B–associated Reye's syndrome: Clinical vs. pathologic criteria. Pediatrics 60:702–708, 1977.

Corey, L., Rubin, R. J., Hattwick, M. A. W., Noble, G. R., and Cassidy, E.: A nationwide outbreak of Reye's syndrome. Its epidemiologic relationship to influenza B. Am. J. Med. 61:615–625, 1976.

Cullity, G. J., and Kakulas, B. A.: Encephalopathy and fatty degeneration of the viscera: An evaluation. Brain 93:77–88, 1970.

DeVivo, D. C.: Reye syndrome: A metabolic response to an acute mitochondrial insult? Neurology 28:105–108, 1978.

DeVivo, D. C., and Keating, J. P.: Reye's syndrome. Adv. Pediat. 22:175–229, 1976.

DeVivo, D. C., Keating, J. P., and Haymond, M. W.: Reye syndrome: Results of intensive supportive care. J. Pediat. 87:875–880, 1975.

Dorman, J. M., Glick, T. H., Shannon, D. C., Galdabini,

J., and Walker, W. A.: Complications of infectious mononucleosis. A fatal case in a 2-year-old child. Am. J. Dis. Child. 128:239–243, 1974.

Ellis, G. H., Mirkin, L. D., and Mills, M. C.: Pancreatitis and Reye's syndrome. Am. J. Dis. Child. 133:1014–1016, 1979.

Evans, H., Bourgeois, C. H., Comer, D. S., and Keschamras, N.: Brain lesions in Reye's syndrome. Arch. Path. 90:543–546, 1970.

Fox, D. W., Hart, M. C., Bergeson, P. S., Jarrett, P. B., Stillman, A. E., and Huxtable, R. J.: Pyrrolizidine (Senecio) intoxication mimicking Reye syndrome. J. Pediat. 93:980–982, 1978.

Freed, M. D., and Keane, J. F.: Cardiac output measured by thermodilution in infants and children. J. Pediat. 92:39–42, 1978.

Gall, D. G., Cutz, E., McClung, H. J., and Greenberg, M. L.: Acute liver disease and encephalopathy mimicking Reye syndrome. A report of three cases. J. Pediat. 87:869–874, 1975.

Glasgow, A. M., Cotton, R. B., Bourgeois, C. H., and Dhiensiri, K.: Reye's syndrome. II. Occurrence in the absence of severe fatty infiltration of the liver. Am. J. Dis. Child. 124:834–836, 1972.

Glasgow, A. M., Cotton, R. B., and Dhiensiri, K.: Reye's syndrome. I. Blood ammonia and consideration of the nonhistologic diagnosis. Am. J. Dis. Child. 124:827–833, 1972.

Glasgow, A. M., Cotton, R. B., and Dhiensiri, K.: Reye syndrome. III. The hypoglycemia. Am. J. Dis. Child. 125:809–811, 1973.

Glasgow, J. F. T., and Ferris, J. A. J.: Encephalopathy and visceral fatty infiltration of probable toxic aetiology. Lancet 1:451–453, 1968.

Glick, T. H., Ditchek, N. T., Salitsky, S., and Friemuth, E. J.: Acute encephalopathy and hepatic dysfunction. Associated with chickenpox in siblings. Am. J. Dis. Child. 119:68–71, 1970.

Glick, T. H., Likosky, W. H., Levitt, L. P., Mellin, H., and Reynolds, D. W.: Reye's syndrome: An epidemiologic approach. Pediatrics 46:371–377, 1970.

Golden, G. S., and Duffell, D.: Encephalopathy and fatty change in the liver and kidney. Pediatrics 36:67–74, 1965.

Griffin, N., Keeling, J. W., and Tomlinson, A. H.: Reye's syndrome associated with respiratory syncytial virus infection. Arch. Dis. Childh. 54:74–76, 1979.

Hanson, P. A., and Urizar, R. E.: Ultrastructural lesions of muscle and immunofluorescent deposits in vessels in Reye's syndrome: A preliminary report of serial muscle biopsies. Ann. Neurol. 1:431–437, 1977.

Hilty, M. D., McClung, H. J., Haynes, R. E., Romshe, C. A., and Sherard, E. S., Jr.: Reye syndrome in siblings. J. Pediat. 94:576–579, 1979.

Hilty, M. D., Romshe, C. A., and Delamater, P. V.: Reye's syndrome and hyperaminoacidemia. J. Pediat. 84:362–365, 1974.

Huttenlocher, P. R.: Reye's syndrome: Relation of outcome to therapy. J. Pediat. 80:845, 1972.

Huttenlocher, P. R., Schwartz, A. D., and Klatskin, G.: Reye's syndrome: Ammonia intoxication as a possible factor in the encephalopathy. Pediatrics 43:443–454, 1969.

Huttenlocher, P. R., and Trauner, D. A.: Reye's syndrome in infancy. Pediatrics 62:84–90, 1978.

Jenkins, R., Dvorak, A., and Patrick, J.: Encephalopathy and fatty degeneration of the viscera associated with chickenpox. Pediatrics 39:769–771, 1967.

Karpati, G., Carpenter, S., Engel, A. G., Watters, G., Allen, J., Rothman, S., Klassen, G., and Mamer, O.

A.: The syndrome of systemic carnitine deficiency. Clinical, morphologic, biochemical, and pathophysiologic features. Neurology 25:16–24, 1975.

Kindt, G. W., Waldman, J., Kohl, S., Baublis, J., and Tucker, R. P.: Intracranial pressure in Reye syndrome. Monitoring and control. J.A.M.A. 231:822–825, 1975.

LaBrecque, D. R., Latham, P. S., Riely, C. A., Hsia, Y. E., and Klatskin, G.: Heritable urea cycle enzyme deficiency-liver disease in 16 patients. J. Pediat. 94:580–587, 1979.

Linnemann, C. C., Jr., Shea, L., Kauffmann, C. A., Schiff, G. M., Partin, J. C., and Schubert, W. K.: Association of Reye's syndrome with viral infection. Lancet 2:179–182, 1974.

Linnemann, C. C., Jr., Shea, L., Partin, J. C., Schubert, W. K., and Schiff, G. M.: Reye's syndrome: Epidemiologic and viral studies, 1963–1974. Am. J. Epidemiol. 101:517–526, 1975.

Lovejoy, F. H., Jr., Bresnan, M. J., Lombroso, C. T., and Smith, A. L.: Anticerebral oedema therapy in Reye's syndrome. Arch Dis. Childh. 50:933–937, 1975.

Lovejoy, F. H., Jr., Smith, A. L., Bresnan, M. J., Wood, J. N., Victor, D. I., and Adams, P. C.: Clinical staging in Reye syndrome. Am. J. Dis. Child. 128:36–41, 1974.

Lyon, G., Dodge, P. R., and Adams, R. D.: The acute encephalopathies of obscure origin in infants and children. Brain 84:680–708, 1961.

Morens, D. M., Hammar, S. L., and Heicher, D. A.: Idiopathic acute pancreatitis in children. Association with a clinical picture resembling Reye syndrome. Am. J. Dis. Child. 128:401–404, 1974.

Nicholls, S., Gill, D., and Craske, J.: Reye's syndrome associated with acute tubular necrosis. Arch. Dis. Childh. 50:960–962, 1976.

Nogen, A. G., and Bremner, J. E.: Fatal acetaminophen overdosage in a young child. J. Pediat. 92:832–833, 1978.

Norman, M. G.: Encephalopathy and fatty degeneration of the viscera in childhood: I. Review of cases at the Hospital for Sick Children, Toronto (1954–1966). Arch. Neurol. 29:135–139, 1973.

Olson, L. C., Bourgeois, C. H., Jr., Cotton, R. B., Harikul, S., Grossman, R. A., and Smith, T. J.: Encephalopathy and fatty degeneration of the viscera in northeastern Thailand. Clinical syndrome and epidemiology. Pediatrics 47:707–716, 1971.

Olson, L. C., Bourgeois, C. H., Jr., Keschamras, N., Harikul, S., Sanyakorn, C. K., Grossman, R. A., and Smith, T. J.: Encephalopathy and fatty degeneration of the viscera in Thai children. Am. J. Dis. Child. 120:1–2, 1970.

Orlowski, J. P., Johannsson, J. H., and Ellis, N. G.: Encephalopathy and fatty metamorphosis of the liver associated with cold-agglutinin autoimmune hemolytic anemia. J. Pediat. 94:569–575, 1979.

Partin, J. C., Partin, J. S., Schubert, W. K., and McLaurin, R. L.: Brain ultrastructure in Reye's syndrome (encephalopathy and fatty alteration of the viscera). J. Neuropath. Exp. Neurol. 34:425–444, 1975.

Partin, J. C., Schubert, W. K., and Partin, J. S.: Mitochondrial ultrastructure in Reye's syndrome (encephalopathy and fatty degeneration of the viscera). New Eng. J. Med. 285:1339–1343, 1971.

Partin, J. C., Schubert, W. K., Partin, J. S., Jacobs, R., and Saalfeld, K.: Isolation of influenza virus from liver and muscle biopsy specimens from a surviving case of Reye's syndrome. Lancet 2:599–602, 1976.

Partin, J. S., McAdams, A. J., Partin, J. C., Schubert, W. K., and McLaurin, R. L.: Brain ultrastructure in Reye's disease. II. Acute injury and recovery processes in three children. J. Neuropath. Exp. Neurol. 37:796–819, 1978.

Pegelow, C., Goldberg, R., Turkel, S., and Powars, D.: Severe coagulation abnormalities in Reye syndrome. J. Pediat. 91:413–416, 1977.

Pichichero, M. E., and McCabe, E. R. B.: Recurrent Reye's syndrome. Am. J. Dis. Child. 132:1097–1099, 1978.

Pickering, R. J., Urizar, R. E., Hanson, P. A., and Laffin, R. J.: Abnormalities of the complement system in Reye syndrome. J. Pediat. 94:218–222, 1979.

Pitel, P. A., McCormick, K. L., Fitzgerald, E., and Orson, J. M.: Subclinical hepatic changes in varicella infection. Pediatrics 65:631–633, 1980.

Pizzi, F. J., Schut, L., Berman, W., and Holtzapple, W.: Intracranial pressure monitoring in Reye's syndrome. Child's Brain 2:59–66, 1976.

Powell, H. C., Rosenberg, R. N., and McKellar, B.: Reye's syndrome: Isolation of parainfluenza virus. Report of three cases. Arch. Neurol. 29:135–139, 1973.

Pross, D. C., Bradford, W. D., and Krueger, R. P.: Reye's syndrome treated by peritoneal dialysis. Pediatrics 45:845–847, 1970.

Rahal, J. J., Jr., and Henle, G.: Infectious mononucleosis and Reye's syndrome: A fatal case with studies for Epstein-Barr virus. Pediatrics 46:776–779, 1970.

Randolph, M., and Gelfman, N. A.: Acute encephalopathy in children associated with acute hepatocellular dysfunction. Reye's syndrome revisited. Am. J. Dis. Child. 116:303–307, 1968.

Randolph, M., Kranwinkel, R., Johnson, R., and Gelfman, N. A.: Encephalopathy, hepatitis and fat accumulation in viscera. Am. J. Dis. Child. 110:95–99, 1965.

Reye, R. D. K., Morgan, G., and Baral, J.: Encephalopathy and fatty degeneration of the viscera. A disease entity in childhood. Lancet 2:749–752, 1963.

Reynolds, D. W., Riley, H. C., Jr., LaFont, D. S., Vorse, H., Scout, L. C., and Carpenter, R. L.: An outbreak of Reye's syndrome associated with influenza B. J. Pediat. 80:429–432, 1972.

Riley, H. D., Jr.: Reye's syndrome. J. Infect. Dis. 125:77–81, 1972.

Roe, C. R., Schonberger, L. B., Gelbach, S. H., Wies, L. A., and Sidbury, J. B., Jr.: Enzymatic alterations in Reye's syndrome: Prognostic implications. Pediatrics 55:119–126, 1975.

Rosenfeld, R. G., and Liebhaber, M. I.: Acute encephalopathy in siblings. Reye syndrome vs. salicylate intoxication. Am. J. Dis. Child. 130:295–297, 1976.

Rumack, B. H., and Peterson, R. G.: Acetaminophen overdose: Incidence, diagnosis, and management in 416 patients. Pediatrics 62(Suppl.):898–903, 1978.

Samaha, F. J., Blau, E., and Berardinelli, J. L.: Reye's syndrome. Clinical diagnosis and treatment with peritoneal dialysis. Pediatrics 53:336–340, 1974.

Schubert, W. K.: Commentary: The diagnosis of Reye syndrome. J. Pediat. 87:867, 1975.

Schubert, W. K., Partin, J. C., Bobo, R., and Partin, J. S.: Exchange transfusion in Reye's syndrome. *In:* Pollack, J. D.: Reye's Syndrome. Grune and Stratton, New York, 1975.

Schwartz, A. D.: The coagulation defect in Reye's syndrome. J. Pediat. 78:326–328, 1971.

Shannon, D. C., De Long, R., Bercu, B., Glick, T., Herrin, J. T., Moylan, F. M. B., and Todres, I. D.: Studies on the pathophysiology of encephalopathy in

Reye's syndrome: Hyperammonemia in Reye's syndrome. Pediatrics 56:999–1004, 1975.

Shield, L. K., Coleman, T. L., and Markesbery, W. R.: Methyl bromide intoxication: Neurologic features, including simulation of Reye syndrome. Neurology 27:959–962, 1977.

Snodgrass, P. J., and DeLong, G. R.: Urea-cycle enzyme deficiencies and an increased nitrogen load producing hyperammonemia in Reye's syndrome. New Eng. J. Med. 294:855–860, 1976.

Stover, S. L., Wanglee, P., and Kennedy, C.: Acute hemorrhagic pancreatitis and other visceral changes associated with acute encephalopathy. Report of three cases. J. Pediat. 73:235–241, 1968.

Tanaka, K., Kean, E. A., and Johnson, B.: Jamaican vomiting sickness. Biochemical investigation of two cases. New Eng. J. Med. 295:461–467, 1976.

Tang, T. T., Siegesmund, K. A., Sedmak, G. V., Casper, J. T., Varma, R. R., and McCreadie, S. R.: Reye syndrome. A correlated electron-microscopic, viral, and biochemical observation. J.A.M.A. 232: 1339–1346, 1975.

Thaler, M. M.: Metabolic mechanisms in Reye syndrome. End of a mystery? Am. J. Dis. Child. 130:241–243, 1976.

Thaler, M. M., Bruhn, F. W., Appelbaum, M. N., and Goodman, J.: Reye's syndrome in twins. J. Pediat. 77:638–646, 1970.

Thaler, M. M., Hoogenraad, N. J., and Boswell, M.: Reye's syndrome due to a novel protein-tolerance variant of ornithine-transcarbamylase deficiency. Lancet 2:438–440, 1974.

Trauner, D. A., Brown, F., Ganz, E., and Huttenlocher, P. R.: Treatment of elevated intracranial pressure in Reye syndrome. Ann. Neurol. 4:275–278, 1978.

Trauner, D. A., Nyhan, W. L., and Sweetman, L.: Short-chain organic acidemia and Reye's syndrome. Neurology 25:296–298, 1975.

Trauner, D. A., Stockard, J. J., and Sweetman, L.: EEG correlations with biochemical abnormalities in Reye's syndrome. Arch. Neurol. 34:116–118, 1977.

Trauner, D. A., Sweetman, L., Holm, J., Kulovich, S., and Nyhan, W. L.: Biochemical correlates of illness and recovery in Reye's syndrome. Ann. Neurol. 2:238–241, 1977.

Turel, A. P., Jr., Levinsohn, M. W., Derakhshan, I., and Gutierrez, Y.: Reye syndrome and cerebellar intracytoplasmic inclusion bodies. Arch. Neurol. 32:624–628, 1975.

Van Caillie, M., Morin, C. L., Roy, C. C., Geoffroy, G., and McLaughlin, B.: Reye's syndrome: Relapses and neurological sequelae. Pediatrics 59:244–249, 1977.

Varma, R. R., Riedel, D. R., Komorowski, R. A., Harrington, G. J., and Nowak, T. V.: Reye's syndrome in nonpediatric age groups. J.A.M.A. 242:1373–1375, 1979.

Venes, J. L., Shaywitz, B. A., and Spencer, D. D.: Management of severe cerebral edema in the metabolic encephalopathy of Reye-Johnson Syndrome. J. Neurosurg. 48:903–915, 1978.

Ware, A. J., Burton, W. C., McGarry, J. D., Marks, J. F., and Weinberg, A. G.: Systemic carnitine deficiency. Report of a fatal case with multisystemic manifestations. J. Pediat. 93:959–964, 1978.

Yamada, T., Young, S., and Kimura, J.: Significance of positive spike bursts in Reye syndrome. Arch. Neurol. 34:376–380, 1977.

Chapter Twenty-Five

GUILLAIN-BARRÉ SYNDROME

Described as an illness easy to diagnose but impossible to define, the Guillain-Barré syndrome refers to an acute symmetrical polyneuropathy in which motor dysfunction predominates over sensory disturbances and in which there is usually bilateral facial paresis or paralysis and, occasionally, weakness of the bulbar and respiratory musculature. Its onset characteristically but not invariably occurs one to three weeks after an upper respiratory infection or other form of viral illness and it is notably associated with an elevated cerebrospinal fluid protein content without a significant cellular response.

Confusion continues to exist as to the precise criteria needed for the diagnosis of the Guillain-Barré syndrome and what to include in regard to etiologic factors. Some investigators have proposed rather exact diagnostic criteria (Osler and Sidell). Others have required the identification of an elevated cerebrospinal fluid protein content (Guillain et al.), and certain authors have accepted the diagnosis only when no etiologic source could be identified (Marshall, McFarland and Heller). Still other authors have included cases with symmetrical polyneuropathy due to metabolic disorders such as porphyria or resulting from exogenous intoxications. Acute symmetrical neuropathies of the Guillain-Barré type have also been described following immunizations (Gunderman) or the administration of tetanus antitoxin (Midlets et al.). In addition, a variety of viral and other infectious agents have now been associated with this illness, even though the pathogenesis of the neurologic dysfunction has not been entirely clarified.

In order to preserve the term Guillain-Barré syndrome and for it to have meaning, it seems reasonable to define it on the basis of a compatible clinical picture, not due to an underlying, identified disease well known to be commonly associated with peripheral neuropathy. In view of the increasing evidence that the disorder represents an immunologic response of peripheral nerve tissue to hypersensitive cells, the identification of a specific infectious illness or the recognition of a viral or other infectious agent should not be viewed as incompatible with the diagnosis. Restricting the definition in this fashion, it can be assumed that in the great majority of cases, the Guillain-Barré syndrome is an immune reaction, triggered by recent exposure to an exogenous agent, usually infectious, which leads to certain cellular changes eventuating in attack on the spinal rootlets and peripheral and cranial nerves.

The first widely recognized description of this form of acute polyneuropathy was by Landry in 1859. Onset of weakness in the lower extremities followed by progression in an ascending fashion was emphasized in this early report, and in 1876, Westphal referred to the syndrome as "Landry's ascending paralysis." In 1892, Osler wrote of "acute febrile polyneuritis," pointing out the association of a preceding infectious illness followed by the subsequent development of weakness of the facial and limb musculature. The contribution of Guillain, Barré, and Strohl in 1916 was made possible by the earlier introduction of the technique of lumbar puncture by Quincke in 1891. Guillain and colleagues directed attention to the high cerebrospinal fluid protein content and popularized the "albuminocytologic dissociation" which they believed was constantly present with this illness. Perhaps because of the relatively limited number of patients in their series, the authors did underestimate its potential seriousness, stating that it was invariably benign and not to be considered a potentially fatal disorder. Draganesco and Claudian in 1927 introduced the eponym Guillain-Barré syndrome, thus obscuring the memorable contributions of Strohl and of Landry.

Mills provided one of the early descriptions of the pathology of the disorder in 1898. Because of the degenerative peripheral nerve lesions, he proposed the term "neuronitis," one still used by some writers. The study by Haymaker and Kernohan in 1949, however, established our present concepts of the primary site of the disease. Fifty fatal cases were examined pathologically in which death occurred at variable times after onset of symptoms. Lesions were concentrated in the anterior and posterior rootlets and the proximal portion of the peripheral nerves. Comparing duration of illness to histologic findings, the authors concluded that edema of the rootlets develops in the first few days after onset and irregularity of myelin sheaths and axons appears by the fifth or sixth day. Infiltration with lymphocytes occurs on approximately the ninth day, with the appearance of phagocytes about 12 days after onset. The most profound degenerative changes of the rootlets and peripheral nerves were observed in a patient who survived 46 days before death. Myelin and axons were both badly damaged, and in certain areas were virtually destroyed. Except for some anterior horn cell changes which the authors considered to be retrograde in origin, no significant spinal cord, brain stem, or cerebral abnormalities were identified. Subsequently, ultrastructural studies of the rootlet pathology in Guillain-Barré syndrome have demonstrated primary myelin disruption with infiltration of macrophages, large mononuclear cells, plasma cells, and small lymphocytes (Wisniewski et al.). Such histologic findings have been compared with those of experimental allergic neuritis (Waksman and Adams), adding emphasis to the now-popular concept that Guillain-Barré syndrome is an immunologic process in which the primary target is the proximal portion of the peripheral nervous system.

While there is uniform agreement that the main impact of the illness is on the rootlets and peripheral nerves, whether there is a primary effect within the spinal cord or brain stem has been a matter of dispute for years. Haymaker and Kernohan attributed chromatolysis of anterior horn cells to retrograde damage and Rosenblum et al. described severe spinal cord damage which included demyelination within the posterior columns, believed to be secondary to chronic and extensive dorsal root involvement. Ataxia has occasionally been observed in patients with the Guillain-Barré syndrome, and in some cases it occurs without sufficient sensory disturbances to account for its presence. Richter referred to this variation as the "ataxic form of polyradiculoneuritis" and demonstrated damage of the spinal component of the spinocerebellar pathways in such a patient. Evidence of "central" involvement was postulated by Jampel and Haidt because of the preservation of Bell's phenomenon in a patient who exhibited bilateral external ophthalmoplegia as well as other customary findings of Guillain-Barré syndrome. While exceptional cases may reveal some central nervous system involvement, the hallmark of the Guillain-Barré syndrome is the presence of peripheral nerve, and especially anterior rootlet, dysfunction.

Clinical Manifestations

The Guillain-Barré syndrome occurs in either sex but with a slight male predominance (Lesser et al., Pleasure et al., Wiederholt et al.), shows no particular seasonal incidence, and may affect any age group. The mean annual incidence rate has been estimated at 1.7 cases per 100,000 when all age groups are considered (Kennedy et al., Lesser et al.). There are now many reports of the illness in children (Aylett, Low et al., Markland and Riley, Paulson, Peterman et al.), among which most patients have been older than two years of age. Patients under a year of age have only rarely been described (Carroll et al., Eden), perhaps partly reflecting the diagnostic importance of a gait abnormality signaling the existence of muscle weakness. Among 97 patients of all ages reviewed by Wiederholt and colleagues, 20 were children ten years of age or younger, an incidence unequaled in this series by any single decade except for the sixth. In general, the clinical features, laboratory findings, and eventual outcome appear to be approximately the same in children with this illness compared with their older counterparts.

In more than 50 percent of patients with Guillain-Barré syndrome in most series, the neurologic abnormalities are preceded one to three weeks by an infectious illness, most often a mild upper respiratory infection presumed to be viral in type. The first manifestation of the disorder in approximately one-half of the patients is muscle weakness, most often of the lower extremities. The other half will first describe pain or paresthesias, especially distally, with evidence of weakness developing soon thereafter. Very rarely, the illness begins with bulbar dysfunction, facial weakness, or extraocular muscle dysfunction. Once noticed, weakness of the lower extremities usually progressively worsens in association with decreased strength in the upper limbs, in addition to bilateral weakness of the facial musculature. Progression continues for one to several days, with the ultimate degree of weakness varying from mild to virtual complete flaccid paralysis of all four extremities as well as intercostal weakness, which may require ventilatory assistance. In a large series of patients with Guillain-Barré syndrome, McFarland and Heller found significant respiratory muscle weakness in 20 percent. The duration from onset of symptoms until the peak of paralytic involvement may be as short as one or two days or as long as three weeks, but most patients reach their maximum degree of weakness within a few days after onset.

Facial muscle weakness is present in most with Guillain-Barré syndrome but frequently results in no abnormalities which the patient recognizes. Because of the bilateral and symmetrical involvement, its presence may not be initially identified by the examiner unless special attention is directed to the strength of eyelid closure (Fig. 25–1). Less often, lower cranial nerve dysfunction gives rise to dysarthria or dysphagia, and, in general, tends to be associated with significant respiratory compromise. Other cranial nerves can be affected but are involved much less frequently than the seventh or the lower cranial nerves. External ophthalmoparesis is unusual but can occur (Gibberd, Marshall) and trigeminal sensory loss is even more infrequent.

Findings on physical examination depend on the degree and extent of involvement but consist of decrease of muscle tone and strength in a roughly symmetrical distribution, in addition to diminished to absent deep tendon reflexes. Occasionally, in the first few days after onset, one is surprised to find reasonably intact stretch reflexes despite the existence of considerable loss of strength. This is ordinarily temporary, as reflex loss develops if progression of weakness continues. Sensory findings are extremely variable and are nearly always far less impressive than the motor deficits. Muscle tenderness is observed in some, while others exhibit either pain or proprioceptive disturbances, especially distally and more often in the lower extremities than in the hands. Although an occasional patient may have diminished superficial sensation in a "glove and stocking" distribution, a well-established sensory level with profound sensory loss to all modalities below the level should not be accepted to be consistent with this disorder and is more suggestive of a spinal cord compressive lesion. Bladder and bowel function are unaffected in the majority of patients, even in those with marked peripheral muscle weakness. Among those with bulbar and intercostal muscle weakness, speech becomes diminished in volume and is poorly articulated, while disturbed swallowing results in nasal regurgitation. The force of the cough becomes notably reduced, and the depth of maximal inspiration gets progressively more shallow. Meningeal signs, including mild neck stiffness or some degree of limitation on straight leg raising, are occasionally present in the first few days after onset. This seems to be more common in children than in adults and is usually transient (Paulson).

Less well known clinical features in the Guillain-Barré syndrome are a variety of vasomotor disturbances (Appenzeller and Marshall) and autonomic abnormalities, manifested by either orthostatic hypotension or systemic hypertension (Birchfield and Shaw, Haymaker and Kernohan). Papilledema is a rare complication which has received considerable attention in the literature (Buchsbaum and Gallo, Janeway and Kelly, Joynt, Morley and Reynolds), especially relative to its pathogenesis. In certain cases, increased intracranial pressure has been ascribed to brain swelling occurring simultaneously with peripheral neuropathy (Joynt). A more popular concept has attributed increased pressure and subsequent papilledema to a cerebrospinal fluid absorptive defect, somehow secondary to the high cerebrospinal fluid protein content (Janeway and Kelly). In addition to the rare occurrence of papilledema in older persons, Gilmartin and Ch'ien have reported an infant with Guillain-Barré syndrome with a very high CSF protein with progressive head enlargement resulting from communicating hy-

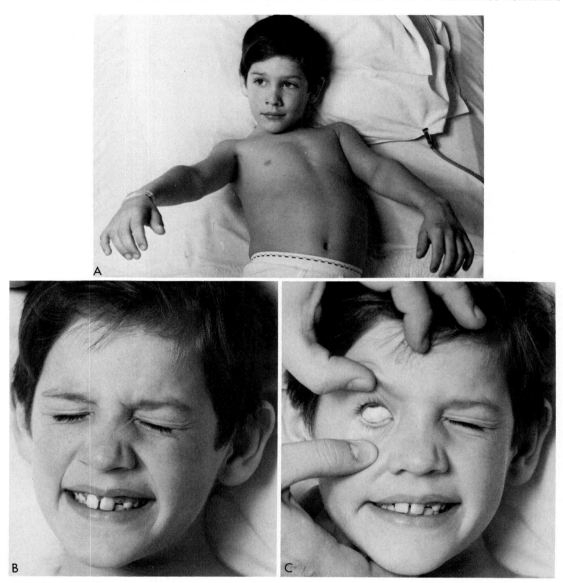

Figure 25–1. Guillain-Barré syndrome. This 7-year-old boy was well until 3 days before admission to the hospital when he complained of tingling in both feet, followed by progessive weakness, first in the legs and subsequently in the arms. Examination on admission revealed the child to be unable to sit or stand because of severe hypotonic weakness of the limbs and trunk. Deep tendon reflexes were absent in all limbs. His cough was diminished in force and voice was decreased in volume. Sensory examination was normal. CSF protein content was 150 mg. per 100 ml. and no cells were present. *A,* Child could not elevate the arms to a horizontal position. *B,* Because the facial muscle weakness is bilateral, the facial grimace is symmetical and thus weakness is easily overlooked. *C,* Ease of opening the eyelid during attempted forced closure indicates the presence of facial muscle weakness. Note the Bell's phenomenon (upward and lateral deviation of the eye) which provides evidence of attempted forced closure.

drocephalus. Neither theory has acquired universal support, and it is possible that other factors yet to be clarified may also be operative. Still another poorly understood manifestation of the Guillain-Barré syndrome is a form of acute glomerulonephritis (Behan et al.). Rodríquez-Iturbe et al. found histologic evidence of an immune nephritis in eight of nine patients with this illness, several of whom had microscopic hematuria or systemic hypertension, identified only by repeated urine examinations.

Guillain-Barré syndrome occurs in all degrees of severity, ranging from a very mild degree of muscle weakness not requiring hospitalization to complete flaccid paralysis of all extremities with sufficient respiratory muscle weakness that artificial ventilation is required. It is probable that mildly affected cases are diagnosed with considerably less frequency than those with greater deficits. Since most published series deal primarily with hospitalized cases, information regarding morbidity and mortality is probably somewhat biased in the direction of the more severely affected individual. As a generalization, it can be said that patients whose weakness is not more than mild at its greatest degree can be expected to achieve complete recovery. Those with more extensive involvement may or may not recover completely. Among 25 children with Guillain-Barré syndrome, Peterman et al. found complete recovery in 17. In a number of these cases, improvement continued for over a year. Markland and Riley observed complete recovery in 14 of 19 children with the illness, while Wiederholt et al. noted complete recovery in 61 of 97 patients in all age groups. Among 47 children with Guillain-Barré syndrome, Eberly et al. classified 36 as recovered when examined three years after onset of the illness, while 11 retained some degree of residual deficits.

Of patients left with permanent disability, most show gradual improvement for one or more years after the onset of the disorder but a small percentage are left with profound limb weakness which is associated with extensive muscle atrophy. Even those who achieve complete functional recovery may remain areflexic indefinitely. An unusual pattern described more often in adults than children is recurrent polyneuropathy, often with recovery occurring between relapses (Novak and Johnson, Thomas et al.). Little is known as to why recurrence affects a few while most patients with this disorder experience the illness only once. The most remarkable example is that published by Austin in which an adult had 20 episodes of polyneuropathy over a five-year period.

A mortality rate of 20 percent has often been quoted for this disease but is clearly too high, especially since the advent of adequate respirator care. Death rates between 2 and 6 percent published recently would seem to be more accurate estimates (McFarland and Heller, Peterman et al., Pleasure et al., Wiederholt et al.).

Fisher Syndrome

A syndrome believed by most authorities to be an unusual variation of the Guillain-Barré syndrome was first described by Fisher in 1956 and has subsequently been called the Fisher syndrome. Numerous cases have now been identified and reported (Elizan et al., Goodwin and Poser, Hynes, Patel et al., Smith and Walsh), but only a few have been children (Bell et al., Marks et al., Qaqundah and Taylor). The cardinal manifestations of this disorder are external ophthalmoplegia of variable type and degree, ataxia which appears to be cerebellar in type, and diffuse areflexia. The illness is usually of sudden onset and, like the Guillain-Barré syndrome, an upper respiratory infection often precedes the onset of the neurologic signs. The cerebrospinal fluid protein content is often normal but can be mildly elevated. In the child reported by Price et al., the illness occurred coincident with heterophil-positive infectious mononucleosis. The Fisher syndrome is transient in most cases, with recovery expected within several weeks or a few months after onset. Peripheral limb weakness may accompany the other signs in some patients (Fig. 25–2).

Several authors have commented upon the presence of lethargy or drowsiness in the initial stages, a point suggestive of at least some "central" involvement, perhaps at the level of the brain stem, in view of the other associated signs. Fisher noted total external ophthalmoplegia with relative sparing of the levator palpebrae function and suggested the possibility of central nervous system dysfunction on this basis. Since the disease has been benign in reported cases, pathologic confirmation of the site or sites of pathology has not been available.

Laboratory Studies

Except for the cerebrospinal fluid examination, laboratory biochemical studies are usually non-revealing in patients with the Guillain-Barré syndrome. Transient diabetes insipidus has been described (Pessin) and also hyponatremia secondary to inappropriate release of antidiuretic hormone has been reported (Posner et al.) in this illness, but such metabolic disorders are rare. Laboratory tests that should be accomplished to attempt to establish an etiologic source include a hetero-

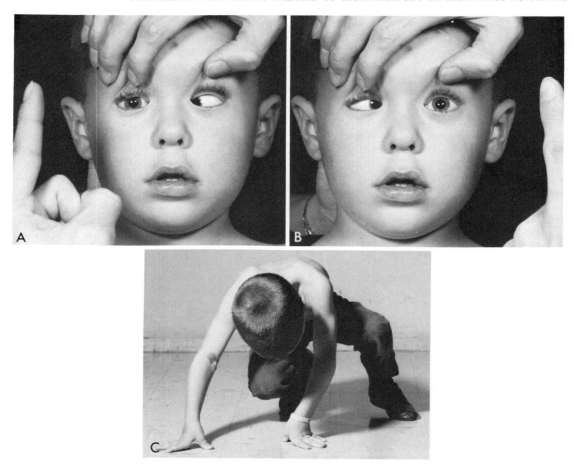

Figure 25–2. Fisher syndrome. Five-year-old boy with a 6-day history of lethargy, ataxia, and diplopia. CSF protein content was 222 mg. per 100 ml. Physical examination demonstrated muscle weakness with hyporeflexia, ataxia, and partial ophthalmoplegia. *A,* Attempted gaze to the right shows a right sixth nerve paralysis, hyperadduction of the left eye, and dilated pupils. *B,* Attempted gaze to the left reveals nearly complete left sixth nerve paralysis, hyperadduction of the right eye, and dilated pupils. *C,* The child is unable to rise from a sitting position without using his upper extremities. The clinical course was one of gradual improvement and eventual recovery except for mild, persistent ocular deficits.

phil agglutination test, serologic tests for Mycoplasma pneumoniae and the cytomegaloviruses, and collection of stool and CSF specimens in an effort to isolate an enterovirus.

Cerebrospinal fluid examination is the most valuable ancillary diagnostic procedure, with the primary abnormality being an elevated protein content between 50 and 250 mg. per 100 ml. and occasionally even higher. A significant cellular response is usually absent, and the Queckenstedt test demonstrates a normal rise and fall of the fluid column. Wiederholt and Mulder analyzed the CSF findings of 93 patients with the Guillain-Barré syndrome and found that 89 had elevated protein values while only four had

normal levels. Their study indicated that the protein content is not always increased in the initial stages of the illness but can become elevated at a later date. Thus, a single examination revealing a normal protein soon after onset is not incompatible with the diagnosis. Peterman et al. found the CSF protein to be elevated in all of 25 children with the disease, the highest level being 800 mg. per 100 ml. In several, the increased protein content persisted for a number of months, and according to McFarland and Heller, it can remain high for years.

Electrodiagnostic studies are of decided value in this disorder, although the anticipated findings of denervation on electromyography and slowed motor conduction velocity are not always present. In the very early stages, nerve conduction velocities may still be normal and can, therefore, be misleading. In the study of 25 patients by Eisen and Humphreys, almost 20 percent had entirely normal electrodiagnostic studies throughout the course of the illness. Within a few days after onset of the illness, motor nerve conduction is usually slowed (Banerji and Millar), with improvement often lagging behind clinical recovery. Study of the F-wave responses frequently provides additional diagnostic information, and may indicate slowing over the proximal portions of the spinal rootlets and nerve trunks (Kimura).

Differential Diagnosis

Differential diagnostic considerations with this form of acute polyneuropathy include a wide spectrum of disorders, but a few are notable because of their similarity to this illness. Historically, poliomyelitis held first place in the differential list but its decline has reduced it from common consideration. Spinal cord or bulbar involvement in polio precipitates a cellular response in the CSF in most cases and the illness is usually associated with more asymmetrical weakness than occurs with the Guillain-Barré syndrome. Botulism is uncommon but bears many similarities to the Guillain-Barré syndrome and can easily be confused with it. Blurred vision or diplopia and lower cranial nerve involvement are the common first symptoms in botulism, and only later does weakness of the extremities supervene. The CSF protein is generally normal and cases of botulism usually occur in clusters. It is the first case in an outbreak or the isolated case, such as with wound botulism, that is especially likely to result in diagnostic confusion. Infantile botulism is characterized by diffuse hypotonic weakness but the age of its occurrence is an unusual one for the Guillain-Barré syndrome (Arnon et al., Pickett et al.). Otherwise, however, the infant with botulism could readily be assumed to have an acquired polyneuropathy unless one is aware of this unusual disorder. Diagnosis of botulism can be confirmed by identification of toxin in blood and stool or recovery of the organism from gastric washings or stool in patients ill from ingestion of infected food.

Periodic paralysis of either the hypokalemic or hyperkalemic types are additional disorders which can mimic this syndrome but

can usually be separated on the basis of periodic recurrences, rapidity of recovery from muscle weakness, and identification of the underlying metabolic disorder, either primarily of potassium metabolism or secondary to renal tubular dysfunction. In young children especially, differentiation of the Guillain-Barré syndrome from acute cerebellar ataxia can be particularly difficult. A mild degree of muscle weakness often manifests itself as incoordination of gait in this age group in which cooperation on examination is often limited. An important differentiating point is that the child who is ataxic can generally rise from sitting on the floor without difficulty if supported but one who has limb weakness cannot. A significant elevation of the CSF protein content also is more consistent with acute polyneuropathy and is much less often present with acute cerebellar ataxia. Polymyositis shares many features in common with the Guillain-Barré syndrome but can usually be distinguished on the basis of elevated muscle enzymes, characteristic electromyographic abnormalities, and a normal CSF protein content. Myopathy secondary to corticosteroid treatment, so-called "steroid myopathy," also can be confused with this illness because of the similarity of the physical findings. In rare instances, rabies will present with spinal cord involvement before clear-cut encephalitic features emerge. In such patients, the illness begins with flaccid paresis of the limbs, which can be followed by bulbar paresis and bilateral facial weakness (Houff et al.). Unless a history of an animal bite is elicited, the disorder is readily confused with the Guillain-Barré syndrome on the basis of the clinical findings.

Mercury poisoning (Swaiman and Flagler), tick paralysis, and porphyria are other disorders associated with neuropathy or muscle weakness that resemble the Guillain-Barré syndrome but are not primary considerations in most cases. A practical consideration in every case, however, relates to the possibility of a spinal cord or cauda equina compressive lesion as the cause of acquired lower extremity weakness. This is particularly applicable to the younger childhood group in which cooperation on examination usually diminishes with decreasing age. The presence of cranial nerve deficits in the Guillain-Barré syndrome will place the level of highest involvement above the spinal cord but such findings may be absent initially. Clinical features that should be considered incompatible with the diagnosis of Guillain-Barré syndrome include significant back pain or spinal percussion tenderness, hyperactive deep reflexes in the lower extremities, a well-established sensory level on the trunk, or xanthochromic spinal fluid with evidence of a block on the Queckenstedt test. Findings such as these in a child with acquired weakness of the lower extremities warrant further diagnostic studies, including spine x-rays and, perhaps, myelography.

Etiology and Pathogenesis

Although much remains to be clarified in regard to the pathogenesis of the Guillain-Barré syndrome, numerous associations have been made with its occurrence in relationship to infectious agents, immunizing agents, and specific infectious illnesses. The disorder has followed tetanus antitoxin injection (Midlets et al.), antirabies vaccination (Appelbaum et al.), smallpox vaccination (Winkelman), typhoid vaccination (Miller and Stanton), and administration of mumps-rubella vaccine (Gunderman). Guillain-Barré syndrome has complicated immunization with live measles vaccine (Grose and Spigland) and has been attributed to an otherwise asymptomatic measles virus infection in a patient receiving long-term hemodialysis for chronic renal failure (Drüeke et al.). Influenza immunization, most notably the program in this country in 1976, provoked a number of cases of this type of polyneuropathy (Furlow, Schonberger et al., Seyal et al.). The illness has also complicated varicella and other childhood exanthems (Welch), has been associated with influenza virus and Coxsackie virus infections (Jackson, Wells et al.), and, rarely, with Herpes simplex virus infection (Olivarius and Buhl). Guillain-Barré syndrome has occurred in a child in whom Echo virus type 7 was isolated from stool and CSF (Urano et al.) and in an adult with parainfluenza virus isolated from the CSF (Roman et al.). Several cases have been described in relationship to infectious mononucleosis (Creaturo, Davie et al., Ricker et al., Silverstein et al.) and, in some, the disease has developed in the absence of clinical evidence of mononucleosis but with elevated antibody titers to the Epstein-Barr virus (Boyce, Grose and Feorino). In other patients with Epstein-Barr virus–related Guillain-Barré syndrome, the heterophil antibody tests do not become positive and are recognized only by specific serodiagnostic procedures (Grose et al.).

Evidence has also been compiled to relate the occurrence of acute, symmetrical polyneuropathy to infection with Mycoplasma pneumoniae (Steele et al.) and to cytomegalovirus infections (Jordan et al., Kabins et al., Klemola et al., Leonard and Tobin). Findings in recent studies suggest that the cytomegaloviruses are, perhaps, among the most common viral precipitants of the Guillain-Barré syndrome. Dowling et al. found significant cytomegalovirus titer elevations in approximately one-third of 92 patients with this disorder. In a series of 94 patients with Guillain-Barré syndrome, Schmitz and Enders demonstrated serologic evidence of a recently preceding cytomegalovirus infection in 10 cases, in most instances on the basis of the presence of virus-specific IgM antibodies.

Thus, many different antigenic factors appear capable of provoking a common response in which the primary target organ is the proximal portion of the peripheral nervous system. As the result of many experimental studies coupled with a variety of clinical observations, the prevailing opinion at present is that the Guillain-Barré syndrome is an immunopathologic disorder which develops when lymphocytes somehow become sensitized to peripheral nerve antigen and attack myelin of the peripheral nerve tissue (Currie and Knowles, Knowles et al.). With this concept in mind, the significance of the parallel made by previous investigators of the histologic findings in this disease to those of experimental allergic neuritis becomes obvious. This immune-mediated experimental lesion was produced in rabbits by Waksman and Adams in 1955 by injections of peripheral nerve with Freund's adjuvant which resulted in segmental demyelination with mononuclear cell infiltration. The mononuclear cell infiltration of involved rootlets in the Guillain-Barré syndrome is believed to be analogous to that in experimental allergic neuritis.

Recent studies have also demonstrated the presence of atypical basophilic mononuclear cells circulating in the peripheral blood in the acute stage of the Guillain-Barré syndrome (Cook et al., Whitaker et al.). These circulating cells, referred to as "immunocytes," have been shown to be active in DNA synthesis and are indistinguishable from those that are in intimate contact with the affected rootlets and nerves. According to Cook et al., patients with the highest number of circulating "immunocytes" have the greatest degree of morbidity compared to those with a lesser number of such cells. Additional in vitro experiments have shown that lymphocytes obtained from patients with Guillain-Barré syndrome exhibit hypersensitivity to peripheral nervous system antigen (Abramsky et al., Sheremata et al.). Cook and colleagues and Hirano et al. have also demonstrated that in a high percentage of patients with Guillain-Barré syndrome, the serum contains a complement-dependent myelinotoxic factor. The identification of an immune nephritis in some patients with this illness (Behan et al., Rodríquez-Iturbe et al.) has been an additional impetus to the theory that the neurologic damage is on the basis of an immune process.

Although the above discoveries would appear to provide strong support for an immunologic basis for this disease, certain other observations indicate that continued investigations are needed before complete understanding of the pathogenesis is available. For example, Drachman et al. described an adult who developed the Guillain-Barré syndrome while immunosuppressed with drug therapy following renal transplantation, and other reports have documented the condition in immunosuppressed patients with Hodgkin's disease (Lisak et al.).

Treatment

Management of the child with the Guillain-Barré syndrome depends on the stage of the illness when seen and the extent of involvement. In the acute stage when progressive weakness is still evolving, the most important aspect of management is frequent observations of respiratory and bulbar function. It is most important that the need for intubation, tracheotomy, or respirator care be anticipated and accomplished before hypoxia or respiratory arrest occurs. Careful and expert judgment are required for this decision, and no absolute guidelines are applicable to a given patient. When it becomes reasonably predictable that respiratory muscle function will become insufficient to maintain ventilation, ventilatory support should be initiated.

Less severely affected patients who have little or no respiratory problem should be kept in bed in the acute stage. Physical therapy of the passive type can be delayed for a short period until the course of the disease becomes apparent. When weakness is moderate to severe, nursing care, physical therapy, and an eventual rehabilitation program represent the hallmarks of management. The development of systemic hypertension in the child with the Guillain-Barré syndrome sometimes warrants evaluation of the renin-angiotensin system and measurement of catecholamine excretion (Stapleton et al.). Specific treatment depends on the degree of the blood pressure elevation and the results of the laboratory studies.

The value of corticosteroid therapy has been a point of dispute among authors for years and remains unresolved. Some have described favorable results when compared to an untreated control series (Heller and DeJong, Swick and McQuillen), but no study has shown spectacular effects of corticosteroid treatment. Goodall and colleagues, in a retrospective study, concluded that treatment with corticosteroids was not beneficial in patients with Guillain-Barré syndrome and was not indicated for this illness. A current opinion held by many is that corticosteroid therapy is warranted if the patient is seen in the acute stage of illness and has significant motor deficits which are still in the progressively worsening phase. The usual approach is to give an intensive intravenous course with corticosteroids in a high dose initially, with the hope that discontinuation of therapy can be achieved within one to three weeks.

REFERENCES

Abramsky, O., Webb, C., Teitelbaum, D., and Arnon, R.: Cell-mediated immunity to neural antigens in idiopathic polyneuritis and myeloradiculitis. Clinical-immunologic classification of several autoimmune demyelinating disorders. Neurology 25:1154–1159, 1975.

Appelbaum, E., Greenberg, M., and Nelson, J.: Neurological complications following antirabies vaccination. J.A.M.A. 151:188–191, 1953.

Appenzeller, O., and Marshall, J.: Vasomotor disturbance in Landry-Guillain-Barré syndrome. Arch. Neurol. 9:368–372, 1963.

Arnon, S. S., Midura, T. F., Clay, S. A., Wood, R. M., and Chin, J.: Infant botulism. Epidemiological, clinical, and laboratory aspects. J.A.M.A. 237:1946–1951, 1977.

Austin, J. H.: Recurrent polyneuropathies and their corticosteroid treatment. With five-year observations of a placebo-controlled case treated with corticotropin, cortisone, and prednisone. Brain 81:157–192, 1958.

Aylett, P.: Five cases of acute infective polyneuritis (Guillain-Barré syndrome) in children. Arch. Dis. Childh. 29:531–536, 1954.

Banerji, N. K., and Millar, J. H. D.: Guillain-Barré syndrome in children, with special reference to serial nerve conduction studies. Dev. Med. Child Neurol. 14:56–63, 1972.

Behen, P. O., Stilmant, M., Lowenstein, L. M., and Sax, D. S.: Landry-Guillain-Barré-Strohl syndrome and immune-complex nephritis. Lancet 1:850–854, 1973.

Bell, W., Van Allen, M., and Blackman, J.: Fisher syndrome in childhood. Dev. Med. Child Neurol. 12:758–766, 1970.

Birchfield, R. I., and Shaw, C.: Postural hypotension in the Guillain-Barré syndrome. Arch. Neurol. 10:149–157, 1964.

Boyce, M. J.: E. B. virus and the Guillain-Barré syndrome. Lancet 2:1028–1029, 1972.

Buchsbaum, H. W., and Gallo, A. E., Jr.: Polyneuritis, papilledema, and lumboperitoneal shunt. Arch. Neurol. 21:253–257, 1969.

Carroll, J. E., Jedziniak, M., and Guggenheim, M. A.: Guillain-Barré syndrome. Another cause of the "floppy infant." Am. J. Dis. Child. 131:699–670, 1977.

Cook, S. D., Dowling, P. C., Murray, M. R., and Whitaker, J. N.: Circulating demyelinating factors in acute idiopathic polyneuropathy. Arch. Neurol. 24:136–144, 1971.

Cook, S. D., Dowling, P. C., and Whitaker, J. N.: The Guillain-Barré syndrome. Relationship of circulating immunocytes to disease activity. Arch. Neurol. 22:470–474, 1970.

Creaturo, N. E.: Infectious mononucleosis and polyneuritis (Guillain-Barré syndrome). J.A.M.A. 143:234–236, 1950.

Currie, S., and Knowles, M.: Lymphocyte transformation in the Guillain-Barré syndrome. Brain 94:109–116, 1971.

Davie, J. C., Ceballos, R., and Little, S. C.: Infectious mononucleosis with fatal neuronitis. Arch. Neurol. 9:265–272, 1963.

Dowling, P., Menonna, J., and Cook, S.: Cytomegalovirus complement fixation antibody in Guillain-Barré syndrome. Neurology 27:1153–1156, 1977.

Drachman, D. A., Paterson, P. Y., Berlin, B. S., and Roguska, J.: Immunosuppression and the Guillain-Barré syndrome. Arch. Neurol. 23:385–393, 1970.

Draganesco, S., and Claudian, J.: Sur un cas de radiculonevrite curable (syndrome de Guillain-Barré) apparue au cours d'une osteomyelite du bras. Rev. Neurol. 2:517–521, 1927.

Drüeke, T. B., Pujade-Lauraine, E., Poisson, M., Zingraff, J., Ulmann, A., and Crosnier, J.: Measles virus and Guillain-Barré syndrome during long-term hemodialysis. Am. J. Med. 60:444–446, 1976.

Eberle, E., Brink, J., Azen, S., and White, D.: Early predictors of incomplete recovery in children with Guillain-Barré polyneuritis. J. Pediat. 86:356–359, 1975.

Eden, A. N.: Guillain-Barré syndrome in a six-month-old infant. Am. J. Dis. Child. 102:224–227, 1961.

Eisen, A., and Humphreys, P.: The Guillain-Barré syndrome. A clinical and electrodiagnostic study of 25 cases. Arch. Neurol. 30:438–443, 1974.

Elizan, T. S., Spire, J. P., Andiman, R. M., Baughman, F. A., Jr., and Lloyd-Smith, D. L.: Syndrome of acute idiopathic ophthalmoplegia with ataxia and areflexia. Neurology 21:281–292, 1971.

Fisher, M.: An unusual variant of acute idiopathic polyneuritis (syndrome of ophthalmoplegia, ataxia and areflexia). New Eng. J. Med. 255:57–65, 1956.

Furlow, T. W., Jr.: Neuropathy after influenza vaccination. Lancet 1:253–254, 1977.

Gibberd, F. B.: Ophthalmoplegia in acute polyneuritis. Arch. Neurol. 23:161–164, 1970.

Gilmartin, R. C., and Ch'ien, L. T.: Guillain-Barré syndrome with hydrocephalus in early infancy. Arch. Neurol. 34:567–569, 1977.

Goodall, J. A. D., Kosmidis, J. C., and Geddes, A. M.: Effect of corticosteroids on course of Guillain-Barré syndrome. Lancet 1:524–526, 1974.

Goodwin, R. F., and Posner, C. M.: Ophthalmoplegia, ataxia, and areflexia. Fisher's syndrome. J.A.M.A. 186:258–259, 1963.

Grose, C., and Feorino, P. M.: Epstein-Barr virus and Guillain-Barré syndrome. Lancet 2:1285–1287, 1972.

Grose, C., Henle, W., and Feorino, P. M.: Primary Epstein-Barr virus infections in acute neurologic diseases. New Eng. J. Med. 292:392–395, 1975.

Grose, C., and Spigland, I.: Guillain-Barré syndrome following administration of live measles vaccine. Am. J. Med. 60:441–443, 1976.

Guillain, G.: Radiculoneuritis with acellular hyperalbuminosis of the cerebrospinal fluid. Arch. Neurol. Psychiat. 36:975–990, 1936.

Guillain, G., Barré, J. A., and Strohl, A.: Sur un syndrome de radiculo-névrite avec hyperalbuminose du liquide céphalo-rachidien sans réaction cellulaire. Remarques sur les caractéres cliniques et graphiques des réflexes tendineux. Bull. Mém. Soc. Med. Hop. Paris 40:1462–1470, 1916.

Gunderman, J. R.: Guillain-Barré syndrome. Occurrence following combined mumps-rubella vaccine. Am. J. Dis. Child. 125:834–835, 1973.

Haymaker, W., and Kernohan, J. W.: The Landry-Guillain-Barré syndrome: a clinicopathologic report of fifty fatal cases and a critique of the literature. Medicine 28:59–141, 1949.

Heller, G. L., and DeJong, R. N.: Treatment of the Guillain-Barré syndrome. Use of corticotropin and glucocorticoids. Arch. Neurol. 8:179–193, 1963.

Hirano, A., Cook, S. D., Whitaker, J. N., Dowling, P. D., and Murray, M. R.: Fine structural aspects of demyelination in vitro. The effects of Guillain-Barré serum. J. Neuropath. Exp. Neurol. 30:249–265, 1971.

Houff, S. A., Burton, R. C., Wilson, R. W., Henson, T. E., London, W. T., Baer, G. M., Anderson, L. J., Winkler, W. G., Madden, D. L., and Sever, J. L.: Human-to-human transmission of rabies virus by corneal transplant. New Eng. J. Med. 300:603–604, 1979.

Hynes, E. A.: Syndrome of Fisher. Ophthalmoplegia, ataxia and areflexia. Am. J. Ophthal. 51:701–704, 1961.

Jackson, A. L.: A clinical study of the Landry-Guillain-Barré syndrome with reference to aetiology, including the role of Coxsackie virus infections. S. Afr. J. Lab. Clin. Med. 7:121–137, 1961.

Jampel, R. S., and Haidt, S. J.: Bell's phenomenon and acute idiopathic polyneuritis. Am. J. Ophthal. 74:145–153, 1972.

Janeway, R., and Kelly, D. L., Jr.: Papilledema and hydrocephalus associated with recurrent polyneuritis. Guillain-Barré type. Arch. Neurol. 15:507–514, 1966.

Jordan, M. C., Rousseau, W. E., Stewart, J. A., Noble, G. R., and Chin, T. D. Y.: Spontaneous cytomegalovirus mononucleosis. Ann. Intern. Med. 79:153–160, 1973.

Joynt, R. J.: Mechanism of production of papilledema in the Guillain-Barré syndrome. Neurology 8:8–12, 1958.

Kabins, S., Keller, R., Peitchel, R., and Ali, M. A.: Acute idiopathic polyneuritis caused by cytomegaloviruses. Arch. Intern. Med. 136:100–101, 1974.

Kennedy, R. H., Danielson, M. A., Mulder, D. W., and Kurland, L. T.: Guillain-Barré syndrome. A 42-year epidemiologic and clinical study. Mayo Clin. Proc. 53:93–99, 1978.

Kimura, J.: Proximal versus distal slowing of motor

nerve conduction velocity in the Guillain-Barré syndrome. Ann. Neurol. 3:344–350, 1978.

Klemola, E., Weckman, N., Haltia, K., and Kaariainen, L.: The Guillain-Barré syndrome associated with acquired cytomegalovirus infection. Acta Med. Scand. 181:603–607, 1967.

Knowles, M., Currie, S., Saunders, M., Walton, J. N., and Field, E. J.: Lymphocyte transformation in the Guillain-Barré syndrome. Lancet 2:1168–1170, 1969.

Landry, O.: Note sur la paralysie ascendante aigue. Gaz. Hébd. Méd. Chir. 6:472–474, 468–488, 1859.

Leonard, J. C., and Tobin, J. O.: Polyneuritis associated with cytomegalovirus infections. Quart. J. Med. 40:435–442, 1971.

Lesser, R. P., Hauser, W. A., Kurland, L. T., and Mulder, D. W.: Epidemiologic features of the Guillain-Barré syndrome. Experience in Olmsted County, Minnesota, 1935 through 1968. Neurology 23:1269–1272, 1973.

Lisak, R. P., Mitchell, M., Zweiman, B., Orrechio, E., and Asbury, A. K.: Guillain-Barré syndrome and Hodgkin's disease: Three cases with immunological studies. Ann. Neurol. 1:72–78, 1977.

Low, N. L., Schneider, J., and Carter, S.: Polyneuritis in children. Pediatrics 22:972–990, 1958.

Markland, L. D., and Riley, H. D., Jr.: The Guillain-Barré syndrome in childhood. A comprehensive review, including observations on 19 additional cases. Clin. Pediat. 6:162–170, 1967.

Marks, H. G., Augustyn, P., and Allen, R. J.: Fisher's syndrome in children. Pediatrics 60:726–729, 1977.

Marshall, J.: The Landry-Guillain-Barré syndrome. Brain 86:55–77, 1963.

McFarland, H. R., and Heller, G. L.: Guillain-Barré disease complex. A statement of diagnostic criteria and analysis of 100 cases. Arch. Neurol. 14:196–201, 1966.

Midlets, A. W., Bartlett, W. G., Arbesman, C. A., and Loeser, W. E.: Guillain-Barré syndrome resulting from tetanus antitoxin injection. Second reported case with immunologic studies. Neurology 10:658–661, 1960.

Miller, H. G., and Stanton, J. B.: Neurological sequelae of prophylactic inoculation. Quart. J. Med. 23:1–27, 1954.

Mills, C. K.: The reclassification of some organic nervous diseases on the basis of the neuron. J.A.M.A. 31:11–13, 1898.

Morley, J. B., and Reynolds, E. H.: Papilledema and the Landry-Guillain-Barré syndrome. Case reports and a review. Brain 89:205–222, 1966.

Novak, D. J., and Johnson, K. J.: Relapsing idiopathic polyneuritis during pregnancy. Immunological aspects and literature review. Arch. Neurol. 28:219–223, 1973.

Olivarius, B., and Buhl, M.: Herpes simplex virus and Guillain-Barré polyradiculitis. Brit. Med. J. 1:192–193, 1975.

Osler, L. D., and Sidell, A. D.: The Guillain-Barré syndrome. The need for exact diagnostic criteria. New Eng. J. Med. 262:964–969, 1960.

Osler, W.: The Principles and Practice of Medicine. Ed. 1. Appleton Co., New York, 1892.

Patel, A., Pearce, L., and Hairston, R.: Miller Fisher syndrome (variant of Landry-Guillain-Barré-Strohl syndrome—ophthalmoplegia, ataxia, areflexia). South. Med. J. 59:171–175, 1966.

Paulson, G. W.: The Landry-Guillain-Barré-Strohl syndrome in childhood. Dev. Med. Child Neurol. 12:604–607, 1970.

Pessin, M. S.: Transient diabetes insipidus in the Landry-Guillain-Barré syndrome. Arch. Neurol. 27:85–86, 1972.

Peterman, A. F., Daly, D. D., Dion, F. R., and Keith, H. M.: Infectious neuronitis (Guillain-Barré syndrome) in children. Neurology 9:533–539, 1959.

Pickett, J., Berg, B., Chaplin, E., and Brunstetter-Shafer, M-A.: Syndrome of botulism in infancy. Clinical and electrophysiologic study. New Eng. J. Med. 295:770–772, 1976.

Pleasure, D. E., Lovelace, R. E., and Duvoisin, R. C.: The prognosis of acute polyradiculoneuritis. Neurology 18:1143–1148, 1968.

Posner, J. B., Ertel, N. H., Kossmann, R. J., and Scheinberg, L. C.: Hyponatremia in acute polyneuropathy. Four cases with the syndrome of inappropriate secretion of antidiuretic hormone. Arch. Neurol. 17:530–541, 1967.

Price, R. L., O'Conner, P. S., and Rothner, A. D.: Acute ophthalmoplegia, ataxia, and areflexia (Fisher syndrome) in childhood. Cleveland Clin. Quart. 45:247–252, 1978.

Qaqundah, B. Y., and Taylor, W. F.: Miller Fisher syndrome in a 22-month-old child. J. Pediat. 77:868–870, 1970.

Quincke, H.: Die Lumbalpunction des Hydrocephalus. Berlin Klin. Wchnschr. 28:929–933, 965–968, 1891.

Richter, R. B.: The ataxic form of polyradiculoneuritis (Landry-Guillain-Barré syndrome). Clinical and pathologic observations. J. Neuropath. Exp. Neurol. 21:171–184, 1962.

Ricker, W., Blumberg, A., Peters, C. H., and Widerman, A.: The association of the Guillain-Barré syndrome with infectious mononucleosis. Blood 2:217–226, 1947.

Rodríquez-Iturbe, B., García, R., Rubio, L., Zabala, J., Moros, G., and Torres, R.: Acute glomerulonephritis in the Guillain-Barré-Strohl syndrome. Report of nine cases. Ann. Intern. Med. 78:391–395, 1973.

Roman, G., Phillips, A., and Poser, C. M.: Parainfluenza virus type 3. Isolation from CSF of a patient with Guillain-Barré syndrome. J.A.M.A. 240:1613–1615, 1978.

Rosenblum, W. I., Budzilovich, G., and Feigin, E.: Lesions of the spinal cord in polyradiculoneuropathy of unknown aetiology and a possible relationship with the Guillain-Barré syndrome. J. Neurol. Neurosurg. Psychiat. 29:69–76, 1966.

Schmitz, H., and Enders, G.: Cytomegaloviruses as a frequent cause of Guillain-Barré syndrome. J. Med. Virol. 1:21–27, 1977.

Schonberger, L. B., Bregman, D. J., Sullivan-Bolyai, J. Z., Keenlyside, R. A., Ziegler, D. W., Retailliau, H. F., Eddins, D. L., and Bryan, J. A.: Guillain-Barré syndrome following vaccination in the national influenza immunization program, United States, 1976–1977. Am. J. Epidemiol. 110:105–123, 1979.

Seyal, M., Ziegler, D. K., and Couch, J. R.: Recurrent Guillain-Barré syndrome following influenza vaccine. Neurology 28:725–726, 1978.

Sheremata, W., Colby, S., Lusky, G., and Cosgrove, J. B. R.: Cellular hypersensitization to peripheral nervous antigens in the Guillain-Barré syndrome. Neurology 25:833–839, 1975.

Silverstein, A., Steinberg, G., and Nathanson, M.: Nervous system involvement in infectious mononucleosis. Arch. Neurol. 26:353–358, 1972.

Smith, J. L., and Walsh, F. B.: Syndrome of external ophthalmoplegia, ataxia, and areflexia (Fisher). Ocular manifestations in acute idiopathic polyneuritis (Guillain-Barré syndrome); report of two cases. Arch. Ophthal. 58:109–114, 1957.

Stapleton, F. B., Skoglund, R. R., and Daggett, R. B.: Hypertension associated with the Guillain-Barré syndrome. Pediatrics 62:588–590, 1978.

Steele, J. C., Thanasophon, S., Gladstone, R. M., and Fleming, P. C.: Mycoplasma pneumoniae as a determinant of the Guillain-Barré syndrome. Lancet 2:710–713, 1969.

Swaiman, K. F., and Flagler, D. G.: Mercury poisoning with central and peripheral nervous system involvement treated with penicillamine. Pediatrics 48:639–642, 1971.

Swick, H. M., and McQuillen, M. P.: The use of steroids in the treatment of idiopathic polyneuritis. Neurology 26:205–212, 1976.

Thomas, P. K., Lascelles, R. G., Hallpike, J. F., and Hewer, R. L.: Recurrent and chronic relapsing Guillain-Barré polyneuritis. Brain 92:589–606, 1969.

Urano, T., Kawase, T., Kodaira, K., Takeuchi, Y., Kikuchi, T., and Kimura, M.: Guillain-Barré syndrome associated with Echo virus type 7 infections. Pediatrics 45:294–295, 1970.

Waksman, B. H., and Adams, R. D.: Allergic neuritis: An experimental disease of rabbits induced by the injection of peripheral nervous tissue and adjuvants. J. Exp. Med. 102:213–235, 1955.

Welch, R. G.: Chicken-pox and the Guillain-Barré syndrome. Arch. Dis. Childh. 37:557–559, 1962.

Wells, C. E. C., James, W. R. L., and Evans, A. D.: Guillain-Barré syndrome and virus of influenza A (Asian strain). Report of two fatal cases during the 1957 epidemic in Wales. Arch. Neurol. Psychiat. 81:699–705, 1959.

Westphal, C.: Ueber einige Fälle von acuter, todlicher Spinallähmung (sogenannter acuter aufsteigender Paralyse). Arch. Psychiat. 6:765–822, 1873.

Whitaker, J. N., Hirano, A., Cook, S. D., and Dowling, P. C.: The ultrastructure of circulating immunocytes in Guillain-Barré syndrome. Neurology 20:765–770, 1970.

Wiederholt, W. C., and Mulder, D. W.: Cerebrospinal fluid findings in the Landry-Guillain-Barré-Strohl syndrome. Neurology 15:184–187, 1965.

Wiederholt, W. C., Mulder, D. W., and Lambert, E. H.: The Landry-Guillain-Barré-Strohl syndrome or polyradiculoneuropathy: Historical review, report on 97 patients, and present concepts. Mayo Clin. Proc. 39:427–451, 1964.

Winkelman, N. W.: Peripheral nerve and root disturbances following vaccination against smallpox. Arch. Neurol. Psychiat. 62:421, 1949.

Wisniewski, H., Terry, R. D., Whitaker, J. N., Cook, S. D., and Dowling, P. C.: Landry-Guillain-Barré syndrome. A primary demyelinating disease. Arch. Neurol. 21:269–276, 1969.

Chapter Twenty-Six

ACUTE CEREBELLAR ATAXIA OF CHILDHOOD

The term "acute cerebellar ataxia of infancy or childhood" is fundamentally descriptive, indicating that the neurologic disorder is recent in onset, characterized by ataxia, and of diverse etiologies. The descriptive phrase, however, is also used in reference to a poorly understood illness which usually follows a variety of childhood exanthems or nonspecific respiratory infections. Children between one and five years of age are chiefly affected, although the illness is not restricted to this age group. The disease designated as acute cerebellar ataxia of infancy or childhood is now widely accepted as a post-viral syndrome but this is partially misleading because certain patients exhibit signs not explained solely on the basis of cerebellar dysfunction. As early as 1905, Batten described acute ataxic syndromes following exanthematous diseases in children and pointed out that such cases had been reported periodically since the early part of the nineteenth century, mostly subsequent to viral respiratory illnesses, pertussis, or typhoid. Batten and many subsequent authors emphasized the lack of localizing anatomic specificity of ataxia plus the presence in some of other signs suggesting cerebral or brain stem involvement. It is probable that certain cases previously described as acute cerebellar ataxia in which coma, convulsions, or other distinct cerebral signs occurred were examples of other disorders, perhaps better categorized as encephalopathies or encephalitis. The outstanding component of this disorder is truncal ataxia, manifested in one form or another, in part depending on the age of the patient and the severity of involvement.

Clinical Manifestations

The post-viral ataxic syndrome occurs in either sex and, as mentioned, shows a predilection for children between one and five years of age. At least one-half of the reported patients have had a preceding mild infectious illness a week or so before the onset of neurologic signs (Weiss and Carter). Other children develop the syndrome in association with or following recognizable infections such as varicella or other exanthems, or infectious mononucleosis. Except that the first group remains "idiopathic" and the second group represents a complication of an identified childhood infection, there seems no justification for separation of the groups into different categories since the clinical features are the same and the pathogenesis remains unestablished regardless of the preceding illness.

The onset of the disorder is characteristically abrupt and the outstanding initial manifestation is a rapid deterioration of gait in the form of staggering and frequent falling. Truncal ataxia varies from mild instability while standing or sitting to total inability to stand alone or walk. In most affected children, the degree of incoordination reaches its zenith within 24 to 48 hours after onset but, occasionally, progressive worsening is gradual over the course of several days (Blaw and

Sheehan). Irritability or vomiting may develop simultaneously with the coordination disturbances or even precede them by several hours.

Tremulousness of the head and trunk in the upright position or of the extremities when the child attempts to reach for objects is a prominent feature in some ataxic patients. Nystagmus or other types of ocular gaze abnormalities are less commonly observed than the above findings. Other signs described in some include dysarthria, slight nuchal rigidity, hypotonia, and either slightly enhanced or diminished deep stretch reflexes.

The degree of the gait abnormality extends from mild to severe and the duration of the illness varies from three to four days to several weeks or even months before recovery is complete. Complete restoration of function is the rule, but when ataxia is profound early in the illness, persistent cerebellar deficits can remain permanently. Among eight patients with acute cerebellar ataxia, King et al. noted less than total recovery in three. Weiss and Carter stressed the possibility of lasting neurologic sequelae because eight of their 18 patients pursued such a course. Although there is no doubt that acute cerebellar ataxia in childhood is not always benign, hospital identification and subsequent case reporting is biased toward more severely affected cases. Mildly or transiently affected children probably constitute the majority and complete recovery is the expected pattern in most.

Laboratory Findings

The basic laboratory studies, such as blood count, urinalysis, sedimentation rate, and skull x-rays, are usually unrevealing in children with post-viral acute cerebellar ataxia. The electroencephalogram likewise is helpful in a negative fashion in that it is usually normal or reveals nonspecific, posterior slow activity. Cerebrospinal fluid examination may result in entirely normal findings or show either a mild lymphocytic pleocytosis or a modest increase in protein content. When cells are present, the total number is usually less than 25 per cu. mm. When the CSF pressure can be measured, it is generally normal but, because most patients with this illness are less than five years of age, pressure measurements are usually unreliable because of crying or struggling. The absence of increased intracranial pressure in the young

child with acute cerebellar ataxia is better documented by the visualization of normal optic discs and the presence of normal sutures on skull films. If there is doubt about the presence or absence of intracranial hypertension in the acutely ataxic child, cranial computed tomography will usually clarify the issue by the demonstration of the ventricular size and the presence or absence of a mass lesion in the cerebellum or brain stem. When the diagnosis of acute cerebellar ataxia is evident from the available information, further examinations should include attempts at viral isolation from stool and CSF specimens, heterophil agglutination test, and *Mycoplasma pneumoniae* complement fixation test.

Pathogenesis and Etiology

The pathogenesis of post-viral acute cerebellar ataxia of childhood is unclear, regardless of whether the syndrome follows a nonspecific viral illness or complicates a recognized childhood exanthem. It has been ascribed to a nonsuppurative encephalitis with primary involvement of the cerebellum by some authors (Griffith, Levin), while others have favored a nonspecific toxic or allergic cerebellar response to the preceding viral infection. In view of the known vulnerability of the cerebellum to injury, it is probable that insults of different types associated with various etiologic agents can produce a common syndrome with abrupt onset, cerebellar ataxia, and a transient clinical course.

Of the specific infectious disorders of children that have precipitated this illness, varicella is the best known and the most common (Goldston et al., Levin). Cerebellar signs in such cases usually appear five to ten days after the onset of the rash, with recovery occurring in most within a week or so. An acute cerebellar syndrome may complicate infectious mononucleosis (Bergen and Grossman, Dowling and Van Slyck, Lascelles et al.) and also has occurred in association with *Mycoplasma pneumoniae* infections (Steele et al.). Acute cerebellar ataxia in rare cases can be provoked by Epstein-Barr virus infection with few or no physical signs typical of infectious mononucleosis (Cleary et al.). Viruses isolated from patients with acute ataxic syndromes have included the poliovirus (Berglund et al., Mendez-Cashion et al.), ECHO virus type 9 (McAllister et al.), Coxsackie B (Berg and Jelke), and adenovirus (Sutton et al.).

Differential Diagnosis

Differential diagnosis in the child with acute onset of ataxia includes a number of conditions, some of which are benign and transient, others being serious disorders with a progressive course, while still others prove to be an intermittently recurring illness, often with an underlying metabolic defect. A particular problem concerning differential diagnosis relates to the degree of certainty one has that an illness with an alleged acute onset did, in fact, begin abruptly. The date symptoms first begin and when they are first noticed can be entirely different, a matter which sometimes results in misleading information obtained in the history. This is especially a problem in dealing with gait disorders in younger children who are preverbal and, thus, cannot describe their own observations.

An acute ataxic syndrome can result from drug or alcohol ingestion by young children but creates diagnostic problems primarily when the ingestion was not observed or recognized by a parent or guardian. Other signs of intoxication are usually quite evident. Phenytoin, barbiturates, and other sedatives are the usual offenders in such children. Conversion reactions in childhood can emerge in the form of a gait abnormality resembling ataxia but generally are seen in an older age group compared to the usual age in which post-viral acute cerebellar ataxia of childhood occurs. Head trauma, otherwise uncomplicated, is occasionally followed by ataxic signs for hours or a day or so, and also is a diagnostic dilemma when the traumatic event was not recognized or reported. Acute ataxia is a cardinal sign in the child with a traumatic posterior fossa subdural hematoma but history of injury is nearly always available and increased pressure signs develop quickly. Furthermore, subdural hemorrhage in the posterior fossa is exceedingly uncommon in the age group in which acute cerebellar ataxia of childhood is most common. Acute cerebellar hemorrhage is not common in children but is usually associated with sudden onset of gait ataxia. The child with this lesion rapidly becomes lethargic secondary to obstructive hydrocephalus, and has other signs, including nystagmus, vomiting, and neck stiffness, which signal its presence. Posterior fossa tumors in children are accompanied by a more chronic history than is the case with acute cerebellar ataxia but occasional exceptions are encountered. Problems in differential diagnosis can arise in the young child with a brain stem glioma because of the usual absence of increased intracranial pressure with this lesion. The customary presence of cranial nerve palsies and the progressively worsening course lead to diagnostic studies, which eventually clarify the diagnosis.

On rare occasions, ataxia of gait is the presenting manifestation of acute bacterial meningitis (Schwartz, Yabek) although other more characteristic signs develop soon thereafter. Acute onset of truncal ataxia also is sometimes encountered with otitis media. Most affected children experience vertigo, especially with movement of the head, suggesting that abnormalities of equilibrium are probably secondary to labyrinthine dysfunction precipitated by the middle ear infection.

Of greater importance in differential diagnosis is the disorder referred to as benign paroxysmal vertigo of childhood (Basser, Koenigsberger et al.). The hallmark of this disorder is episodic vertigo believed to be due to recurrent dysfunction of the labyrinth or the vestibular division of the eighth nerve. Inability to walk or a wide-based, ataxic gait accompanies the vertiginous sensation and, thus, may be confused with the syndrome of acute cerebellar ataxia of childhood. Paroxysmal vertigo of childhood usually begins in children between one and four years of age and occurs in episodic and recurrent fashion. Attacks are of sudden onset, and are characterized by true vertigo lasting seconds to a few minutes without tinnitus or hearing loss. Pallor, sweating, or vomiting may occur during the episode and nystagmus sometimes is described by observant parents. Consciousness is not impaired and headaches are not associated with the attack, although some parents misinterpret the initial episodes as such. The intervals between vertiginous attacks vary widely. In some children they recur every four to six weeks, but in others they are separated by intervals of several months. Caloric testing between attacks usually reveals canal paresis, which may be unilateral or bilateral. Auditory function remains unimpaired. The illness is self-limited in most children, with recurrent episodes gradually becoming more infrequent until eventual disappearance by age six to eight years.

Disorders characterized by the acute onset of muscle weakness sometimes resemble ataxia of cerebellar origin but can usually be differentiated by a detailed neurologic examination. Tick paralysis manifested by the abrupt onset of ataxia has been reported (Lagos and Thies) and the Guillain-Barré syndrome, especially in younger children, may present with a gait abnormality due to weakness that simulates that due to cerebellar disease. A variation of this disorder, referred to as the Fisher syndrome, consists of ophthalmoplegia, ataxia, and areflexia of sudden onset (Bell et al.). The condition is rare in children but bears considerable similarity to post-viral acute cerebellar ataxia of childhood.

Another rare disorder considered in differential diagnosis is called myoclonic encephalopathy by some authors (Christoff, Kinsbourne) and infantile polymyoclonia by others (Dyken and Kolar). The onset is sudden, the course protracted, and the main features of the illness include chaotic ocular movements called opsoclonus and irregular bizarre jerky movements of the head, trunk, and extremities. Fever and vomiting often precede the other manifestations and intense irritability has been characteristic of most reported cases. In ambulatory children, the twitching and myoclonus-like body and limb movements disturb the gait, resembling ataxia of cerebellar origin. The presence of cerebrospinal fluid plasmocytosis in some cases (Dyken and Kolar) and a favorable response to corticosteroid therapy have suggested an immunologic basis for the disease. Most cases have been benign and self-limited but permanent sequelae have been described (Chiba et al.). In addition to its spontaneous occurrence, an illness with identical features has been observed in several children with thoracic or intra-abdominal neuroblastoma (Bray et al., Martin and Griffith, Moe and Nellhaus, Solomon and Chutorian), and in some reports has been confused with acute cerebellar ataxia of childhood (Klingman and Hodges). In certain instances, the myoclonic syndrome has preceded the first manifestations indicative of the presence of a neoplasm, and receded with subsequent removal of the lesion. Less often, an acute cerebellar syndrome without opsoclonus can represent the initial indication of a visceral neuroblastoma (Roberts and Freeman).

Acute but recurrent ataxic syndromes are known to occur in children with certain metabolic disorders, such as Hartnup disease. In this rare familial condition, a recurrent pellagra-like rash develops on exposed parts of the body with exposure to sunlight, in addition to severe but reversible cerebellar ataxia. These signs are accompanied by an aminoaciduria involving that group of monoaminomonocarboxylic acids that share a common renal tubular mechanism for reabsorption (Jepson). Acute, but intermittent, cerebellar ataxia in children has also been identified with hyperpyruvic acidemia and hyperalaninemia secondary to pyruvate decarboxylase deficiency (Lonsdale et al., Blass et al.). Ataxia, and often transient choreoathetosis, is precipitated by fever or excitement in these cases, and persists for several days before receding.

Other familial disorders with acute intermittent cerebellar ataxia have been the source of several publications but an underlying metabolic defect has not been identified (Farmer and Mustian, Hill and Sherman, White). The patients in the series of Farmer and Mustian experienced periodic attacks of ataxia in addition to vertigo and diplopia. After several years of recurrent episodes, the illness evolved into a slowly progressive disease resembling one of the spinocerebellar degenerations. Cases described by Hill and Sherman and those reported by White began at an earlier age, were characterized by attacks of ataxia, dysarthria, and nystagmus, and tended to abate as the affected patient advanced into adult life. Autosomal dominant inheritance was postulated and a metabolic disturbance could not be discovered. These rare metabolic disorders are set apart from the syndrome of post-viral acute cerebellar ataxia of childhood by their conspicuous tendency to recur and remit. With the initial or even the second episode, however, the possibility of differential diagnostic confusion is obvious.

Several progressive degenerative brain diseases of infancy and early childhood are associated with ataxia but other signs usually coexist. On occasion, however, the parents will observe gait incoordination in the early stages of the illness and report it to be of abrupt and recent onset. Until the pattern unfolds, such findings may be assumed to be due to acute cerebellar ataxia of childhood. Ataxia represents a prominent sign in some cases of metachromatic leukodystrophy and infantile neuroaxonal dystrophy. Ataxia may also be "suddenly noticed" in the initial stages of ataxia-telangiectasia, long before cutaneous or conjunctival telangiectasia will have developed.

Management

The emphasis on management of an acute ataxic syndrome in a child is primarily oriented toward diagnosis. When other conditions are excluded and the diagnosis of post-viral acute cerebellar ataxia is considered to be established, attempts are made to identify a provocative cause. Until recovery is evident, it is advisable to retain consideration of other possibilities to be certain that other unsuspected disorders are not overlooked.

There is no specific therapy for post-viral acute cerebellar ataxia of childhood. Management is conservative, including attention to fluid and electrolyte balance if vomiting has been frequent, and prevention of injury by proper precautions and appropriate padding of the sides of the bed.

REFERENCES

Basser, L. S.: Benign paroxysmal vertigo of childhood. A variety of vestibular neuronitis. Brain 87:141–152, 1964.

Batten, F. E.: Ataxia in childhood. Brain 28:484–505, 1905.

Bell, W., Van Allen, M., and Blackman, J.: Fisher syndrome in childhood. Dev. Med. Child. Neurol. 12:758–766, 1970.

Berg, R., and Jelke, H.: Acute cerebellar ataxia in children associated with Coxsackie viruses group B. Acta Paediat. Scand. 54:497–502, 1965.

Bergen, D., and Grossman, H.: Infectious mononucleosis as a cause of acute cerebellar ataxia of childhood. Dev. Med. Child. Neurol. 18:799–802, 1976.

Berglund, G., Mossberg, H. O., and Rydenstam, B.: Acute cerebellar ataxia of childhood. Acta Pediat. Scand. 44:254–262, 1955.

Blass, J. P., Kark, R. A. P., and Engel, W. K.: Clinical studies of a patient with pyruvate decarboxylase deficiency. Arch. Neurol. 25:449–460, 1971.

Blaw, M. E., and Sheehan, J. C.: Acute cerebellar syndrome of childhood. Neurology 8:538–542, 1958.

Bray, P. F., Ziter, F. A., Lahey, M. E., and Myers, G. G.: The coincidence of neuroblastoma and acute cerebellar encephalopathy. J. Pediat. 75:983–990, 1969.

Chiba, S., Motoya, H., Shinoda, M., and Nakao, T.: Myoclonic encephalopathy of infants: A report of two cases of 'dancing' eyes syndrome. Dev. Med. Child. Neurol. 12:767–771, 1970.

Christoff, N.: Myoclonic encephalopathy of infants. A report of two cases and observations on related disorders. Arch. Neurol. 21:229–234, 1969.

Cleary, T. G., Henle, W., and Pickering, L. K.: Acute cerebellar ataxia associated with Epstein-Barr virus infection. J.A.M.A. 243:148–149, 1980.

Dowling, M. D., Jr., and Van Slyck, E. J.: Cerebellar disease in infectious mononucleosis. Arch. Neurol. 15:270–274, 1966.

Dyken, P., and Kolar, O.: Dancing eyes, dancing feet: Infantile polymyoclonia. Brain 91:305–320, 1968.

Farmer, T. W., and Mustian, V. M.: Vestibulocerebellar ataxia. Arch. Neurol. 8:471–480, 1963.

Goldston, A. S., Millichap, J. G., and Miller, R. H.: Cerebellar ataxia with pre-eruptive varicella. Am. J. Dis. Child. 106:197–200, 1963.

Griffith, J. P. C.: Acute cerebrocerebellar ataxia. Am. J. Dis. Child. 20:82–88, 1920.

Hill, W., and Sherman, H.: Acute intermittent familial cerebellar ataxia. Arch. Neurol. 18:350–357, 1968.

Jepson, J. B.: Hartnup disease. In: Stanbury, J. B., Wyngaarden, J. B., and Fredrickson, D. S.: The Metabolic Basis of Inherited Disease. McGraw-Hill, New York, 1966, Pp. 1283–1299.

King, G., Schwarz, G. A., and Slade, H. W.: Acute cerebellar ataxia of childhood. Report of nine cases. Pediatrics 21:731–745, 1958.

Kinsbourne, M.: Myoclonic encephalopathy of infants. J. Neurol. Neurosurg. Psychiat. 25:271–276, 1962.

Klingman, W. O., and Hodges, R. G.: Acute ataxia of unknown origin in children. J. Pediat. 24:536–543, 1944.

Koenigsberger, M. R., Chutorian, A. M., Gold, A. P., and Schvey, M. S.: Benign paroxysmal vertigo of childhood. Neurology 20:1108–1113, 1970.

Lagos, J. C., and Thies, R. E.: Tick paralysis without muscle weakness. Arch. Neurol. 21:471–474, 1969.

Lascelles, R. G., Johnson, P. J., Longson, M., and Chiang, A.: Infectious mononucleosis presenting as acute cerebellar syndrome. Lancet 2:707–709, 1973.

Levin, S.: Cerebellar ataxia following chickenpox. Lancet 1:1222–1223, 1960.

Lonsdale, D., Faulkner, W. R., Price, J. W., and Smeby, R. R.: Intermittent cerebellar ataxia associated with hyperpyruvic acidemia, hyperalaninemia, and hyperalaninuria. Pediatrics 43:1025–1034, 1969.

Martin, E. S., and Griffith, J. F.: Myoclonic encephalopathy and neuroblastoma. Report of a case with apparent recovery. Am. J. Dis. Child. 122:257–258, 1971.

McAllister, R., Hummeler, K., and Coriell, L.: Acute cerebellar ataxia. Report of a case with isolation of type 9 ECHO virus from the cerebrospinal fluid. New Eng. J. Med. 261:1159–1162, 1959.

Mendez-Cashion, D., Sanchez-Longo, L. P., Valcarcel, M., and Rosen, L.: Acute cerebellar ataxia in children associated with infection by poliovirus 1. Pediatrics 29:808–815, 1962.

Moe, P. G., and Nellhaus, G.: Infantile polymyoclonia-opsoclonus syndrome and neural crest tumors. Neurology 20:756–764, 1970.

Roberts, K. B., and Freeman, J. M.: Cerebellar ataxia and "occult neuroblastoma" without opsoclonus. Pediatrics 56:464–465, 1975.

Schwartz, J. F.: Ataxia in bacterial meningitis. Neurology 22:1071–1074, 1972.

Solomon, G. E., and Chutorian, A. M.: Opsoclonus and occult neuroblastoma. New Eng. J. Med. 279:475–477, 1968.

Steele, J. C., Gladstone, R. M., Thanasophon, S., and Fleming, P. C.: Acute cerebellar ataxia and concomitant infection with Mycoplasma pneumoniae. J. Pediat. 80:467–469, 1972.

Sutton, R. N. P., Pullen, H. J. M., Blackledge, P., Brown, E. H., Sinclair, L., and Swift, P. N.: Adenovirus type 7; 1971–74. Lancet 2:987–991, 1976.

Weiss, S., and Carter, S.: Course and prognosis of acute cerebellar ataxia in children. Neurology 9:711–721, 1959.

White, J. C.: Familial periodic nystagmus, vertigo, and ataxia. Arch. Neurol. 20:276–280, 1969.

Yabek, S. M.: Meningococcal meningitis presenting as acute cerebellar ataxia. Pediatrics 52:718–720, 1973.

Chapter Twenty-Seven

VOGT-KOYANAGI-HARADA SYNDROME

This unusual and curious multisystem inflammatory disorder is characterized by ophthalmologic, neurologic, and dermatologic manifestations in variable degrees and severity. Bilateral uveitis, meningoencephalitis with cerebrospinal fluid lymphocytic pleocytosis, poliosis, vitiligo, alopecia, and vestibulo-auditory symptoms are the clinical manifestations of the disorder. In addition to the eponym above, the disease has also been designated as the uveomeningoencephalitic syndrome, emphasizing the sites of its most disabling aspects. Originally, the Vogt-Koyanagi syndrome and that described by Harada were considered to be separate entities but are now regarded to be variants of the same condition (Cowper). The Vogt-Koyanagi syndrome included acute anterior uveitis with alopecia and vitiligo, while the term Harada syndrome was used when the signs were those of a posterior uveitis, meningeal irritation, and CSF pleocytosis. Because of the frequent overlap of the clinical manifestations, the currently accepted term is Vogt-Koyanagi-Harada syndrome. The etiology remains speculative, with some favoring a viral cause while others consider it to be an autoimmune response to uveal pigment (Walsh and Hoyt). The Vogt-Koyanagi-Harada syndrome occurs primarily in young adults but has also been described in teen-age children (Johnson). It is more common in people of Oriental extraction than otherwise.

Clinical Manifestations

Ocular Symptoms and Signs. Ophthalmologic symptoms are occasionally the presenting manifestations of the disease or appear soon after the onset of symptoms and signs of meningeal irritation. Less often, cutaneous changes precede ocular involvement by weeks or even months. Photophobia, lacrimation, ocular pain, and visual blurring are usually the initial complaints, which result from a severe anterior and posterior uveitis that is abrupt in onset and generally is or becomes bilateral. Inflammatory involvement of the ciliary body, iris, and retina leads to rapid and occasionally total visual loss. Extensive formation of anterior synechiae often leads to glaucoma (Perry and Font). Other complications that may ensue include retinal detachment and cataracts.

Neurologic Symptoms and Signs. The neurologic aspects of the Vogt-Koyanagi-Harada syndrome are usually mild but in certain cases, the signs are those of severe brain or spinal cord involvement (Pattison). Neurologic signs of the disease are best described as variable from case to case, fluctuating over the course of weeks or months, and with possible involvement of the brain, spinal cord, cranial or peripheral nerves, and meninges (Riehl and Andrews). The most common pattern is for neurologic signs to precede or develop at approximately the same time that ocular signs are noted. Signs of meningeal irritation such as headache and neck stiffness lead the list and are often accompanied by malaise or lethargy. Less common is the occurrence of a rapidly progressive neurologic syndrome manifested by lethargy, confusion, hemiparesis, and papilledema. Spinal cord signs such as paraparesis and neurogenic bladder dysfunction may coexist with cerebral or meningeal signs or can be present in isolated fashion. Cranial nerve and peripheral nerve palsies in concert with the above manifestations tend to complicate localizing neurologic diagnosis unless the disseminated nature of the process is recognized. Tinnitus, episodic vertigo, and hearing loss also occur in various degrees and combinations.

Cerebrospinal fluid findings, like other aspects of the neurologic syndrome, will vary from time to time in the same patient. The CSF pressure is sometimes elevated and the protein content increased. The laboratory hallmark of the syndrome, however, is a lymphocytic pleocytosis with counts from a dozen up to 500 per cu. mm. Even this is not entirely constant, as certain patients with neurologic deficits have no cerebrospinal fluid abnormalities.

Relatively little is known of the neuropathology of this condition since few necropsies have been performed. Arachnoidal thickening with lymphocytic infiltration in meninges as well as in the brain has been described but detailed studies are lacking.

Dermatologic Symptoms and Signs. Poliosis, or the progressive whitening of hair and eyelashes, and vitiligo are usually noted soon after the onset of uveitis but remarkable exceptions in either direction have been described. Depigmentation of the eyebrows and eyelashes can be unilateral and may be associated with progressive iris depigmentation on the same side. The skin depigmentation tends to be splotchy and can remain fairly localized or become widespread. On the trunk, it is frequently bilaterally symmetrical with annoying dysesthesiae in the depigmented areas.

Course of the Disease. The ophthalmologic and neurologic features are characterized by fluctuations in regard to severity during the active stage of the disorder. After weeks or months, the inflammatory process gradually resolves and many patients then experience functional recovery. Reattachment of the retina may be followed by gradual recovery of vision unless precluded by the previous occurrence of cataracts or scarring of the entire globe. Such patients will be left with severe visual deficits or blindness. Resolution of neurologic dysfunction is expected in most, although exceptional patients are disabled by persisting long tract signs or cerebral deficits. Patches of hair loss eventually regrow and even the depigmented cutaneous lesions subsequently may return to their normal condition.

Diagnosis and Treatment

Diagnosis of the Vogt-Koyanagi-Harada syndrome is on the basis of clinical recognition of the presence of severe uveitis of acute onset associated with the characteristic neurologic symptoms and cutaneous lesions. Except for the cerebrospinal fluid pleocytosis, which is not diagnostically specific, there is no laboratory method available to confirm or exclude the diagnosis. Because of the frequent association of visual loss of abrupt onset plus fluctuating neurologic signs, multiple sclerosis is frequently misdiagnosed. Patients with increased intracranial pressure may be erroneously thought to have an intracranial mass lesion, perhaps leading to unnecessary diagnostic tests unless the widespread nature of the illness is recognized. Sarcoidosis and brucellosis are additional differential diagnostic considerations, as well as Behçet's syndrome, which some feel may be somehow related.

Corticosteroid therapy is recommended during the acute stage of the disease. The primary objective of steroid treatment is control of ocular inflammation, thereby preventing loss of vision. Because of the lengthy duration of the illness notable in most cases, progressive decline in steroid dosage and the use of an alternate day regimen would seem desirable.

REFERENCES

Cowper, A. R.: Harada's disease and Vogt-Koyanagi syndrome. Arch. Ophthal. 45:367–376, 1951.

Harada, Y.: Beitrag zur klinischen kenntnis von nichteiteriger choroiditis. Nippon Ganka Gakkai Zasshi 30:356–378, 1926.

Johnson, W. C.: Vogt-Koyanagi-Harada syndrome. Arch. Derm. 88:146–149, 1963.

Koyanagi, Y.: Dysakusis, alopecia und poliosis bei schwerer uveitis nicht traumatischen ursprungs. Klin. Mbl. Augenheilk 82:194–211, 1929.

Pattison, E. M.: Uveomeningoencephalitic syndrome (Vogt-Koyanagi-Harada). Arch. Neurol. 12:197–205, 1965.

Perry, H. D., and Font, R. L.: Clinical and histopathologic observations in severe Vogt-Koyanagi-Harada syndrome. Am. J. Ophthal. 83:242–254, 1977.

Riehl, J-L., and Andrews, J. M.: The uveomeningoencephalitic syndrome. Neurology 16:603–609, 1966.

Vogt, A.: Frühzeitiges ergrauen der zilien und bemerkungen über den sogenannten plötzlichen eintritt dieser veränderung. Klin. Mbl. Augenheilk 44:228–242, 1906.

Walsh, F. B., and Hoyt, W. F.: Clinical Neuro-ophthalmology, Volume 2. Williams and Wilkins Company, Baltimore, 1969.

Chapter Twenty-Eight

LEPROSY (HANSEN'S DISEASE)

Leprosy is perhaps the most common cause of neuropathy in the world today but is little regarded by physicians in this country because of its rare occurrence here. The disease is caused by the acid-fast bacillus *Mycobacterium leprae* and occurs endemically in parts of Mexico, Central and South America, Africa, and the Far East. It is also found in certain European countries and in portions of the Middle East. Leprosy continues to occur occasionally in certain states in the southern region of the United States as well as in Hawaii, and can be seen anywhere in immigrants from endemic zones (Rodriguez and Stevens 1978). The incubation period is usually stated to be one to five years but is probably considerably longer in many instances. It is generally believed that long and close contact with an infected patient is required for one to acquire the disease. It is also assumed that a genetic predisposition accounts for a higher incidence of leprosy in certain races.

Clinical Features

The current classification of leprosy into four types is that which was adopted at the Madrid Congress of 1953. These include the lepromatous type, the tuberculoid type, a dimorphous form, and an ill-defined form referred to as indeterminate. Ridley and Jopling, in 1966, expanded the classification by the addition of three borderline forms. The type of leprosy a given person acquires is determined to a large extent by the degree of the resistance of the host against *Mycobacterium leprae*.

Lepromatous leprosy is characterized by diffuse or local involvement of the skin, subcutaneous tissues, and mucous membranes, eventually associated with a slowly progressive symmetrical neuropathy. Cutaneous lesions are bilateral and often symmetrical, and consist of numerous macules, papules, and nodules, leading to diffuse thickening of soft tissues (Fig. 28–1). Macules are generally small with a smooth surface and are not an-

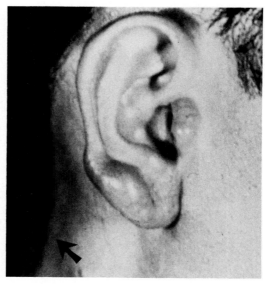

Figure 28–1. Lepromatous leprosy. Lepromatous nodules in the tragus and the pinna of the right ear. Note the enlarged great auricular nerve (arrow). (Courtesy of Dr. Richard Caplan, Iowa City, Iowa.)

esthetic, as occurs in the tuberculoid form. Thickening of skin, loss of eyebrows, and necrosis of nasal cartilaginous structures lead to the facial appearance referred to as the "leonine" facies. Late features of the illness include saddle-nose deformity, ocular involvement with keratitis or iritis, and testicular atrophy in the male (Ridley and Jopling). Histologically, the cellular infiltrate contains many foamy histiocytes abundant with acid-fast organisms but with few if any small lymphocytes. The low resistance to the infection in lepromatous leprosy is evidenced by the negative lepromin skin test, the ease of demonstration of *Mycobacterium leprae* in biopsy of the lesions, and the minimal inflammatory response in the form of lymphocytic infiltration found on microscopic examination of the lesions.

It has been proposed that the susceptibility to develop lepromatous leprosy is on a "constitutional" basis, which may represent a familial characteristic. This concept is an outgrowth of findings by certain investigators that patients with lepromatous leprosy have innate defects in cell-mediated immunity against *Mycobacterium leprae,* allowing active proliferation of the bacillus within tissues with minimal inflammatory reaction to its presence (Turk). Other studies found such patients to have a nonspecific disturbance in other aspects of cell-mediated immunity, including an inability to develop contact sensitivity to dinitrochlorobenzene (Waldorf et al.) and a disturbance in skin homograft rejection (Han et al.). Lymph nodes from patients with lepromatous leprosy have been found in some investigations to be qualitatively similar to those seen in children with congenital thymic dysplasia, suggesting an inherent defect in thymic control of their cell-mediated immune mechanisms (Turk and Waters). Still other workers have reported an increased number of circulating B lymphocytes in the lepromatous form of the disease, postulated to be due to overcompensatory production in the presence of a deficiency of T cells (Gajl-Peczalska et al.).

Among those who identified various types of impairment of cell-mediated immune reactions in lepromatous leprosy, there has been dispute regarding the explanation for their presence. Some have regarded such immune defects to be a predisposing cause for this type of leprosy while others have postulated that such disturbances are the end result of the infectious illness. With equally extensive investigative studies, other workers have shown that patients with lepromatous leprosy have normal immune reactions to antigens other than lepromin, and insignificant changes in the B and T cell circulating lymphocyte populations (Convit et al., Rea et al., Ulrich et al.). The literature compiled in the past two decades, thus, contains many conflicting results that pertain to studies of the immune response in patients with lepromatous leprosy. The single constant defect agreed upon by all is the absence of reaction to lepromin in patients with this form of the disease.

Glomerulonephritis is a well-known feature of lepromatous leprosy (Date et al.) although its pathogenesis is unclear. In at least some cases, it is assumed to represent an immune complex disease associated with low serum complement levels (Drutz and Gutman) and immunoglobulin deposits in glomeruli (Iverson et al.). Long-standing lepromatous leprosy may be complicated by the development of secondary amyloidosis.

Tuberculoid leprosy (previously called the neural or maculoanesthetic type) is the variety most common in children and is characterized by a single or small number of erythematous plaque-like cutaneous lesions which are rough, dry and hairless and are surrounded by slightly elevated margins (Fig. 28–2). They are hypesthetic or anesthetic to external stimulation. Unlike the skin lesions in the lepromatous form, those in tuberculoid leprosy are heavily infiltrated with small lymphocytes. Histiocytic macrophages are abundant but cannot usually be shown to harbor *Mycobacterium leprae*. Palpably thickened peripheral nerves, especially the greater auricular nerves and the large nerve trunks in the upper extremities, are also found in this condition. Peripheral nerve involvement results in an asymmetrical mixed neuropathy, with sensory loss as well as muscle weakness and wasting. In some instances, only one or two major nerve trunks are affected. The great majority of patients with tuberculoid leprosy have cutaneous lesions as well as peripheral neuropathy. On rare occasion, the disease can be manifested only by peripheral neuropathy in the absence of cutaneous disease (Jopling and Morgan-Hughes). Recognition of such cases depends upon the epidemiologic features of the illness, the presence of enlarged nerves on examination, and the characteristic histopathologic changes on biopsy of affected peripheral nerve tissues. The greater degree of resistance associated with this form of leprosy is indicated by the posi-

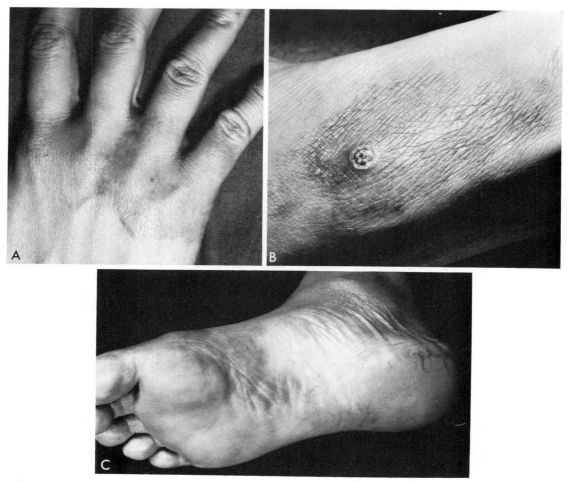

Figure 28–2.   Tuberculoid leprosy, cutaneous lesions. *A,* Thirty-three-year-old student from Thailand with an anesthetic, erythematous, scaly lesion with slightly raised margins of 3 months' duration. Diagnosis was established by biopsy of the lesion. *B,* Twenty-seven-year-old female from Thailand with a dry, scaly, erythematous lesion with slightly elevated borders located on the lateral surface of the forearm. The area was anesthetic and had been gradually enlarging for several months. The circular punctate lesion is the biopsy site from which the diagnosis was established. *C,* Anesthetic depigmented lesion on the medial surface of the right foot. (Courtesy of Dr. Richard Caplan, Iowa City, Iowa.)

tive lepromin skin test and the absence or sparseness of acid-fast bacilli on skin scrapings or biopsy of the lesions. Tuberculoid leprosy is more benign, more slowly progressive, and generally less disfiguring than the lepromatous form.

The dimorphous type of leprosy includes cases which are intermediate between the two polar forms, containing features peculiar to each. The degree of inflammatory response, the rate of progression, and the reaction to the lepromin skin test vary from case to case. Indeterminate leprosy is a type usually seen in the early stages of the illness, at which time the findings are atypical and do not resemble the clinical features of the more common types of leprosy. With the passage of time, the lesions eventually evolve toward either the lepromatous or the tuberculoid type.

In lepromatous leprosy, the white blood cell count is often somewhat elevated while in the tuberculoid type it is usually normal. Cryoglobulinemia and reactive serologic tests for syphilis are also sometimes found in the lepromatous form. Biopsy of cutaneous lesions, and sometimes of involved peripheral nerve, is valuable for diagnosis, especially in geographic regions where the disease is ordinarily considered uncommon. In some cases, *Mycobacterium leprae* can be demonstrated within bone marrow histiocytes by the use of Fite's stain (Lawrence and Schreiber).

The lepromin skin test is not a diagnostic test for the presence or absence of the disease but is one which has been used to denote resistance to the illness. It is performed by the intradermal injection of an autoclaved suspension of *Mycobacterium leprae* in human tissue. There is usually no reaction in patients with low resistance who have lepromatous leprosy, but in those with the tuberculoid form, the formation of an inflammatory nodule one to three weeks after injection, the so-called Mitsuda reaction, indicates relatively high resistance. It is assumed that this reaction is evidence of a high degree of cell-mediated immunity against the mycobacterial antigens. Thus, patients with tuberculoid leprosy have circulating sensitized lymphocytes that can activate macrophages which interact with *Mycobacterium leprae,* thereby accounting for the difficulty in finding organisms in stained tissue preparations. The lepromin test is often positive in persons in endemic zones who do not have leprosy, especially in those with positive tuberculin skin reactions.

Pathology and Pathogenesis

Clinical evidence of peripheral nerve involvement occurs in virtually all cases of leprosy, relatively early in the tuberculoid type and relatively late in the lepromatous variety (Fig. 28–3). In lepromatous leprosy, the classic pattern is a slowly progressive symmetrical sensory polyneuropathy which sometimes occurs with sensory dissociation similar to that with syringomyelia (Rosenberg and Lovelace). In other cases, all sensory modalities are affected. In the acute stages, the nerves are swollen and tender, especially at certain predisposed sites of involvement.

In a detailed study of the peripheral nerve pathology of four patients with lepromatous leprosy, Job and Desikan found a decided predilection for nerve involvement at specific sites. Predisposed areas include the ulnar nerve at the region of the medial epicondyle and at the wrist, the median nerve just proximal to the carpal tunnel, the radial nerve immediately above the elbow and at the wrist, the posterior tibial nerve and the common peroneal nerve at the flexor retinaculum, and the facial nerve as it crosses the zygomatic process of the maxilla. These areas, which reveal the greatest degree of swelling grossly and most marked changes histologically, are at points where the nerves become most superficial in subcutaneous tissues, compatible with the previously suggested concept that inflammation produced by *Mycobacterium leprae* might be a temperature-dependent phenomenon. Swelling of the nerves is secondary to edema and infiltration with bacillus-laden foamy macrophages, perineurial cells, and proliferating Schwann cells. The inflammatory reaction in the affected areas of peripheral nerve is generally minimal compared to the number of bacteria present. Demyelination is out of proportion to axonal degeneration for a period of time, but in the late stages of the illness, individual nerves are converted to thin, fibrous cords.

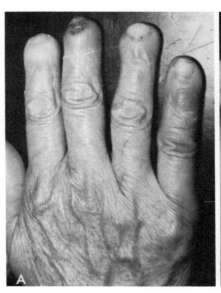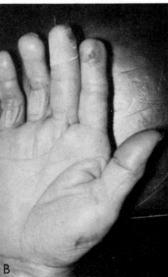

Figure 28–3. A and *B,* Leprosy with peripheral neuropathy leading to extensive soft-tissue damage due to repeated injury to the anesthetic finger tips. There is mild thenar atrophy.

In tuberculoid leprosy, individual peripheral nerves are attacked in asymmetrical fashion. The nerve histopathology includes multiple granulomata containing epithelioid cells and multinucleated giant cells, usually with an intense lymphocytic inflammatory reaction but in the absence of acid-fast bacilli. Myelin and axons are damaged and Schwann cells are severely damaged or even completely destroyed.

The Schwann cell is now believed to be of primary importance in the pathogenesis of the peripheral nerve involvement in leprosy. Clinical and experimental studies have shown multiplication of *Mycobacterium leprae* within Schwann cells in the early stages of the illness. Initial proliferation and swelling of Schwann cells is followed by eventual degenerative changes associated with myelin and axonal destruction (Job 1970, Dastur et al. 1972, Rees and Waters 1972).

Treatment

Leprosy is treated with one of the sulfone preparations (Avlosulfon, dapsone), drugs which are bacteriostatic and thus must be administered over the course of many years. Because sulfone can provoke an acute hemolytic reaction in persons with glucose-6-phosphate dehydrogenase deficiency, this deficiency should be excluded before therapy is begun. Sulfone therapy can dramatically worsen symptoms of leprosy in certain stages of the disease (Trautman 1965). Skin lesions may become acutely edematous and inflamed, peripheral nerve function can deteriorate, and erythema nodosum may develop in some cases. Erythema nodosum leprosum is an acute vasculitis affecting the skin and is sometimes associated with iridocyclitis, arthritis, or glomerulonephritis. Anti-mycobacterial antibodies interact with bacterial antigen circulating in excess as a result of chemotherapy. Antigen-antibody complexes are deposited in small blood vessels, resulting in skin lesions in a fashion resembling the Arthus reaction (Turk).

Some authors recommend discontinuation of the drug and the temporary administration of corticosteroids for acute severe reactions to sulfone therapy (Trautman). Others emphasize the importance of full-dose, continued treatment without interruptions for reactions because of the increased incidence of development of sulfone resistance in patients receiving low-dose or irregular therapy. If sulfone treatment is discontinued, when it is again started, the initial dosage should be reduced followed by gradual increments depending on patient tolerance. Thalidomide has been recommended for severe reactions manifested by erythema nodosum (Vargas 1971) but has the limitation of its known teratogenic properties when used during pregnancy. One of the main problems with treatment of leprosy in underdeveloped countries has been compliance with the therapeutic regimen. This can be alleviated to some degree by the development of a repository sulfone (dapsone) preparation which requires a single intramuscular injection every 70 to 80 days and has been effective in some patients with the disease (Peters et al.).

Sulfone-resistant cases have been described but are believed to be infrequent. This is a problem primarily in lepromatous leprosy, which is the type characterized by heavy infiltration of lesions with *Mycobacterium leprae*. Drug resistance is believed to arise from the presence of a few specific mutants in the bacterial population, and thus a large bacterial population is required for the development of resistance (Pearson et al.). Alternate drugs which have been recommended in sulfone-resistant cases include rifampin, sulfonamides, and clofazimine (Pearson et al. 1975, Wilkinson et al. 1972). Rifampin may prove to be of definite value in the treatment of leprosy since, unlike other available anti-leprosy drugs, it has bactericidal activity against *Mycobacterium leprae* (Rees et al. 1970). The disadvantage of rifampin is the high price of the drug, which, for this disease, must be given for lengthy periods of time.

BCG vaccination has been proposed as a possible preventive measure when given to lepromin-negative non-infected persons in endemic zones (Brown). Studies by Chaussinand in 1948 revealed that, to some extent, leprosy and tuberculosis are mutually antagonistic diseases. Convit et al. in Venezuela found that fewer persons vaccinated with BCG subsequently developed leprosy compared to an unvaccinated group. Other workers showed that BCG vaccine often converted lepromin-negative persons to positive reactors (Brown and Stone). Additional evidence supporting the possible value of BCG vaccine is the finding that vaccination interferes with the multiplication of *Mycobacterium leprae* in the experimentally infected mouse foot pad (Shepard). The full importance of this preventive method has not yet been documented but studies to this date seem consistently favorable.

REFERENCES

Brown, J. A. K., and Stone, M. M.: The depot lepromin test and B.C.G. vaccination. Leprosy Rev. 30:110, 1959.

Brown, R. E.: Prevention of leprosy. New ideas out of Africa. Clin. Pediat. 6:446–450, 1967.

Chaussinand, R.: Tuberculose et lepre, maladies antagoniques. Int. J. Leprosy 16:431, 1948.

Convit, J., Pinardi, M. E., and Rojas, F. A.: Some considerations regarding the immunology of leprosy. Int. J. Leprosy 39:556–564, 1971.

Dastur, D. K., Ramamchan, Y., and Shah, J. S.: Ultrastructure of lepromatous nerves. Neural pathogenesis in leprosy. Int. J. Leprosy 41:47–80, 1972.

Date, A., Thomas, A., Mathai, R., and Johny, K. V.: Glomerular pathology in leprosy. Am. J. Trop. Med. 26:266–272, 1977.

Drutz, D. J., and Gutman, R. A.: Renal manifestations of leprosy. Glomerulonephritis—a complication of erythema nodosum leprosum. Am. J. Trop. Med. 22:496–502, 1973.

Gajl-Peczalska, K. J., Lim, S. D., Jacobson, R. R., and Good, R. A.: B lymphocytes in lepromatous leprosy. New Eng. J. Med. 288:1033–1035, 1973.

Han, S. H., Weiser, R. S., and Kau, S. T.: Prolonged survival of skin allografts in leprosy patients. Int. J. Leprosy 39:1–6, 1971.

Iveson, J. M. I., McDougall, A. C., Leathem, A. J., and Harris, H. J.: Lepromatous leprosy presenting with polyarthritis, myositis, and immune-complex glomerulonephritis. Brit. Med. J. 3:619–621, 1975.

Job, C. K.: Mycobacterium leprae in nerve lesions in lepromatous leprosy: An electron-microscopic study. Arch. Path. 89:195–207, 1970.

Job, C. K., and Desikan, K. V.: Pathologic changes and their distribution in peripheral nerves in lepromatous leprosy. Int. J. Leprosy 36:257–270, 1968.

Jopling, W. H., and Morgan-Hughes, J. A.: Pure neural tuberculoid leprosy. Brit. Med. J. 2:799–800, 1965.

Lawrence, C., and Schreiber, A. J.: Leprosy's footprints in bone-marrow histiocytes. New Eng. J. Med. 300:834–835, 1979.

Madrid Congress. Classification. Technical resolutions. Int. J. Leprosy 21:504–516, 1953.

Pearson, J. M. H., Rees, R. J. W., and Waters, M. F. R.: Sulphone resistance in leprosy. Review of 100 proved clinical cases. Lancet 2:69–72, 1975.

Peters, J. H., Murray, J. F., Gordon, G. R., Levy, L.,

Russell, D. A., Scott, G. C., Vincin, D. R., and Shepard, C. C.: Acedapsone treatment of leprosy patients: Response versus drug disposition. Am. J. Trop. Med. 26:127–136, 1977.

Rea, T. H., Quismorio, F. P., Harding, B., Nies, K. M., DiSaia, P. J., Levan, N. E., and Friou, G. J.: Immunologic responses in patients with lepromatous leprosy. Arch. Dermatol. 112:791–800, 1976.

Rees, R. J. W., Pearson, J. M. H., and Waters, M. F. R.: Experimental and clinical studies on rifampicin in treatment of leprosy. Brit. Med. J. 1:89–92, 1970.

Rees, R. J. W., and Waters, M. F. R.: Recent trends in leprosy research. Brit. Med. Bull. 28:16–21, 1972.

Ridley, D. S., and Jopling, W. M.: Classification of leprosy according to immunity. A five-group system. Int. J. Leprosy 34:255–273, 1966.

Rodriguez, J. M., and Stevens, D. M.: Leprosy: A report of two cases in children. J. Pediat. 93:192–195, 1978.

Rosenberg, R. N., and Lovelace, R. E.: Mononeuritis multiplex in lepromatous leprosy. Arch. Neurol. 19:310–314, 1968.

Shepard, C. C.: Vaccination against experimental infection with Mycobacterium leprae. Am. J. Epidem. 81:150–163, 1965.

Trautman, J. R.: The management of leprosy and its complications. New Engl. J. Med. 273:756–758, 1965.

Turk, J. L.: Cell-mediated immunological process in leprosy. Bull. W.H.O. 41:779–792, 1969.

Turk, J. L., and Waters, M. F. R.: Immunological basis for depression of cellular immunity and the delayed allergic response in patients with lepromatous leprosy. Lancet 2:436, 1968.

Turk, J. L., and Waters, M. F. R.: Immunological significance of changes in lymph nodes across the leprosy spectrum. Clin. Exp. Immunol. 8:363–376, 1971.

Ulrich, M., deSalas, B., and Convit, J.: Lymphocyte transformation with phytomitogens in leprosy. Int. J. Leprosy 40:4–9, 1972.

Vargas, S.: Current treatment of the lepra reaction with thalidomide. Rev. Mex. Dermat. 15:142, 1971.

Waldorf, D. S., Sheagren, J. N., Trautman, J. R., and Block, J. B.: Impaired delayed hypersensitivity in patients with lepromatous leprosy. Lancet 2:773–776, 1966.

Wilkinson, F. F., Gago, J., and Santabaya, E.: Therapy of leprosy with rifampicin. Int. J. Leprosy 40:53–57, 1972.

Chapter Twenty-Nine

BEHÇET'S DISEASE

The symptoms, signs, and clinical pattern of this illness have been recognized as an entity since the report by Behçet in Istanbul in 1937. It is a chronic inflammatory disorder, usually characterized by exacerbations and remissions extending over many years, and with great variability in severity. Oral and genital ulcerations in addition to relapsing uveitis represent the clinical hallmarks of the disease, although it is now recognized that the illness is a systemic one in which many organs can be affected. A relatively small percentage of cases are complicated by neurologic disease, but in those that are, the illness becomes a life-threatening disorder. Although it is generally thought to be a rare condition, the incidence of Behçet's disease is probably greater than generally appreciated, with many cases escaping diagnosis. It is primarily a disease of young adults but can also occur in the elderly. There are a number of reports in which the first symptoms appeared in adolescent or teen-age youngsters (Buckley and Gills, Kalbian and Challis, Mir-Madjlessi and Farmer, Wadia and Williams). In one child, recurrent stomatitis had its onset at two years of age, and was eventually followed by neurologic complications at age 15 years (Mundy and Miller). Behçet's disease is believed to have a worldwide distribution but the majority of reports have come from the Mediterranean basin, the Middle East, and Japan (Chajek and Fainaru, Kawakita et al.). The disorder occurs in either sex but males are affected considerably more often than females.

The etiology of Behçet's disease remains unknown to the present date. Behçet proposed a viral etiology on the basis of the presence of inclusion bodies in smears of oral ulcers, a finding conspicuously absent in more recent studies. Sezer, and subsequently Evans et al., added impetus to the viral theory by reports of the isolation of a virus from affected tissues. Additional support for the viral etiology resulted from studies by Alm and Oberg in which cerebrospinal fluid from patients with Behçet's disease was injected into the spinal fluid of rabbits, producing encephalitis, uveitis, and other inflammatory signs. Despite these observations, many investigators have remained skeptical of a viral origin for this disease and most current authors place it in an autoimmune category. Supporting the immune theory is the commonly observed pathologic evidence of vasculitis (O'Duffy et al.) in addition to the demonstration of antibodies against human mucous membrane in a significant number of patients with Behçet's disease (Oshima et al.). Still another consideration is the possibility that Behçet's disease is the result of an immune deficiency which permits viral persistence.

Clinical Manifestations

Recurrent oral and genital ulcerative lesions are by far the most common initial manifestations of Behçet's disease (Fig. 29–1), although ocular involvement is the customary complaint for which the patient seeks medical attention. The oral ulcerations are recurrent and persist for several days to weeks before healing occurs. Attacks three or four times per year are customary and frequently are present simultaneously with recurrent attacks of genital ulcerations. The oral ulcers may be single or multiple, measure up to one centi-

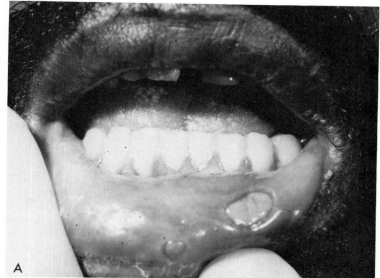

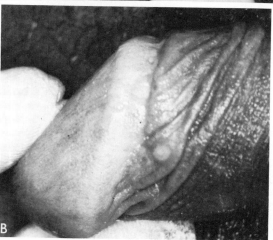

Figure 29–1. Behçet's disease. *A,* Characteristic ulcerative lesion on the buccal mucosa. Such lesions may be single or multiple, persist for days or weeks and recur periodically, and are usually intensely painful. *B,* Penile ulcerative lesion in the same patient. (Courtesy of Dr. Franklin Kozin, Milwaukee, Wisconsin; Neurology, 27:1148–1152, 1977.)

meter in diameter, and usually exhibit a central, yellow necrotic base surrounded by an inflamed border. The ulcers can be on the lip or tongue only or may be widely distributed over the mucosa of the cheek, palate, the base of the tongue, or the gums. They are associated with intense local pain, sometimes sufficient to result in weight loss from diminished food intake. Systemic signs including low-grade fever and malaise may also be present during the exacerbations. The genital ulcerations are similar in appearance to those of the oral mucosa and also cause local discomfort. They generally cause more discomfort in men and less in women, and are usually less painful than those of the oral mucosa. Frequent locations are the glans penis or the scrotum in the male, or the vulva, labia, or vagina of the female.

Even after the repetitive occurrence of crops of oral and genital ulcerative lesions over the course of months or years, the diagnosis of Behçet's disease is not usually suspected until the eventual development of ocular inflammation. Prior to this time, the mucosal ulcers are erroneously attributed to a herpetic etiology, to some form of allergic response, or to a dietary indiscretion. The typical ocular lesion is an inflammatory iritis with hypopyon, but other types include retinal vessel occlusions, optic neuritis, conjunctivitis, and papilledema secondary to increased intracranial pressure. Complications of the various types of ophthalmologic involvement occasionally lead to severe compromise of vision because of cataracts, glaucoma, retinal detachment, or optic atrophy. Enucleation is required in some instances when damage to the eye is extensive (Fenton and Easom). The various inflammatory reactions may be either unilateral or bilateral, and, like other aspects of the illness, tend to remit and relapse. Because of the diverse ways in which the eye can be affected, the complaints of the patient referable to ocular involvement are variable. Since uveitis is the most characteristic lesion, ocular pain, photophobia, lacrimation, conjunctival injection, and blurred vision are the customary symptoms.

Additional manifestations of Behçet's disease are variable from patient to patient and are much less frequent than those already mentioned. Cutaneous eruptions of different types have been described, the best known being recurrent erythema nodosum, which is usually confined to the lower extremities. Indolent cutaneous ulcerations as well as acneiform and pustular lesions may also occur. Recurrent thrombophlebitis is bothersome to some patients, as is relapsing arthralgia. Thrombophlebitis can involve superficial or deep veins in the extremities, or can lead to obstruction of the superior or inferior vena cava, causing hepatic enlargement or profound edema of the extremities (Chajek and Fainaru, Kawakita et al.). Hepatic vein thrombosis with the Budd-Chiari syndrome has also been described (Kawakita et al., Wolf et al. 1977). Gastrointestinal manifestations occasionally develop several years after the onset of the oral and genital ulcerations and, in most cases, resemble either ulcerative colitis or regional enteritis (Mir-Madjlessi and Farmer). Unusual to rare manifestations of Behçet's disease include myocarditis and pericarditis (Kansu et al., Scarlett et al.), and necrotizing glomerulonephritis (Kansu et al.).

The clinical course of Behçet's disease is quite variable, regarding both the frequency with which symptoms recur and the eventual outcome. The illness may persist in remitting and relapsing fashion for 10 to 20 years and then abate spontaneously. Some will have no sequelae while others are left with severe visual deficits. Those with neurologic involvement experience the most severe impact from the disease, regarding both sequelae and mortality. If death results from Behçet's disease, it is usually because of neurologic involvement. Death has occurred secondary to *Pneumocystis carinii* pneumonia (Wolf et al. 1977) and cytomegalovirus pneumonia (Kansu et al.) in patients treated with corticosteroid or immunosuppressive therapy.

Laboratory examinations are usually of little specific diagnostic help except in a negative fashion. The erythrocyte sedimentation rate is elevated during exacerbations but reverts to normal when the process becomes quiescent. Likewise, serum alpha-2-globulin and gamma globulin are increased during the active stages of the illness but are normal during remissions (Chajek and Fainaru). Anticytoplasmic antibodies can be demonstrated by immunofluorescence in some (O'Duffy et al.) but can be done only in research laboratories. Cerebrospinal fluid abnormalities are usually present in patients with neurologic complications.

Neurologic Involvement

The incidence of central nervous system involvement in patients with Behçet's disease has been estimated to be in the range of 10 to 30 percent of cases (Oshima et al., Wolf et al. 1965). Once neurologic signs appear, the prognosis of the illness is altered from a disorder that is intermittently troublesome or even temporarily disabling to one that is potentially life-threatening. Schotland et al. reviewed 37 previously described cases in which the brain was afflicted and found the mortality rate in this group to be 47 percent, a figure higher than in many other reports. Two-thirds of the deaths had occurred within one year after the onset of neurologic signs.

In the great majority of cases, the initial oral, genital, or ocular signs of Behçet's disease occur from several weeks to more than 20 years before neurologic dysfunction becomes evident. The 22-year-old man reported by Strouth and Dyken was a remarkable exception to the more customary evolution of the illness, in that nystagmus, ataxia, long tract signs, and cerebrospinal fluid pleocytosis were the presenting features of the illness. The subsequent development of recurrent uveitis and cutaneous ulcerative lesions led to the correct diagnosis. The same is true of two adult cases described by Kozin et al. in which neurologic signs antedated more typical lesions of Behçet's disease by several months. In view of the usual delayed appearance of neurologic signs for months or even years after the beginning of the disorder, it can be assumed that neurologic involvement in children due to Behçet's disease must be decidedly uncommon.

There is no one common pattern that represents the presenting neurologic symptoms of Behçet's disease or characterizes the subsequent clinical course. The initial neurologic signs are usually abrupt in onset and characterized by a fluctuating course, but in some the onset is gradual and followed by progressive deterioration. Attempts have been made to classify the neurologic features into three types, including a brain stem syndrome, a relapsing meningoencephalitis, and a progressive confusional syndrome highlighted by dementia (Pallis and Fudge). Certain cases fall predominantly into one or the other of these patterns but a blending of different aspects of each pattern in a given patient is more common. In addition to the three types mentioned above, some patients have an increased intracranial pressure syndrome with vomiting, headaches, and papilledema but without localized neurologic signs which, thus, resembles pseudotumor cerebri (Kalbian and Challis, Kawakita et al.). Papilledema secondary to intracranial hypertension can be the result of intracranial venous thrombosis (Masheter), and it is possible that some degree of compromise of intracranial venous drainage is the most common explanation for cases reported with cerebral swelling without localizing neurologic signs. Peripheral neuropathy has been described with Behçet's disease but is believed to be very unusual (O'Duffy et al.).

The varied ways in which the nervous system is affected in Behçet's disease make it difficult to outline the clinical features or the natural history except to say that the illness is a chronic one, that there is a predilection for brain stem involvement, and that meningeal signs are likely to occur sooner or later during the evolution of the illness. In some patients, the onset of neurologic disease is manifested by the "stroke-like" occurrence of a hemiparesis with dysphasia or dysarthria, perhaps associated with acute unilateral visual loss or mental confusion. The signs may gradually recede, later to be followed by recurrence of weakness or complicated by headache and neck rigidity. Of the patients with nervous system involvement reported by O'Duffy and Goldstein, the most common initial neurologic manifestation was aseptic meningitis with fever, meningeal signs, and cells in the CSF. Spastic paraparesis of either sudden or insidious onset represents the mode of onset in still others (Whitty). Regardless of the pattern that is followed, motor deficits are more outstanding than sensory abnormalities, and signs of disseminated

brain disease eventually become apparent. Recurrent convulsions have been the first described neurologic event in certain cases, followed by evidence of widespread cerebral and brain stem pathology (McMenemey and Lawrence). A slow but progressive dementing syndrome characterizes a small percentage of patients with Behçet's disease. Neurologic signs of many types accompany the deteriorating state, including tremor, rigidity, bulbar palsy, and more specific localizing abnormalities. Another common mode of onset is with brain stem signs, acutely or subacutely, resulting in extraocular muscle palsies, nystagmus, diplopia, ataxia, hyperreflexia, and extensor toe signs. Gradual deterioration sometimes follows or improvement may be noted weeks later only to be replaced by recurrence of similar or even remarkably different clinical manifestations. As the neurologic illness progresses, either in a steadily worsening fashion or punctuated by periods of improvement followed by relapse, headache and meningeal signs eventually enter the picture in most, if not present early in the course.

The neurologic complications of Behçet's disease are accompanied by cerebrospinal fluid abnormalities in the majority of cases, but these also fluctuate from time to time. A cellular response in the CSF is the most common finding. Among patients with neurologic signs reviewed by Schotland and colleagues, 81 percent had a cerebrospinal fluid pleocytosis. Both lymphocytes and polymorphonuclear leukocytes are observed, usually numbering between 10 and 200 cells per cu. mm. but considerably higher in some cases. The glucose content is consistently normal but the protein level is generally raised to between 50 and 150 mg. per 100 ml. When brain swelling is present, the CSF pressure is elevated, but this has been the exception in recorded cases rather than the rule.

Knowledge of the neuropathology of Behçet's disease complicated by neurologic involvement is based on relatively few examinations (McMenemey and Lawrence, Rubinstein and Urich, Strouth and Dyken) but the findings have been remarkably consistent in the available descriptions. A diffuse, low-grade meningoencephalitis has been the characteristic observation in virtually all the reports. There is meningeal thickening associated with sparse mononuclear infiltration, in addition to perivascular lymphocytic cuffing within the brain. Considerable gliosis occurs in the cortex and subependymal regions in a widespread fashion but with relatively little morphologic alteration of nerve cells. Focal cerebral lesions were emphasized by Rubinstein and Urich as the most characteristic feature and consist of small, discrete areas of necrosis with subtotal or total loss of all tissue elements, accumulation of microglial phagocytes, and eventual glial scarring. These foci can be observed scattered indiscriminately through the cortex and white matter as well as within the deep nuclear structures and the brain stem. Similar necrotic foci, especially at the junction of the cerebral cortex and white matter, were found by Kawakita et al., in addition to angiitis affecting small and medium-sized arteries and veins in the same regions. Rubinstein and Urich also pointed out the usual sparing of sensory pathways, an observation that correlates with the relative lack of clinical sensory abnormalities in most reported cases.

Diagnosis and Management

Consideration of the diagnosis of Behçet's disease is not common during the stage of recurrent oral and genital ulcers but becomes possible when ocular inflammatory lesions or neurologic dysfunction is engrafted upon the previous events. It is apparent, therefore, that if the patient is first seen because of signs of cerebral or brain stem disease, establishment of the diagnosis is dependent on eliciting the past history of periodic oral and genital ulcerative lesions with or without episodes of uveitis. Such information may not become available unless specifically searched for when the history is obtained. The multiplicity of possible neurologic signs plus the cerebrospinal fluid abnormalities may raise suspicion of either tuberculous meningitis or cryptococcal meningoencephalitis. The persistently normal CSF glucose content in Behçet's disease is one of the more important differentiating features. Sarcoidosis with intracranial involvement can also resemble Behçet's disease, especially since iritis and elevated erythrocyte sedimentation rate are common to both. Multiple sclerosis is an additional consideration in certain patients because of the relapsing nature of the neurologic signs as well as the disseminated distribution of the cerebral and brain stem process. When the onset is sudden with signs suggestive of focal cerebral disease, a cerebral vascular occlusive episode or brain abscess may initially be suspected, or a vascular disorder such as systemic lupus erythematosus might be entertained. In patients with a gradual, progressive dementing syndrome, one of the many presenile dementias is a possible consideration.

Treatment of the disease is controversial, a point made readily evident by the conflicting results in past reports. Topical corticosteroids applied to the oral ulcerative lesions have provided symptomatic relief for some, but oral ulcers have developed and progressed during the course of systemic corticosteroid therapy in others. Ocular inflammation may be diminished by topical application of corticosteroids but does not necessarily prevent severe ocular damage. The effect of corticosteroids on the neurologic aspects of the disease are likewise variable and unpredictable. Certain patients have developed neurologic abnormalities while on therapy whereas others have noted considerable suppression of activity of the illness from corticosteroid treatment (O'Duffy and Goldstein, Wadia and Williams, Wolf et al.). More recently, immunosuppressive therapy with cyclophosphamide, chlorambucil, or azathioprine either alone or in conjunction with corticosteroids has received consideration (Buckley and Gills, Mamo, Tricoulis). Transfer factor has been used in a limited number of patients with Behçet's disease with some favorable responses in the alleviation of mucosal or articular symptoms but with little information to date about its effectiveness for ocular or neurologic lesions (Kozin et al., Wolf et al. 1977). Studies by Abdou et al. have supported the consideration of the use of transfer factor or levamisole as a means of enhancing the T cell system which is essential to host immunocompetence. Although proof of benefit of the various therapeutic methods described above is not yet available, when neurologic involvement complicates Behçet's disease, the seriousness of the condition warrants aggressive treatment measures.

REFERENCES

Abdou, N. I., Schumacher, H. R., Colman, R. W., Sagawa, A., Hebert, J., Pascual, E., Carroll, E. T., Miller, M., South, M. A., and Abdou, N. L.: Behçet's disease: Possible role of secretory component deficiency, synovial inclusions, and fibrinolytic abnormality in the various manifestations of the disease. J. Lab. Clin. Med. 91:409–422, 1978.

Alm, L., and Oberg, L.: Djurforsök vid s. k. Behçet's syndrom. Nord. Med. 25:603–604, 1945.

Behçet, H.: Üeber die rezidivierende, aphthöse durch ein virus verursachte geschwüre am mund, am auge und an den genitalien. Dermat. Wschnschr. 105:1152–1157, 1937.

Buckley, C. E., and Gills, J. P., Jr.: Cyclophosphamide therapy of Behçet's disease. J. Allergy 43:273–283, 1969.

Chajek, T., and Fainaru, M.: Behçet's disease. Report of 41 cases and a review of the literature. Medicine 54:179–196, 1975.

Evans, A. D., Pallis, C. A., and Spillane, J. D.: Involvement of the nervous system in Behçet's syndrome: Report of three cases and isolation of virus. Lancet 2:349–353, 1957.

Fenton, R. H., and Easom, H. A.: Behçet's syndrome. A histopathologic study of the eye. Arch. Ophthal. 72:71–81, 1964.

Kalbian, V. V., and Challis, M. T.: Behçet's disease. Report of twelve cases with three manifesting as papilledema. Am. J. Med. 49:823–829, 1970.

Kansu, E., Deglin, S., Cantor, R. I., Burke, J. F., Jr., Cho, S. Y., and Cathart, R. T.: The expanding syndrome of Behçet syndrome. A case with renal involvement. J.A.M.A. 237:1855–1856, 1977.

Kawakita, H., Nishimura, M., Satoh, Y., and Shibata, N.: Neurological aspects of Behçet's disease. A case report and clinico-pathological review of the literature in Japan. J. Neurol. Sci. 5:417–439, 1967.

Kozin, F., Haughton, V., and Bernhard, G. C.: Neuro-Behçet disease. Two cases and neuroradiologic findings. Neurology 27:1148–1152, 1977.

Mamo, J. G.: Treatment of Behçet's disease with chlorambucil. A follow-up report. Arch. Ophthal. 94:580–583, 1976.

Masheter, H. C.: Behçet's syndrome complicated by intracranial thrombophlebitis. Proc. Roy. Soc. Med. 52:1039, 1959.

McMenemey, W. H., and Lawrence, B. J.: Encephalomyelopathy in Behçet's disease. Report of necropsy findings in two cases. Lancet 2:353–358, 1957.

Mir-Madjlessi, S. H., and Farmer, R. G.: Behçet's syndrome, Crohn's disease and toxic megacolon. Cleveland Clin. Quart. 39:49–55, 1972.

Mundy, T. M., and Miller, J. J., III: Behçet's disease presenting as chronic aphthous stomatitis in a child. Pediatrics 62:205–208, 1978.

O'Duffy, J. D., Carney, J. A., and Deodhar, S.: Behçet's disease. Report of 10 cases, 3 with new manifestations. Ann. Intern. Med. 75:561–570, 1971.

O'Duffy, J. D., and Goldstein, N. P.: Neurologic involvement in seven patients with Behçet's disease. Am. J. Med. 61:170–178, 1976.

Oshima, Y., Shimizu, T., Yokohari, R., Matsumoto, T., Kano, K., Kagami, T., and Nagaya, H.: Clinical studies on Behçet's syndrome. Ann. Rheum. Dis. 22:36–45, 1963.

Pallis, C. A., and Fudge, B. J.: Neurological complications of Behçet's syndrome. Arch. Neurol. Psychiat. 75:1–14, 1956.

Rubinstein, L. J., and Urich, H.: Meningo-encephalitis of Behçet's disease: Case report with pathological findings. Brain 86:151–160, 1963.

Scarlett, J. A., Kistner, M. L., and Yang, L. C.: Behçet's syndrome. Report of a case associated with pericardial effusion and cryoglobulinemia treated with indomethacin. Am. J. Med. 66:146–148, 1979.

Schotland, D. L., Wolf, S. M., White, H. H., and Dubin, H. V.: Neurologic aspects of Behçet's disease. Case report and review of the literature. Am. J. Med. 34:544–553, 1963.

Sezer, F. N.: Isolation of a virus as cause of Behçet's disease. Am. J. Ophthal. 36:301–315, 1953.

Strouth, J. C., and Dyken, M.: Encephalopathy of Behçet's disease. Report of a case. Neurology 14:794–805, 1964.

Tricoulis, D.: Treatment of Behçet's disease with chlorambucil. Brit. J. Ophthal. 60:55–57, 1976.

Wadia, N., and Williams, E.: Behçet's syndrome with neurological complications. Brain 80:59–71, 1957.

Whitty, C. W. M.: Neurologic implications of Behçet's syndrome. Neurology 8:369–373, 1958.

Wolf, R. E., Fudenberg, H., Welch, T. M., Spitler, L. E., and Ziff, M.: Treatment of Behçet's syndrome with transfer factor. J.A.M.A. 238:869–871, 1977.

Wolf, S. M., Schotland, D. L., and Phillips, L. L.: Involvement of nervous system in Behçet's syndrome. Arch. Neurol. 12:315–325, 1965.

Chapter Thirty

"FEBRILE" SEIZURES

A convulsion precipitated by a febrile illness in the absence of meningitis or encephalitis is one of the commonest neurologic disorders of infants and young children. Practitioners widely recognize the ease with which children less than three or four years of age will convulse when febrile and refer to this event as a "febrile" seizure. Although the concept is one of common knowledge, the significance of such convulsions, their relationship to epilepsy, and their management have been subjects of controversy and disagreement. In part, the confusion that prevails is the consequence of studies in which statistics, sequelae, and results of treatment have been described but without sufficient clarification of the definition of "febrile" seizures.

Convulsions in the febrile child may be the result of one of several conditions. The most common explanation is on the basis of what is customarily known as a simple "febrile" seizure, criteria for which are elaborated upon below. Secondly, fever, like emotional upsets, excitement, or even minor head trauma, may precipitate a seizure in the child known to have spontaneous, recurrent convulsions, that is, the child with epilepsy. Seizures in a child with a febrile illness may also be caused by a primary neurologic infection (meningitis, encephalitis, or abscess) or may result from a neurologic complication of the infection, such as cerebral vasculitis with ischemic infarction. Finally, convulsions can be secondary to an identifiable complication of either the infectious illness or its treatment, including hypoglycemia, hypernatremia, or hyponatremia. Many cases will fall rather clearly into one or another of these categories, but some will have characteristics sufficiently atypical that one cannot be sure of the underlying cause, at least without additional studies or prolonged follow-up assessment.

The Concept of "Febrile" Seizures

Most authors set apart a "febrile" seizure from other paroxysmal cerebral disorders in children and categorize it as a phenomenon that is age-related, not secondary to underlying neurologic disease, and provoked by fever rather than some other primary effect of the infectious illness. It is estimated that 2 to 3 percent of children will experience such "febrile" convulsions in their first five years of life (Lennox, Millichap) and that boys are more likely to experience "febrile" seizures than girls in a ratio of between 1.4 and 1.6 to 1. A definition of "febrile" seizures includes features consistent with most examples but with the recognition that variations do exist and occasional exceptions to the rule are to be expected. They are usually brief seizures, not more than a few minutes in duration, are generalized rather than focal, and occur in the absence of a neurologic infection or metabolic abnormalities which could account for their precipitation. They occur in association with a febrile illness but especially soon after rapid temperature elevation, and with an interictal electroencephalogram that does not show epileptogenic activity. Children six months to four years of age are susceptible and only rarely are "febrile" seizures documented in children beyond age five years. The second year of life is the most common time for their occurrence, with the mean age of onset being 18 months (Friderichsen and Melchior).

Fishman (1979) has divided "febrile" seizures into *simple* and *complex* types with *simple* "febrile" seizures having characteristics described immediately above. *Complex* "febrile" seizures are those that occur in young children with fever, are of longer duration, have focal features or postictal focal weakness, and may occur in series with a single febrile illness. He correctly points out that combining the two types and assuming that they have the same significance may result in a distorted concept of the eventual prognosis.

While the above serve as criteria that are consistent with the diagnosis of a simple "febrile" seizure, the pattern described by Fishman as a *complex* "febrile" seizure is associated with an increased risk of subsequent recurrences or raises suspicion about the possibility of underlying cerebral dysfunction which might later be manifested in the form of afebrile seizures, learning disabilities, or other neurologic deficits. A persistent and prolonged convulsion, for example, one lasting 30 minutes or more, is in some instances due to pre-existent cerebral dysfunction. A convulsion that has definite focal implications, and especially if followed by significant unilateral postictal paralysis, is more likely an indication of pre-existent organic brain disease or an acquired disease with a direct cerebral complication of a systemic infection. One disorder of this type in which a febrile illness is associated with abrupt onset of convulsions followed by persistent hemiparesis is referred to as "acute hemiplegia of infancy" and, in some cases, is the result of a cerebral vascular occlusive lesion.

Seizures in the febrile infant under three months of age can rarely be placed in the "febrile" category and are an urgent indication for cerebrospinal fluid examination because of the possibility of a primary neurologic infection. One should also accept the diagnosis of "febrile" seizures with reluctance when a child with a diagnosis of cerebral palsy or another form of significant organic brain disease develops seizures in association with an acquired febrile illness. The reduced seizure threshold in such children is usually secondary to the underlying brain disease and will eventually be manifested by afebrile convulsions in many.

Finally, there is a need for reasonable documentation of a febrile response at the time of the occurrence of a seizure if it is to be placed in the "febrile" category. A convulsion that occurs when the child "felt a little warm," or "probably had an ear infection" may or may not have been secondary to fever but should not be accepted as such without additional confirmation of a febrile illness. Furthermore, a certain degree of temperature elevation, as well as leukocytosis, can result *from* vigorous convulsive activity, adding further difficulty to interpretation in some cases.

"Febrile" convulsions in children may complicate virtually any type of febrile illness. Both the degree of temperature elevation and the rate of rise appear to be important factors in the precipitation of seizures of this type. In general, if a child has had an infectious illness with fever for longer than 24 hours, he probably will not have a "febrile" seizure with that particular illness. In the large series reported by Wolf et al., parents were unaware of the existence of fever prior to the occurrence of a seizure in 30 percent, and in 81 percent the preseizure duration of fever was not over 24 hours. Approximately 70 to 80 percent of such seizures are associated with the common types of upper respiratory infections, including tonsillitis, pharyngitis, or acute otitis media (Millichap, Stokes et al.). Roseola has been mentioned by many authors to be commonly associated with convulsions of the "febrile" type, although this illness accounts for only a small percentage of children who have a febrile convulsion. In a series of 448 children with "febrile" seizures, Möller found that 7.6 percent were secondary to roseola, while Nelson and Ellenberg (1978) noted roseola to be the precipitating factor in only 5 percent of their cases.

Considerable attention has also been devoted to the pathogenesis of convulsions in children with shigella gastroenteritis. Kowlessar and Forbes found that 30 percent of children less than six years of age with shigella enteritis experienced "febrile" seizures. As in "febrile" seizures related to other infections, those with shigella enteritis in this series were age-related, occurred more often in males, and could not be explained on the basis of identifiable metabolic derangements. Certain authors have attributed seizures to the high fever itself while others have postulated a neurotoxin elaborated by shigella which leads to an acute encephalopathy manifested by seizures (Donald et al.).

A notable characteristic of "febrile" convulsions in childhood which can be of some limited diagnostic assistance is the tendency for the condition to have occurred in other members of the family. A positive family history of "febrile" seizures has been obtained in 30 to 58 percent of children with convulsions of the febrile type (Frantzen et al., Livingston, Millichap et al.).

Laboratory Studies

Laboratory and ancillary examinations performed on the child with "febrile" seizures obviously depend on the circumstances prevailing when the child is seen. For example, if the child is first evaluated two weeks after the event and has recovered entirely, perhaps only an electroencephalogram is indicated. More often, however, the judgments must be made when one encounters the febrile child either actively convulsing or immediately postictal in the emergency area of the hospital. While the initial requirements are the establishment of an airway, termination of seizures, and control of hyperthermia, the selection of the appropriate diagnostic studies soon becomes necessary. Each case must be individualized in this regard, and, in part, the examinations indicated will depend on the physical findings and whether a cause of fever is identified. In addition to a blood count and urine examination, laboratory studies that deserve consideration include serum electrolytes, glucose, urea nitrogen, and blood culture. If the child had experienced recurrent attacks of vomiting with progressive lethargy before the onset of seizures, liver enzymes in serum and serum ammonia should be determined, although seizures are not a prominent feature in most cases of Reye's syndrome. Not every child will need such studies, which entail considerable expense, but some will require laboratory tests in order to properly identify the cause of the convulsion.

The need for lumbar puncture and CSF examination, likewise, is determined by the circumstances, which include many variables. The procedure should be done if from the history and physical examination one cannot otherwise exclude the possibility of meningitis or encephalitis. If the child is one known to have had previous "febrile" seizures, has fever secondary to otitis or tonsillitis that is unequivocal, and is rapidly demonstrating progressive improvement after a brief seizure, it is often possible to avoid lumbar puncture, assuming that meningeal signs are absent and that his course can be observed for a period of time. In reality, when the child is seen just after having had a seizure associated with an acute febrile illness, lumbar puncture is advised in the great majority of instances. It is important to keep in mind that experienced clinicians have observed children with either tuberculous meningitis or lead encephalopathy, as well as acute bacterial meningitis, in whom the first manifestation of illness was a convulsion, initially believed to be "febrile" in type.

Performance of an electroencephalogram after the first seizure associated with fever is indicated, but to obtain the maximum amount of information the procedure should be postponed for a minimum of seven days after the seizure because of diffuse electrical slowing that temporarily follows a convulsive episode (Frantzen et al.). In the child with simple "febrile" seizures as described herein, the electroencephalogram should be normal or not more than minimally abnormal between seizures and at least should not contain paroxysmal dysrhythmic activity which is more indicative of epilepsy.

Course and Prognosis

In the series compiled by Lennox, almost 42 percent of patients had only one "febrile" seizure while 13 percent had two and 11 percent experienced three. The remainder had more than three seizures of this type. In a more recent series, Gates found that 66 percent of 98 children with seizures of the "febrile" type had only a single such episode. Among 1706 children with "febrile" seizures, Nelson and Ellenberg (1978) observed that one-third had recurrence of "febrile" seizures at some time following the initial one and that 9 percent had three or more such attacks. The probability of recurrence was higher when the first attack occurred in infants less than one year of age. In this group, one-half experienced recurrent "febrile" seizures.

The subsequent occurrence of afebrile or spontaneous convulsions in the child who earlier had "febrile" seizures appears to be infrequent but is higher than in the population generally. This is especially true in studies in which children are included whose "febrile" convulsions were *complex,* that is, were of prolonged duration or had focal implications, or in which children had shown prior evidence of neurologic dysfunction (Annegers et al.). Among children with the latter characteristics, Nelson and Ellenberg (1976) found that subsequent afebrile seizures occurred at a rate 18 times higher than in children with no history of febrile seizures. Livingston found that only 2.9 percent of children with simple "febrile" seizures subsequently developed recurring afebrile seizures, a figure similar to that recorded by other authors (Friderichsen and Melchior, Gates). A concept of particular interest is that convulsions in the febrile child with the attendant "convulsive hypoxia" might lead to medial temporal lobe injury which subsequently becomes epileptogenic, giving rise to psychomotor epilepsy in the older child (Falconer, Falconer et al., Taylor and Ounsted). The possibility has neither been proved nor disproved to the present date and deserves further consideration in future studies. Diffuse and severe brain damage secondary to hypoxia has been described with seizures associated with a non-neurologic febrile illness (Fowler). These cases have generally been complicated ones with prolonged convulsions, often lasting several hours. It is possible that convulsions in such cases are initially precipitated by fever but perpetuated by secondary factors such as airway obstruction or diminished cerebral perfusion leading to hypoxic and ischemic cerebral injury.

Management

Treatment in the acute stage includes immediate attention to the airway and respiratory function, termination of convulsive activity with the use of appropriate medication, control of hyperthermia, and management of the infectious illness causing fever. Cessation of the seizure often occurs spontaneously, but, if not, intravenous administration of diazepam or a short-acting barbiturate is usually sufficient.

Long-term management of the child with "febrile" seizures is the point of greatest divergence of opinion. Some authors have recommended that all such children be placed on anticonvulsant medication after the first seizure and be retained on therapy until five or six years of age (Hammill and Carter). Others recommend no drug therapy, assuming that seizures can be assigned to the simple "febrile" category and that the child does not exhibit a tendency, either clinically or electroencephalographically, to have spontaneous, afebrile convulsions (Livingston). Still others advise the use of intermittent phenobarbital therapy whenever fever occurs.

Intermittent drug therapy, or the use of phenobarbital only during a febrile illness, seems of doubtful value because of the tendency for "febrile" seizures to occur soon after an abrupt rise in temperature and also because of the time period required to achieve therapeutic blood levels following oral administration. Among the approximately 30 percent of children whose seizures occur before parents are aware of the existence of fever, intermittent anticonvulsant therapy could have no beneficial effect (Wolf et al.). Despite this expected improbability of benefit, certain studies have suggested a reduction in recurrences with such prophylactic treatment (van den Berg and Yerushalmy). Continuous anticonvulsant treatment for this problem has also been a point of dispute, with some investigations indicating that persistent, daily therapy does not significantly decrease the risk of recurrences (Faero et al., Melchior et al., Millichap), while others reveal a decided improvement among children treated with phenobarbital (Wolf et al.). Whether continuous treatment decreases the severity of seizures that occur is unknown. Virtually all authors agree that when phenobarbital is used on a daily basis for treatment of febrile seizures, compliance is often poor and behavioral side effects are disturbingly high (Fishman, Wolf and Forsythe, Wolf et al.).

It is apparent, then, that no universal approach is applicable to all children who convulse with a febrile illness and that patients should be individualized in regard to the advisability of anticonvulsant therapy. Treating all children with one febrile seizure with phenobarbital would mean that 2 to 3 percent of all children in this country would receive the drug for a prolonged period, and that 65 to 70 percent would receive it unnecessarily because this is the estimate of those that have only one such attack. A more logical approach would be to attempt to identify those children at greater risk for recurrence of seizures after the first "febrile" seizure in whom constant therapy would be appropriate. Indications for treatment would include the child with a "febrile" seizure who is under 15 months of age, the one who has a second such attack and is still less than 36 months of age, and the one with a clearly dysrhythmic electroencephalogram performed in the interictal period and interpreted by one experienced in reading children's records. The child with prolonged seizures, over 15 minutes in duration, the child with focal convulsive activity or a postictal transient focal paresis, or the one with a history of neurologic abnormality or developmental retardation prior to the ictal event would also be a candidate for daily phenobarbital therapy. Conversely, the occurrence of a single, brief, generalized seizure with fever in an otherwise normal young child over 15 months of age with a normal electroencephalogram can be managed conservatively without medication. Parents should be advised of the possible good prognosis and advised of methods to recognize and control fever associated with infectious illnesses.

Among those placed on phenobarbital, the period of time to continue treatment will depend on many circumstances, but in most it would range from one to two years, unless subsequent afebrile seizures were to occur. Periodic monitoring of serum levels to keep the serum concentration between 15 and 20 μg/ml. would, perhaps, improve compliance as well as ensure that the dosage is proper. This determination could be done at four- to six-month intervals with only minor inconvenience to patient or family. In those intolerant of phenobarbital, phenytoin or valproic acid (Depakene) could be used, although experience with these drugs for this purpose is limited.

REFERENCES

Annegers, J. F., Hauser, W. A., Elveback, L. R., and Kurland, L. T.: The risk of epilepsy following febrile convulsions. Neurology 29:297–303, 1979.

Donald, W. D., Winkler, C. H., Jr., and Bargeron, L. M., Jr.: The occurrence of convulsions in children with shigella gastroenteritis. J. Pediat. 48:323–327, 1956.

Faero, O., Kastrup, K. W., Melchior, J. C., and Thorm, J.: Phenobarbital as prophylaxis for febrile convulsions. A preliminary report. Epilepsia 12:109–112, 1971.

Falconer, M. A.: Genetic and related aetiological factors in temporal lobe epilepsy. Epilepsia 12:13–31, 1971.

Falconer, M. A., Serafetinides, E. A., and Corsellis, J. A. N.: Etiology and pathogenesis of temporal lobe epilepsy. Arch. Neurol. 10:233–248, 1964.

Fishman, M. A.: Febrile seizures. The treatment controversy. J. Pediat. 94:177–184, 1979.

Fowler, M.: Brain damage after febrile convulsions. Arch. Dis. Childh. 32:67–76, 1957.

Frantzen, E., Lennox-Buchthal, M., and Nygaard, A.: Longitudinal EEG and clinical study of children with febrile convulsions. Electroenceph. Clin. Neurophysiol. 24:197–212, 1968.

Friderichsen, C., and Melchior, J.: Febrile convulsions in children, their frequency and prognosis. Acta Paediat. 43(Suppl. 100):307–317, 1954.

Gates, M. J.: Prognosis of febrile seizures. NINDS Monograph No. 14, 123–128, 1972.

Hammill, J. F., and Carter, S.: Febrile convulsions. New Eng. J. Med. 274:563–565, 1966.

Kowlessar, M., and Forbes, G. B.: The febrile convulsion in shigellosis. New Eng. J. Med. 258:520–526, 1958.

Lennox, W. G.: Significance of febrile convulsions. Pediatrics 11:341–356, 1953.

Livingston, S.: Infantile febrile convulsions. Dev. Med. Child Neurol. 10:374–376, 1968.

Melchior, J. C., Buchthal, F., and Lennox-Buchthal, M.: The ineffectiveness of diphenylhydantoin in preventing febrile convulsions in the age of greatest risk, under three years. Epilepsia 12:55–62, 1971.

Millichap, J. G.: Febrile Convulsions. The Macmillan Company, New York, 1968.

Millichap, J. G., Madsen, J. A., and Aledort, L. M.: Studies in febrile seizures. V. Clinical and electroencephalographic study in unselected patients. Neurology 10:643–653, 1960.

Möller, K. L.: Exanthema subitum and febrile convulsions. Acta Paediat. 45:534–540, 1956.

Nelson, K. B., and Ellenberg, J. H.: Prognosis in children with febrile seizures. Pediatrics 61:720–727, 1978.

Nelson, K. B., and Ellenberg, J. H.: Predictors of epilepsy in children who have experienced febrile seizures. New Eng. J. Med. 295:1029–1033, 1976.

Stokes, M. J., Downham, M. A. P. S., Webb, J. K. G., McQuillin, J., and Gardner, P. S.: Viruses and febrile convulsions. Arch. Dis. Childh. 52:129–133, 1977.

Taylor, D. C., and Ounsted, C.: Biological mechanisms influencing the outcome of seizures in response to fever. Epilepsia 12:33–45, 1971.

van den Berg, B. J., and Yerushalmy, J.: Studies on convulsive disorders in young children. II. Intermittent phenobarbital prophylaxis and recurrence of febrile convulsions. J. Pediat. 78:1004–1012, 1971.

Wolf, S. M., Carr, A., Davis, D. C., Davidson, S., Dale, E. P., Forsythe, A., Goldenberg, E. D., Hanson, R., Lulejian, G. A., Nelson, M. A., Trietman, P., and Weinstein, A.: The value of phenobarbital in the child who has had a single febrile seizure: A controlled prospective study. Pediatrics 59:378–385, 1977.

Wolf, S. M., and Forsythe, A.: Behavioral disturbance, phenobarbital, and febrile seizures. Pediatrics 61:728–731, 1978.

Index

Page numbers in *italics* indicate illustrations;
page numbers followed by the letter *t* refer to tables.

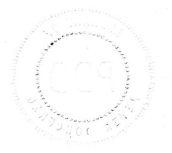

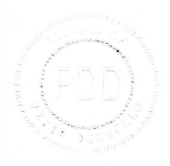

TABLE III.

FUNGI AND ACTINOMYCETES
THAT CAUSE NEUROLOGIC DISEASE IN MAN

Actinomyces

    Actinomyces
    Nocardia

Phycomycetes (Zygomycetes)

    Mucor
    Rhizopus
    Absidia

Ascomycetes

    Histoplasma
    Candida
    Blastomyces
    Allescheria (Petriellidium)

Basidiomycetes

    Cryptococcus neoformans

Deuteromycetes (Fungi Imperfecti)

    Coccidioides
    Aspergillus
    Penicillium
    Cladosporium
    Sporothrix